Otolaryngology— Head and Neck Surgery

William L. Meyerhoff, M.D., Ph.D.
Professor and Chairman
Department of Otorhinolaryngology
University of Texas
Southwestern Medical Center
Dallas, Texas

Dale H. Rice, M.D.
Professor and Chairman
Department of Otolaryngology—Head and Neck Surgery
University of Southern California
School of Medicine
Los Angeles, California

W. B. SAUNDERS COMPANY
Harcourt Brace Jovanovich, Inc.
Philadelphia   London   Toronto   Montreal   Sydney   Tokyo

W. B. SAUNDERS COMPANY
Harcourt Brace Jovanovich, Inc.

The Curtis Center
Independence Square West
Philadelphia, Pennsylvania 19106

Library of Congress Cataloging-in-Publication Data

Otolaryngology—head and neck surgery / [edited by] William L. Meyerhoff, Dale H. Rice.

p. cm.

ISBN 0–7216–3623–3

1. Otolaryngology.   2. Head—Surgery.   3. Neck—Surgery.
I. Meyerhoff, William L.   II. Rice, Dale H.
[DNLM: 1. Head—surgery.   2. Neck—surgery.
3. Otorhinolaryngologic Diseases—surgery.   WV 168 0879]

RF46.0754   1992

617.5′1059—dc20

DNLM/DLC   91–33827

for Library of Congress   CIP

Editor: Jennifer Mitchell

Designer: Dorothy Chattin

Production Manager: Peter Faber

Manuscript Editors: Anne Ostroff and Rose Marie Klimowicz

Illustration Coordinator: Brett MacNaughton

Indexer: Mark Coyle

Cover Designer: Michelle Maloney

OTOLARYNGOLOGY—HEAD AND NECK SURGERY   ISBN 0–7216–3623–3

Last digit is the print number: 9   8   7   6   5   4   3   2   1

Contributors

William C. Ardary, MD, DDS

Clinical Associate Professor, Department of Oral and Maxillofacial Surgery, University of Southern California School of Dentistry; Staff, Arcadia Meramiss Hospital; Staff, Los Angeles County—University of Southern California Medical Center, Los Angeles, California
Anatomy and Physiology of the Oral Cavity

H. Alexander Arts, MD

Instructor, Department of Otolaryngology—Head and Neck Surgery, University of Virginia School of Medicine, Charlottesville, Virginia
Anatomy and Embryology of the Ear

Paul R. Bergstresser, MD

Professor and Chairman, Department of Dermatology, University of Texas Southwestern Medical Center; Staff, Parkland Memorial Hospital; Staff, Zale Lipshy University Hospital; Staff, Children's Medical Center; Staff, Veterans Administration Medical Center, Dallas, Texas
Cutaneous Lesions

Gerald S. Berke, MD

Associate Professor of Head and Neck Surgery, University of California, Los Angeles (UCLA), School of Medicine; UCLA Acting Chief, Division of Head and Neck Surgery, Wadsworth Veterans Administration Medical Center, Los Angeles, California
Hoarseness, Nonspecific Voice Disorders, and Chronic Inflammatory Disorders of the Larynx and Cervical Esophagus

Forrest C. Brown, MD

Associate Clinical Professor, Department of Dermatology, University of Texas Southwestern Medical School; Attending Physician, Parkland Hospital and Humana Medical Center, Dallas, Texas
Cutaneous Lesions

Orval E. Brown, MD

Associate Professor, Department of Otorhinolaryngology, University of Texas Southwestern Medical Center; Staff, Children's Medical Center, Dallas, Texas
Pediatric Otolaryngology; Tonsillectomy and Adenoidectomy

Phillip Mark Brown, MD

Chief Resident, Department of Otolaryngology, University of Texas Southwestern Medical Center; Chief Resident, Parkland Memorial Hospital, Zale Lipshy University Hospital, Dallas, Texas
Trauma to the Larynx, Cervical Esophagus, and Neck

Vincent G. Caruso, MD

Assistant Professor of Clinical Otolaryngology, Columbia University College of Physicians and Surgeons, New York City; Attending Physician, Southampton Hospital, Southampton; Attending Physician, Central Suffolk Hospital, Riverhead, New York
Acquired Lesions of the Auricle and Ear

Lanny Garth Close, MD

Professor and Vice-Chairman, Department of Otorhinolaryngology; Chairman,

Division of Head and Neck Surgery, University of Texas Southwestern Medical Center, Dallas; Active Staff, Zale Lipshy University Hospital; Chief, Otorhinolaryngology, Veterans Administration Medical Center; Active Staff, Parkland Memorial Hospital, Children's Medical Center, St. Paul Medical Center, Dallas, Texas
Cancer of the Oral Cavity and Oropharynx

Barbara Cone-Wesson, PhD
Associate Professor, Clinical Otolaryngology—Head and Neck Surgery, University of Southern California (USC) School of Medicine; Audiology Director, Los Angeles County and USC Medical Center, USC Health Care Consultation Center University Hospital, Los Angeles, California
Auditory System Tests

Ted A. Cook, MD
Chief, Division of Facial Plastic and Reconstructive Surgery, Oregon Health Sciences University, Portland, Oregon
Facial Plastic and Reconstructive Surgery

Stanley W. Coulthard, MD
Chief Otolaryngology/Head and Neck Surgery, University of Arizona Health Sciences Center; Staff, University Medical Center, Tucson Medical Center, Northwest Hospital, El Dorado Medical Center, St. Joseph's Medical Center, Tucson, Arizona
Nonneoplastic Salivary Gland Diseases

Dennis M. Crockett, MD
Assistant Professor, Department of Otolaryngology—Head and Neck Surgery, University of Southern California School of Medicine; Staff, Los Angeles County—University of Southern California Medical Center; Children's Hospital of Los Angeles, University of Southern California University Hospital, Los Angeles, California
Congenital Aural Atresia and Microtia; Congenital Lesions

Roberto A. Cueva, MD
Assistant Clinical Professor, Division of Otolaryngology—Head and Neck Surgery, University of California, San Diego; Faculty Physician, University of California, San Diego, Medical Center; Staff Physician, Veterans Administration Medical Center, La Jolla, California
Conductive Hearing Loss: Inflammatory and Noninflammatory Causes

Richard J. De Angelis, MD
Private Practice; Consulting Dermatologist, Anderson Memorial Hospital, Anderson, South Carolina
Mohs Micrographic Surgery

Isaiah W. Dimery, MD
Assistant Professor of Medicine, University of Texas, M. D. Anderson Cancer Center, Section of Head, Neck and Thoracic Medical Oncology, Houston, Texas
Chemotherapy in Head and Neck Cancer

Paul J. Donald, MD, FRCS(C)
Professor, Department of Otolaryngology—Head and Neck Surgery, University of California, Davis, Medical Center; Director, Skull Base Surgery, University of California, Davis, Medical Center, Sacramento, California
Reconstruction of the Head and Neck

Larry G. Duckert, MD, PhD
Professor, Department of Otolaryngology—Head and Neck Surgery, University of Washington; Staff, University of Washington Medical Center, Harborview Medical Center, Veterans Administration Hospital, and Children's Orthopedic Hospital, Seattle, Washington
Anatomy and Embryology of the Ear

David N. F. Fairbanks, MD
Clinical Professor, Otolaryngology—Head and Neck Surgery, George Washington University School of Medicine and Health Sciences, Washington, D.C.; Active Staff, Sibley Memorial Hospital, Washington, D.C.
Management of Patients with Snoring and Obstructive Sleep Apnea

David W. Fairbanks, MD
Resident, Otolaryngology—Head and Neck Surgery, University of Louisville; Resident Staff, University of Louisville Medical Center, Louisville, Kentucky
Management of Patients with Snoring and Obstructive Sleep Apnea

George M. Gerken, PhD
Professor, University of Texas at Dallas, Dallas, Texas
Central Auditory Physiology

G. E. Ghali, DDS
Chief Resident, Department of Surgery, Division of Oral and Maxillofacial Surgery, University of Texas Southwestern Medical Center, Dallas; Resident, Parkland Memorial Hospital, Dallas; Resident, John Peter Smith Hospital, Ft. Worth; Resident, Dallas Veterans Administration Hospital, Dallas, Texas
Neoplastic and Nontraumatic Lesions of the Maxillofacial Skeleton; Orthognathic Surgery

Jeffrey E. Goldberg, MD
Resident, Department of Otolaryngology, New York Eye and Ear Infirmary—New York Medical College, New York, New York
Headache and Facial Pain

David G. Hanson, MD, FACS
Professor and Chairman, Department of Otolaryngology—Head and Neck Surgery, Northwestern University Medical School; Chairman, Department of Otolaryngology—Head and Neck Surgery, Northwestern Memorial Hospital, Chicago, Illinois
Physiology of Pharynx and Larynx

Jeffrey P. Harris, MD, PhD
Professor, Division of Otolaryngology—Head and Neck Surgery, University of California, San Diego (UCSD), Medical Center, San Diego; Professor and Chief, Head and Neck Surgery, UCSD Medical Center, San Diego; Staff Physician, Veterans Administration Hospital, La Jolla, California
Conductive Hearing Loss: Inflammatory and Noninflammatory Causes

Malcolm H. Hast, PhD
Professor of Otolaryngology—Head and Neck Surgery; Professor of Cell, Molecular, and Structural Biology, Northwestern University Medical and Dental Schools; Health Professional, Northwestern Memorial Hospital, Chicago, Illinois
Physiology of Pharynx and Larynx

Donald B. Hawkins, MD
Professor of Otolaryngology—Head and Neck Surgery, University of Southern California School of Medicine; Director of Pediatric Otolaryngology, Los Angeles County—University of Southern California Medical Center, Los Angeles, California
Cysts, Primary Tumors, and Infections of the Neck; Intubation, Tracheotomy, and Cricothyrotomy; Rigid and Flexible Endoscopy of the Airway

John F. Hoffman, MD
Assistant Professor, Division of Otolaryngology—Head and Neck Surgery, University of Utah, Salt Lake City, Utah
Facial Plastic and Reconstructive Surgery

Michael E. Johns, MD
Dean of the Medical Faculty and Vice President for Medicine, The Johns Hopkins University School of Medicine; Professor, Department of Otolaryngology—Head and Neck Surgery, The Johns Hopkins Hospital, Baltimore, Maryland
Salivary Glands: Anatomy and Physiology

Gary D. Josephson, MD
Staff, Beth Israel Hospital, New York, New York
Inflammatory and Granulomatous Diseases of the Nose and Paranasal Sinuses

Jordan S. Josephson, MD
Assistant Professor, State University of New York Downstate Medical Center; Attending Physician, Long Island College Hospital, Brooklyn, New York
Inflammatory and Granulomatous Diseases of the Nose and Paranasal Sinuses

Jack M. Kartush, MD
Michigan Ear Institute, Farmington Hills; Providence Hospital, Southfield, Michigan
Facial Nerve Paralysis

Daniel Kempler, PhD
Assistant Professor, University of Southern California; Chief Speech Pathologist, Los Angeles County—University of Southern California Medical Center, Los Angeles, California
Speech Pathology: Evaluation and Treatment of Speech, Language, Cognitive, and Swallowing Disorders

Eugene B. Kern, MD

Professor of Rhinology and Otolaryngology, Mayo Clinic, Mayo Foundation and Mayo Medical School, Rochester, Minnesota
Nasal Obstruction

Theda C. Kontis, MD

Staff, Department of Otolaryngology—Head and Neck Surgery, The Johns Hopkins Hospital, Baltimore, Maryland
Salivary Glands: Anatomy and Physiology

Charles F. Koopmann, Jr., MD, FACS

Associate Professor, Department of Otolaryngology—Head and Neck Surgery, University of Michigan Medical School; Staff, University of Michigan Hospitals, Ann Arbor; C. S. Mott Children's Hospital, Detroit; Veterans Administration Hospital, Ann Arbor; Chelsea Community Hospital, Chelsea, Michigan
Geriatric Otolaryngology

Rodney F. Kovach, MD

Associate Professor, Section of Dermatology, Departments of Medicine and Otolaryngology/Head and Neck Surgery, West Virginia University, School of Medicine; West Virginia University Hospitals, Inc.—Ruby Memorial Hospital, Morgantown, West Virginia
Mohs Micrographic Surgery

Michael J. LaRouere, MD

Michigan Ear Institute, Farmington Hills: Providence Hospital, Southfield, Michigan
Facial Nerve Paralysis

Joseph L. Leach, MD

Assistant Professor, Department of Otorhinolaryngology, University of Texas Southwestern Medical School, Dallas, Texas
Vertigo

Norris K. Lee, MD

Assistant Professor, Department of Otorhinolaryngology—Head and Neck Surgery, University of Texas Southwestern Medical Center; Active Staff, Zale Lipshy University Hospital, Parkland Memorial Hospital, Veterans Administration Medical Center, St. Paul Medical Center, Dallas, Texas
Cancer of the Oral Cavity and Oropharynx

Jeri A. Logemann, PhD

Professor, Departments of Communication Sciences and Disorders, Otolaryngology—Head and Neck Surgery and Neurology, Northwestern University; Associate Staff, Northwestern Memorial Hospital, Chicago; Children's Memorial Hospital, Chicago; Evanston Hospital, Evanston, Illinois
Physiology of Pharynx and Larynx

Frank E. Lucente, MD, FACS

Chairman, Department of Otolaryngology, State University of New York—Health Science Center at Brooklyn; Chairman, Department of Otolaryngology, Long Island College Hospital; Chairman, Department of Otolaryngology, University Hospital of Brooklyn; Attending Physician, Department of Otolaryngology, Brooklyn Veterans Administration Hospital; Chairman, Department of Otolaryngology, Kings County Medical Center, Brooklyn, New York
Headache and Facial Pain

Carolyn B. Lyde, MD

Assistant Professor of Dermatology, University of Texas Southwestern Medical School; Staff, Parkland Memorial Hospital, Zale Lipshy University Hospital, St. Paul Hospital, Children's Medical Center, Dallas, Texas
Cutaneous Lesions

Richard L. Mabry, MD, FACS, FAAOA

Clinical Professor of Otorhinolaryngology, University of Texas Southwestern Medical Center; Active Staff (Private Practice of Otorhinolaryngology), Charlton Methodist Hospital, Dallas, Texas
Epistaxis; Otolaryngologic Allergy: Evolution of a Discipline

Dennis R. Maceri, MD

Assistant Professor, University of Southern California School of Medicine; Staff, Los Angeles County—University of Southern California Medical Center, Huntington Memorial Hospital, University of Southern California University Hospital, Children's Hospital of Los Angeles, Los Angeles, California
Sensorineural Hearing Loss: Sudden, Fluctuating, and Gradual; Congenital Aural Atresia and Microtia

Abraham M. Majchel, MD
Research Fellow, Department of Otolaryngology, The Johns Hopkins University School of Medicine, Baltimore, Maryland; Staff, Department of Otolaryngology, Hospital San Juan de Dios, San Jose, Costa Rica
Allergy and Immunology in the Ear, Nose, and Throat

Anthony A. Mancuso, MD
Professor of Radiology, University of Florida College of Medicine; Neuroradiology/ENT Section, Shands Hospital at the University of Florida, Gainesville, Florida
Diagnostic Imaging

Scott C. Manning, MD
Assistant Professor, Department of Otorhinolaryngology, University of Texas Southwestern Medical Center; Active Attending Staff, Children's Medical Center, Parkland Memorial Hospital, Zale Lipshy University Hospital, St. Paul Hospital, Dallas, Texas
Pediatric Otolaryngology; Tonsillectomy and Adenoidectomy

Michael D. Maves, MD, FACS
Professor and Chairman, Department of Otolaryngology—Head and Neck Surgery, St. Louis University School of Medicine; Chairman, Department of Otolaryngology—Head and Neck Surgery, St. Louis University Medical Center; Attending Staff, Cardinal Glennon Children's Hospital; Attending Staff, St. Mary's Health Center; St. John's Mercy Medical Center, St. Louis, Missouri
Congenital Lesions of the Oral Cavity, Oropharynx, Hypopharynx, and Salivary Glands

Dorothy L. Mellon, MD
Assistant Professor of Otolaryngology, University of Miami School of Medicine; Staff, Jackson Memorial Hospital, Bascom-Palmer Eye Institute, Veterans Administration Medical Center, Sylvester Comprehensive Cancer Center, Miami, Florida
History and Physical Examination: Head and Neck

William M. Mendenhall, MD
Associate Professor, Department of Radiation Oncology, University of Florida College of Medicine; Clinic Director, Department of Radiation Oncology, Shands Hospital, Gainesville, Florida
Radiation Therapy in the Management of Head and Neck Cancer

William L. Meyerhoff, MD, PhD
The Arthur E. Meyerhoff Professor and Chairman, Department of Otorhinolaryngology, University of Texas Southwestern Medical Center; Staff, Zale Lipshy University Hospital, St. Paul Medical Center, Parkland Memorial Hospital, Dallas, Texas
Geriatric Otolaryngology; Otalgia; Vertigo; Tinnitus

Bruce E. Mickey, MD
Associate Professor of Neurosurgery, University of Texas Southwestern Medical School, Dallas, Texas
General Principles of Skull Base Surgery

Robert H. Miller, MD, FACS
Professor and Chairman, Department of Otolaryngology—Head and Neck Surgery, Tulane University School of Medicine; Chief of Otolaryngology—Head and Neck Surgery, Tulane University Hospital; Chief of Tulane Otolaryngology Service Charity Hospital of New Orleans, New Orleans, Louisiana
Congenital Defects of the Larynx and Cervical Esophagus

Rodney R. Million, MD
John P. Cofrin Chairman's Professorship of Radiation Oncology, University of Florida College of Medicine; Medical Director, Department of Radiation Oncology, Shands Hospital, Gainesville, Florida
Radiation Therapy in the Management of Head and Neck Cancer

Carolyn H. Musket, MA
Clinical Instructor in Communication Disorders, University of Texas at Dallas—Callier Center for Communication Disorders, Dallas, Texas
Hearing Aids and Aural Rehabilitation

Robert M. Naclerio, MD
Associate Professor of Otolaryngology—Head and Neck Surgery and Medicine, The Johns Hopkins University School of Medicine; Staff, The Johns Hopkins Hospital, Baltimore, Maryland
Allergy and Immunology in the Ear, Nose, and Throat

Dennis P. O'Leary, PhD
Professor, Department of Otolaryngology, University of Southern California School of Medicine; Director, Center for Balance Disorders, University of Southern California University Hospital, Los Angeles, California
Vestibular Physiology

Robert H. Ossoff, DMD, MD
Guy M. Maness Professor and Chairman, Department of Otolaryngology, Vanderbilt University Medical Center, Nashville, Tennessee
Lasers in Otolaryngology—Head and Neck Surgery

James T. Parsons, MD
The Rodney R. Million, M.D., Professor of Radiation Oncology and Associate Professor, Department of Radiation Oncology, University of Florida College of Medicine; Radiation Oncologist, Shands Hospital, Gainesville, Florida
Radiation Therapy in the Management of Head and Neck Cancer

Bradford S. Patt, MD
Chief Resident, Department of Otolaryngology—Head and Neck Surgery, University of Texas Southwestern Medical Center, Dallas, Texas
Geriatric Otolaryngology

Steven P. Peskind, MD
Resident, Department of Otolaryngology—Head and Neck Surgery, University of Southern California School of Medicine, Los Angeles, California
Congenital Lesions

George H. Petti, Jr., MD, FACS
Professor, Surgery Division, Head and Neck Surgery, Loma Linda University Medical Center, Loma Linda; Chief, Head and Neck Surgery, Loma Linda University Medical Center, Loma Linda; Attending Physician, Jerry L. Pettis Veterans Administration Hospital, Loma Linda; Chief Otolaryngology—Head and Neck Surgery, Riverside General Hospital, University Medical Center, Riverside, California
Thyroid and Parathyroid

Harold C. Pillsbury III, MD
Professor of Surgery, Otolaryngology—Head and Neck Surgery, University of North Carolina, Chapel Hill, School of Medicine; Attending Physician, University of North Carolina Hospitals, Chapel Hill, North Carolina
Peripheral Auditory Physiology

Patrick H. Pownell, MD
Resident, Department of Otolaryngology, University of Texas Southwestern Medical Center, Dallas, Texas
Otalgia

Terry D. Rees, DDS, MSD
Professor and Chairman, Department of Periodontics; Director, Stomatology Center, Baylor College of Dentistry; Associate Attending Physician, Baylor University Medical Center, Dallas, Texas
Diseases of the Oral Mucous Membranes

Dale H. Rice, MD
Tiber/Alpert Professor and Chairman, Department of Otolaryngology—Head and Neck Surgery, University of Southern California School of Medicine, Los Angeles, California
Neoplastic Diseases; Neoplasms of the Salivary Glands; Staging of Head and Neck Cancer

Brock D. Ridenour, MD
Acting Instructor, Department of Otolaryngology—Head and Neck Surgery, University of Washington, Seattle, Washington
Tinnitus

Ross J. Roeser, PhD
Professor, University of Texas at Dallas—Callier Center for Communication Disorders, Dallas, Texas
Hearing Aids and Aural Rehabilitation

Peter S. Roland, MD
Associate Professor, Department of Otorhinolaryngology, University of Texas Southwestern Medical Center; Chief of Otolaryngology, Parkland Memorial Hospital; Chief of Medical Services, Callier Center for Communicative Disorders, University of Texas at Dallas; Zale Lipshy University Hospital; St. Paul Medical Center; Veterans Administration Medical Center, Dallas, Texas
History and Physical Examination: Ear; Noninflammatory Lesions of the Ear and Skull Base; General Principles of Skull Base Surgery

Robert O. Ruder, MD
Private Practice, Beverly Hills, California
Congenital Aural Atresia and Microtia

Steven D. Schaefer, MD
Professor of Otorhinolaryngology, University of Texas Southwestern Medical Center; Adjunct Professor of Communicative Sciences, Callier Center, University of Texas at Dallas; Staff, Zale Lipshy University Hospital, Parkland Memorial Hospital, Veterans Administration Medical Center, St. Paul Medical Center, Dallas, Texas
Anatomy and Physiology of the Nose and Paranasal Sinuses; Trauma to the Larynx, Cervical Esophagus, and Neck

Maher Sesi, MD
Chief Resident, Department of Otorhinolaryngology, University of Texas Southwestern Medical Center, Dallas, Texas
Anatomy and Physiology of the Nose and Paranasal Sinuses

Douglas P. Sinn, DDS
Professor and Chairman, Department of Surgery, Division of Oral and Maxillofacial Surgery, University of Texas Southwestern Medical Center; Staff, Parkland Hospital, Children's Medical Center, Zale Lipshy University Hospital, Veterans Administration Hospital, St. Paul Medical Center, Baylor Medical Center, Dallas; John Peter Smith Hospital, Fort Worth, Texas
Orthognathic Surgery

Robert B. Stanley, Jr., MD, DDS
Associate Professor and Vice Chairman, Department of Otolaryngology—Head and Neck Surgery, University of Southern California School of Medicine; Active Staff, University of Southern California University Hospital, Los Angeles County—University of Southern California Medical Center, Los Angeles, California
Management of Fractures of the Facial Skeleton

Charles M. Stiernberg, MD, FACS
Associate Professor of Otolaryngology and Deputy Chairman, Department of Otolaryngology, University of Texas Medical Branch at Galveston; Full-Time Staff, Department of Otolaryngology, University of Texas Medical Branch Hospitals, Galveston, Texas
Dysphagia and Odynophagia

John A. Stith, MD
Assistant Professor and Director, Division of Pediatric Otolaryngology, Department of Otolaryngology—Head and Neck Surgery, St. Louis University School of Medicine; Director, Pediatric Otolaryngology, Cardinal Glennon Children's Hospital; Attending Staff, St. Louis Medical Center; Attending Staff, St. Mary's Hospital; Consulting, St. John's Mercy Medical Center, St. Louis, Missouri
Congenital Lesions of the Oral Cavity, Oropharynx, Hypopharynx, and Salivary Glands

Scott P. Stringer, MD
Assistant Professor, Department of Otolaryngology, University of Florida College of Medicine; Staff, Shands Hospital, Gainesville, Florida
Neoplasms and Cysts of the Larynx and Cervical Esophagus

Jonathan M. Sykes, MD
Assistant Professor, Department of Otolaryngology—Head and Neck Surgery, University of California, Davis; Facial Plastic Surgeon, Department of Otolaryngology—Head and Neck Surgery, University of California, Davis Medical Center, Sacramento, California
Reconstruction of the Head and Neck

Robert V. Walker, DDS

Professor, Department of Surgery, Division of Oral and Maxillofacial Surgery, University of Texas Southwestern Medical Center; Active Attending Member, Medical Staff, Department of Surgery, Division of Oral Surgery, Zale Lipshy University Hospital; Attending Physician, Parkland Memorial Hospital, Dallas, Texas

Neoplastic and Nontraumatic Lesions of the Maxillofacial Skeleton

Jay A. Werkhaven, MD

Assistant Professor, Pediatric Otolaryngology, Vanderbilt University Medical Center, Nashville, Tennessee

Lasers in Otolaryngology—Head and Neck Surgery

Adam S. Wilson, MD

Resident, Department of Otolaryngology/Head and Neck Surgery, Georgetown University Medical Center, Washington, D.C.

Peripheral Auditory Physiology

Gayle E. Woodson, MD, FACS, FRCS(C)

Associate Professor in Residence, Division of Head and Neck Surgery, University of California, San Diego; Staff, University of California, San Diego, Medical Center; Chief of Head and Neck Surgery, Veterans Administration Medical Center, San Diego, California

Anatomy of the Neck and Larynx

Preface

The editors of this text have been frequent contributors to books in their areas of interest and have long felt the need for a text that covers the specialty more thoroughly than the currently available single volumes, while simultaneously being more manageable than the multivolume sets. This was an impossible task for two authors, and so they recruited a cadre of experts whose charge was to target each assigned topic to both the resident-in-training and the otolaryngologist–head and neck surgeon in practice. The book should also serve as a more comprehensive reference for the medical student with a deeper interest in the specialty as well as for the non–otolaryngologist–head and neck surgeon.

Rather than provide the typical review of the literature, each author was asked instead to give his or her philosophy and approach to the topic. Thus although a list of recommended readings follows each chapter, there is no formal bibliography. For each topic, a single expert's opinion prevails. We recognize that there may be other credible approaches, and the reader who wishes to determine those approaches should consult the current literature for appropriate review articles. The approach of this book—no literature review and no references—was chosen so the maximal amount of information could be included in each chapter and yet all the chapters could fit into a single volume.

The editors thank the contributors for their diligence, thoroughness, and promptness. Finally, they hope the reader will find the book both educational and enjoyable.

Contents

PART ONE

General Considerations

History and Physical Examination

Head and Neck

Dorothy L. Mellon, MD

The history and physical examination in head and neck surgery in otolaryngology, as in other specialties, form the data base by which clinical decisions and treatment plans are formulated. The ability to take a concise specialty-oriented history, in addition to a systemically oriented history, is not an easily learned skill; however, the reader is encouraged to become familiar with basic techniques described here and in the referenced texts.

As specialization within areas of head and neck surgery in otolaryngology becomes more common, history taking becomes weighted to these areas of special interest. One seeks different information from a patient desiring facial plastic surgery than from a patient requiring otovestibular evaluation, head and neck oncologic workup, or allergic work-up. While the history is being taken, the physician begins to correlate symptoms and signs, often opening new lines of questioning. Once the initial interview is complete, the historical interchange is not terminated; the flow of information continues on subsequent visits, which often clarifies subtle diagnostic criteria. Only after adequate historical background is gathered and the physical examination completed should one proceed with diagnostic tests. Because of concerns about cost containment and medicolegal controversy, the number and detail of ancillary tests must be carefully considered and justified.

Questionnaires may serve as information-gathering guidelines but should never displace the personal interdigitation that is gained through history taking.

OTOLARYNGOLIC HISTORY

A problem-oriented approach to a patient's history is recommended; the examiner starts with definition of the chief complaint, followed by a concise narrative of the present illness. These are clarified by the ensuing patient-physician interchange and supplemented by information about past medical and surgical histories, current or recent medications, pharmacologic allergies, and social and family histories. In particular, evidence of nicotine, alcohol, cocaine, or intravenous drug abuse, as well as homosexual or bisexual lifestyles, should be sought because all these may contribute significantly to pathologic conditions of the head and neck. Medication history often reveals an illness that was perhaps forgotten or not mentioned by the patient, or it actually may uncover an unrecognized drug side effect or untoward reaction manifesting in the head and neck region. The family history may suggest inherited conditions, such as otosclerosis, or transmitted infections, such as syphilis or tuberculosis. Major familial illnesses, such as diabetes and hypertension, may play a role in head and neck disorders.

As emphasized in the introduction to this chapter, the clinical history accumulation extends beyond the first encounter between physician and patient and becomes more detailed as the data base accrues. The narrative often must be supplemented by answers to direct questions about associated symptoms or related factors; these expansions of the history often require the experience of the examiner to guide the interview to the needed conclusion. An example of a possible line of questioning for an adult with a jugulodigastric neck mass is given in Table 1A–1.

By the completion of the historical narrative, most patients have revealed their own diagnosis or, at minimum, a differential diagnosis—if the physician has listened carefully. It should be rare for the physical examination to uncover any surprises.

OTOLARYNGOLIC EXAMINATION

A *standard format* for each head and neck examination is strongly recommended because it avoids omission of valuable data. Regardless of format, however, the initial evaluation should be *comprehensive* because head and neck disorders are commonly as-

TABLE 1A–2. One Protocol for Head and Neck Examination

General inspection/observation
Ears
Nose
Throat
  Oropharynx
  Nasopharynx
  Hypopharynx
  Larynx
Neck and face (bimanual examination, auscultation)
Cranial nerves

sociated. Some authors suggest deferring the region of interest to the end of the examination to avoid overlooking other abnormalities. Once a standard method of organization is learned, however, this is usually unnecessary. A suggested protocol is listed in Table 1A–2.

Most patients, even children as young as 4 or 5 years of age, may be adequately evaluated once their cooperation is established. A physician's calm, confident attitude lends more to a successful examination than does specialized instrumentation. A moment to explain the examination process does much to allay a patient's fears and elicit compliance.

Instrumentation

The basic instruments required are listed in Table 1A–3. Most physicians find that a uniform method of instrument storage facilitates

TABLE 1A–1. Directed History-Taking Questions

Chief Complaint: Neck Mass
Location?
Time period present?
Age of patient?
Change in size of mass?
Painful or nonpainful?
Associated signs or symptoms?
  Weight loss
  Fever or chills
  Erythema of mass
  Dysphagia
  Odynophagia
  Otalgia
  Hoarseness
  Sore throat
  Cough
  Nasal drainage, epistaxis, or obstruction
Previous therapies or evaluation with their success
  or failure?
Tobacco or alcohol abuse?
Tuberculosis or syphilis exposure or treatment?
Human immunodeficiency virus risk?
History of cancer of *any* type?
Exposure to cats, wild animals?

TABLE 1A–3. Basic Instrumentation for Otolaryngologic Examination

Source of illumination
Nasal speculum
Two tongue blades
4 × 4 inch gauze sponges
No. 5 laryngeal mirror
No. 0 nasopharyngeal mirror
Gloves
Sources of heat or defogger
Instruments Available as Required
  Bayonette forceps
  Suction tips (nasal)
  Cotton-tipped applicators
  Suction trap and atomizer
Medications Available
  Topical vasoconstrictor
  Topical anesthetic
  Antibiotic ointment
  Hydrogen peroxide
  Silver nitrate applicators

Note: Otologic instruments are discussed in Chapter 1B.

the evaluation, particularly when several examination rooms are being used. Instruments may be kept in a self-contained unit that includes suction and pressurized air for administering atomized medications.

Before beginning the examination—touching either the patient or instruments—the physician washes his or her hands with an antibacterial soap. This not only protects patients from contagion but also reassures them of concern for their health and well-being. Only then should clean instruments be removed from storage. All necessary instruments should be readied *before* the physical examination is started, and the storage drawers should be closed to avoid contamination. Some authors have recommended that the physician wear glasses or goggles, gloves, and a mask to avoid "splash" contamination (universal precautions for human immunodeficiency virus [HIV] and hepatitis B virus transmission) for *any* head and neck examination. In addition, cleaning and sterilization of instruments should adhere to current recommended guidelines to prevent the transmission of disease.

Adequate lighting, whether from the traditional head mirror or from newer headlights, is necessary for inspection of most portions of the head and neck. Some authors believe that the indirect light from the head mirror may be focused more sharply for posterior or deep examinations than is the direct light of the headlamp. However, in most cases, individual preference rules.

The ideal head mirror has a fixed focal length of 10 to 12 inches (25.4 to 30.5 cm) when reflecting light from a 150-W clear bulb. The most difficult aspect of learning head mirror use seems to be sighting through the central aperture while still keeping the light beam brightly focused. The mirror may be placed over either eye but preferably over the dominant eye (the one that focuses on distant objects so that when alternate eye closure is performed, the object does not appear to move when the dominant or "sighting" eye is open). Both eyes, however, remain open and are used in the visual inspection, and the mirror is further adjusted so that the vision is comfortably parfocal. The examiner must move his or her head to maintain the focal distance and thus keep the light brightly focused on the area of interest.

Patient and Examiner Position

Proper positioning for examination of the head and neck cannot be overemphasized. Most patients understand the instruction to "sit at attention" but tend to slump or back away as the examination progresses. Most modern examination chairs have a platform for the patient's feet, which helps maintain erect posture; the small of the back should be almost pressed into the chair and the shoulders positioned slightly anterior. The head should be positioned forward on the shoulders. The headrest when present should also be positioned forward, not to allow the patient to recline comfortably but to prevent retraction of the head during examination. The examiner's nondominant hand is used to turn and reposition the patient's head as necessary.

The examiner may either sit or stand; this is more a matter of preference than of adequacy of visualization. The examiner may prefer to sit with the patient's knees between his or her knees or to sit to the side; the standing examination position may be directly anterior to the patient or to the side as well.

Control of Instruments

The gag reflex or even pain and injury to the patient may result from failure to brace instruments properly. This is especially important when cleaning ears, using intranasal implements, or using indirect mirrors. It is best to brace instruments and hands *on the patient* so that if the patient moves, he or she will move as a unit with the instrument. This technique is demonstrated in subsequent sections.

The otolaryngologist relies heavily on visual inspection but also on palpation of the structures of the head and neck. The eyes and the fingertips work in unison; palpation often reveals a lesion that is submucosal and undetectable by the eye alone.

General Inspection/Observation

The physical examination begins with a general inspection, which includes noting the patient's habitus and attitudes. Body habitus is known to contribute to disease, as in morbid obesity complicating obstructive sleep apnea. Mouth breathing and periorbital "shiners" may guide the examiner to the

diagnosis of allergic rhinitis. Cachexia and temporal muscle wasting can be clues to chronic or severe illness, such as a head and neck malignancy. The physician notes the patient's apparent nutritional status, physiologic age in comparison with chronologic age, and mental status, particularly in relation to ability to cooperate with the examination. At this time dermatologic conditions and major deformities may be recorded.

The otologic examination is outlined in Chapter 1B.

Nose

The external and internal framework of the nose is quite complex. Occupying the central portion of the face, the nose plays a prominent cosmetic role as well as a functional role.

Examination of the external nose requires palpation in addition to inspection. The upper portion of the nose is bony; the lower portion, cartilaginous. As a result of trauma, either the bony or the cartilaginous framework, or both, may be displaced and de-

formed, even twisted. Overlying external deviations, however, may or may not result in or contribute to functional problems with airway obstruction. There are now cosmetically accepted standards for the male and female nose: what shapes and forms are considered to be esthetic. Although these norms are beyond the basic examination, the physician should be familiar with them. Frequent abnormalities noted are cartilaginous or bony humps, dorsal saddling, and tip droop. Rarer are nasal dermoids and other congenital abnormalities.

Nasal airway obstruction and epistaxis are complaints commonly encountered in otolaryngologic practice, and these symptoms require a thorough intranasal evaluation. Although not used in every case, topical decongestant and anesthetic solutions should be available.

The patient usually tilts the head back to allow the examiner to first observe the "basal" view of the nostrils. Any asymmetry is noted; the feet of the medial crura and caudalmost cartilaginous septum should align. The nasal "valve" or junction of the upper lateral cartilage with the septum is

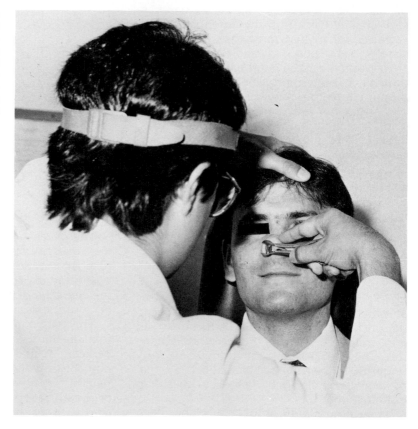

Figure 1A–1. The nasal speculum is opened gently with the blades placed superiorly and inferiorly to avoid pressure on the nasal septum. The examiner's nondominant hand is used to position the patient's head. The nasal speculum and the examiner's dominant hand are braced on the patient's face.

usually a 15° angle; larger or smaller angulations result in a sensation of nasal obstruction. The physician then holds the nasal speculum, bracing one hand on the patient's cheek if necessary, to spread the nasal ala (nostrils). This is best done gently, avoiding pressure on the septum, which can cause discomfort (Fig. 1A–1). The physician inspects first the vestibular skin and then the cartilaginous (anterior) and bony (posterior) septum, the lateral wall of the nasal cavity, and the posterior choanae if visible. The nasal vestibule is frequently a site of folliculitis and even skin cancer. The anterior portions of the septum may be extensively deviated even without external deformity because of the springy cartilaginous nature, which enables the septum to absorb most trauma. Septal deviations may or may not contribute to airway obstruction, depending on degree and location. A useful test for significant obstruction is Cottle's sign: a gentle pull laterally that opens the nasal passage may indicate a significant septal deviation. In addition, collapse of the cartilaginous vault during deep inspiration indicates a weakness of the upper lateral or lower lateral cartilages or a restriction at the nasal valve. Kiesselbach's plexus, a collection of prominent blood vessels (erectile tissue) on the anterior septum, is important in that most cases of epistaxis arise in this region.

Inspection of the lateral nasal wall is more difficult. Usually the turbinates are the most prominent feature, and the inferior and middle turbinates are readily identified. Their color should be pale pink; flame red usually indicates inflammation, and blue-gray indicates allergy. The meati are the openings immediately beneath the turbinates; the most significant pathologically is the middle meatus beneath the middle turbinate. The anterior ethmoids, frontal sinuses, and maxillary sinuses open into this meatus; discharge of purulent matter or overgrowth of pale, boggy mucosa (polyps) can frequently be seen to originate from this meatus, as can a large variety of nasal tumors. The posterior ethmoids drain usually in the superior meatus and the sphenoid via an ostium posterior to the posterior tip of the middle turbinate, an area collectively called the *sphenoethmoid recess*. The nasolacrimal duct drains anteriorly underneath the inferior turbinate. The actual ostia are usually not visible by speculum examination.

Transillumination of the sinuses has been replaced in large part by paranasal sinus radiographs and is mentioned here only because of its classic role. The facial surfaces overlying the sinuses are palpated to elicit point tenderness or edema; the maxillary molar and premolar teeth are percussed to elicit any referred pain or dental origin of sinus pathologic conditions.

The normal nasal cycle usually allows one nasal passage to congest and the opposite to dilate over a fairly constant time course; other conditions such as allergies or infections cause vasodilation and persistent nasal congestion. A great aid to intranasal examination is the abolition of this reflex or pathologic mucosal congestion by the use of topical vasoconstrictors such as oxymetazoline or ephedrine.

Nasal endoscopy with the use of nasal telescopes is an innovation in the assessment and treatment of nasal/paranasal sinus pathologic conditions. Not only are the turbinates visible, but the meati and sinus ostia are accessible, enabling a thorough diagnostic examination not before possible.

Oral Cavity/Oropharynx

The oropharyngeal examination is the most familiar portion of the head and neck evaluation. Adequate lighting again is stressed, as is also exposure by the use of tongue blades and retractors when necessary. The examination with two tongue blades is preferred; the blades are used to gently roll the lips outward first to inspect both inner and outer surfaces and then to evaluate dentition and the alveoli (Fig. 1A–2). Dentures should be *removed*. Caries and inflammation of gingiva (gingivitis) are common abnormalities. The patient's occlusion should also be assessed because of frequent cosmetic or functional disturbances.

The cheeks and lips are retracted laterally to reveal any abnormality of the buccal mucosa or parotid (Stensen's) duct orifice opposite the maxillary second molar. To assess the character of saliva, the parotid gland may be gently massaged to express fluid.

The patient's head is tilted posteriorly so that the hard and then the soft palates can be seen. A midline bony growth frequently noted to involve the hard palate is a torus palatine. A bifid uvula is seen in about 10% of the normal population but may be associated with a submucosal cleft palate.

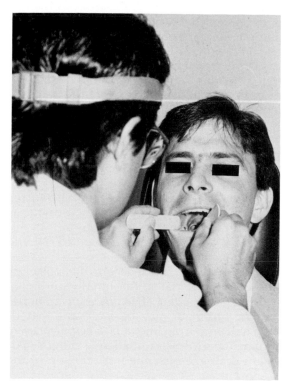

Figure 1A–2. Two tongue blades are used for wide exposure in oral/oropharyngeal evaluation.

The tongue is elevated in order to examine the anterior floor of the mouth, which contains, on either side of the frenulum, the submandibular (Wharton's) duct orifices. The tongue itself is then inspected; the physician should make sure to retract the patient's tongue laterally in both directions so that the posterior sulci of the floor of the mouth and the retromolar trigone (the ascending mandibular ramus posterior to the last molar tooth) can be examined. The ventral and then dorsal surfaces of the tongue are inspected, and the character of the papillae and any masses or alterations in tongue mobility are noted. The tongue is a powerful muscular organ, and adequate evaluation requires the patient's cooperation, regardless of the number of tongue blades used. Gentle pressure with the tongue blades or retractor to pull the tongue anteriorly as well as to depress it usually gives the best exposure of the posterior tongue and pharynx (Fig. 1A–3). The strongest gag reflex is triggered by manipulation of the posterior and posterior-central portions of the tongue, and so instruments are best used on the middle portion anterior to the circumvallate papillae. Having the pa-

tient breathe slowly through the open mouth with eyes open often makes the use of topical anesthetic unnecessary.

The palatine tonsils are then visualized by depressing the tongue, first on one side, then if necessary the other. The tonsils may be considered enlarged if they extend beyond the level of the anterior and posterior pillars with enlargement scaled up to 4+ (touching in midline), but this is only an approximation because tonsils frequently are largest in their inferior poles. The surface characteristics are carefully noted; deep crypts and white, malodorous debris are often present in cases of recurrent tonsillitis. A superficial erosion may be the earliest sign of tonsillar carcinoma.

The posterior pharyngeal wall is examined at this time. Frequently noted are prominent vessels and patches of lymphoid tissue (a part of Waldeyer's ring) covering the posterior pharyngeal wall. These are most indicative of posterior nasal drainage, a frequent component of allergic rhinitis. Palatal petechiae are also seen with some frequency in

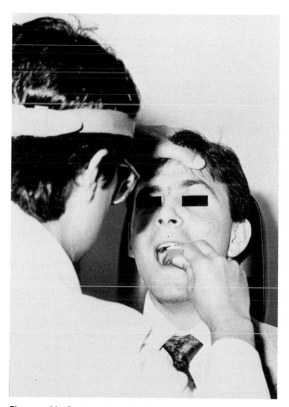

Figure 1A–3. Anterior displacement and downward pressure on the tongue are required for evaluation of the posterior tongue and pharynx.

patients with posterior rhinorrhea. Having the patient say "ah" allows assessment of palatal and pharyngeal wall motion, but it is also a concentration task to decrease gagging.

Of special mention is the varied presentation of mucosal carcinoma, usually squamous cell carcinoma, in the head and neck. Any nonhealing erosion is suspect, even in nonsmokers. In addition, carcinoma may present as a friable exophytic lesion or a deep burrowing ulcer much like an iceberg—larger under the surface than visible above. Another presentation of head and neck carcinoma that is uncommon but particularly difficult to diagnose is the entirely submucosal mass, which is seen most frequently in the tongue and supraglottis with no mucosal abnormality. This example underscores the need for palpation as part of the evaluation, especially when there are symptoms that are not explained by visual inspection. This situation is discussed later.

INDIRECT EXAMINATIONS

Nasopharynx

The nasopharynx is the superiormost portion of the pharynx, lying above the margins of the soft palate. The nasopharynx is accessible for evaluation through use of either indirect technique or flexible or rigid nasal endoscopy.

Most patients will cooperate with the indirect examination as long as they understand what is being accomplished and the physician carefully and deliberately uses instruments and hand bracing to avoid producing a gag reflex. In rare instances, topical anesthetic sprays may be required, but their use is discouraged because they may induce gagging or later aspiration.

A strong light source is required, as is some mechanism to either warm the indirect mirror to body temperature or coat the surface to prevent condensation. An alcohol lamp, an electric bead sterilizer, or a tray-type warmer are all good alternatives, but hot water or even the patient's saliva may be used to prevent mirror fogging. Soap may be used to coat the mirror but tastes unpleasant. When the mirror is heated, it is brought to body temperature and tested against the examiner's own hand or wrist before being inserted into the patient's mouth. The tongue

is depressed by two tongue blades stacked one on the other; a No. 0 nasopharyngeal mirror warmed to body temperature (or coated) is introduced along the surface of the tongue blades to the region of the uvula. The mirror is braced in the corner of the patient's mouth. The patient is requested to breathe through the nose, which allows the soft palate to separate from the posterior pharyngeal wall; this creates enough space to twist the tiny mirror into the nasopharyngeal inlet without touching the posterior pharyngeal wall, which would cause gagging. The mirror is slowly turned to visualize the structures within the nasopharynx (Fig. 1A–4).

The posterior choanae separated by the usually stark-white vomer are first visualized. Within the choanae are the posterior tips of the turbinates; the inferior turbinate is usually the largest. The posterior tip of the inferior turbinate may be large and pitted, with a deep purple hue; it is called a *mulberry turbinate* and is seen in allergic rhinitis. Purulent drainage over the posterior tip of the

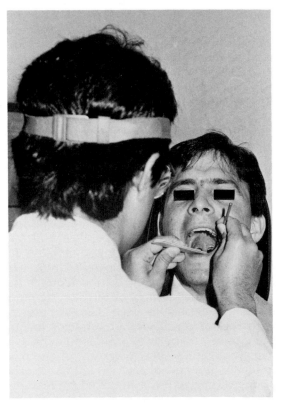

Figure 1A–4. The nasopharyngeal mirror is braced at the corner of the patient's mouth and introduced into the nasopharynx as the patient, with eyes open, breathes through the nose.

inferior turbinate has classically been attributed to maxillary sinusitis; however, evaluation of drainage from the nasopharynx is less accurate than direct inspection of the lateral nasal wall. Purulent drainage from high in the nasopharynx can be caused by sphenoid sinusitis or posterior ethmoid disease. Laterally, the eustachian tube orifices can be identified with the torus tubarius superiorly and the fossae of Rosenmüller, the fold of mucosa just superior to the torus cartilage. The superior surface of the soft palate is also seen.

In children much of the nasopharynx may be obliterated by a hypertrophied adenoid pad; there is usually a large central pad on the posterior wall flanked by two smaller lateral bands. By adulthood the adenoid should be vestigial if present at all. However, Tornwaldt's cyst or a midline dimple representing a remnant of Rathke's pouch may be visible.

Soft palate retractors and red rubber catheters slipped through the nose and pulled out through the mouth have been used to retract the soft palate in cases in which mirror examination has been unsuccessful. In these difficult cases, a preferable method may be the nasal telescope or a flexible endoscope after nasal vasoconstriction and administration of topical anesthetic. The nasopharynx is approached along the floor of the nose; septal spurs may necessitate entrance through the middle meatus. The same structures are identified, although from a different and less stereotypic view.

Larynx and Hypopharynx

A larger mirror (usually No. 5.0) is used to assess the larynx and hypopharynx. Attention to proper patient position and adequate lighting again is given. Use of topical anesthetic is usually unnecessary.

The mirror is warmed to body temperature (or coated) to prevent fogging, as noted in the previous section. Two techniques can be used to perform the indirect laryngoscopy. In the first, two tongue blades are used to push the tongue downward and forward as the mirror is introduced into the oral cavity. The warmed mirror is introduced slowly over the blades; the mirror handle is braced in the corner of the patient's mouth, or the hands are braced on the patient's cheek. When the soft palate is reached, the uvula is lifted

carefully, and the mirror is turned slightly first to one side and then to the other to visualize the hypopharyngeal and laryngeal structures. The patient, with eyes open, concentrates on breathing purposely through the mouth (Fig. 1A–5). In the second technique, the patient's tongue is grasped with a gauze sponge and pulled forward, with the examiner's nondominant hand braced on the face. This, of course, is done gently, and care is taken not to cut the tongue on the lower incisors (Fig. 1A–6). Some patients find this technique unpleasant; however, this method may expose the anterior larynx better than the aforementioned technique.

First the base of the tongue is visualized with the prominent circumvallate papillae and sometimes visible midline foramen cecum. The vallecula may be filled with a symmetric overgrowth of the lingual tonsils; any asymmetry should be noted. A large venous plexus or inclusion cysts are frequent

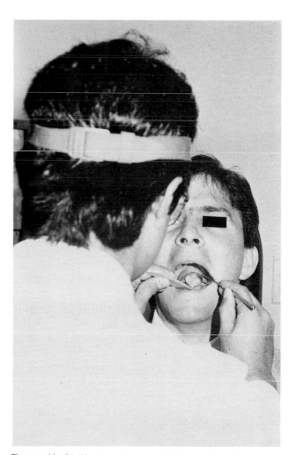

Figure 1A–5. The two–tongue blade indirect laryngoscopy. This technique may fail to adequately reveal the anterior confines of the larynx.

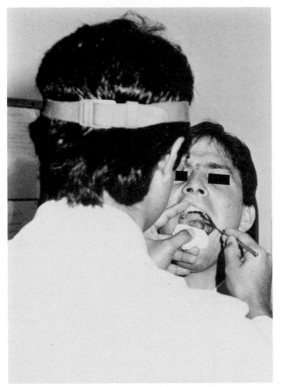

Figure 1A–6. The tongue-grasp technique of indirect laryngoscopy. Note techniques for hand and mirror bracing.

normal variants. The indirect mirror is also excellent for inspecting the inferior poles of the tonsils. The epiglottis is seen below the tongue base; it is usually quite thin and rigid and is attached to the base of the tongue by the median glossoepiglottic fold and to the lateral pharyngeal walls by the lateral pharyngoepiglottic folds. One may readily examine its superior or lingual surface, but evaluation of its inferior or laryngeal surface is much more difficult. For the examination to be complete, however, the base of the laryngeal surface (epiglottic tubercle) should be seen. The lateral and posterior pharyngeal walls are next inspected. Bulging may indicate a space-occupying tumor, an aneurysm, an infection, or a cervical osteophyte. The pyriform sinuses (extensions of the hypopharynx laterally and posteriorly) are usually not entirely seen in indirect examination, but pathologic conditions are hinted at by pooling of secretions, subtle bulging, or asymmetry. The endolarynx is next brought into view. The true vocal folds or cords themselves are stark white; the remainder of the

endolarynx and hypopharynx is pale pink. The anterior commissure (the fixed attachment to the thyroid cartilage) may be difficult to visualize; again, complete examination requires visualization of this region.

Checking patient position, allowing the patient to swallow, and regrasping or positioning the tongue in a more anterior position are at times all that is necessary to view the anterior confines of the larynx and epiglottic base. Having the patient vocalize a high-pitched "eeee" usually causes the epiglottis to be lifted forward and the anterior commissure to come into view. The arytenoid (mobile) cartilages to which the fibrous vocal folds attach are located posteriorly, articulating with the cricoid; they should be symmetric in size and also in level of placement. Erythema of the arytenoids without other findings may indicate gastroesophageal reflux.

The vocal process describes a pale, slightly depressed area at the attachment of the vocal fold with the arytenoid, the site of contact ulcers or granulomas. The posterior commissure describes the crease between the arytenoids. Just superior to the true vocal folds are the false vocal folds. Between the true and false folds lie the laryngeal ventricles or a lateral crease in the laryngeal mucosa. The aryepiglottic folds, containing ligaments of attachment for the epiglottis and the cuneiform and corniculate cartilages, lie further superiorly.

The vocal folds are assessed for asymmetry of structure and movement. A detailed analysis of cord paralysis is to be presented in subsequent chapters; however, delineating fixation from paralysis may not be possible without direct palpation of the arytenoid mass.

The subglottis and trachea may be seen in the indirect mirror examination, but visualization is usually a function more of glottic size than of the examiner's skill. Nonetheless, in large larynges, several tracheal rings and occasionally the carina may be clearly seen.

The flexible endoscope or the rigid telescope may be a useful instrument for examining the larynx, the hypopharynx, and the trachea. Certainly when prolonged study such as for cord mobility abnormalities or photodocumentation is required, endoscopy may be the examination method of choice.

Nasal decongestion and topical anesthesia are required. As the telescope is passed along the nasal floor, the patient is asked to breathe through the nose to open the nasopharyngeal inlet; the flexible telescope is manipulated to pass gently through the nasopharynx until the epiglottis and then the larynx come into view (Fig. 1A–7). Not only are lesions of the endolarynx readily visualized, but the patient may be instructed to perform Valsalva's maneuver as the nostrils are pinched closed to "blow out" the piriform sinuses, so that lesions in their far recesses can be seen. The anterior commissure and subglottis are particularly well seen by this technique, and with topical anesthesia of the larynx and trachea, flexible tracheoscopy is possible.

Neck, Including Bimanual Examination

For cervical palpation, most examiners prefer the "from behind" stance for side-to-side comparison of anatomic detail. Obstructive collars and ties require loosening or removal. An almost massaging motion is required to roll the structures of the neck under the examiner's fingers.

The midline structures are evaluated in side-to-side comparison. The thyroid and cricoid cartilages are usually readily identifiable: the thyroid is most prominent in adult males, and the cricoid is most prominent in prepubescent males and all females. The thyroid cartilage is shieldlike in form, and the cricoid

has a signet ring shape. The cricoid is the only complete ring in the laryngotracheal complex, which makes it most important for structural support.

A normal grinding sensation, or *laryngeal crepitance*, is elicited by rolling the thyroid-cricoid complex against the vertebral column. Lack of crepitance indicates inflammation or tumor involvement posterior to the larynx (postcricoid involvement). It is important, particularly after trauma, to identify the normal laryngeal landmarks and to ensure that the laryngeal skeleton is stable. When laryngeal, esophageal, and thyroid tumors are suspected, the examiner must note any expansion, abnormal soft tissue, or extralaryngeal masses.

The junction between the thyroid and cricoid cartilages is quite superficial (cricothyroid membrane), and so emergency tracheal access is possible here. A Delphian node may be found here in thyroid tumors or in laryngeal tumors. The examiner may palpate the hyoid by grasping it between the thumb and forefinger and gently rocking it back and forth. The greater cornu is directly proximal to the first part of the external carotid artery. Between the thyroid notch and the body of the hyoid is a potential space called the thyrohyoid space, a common site of thyroglossal duct cysts. The thyroid gland usually lies along the tracheoesophageal groove; its isthmus crosses anteriorly on the cricoid or upper tracheal rings. The patient may be

Figure 1A–7. After a topical nasal decongestant and anesthesia are applied, the flexible nasopharyngoscope is passed under direct visualization through the nose, usually via the inferior meatus.

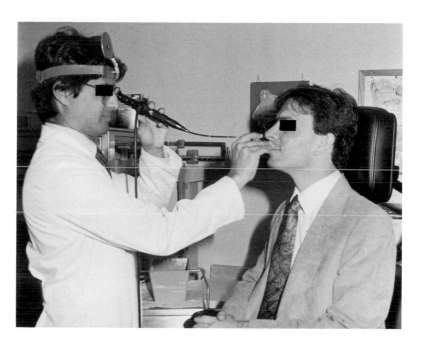

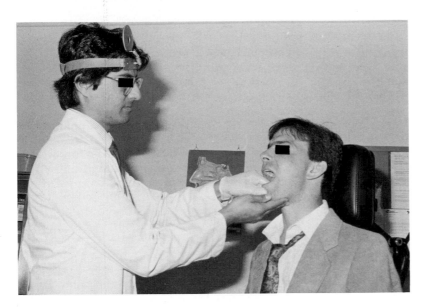

Figure 1A–8. Bimanual examination may reveal subtle masses or sialoliths.

asked to swallow to elevate the gland so that it can be rolled underneath the examiner's fingers.

Next, the clavicles and then the supraclavicular fossae may be identified. Subtle adenopathy in this region is detected through gentle massage against the floor of the fossae. The sternomastoid muscle is identified with its two insertions on the sternum and medial clavicle. This muscle is followed superiorly to its origin on the mastoid tip. Adenopathy frequently lies deep to the sternomastoid, and having the patient flex the neck will relax the muscle so that the examiner may palpate deep to it. Caution should be used in deep palpation along the carotid sheath because syncope may be elicited through a baroreceptor response. Carotidodynia, or tenderness of the carotid vessels, is frequently seen in older patients. Next, one may palpate the submandibular triangles. Here, as well as under the sternomastoid, are frequent sites of adenopathy. The submandibular glands may be ptotic, particularly in older persons, and may be mistaken for a mass in this region; however, the symmetric nature of this finding usually leads the examiner to the correct conclusion. The glands themselves should be assessed for unilateral enlargement or mass.

The examiner may then palpate the posterior confines of the neck (including suboccipital regions) and search for asymmetry or adenopathy. If any masses are found, their location, consistency (whether stony, rubbery, soft, or fluctuant), tenderness, and fixation (to skin or deeper structures) are recorded. Whether the mass is warm or has a coloration is noted. Transillumination may be helpful in examination of fluid-containing lesions such as cystic hygroma or lymphangioma; change in size of the mass with straining may indicate a vascular or lymphatic anomaly, classically a cystic hygroma. Auscultation may be useful if a vascular mass is suspected.

The parotid glands and finally the temporomandibular joints are palpated for mass or tenderness. Of note, temporomandibular joint dysfunction is a frequent cause of head and neck pain. Pressing lightly into the joint anterior to the tragus or within the external canal while the patient widely opens and then closes the jaw may reveal grinding, clicking, or discomfort. Intraoral palpation may reveal tenderness of the tendinous insertion of the temporal muscle. Occlusal abnormalities or unusual wear facets may be further clues.

Bimanual examination, although not required for all cases, is helpful should no cause of a patient's complaints be apparent; it is mandatory to help outline the margins of tumor involvement of the head and neck. Topical anesthesia may be required. Wearing protective gloves, the examiner uses one hand to gently palpate the floor of mouth and tongue, even as far as the tongue base and vallecula, and the opposite hand to feel from outside against the neck (Fig. 1A–8).

Both tonsils and the posterior pharynx may also be palpated in this fashion. Submucosal tumors are usually more apparent through bimanual palpation; stones within the submandibular glands may be detected only by bimanual palpation. Tenderness of the styloid process felt through the tonsillar fossa is known as Eagle's syndrome.

AUSCULTATION OF THE HEAD AND NECK

As noted in the previous section, auscultation of a neck mass may be revealing if a vascular lesion is suspected. The bell of the stethoscope is used for this portion of the examination to hear the low-frequency vascular vibrations or bruits. The course of the carotid is followed from the supraclavicular region to the skull base. Carotid body tumors generally exhibit an audible bruit in sequence with the patient's pulse; indeed, many pulsate against the examiner's hand. Arteriovenous malformations may likewise pulsate and exhibit an audible bruit but also tend to be warm to the touch.

A carotid-cavernous fistula with proptosis and chemosis may also exhibit an audible high-pitched bruit with auscultation over the affected globe. After trauma, the bruit may precede the eye signs.

Auscultation over the ear and temporal region is also performed, particularly in otovestibular evaluations in which a cause of tinnitus is sought.

NEUROLOGIC ASSESSMENT

Neurologic evaluation, particularly of the cranial nerves, becomes a part of many head and neck examinations. Olfaction (cranial nerve I) may be tested with readily available odorants such as coffee or perfume. Vision and eye movements are noted for asymmetry, field cuts, and nystagmus (cranial nerves II, III, IV, and VI) and are usually assessed with an eye chart or by having the patient read small print, followed by confrontational fields and extraocular motility testing. Sensation of the three branches of the trigeminal nerve (V) is assessed by light touch, usually with a cotton wisp stroking the forehead, cheek, and jaw. Corneal sensation is tested as well. Loss of reflex blink may be the first

evidence of a cerebellopontine angle lesion. To assess masticatory function (motor nerve V), the patient bites down and the masseter and temporalis muscles are palpated. To assess motor function of the facial nerve, the patient grimaces, puckers the lips, smiles, or closes the eyes tightly—whatever combination will allow the examiner to compare movements of all branches. Assessing taste on the anterior two thirds of the tongue and stapedius reflex requires more detailed testing. Asymmetry can indicate a peripheral or a central lesion, and testing may help to define the site of the lesion (topognostic testing). The statoacoustic cranial nerve (VIII) is discussed in more detail in other sections, but gross integrity may be assessed with tuning forks and medical history. The gag reflex and elevation of the soft palate are thought to be combined functions of the glossopharyngeal nerve (IX) and vagus nerve (X). Laryngeal movement and sensation are mediated through the vagus. The sternomastoid and trapezius muscles are innervated by the accessory nerve (XI) and are assessed by resistance to head turning, shoulder shrugging, and arm raising. The hypoglossal nerve (XII) mediates tongue motion; in complete paralysis, the tongue deviates toward the site of lesion. Partial paralysis will lead to atrophy and fasciculation of the involved side before deviation.

Autonomic functions may also be evaluated. Unilateral ptosis, miosis, and anhidrosis (Horner's syndrome) indicate a cervical sympathetic chain lesion. Parasympathetic functions such as lacrimation may be assessed by Schirmer's tear test; salivation, by the lemon-drop stimulation test.

Depending on the patient's history and findings involving the cranial nerves, a more detailed neurologic evaluation that includes assessment of the peripheral nervous system may be required; the reader is referred to the referenced neurology texts for more detailed evaluations.

SUGGESTED READINGS

Adams RD, Victor M: Principles of Neurology, 4th ed. New York, McGraw-Hill Information Services, 1989.
Bailey BJ, Strunk CL, Jones JK: Methods of examination (the larynx, trachea, bronchi, and lungs). *In* Bluestone CD, Stool SE (eds): Pediatric Otolaryngology, 2nd ed (pp 1064–1077). Philadelphia: WB Saunders, 1990.
Ballenger JH: Anatomy of the larynx. *In* Ballenger JH

(ed): Diseases of the Nose, Throat, Ear, Head and Neck, 13th ed (pp 376–385). Philadelphia: Lea & Febiger, 1985.

Ballenger JJ: The clinical anatomy and physiology of the nose and accessory sinuses. *In* Ballenger JH (ed): Diseases of the Nose, Throat, Ear, Head and Neck, 13th ed (pp 1–25). Philadelphia: Lea & Febiger, 1985.

Hamilton WJ, Harrison RJ: Anatomy of the nose, nasal cavity and paranasal sinuses. *In* Ballantyne J, Groves J (eds): Scott-Brown's Diseases of the Ear, Nose and Throat, 4th ed, vol. I (pp 133–156). Boston: Butterworths, 1979.

Healy GB: Methods of examination (the nose, paranasal sinuses, face, and orbit). *In* Bluestone CD, Stool SE (eds): Pediatric Otolaryngology, 2nd ed, vol. I (pp 643–656). Philadelphia: WB Saunders, 1990.

Lima JA, Graviss ER: Methods of examination (the neck). *In* Bluestone CD, Stool SE (eds): Pediatric Otolaryngology, 2nd ed, vol. II (pp 1282–1293). Philadelphia: WB Saunders, 1990.

Mayo Clinic, Department of Neurology: Clinical Examinations in Neurology, 5th ed. Philadelphia: WB Saunders, 1981.

McNab Jones RF: Anatomy of the mouth, pharynx and oesophagus. *In* Ballantyne J, Groves J (eds): Scott-Brown's Diseases of the Ear, Nose and Throat, 4th ed, vol. I (pp 263–311). Boston: Butterworths, 1979.

Perkin D, Rose FC, Blackwood W, Shawdon HH: Atlas of Clinical Neurology. Philadelphia: JB Lippincott, 1986.

Potsic WP, Handler SD: Methods of examination (the mouth, pharynx, and esophagus). *In* Bluestone CD, Stool SE (eds): Pediatric Otolaryngology, 2nd ed, vol. II (pp 823–836). Philadelphia: WB Saunders, 1990.

Powell N, Humphreys B: Proportions of the Aesthetic Face. New York: Thieme Medical Publishers, 1983.

Rowland, LP (ed): Merritt's Textbook of Neurology, 8th ed. Philadelphia: Lea & Febiger, 1989.

Saunders WH: Physical examination of the head and neck. *In* Paparella M, Shumrick D (eds): Otolaryngology, 2nd ed, vol. III (pp 1929–1943). Philadelphia: WB Saunders, 1980.

Stell PM, Bickford BJ: Anatomy of the larynx and tracheobronchial tree. *In* Ballantyne J, Groves J (eds): Scott-Brown's Diseases of the Ear, Nose and Throat, 4th ed, vol. I (pp 385–431). Boston: Butterworths, 1979.

Ballenger JH: Surgical anatomy of the pharynx. *In* Ballenger JH (ed): Diseases of the Nose, Throat, Ear, Head and Neck, 13th ed (pp 281–289). Philadelphia: Lea & Febiger, 1985.

Walker HK, Hall WD, Hurst JW (eds): Clinical Methods: The History, Physical and Laboratory Examinations, 2nd ed. Boston: Butterworths, 1980.

Weiner HL, Levitt LP: Neurology for the House Officer, 3rd ed. Baltimore: Williams & Wilkins, 1983.

Wood, RP, Northern JL (eds): Manual of Otolaryngology—A Symptom Oriented Text. Baltimore: Williams & Wilkins, 1979.

History and Physical Examination

Ear

Peter S. Roland, MD

AURICLE

The auricle, or pinna, is a complex cartilaginous structure covered with skin. Embryologically, it is derived from the six hillocks of His. Its innervation and vascular supply are complex. When one is examining the auricle, attention should be given to its size, shape, and position, and it must be remembered that the auricle itself may be hiding postauricular lesions (Figs. 1B–1, 1B–2). An abnormally positioned auricle may be part of a congenital syndrome that involves multiple organ systems. Down's syndrome, in which the external ear is in an abnormally low position, is a good example. Abnormally sized and shaped external ears may also be part of a congenital syndrome but frequently occur as isolated findings. Such abnormalities may be bilateral or unilateral. Very small external ears (microtia) may occur alone or may be associated with atresia of the external auditory canal and congenital malformation of the tympanic membrane, ossicles, or cochleovestibular organs (Fig. 1B–3). In general, minimal auricular deformities are associated with a normally formed membranous labyrinth, middle ear, and mastoid. The more severe the auricular deformity, the greater the likelihood that the middle or the inner ear, or both, are malformed (Fig. 1B–4). Small dimples, pits, or tracks may be isolated manifestations of faulty fusion of the hillocks of His or may be the surface manifestations of

more complex branchial cleft anomalies. Their positions should be noted, and minimal attempts at probing their depths should be undertaken. Thickening and twisting of the cartilage, as in cauliflower ears, may indicate old injury.

A variety of systemic conditions may be manifested in abnormalities of the auricle. A variety of nodules may occur on the auricle. Darwin's tubercle, a developmental nodule on the upper third of the posterior helix, should be distinguished from pathologic nodules. The subcutaneous deposition of uric acid crystals (*tophi*) may occur in gout. Subcutaneous amyloid may also accumulate in the presence of systemic disease. The auricle is subject to a variety of conditions common to skin in general, including herpes zoster oticus (Ramsey Hunt syndrome), impetigo, psoriasis, erysipelas, and fungal dermatitis. Neoplastic lesions occur with considerable frequency on the external ear. The usual cutaneous neoplasms (squamous cell and basal cell) are the most frequent. These lesions, although often small, should be treated carefully because inadequate removal of them can ultimately result in the patient's demise. Most cystic lesions of the external ear are sebaceous inclusion cysts, but benign pseudocysts and cystic neoplasms may also occur. Obvious inflammation of the external ear may indicate a bacterial dermatitis (impetigo, erysipelas) or inflammation of the underlying cartilage. Bacterial inflammation

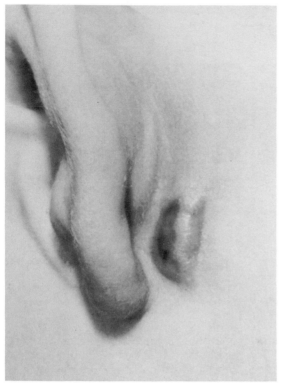

Figure 1B–1. This postauricular keloid could have easily been missed if care had not been taken to look behind the ear.

of the underlying cartilage (chondritis or perichondritis) is usually an isolated finding. Autoimmune inflammation (relapsing polychondritis) is generally associated with inflammation of the nasal and laryngeal cartilages and a very high rate of erythrocyte sedimentation. Other signs of autoimmune dysfunction may also be associated with relapsing polychondritis. Allergic reactions may involve the auricle. Allergy to topical antibiotics (especially neomycin) or to their vehicles is not uncommon, and these allergic reactions may be much worse than the initial bacterial infection (Fig. 1B–5). Quite commonly seen on the lobule is the topical reaction to nickel, which is caused by inexpensive pierced earrings.

EXTERNAL AUDITORY CANAL AND TYMPANIC MEMBRANE

To adequately evaluate the external auditory canal and tympanic membrane, the tragus must be pulled anteriorly and the auricle drawn upward and backward. This maneuver straightens the external auditory canal. This preliminary manipulation of the external ear also rapidly elicits signs of any tenderness. Such tenderness on movement of the auricle is a reliable symptom of external otitis but is not found in acute otitis media. The position of the patient's head is of considerable importance in examining the external auditory canal and the tympanic membrane. The head should not be left upright but should be tilted toward the opposite shoulder to compensate for the normal inclination of the ear canal. The novice examiner usually fails to tilt the head sufficiently and finds visualization of the tympanic membrane very difficult. For some patients, manipulation of the tragus and auricle alone yields an adequate view of the external auditory canal and tympanic membrane. However, for many patients it is necessary to use an aural speculum. The hand that holds the speculum must also grasp the auricle and stretch it upward and posteriorly (Fig. 1B–6). The examiner's other hand is thus free to hold

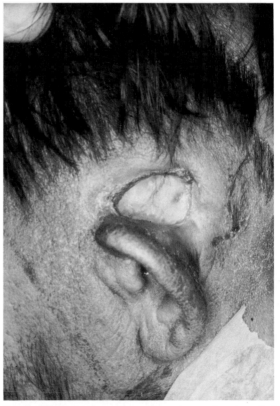

Figure 1B–2. A squamous cell carcinoma has invaded down to bone in the supra-auricular area.

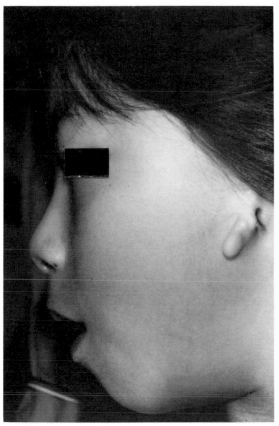

Figure 1B–3. Microtia. This child had complete agenesis of the external auditory canal and middle ear. She had a badly deformed cochlea and was completely deaf in the involved ear. The contralateral ear was normal.

canal laceration or a tympanic membrane injury.

Although the tympanic membrane can be evaluated with only a light source and speculum, magnification is now routinely used. The device most commonly used for magnification of the tympanic membrane is the hand-held otoscope. A magnifying lens is attached to the device and can be inserted between the examiner's line of vision and the end of the speculum to provide a moderate amount of magnification. The otoscope has the advantage of being portable and relatively easy to use. The other method of obtaining a magnified image of the tympanic membrane is the use of the operating microscope. Otolaryngologists routinely use otomicroscopy, which they believe is more accurate than otoscopy. Available magnification is much higher (up to 22 times) and can be varied. The light source is usually brighter, and the optics are significantly better. Otomicroscopy, however, requires months of training and takes a relatively long time (5 to 15 minutes) to perform. Another disadvantage is that the operating microscope is essentially nonportable. When one examines

instruments. One should learn to use the nondominant hand to hold the speculum so that the dominant hand is free to hold instruments. After straightening the ear canal as much as possible by moving the auricle, the examiner should insert the largest speculum that will fit into the canal. In general, an oval speculum fits better than a round one. The speculum should be inserted no farther than the cartilaginous portion of the external auditory canal because any pressure on the bony inner third of the ear canal is quite painful. When an otoscope tip, a speculum, or an instrument is inserted into the ear, the examiner's hand should be stabilized against the patient's head. This helps to prevent injury from abrupt head movement. As the patient's head moves, the hand resting on it moves with it. When the hand is not stabilized against the patient's head, abrupt or unexpected head movement may result in a

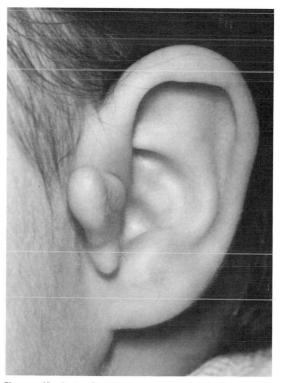

Figure 1B–4. A skin tag associated with the tragus, indicative of faulty fusion of the hillocks of His.

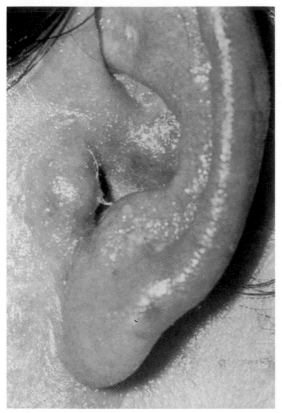

Figure 1B–5. Marked allergic reaction to polymyxin B-sulfate (Cortisporin) drops. This patient's allergic reaction was much more serious than the original episode of external otitis.

causes pain and bleeding. Although unexpected head movement still presents difficulty, the better visualization afforded by the operating microscope makes direct removal of cerumen much easier and, therefore, safer. The light source is generally brighter, magnification is retained, and binocular vision permits accurate depth perception. With a nonreflective speculum, a variety of small suction tips, cerumen spoons, hooks, and alligator forceps can be used to safely remove cerumen and debris (Fig. 1B–7).

Gentle irrigation by an ear syringe or a water pick is an acceptable alternative to manual removal of cerumen. This technique is effective if the cerumen is not tightly packed within the external auditory canal. Successful removal of cerumen by irrigation requires that some of the stream of water get behind the obstructing cerumen in order to push it laterally and out of the external auditory canal. Although water pick irrigators are generally safe, tympanic membrane perforation and even more serious otologic injuries from these instruments have been reported; therefore, the lowest effective pressure should be used to prevent mechanical trauma. If pre-existing tympanic membrane perforation lurks behind the cerumen impaction, water may enter the middle ear space. The infusion of cool water into the middle ear can produce acute vertigo by inducing

the external auditory canal and tympanic membrane, it is possible to apply negative and positive pressure on the tympanic membrane, using either technique, to assess its mobility. Assessment of tympanic membrane mobility is an integral aspect of the complete physical examination of the tympanic membrane.

It is frequently necessary to remove cerumen before completion of the examination. Removal of cerumen from uncooperative children or adults can be a difficult and potentially morbid procedure. One may remove cerumen with a hand-held otoscope by taking off the magnifying lens and manipulating the instrument through the attached speculum. It is, however, difficult to see well when the magnifying lens has been removed, and the view is frequently obstructed by the hand or instrument being manipulated. Abrupt or unexpected movement by the patient may cause the instrument to lacerate the ear canal or tympanic membranes, which

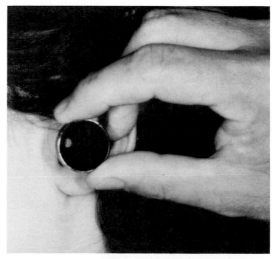

Figure 1B–6. The auricle can be retracted posteriorly with the third and fourth fingers while the index finger and thumb hold the speculum firmly in the external auditory canal. The fourth and fifth fingers rest on the bone posterior to the auricle in order to stabilize the speculum.

Figure 1B–7. With the patient's head tilted toward the opposite shoulder and the speculum held in the examiner's nondominant hand, the operating microscope can be used to evaluate the ear. Instruments should be held in the dominant hand in order to gain finer control.

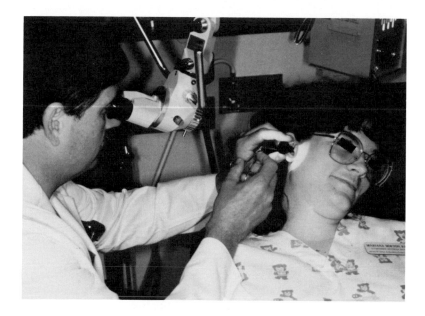

thermal convection currents in the semicircular canals. Contamination of the middle ear with water may produce infection not only by the introduction of bacteria but also by washing out the normal acid milieu of the external auditory canal. Irrigation of the external auditory canal has also been shown to be an important cause of malignant external otitis (temporal bone osteomyelitis) in elderly diabetics. If it is necessary to perform aural irrigation in diabetic patients, sterile solutions should be used.

In very difficult cerumen impactions, one may fill the ear with a solution of 3% hydrogen peroxide two or three times a day for several days before evaluation. If the cerumen is extremely hard and tightly impacted, the instillation of mineral oil on a daily basis for several days before attempted removal may also be helpful. Although most adults and a great many children will cooperate during otologic examination, it is occasionally necessary to forcefully immobilize an infant or a very young child. This can be accomplished either by use of the papoose board or through the assistance of one parent. It is surprising how difficult it can be to eliminate head movements completely in even a very young child. It is frequently necessary to have a second assistant just to hold the child's head still. If very great difficulty is experienced in an attempt to examine the ear or to remove impacted cerumen or mucopurulent debris, it may be better to administer a short general anesthetic rather than persist

in a protracted, potentially injurious attempt to physically restrain a panicked child.

In evaluating the external auditory canal, one should note the presence or the absence of cerumen. Cerumen is normally present in at least small quantities. The complete absence of cerumen when it has not been removed (asteatosis) is abnormal. Dry, flaking skin in the meatus and conchal bowl with minimal cerumen suggests chronic seborrheic dermatitis, which predisposes the patient to external otitis. During examination, the caliper of the canal should be assessed. The lateral cartilaginous external auditory canal should be inspected for furuncles and sebaceous cysts. The former are tender; the latter are painless unless infected. The presence or the absence of cutaneous lesions, especially vesicular ones, should be noted. Vesicular lesions of the external auditory canal and tympanic membrane may represent herpetic infection or bullous myringitis. The presence of granulation tissue or exposed bone in the external auditory canal may be associated with very aggressive infections (malignant otitis externa) or with a true neoplasm. Marked narrowing of the ear canals can be a consequence of previous surgery, recurrent canal infections, or congenital anomalies. The medial portions of the canal should be examined for the presence of a sagging posterior canal wall, because this suggests bony erosion from mastoid or antral cholesteatoma. Foreign objects are found with some frequency in the ears of preschool children and, occasionally, mentally impaired adults. External otitis, or swimmer's ear, is a common affliction and may be exquisitely painful. It may be associated with marked edema of the external auditory canals and complete closure of the meatus or with a voluminous mucopurulent exudate. Marked accumulation of keratinous debris may represent disease limited to the external auditory canal, such as keratosis obturans or canal cholesteatoma. It may also, however, represent desquamated epithelium resulting from a cholesteatoma of the middle ear or the mastoid process. Only meticulous and careful cleaning of the external auditory canal permits differentiation. Polyps of the external auditory canal may be gently manipulated to determine their point of origin. Some arise from the external canal and are secondary to chronic external otitis. Others arise from the middle ear and present through a tympanic membrane perforation, and they are indicative of chronic middle ear disease, very often cholesteatoma. It is unwise to attempt to remove these polyps outside the operating room unless the point of origin can be clearly determined; otherwise, inadvertent avulsion of the ossicles, especially the stapes, or damage to the facial nerve may occur. Limited biopsy is recommended if surgery is not warranted.

A variety of fungi may reside within the auditory canal as either primary or secondary pathogens. Infections by both *Aspergillus niger* and *Candida albicans* occur with some frequency, especially after prolonged instillation of antibiotic otic drops. Otomycosis caused by aspergillosis usually appears as either black or white fluffy, cottonlike growths. Other fungal organisms are less common but, when present, are more likely to produce active infections. Tumors of the external auditory canal are uncommon and include both benign and malignant varieties. They should not, however, be confused with bony exostosis, which frequently occurs at suture lines and is of no clinical significance unless it blocks the egress of desquamated epithelium and cerumen.

TYMPANIC MEMBRANE AND MIDDLE EAR

The status of the middle ear has been inferred from examination of the tympanic membrane

for hundreds of years. No examination of the tympanic membrane is complete unless the pars flaccida has been specifically visualized. Systematic evaluation of the tympanic membrane includes notation of its color, its position, and what conditions (if any) induce visible movement in it. The color of the normal tympanic membrane varies from a somewhat dusky off-white through shades of gray to silver. It is frequently possible to see the shadows of the round window niche, the long process of the incus, and the chorda tympani through a normal drum. When middle ear structure can be seen through the tympanic membrane, it is fairly certain that the middle ear is normal (Fig. 1B–8).

Classically, acute otitis media is said to produce fiery redness of the tympanic membrane. However, a dark, dusky tympanic membrane is also associated with acute middle ear infection. In subacute stages the tympanic membrane can actually be a fairly intense white as a result of the presence of accumulated pus behind the drum head. Chronic middle ear effusion is traditionally described as giving the tympanic membrane an "amber" appearance and frequently does so. Occasionally, bubbles can be seen behind the tympanic membrane, and this finding is an extremely reliable physical sign of the presence of the middle ear fluid. The position of the tympanic membrane is an important diagnostic feature but can be difficult to appreciate. In many cases of middle ear effusion, the tympanic membrane is only slightly or moderately retracted. When the tympanic membrane is pulled inward, toward the medial wall of the middle ear, the long process of the malleus is pulled inward with it. Optical foreshortening in visual inspection of the tympanic membrane results in the appearance of apparent shortening of the long process of the malleus. Thus a long process of the malleus that appears very short is a fairly frequent, and often useful, finding when the tympanic membrane is retracted. Visualization of the incudostapedial joint may be indicative of retraction of the eardrum. If the tympanic membrane adheres to the incudostapedial joint (an anatomic arrangement termed a *myringostapediopexy*, chronic retraction can be assumed. When retraction is sufficiently severe to cause draping of the attenuated eardrum over the incudostapedial joint with adhesion of the tympanic membrane to the promontory, *atelectasis* of the tympanic membrane is said to

Posterior Superior Quadrant | Anterior Superior Quadrant

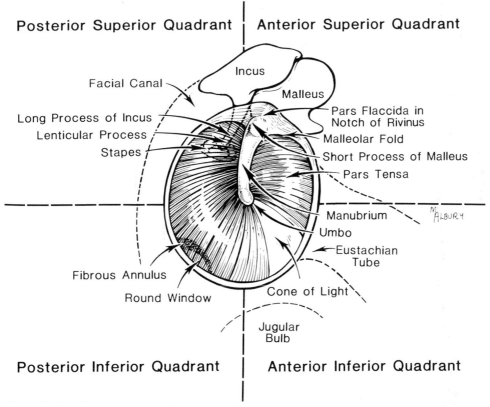

Facial Canal

Incus

Malleus

Pars Flaccida in Notch of Rivinus

Long Process of Incus

Lenticular Process

Stapes

Malleolar Fold

Short Process of Malleus

Pars Tensa

Manubrium

Umbo

Eustachian Tube

Fibrous Annulus

Round Window

Cone of Light

Jugular Bulb

Posterior Inferior Quadrant | Anterior Inferior Quadrant

Figure 1B–8. The important landmarks of the tympanic membrane and what they represent are illustrated by quadrant. Each of these landmarks should be noted in every physical examination of the tympanic membrane. (From Meyerhoff L: Diagnosis and Management of Hearing Loss. Philadelphia: WB Saunders, 1984.)

be present. Such severe, permanent retraction of the tympanic membrane is generally due to irremediable dysfunction of the eustachian tube.

A normal tympanic membrane can be induced to move both inward and outward with applied positive and negative pressure. The hand-held otoscope can be used to perform this examination if a pneumatic bulb is attached to it. The Arnold-Bruening otoscope can be used in conjunction with the operating microscope. One should test with both positive and negative pressures. The normal tympanic membrane moves freely with applied positive and negative pressures. Both the bulging drum of otitis media and the atelectatic drum adherent to the medial wall of the middle ear are immobile. When simple retraction is present, however, positive pressure frequently produces no visible movement, whereas negative pressure may result in outward displacement of the drum.

Perforations of the tympanic membrane are categorized as central perforations and marginal perforations. Central perforations are those that have any rim (however narrow) of normal drum between the edge of the perforation and the bony annulus. Marginal perforations are those with no drum between them and the bony annulus. The distinction is important because marginal perforations are thought to be more likely to produce cholesteatomas. This is especially true of posterior marginal perforations. Many anterior perforations appear to be marginal when examined in the physician's office because the bulge of the anterior bony canal obscures the anterior drum remnant. In many cases, a rim of retained tympanic membrane may be found during surgery.

Care should be taken to determine that apparent perforations are real. Perforations may heal as thin, "secondary," or "dimeric" membranes that may be difficult to identify, especially if retracted. Careful examination with the binocular microscope and pneumatic otoscopy may be required to identify a secondary membrane. The size and position of the perforation, when present, should be noted. It is difficult to estimate the size of perforations in millimeters, especially when magnification is being used. Thus size is often estimated as a percentage of the involved drum. For example, a posterior central perforation may be described as involving approximately 25% of the drum. It is especially important to notice apparent perforations of the pars flaccida. It is an axiom of otology that these apparent perforations are, in fact, the open ends of cholesteatoma sacs. Thus all "perforations" of the pars flaccida are to be considered cholesteatomas until absolutely proved otherwise.

When perforations are present in the posterior quadrant, some notation about the status of the ossicular chain is frequently possible. Absence of the long process of the incus or erosions of the stapes may be seen. Chronic perforations, especially when associated with cholesteatoma, may also be associated with marked mucopurulent exudate and debris. Such debris should be suctioned clean and every attempt made to inspect the cleansed external auditory canal and the middle ear space. The mucosa may vary from a thin, healthy, and glistening one to a markedly thickened mucosa with associated granulation tissue and mucopurulent exudate. When granulation tissue polyps are seen coming from the middle ear space, it is unwise to attempt avulsion or blind manipulation. These polyps may be attached to portions of the stapes or facial nerve. When it is necessary to remove these polyps in order to fully examine the ear, a sharp excision of clearly visible portions is preferable to avulsion.

Occasionally, a mass lesion can be seen behind an intact tympanic membrane. Its color and balance should be noted. The color of any mass behind the tympanic membrane provides important information for differential diagnosis. A white, glistening mass is most likely cholesteatoma but may represent tympanosclerosis, an adenoma, a neuroma, or in rare cases a bony middle ear osteoma. Gray neoplasms may represent mensenchymal tumors or neuromas. Sometimes palpation with a blunt hook helps in distinguishing masses. A high jugular bulb generally presents as a very dark, blue mass with a clear superior margin arising from the hypotympanum. Vascular tumors such as paragangliomas vary in color from red to dark blue and are dusky in nature. Highly vascular neoplasms may blanch with the application of positive pressure from a pneumatic otoscope, a phenomenon termed *Brown's sign*. Exploratory tympanotomy and biopsy are required for definitive diagnosis after appropriate radiologic imaging. Biopsy should be preceded by arteriography if there is any suspicion that the lesion is vascular or if the carotid artery is exposed.

PHYSICAL EXAMINATION OF THE POSTOPERATIVE EAR

Otologic examination in patients who have had previous surgery is especially difficult. Normal landmarks are often absent. The type of incision used should be noted; this may give some clues as to the type of operation performed. Inspection should be made for the presence or the absence of the posterior bony canal wall. Although this is generally easy, a few patients who have had very small, sclerotic preoperative mastoids have undergone a canal-wall–down mastoidectomy, and they have what appears to be only a very large external auditory canal. When the posterior canal wall has been removed, one should note the adequacy of meatal size. In most problem-free canal-wall–down mastoid cavities, portions of the conchal cartilage have been removed in order to create a large meatus. When cleansing of the mastoid cavity is difficult, it is generally because an inadequate meatoplasty has been performed (Fig. 1B–9).

The facial ridge should be identified and its height noted. In most well-crafted mastoid cavities, the facial ridge has been lowered to the level of the nerve itself. Inspection should be made for the presence or the absence of the lateral wall of the epitympanum. Retention of this structure should raise suspicions that residual disease may be concealed in the epitympanum or in the anterior epitympanic recess. In general, a problem-free mastoid cavity is seen as a relatively smooth, contoured bowl free of obvious landmarks. The presence or the absence of a grafted tympanic membrane is noted; if present, the membrane is inspected for lateralization, retraction, perforation, and ossicular landmarks. In many cases, only a thick, opaque tympanic membrane graft can be seen, and the arrangement of the underlying ossicular chain, if any, cannot be inferred.

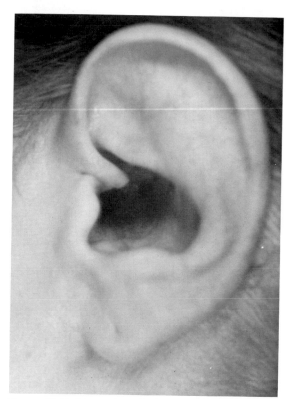

Figure 1B–9. Illustration of a large, well-crafted meatoplasty associated with a problem-free cavity.

Some patients who have undergone a canal-wall–down mastoidectomy have had labyrinthine fistulas. Such fistulas can arise as complications of cholesteatoma, as the result of inadvertent operative injury, or, in patients operated on before 1960, as a deliberately created surgical fenestra. Insertion of instruments in, or irrigation of, such cavities is likely to produce severe vertigo. Suctioning directly on the fistulas could produce irreversible, serious otologic injury. Other patients have had natural or surgically created dehiscences in the facial nerve, the jugular bulb, or the dura mater. Thus cleansing of and insertion of instruments in the previously operated ear must be done with caution, and possible pitfalls must be kept in mind. It is best to attempt to identify the horizontal semicircular canal in canal-wall–down mastoidectomies before instruments are inserted. This identification provides rapid anatomic orientation and minimizes the chances of inadvertent injury to important structures. If the posterior canal wall has been left intact, then the state of the ear must be inferred from evaluation of the tympanic

membrane. When the eardrum is intact, the sharpness of the anterior angle can be assessed. The presence of marked anterior blunting, especially when associated with a conductive hearing loss, suggests lateralization of the grafted tympanic membrane. The presence of a white mass behind the tympanic membrane may represent recurrent cholesteatoma, deliberately placed homograph cartilage, or an ossicular prosthesis. Sometimes differentiation among these various situations is not possible without exploratory tympanotomy. The examiner should always remember that the presence of clear fluid, either behind an intact tympanic membrane or within a mastoid cavity, may represent cerebrospinal fluid and that soft tissues present in these areas may represent a herniated brain.

TUNING FORK TEST

No otologic evaluation is complete without some assessment of hearing. Although the definitive test of auditory acuity is the formal audiogram, rapid assessment of hearing acuity by the use of tuning forks can alert the examiner to unknown difficulties, verify suspected problems, and confirm audiologic tests. The 512-Hz tuning fork is used most frequently. However, the 1024-Hz and 2048-Hz forks can also yield useful information. As a general rule, frequencies below 512 Hz are so easily perceived as vibrotactile stimulation that they are not useful in the assessment of hearing.

The Weber test is performed by placing the vibrating tuning fork firmly on a solid, midline bony facial structure, such as the forehead or the central incisors of the mandible or maxilla (Fig. 1B–10A). The patient who hears the tuning fork more clearly in one ear than in the other is said to lateralize the Weber test to the ear in which he or she hears it best. When the patient has a unilateral conductive hearing loss, the tuning fork is lateralized to the ear with the loss. When the patient has a sensorineural loss, the test is lateralized to the ear opposite the hearing loss. In mixed losses or when losses are present in both ears, the Weber test yields a less exact result.

In the Rinne test, bone conduction is compared with air conduction in a given ear. The test is performed by first placing the rapidly

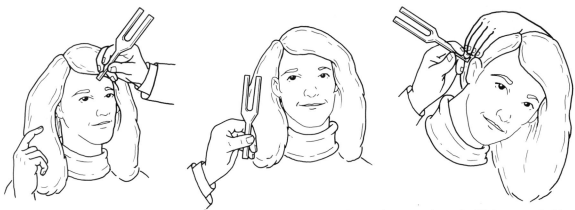

Figure 1B–10. *A.* The vibrating tuning fork is placed on the forehead in order to perform the Weber test. *B.* The Rinne test. The tuning fork is held 1 to 2 cm from the external auditory canal. *C.* The tuning fork is placed firmly onto the mastoid bone. Normally, the tuning fork is heard better in position *B* than in *C.* If the opposite is true, the Rinne test is said to have "converted." (Redrawn from Meyerhoff L: Diagnosis and Management of Hearing Loss. Philadelphia: WB Saunders, 1984.)

vibrating tuning fork firmly on the mastoid tip behind the auricle. In this position the tuning fork is heard principally by bone conduction. After a couple of seconds, the tuning fork is shifted to a position just outside the external auditory canal (Figs. 1B–10*B,* 1B–10*C*). The patient is asked to determine whether the sound was louder in the first or second position. Alternatively, one can allow the tuning fork to rest on the mastoid tip until the patient can no longer hear the sound and then immediately shift the vibrating fork to a position just outside the external auditory canal and ask the patient if he or she can now perceive any sound. When bone conduction is greater than air conduction, the patient has a conductive hearing loss in that ear. If air conduction is greater than bone conduction, one infers that the patient has a sensorineural loss. Careful attention should be given to the terminology when one is discussing Rinne test results. A positive Rinne result is the *normal* response. This is the very opposite of almost every other test, for which a positive result is an *abnormal* result. It is often better to record results simply as "air conduction greater than bone conduction" (ac > bc) or vice versa (bc > ac); this eliminates confusion. A patient whose bone conduction is greater than air conduction is said to have converted the Rinne test. Approximately 20 db of conductive hearing loss is required before bone conduction is greater than air conduction and the Rinne test is converted. A combination of Weber and Rinne test results provides a significant amount of qualitative information about hearing. It is important to note that accurate information from tuning fork tests is dependent on generating bone vibration, a condition that can be assumed only if adequate pressure has been applied.

THE CRANIAL NERVES

As alluded to in Chapter 1A, no otologic examination is complete without evaluation of the cranial nerves. The first cranial nerve may be evaluated, one side at a time, either by a commercially available scratch test system or by household aromatic substances. Tobacco and coffee aromas are frequently used and are readily available. Caustic substances, such as ammonia, should not be used because they stimulate the fifth nerve and do not test for olfactory function.

To assess gross vision, the patient reads with each eye. In patients unable to read or in whom vision is so poor as to preclude reading, one should test for the ability to count fingers. In comatose or otherwise severely mentally impaired patients, one should check for pupillary constriction in response to light. Both the ipsilateral and the contralateral reflexes should be checked. Even if the efferent limb of the pupillary restrictive reflex is injured in the ipsilateral eye, contralateral pupillary constriction should occur if the vision is present.

The third or ocular motor nerve provides innervation to all the extraocular muscles except the superior oblique and lateral rectus muscles. Therefore, severe injury to the ocular motor nerve will produce severe ptoses, mydriasis, and outward displacement of the eye with diplopia.

The fourth cranial nerve (trochlear) supplies the superior oblique muscle, and injury to it produces vertical displacement of the affected eye with vertical diplopia and cyclotorsion (image tilting).

Damage to the sixth cranial nerve (abducens), which supplies the lateral rectus muscle, produces a marked inward displacement of the globe and diplopia in all fields of vision. Even very subtle weakness of the extraocular muscles may produce diplopia. When diplopia is present, dysfunction of cranial nerve III, IV, or VI may be suspected even when gross examination reveals no obvious deficit. Ophthalmologic consultation may be required to fully characterize more subtle deficits.

The fifth cranial nerve (trigeminal) provides sensation to the face, including the cornea, and innervation to the muscles of mastication. The face should be tested for sensation to pinprick and light touch. Anesthesia of the cornea is generally readily detected by having the patient look to the opposite side and placing a wisp of cotton on the lateral conjunctiva of the globe. Contact with the global conjunctiva rarely produces significant discomfort. As the cotton wisp is moved toward the midline, contact with the cornea occurs and induces a brisk blink. Whenever cranial nerve V is tested, careful comparison should be made between the two sides. This permits detection of relatively subtle defects. The motor fibers are carried in the third or inferior division of the fifth nerve, and severe injury to the motor fibers, which produces paralysis of the ipsilateral muscles of mastication, also produces significant malocclusion with shifting of the jaw to the opposite side.

Assessment of the seventh cranial nerve is crucial to the complete neuro-otologic examination. The patient should be asked to wrinkle the forehead, close the eyes, sniff, smile, show the teeth, and wrinkle the skin of the neck so that the examiner can fully assess the facial nerve. The examiner's hand should be rapidly moved toward the patient's eye unexpectedly in order to produce a blink reflex, which may demonstrate subtle lagophthalmos. This is the most subtle sign of facial weakness. The patient should also be asked to hold the eyes shut against the examiner's attempt to forcibly open them. The result of this test may also reveal subtle facial nerve weakness not demonstrated by passive examination. Sophisticated topographic testing is dealt with in Chapter 17.

At the very minimum, crude estimates of hearing acuity should be used to assess the auditory function of the eighth cranial nerve. Formal audiometry is preferable. A Romberg test should be used to grossly assess the vestibular system. The patient is asked to place the feet completely together, stretch the arms in front of him or her, and close the eyes. Even in the absence of visual input, a person with normal vestibular function is easily able to maintain this position indefinitely. Falling or staggering constitutes a positive test result and raises suspicion of vestibular dysfunction.

The ninth cranial nerve (glossopharyngeal) should be evaluated by examining the position of the uvula. Ninth cranial nerve dysfunction with paralysis of one side of the palatal musculature may produce deviation of the uvula to the opposite side. A tongue blade should be used to scrape the posterior soft palate and the posterior pharynx in order to elicit a gag reflex. A brisk drag reflex on one side without a gag reflex on the other should raise suspicion of a ninth nerve dysfunction.

The tenth nerve (vagus) supplies pharyngeal muscle innervation and vocal fold motor function. The vagus is most readily assessed by evaluating vocal cord movement either directly or indirectly, as discussed earlier in this chapter. The type of disability incurred as a consequence of vagal dysfunction depends on the level of injury. "High" vagal injuries, which occur close to the cranial base, result in dysfunction of pharyngeal fibers and produce disruption of the orderly swallowing sequence. Most important, the cricopharyngeal muscle will not open the esophageal inlet at the appropriate time. The descending food bolus then meets an esophagus that is closed and a larynx that is open (as a result of vocal fold paralysis), and aspiration results. The combination of hoarseness with dysphasia and aspiration should always raise suspicion of vagal lesions.

Long-standing injury to the eleventh nerve (accessory) produces noticeable atrophy of the ipsilateral sternocleidomastoid and trapezius muscles. When dysfunction is recent, visible atrophy may not yet be apparent. Therefore, the patient should be asked to elevate the shoulders against the examiner's resistance. A difference between one side and the other side should raise suspicion of eleventh nerve paralysis.

Injury to the twelfth cranial nerve (hypoglossal) produces paralysis of the ipsilateral tongue. The strong action of the tongue muscles of the opposite side causes the tongue to deviate toward the paralysis. Peripheral nerve injury produces atrophy and fasciculation of the involved side that are readily visible simply by asking the patient to show the tongue.

SUGGESTED READINGS

Bluestone CD, Klein JO: Diagnosis. *In* Bluestone CD, Klein JO: Otitis Media in Infants and Children (pp 69–121). Philadelphia: WB Saunders, 1988.

DeGowin, EL, DeGowin RL: Bedside Diagnostic Examinations (pp 173–196). New York: Macmillan, 1969.

Hawke M, John AF: Diseases of the Ear. Philadelphia: Lea & Febiger, 1987.

CHAPTER 2

Diagnostic Imaging

Anthony A. Mancuso

ROLE OF MODERN IMAGING

Modern imaging methods can provide an extraordinary amount of useful data to those who must diagnose and manage head and neck disorders. A good deal of the potential of the newer tools, computed tomography (CT) and magnetic resonance imaging (MRI), is still unrealized. Most of the information that could lead to optimal use of these powerful imaging tools is available; it must now be dispersed and applied. The single most important factor in this educational process is mutual cooperation between the diagnostic imaging specialist and the physicians in charge of patient care, assuming that there is an active interest on the part of the diagnostic imager in solving the problems unique to head and neck disorders. Such a two-way commitment is essential if the costs and small risks of diagnostic imaging are to be justified. With the basic requirement of such mutual cooperation held as a central premise, this chapter aims to

1. Define the various imaging techniques available.

2. Describe which techniques are currently useful and which are obsolete.

3. Define the role of the diagnostic radiologist in the treatment team.

4. Suggest efficient algorithms for imaging of commonly encountered clinical problems.

5. Propose guidelines for the relative use of imaging modalities in disorders of each of the head and neck subregions.

6. Help anticipate what technical innovations will lead to changes in the next 3 to 5 years.

The overall goal of this chapter is to suggest how the full potential of modern imaging may be realized in the diagnosis, determination of extent, and follow-up of treatment in ear, nose, and throat (ENT)–related disorders, the unifying theme being how to obtain all of the information that matters for the care of the patient at the least cost and risk.

Diagnostic Imager as a Consultant

Service Versus Consultation

Some imaging studies are virtually risk free, are relatively inexpensive, and require little physician supervision. In this situation, the diagnostic imager needs to provide only general supervision and accurate interpretation of the examination; in other words, diagnostic imagers are a service organization. Plain radiographs and routine survey studies, such as bone scan or brain CT or MRI for determining metastatic disease, might come under this heading. The vast majority of head and neck imaging studies, however, *require* careful planning of the examination if the full benefits of imaging are to be realized. Few of the studies pose significant risk; however, most are expensive. It is essential whenever there is significant risk or expense involved in a study that the diagnostic imager be considered a consultant, rather than provider of a service. It is not uncommon to see $600 to $1200 (with a $100 to $150 physician component of that fee) spent on a diagnostic examination that adds little or no useful information (Fig. 2–1). The fault is usually *not* in the technology per se. It usually lies in

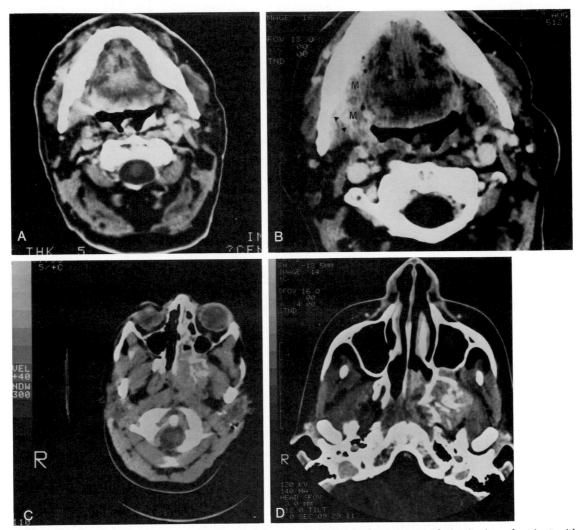

Figure 2–1. Images from CT studies of the same patient. *A.* CT study from an outside institution of patient with retromolar trigone carcinoma. The field of view is too large, and the patient was not instructed to suspend respiration; the result is a diagnostically useless image on which the cancer is not even visible. *B.* The same patient as in *A* restudied within 1 week at the University of Florida. Correction of the technical errors leads to a much more informative image showing an aggressive mass lesion (M) infiltrating the parapharyngeal space and adjacent medial pterygoid muscle (arrowheads) and spreading into the posterior floor of the mouth along the posterior edge of the mylohyoid muscle and lingual surface of the mandible (more anterior M). Attention to technical detail is of paramount importance in head and neck imaging. *C.* Patient with a juvenile angiofibroma studied at another institution. The scan is made oblique to the infraorbital meatal line, with distortion of the relationship of the mass to the orbits and ethmoids. The field of view is suboptimal, and there is motion artifact (note blurring around mandibular heads). *D.* Same patient as in *C;* technical errors have been corrected. A more aesthetic *and* anatomically accurate image results. (The rest of this patient's images are shown in Fig. 2–4.)

improper sequencing of studies, suboptimal technique, or underinformed interpretation of the images. Referring clinicians must be sure that the imaging consultants are providing safe and highly informative studies. This can best be judged by the image quality and content of the report. Modern imaging should have a positive impact on diagnosis and treatment planning in the vast majority of patients studied. If this is not true, the cause is in one of three general spheres of influence: (1) patient selection, (2) providing sufficient information to the imaging consultant, and (3) choice, execution, and interpretation of the study. The first two of these are within the realm of the referring clinician, and the third is the responsibility of the diagnostic imager (Fig. 2–1).

Clinician Responsibilities

The referring clinician *must* provide a well-screened population. The relative roles of clinical diagnostic testing and imaging in "screening" are shifting constantly. The shifts are often subtle and debatable. Algorithms, such as those suggested throughout this chapter, for sequencing imaging examinations and clinical testing should be re-examined and revised occasionally by mutual agreement of the referring clinicians and diagnostic imagers. If local expertise is not sufficient for making these decisions, perhaps the framework provided in this chapter and other sources can help in the process.

Once a patient has been triaged to imaging, it is *absolutely essential* that a good data base concerning the problem at hand, as well as one or more medical conditions of the patient that might affect the imaging approach, be transmitted to the diagnostic imagers. Information such as contrast allergy or the status of renal function may greatly affect the safety of the study. Data concerning the nature and extent of a suspected pathologic process are essential to ensure that the study is tailored to each patient. At a minimum, the specific area of anatomic interest, the pertinent symptoms and physical findings, and the top two or three diagnoses of exclusion should be provided. "Rule out cancer" and "hearing loss," for example, are not sufficient data bases for performing a $600 to $1500 diagnostic study, whereas "carcinoma of the pyriform sinus; evaluate extent of the primary and for cervical metastases" and "conductive hearing loss; please evaluate for ossicular fixation or discontinuity" are minimally sufficient. The amount and quality of data that the referring clinician supplies should have a positive impact on image quality and yield of clinically useful information. If this does not occur, the level of competency of the diagnostic imager in the realm of ENT and head and neck disorders should be questioned and, if necessary, improved.

Finally, there should be wide-open lines of communication between referring clinicians and diagnostic imagers. Feedback, both positive and negative, concerning the quality of images and accuracy of interpretation is essential to the diagnostic imagers who aim to continually refine their skills. Most important, a clinician who is uncertain about whether imaging can help or which study best fits the clinical problem should ask another physician rather than order an expensive, potentially risky study that may not be the one best suited to the problem at hand.

Diagnostic Imager's Responsibilities

Diagnostic imagers must view themselves as patient advocates. If an unnecessarily risky, inappropriate, or obsolete study has been requested, a more suitable alternative should be found. To this end, the diagnostic imager must have a basic framework, preferably in algorithm form, for dealing with clinical problems that require imaging. In this approach to specific problems, the imager should consider the sequencing of imaging studies in relation to clinical diagnostic methods, such as audiometry, aspiration biopsy, and endoscopy. The diagnostic imager should *refuse* to perform a nonemergent study unless a sufficient data base is available to aid in choosing the correct examination that is properly tailored to the individual patient's problem. Although this may cause some delay and disagreement, it is in the best interest of the patient.

The diagnostic imager is completely responsible for the quality and interpretation of the study. The physician fees, especially for CT, MRI, and angiography, justify a high level of physician supervision and competence. Anything less than good to excellent quality of images is acceptable only under unusual circumstances (e.g., an uncooperative patient or unavoidable artifacts) (Fig. 2–2). The factors involved in quality control of images are discussed in later sections. Quality interpretation mandates a special interest in head and neck imaging. Interpreters of these highly specialized studies are most valuable when they have a thorough understanding of the anatomy and natural history of head and neck disorders as well as at least a basic working knowledge of the clinical aspects of ENT and head and neck disorders that require imaging.

In summary, the diagnostic imager must get the answers that make a difference in the patient's care both efficiently and for the least cost possible. The imagers must view themselves as consultants and patients' advocates and stimulate a level of communication and cooperation that serves those purposes.

Organization of Chapter

The remainder of this chapter is organized in two main blocks; the first is by diagnostic

oroscopic examination with orally administered contrast agents in this setting. There
are still some indispensable uses of plain
radiography and fluoroscopy in radiotherapy
planning and in the guidance of certain surgical procedures (e.g., 6-foot Caldwell template for osteoplastic frontal flap).

Obsolete Uses. Assuming that modern
imaging techniques are available, the use of
plain radiography seems unwarranted in the
evaluation of (1) patients who may be suffering from orbital or intracranial complications
of inflammatory sinus disease or who are
considered at high risk for such complications, (2) patients who have sustained significant head or facial trauma and are likely to
have either intracranial injuries or complex
facial fractures, or (3) patients who have
deformities of the craniofacial region. All of
these patients should have CT examinations
rather than plain film studies. Plain film
studies in these situations usually add needless expense and may delay an urgent need
for more advanced imaging in some circumstances.

Contraindications to Plain Radiography.
There are no real medical contraindications
to the use of plain films. Needless plain
radiography should definitely be avoided in
the pediatric population because it can deliver unnecessary dosage to radiosensitive
structures, such as the lens and the thyroid
gland.

Conventional Tomography

Conventional tomographic techniques entered a rapid phase of development in the
1960s, which continued into the early 1970s.
There was still widespread application of
these techniques into the late 1970s; however, in the late 1970s and early 1980s, CT
techniques were refined to the point at which
it became apparent that conventional tomographic techniques were relatively obsolete.
Units capable of complex motion are still
available, and they can be used in some
circumstances when the more advanced techniques are not available or for patients who
are unable to undergo CT or MRI.

These studies are performed with standard x-ray tubes and film/screen combinations. The techniques are based on the principle of moving the x-ray tube in relation to
the film either in a simple one-dimensional
arc or in a more complex manner, such as a
trispiral or hypocycloidal pattern. The effect
of moving the tube and keeping the film and
the patient stationary is to blur structures
that are out of the focal plane. In general, a
more complex motion results in thinner sections and fewer artifacts. Most radiology departments still have tomographic equipment
available; however, many of these specialized
units, such as those capable of complex motion, have been removed to make way for
newer technologies. The most common, and
still very useful, tomographic technique in
practice is orthopantomography for dental
practices. Beyond this, the studies that previously used conventional tomographic
methods have been virtually completely supplanted by CT and MRI.

Current Indications. There are few, if any.
At the University of Florida, the main use of
conventional tomographic procedures is to
study the cervical spine and craniocervical
junction in the coronal and sagittal planes.
The detail available with conventional tomography is sometimes superior to that available
with axial CT and reformations of this area.
Occasionally, coronal views of the sinuses
are done in lieu of coronal reformation of
axial CT data or if, for some reason, CT is
not available and a timely study of the facial
region is necessary. Occasionally, conventional tomography is used to survey the bone
detail of the TMJ.

**Obsolete Uses of Conventional Tomog-
raphy.** Assuming that modern imaging techniques are available, conventional tomography should not be used for studying the
temporal bone. Plain radiographic or tomographic evaluation of the internal auditory
canals is obsolete in the evaluation of patients
for acoustic schwannoma or other cerebellopontine angle masses. Any disease affecting
the temporal bone, which requires specialized study, demands CT, MRI, or both. Conventional tomography is simply not adequate
or comparable with CT in detail, if CT is
being properly used. Conventional tomography should likewise not be used for evaluating laryngeal cancer. Such an examination
provides only gross assessment of the air–
soft-tissue interface and cartilages. If an imaging examination of the larynx is required,
either CT or MRI should be done. CT is

clearly preferable to conventional tomography for evaluating the sinonasal region, the skull base, and the airway.

Contraindications. There are really no medical contraindications to the use of conventional tomography. These techniques should absolutely be avoided in pediatric patients, in whom they deliver unnecessarily high radiation doses to tissue, such as the lens and thyroid gland. Combinations of CT, MRI, and ultrasonography can be used for virtually all diagnostic imaging problems in pediatric patients, and unnecessary x-ray exposure is thus avoided.

Fluoroscopy

Fluoroscopic techniques basically employ an image intensifier with links to videotape recording of the data, cineradiographic techniques, or plain film techniques (usually called *spot filming*). Most fluoroscopic examinations are performed with the addition of orally administered contrast material, either barium or a water-soluble contrast. Selected studies of the airway, including those related to speech disorders and possibly airway patency, are often done without contrast.

Current Indications. Fluoroscopic techniques in conjunction with barium administration are most often used for evaluating swallowing physiology and for screening the mucosa of the esophagus and, to a lesser extent, the hypopharynx for lesions. These studies produce little or no information about deep infiltrating lesions, except for occasional displacement of the hollow viscus. If the main aim of the study is to evaluate physiology, certainly some method of recording motion, such as a videotape system or a cineradiographic technique, is necessary. Cineradiography requires a much larger dose to the patient, less convenient viewing, and more processing time than does videotaping. Fluoroscopic studies with water-soluble contrast agents are preferred whenever a leak into the soft tissues, mediastinum, or elsewhere is possible. Therefore, water-soluble contrast, rather than barium, is also suggested for use in fistulograms. In the past, there was some concern over the use of water-soluble contrast when there was a potential for aspiration. In general, aspiration of barium, which is rather inert, is safer than

aspiration of the earlier generation of water-soluble contrast agents, which could result in a severe chemical pneumonitis. The danger associated with aspiration of water-soluble contrast has been lessened by the development of newer nonionic and less hyperosmolar contrast agents. Certainly the mucosal detail available with barium is better because of its superior coating of mucosal surfaces. Barium, rather than water-soluble contrast, should be used whenever these safety considerations are not operative.

Few institutions still employ tracheography as a diagnostic tool; however, in institutions in which large volumes of tracheal surgery are done, positive contrast tracheography might be useful in evaluating dynamic changes in the airway, which identify tracheomalacic segments. Over the years, at the University of Florida, excellent success has been obtained in predicting the significantly diseased segments of the trachea on the basis of the clinical evaluation, including bronchoscopy, along with static CT images.

Obsolete Uses. Study of the larynx and hypopharynx with these techniques, usually referred to as laryngography, is clearly obsolete if modern imaging techniques are available. Laryngography merely produces the same information available from the endoscopic evaluation of the patient. Laryngography is largely a study of the mucosa and gives only indirect assessment of the deep extension of tumors and other diseased processes that affect the larynx and hypopharynx. Its use could conceivably be justified for patients who, for some reason, cannot undergo CT or MRI. The combination of modern endoscopy and advanced imaging techniques makes these older studies unwarranted for screening. Bronchography, likewise, has been rendered obsolete by this combination of modern bronchoscopy and imaging.

Contraindications. It is imperative that barium not be used in a situation in which it could leak into a potentially infected space. Such an occurrence could lead to potential worsening and render an otherwise controllable infection incurable. Water-soluble contrast should be used with caution in patients at risk for aspiration.

Special Contrast Studies

Sialography

The role of sialography, in relation to other imaging studies and needle biopsy, is outlined in Figure 2–3. Basically, sialography should be done only to evaluate the ductal systems of the parotid and submandibular glands. One exception to this is the visualization of an abnormal parenchymal pattern, which may be observed in patients with chronic punctate sialadenitis, and of some of the more diffusely infiltrative, inflammatory processes. There are two major precautions when one is considering sialography. The first is never to study a patient with acute sialadenitis, especially if it is infectious. The infection can be worsened and may progress to abscess or gross necrosis of the gland if contrast is injected into the ductal system. Suggestions for evaluation of such patients are included in Figure 2–3. The second precaution is relative and related to the type of contrast used. For years, oil-based contrast media were used for studying the salivary ductal systems. This contrast is necessarily injected under some pressure, and if it is not cleared from the gland, it appears to incite a chronic granulomatous response within the gland. The advantage of this contrast was better ductal detail; however, newer contrast agents provide excellent ductal detail and do not run the risk of inciting such a chronic granulomatous response. Therefore, oily contrast media should not be used in this study if alternative contrast media are available.

Dacryocystography

This study is done by cannulating the inferior canaliculus of the nasolacrimal system. Contrast is then injected, and films are usually made with static plain radiographic techniques. This is an excellent means of studying the nasolacrimal system and is still a useful study in well-screened patients with epiphora of uncertain etiology or other potential abnormalities of the lacrimal drainage system.

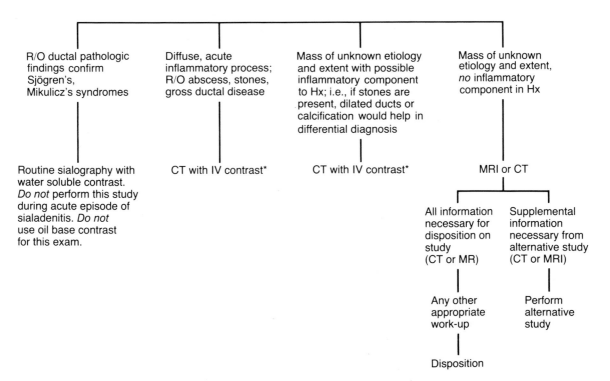

*N.B. CT assisted sialography (i.e., contrast injected into the parotid duct) is no longer performed for mass lesions and is contraindicated in an acutely inflamed salivary gland.

Figure 2–3. Imaging options for parotid abnormalities after clinical triage. (From Mancuso A: Workbook for MRI and CT of the Head and Neck, 2nd ed. Baltimore: Williams & Wilkins, 1989.)

Temporomandibular Joint Arthrography

Under fluoroscopic control, this study is usually done as a single-contrast examination by the injection of water-soluble contrast into the inferior joint space. The major advantages of TMJ arthrography include the ability to recognize perforations of the articular disk and to study the joint dynamics. Although this is still a generally accepted and fairly widely used examination, it is rapidly being replaced by MRI. MRI remains incapable of detecting disk perforation; however, newer techniques are allowing joint motion studies. The number of patients undergoing TMJ arthrography will probably continue to decrease over the next several years to a relatively small, highly selected subset of patients with TMJ dysfunction.

Orbitography

For a short time, injection of contrast into the orbit was used as a diagnostic examination. This examination is basically not used any longer. The risks of the examination do not justify its use.

General Contraindications of Contrast Studies

Whenever iodinated contrast is injected into any part of the body, one must consider the potential for an allergic reaction or a local toxic response. Allergic reactions can be minimized by the use of nonionic, less hyperosmolar agents, which have been developed over the last several years. Any time a patient has a history of severe allergy (e.g., hypotension, upper airway obstruction) to iodinated contrast, these newer contrast agents should be used, probably in combination with premedication. For more minor allergic histories (e.g., hives), either premedication or the newer agents may be used. Also, whenever an infectious process is present in a closed space or system, one must consider the possibility that the injection of contrast may worsen the inflammatory response and potentially spread or worsen the infection. In the worst case scenario, injecting under pressure into an abscess cavity or infected space can lead to generalized sepsis. Such occurrences are uncommon in the head and neck region; however, one must consider the possibility. If alternative imaging is available without such risk, it should be substituted for the more potentially risky study. In the head and neck region, the most important of these situations is probably the avoidance of using contrast sialography in an acutely inflamed gland.

Angiography

General Technique

The arterial, venous, and lymphatic systems may all be studied by injecting an iodinated contrast agent and recording images with any one of a number of available devices. Lymphangiography is not used in the head and neck region and is therefore not discussed any further. Venography is used relatively infrequently, but some selected venous side studies are discussed. The most commonly used angiographic study is, of course, arteriography. This may be done with standard rapid filming (cut-film), digital recording, or cineradiographic recording techniques. Digital recording is frequently used in the head and neck region (Fig. 2–4). With the invention of higher resolution digital recording equipment, there should be a gradual decrease in the use of cut-film techniques and eventually complete replacement of these older methods by digital subtraction angiography. When a digital recording device is used, an injection of contrast may be administered either intravenously or intraarterially. Intravenous injection studies are generally used for more survey type indications, whereas arterial injections are used for those studies that require a more detailed and selective study of the various portions of the arterial and venous system in the head and neck region.

All of these examinations are relatively safe and low risk, with the use of modern catheter techniques. Arteriography has perhaps the largest potential risk for significant complications. Minor complications at the site of femoral puncture are not unusual and have little or no long-term consequences for the patient. Femoral artery occlusion due to dissection or thrombosis is a serious but usually treatable local complication. Hematomas usually pose no particular long-term danger. Excessive bleeding can occur at the puncture site in patients who have clotting disorders. When selective catheterization of the arteries in the carotid system is carried

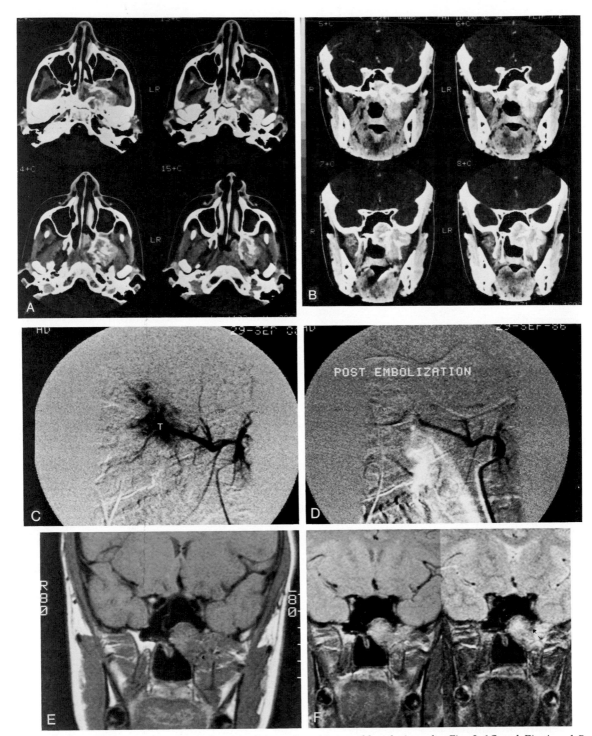

Figure 2–4. Juvenile angiofibroma of the nasopharynx in a 14-year-old male (see also Fig. 2–1C and D). A and B. Four axial (A) and coronal images (B) show the extent of tumor in the nasopharynx, sphenoid sinus, skull base, pterygopalatine and pterygoid fossa, and infratemporal fossa. C. Midway through preoperative embolization, the tumor (T) is reduced to approximately half its original volume. D. At the completion of embolization, no external carotid supply is present. The tumor was removed with 250 to 500 mL of blood loss. E. The tumor regrew postoperatively and was treated with radiotherapy. The T1-weighted image shows minimal residual flow voids (arrow) within the obvious tumor mass. F. On this spin density and T2-weighted pair, zones of decreased intensity (arrow) probably are more solid stromal (?fibrous) and cellular elements; brighter areas may represent slow-flow vascular spaces or necrosis. This mass, which received 35 Gy, has been stable for 3 years.

out, there is always the potential risk of neurologic deficit due to dissection, embolism, or other transient circumstances that produce vascular occlusion. The chances of such occurrences go up significantly in therapeutic embolization procedures and, to a lesser extent, in test occlusions of the carotid system. Because risks are *potentially* serious, the risks/benefits of all of these procedures should be considered carefully in formal consultation with the diagnostic imager. All prior diagnostic studies must be available for review before the angiographic examination. A specific plan for obtaining the information needed, or therapeutic effect desired, should be agreed upon by the referring physician and the diagnostic imager *before* the study starts. In cases of therapeutic embolization, it is most effective if the clinical and imaging teams are following the patient together and, at times, performing the procedure as a team.

Arteriography

Diagnostic Indications
Virtually all arteriography in ENT-related head and neck disorders are preceded by CT or MRI. It is therefore essential to review high-quality diagnostic imaging studies before the angiographic procedure. Frequently, all of the information that is necessary may be obtained by simply repeating an otherwise unsatisfactory imaging study. At the very least, a review of the study usually focuses the diagnostic issues at hand and, therefore, the examination. This critically reduces the catheterization time and perhaps avoids needless injection of vessels that are not related to the pathologic process under study. These diagnostic studies should always be available at the time of the angiographic procedure. Arteriography should be integrated into the algorithms for approaches of various clinical problems; this should be apparent from reviewing the algorithms presented in this chapter.

The main purpose for diagnostic angiography is to characterize and confirm the diagnosis of a mass lesion seen on other imaging studies (Fig. 2–4). Most commonly, angiography is done to confirm a paraganglioma. This is usually not necessary in the glomus tympanicus type paraganglioma; however, in glomus jugulare, glomus vagale, and carotid body tumors, it may prove necessary. Juvenile angiofibromas are also studied for this purpose. In the proper clinical setting, a typical arteriogram may be considered equivalent to a biopsy of a paraganglioma or an angiofibroma for treatment purposes. In rare instances, other vascular masses mimic these tumors, but there is usually atypical imaging or clinical features suggestive of some other etiologic factors for the hypervascular mass. Hemangiopericytoma and hypervascular metastatic lesion, although rare, are perhaps the most common vascular masses affecting the head and neck other than those just mentioned.

The other common indication for arteriography in ENT-related disorders is to identify vascular malformations or vascular lesions as a source of some symptom. This is most usually a symptom such as pulsatile tinnitus or, more rarely, one that produces an audible or palpable bruit. Even for these indications, it is essential to sequence arteriography properly, in relation to other imaging techniques. In most situations, it is appropriate to proceed with either CT or MRI as a screening examination before an arteriogram is performed. There are very few exceptions to this. Moreover, lesions at the junction of the head and neck or in the neck are amenable to the evaluation with duplex sonography. This method can, in selected cases, provide rapid and effective way of screening abnormality to either another imaging study or arteriography as the next most appropriate step. Also, magnetic resonance angiography (MRA) is now available and may be a useful adjunct to standard MR studies, and it certainly has the potential to eliminate some diagnostic angiography now and probably more so as these new MR techniques are refined (Fig. 2–5). CT, even with further advances, will likely remain inferior to MRI in this regard.

Finally, diagnostic angiography is often done as a prologue to definitive endovascular therapy of head and neck lesions or to endovascular therapy as an adjunct to definitive surgical management of a lesion (Fig. 2–4). In this regard, the diagnostic portion of the examination should be separated in time from the therapeutic endovascular procedure. This is important for two reasons. First, patients frequently become fatigued if they must cooperate for both diagnostic and therapeutic procedures at one sitting. Patients' cooperation is essential in the often protracted period it takes to perform an endovascular therapeutic procedure. Second, the

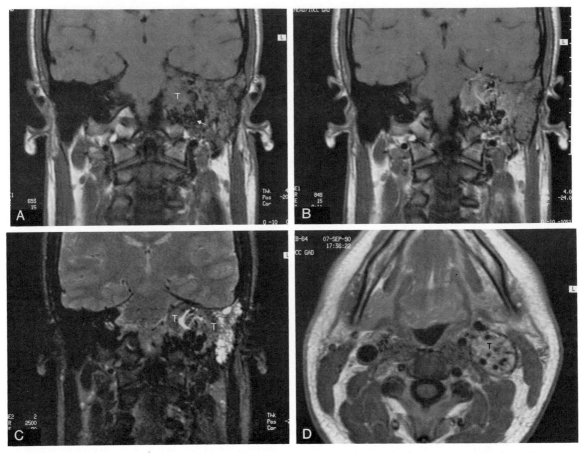

Figure 2–5. Glomus vagale type of paraganglioma in a 35-year-old male. *A.* Coronal noncontrast MR shows the tumor (T), numerous flow voids representing a large vascular pedicle (arrow), and cerebellopontine angle (CPA) extension but does not differentiate tumor from obstructive mastoid disease. *B.* Contrast-enhanced MR in same plane as *A;* tumor, vascular pedicle, and tentorial involvement (arrow) are better defined. *C.* Heavily T2-weighted MR differentiates tumor (T) from the brighter, more lateral, obstructive, and inflammatory mastoid disease with greater clarity than in *A* or *B;* the vascular pedicle is a little harder to detect. *D.* Axial contrast-enhanced MR shows tumor (T) in the jugular vein.

diagnostic study usually needs to be evaluated in detail and, in light of other diagnostic imaging studies, in order to plan the safest approach to obtaining the desired therapeutic effect. The patient is best served when the treatment team gathers all of the information available from imaging and diagnostic arteriographic studies and decides on the best management approach before embarking on either a definitive endovascular or combined endovascular-surgical approach.

Therapeutic Indications

Endovascular therapeutic procedures are becoming more widely available. Most often, these are done for hypervascular lesions either as a definitive procedure or as an adjunct to surgery. The major benefit of preoperative embolization is reduction of blood loss during the operative procedure. Almost all surgeons would agree that preoperative embolization is mandatory in a juvenile angiofibroma. Opinions concerning the value of preoperative embolization and management of paragangliomas are mixed, but there seems to be more general acceptance of these procedures as the catheter systems and expertise of interventional angiographers improve.

One of the more gratifying uses of endovascular therapy is in treating vascular lesions that involve the skin of the face. Staged endovascular procedures may produce complete obliteration of a lesion or at least make surgical approach a viable option. Arteriovenous malformations of the extracranial head and neck are unusual, but endovascular therapy of such abnormalities is rapidly becoming the primary and definitive means of

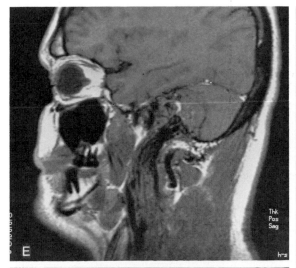

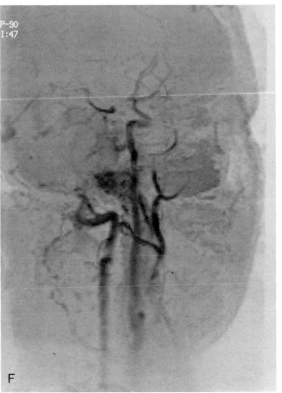

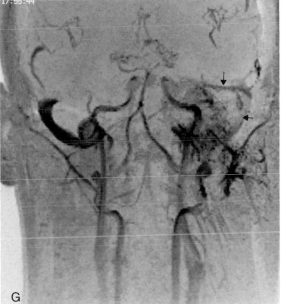

Figure 2–5 *Continued E.* Sagittal noncontrast MR shows tumor growing down the neck within the jugular vein; location in the vein is better appreciated on the axial view. *F.* Sagittal slab MR angiogram view from a left-sided posterolateral vantage point showing the hypervascular tumor. *G.* Coronal slab MR angiogram viewed anteriorly shows the tumor and partial occlusion of the transverse and sigmoid sinuses (arrows).

treating these often difficult problems. Uncontrolled epistaxis may also be treated with therapeutic embolization.

Test balloon occlusion of the internal carotid artery is becoming an increasingly important adjunct to the head and neck surgeon. This is used mainly in surgery for lesions of the skull base, but it is occasionally used in patients with advanced metastatic disease in the neck with carotid fixation and in whom carotid sacrifice is being considered as part of a palliative surgical procedure. The endovascular interventional radiologist should oversee this procedure. It has become commonplace to integrate this procedure with xenon CT blood flow studies of the

brain. Perhaps in the near future, single photon emission computed tomography (SPECT) or positron emission tomography (PET) studies of the brain will be used in identifying patients at risk for significant neurologic deficit if carotid sacrifice is undertaken. Careful coordination between the angiographic techniques and the adjunctive blood flow studies is essential for ensuring patient safety and useful results.

Venography

Diagnostic Indications

Venography is predominantly used to study the dural venous sinuses of the brain. This is probably best done with intra-arterial injection into the carotid system and digital recording. CT is a reasonable screening examination for dural venous sinus occlusion, and MRI is potentially better, especially when coupled with MRA capabilities (Fig. 2–5). In fact, MRI and MRA may obviate the need for traditional angiographic study in selected patients. In the past, retrograde jugular studies were sometimes done to evaluate the extent of paragangliomas that might be growing within or adjacent to the jugular vein. MRI and CT usually clearly show the extent of tumor within the vein (Fig. 2–5). For a short time, orbital venography was used to study the cavernous sinus. Currently, a combination of CT and MRI, with the use of iodinated and paramagnetic contrast, respectively, can usually sort out any diagnostic problem related to the cavernous sinus. Orbital venography is a difficult study to perform and is frequently nondefinitive even in experienced hands.

Therapeutic Indications

Endovascular neuroradiologists sometimes use venous side approaches for dealing with various intracranial lesions; complete discussion is beyond the scope of this text. Occasionally, venous sampling is used to evaluate patients with hyperparathyroidism; this is usually done for patients who have been operated on previously and have evidence of recurrent hyperparathyroidism. Similar venous sampling techniques may occasionally be used to confirm the presence of cortisol-producing pituitary tumors, but this is not within the realm of the ENT surgeon.

Contraindications

There are very few patients who cannot undergo a diagnostic or therapeutic angiogram if necessary. Precautions are necessary in patients who have demonstrated hypersensitivity to iodinated contrast. Untoward reactions are much less common during injections into the arterial system than during those into the venous system. The exact reason for this is not certain, but empirically it is true. Even in the case of severe contrast allergy, risks can be minimized by the use of nonionic contrast, premedication, and anesthesia standby, if necessary. In therapeutic endovascular procedures, one must be very careful to analyze the patient's vascular anatomy in order to identify potential con-

traindications to injection of specific vessels. Relative contraindications to elective angiographic procedures on the arterial side might include uncontrolled high blood pressure or clotting disorder. Also, the patient's renal status may restrict the contrast load. All these factors must be considered by the consultant radiologist in any angiographic procedure. Another relative contraindication to an angiographic procedure is the unavailability of prior imaging studies. Any elective study should be delayed until one can determine whether, on the basis of these studies, the procedure is necessary and what specific questions need to be answered by the angiogram. Careful preplanning minimizes catheter time, the number of injections, and, therefore, the risk of complications.

In light of these potential complications and possible contraindications, both the clinician and diagnostic imager must realize, when analyzing the use of an angiographic procedure, that there are alternatives to obtaining some of this information. These may not be classically accepted alternatives, and the images may not be of optimal quality; however, the emerging role of MRA and duplex sonography (with color-flow Doppler imaging) may provide all of the information truly necessary for patient care. Of course, angiography will remain indispensable for some indications.

Ultrasonography

Development/General Technique

Diagnostic ultrasonography went through its most rapid phase of development during the 1970s. In the early 1970s, A-mode ultrasonography was used for ocular studies and to look for midline shifts of the ventricular system of the brain. Bi-stable ultrasonography produced relatively crude images with no gray scale; however, this led to the development of imaging with gray scale, static B-mode techniques. Early on, this was done with analog equipment and transducers that were attached to mechanical arms. In the mid- to late 1970s, technology rapidly improved to include high-resolution, real-time studies with continued improvement in the gray scale of the images. This was greatly aided by the switch from analog to digital systems in the late 1970s. During the 1980s, vast improvements were made in these instruments, perhaps the most notable being the introduction of duplex sonography, which combines imaging and Doppler techniques. This method has been refined by the introduction of color-flow Doppler techniques, which in general makes the Doppler portion of the examination much more user friendly. Currently, ultrasonography is an extremely important imaging tool in many organ systems, including the head and neck region.

Basically, ultrasonography works by sending sound waves into the body and almost instantaneously reading the reflections of the sound waves that come from anatomic interfaces with various degrees of acoustic impedance and reflectivity. The quality of the image depends on the equipment used. The resolving power of the transducer must be matched to the patient's anatomy as well as to the imaging task at hand. In general, the highest resolution techniques are capable of relatively limited depths of penetration in the body. Fortunately, this does not seriously impede the examination of the pathologic disorders of the head and neck region because most of the structures of interest are superficial (in comparison with the requirements for penetration in abdominal and pelvic studies). Ultrasonography is also highly user dependent, and it takes a fairly long time to train technologists or physician users. Moreover, the anatomy as seen on ultrasonography is not as inherently obvious as it is on other modern imaging techniques, such as CT and MRI. This sometimes leads to less acceptance by clinicians of ultrasonography, in comparison with other techniques.

There has always been some enthusiasm among ultrasonographers for "tissue characterization" that is based on the acoustic profiles of various tissues. This interest probably developed because of the ability of ultrasonography, at times, to differentiate fluid areas from solid structures. To date, the status of ultrasonography in this regard remains basically the same as it was in the 1970s and 1980s. Evaluation of gross morphologic features, such as zones of simple and complex cystic change within masses, can be defined, and certainly exquisite studies of the anatomic relationships of pathologic processes to the various involved or adjacent structures are available. Ultrasonography is still, however, not a histologically specific tool.

Current Indications

In general, it is useful to be confident that ultrasonography will contribute potentially definitive or at least unique incremental data to the clinical diagnosis before the time and expense of the examination are incurred. Too often, ultrasonographic examinations really have no significant impact on decision making; in these situations, ultrasonography becomes cost additive. The most common of these situations is when there is an obviously palpable mass in the upper neck or parotid region. The ultrasonographic examination usually does not define the full extent of a mass or its nature beyond that supposed by the physical examination, other than to exclude a vascular nature or origin (Figs. 2–6, 2–7). Sometimes this information is critical; however, it is seriously questioned only occasionally, and this aspect alone cannot justify the use of ultrasonography in all neck and parotid masses. The patient then goes on to have an additional study, such as CT or MRI, for defining the full extent of the lesion. One of the obvious situations in which this occurs is in patients with cystic hygromas of the neck. The diagnosis is usually clinically obvious, especially in pediatric patients. An ultrasonographic study confirms the cystic nature of the mass, which is usually suspected clinically, and then CT or MRI is still needed for defining the full extent of the mass before surgical therapy. The ultrasonographic examination can clearly be eliminated from the diagnostic loop for these patients. In other situations, ultrasonography can be indispensable, such as the infrequent occasions when there is a mass in the upper neck or thoracic inlet that is suspected of being vascular in origin. Here, the duplex ultrasonographic examination can usually definitively show whether the mass is arising from the vessel, whether the mass is vascular, or whether it is merely adjacent to and displacing surrounding vessels (Fig. 2–8). This can be very useful in deciding whether to examine the lesion by needle biopsy or continue with other diagnostic procedures (Fig. 2–7). The aim of this discussion is to sensitize the clinician to the importance of sequencing examinations properly so that costs can be kept at a minimum. Clinicians should be aware that imagers who are very experienced in ultrasonography sometimes suggest that it can be a definitive study in a majority of cases; however, in less experienced hands or

TABLE 2–3. CT Technique for Oral Cavity and Oropharynx Cancer

Area Under Study	Extent of Study	Gantry Angle	Slice Thickness	Field of View	Coronals	Algorithm	Contrast/Comment
Oral Cavity Cancer*							
Upper gingivobuccal sulcus, hard palate	Floor of orbit to angle of mandible	Basically parallel to HP, but angle to avoid fillings as necessary	3–4 mm contiguous	15–18 cm	Always for hard palate; otherwise not necessary	Bone for coronal hard palate and selected axials; otherwise ST	Coronals are essential and of prime importance if hard palate is potentially involved; contrast used; survey nodes
Lower gingivobuccal sulcus	Midaxillary antrum to hyoid	Parallel to MB	3–4 mm contiguous	15–18 cm	Rarely	Bone for lingual plate mandible; otherwise ST	Higher sections may be eliminated in smaller lesions limited to lower gingivobuccal sulcus; contrast used; survey nodes
Retromolar trigone	Midaxillary antrum to hyoid	Parallel to HP, then reangle parallel to MB at top mandibular alveolar ridge	3–4 mm contiguous	15–18 cm	Rarely	Bone for lingual plate mandible; otherwise ST	Watch for subtle retroantral and floor of mouth spread; contrast used; survey nodes
Oral tongue	Midoral cavity to hyoid	Parallel to MB below fillings, otherwise angle to avoid fillings	3–4 mm contiguous	15–18 cm	Rarely	Bone if primary near mandible	Watch for spread to floor of mouth and base of tongue; contrast used; survey nodes
Floor of the mouth	Top mandibular alveolar ridge to hyoid	Parallel to MB	3–4 mm contiguous	15–18 cm	Rarely	Bone if primary near lingual plate (e.g., lateral floor of mouth); otherwise ST	Watch for obstructed SMG mimicking primary spread; contrast used; survey nodes

Oropharynx Cancer*

Site	Superior/inferior extent	Angulation	Slice	Length	Bone	Tissue	Comments
Anterior tonsillar pillar, faucial tonsil, soft palate	Midantrum (midnasopharynx) to hyoid	Parallel to IOML (HP) to midoral cavity then parallel to MB; change sooner to avoid fillings as necessary	3–4 mm contiguous	15–18 cm	Only if HP involvement is known or suspected	ST; bone only when tumor is adjacent to bone	Spread to nasopharynx, retropharyngeal nodes, soft tissues of neck possible; may have to alter sections to avoid fillings; contrast used; survey nodes
Tongue base, glossotonsillar sulcus	Mandibular alveolar ridge to 1 cm below hyoid. Cephalad spread of tumor may require higher sections	Parallel to MB. Parallel to IOML (HP) if higher sections required	3–4 mm contiguous	15–18 cm	No	Bone for lingual plate; mandible if tumor adjacent, otherwise ST	Look for unsuspected anterior spread via mylohyoid, sublingual space, direct spread to pre-epiglottic space; check status of midline
Lateral and posterior pharyngeal wall	Midantrum to mandibular alveolar ridge	Parallel to IOML (HP) to midoral cavity, then parallel to mandibular body	3–4 mm contiguous	15–18 cm	No	ST; bone rarely necessary	Most lesions occur from midoropharynx to level of arytenoids; contrast used; survey nodes

Node Survey†

Site	Superior/inferior extent	Angulation	Slice	Length	Bone	Tissue	Comments
	Continue inferiorly from last section	Parallel to MB	3–4 mm contiguous or 5-mm increments	14–16 cm	No	ST	Must evaluate all retropharyngeal nodes carefully C1–C3

From Mancuso A: Workbook for MRI and CT of the Head and Neck, 2nd ed. Baltimore: Williams & Wilkins, 1989.

*Intravenous contrast is always used; if contrast cannot be used, consider MR first; however, CT is the preferred imaging examination.

†Node survey is included in all cases and is continued inferiorly from the last section done for primary site.

HP = hard palate; MB = mandibular body; ST = soft tissue; IOML = infraorbital meatal line; SMG = submandibular gland.

TABLE 2–4. CT Techniques for Temporal Bone and Related Disorders

Area Under Study	Extent of Study	Gantry Angle	Slice Thickness	Field of View	Coronals	Algorithm	Contrast/Comment
Temporal Bone (by Indication)							
a. Acquired cholesteatoma and other inflammatory diseases	Axials: from about 6 mm above to about 6 mm below EAC Coronals: 6 mm in front of 6 mm in back of EAC	Parallel to IOML (axials); approximately perpendicular to IOML (coronals)	1.5 mm (1.0–2.0 mm) contiguous	9–12 cm on side of interest	Almost always, but decide on case by case basis	Always bone; ST and brain on case by case basis	Usually noncontrast, but contrast if intracranial complication suspected; *look at nasopharynx,* especially in all adults with unilateral disease
b. Benign mass or mass of unknown etiology in external canal, middle ear; include congenital cholesteatoma, facial neuroma, hemangioma, etc.	As in *a*; extend as necessary, depending on extent of mass	As in *a*	1.5 mm, sometimes 3 mm in large lesions	9–12 cm on side of interest	Almost always	May be primary bone or ST, usually both	Axial noncontrast to start; coronal with or without contrast depending on history and axial findings Consider three-dimensional reconstruction in complex cases
c. "Noise in ear"/ pulsatile tinnitus; rule out glomus jugulare/ tympanicus, ectopic carotid, dural vascular malformation, etc.	Temporal bone as above; entire posterior fossa to C1–C2 level; survey to carotid bifurcation depending on above; sometimes finish head See pulsatile tinnitus algorithm	As in *a* for posterior fossa, for temporal bone, and to hard palate as necessary If lower sections necessary, avoid fillings and switch to parallel to mandibular body	3 mm to tegmen tympani; 1.5 mm to hypotympanum; finish posterior fossa by 3 mm If survey to carotid necessary, do 3-mm thick by 5-mm increments	14–18 cm; selectively smaller for temporal bone as necessary	As necessary depending on axials	ST/brain for posterior fossa and below skull base; bone for temporal bone	Contrast used mainly for posterior fossa (e.g., dural vascular malformation); if ectopic carotid, glomus typanicus main diagnoses, can do without Contrast necessary below skull base for arteriovenous malformation, etc. and carotid bifurcation (see pulsatile tinnitus algorithm)
d. Malignant tumor, unknown extent of temporal bone involvement (usually squamous cell carcinoma of pinna or parotid primary)	Depends on tumor size, location; usually from zygoma to at least angle of mandible and neck survey for nodes	As in *a* for temporal bone; through parotid angle only for avoidance of fillings; parallel to mandible for remainder	3 mm to tegmen tympani; 1.5 mm to mastoid tip; 3 mm to hyoid 3-mm by 5-mm increments if neck survey necessary	14–18 cm; zoom (retro) 9–12 cm for temporal bone as necessary	As necessary depending on axials	Acquire in ST; retro bone, view brain	Contrast used for axials, very helpful for nodes; contrast for coronals usually not necessary
e. Cochlear implant, otosclerosis, labyrinthitis ossificans	Axials: about 6 mm above to about 6 mm below EAC Coronals: 6 mm in front to 6 mm in back of EAC	Parallel to IOML (axial); approximately perpendicular to IOML (coronals)	1.5 mm (1.0–2.0 mm) contiguous	9–12 cm	Most cases *all* cochlear implants and otosclerosis	Primarily bone but view brain	No contrast; consider contiguous 1.0 or 1.0–2.0 mm at 1-mm increments for stapes/oval window detail

f. Congenital malformation of middle ear, inner ear	As in *e*; consider 1.5 × 1 mm overlap in middle ear for subtle ossicular cases (stapes evaluation)	As in *e*	1.5 mm (1.0–2.0 mm) Consider 1-mm increments for evaluation of ossicles (stapes)	9–12 cm	Almost always	Primarily bone but view brain	Sometimes will include contrast and standard brain views in posterior fossa at request of clinical staff
g. Trauma, excluding cerebrospinal fluid otorrhea (see *h*)	As in *e*	As in *e*	1.5 mm (1.0–2.0 mm)	9–12 cm	Almost always	Bone and ST (for brain)	Usually noncontrast
h. Cerebrospinal fluid otorrhea or leak into temporal bone suspected for other reasons	As in *e*; begin with *prone* axial following C1–C2 puncture; follow with *prone* coronals if intrathecal contrast is used	As in *e*	1.5 mm	9–12 cm	Almost always; mandatory for tegmen leak	ST and bone	Water-soluble contrast via C1–C2 with prone axial (for posterior leak) and prone coronals (for tegmen leak) probably best overall yield. Intravenous contrast for ruling out infection at separate siting as necessary. Lumbar puncture okay. Leak site found without intrathecal contrast
i. Peripheral VII nerve palsy; combined with MRI-MR or CT first, depending on circumstances (see diagnostic algorithms for cranial nerves)	As in *e*; include parotid	As in *e*	1.5 mm temporal bone; 3 mm parotid	9–12 cm temporal bone; 14–18 cm parotid	Frequently depends on axials	ST and bone	Intravenous contrast usually unnecessary; study is complementary to MRI
j. Cranial nerves IX–XII, Horner's syndrome, jugular fossa syndrome	See diagnostic algorithms. MRI is done first in almost all cases; if CT is necessary, proceed to appropriate area for specifics (e.g., skull base, temporal bone, facial nerve).						
k. Sensorineural hearing loss; rule out acoustic or recurrence	MR with paramagnetic contrast gadolinium-DTPA is done first. If CT follows, technique similar to *c* is used, omitting "lower sections" and using contrast at outset. See posterior fossa. Air CPA cisternography is rarely used if high-resolution MR is available.						

From Mancuso A: Workbook for MRI and CT of the Head and Neck, 2nd ed. Baltimore: Williams & Wilkins, 1989. EAC = External auditory canal; IOML = infraorbital meatal line; ST = soft tissue.

major factor affecting pixel size and, therefore, spatial resolution (Table 2–2). The xy dimensions of a voxel can be derived by dividing the field of view by the matrix size. If a 512×512 matrix and a 12- to 18-cm field of view are used routinely, one can see that approximately a 0.25- to 0.35-mm pixel size is now the rule in the head and neck region (Figs. 2–11, 2–13). Every effort should be made to reduce the field of view to the smallest practical limit because of the improved spatial resolution that results. On current systems this can now be done easily, but unfortunately, one of the most common faults in images of poor quality is lack of an optimized field of view (Figs. 2–1, 2–13). If images appear to be small and surrounded by a lot of black areas on the hard copy or as they appear on the screen, the field of view and, therefore, spatial resolution have not been optimized.

The last major factor that affects the spatial resolution of an image is the way it is processed in the computer (Table 2–2). The raw CT data obtained can be put through various filters, which are capable of producing images that in general emphasize bone or soft tissue detail. It is often appropriate for the raw data to be put through two different algorithms for optimizing the information content of the study (Fig. 2–14).

Contrast Resolution

Anything that is done to optimize spatial resolution potentially affects contrast resolution. Using thinner sections or smaller fields of view makes the voxel smaller. This potentially reduces contrast resolution. As a practical matter, this poses no particular difficulty with modern CT equipment. Some increased dose of radiation to the patient might be required to improve the contrast resolution in a highly spatial resolved image on older units; however, in the 1980s there was marked improvement in both x-ray tubes and detector systems, which makes increased dose of little practical significance if the newer equipment is available. The trade-offs between contrast resolution and spatial resolution are more acutely evident in MRI.

Intravenous Contrast

Iodinated contrast is an extremely valuable tool when used properly in conjunction with intra- and extracranial studies of the head and neck. Its use involves risk. Currently, the risks are minimal, but it is still useful to do a risk/benefit analysis for each patient. This decision should largely be left to the diagnostic imager. If contrast injection is con-

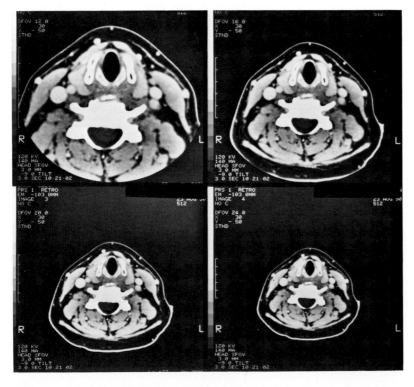

Figure 2–13. The same image is reconstructed from raw CT data (not photographically magnified) at an increasingly larger field of view: upper left, 12 cm; upper right, 16 cm; lower left, 20 cm; lower right, 24 cm. The black area around the image represents wasted spatial resolution. This also illustrates optimal opacification of vessels with contrast.

Figure 2-14. Importance of selecting the correct reconstruction algorithm. In the upper left is a bone *window* of a data set processed with a soft tissue *algorithm;* the bone detail is not much improved even by reprocessing the data at a smaller field of view (lower left). The same data, on the right, are processed with use of a bone algorithm that improves edge detection at the expense of contrast resolution. Note the improvement in the quality of bone detail at the lower right.

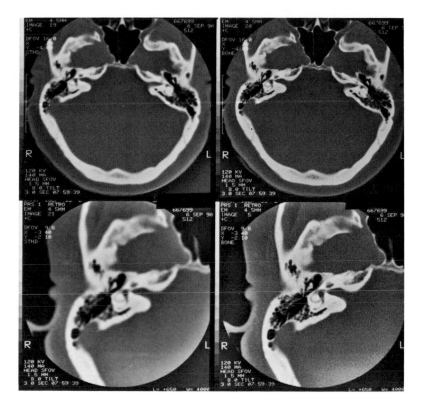

sidered too dangerous, one might consider performing MRI rather than CT. The contrast used with MRI poses virtually no risk of untoward reaction. Newer, nonionic/low-osmolality products are making iodinated contrast use much safer, and these relative risk considerations are therefore becoming much less critical.

The aims of contrast infusion in the extracranial head and neck are to (1) determine the vascularity of a lesion, (2) see the margins of a lesion with greater clarity, (3) distinguish normal vessels from a pathologic process (primary tumor and lymph nodes) and study the effects of disease on these same vessels, and (4) aid in a differential diagnosis. These goals require that the iodine be in the vascular phase throughout image acquisition. In general, this means that in the images, the major vessels such as the carotid artery and jugular vein should be obviously different in density from surrounding tissue (Fig. 2–13). If this is not true, contrast has not been used effectively in the extracranial head and neck structures (Fig. 2–1C). It is the diagnostic imager's responsibility to optimize injection techniques for safety and effectiveness. Several strategies available today can virtually ensure optimal contrast use in 90% or more of patients.

Special Techniques

Dynamic intravascular CT studies are done by injecting contrast, usually with a power injector, and scanning the area of interest rapidly. This was previously thought to be potentially useful in diagnosis of vascular masses and other uses primarily related to neuroradiologic applications. Currently, dynamic scanning serves basically as an option for obtaining images while vessels are maximally opacified. The use of such techniques in differential diagnosis of vascular masses has largely been supplanted by MRI, supplemented with MRA when necessary (Fig. 2–5). If there is still a need for additional information, angiography is performed.

There are a limited number of CT scanners capable of obtaining images in very rapid sequence. This technology is being applied but still should be considered developmental; it is not generally available. This can be used for cineradiographic studies of the airway and the temporomandibular joint.

Advances in computer hardware and software have led to widespread applications of reformation of CT data in multiple planes. This in turn has led to development of three-dimensional reconstruction of these data. One may expect further improvements in the ease of such reconstructions and the user interface with three-dimensional CT data (Figs. 2–10, 2–26, 2–28, 2–33).

CT-guided biopsies are very useful in selected patients. They prove especially helpful in lesions of the masticator space, the infratemporal fossa, the parapharyngeal space, and the skull base. Cytologic or histologic samples can be obtained, depending on the circumstances, the nature of the lesion, and the location. These procedures are safe and relatively simple (Fig. 2–15).

Advantages of CT (Versus MRI) and Current Indications

There is some competition between CT and ultrasonography in evaluating head and neck problems. These problems are relatively infrequent and are discussed in the following sections on specific anatomic subregions of interest. They occur mainly in the evaluation of lesions in the parotid region and neck. The choice between CT and MRI as a primary modality for a given anatomic area, or diagnostic problem, can be more subtle and perhaps controversial. In general, there are some basic advantages for each modality; CT is generally more available than is MRI. Throughput on CT scanners is generally faster than on MRI, and there are more CT scanners in the field. Also, demand for MRI studies for traditional neuroradiologic and orthopedic problems is high, and backlogs are not uncommon; these problems limit the availability of these units for other studies. Study failures related to claustrophobia are almost nil with CT, whereas a 2% to 5% rate of failure is not uncommon with MRI. Failure rates due to motion artifacts may approach 20% to 25% in patients with laryngeal and hypopharyngeal cancers. Some patients cannot undergo MRI examination because of implanted objects that might unfavorably interact with the strong magnetic and radiofrequency fields of these imaging units. CT is typically 30% to 50% lower in cost than is MRI. These represent the basic socioeconomic differences between the two studies.

Technically, CT is a much simpler study to perform. In general, the examinations are completed within 20 to 30 minutes and can be done on even marginally cooperative patients. Bone detail is much better on CT than on MRI, and spatial resolution is still typically better on most CT units.

The morphologic characteristics of some disease processes may be more obvious on CT than on MRI; this is especially true of abscesses and inflammatory lesions. In addition, CT shows calcification better than does MRI, and this may significantly aid differential diagnosis (Fig. 2–16). In the early 1980s, CT proved capable of detecting metastases in normal-sized lymph nodes. There are no good data available for suggesting that MRI can match the accuracy of CT in staging cervical metastatic disease.

Current indications for CT in head and neck disorders are many and varied, and they are outlined in detail in the following sections. The relative roles of CT, MRI, and ultrasonography as well as radionuclide studies must be considered for each diagnostic problem. The relative use of these tests is constantly evolving, sometimes shifting in response to technologic advances. No blanket statements or assumptions should be made concerning whether one or another test should be used *all* of the time for a particular head and neck subregion. Such a dogmatic approach might lead to unnecessarily restrictive policies regarding the use of these powerful imaging tools.

Contraindications

The only medical contraindications to the use of CT are related to contrast allergy; these were discussed in detail in the angiography section. Contrast allergy is a relative contraindication that may be overcome in many instances; however, MRI may be reasonably substituted for a contrast-enhanced CT in certain situations and should always be considered a viable option. Few patients are so claustrophobic that they cannot undergo a CT examination without sedation. Sedation short of general anesthesia works in virtually all these patients except some children. CT studies are frequently done on patients who are critically ill or who require general anesthesia. The studies require only routine anesthesia equipment as opposed to the specialized equipment necessary for MRI procedures on such patients.

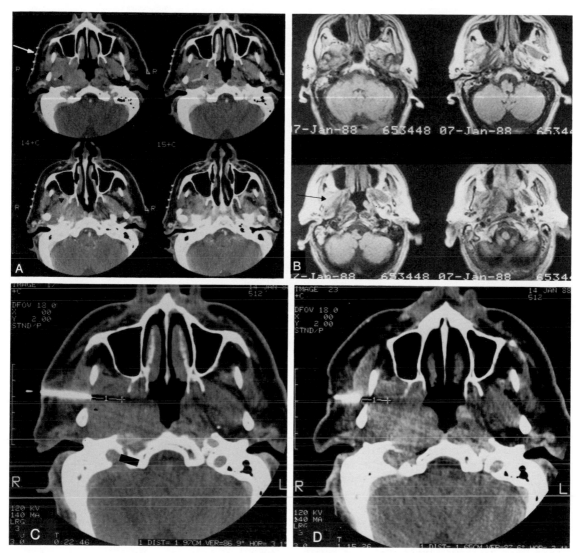

Figure 2–15. General procedure for CT-guided biopsy. *A.* Four views with localizing catheters in place. Dynamic study with contrast infusion localizes the maxillary artery (arrowheads). *B.* Correlation with four views from MR study shows target area of tumor (arrow) different in signal from surrounding muscle; this aids site selection and reduces chances of false sampling of muscle. *C.* A 19-gauge guide needle in place. After access has been established, a 22-gauge needle is passed coaxially. In this case, fine-needle aspiration was nondiagnostic. *D.* An 18-gauge ABC needle positioned so that cutting action begins deep to the facial nerve (note tip is in masseter) and distal excursion is directed away from the maxillary artery (see *A*). Depth was also controlled for avoidance of arterial injury. Core sample, obtained without complications, was hand-carried to surgical pathology. Histologic diagnosis was poorly differentiated carcinoma.

Magnetic Resonance Imaging

Development

MRI, like CT, was introduced in the United States after its initial development in Great Britain. The first units in the United States became operational in 1982 and 1983. There has been very rapid dispersion of the technology between 1985 and 1990. Currently, MRI has reached a reasonably stable level of technologic development. Most manufacturers now have available specialized coils for the study of the head and neck region. Popular imaging field strengths vary from 0.2 to 1.5 tesla (T). Head and neck imaging may be done successfully at any of these field strengths, and perhaps some at slightly lower for limited indications. In general, most of the units have the same basic capabilities, but image quality is best on units in the 0.5-

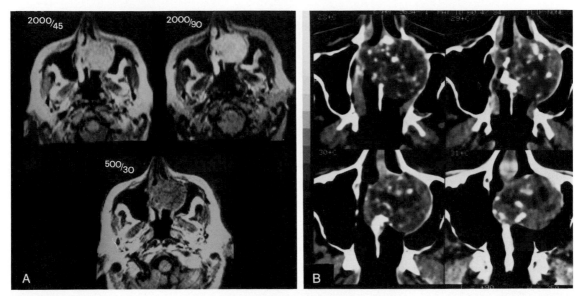

Figure 2–16. Patient with mass in nasal cavity. *A.* T1- and T2-weighted MR images show the mass but no evidence of calcification and no definite evidence that it arises from the nasal septum. *B.* CT examination clearly shows the chondroid matrix (stippled and ring calcification) of the mass and its origin from the nasal septum. Diagnosis of septal enchondroma versus chondrosarcoma is certain on CT but was not even anticipated on MRI.

to 1.5-T range. Imaging for the most part is done with standard T1- and T2-weighted images. Fat suppression imaging has begun to play an important role in studies of the extracranial head and neck, but the techniques are still in a developmental stage and must be standardized in order for them to be as useful as the more proven pulse sequences. Paramagnetic contrast is used in many studies that require detailed evaluation of the intracranial structures; it is less effective in the extracranial head and neck region because it decreases the contrast between fat and pathologic processes. The development of fat suppression techniques that can be used together with these intravenous paramagnetic contrast agents might be the answer to this problem.

More recently, MRA has been developed. This technique is already useful in selected diagnostic circumstances and certainly may eliminate some diagnostic angiographic procedures. It will not completely replace standard angiography at its current state of development, and it is unlikely to do so over the 1990s. MRI is already capable of rudimentary types of cineradiographic studies; in the head and neck region, these have been mainly applied to TMJ function. Improvements in rapid scanning techniques may lead to further development of such motion studies. These as well as MRA techniques are also useful in studying cerebrospinal fluid flow. This is all currently in the phase of late development and early clinical application.

Basic Imaging Principles

It is almost essential to understand basic MRI physics in order to use this imaging tool to its fullest advantage, and there are many excellent sources of this information (see Suggested Readings). Acquiring a working knowledge of MRI physics that is good enough to aid in imaging interpretation is not easy. Observing a large number of images, a basically empiric approach, is probably as good as any for those seeking to acquire basic interpretive skills. From the author's personal experience, learning to interpret MRI studies involves progressing along a much steeper and longer learning curve than does learning to interpret CT studies, but the climb is certainly worth the study required.

For obtaining the MRI image, the patient must be placed in a large magnet. The magnet is equipped with several sets of radiofrequency coils, which are used to transmit radio waves into the body and localize the return signal. The return signal is usually picked up by a radiofrequency coil placed on or near the body so that it is most closely coupled with the region of anatomic interest. In the head and neck region, these coils are usually the standard head coil, which fits snugly around the patient's head, or a coil that covers the region from the low face to low neck and thoracic inlet. Such volume coils are highly efficient, and one can see the full thickness of the area under study. Sometimes smaller coils are placed on the surface of the body. These are also highly efficient receivers for structures that lie no deeper than 3 to 4 cm. Such coils have been used to study the TMJ and orbits but are generally unsuitable for evaluating deeper structures. This series of coils and antennas has the ability to deposit the radiofrequency in the body, spatially encode this information, and then receive the spatially encoded information from the body after it interacts with the volume of tissue under study. The spatially encoded radiofrequency waves coming out of the body are then unscrambled, as in CT, by Fourier mathematical analysis for building an image made out of voxels. For CT, the information in each voxel is determined basically by the interaction of the x-ray photons with the electrons, in the volume of tissue represented by the voxel (Fig. 2–11). The strength and character of the CT signal is, therefore, influenced by just one variable. In MRI, the signal that represents the tissue in each voxel is determined by the interaction of protons and local magnetic fields altered by gradients, and the radiofrequency pulse is applied. Therefore, the intensity of the signal in the MRI voxel is influenced by several variables rather than one variable; these include (1) proton density, (2) longitudinal (T1) and transverse relaxation (T2) times (intrinsic tissue values), and (3) flow (motion). Each of these variables can be influenced by exactly how the operator chooses to design the pulsing sequence that produces the MR image. This inherent complexity is what makes MRI somewhat more difficult to understand than CT on a fundamental as well as an operational basis.

The overall concept of resolution, both spatial and contrast, was discussed in the section on CT. If necessary, this section should be reviewed at this time because it presents a basic discussion of the tissues that follow as well as a definition of the basic terms that are related to resolution.

Basic Technique

An MRI instrument used for studying both intra- and extracranial manifestations of head and neck disorders should be capable of a certain basic range of techniques. The following are guidelines for performing MRI techniques for ENT-related abnormalities.

1. Slice thickness: 4 to 6 mm routine (2 to 3 mm is desirable in selected circumstances) for two-dimensional Fourier transform (FT) studies.
2. Field of view: 10 to 16 cm for T1-weighted images and 16 to 20 cm for T2-weighted images.
3. Acquisition matrix: variable from 128×128 to 256×256.
4. Pixel size: 0.75 to 1×1 mm (0.5 mm desirable).
5. Acquisition time: no more than 10 to 15 minutes per acquisition, and preferably acquisitions on the order of 2 to 8 minutes.
6. Paramagnetic contrast available.
7. MRA fat suppression techniques, and three-dimensional FT techniques available.
8. Receiver coils specially designed for head and neck use available.

Spatial Resolution

The basic concepts of the voxel and the relative impact of image contrast, spatial resolution, and SNR on resolution were introduced in the section on computed tomography. These should be reviewed at this point, if necessary. SNR is generally reflected in image quality. If the signal decreases or the noise increases beyond certain acceptable limits, pictures are of poor quality. In general, artifacts become more prominent, and the pictures look fuzzy or grainy. The need for some finite amount of spatial resolution, in large part, determines the lower limits of acceptable SNR in any imaging system. Because the image is built of voxels, it is really the SNR per voxel that must be considered. As the voxel volume decreases, the SNR decreases as well.

In comparison with CT, MR techniques that reduce voxel size, for the benefit of increased spatial resolution, can more profoundly decrease image quality. There are ways of compensating for the losses, such as increasing the number of signal averages at the cost of increased data acquisition time. Currently, voxel volumes of a fraction of a cubic millimeter on CT do not create any significant degradation of image quality in the head and neck region. Comparatively, MR voxel volumes must stay at or over a cubic millimeter in size for maintaining good image quality. This problem can be somewhat overcome by use of higher field strength instruments; however, this reaches a point of diminishing return at approximately a 1-T field strength in human whole-body systems. It is also, for technical reasons, easier to maintain SNR on T1- than on T2-weighted images. There are always trade-offs in MRI, and the sacrifice here is that certain tissue contrast characteristics are better on T2-weighted pulse sequences than on T1-weighted sequences.

In general, with MRI systems, one should be striving for a voxel volume that at least begins to approximate those available on CT (depending on the anatomic area of interest). As discussed in the CT section, this is done by keeping the field of view as small as possible and using as thin a section as possible. In MRI, as in CT, thin sections somewhat limit the area that can be studied in a time-efficient manner if thin sections are required through an anatomic region that has a long cephalocaudal extent. With MRI, the addition of extra slices is more time-consuming because it often requires another acquisition. The clinician should be aware that many technical nuances are involved in the selection of the field of view and slice thickness. The technical trade-offs that influence the selection of slices and slice intervals profoundly affect the quality of the MR image. These technical choices are all under operator control. Significant artifacts can occur or detail can be lost if techniques are not chosen appropriately. As in CT, this requires the studious development of imaging protocols that fit the equipment available as well as the clinical problems that are under study.

Contrast Resolution and Paramagnetic Contrast Agents

Electron density alone influences contrast in CT. In the case of MRI, proton density, relaxation times (T1 and T2), and flow are the determinants of the image contrast. No matter how the MR image is obtained, these three basic factors interact to influence the tissue contrast seen on the image. There are a tremendous number of options available for obtaining an MR image. The pulse sequences are basically designed to trade off spatial and contrast resolution. The operator can directly control the pulse repetition time,

the echo delay time, and the flip angle; this makes three operator-controlled variables that influence the three basic determinants of image contrast. The possible combinations are myriad. They are almost too numerous to understand individually, so one must take a more simplistic view and understand the reasons for wanting more T1- versus T2-weighting in the image. The specific reasons vary with the clinical questions at hand, the need for spatial resolution versus image contrast, and the region of anatomy versus pathology under study.

A complete discussion of the influences of all of these parameters on image contrast is beyond the scope of this text; however, some generalizations are possible. With spin echo pulse sequences, T1-weighted images are generally the best spatially resolved images. T1-weighted images do well at showing differences among fat, muscle, bone, air, and fluid. In general, the contrast between lymphoid tissue and muscle, or tumor and muscle, is marginal; however, this is somewhat dependent on field strength (Fig. 2–17). Contrast of these various tissues with one another on T1-weighted images can be influenced by the injection of paramagnetic contrast agents. In general, these make tumor contrast better with muscle, but less well with fat. There is a great deal of current interest in using fat suppression MR images together with paramagnetic contrast for resolving this difficulty (Figs. 2–18, 2–19). T2-weighted images generally show pathologic brain changes with much greater sensitivity than do T1-weighted images. In the extracranial head and neck, T2-weighted imaging improves tumor-muscle contrast. Tumor-fat contrast is usually adequate; however, the contrast between tumor and lymphoid tissue may be poor (Fig. 2–17). T2-weighted images are not significantly influenced by the injection of currently available paramagnetic contrast agents. Paramagnetic contrast agents are also very useful for assessing the interface between extracranial disease and the dura, leptomeningeal disease, and any pathologic process that results in blood-brain barrier breakdown.

Special Techniques

Currently, some new applications of MR have reached the status of clinical trials and early use. Fast imaging techniques (e.g., echo

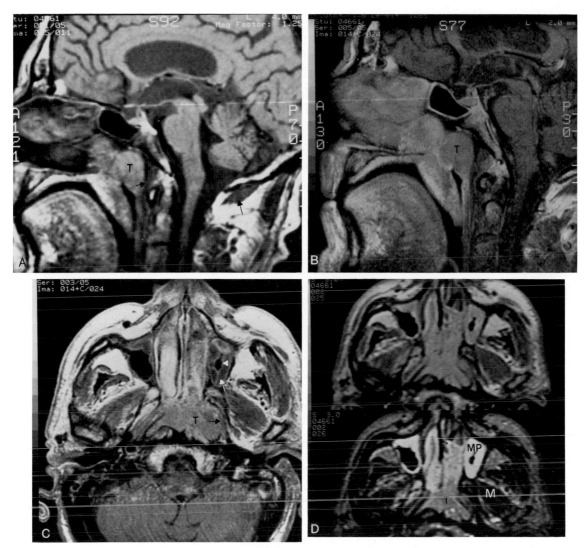

Figure 2–17. Patient with nasopharyngeal carcinoma. *A.* T1-weighted image without contrast shows tumor (T) to be brighter than muscle of posterior pharyngeal wall and neck muscle (arrows). By its signal, however, this could also be normal lymphoid tissue; note that it differs little from the soft palate, which was uninvolved. *B.* Contrast-enhanced MR (T1-weighted) tumor (T) enhances, but so would normal lymphoid tissue. Tumor muscle contrast is still good. Tumor is adjacent to the clivus, but not definitely invading it. *C.* Axial, contrast-enhanced MR shows tumor (T) invading pharyngeal wall (black arrow). If it were not invasive, the study could not distinguish this from a hypertrophic adenoidal pad. Note the submucosal edema (white arrow) and mucosal enhancement (arrowhead) in the obstructed but not invaded maxillary sinus. *D.* Spin density (upper) and T2-weighted (lower) pair shows tumor (T) distinctly different in signal from muscle (M) and mucosal thickening in maxillary antra (MP). Normal adenoids would be the same signal as tumor on both; in fact, part of the mass in the nasopharynx was normal lymphoid tissue.

Illustration continued on following page

planar imaging, turbo FLASH) are being developed, and these may aid in dynamic studies of the airway or TMJ. They definitely aid in the evaluation of cerebrospinal fluid motion.

Flow-sensitive imaging techniques are now fairly well developed. These techniques are becoming generally available on imaging equipment and should be fairly well dispersed by late 1991 or early 1992. There will undoubtedly be continued improvements in these techniques. Currently, flow-sensitive MRI techniques and MRA can be used for confirming the hypervascularity of a lesion and general angiographic mapping (Fig. 2–20). They have some value in the diagnosis

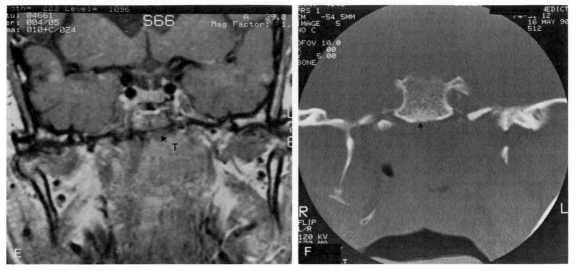

Figure 2–17 *Continued E.* Coronal MR suggests clival invasion (arrow). *F.* CT done to confirm bone invasion shows cortical thinning (arrow), a medullary space sclerosis (just above arrow), as evidence of early bone invasion.

of venous sinus thrombosis. With further improvements, MRA may even become a reasonable gross screening study for cerebral aneurysms and possibly carotid occlusive disease. However, the high cost of MRI will probably keep it from being routinely used to detect carotid occlusive disease. MRA will undoubtedly replace some routine diagnostic angiography; however, it is highly unlikely that it will totally replace diagnostic angiography.

Fat suppression techniques, sometimes referred to as chemical shift imaging, are being developed by all manufacturers (Figs. 2–18, 2–19). There are various approaches to the problem, all of which currently have some drawbacks. It is likely that fat suppression imaging will have either a primary or an adjunctive role in evaluating the orbits and other extracranial head and neck structures. These techniques are likely to be used in combination with already developed and newer paramagnetic contrast agents (Fig. 2–18).

Advantages of MRI (versus CT) and Current Indications*

The choice of whether to use CT or MRI for a particular diagnostic problem is based on many factors. It is sometimes necessary to

---

*See also correlating discussion under computed tomography section.

use both studies, but this should only occur in 10% (or less) of patients. The author's personal view is that MRI is best used when it is focused on a relatively confined area of anatomic interest for answering a specific clinical question. There are many choices to be made when an MRI study is designed for a specific use. The basic decisions include the pulse sequences to be used, which planes should be imaged, what anatomic areas need to be covered, and whether a paramagnetic contrast agent should be used. Paramagnetic contrast agents have complicated matters somewhat because they raise the additional question of whether scans should be done both with and without paramagnetic contrast. The options available become a strength when they are focused on a particular clinical problem; however, they are sometimes a weakness when one is asked to survey a relatively large anatomic area of interest.

In general, MRI is the primary examination for any head and neck problem that might involve the brain, the leptomeninges, or a process that interfaces between the brain and extracranial head and neck structures (Fig. 2–21). Most cranial nerve problems should be studied primarily with MRI. In examination of the extracranial head and neck, the choices are less clear-cut and highly dependent on the clinical situation and, to a lesser extent, the condition of the patient, availability of equipment, and finances.

In choosing between MRI and CT, it is

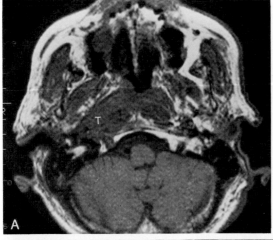

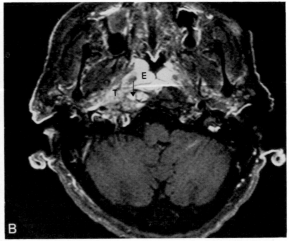

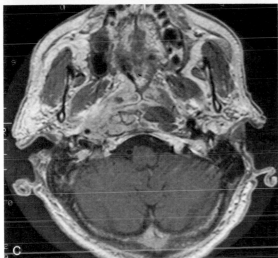

Figure 2–18. *A.* T1-weighted MR image of recurrent carcinoma after total laryngopharyngectomy. No mucosal lesion was visible. Deficits of cranial nerves IX, X, and XII were present. Contrast between tumor (T) and muscle is poor. *B.* Fat-suppressed image with gadolinium enhancement shows tumor (T) to be obviously brighter than muscle and slightly brighter than fat. Tumor in the prevertebral muscles (arrow) is more obvious than in *A*. The nasopharyngeal edema (E) is very bright. *C.* Contrast-enhanced MR also shows the better tumor-muscle contrast than that seen in *A*. It is more difficult to distinguish the reactive changes in the nasopharynx from tumor than in *B*.

useful to have the basic advantages of each technique in mind. Those for CT were discussed in a previous section. The advantages of MRI include the following.

1. MRI involves the use of nonionizing radiation. This is especially important in pediatric patients.

2. The intravenous injection of contrast is often unnecessary; if used, it is probably an order of magnitude or more safer than is the iodinated contrast used in CT studies.

3. MRI can image the body easily in any plane.

4. The contrast between tissue and a pathologic process can be manipulated to a far greater degree with MRI than with CT. Imaging can be further aided by the injection of paramagnetic contrast agents.

5. MRI is more sensitive than is CT in the detection of intra-axial brain and leptomeningeal pathologic processes.

6. MRI is better at determining whether sinuses are obstructed or invaded by tumors.

7. MRI can better differentiate recurrent tumor from *end-stage* fibrosis (but not active scar-granulation tissue).

8. Flow-sensitive imaging techniques can be used in MRI to eliminate some angiographic procedures.

9. Flow-sensitive and fast imaging techniques can be used to study dynamic processes, such as TMJ function and cerebrospinal fluid flow.

There are many indications for MRI in the realm of ENT-related imaging. Some of the basic methods for triage to MRI versus CT were discussed earlier in this section. Specific indications are discussed later in the chapter

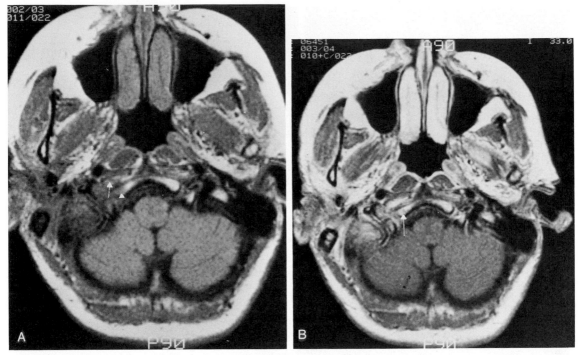

Figure 2–19. Patient with recurrent squamous cell carcinoma of the pinna with invasion of the parotid, mastoid, and basiocciput. *A.* Noncontrast T1-weighted image shows tumor in upper parotid gland (both deep and superficial). Tumor is also in the digastric groove, hypoglossal canal, fat between the prevertebral muscles and clivus (arrow), and clivus (arrowhead). *B.* Contrast-enhanced MR makes it more difficult to distinguish between tumor and fat. Compare with each area mentioned in *A,* and note that tumor is less conspicuous; this is most apparent in the parotid gland and digastric groove regions. The clival invasion (arrow) can no longer be diagnosed because enhancing tumor is isointense to clival fatty marrow.

under each subregion of the head and neck. In general, the diagnostic imager should maintain a flexible attitude about the relative use of MRI, CT, and other imaging techniques. This is probably best accomplished by establishing basic algorithms for given clinical problems and altering these approaches based on technical developments, patient needs, and availability of technology and interpretive expertise. This is reflected in the previous discussions and in the following discussions of different anatomic subregions of the head and neck.

Contraindications

MRI is contraindicated in patients who have certain implanted devices or objects that might be sensitive to the radiofrequencies used or the strong magnetic fields. The most well known of these includes certain aneurysm clips that may torque in the magnetic field and be dislodged. Other implanted ferromagnetic objects may also experience torque in the magnetic field. The ones that most commonly affect the work of the ENT surgeon are cochlear implants and certain stapes prostheses. Several publications that list objects that are implanted in the body and pose a danger are available (see Suggested Readings).

There are no real medical contraindications to MRI; however, some patients may not be able to undergo the study because of extreme claustrophobia. This may be overcome by sedation and encouragement, but still the failure rate for MRI is much higher than that for CT. It is possible to scan patients under anesthesia in MRI units, but this task is greatly complicated by the MRI instrument. Specially designed anesthesia equipment must be used, and some of this is still under development. In particular, pulse oximeters that are compatible with MRI and do not interfere with image quality still need to be developed. The basic requirements for safe studies under general anesthesia will likely be an arterial line, a pulse oximeter,

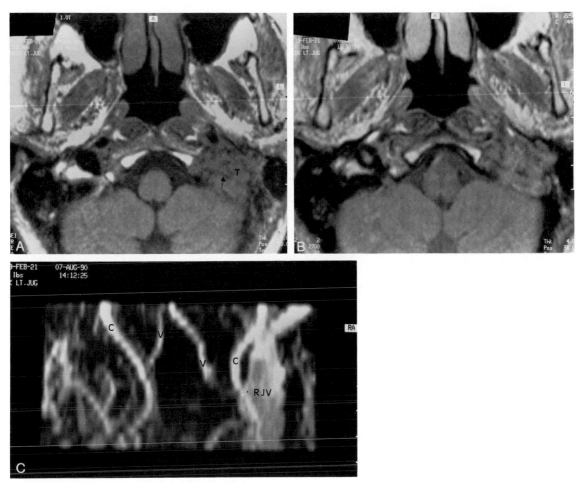

Figure 2–20. Patient with paraganglioma (glomus jugulare) under treatment with radiotherapy. *A.* Standard T1-weighted image showing tumor (T) and only very subtle suggestion of flow voids (arrow). *B.* Contrast-enhanced MR shows minimal uptake of gadolinium-DTPA, suggesting diminished vascularity. *C.* MR angiogram viewing patient from posterior. Right jugular vein (RJV) is patient. Note also vertebral (V) and carotid arteries (C). Left internal jugular vein is not visible, being occluded by tumor or thrombus.

Illustration continued on following page

and an electrocardiogram as well as an MR-compatible respirator.

Radionuclide Studies

Current Development and Basic Technique

Radionuclide studies are experiencing a rebirth because of advances in camera and computer technology. These technologic advances have led to the development of a new imaging technique referred to as single photon emission computed tomography (SPECT). This is basically a sectional imaging technique. SPECT has vastly improved the quality of certain studies done in the head and neck region by allowing more precise and sensitive localization of abnormal accumulations of tracer (Fig. 2–22). This superior image quality has been coupled with newer technetium-labeled agents to allow some basic physiologic and flow-related imaging of the brain, which competes in some respects with positron emission tomography (PET). PET is technically far more complex and requires a greater capital investment in equipment and personnel. Basically, nuclear medicine is in an era of rapid clinical testing of technologic advances that have occurred since 1980 or earlier. These advances will improve the imaging and physiologic studies

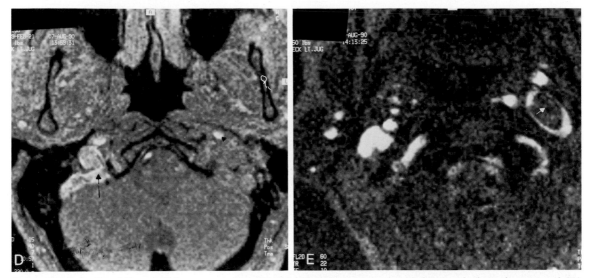

Figure 2–20 *Continued D* and *E*. Images used to generate the MR angiogram in *C* done with three-dimensional *(D)* and two-dimensional *(E)* techniques. Bright areas represent flow. Note patent internal jugular vein–sigmoid sinus junction on right (arrow); only the carotid (arrowhead) is seen on the left. In *E*, clot or tumor (arrow) fills the partially patent internal jugular vein. These images are noisy because they are made for flow imaging rather than for anatomic detail.

already indicated in head and neck disorders and possibly expand the uses of radionuclide studies in the near future.

The general technique involved with radionuclide studies is the injection of a radiotracer that has been tagged to an agent, which will localize in a specific disease process or anatomic site. Depending on the mode of injection and data desired, the radiotracer may be studied in its accumulation, static, and wash-out phases. Curves reflecting the wash-in and wash-out of the radiotracer can be generated. Images may be obtained at one or more points in this cycle as deemed appropriate for the clinical problem and agent being used.

Current Applications

Radionuclide studies remain integral to the evaluation of thyroid disease in a selected group of patients. They may be used either diagnostically or therapeutically in thyroid disease. The basic scheme for integrating radionuclide studies in evaluating thyroid-related disorders is outlined in Figure 2–9.

The use of radionuclide studies for the localization of parathyroid adenomas is discussed later in the chapter.

Gallium scanning or combined techniques with gallium and bone scanning are ex-tremely useful in evaluating patients with inflammatory conditions involving the sinuses, the skull base, and occasionally the deep soft tissues of the face and neck. These studies may be used both for diagnostic purposes and to follow the course of medical therapy. Gallium and bone scans, in particular, have benefited from the newer SPECT techniques.

Radionuclide studies remain critical for patients at risk for metastatic disease. The bone scan remains an integral part of this work-up; however, this must be applied selectively and patients triaged for high risk in order that maximal cost effectiveness be obtained. Liver/spleen scanning may also be used for detecting metastatic disease; however, because patients often have a chest CT as part of the metastatic work-up, it may be more cost effective to continue the CT examination to include the liver and eliminate the radionuclide study of the liver as part of the metastatic work-up.

Less frequent uses of radionuclide studies include blood pool imaging for hemangiomas. Studies done to identify cerebrospinal fluid leaks are still used in diagnostically difficult cases. In rare cases, radionuclide techniques are used to confirm functional abnormalities in the salivary glands and Warthin's tumor in elderly patients who are not particularly good candidates for surgery.

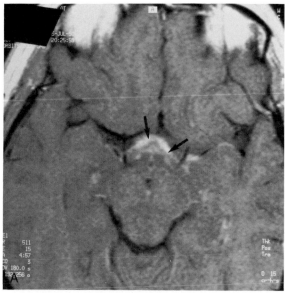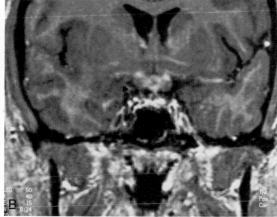

Figure 2–21. Patient with visual disturbances and third cranial nerve palsy. Axial *(A)* and coronal *(B)* T1-weighted images done with paramagnetic contrast show leptomeningeal enhancement surrounding the optic chiasm and tracts (arrows) and involving the course of the right third nerve (arrowhead).

Future Applications

Currently, many techniques are being developed in nuclear medicine. This progress involves software development, multiheaded cameras for improved tomographic imaging, and development of new agents. Much of this work will refine imaging capabilities and lead to improved physiologic applications of radionuclide studies. Currently, much attention is being focused on radiolabeling of monoclonal antibodies, which can be used for tumor localization. It is probably reasonable to assume that nuclear medicine techniques are the ones most liable to be sensitive enough to detect a small amount of tracer accumulation at tumor sites. These techniques may be combined with agents capable of studying flow and metabolic activity of tumor (e.g., use of radiolabeled metabolites in the diagnosis and treatment of paraganglioma). Taken together, these techniques certainly provide the basis for the involvement of diagnostic imagers in the in vivo study of biologic activities of head and neck tumors. Some might argue that this is within the realm of MR spectroscopy. Proton spectroscopy is somewhat promising in this regard. At the currently available field strengths, phosphorus spectroscopy is less likely to be successful because of the tumor volumes necessary for acquisition of data in a reasonable amount of time. Currently,

radionuclide studies are competitive with MRI as a research tool in studying the biologic activity of tumors and their response to therapy.

These technical improvements are also leading to constantly better methods of evaluating brain metabolism and flow. These methods have tremendous applications in the neurosciences. In the realm of head and neck imaging, such studies can be useful in evaluating patients in whom sacrifice of part of the cerebral circulation may be required for treatment of a tumor or other abnormalities. Currently, such studies are done in a relatively gross fashion with use of clinical monitoring during angiographic studies sometimes combined with xenon-assisted CT.

Contraindications

There are really no medical contraindications to radionuclide studies. These studies do require relatively cooperative patients.

USE OF DIAGNOSTIC IMAGING IN SPECIFIC SUBREGIONS OF THE HEAD AND NECK

Orbit and Visual Pathways, Including Cranial Nerves II, III, IV, and VI

In general, there is a very limited role for plain films in evaluating disease involving

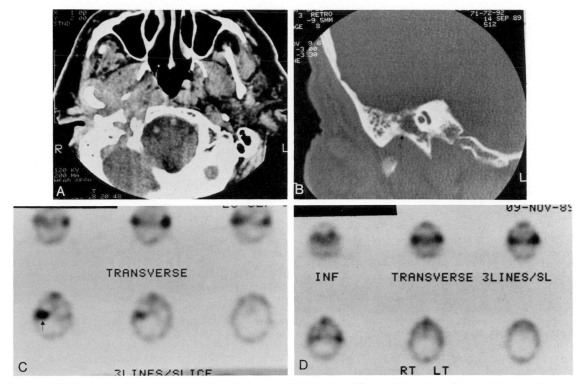

Figure 2–22. Diabetic with malignant otitis externa. *A.* CT showing diffuse obliteration of the soft tissue planes in the masticator, parotid, and pre- and poststyloid parapharyngeal spaces on the right; this finding is highly suggestive of an inflammatory process. *B.* Coronal CT showing subtle erosion of anterior superior external auditory canal (arrow). *C.* SPECT gallium study before therapy shows marked increase in activity in the region of the temporal bone (arrow). *D.* Following 3 weeks of antibiotic therapy, SPECT gallium study reveals dramatic response. The patient was treated for another 3 weeks and cured.

the orbits and visual pathways. The choice of imaging examination is usually between CT and MRI. For the globe, ultrasonography is often useful. Angiography is used occasionally for further evaluation of a pathologic process discovered on CT and MRI. Radionuclide studies have limited applications (Table 2–5).

The Globe

There is little or no role for plain radiography in evaluating ocular abnormalities. On occasion, plain films may be used to look for intraocular foreign bodies. Ultrasonography is the primary tool for evaluating ocular disease when imaging is necessary. Occasionally, MRI or CT is used to determine the nature and extent of a congenital abnormality, the status of the retina, or the extent of a neoplasm. Injuries to the globe are normally evaluated with CT.

Optic Nerve and Posterior Visual Pathways

Assessment of the visual pathways beyond the retina requires a study that can show the optic nerve, chiasm, and tracts; the entire course of cranial nerves III, IV, and VI; and the visual pathways within the brain (Fig. 2–21), inlcuding the optic radiations, visual cortex, and brain stem. MRI is ideally suited to studies of the visual pathways. There are some limitations. Chemical shift artifacts impede subtle diagnosis of lesions involving the intraorbital course of the optic nerve. This is largely being overcome by the use of fat suppression techniques and paramagnetic contrast enhancement. Still, the lack of detection of calcifications can make evaluation of optic sheath meningiomas difficult on rare occasions. Evaluation of these structures should be primarily by MRI. If it is not available, CT is certainly a useful adjunct or, if necessary, primary examination.

Other imaging techniques offer very little

**TABLE 2–5. Comparison Between Magnetic Resonance Imaging
and Other Noninvasive Imaging Tools for Head and Neck Disorders**

Site/Disorder	Ultrasound	Radionuclide	Computed Tomography	Magnetic Resonance Imaging
Orbit				
Ocular	+ + + +	±	+ +	+ +
Orbit	+ +	±	+ + + +	+ + +
Visual pathways	+	±	+ + +	+ + + +
Sinonasal and Facial				
Trauma	0	+	+ + + +	+
Inflammatory disease	0	+	+ + +	+ +
Benign and malignant tumors	0	+	+ + + +	+ + + +
Temporomandibular Joint				
Bone detail	0	0	+ + +	+
Internal derangement	0	±	+	+ + + +
Major Salivary Glands				
Parotid region mass	±	±	+ + +	+ + +
Inflammatory disease	±	±	+ +	+
Submandibular gland region mass	±	±	+ + +	+ + +
Skull Base Cavernous Sinus	0	+ +	+ + +	+ + + +
Temporal Bone				
Acoustic neruoma and other cerebellopontine angle masses	0	0	+ +	+ + + +
Masses—petrous/mastoid	0	0	+ + +	+ + +
Acquired cholesteatoma–middle ear disease	0	0	+ + + +	+
Congenital malformation	0	0	+ + + +	+
Pulsatile tinnitus	±	0	+ + + +	+ + +
Malignant tumor	0	+	+ + + +	+ +
Aggressive inflammation	0	+ +	+ + + +	+ +
Trauma	0	0	+ + + +	+
Precochlear implant	0	0	+ + + +	±
Nasopharynx and Parapharyngeal Space	0	±	+ + +	+ + + +
Oral Cavity, Oropharynx, and Floor of Mouth	±	±	+ + + +	+ +
Larynx and Hypopharynx				
Benign masses	0	0	+ + + +	+ + +
Malignant tumors	±	±	+ + + +	+ +
Trauma	0	0	+ + + +	±
Neck				
Cervical metastatic disease	+	+	+ + + +	+ +
Miscellaneous masses	+	±	+ + + +	+ + +
Thyroid				
Benign masses	+ +	+ + +	+ +	+ +
Malignancies	+	+ + + +	+ +	+ + +
Parathyroid	+ + +	+ + +	+	+ +

0 indicates of no value at present and no obvious potential for the future; ± of questionable value; + of some value but second-line, other technologies are definitely superior; + + of moderate value but second-line, at present frequently competitive with other technologies, but should not be considered as the initial approach; + + + of definite value, usually second-line, but occasionally first line; and + + + + of definite value (first-line).

From Mancuso A: Workbook for MRI and CT of the Head and Neck, 2nd ed. Baltimore: Williams & Wilkins, 1989.

in evaluating the vast majority of disorders affecting visual pathways. Plain films may be done after CT or MRI; they contribute significant information but are almost useless as a first step in evaluating diseases that affect the visual pathways. If used as the first study, they usually are an unnecessary, cost-additive step. Angiography or radionuclide studies, or both, are done as indicated by other imaging studies.

Orbit

The orbit is frequently involved by disease processes that are primarily within the treatment domain of the otolaryngologist and the head and neck surgeon, either because the pathologic process has arisen in the sinonasal region and extended into the orbit or because the head and neck surgeon is part of the treatment team caring for primary craniofacial or neurosurgical problems.

CT and MRI are the studies of choice in evaluating most orbital problems (Table 2–5). Ultrasonography is used for evaluating the globe; in many cases, it is the definitive and only study necessary. In orbital disease, ultrasonography is potentially useful, but in most instances, additional study with CT and MRI is required regardless of the ultrasonographic findings. Plain films are, in general, reserved for evaluating trauma and perhaps for localization of radiodense foreign bodies. They may also be used as an adjunctive study for patients with craniofacial anomalies. Angiography and radionuclide studies are only very infrequently used in orbital work, and then only as an adjunct to other imaging studies.

Developmental Abnormalities

Patients presenting for reconstructive surgery or with mass lesions related to abnormal development may have plain films as the initial study. These may be suitable for gross diagnostic purposes but are usually not sufficient for planning management. Most craniofacial anomalies now receive highly detailed CT studies, wherein the data are reconstructed to produce a three-dimensional image. This image can occasionally be supplemented by MRI if a related developmental abnormality of the central nervous system, such as a meningocele or an encephalocele, is likely to be present (Fig. 2–23).

Infectious and Noninfectious Inflammatory Lesions

A host of inflammatory or infectious conditions may involve the orbit. In the acute setting, these are usually investigated by CT. This is especially true of patients presenting with orbital cellulitis and possible orbital or cranial complications of inflammatory sinus disease. One could begin with MRI in this setting and in other inflammatory lesions of the orbits; however, bone detail is frequently of prime interest in this setting, and MRI assessment of bone is inadequate. Either MRI or CT may be used to evaluate patients with thyroid ophthalmopathy. In general, evaluating inflammatory conditions of the nasolacrimal drainage apparatus requires CT, dacryocystography, or both.

Cancer and Other Mass Lesions

The evaluation of an orbital mass lesion of unknown etiology may begin with plain films, but this is usually not definitive and is unnecessarily cost additive. It is the policy at the University of Florida to do plain films retrospectively, if they are deemed necessary, on the basis of findings of other imaging studies. Ultrasonography may be useful, in experienced hands, for evaluating orbital masses of unknown etiology, but this technique is rarely definitive, and some other imaging with CT and MRI is usually required before a final disposition is reached. One can rationally begin with either MRI or CT in evaluating orbital mass lesions. Depending on the clinical situation, the study not chosen as the primary examination needs to be done as an additional examination in a small percentage of patients (Table 2–5). The same approach holds for patients with cancer, either primarily or secondarily involving the orbit. At this time, patients with malignancies involving the orbit frequently undergo both imaging studies, and such an approach is justified. MRI is particularly well suited to tracing perineural spread of tumor involving the cavernous sinus; for detecting early invasion of the dura, leptomeninges, and brain; and for differentiating tumor invasion from obstructive sinus disease. CT is better suited to showing the bony architecture that is often important in making decisions on the surgical approach to en bloc removal of a cancer.

Angiography and radionuclide studies are used only adjunctively in evaluating orbital mass lesions. Therapeutic endovascular procedures can be very beneficial in devascularizing selected lesions before surgical removal.

Trauma

Orbital trauma is common. Plain films remain the initial examination of choice in most patients; however, many patients undergo CT as a primary examination because of combined craniofacial injuries. Whenever there is craniofacial injury, it is useful to do at least a screening CT examination of the facial region. The screening protocol should include sections that are suitable for evaluating facial trauma; generally acceptable scanning parameters are outlined in the earlier CT section of the chapter.

In severe craniofacial trauma, CT studies should normally be obtained in the axial plane and the direct coronal plane. Examination in the direct coronal plane on CT requires marked hyperextension of the neck

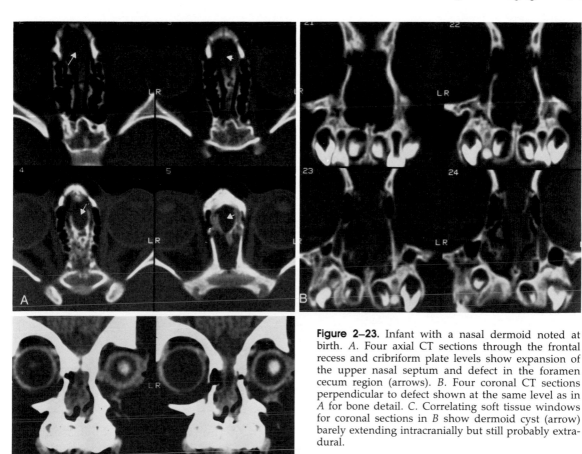

Figure 2–23. Infant with a nasal dermoid noted at birth. *A.* Four axial CT sections through the frontal recess and cribriform plate levels show expansion of the upper nasal septum and defect in the foramen cecum region (arrows). *B.* Four coronal CT sections perpendicular to defect shown at the same level as in *A* for bone detail. *C.* Correlating soft tissue windows for coronal sections in *B* show dermoid cyst (arrow) barely extending intracranially but still probably extradural.

and, therefore, should be done only for patients free of neck injury. If there is any doubt about a neck injury, direct coronal sections should not be done, and reformatted images should be substituted. Also, it is useful to consider obtaining data suitable for three-dimensional reconstruction if the injury is particularly extensive.

Penetrating orbital trauma should usually be investigated with CT alone. Plain films may be used to screen for radiodense foreign bodies but are usually unnecessary and,

therefore, cost additive for little additional yield over CT examination. In general, this examination should be done in two planes so as not to miss foreign bodies that may be far superior or inferior in the globe or the orbital soft tissues. When foreign bodies are present, two planes are necessary for proper localization. Reformatted images of that obtained in a single plane may also be quite useful for this purpose. CT for orbital trauma can also determine whether there has been significant injury to the globe.

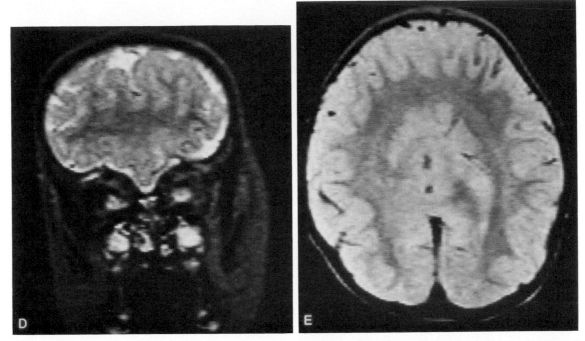

Figure 2–23 *Continued D.* Coronal CT reveals prosencephaly (associated forebrain anomaly) manifest by absence of falx and "fusion" of frontal lobes as well as relationship of brain to cribriform plate region and dermoid shown in *A* to *C. E.* Axial image of the brain anomaly.

Paranasal Sinuses, Nasal Cavity, Anterior Skull Base, and Facial Bones (Excluding the Mandible, Teeth, and TMJ)

General Indications

The relative value of the various imaging modalities available for evaluating disease in this subregion was discussed in detail under each individual imaging modality section. In general, CT and MRI are used for the majority of imaging in the sinonasal and facial region (Table 2–5). Plain films have been a standard study for evaluating patients with signs and symptoms suggestive of sinusitis; this may be changing. Plain films are also used in evaluating patients with trauma and congenital abnormalities; otherwise, the primary imaging studies are CT and MRI. Radionuclide studies, particularly SPECT gallium and bone scanning, are useful in selected cases. Angiography is an infrequently used adjunctive procedure. Ultrasonography plays little or no role in this subregion of the head and neck.

Developmental Abnormalities

The applications of various imaging modalities in developmental abnormalities of this region are the same as those discussed in the preceding section on the orbit. At the University of Florida, this evaluation is begun with CT because bone detail is often critical, especially in three-dimensional planning of craniofacial reconstruction. Some specific conditions warrant particular comment. Dermoid cysts in the nasal region may be investigated by CT or MRI. At the University of Florida, CT is followed by MRI only if there is any evidence suggesting extension of the cyst or tract into the cranial vault, which would require an intracranial approach for closure of the operative defect, or if there is any suggestion of an associated meningocele or encephalocele (Fig. 2–23). Choanal atresia is best evaluated by a combination of axial and coronal CT sections done with 1.5- or 2-mm thick sections.

Infectious and Noninfectious Inflammatory Conditions

There are a myriad of conditions that can involve the sinonasal region. In the past, the mainstay of imaging for routine inflammatory disease was plain radiography. Over the years, it has become increasingly evident with use of both conventional tomography and CT that plain films fail to recognize a significant amount of disease in inflammatory sinonasal conditions and frequently miss more aggressive processes masquerading as benign sinus disease. The latter situation leads to delays in diagnosis of cancers or aggressive inflammatory lesions.

It has been suggested by several groups that in a well-screened clinical population, a survey type CT study can be substituted for plain radiography. This is a reasonable hypothesis; however, some groups propose that such studies be done with approximately four sections made through the entire sinonasal region. *Such technique is entirely suboptimal.* The reasons for this are discussed in the section on plain radiography. Relatively low-cost survey CT examinations that are efficient and more complete are easy to design. If a decision is made to go to a survey type CT examination rather than "full" CT study, the survey should be done with coronal sections and slice intervals no greater than 5 mm and cover the entire sinonasal region. Optimally, these studies should be processed for both bone and soft tissue detail (Fig. 2–24). In more complex sinus disease, both axial and coronal CT sections done with more detailed techniques are indicated. These should include 3- to 4-mm thick contiguous sections in at least a coronal plane and perhaps the axial plane as well. In cases in which intracranial complications or aggressive sinus disease is likely, intravenous contrast may also be used. Supplementary MRI is sometimes necessary but should usually be done only after CT and only in selected cases in which the use of MRI will somehow alter management. MRI is not suitable as a screening examination for the sinuses because of its high cost and lack of bone detail. Also, MRI has a problem demonstrating sinuses that contain dessicated or impacted material (Fig. 2–25). This can lead to serious misdiagnosis.

The bone detail available with CT is indispensable in looking for osteomyelitis. MRI is probably slightly superior to CT for evaluating intracranial complications of inflammatory sinus disease, but this does not justify its routine use because contrast-enhanced CT is certainly an adequate screening test for such intracranial complications, especially if it is done with techniques outlined previously in this chapter and done in two planes.

Functional endoscopic surgery requires preliminary CT for planning. This may be adequately accomplished with contiguous 3- to 4-mm thick sections processed for bone detail. Processing with a bone algorithm reconstruction routine eliminates any significant problems caused by dental fillings or hardware (Fig. 2–24).

Invasive fungal disease is becoming more common because there are more immunocompromised patients. CT is an excellent starting point in evaluating patients suspected of having invasive fungal disease of the sinuses. These studies should be done with contrast infusion because one is searching for intracranial complications as well as the extent of sinonasal disease. Supplemental MRI is occasionally necessary. Once a diagnosis is established, gallium SPECT imaging is a very useful tool for following therapeutic response.

A fairly wide variety of uncommon non-infectious inflammatory conditions involve the paranasal sinuses. These include the granulomatoses, granulomatous responses to trauma and other stimuli such as recurrent hemorrhage, and the idiopathic histiocytoses. Frequently it is difficult to distinguish these processes from neoplastic ones. Evaluation usually begins with CT for reasons discussed previously. If leptomeningeal spread or other intracranial involvement is suspected, then supplemental MRI may be done. Other reasons for supplementary MRI have been outlined previously.

Trauma

The relative use of plain films, CT, and MRI in evaluating facial trauma is basically the same as that described in the previous section on the orbit. Plain films are a reasonable starting point; however, very often supplemental CT with three-dimensional reconstruction is done in selected, complex cases (Fig. 2–26). MRI is rarely necessary.

Tumor

Both benign and malignant tumors usually present with signs and symptoms suggestive of sinonasal inflammatory disease. For this reason, the patient has already often had plain films and usually CT by the time the diagnosis is confirmed by biopsy. At the University of Florida, if the patient is known to have or is suspected of having a tumor of the sinonasal region, CT is done as first

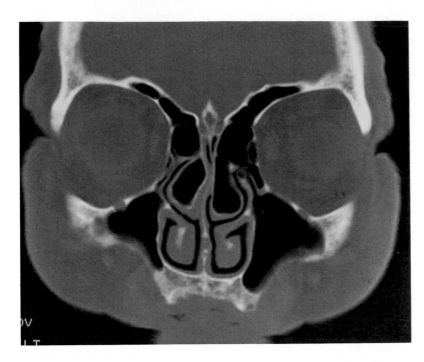

Figure 2–24. Single CT section taken from a coronal survey study of the sinuses. This is processed for bone detail, and if artifacts due to dental work were present, they would not reduce the diagnostic accuracy of the image. On modern CT equipment, it takes 10 to 15 minutes total time to do a 12- to 15-section study of the sinuses with images routinely of this quality. Note the large concha bullosa bilaterally.

choice. If, after CT, any additional information is necessary for management decisions, a supplemental, focused MRI study is done. This occurs in approximately one half to three quarters of the patients who have sinonasal cancer and in a smaller percentage of those who have benign lesions. Usual reasons for supplemental MRI studies are to define the extent of intracranial spread and to help evaluate whether opacification of sinuses is due to tumor invasion or secondary obstruction by the tumor (Figs. 2–17, 2–27). The use of paramagnetic contrast in such supplemental MRI studies is necessary for evaluating the extent of intracranial disease. One must be aware that paramagnetic contrast-enhanced MRI is very sensitive to dural reaction. Purely "reactive" enhancement adjacent to sites of bone, but not true dural invasion, is possible. Also, reaction of dura somewhat remote from the actual point of involvement may occur. In these instances, reactive dural changes often cannot be discerned from those due to actual dural involvement (Fig. 2–28). Also, after surgery, such enhancement may be present for months or years after surgery and not *necessarily* be indicative of recurrent or persistent tumor.

If MRI or CT suggests that the lesion in question is hypervascular, then angiography may be done to confirm this impression. If the lesion is excessively vascular (e.g., juvenile angiofibroma, paraganglioma, hemangiopericytoma, renal cell metastases), then therapeutic embolization as an adjunct to surgical removal might be helpful in the management of the patient (Figs. 2–4, 2–5, 2–20). Radionuclide studies play little or no role in evaluating primary cancers of the sinonasal region. They are sometimes used to evaluate patients for metastatic disease in advanced cases.

Mandible, Temporomandibular Joint, and Teeth

General Indications

Plain films and orthopantomography still play a central role in evaluating the mandible and teeth and, to a lesser extent, the TMJ. This is true for virtually all indications. In contradistinction to most other areas in head and neck imaging, plain films for these anatomic studies frequently are the beginning and ending points of the diagnostic evaluation. Until the late 1980s, CT played only an adjunctive role for pathologic conditions in these locations. More recently, specially designed programs for aiding in dental implants have led to some increased CT usage;

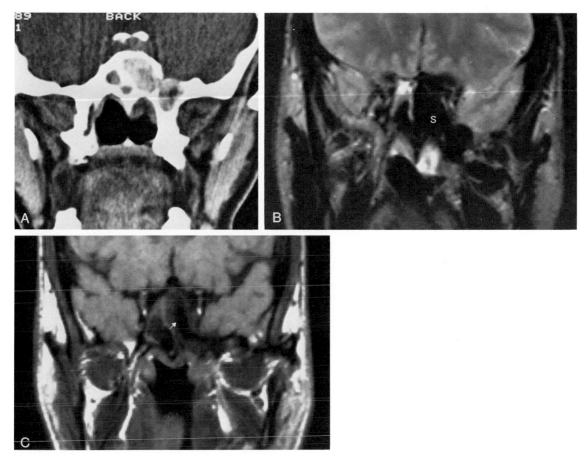

Figure 2–25. Patient with chronic allergic sinusitis and rhinopolyposis. *A*. CT shows sphenoid sinus mucocele with impacted, dried secretions; the desiccation is manifested by increased CT density. Such dense secretions are also usually colonized with fungi. *B*. T2-weighted MR shows the sphenoid sinus (S) to be black, which suggests that it is filled with air; it is, in fact, filled with material seen in *A*. *C*. T1-weighted MR at same level as in *B* shows relatively subtle evidence (in comparison with CT) that the sinus is diseased. Note that the central part of the sinus (arrow) is nearly black owing to the extreme desiccation of secretions and lack of mobile water protons. The appearance mimics the presence of air centrally when the sinus, in fact, is completely opacified.

the volume of such studies is likely to increase. Outside of its use for TMJ disorders, MRI plays a relatively limited role in evaluating abnormalities of the mandible and teeth. Ultrasonography plays virtually no role in these disease processes. Radionuclide studies are used occasionally, but their value is somewhat limited because of the high rate of incidental and inflammatory disease, which frequently causes false-positive results when patients are being evaluated for neoplastic processes. Angiography is rarely used for the diagnostic evaluation of abnormalities at this location. It can be extremely valuable when it is indicated diagnostically and as a therapeutic adjunct.

Developmental Abnormalities

Plain radiography and orthopantomography usually precede CT evaluation in patients with developmental abnormalities of the teeth and jaw. In complex cases, CT is virtually always done and reconstructed by use of three-dimensional techniques. The use of this was discussed in detail in the orbital and facial sections, which preceded this section. MRI is an infrequently used adjunctive study; it is done not so much for looking at the pathologic disorder in this location as for evaluating possible related central nervous system abnormalities.

Infectious and Noninfectious Inflammatory Conditions

The vast majority of patients with the inflammatory lesions have a radiographic evaluation consisting of plain dental views and orthopantomography. CT is indicated for

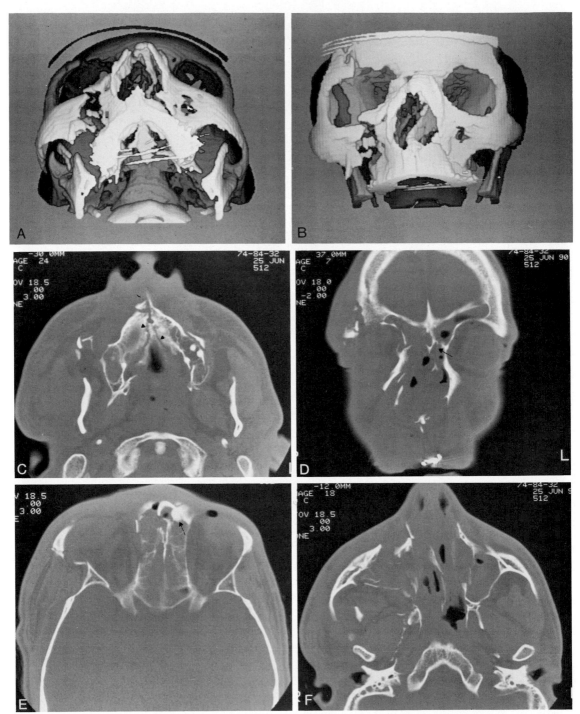

Figure 2–26. Patient suffering craniofacial trauma due to a motor vehicle accident. *A* and *B*. Three-dimensional reformations of CT data provide a good global perspective of this complex injury, basically right LeFort III and left LeFort I fractures. However, some findings are better appreciated on the standard sectional images in *C* through *F*, such as the extent of hard palatal injury (arrowheads), possibility of left nasofrontal recess obstruction (arrows), and status of the posterior right antral wall in relation to the fractured coronoid process.

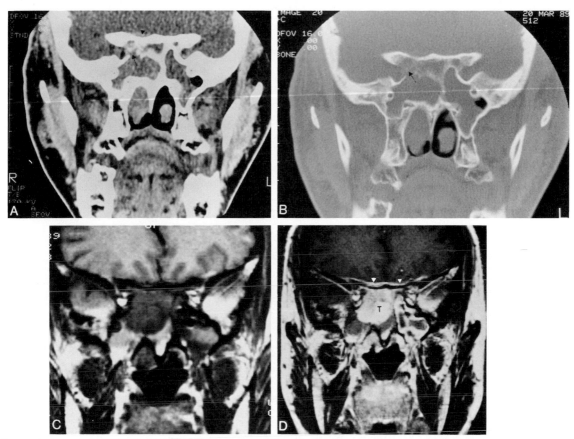

Figure 2–27. Patient with rhabdomyosarcoma of ethmoids. *A.* Contrast-enhanced CT suggests bone erosion (arrow) and dural involvement (arrowhead). *B.* Bone window to correlate with *A* confirms bone erosion near optic canal (arrow). *C.* MR without contrast at same level as in *A* and *B;* bone erosion, tumor, or dural involvement is not obvious. *D.* Contrast-enhanced MR tumor (T) is well seen. Extensive dural enhancement (arrowheads) strongly suggests at least epidural spread of tumor (known to occur in these lesions) and suggests that leptomeningeal involvement may be present. Cerebrospinal fluid study did not confirm leptomeningeal disease.

those patients, who possibly have abscesses in the spaces surrounding the mandible. CT is preferred to MRI for this purpose because it provides a combination of bone and soft tissue detail, which is unmatched by MRI, and is also a study that is somewhat easier to do for an uncomfortable, acutely ill patient. CT clearly maps abscesses involving the masticator, sublingual, submandibular, and parapharyngeal spaces as well as the deep neck. CT is a valuable and frequently essential tool in planning the operative approach to the drainage of dental-related abscesses. It is also very useful for looking for advanced osteomyelitis involving the mandible.

Trauma

Plain radiography is the mainstay of diagnosis in trauma to the mandible. The basic evaluation usually includes standard mandibular views, orthopantomography, and dental views as necessary. In complex cases, CT may be done with or without three-dimensional reconstructions of the CT data. The CT study is more commonly used in the setting in which there has been unsatisfactory reduction of mandibular fractures and reconstructive surgery is required. Most commonly, CT study of mandibular fractures is performed as part of an overall survey of patients with craniofacial injuries (Fig. 2–26). It should always be remembered that patients with mandibular fractures have a relatively high incidence of significant injury of the cervical spine. This means that appropriate plain films and, if necessary, CT examinations be carried out. It also means that in the acute phase of injury these patients not be positioned in such a way that the cervical

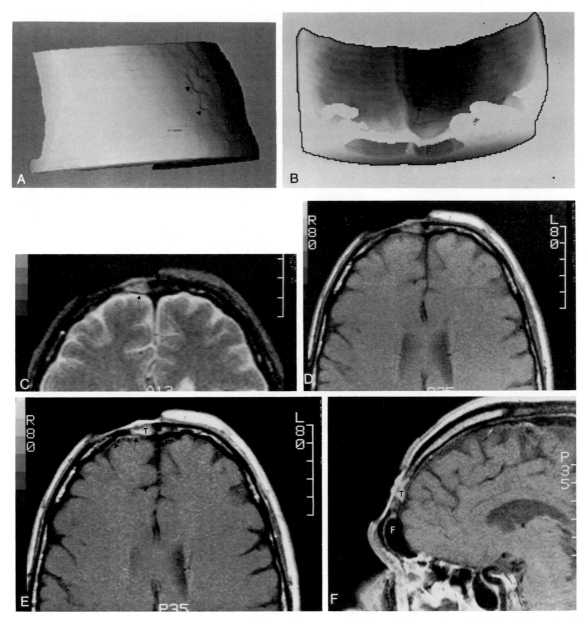

Figure 2–28. Patient with recurrent skin cancer of frontal bone near the frontal sinus. *A* and *B*. Three-dimensional reformations of the CT data for showing outer (arrowhead) and inner table bone defects (arrow), respectively. Note how *B* relates the defect to the midline and frontal sinus (F). *C*. Heavily T2-weighted MR suggests that dura is intact; note the fine black line (arrow). There is no brain involvement. *D*. T1-weighted MR without contrast indicates bone erosion and probable intact dura (as in *C*). *E*. Contrast-enhanced MR shows tumor (T) and adjacent dura (arrow) enhancing. Dura enhancement away from bone defect (arrowhead) was reactive; tumor cells could well have been present in this zone of fibrovascular response to adjacent tumor invasion. *F*. Sagittal contrast-enhanced MR clearly shows relationship of tumor (T) to frontal sinus (F), brain, and dura.

spine is put at risk if it has not been cleared for significant injury.

Tumor

A wide variety of odontogenic and nonodontogenic tumors may involve the mandible.

Plain films and orthopantomography are used in the initial evaluation of these lesions and are indispensable for differential diagnostic and treatment purposes. Adjunctive CT may be done for some lesions. Adjunctive MRI is only rarely necessary. Angiography

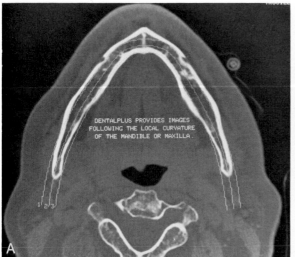

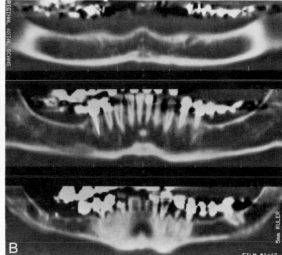

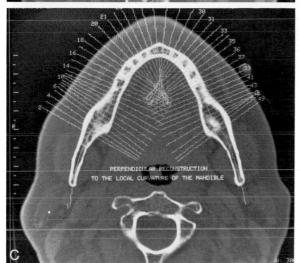

Figure 2–29. Demonstration of how oblique and curved planar two-dimensional reformation of CT data can be useful in evaluating the mandible and maxilla. Curved reformation planning view *A* shows position of orthopantomography-like sections seen in *B*. Radially oriented reformations are planned in *C*.

may be done if a highly vascular tumor is suspected. This is especially important before biopsy if the vascular nature of the mass can be appreciated by other imaging studies or anticipated clinically. Study with CT and the newer software that has been developed primarily for implant surgery may be very useful in evaluating the status of the bone stock of the maxillary and mandibular alveolar ridges as well as the relative position of tumor and the inferior alveolar canal (Fig. 2–29). MRI may be used in the occasional circumstance in which a lesion may be spreading within the marrow space and its spread is undetectable by other means. The value of MRI in this setting has been somewhat overstated in the literature to date.

Cancers arising in the oral cavity and the floor of the mouth frequently involve the mandible. Orthopantomography, standard mandibular views, and dental type radiographs should be used for evaluation of the alveolar ridge and as a gross evaluation of the remaining portions of the mandible. The lingual and buccal surfaces of the mandible are best evaluated by 1.5- to 3-mm CT sections done in the axial plane through the mandible. These should *always* be processed for bone detail. Reformations with the new software described before may also be useful in selected cases (Fig. 2–29). MRI is only occasionally used to evaluate the spread of tumor within the marrow space of the mandible and to detect the retrograde spread of tumor along the fifth nerve intracranially. Radionuclide studies are of very limited value

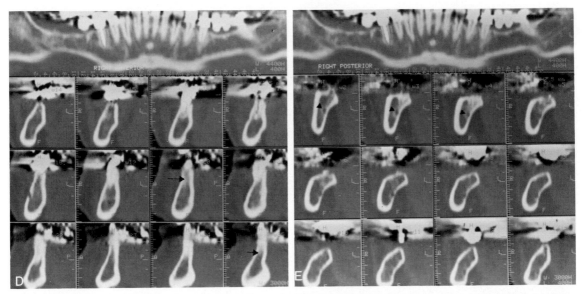

Figure 2–29 *Continued* Curved planar views at the top of *D* and *E* serve as an index for position of each section made perpendicular to lingual and buccal surfaces of the mandible. These views can help evaluate alveolar ridge bone stock (arrow), lingual and buccal surfaces, and extent of lesions relative to the inferior alveolar canal (arrowheads).

in evaluating cancer patients because of the large number of false-positive results caused by incidental inflammatory disease.

Temporomandibular Joint

The study of the TMJ merits some special consideration. It may be evaluated with the diagnostic imaging approach outlined in the preceding section as merely an additional portion of the mandible. However, when the diagnostic evaluation is aimed primarily at the TMJ, some additional factors need to be considered. Patients with possible internal derangement of the TMJ present with varied complaints. Some of these patients have myofacial pain syndromes, some have otalgia and deep face pain, and some actually have TMJ dysfunction. Once it has been determined that an internal derangement of the TMJ is the likely cause of the complaints, the diagnostic imager may become involved. A reasonable screening approach includes standard mandibular views supplemented by lateral views through the TMJ with use of conventional tomography. This is a very effective and inexpensive screen for bone abnormalities. Unfortunately, many radiology departments are no longer equipped to perform high-quality conventional tomography

or lack the trained personnel to do so. For this reason, some are using CT with sagittal and coronal reformatted images as a substitute for conventional tomograms in evaluating the bony detail of the TMJ. This is expensive, but it may be all that is available. A possible benefit of this approach is that these CT data may be used to do multiplanar and three-dimensional reconstructions. Also, the CT study serves as a good screening test for mass lesions of the deep face that mimic TMJ dysfunction.

If a more complete study of the internal anatomy of the TMJ is necessary, then either arthrography or MRI is indicated. Both tests should clearly be used in only highly select segments of the population of patients presenting with TMJ dysfunction. Arthrography remains the only diagnostic method capable of excluding subtle articular disk perforation with a high degree of confidence. The presence of a perforated disk may be implied by MRI findings. Arthrography, until the late 1980s, was also considered superior to MRI because of its being able to provide functional information about joint motion. Advances in MR technology allow cineradiographic studies in cooperative patients. The ability to do such studies will likely improve in the future with the advent of faster imaging techniques. MRI, however, is probably even at this point considered preferable to TMJ arthrography in patients who require more advanced imaging studies for evaluating possible internal derangements. The relative roles of MRI and arthrography are bound to be established over the 1990s.

Temporal Bone, Posterior Fossa, and Cranial Nerves VII and VIII

General Indications

Diagnostic problems related to the temporal bone, posterior fossa, and related neurovascular structures represent a fairly large proportion of imaging done by the otolaryngologist and head and neck surgeon. There are a myriad of problems that may arise from or involve structures in this region. The sequencing of imaging studies, as well as techniques used for each of these studies, is highly dependent on the clinical problems at hand (Table 2–5). This complexity is reflected in the triage factors, differential diagnoses, and algorithms shown in Figures 2–30 and 2–31 and in the protocols outlined in Table 2–4, which deal with just two of the uses of temporal bone imaging. In general, plain films are of very limited value and now are basically used to provide a survey of the state of aeration of the mastoid. CT, MRI, or both usually provide all the diagnostic information necessary. Angiography plays a limited but definitely useful role. Radionuclide studies are occasionally helpful, especially SPECT studies for following the response of inflammatory disease to medical therapy. Ultrasonography has virtually no role in evaluating temporal bone disease.

The following sections present a combination of common clinical problems and pathoanatomic categorization of diseases that require imaging as part of the diagnostic scheme.

Hearing Loss

The diagnostic imager must receive a patient who is very well screened clinically in order to apply CT or MRI efficiently. Those patients with retrocochlear sensorineural hearing loss should be studied with MRI. The examination should be done with high-resolution thin-section techniques, and paramagnetic contrast agent should be used. There are other approaches; however, the author feels that the combination of postcontrast axial and coronal thin-section images through the internal canals and cerebellopontine angle with detailed T2-weighted images represents a very practical and complete approach to this problem. CT is used only adjunctively. Some surgeons still require non–contrast-enhanced CT before surgery in order to define the bony anatomy in the posterior fossa and especially to define the relationship of the jugular fossa to the internal auditory canal. Adjunctive CT is also sometimes useful in cases in which the differential diagnosis of a mass in the cerebellopontine angle is uncertain after MRI.

MRI is so sensitive to pathologic processes involving the eighth nerve that some caution is now in order. Enhancement of the eighth (and seventh) cranial nerves is not necessarily indicative of a schwannoma or neoplastic process. It has become clear that inflammatory conditions, usually virus-induced, can cause enhancement of the cranial nerves. The enhancement is usually transient and correlates fairly well with the onset and resolution of symptoms, although it is not necessarily predictive of return of function or resolution of symptoms in all cases. It is most important that such inflammatory enhancement not be mistaken for tumoral condition (Fig. 2–32). It is sometimes impossible in one MRI examination to determine whether the enhancement is related to inflammation or tumor. Depending on the clinical situation, it is probably wise to wait 3 to 6 months and repeat the imaging studies rather than erroneously operate on an inflammatory lesion of the eighth nerve (or others). Similarly, in a very small number of patients, enhancement of the membranous labyrinth within the cochlea or vestibule may be visible on contrast-enhanced MRI examinations. This enhancement almost always indicates inflammation. Relatively rare cases of vestibular and cochlear schwannomas have been reported, and, again, a repeat study in 3 to 6 months will probably differentiate an inflammatory lesion from tumor.

It is the habit of many surgeons to close the site of removal of an acoustic schwannoma or other mass in the posterior fossa with a tissue graft. Currently, contrast-enhanced MRI is usually used for following these patients. These tissue grafts and adjacent dura frequently show enhancement for months to years after surgery. This should not be taken as definite evidence of recurrent or residual tumor. Also, fat placed in these

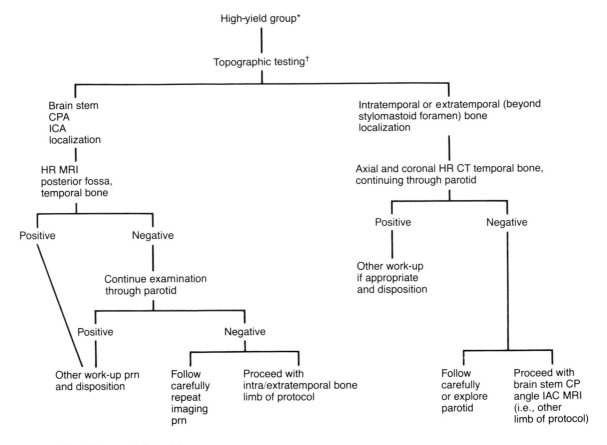

*High- and low-yield groups in Table 2–6.

†Appropriate clinical testing may localize segment of nerve involved and allow a more focused imaging approach.

Figure 2–30. Imaging of facial nerve after clinical triage and topographic testing. (From Mancuso A: Workbook for MRI and CT of the Head and Neck, 2nd ed. Baltimore: Williams & Wilkins, 1989.)

defects may mimic recurrent tumor on non–fat-suppressed, gadolinium-enhanced, T1-weighted images. The first postoperative study should serve as a baseline, and then the follow-up examinations can reasonably be compared with this baseline for determining whether the changes seen represent reactive postoperative or progressive changes related to persistent or recurrent tumor.

Patients with conductive hearing loss who require imaging are best studied with CT because of its superior depiction of bone detail (Tables 2–4, 2–5). On occasion, supplementary MRI is done for evaluation of unusual circumstances such as encephaloceles extending into the middle ear cavity. Such supplemental MRI is necessary for less than 5% of patients (Fig. 2–33).

Cochlear implant candidates should be studied with CT rather than MRI. The main interest for these patients is the status of the bony labyrinth (Fig. 2–34). All adjunctive information necessary for surgery is usually present on the CT studies. To date, at the University of Florida, supplemental MRI has not been found necessary in any of these patients. Such a need could arise, but it would be anticipated only in highly selected circumstances.

Pulsatile Tinnitus

The evaluation of patients with pulsatile tinnitus requires careful clinical screening. After such triage (Table 2–6), an algorithm such as that in Figure 2–31 helps direct the course of the evaluation. Pulsatile tinnitus is a fairly common complaint. Modern imaging techniques can be a great aid in determining the cause as well as for assuring patients that no significant disease is present. These studies, however, require careful monitoring by the physician, excellent technique, and expert

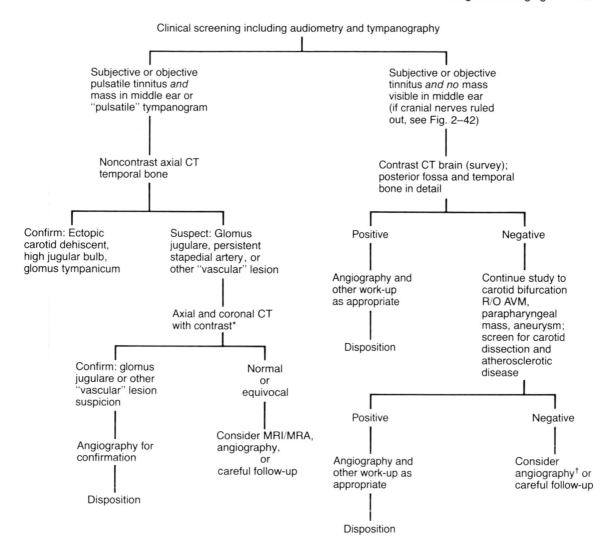

*Contrast and angiography not necessary for confirmation of persistent stapedial artery.

†In highly selected cases (e.g., classical history suggesting dissection) it may be appropriate to start with angiography, although that diagnosis can be made on well-done CT and MR in most patients with acute or subacute dissections.

Figure 2–31. Imaging evaluation of pulsatile tinnitus based on clinical triage. (From Mancuso A: Workbook for MRI and CT of the Head and Neck, 2nd ed. Baltimore: Williams & Wilkins, 1989.)

interpretation in order for their full potential to be realized (Fig. 2–35).

Facial Nerve Palsy and Hemifacial Spasm

The evaluation of each cranial nerve requires an algorithmic approach. Specific recommendations for whether imaging is helpful and how to proceed with the sequencing of imaging studies is highly dependent on careful clinical triage. Suggestions for such an algorithmic approach and triage of patients with

facial nerve problems to high- and low-yield groups are outlined in Table 2–7.

MRI is the mainstay of diagnosis in patients with cranial nerve disease. CT is used adjunctively in evaluating these problems, especially when the course of the facial nerve through the temporal bone needs to be studied in detail. It has been observed that patients with abrupt onset of a peripheral seventh nerve paralysis (typical Bell's palsy) show enhancement of the seventh nerve on contrast-enhanced MRI studies. Early reports suggested some predictive value for linking the degree and extent of enhancement to the

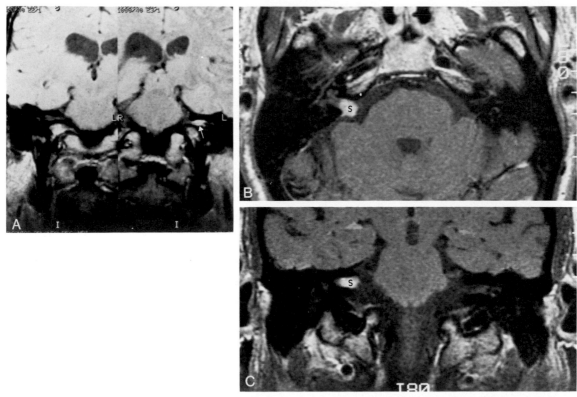

Figure 2–32. Patient with sensorineural hearing loss. *A.* The left eighth nerve is enhanced (arrow). Right eighth nerve (opposite) is normal on the contrast-enhanced MR study. Inflammatory enhancement was suspected because of the morphologic features seen on the scan; the cleft in the center of the enhancing mass was thought to possibly represent the separation between the superior and inferior divisions of the vestibular nerve. Repeat study (not shown) some months later showed complete resolution. (Courtesy of Robert Anderson, M.D., Orlando Regional Medical Center, Orlando, Florida.) Axial *(B)* and coronal *(C)* contrast-enhanced MR images through the internal auditory canal show a surgically proven eighth nerve schwannoma (S). Contrast this to lesion seen in *A.*

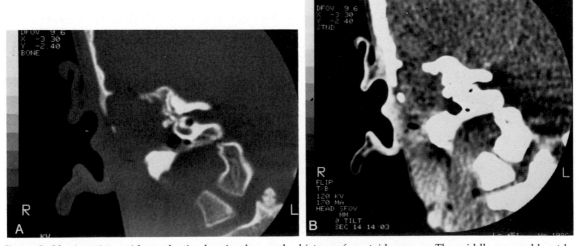

Figure 2–33. A patient with conductive hearing loss and a history of mastoid surgery. The middle ear could not be evaluated clinically. *A.* Coronal CT for bone detail showing mastoid and middle ear mass and large tegmen defect (arrow). *B.* Coronal CT, same level as in *A,* for soft tissue detail cannot identify whether brain is herniated through bone defect.

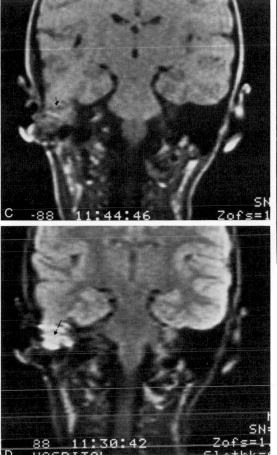

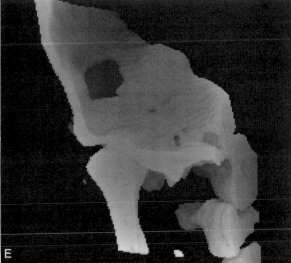

Figure 2–33 *Continued C.* T1-weighted MR shows encephalocele (arrow) and other tissue in mastoid and middle ear. *D.* T2-weighted MR shows that part of "other" tissue (arrow) is most likely inflammation, fluid, cholesteatoma, or a combination. *E.* Three-dimensional reformation of CT data shows size and position of tegmen tympani/mastoid defect. Surgery confirmed encephalocele, cholesteatoma, and granulation tissue in middle ear and mastoid.

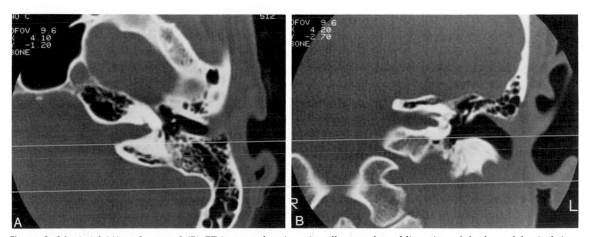

Figure 2–34. Axial *(A)* and coronal *(B)* CT images showing virtually complete obliteration of the bony labyrinth in a cochlear implant candidate. Findings were identical bilaterally and presumably due to prior bacterial meningitis.

TABLE 2–6. Differential Diagnosis in Patients with Pulsatile Tinnitus due to Structural Lesion

*Temporal Bone–Middle Ear**
  High and/or dehiscent jugular bulb (normal variant)†
  Ectopic carotid artery in middle ear
  Persistent stapedial artery
  Carotid aneurysm
  Arteriovenous malformation or fistula
  Paraganglioma (glomus tympanicus or jugulare)
  Other vascular neoplasm (e.g., hemangioma)
  Osteolytic phase of otosclerosis (rare)
  Granulation tissue, cholesterolosis (rare)

Posterior Fossa and Supratentorial Origin
  Arteriovenous malformation or fistula
  Dural venous malformation
  Large draining vessels from vascular malformation/
    neoplasm
  Neoplasm (e.g., meningioma)

Extracranial–Skull Base to Carotid Bifurcation
  Paraganglioma
  Other vascular neoplasm
  Arteriovenous malformation or fistula, acquired or
    congenital
  Carotid aneurysm
  Atherosclerotic disease, fibromuscular dysplasia,
    dissection

From Mancuso A: Workbook for MRI and CT of the Head and Neck, 2nd ed. Baltimore: Williams & Wilkins, 1989.
  *Some may present as middle ear masses rather than as pulsatile tinnitus.
  †A cause and effect between this *common* normal variant and the tinnitus usually cannot be absolutely established.

need for decompression of the nerve. At present, this is speculative, and many more patients need to be studied in a controlled manner before such findings can be used to justify facial nerve decompression. In general, the degree and the extent of enhancement of the facial nerve correlate with the symptoms. Prompt resolution of the enhancement seems to be predictive of return of function. A central issue remains, however, concerning whether these patients should be imaged at all. In general, the symptoms in 85% of patients with Bell's palsy resolve within 6 weeks. Currently, it is not clear whether scanning of all these patients with contrast-enhanced MRI is cost justified. If clinical trials suggest that contrast-enhanced MRI is effective at triaging patients into different categories of treatment, then such study may be warranted. Currently, at the University of Florida, the policy is not to study patients with acute onset peripheral seventh nerve paresis with MRI. Patients who have a slow, progressive onset of seventh nerve paresis or those with a paresis or paralysis that persists beyond 6 weeks are

studied. As with the eighth nerve problems, great care must be exercised not to confuse inflammatory enhancement of the seventh nerve with that related to neoplasm. This problem was discussed in detail in the previous section on hearing loss (Fig. 2–32). Depending on the clinical circumstances, it may be best to wait a clinically appropriate length of time and restudy the patient for help in determining whether the situation is more likely related to inflammation than to neoplasm. As a reminder, the diagnostic imager should always study the parotid gland as well as the posterior fossa and temporal bone in patients with disorders of the seventh nerve.

Patients with hemifacial spasm rarely have tumors as the cause of seventh nerve irritation. More likely the symptoms are related to microvascular compression of the facial nerve. Whereas MRI can occasionally identify abnormal vascular loops adjacent to the seventh nerve, such loops are also seen in a large number of asymptomatic patients. The positive predictive value of linking a vascular loop adjacent to the seventh nerve to the symptoms, therefore, is limited; however, the purpose of an MRI or CT examination in these patients is usually for exclusion of a lesion other than a vascular loop. If the patient has typical symptoms and no other offending mass lesion, then a presumptive diagnosis of microvascular compression can be made. Perhaps CT or MRI showing an ipsilateral tortuous vertical basilar system can be thought of as a minor confirmatory criterion of vascular compression in such patients. Angiography is not indicated in these patients unless CT or MR suggests an aneurysm or other vascular lesion as the etiologic factor.

Developmental Abnormalities

There is little or no role for plain films in the evaluation of developmental abnormalities of the temporal bone. Plain films may be used as a survey in patients with craniofacial anomalies and related temporal bone and TMJ abnormalities; however, their usefulness is limited in evaluation of the temporal bone itself. Plain films may be obtained as a general overview of the mastoid before a planned surgical procedure.

The mainstay of diagnosis in patients with anomalies of the external, middle, and inner ear or those with mixed anomalies is CT. CT

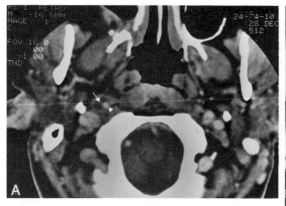
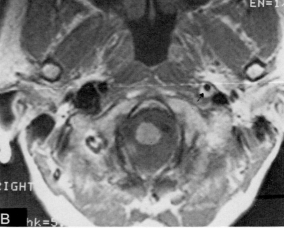
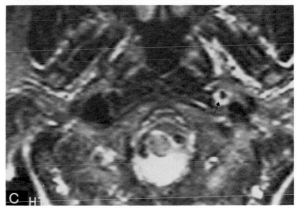

Figure 2–35. *A.* A 45-year-old male presenting with a complaint of right-sided pulsatile tinnitus. There are no other symptoms, and no mass is visible in the middle ear. CT evaluation according to the protocol in Figure 2–31 shows dissection of right internal carotid artery. Note the patent lumen (arrowhead) and clot (arrow). *B* and *C.* A 67-year-old female with acute onset of headache, neck pain, Horner's syndrome, and pulsatile tinnitus. T1-weighted *(B)* and heavily T2-weighted *(C)* MR images show carotid dissection (arrow). The patent lumen is dark, and thrombus within the dissection is bright.

studies should be done with 1.5- to 2-mm thick sections, sometimes done at 1-mm increments. This study should almost always be done in both the axial and coronal planes. Direct coronal sections are preferred to reformatted images. At the University of Florida,

TABLE 2–7. Facial Nerve—Clinical Triage

High-Yield	Low-Yield
Peripheral paresis/palsy of gradual onset with progression	Acute onset of typical Bell's palsy*
Additional cranial nerve deficits	Hemifacial spasm†
Possible parotid mass	Otherwise negative past medical history
History of skin cancer (cheek, ear) or more remote primary site	

From Mancuso A: Workbook for MRI and CT of the Head and Neck, 2nd ed. Baltimore: Williams & Wilkins, 1989.

*The facial nerve enhances the paramagnetic contrast on MRI in a high percentage of these patients. The value of this information is questionable at present.

†This can be associated with structural lesions other than microvascular compression, and imaging is not unreasonable; patients considered to be candidates for microvascular decompression should be studied.

MRI is rarely done as an adjunctive study in this group of patients. MRI is mainly used to look for associated intracranial anomalies or to confirm the presence of an associated or incidental meningoencephalocele, encephalocele, or epidermoid tumor. Adjunctive three-dimensional reconstruction of CT and MRI data is sometimes useful.

Developmental anomalies of vascular origin usually present as pulsatile tinnitus; however, they may present as a "vascular mass" visualized on physical examination. The diagnostic approach to these abnormalities is discussed in the section on pulsatile tinnitus. Angiography is occasionally used to confirm a vascular anomaly suspected on imaging studies. More frequently, the imaging study can make a definitive diagnosis, and angiography is unnecessary.

Infectious and Noninfectious Inflammatory Conditions

The vast majority of patients presenting with acute or chronic otomastoiditis do not require

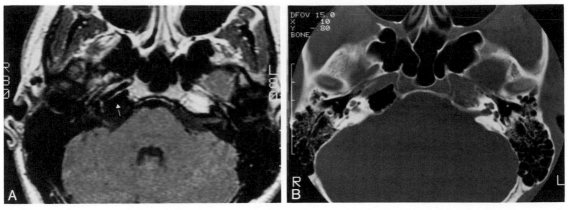

Figure 2–36. Patient undergoing MR for sensorineural hearing loss. *A.* MR exam shows the left petrous apex to be bright, whereas the right (arrow) is dark. An unschooled interpreter took this as evidence of a left petrous apex mass. *B.* CT was ordered, by the unschooled observer, and showed asymmetric aeration of the petrous apices (a normal variation); the "mass" on the right on the MR study is normal fatty marrow in the nonaerated petrous apex.

any diagnostic imaging. Occasionally, in the acute setting, plain films are done for confirmation of the clinical impression of mastoiditis. In the acute setting, CT may be done to look for evidence of coalescent mastoiditis or possibly intracranial complications of middle ear and mastoid disease. CT is preferred to MRI for the initial investigation of these patients because of its superior bone detail. If there is strong evidence of intracranial complications and if CT is negative, then a supplemental MRI may be done because this is potentially more sensitive to dural venous sinus thrombosis, early subdural empyema, and early parenchymal brain changes indicative of intracranial complications of acute or subacute otomastoiditis.

Patients with acquired cholesteatoma sometimes require preoperative evaluation with CT. The relative value of CT in this setting is highly dependent on the experience and desires of the referring clinician. At the University of Florida, CT is only occasionally used routinely for cholesteatoma patients. On the other hand, it is very frequently used in previously operated patients or for those with signs and symptoms suggestive of complications involving the bony labyrinth, facial nerve, or intracranial compartments (Fig. 2–33). The study of these more complex patients requires careful technique as outlined in Table 2–4. Study in two planes is often required, but intravenous contrast usually is not. MRI is used as an adjunct in less than 5% to 10% of patients at the University of Florida.

Cholesterol granuloma or cholesterolosis is not an uncommon pathologic process involving aerated segments of the temporal bone (as well as other head and neck sites) and may present as a petrous apex mass. A combination of MRI and CT is usually necessary to confirm the diagnosis with certainty. Differentiation between this disease process and congenital cholesteatoma (epidermoid and dermoid tumors) may not be possible in all cases. Some caution is in order in regard to abnormalities of the petrous portion of temporal bone and the skull base in general. With the coming of MRI, there has been a tendency to misdiagnose areas of increased signal intensity in and about the petrous portion of the temporal bone as pathologic processes. In some cases, this has led to unnecessary surgical procedures. Often the "abnormalities" seen are, in fact, related to variations in content of marrow within this portion of the temporal bone (Fig. 2–36). Interpretive difficulties are compounded by asymmetric aeration of various portions of the temporal bone and because of flow-related artifacts in the jugular fossa region. Occasionally, minor amounts of mucosal thickening or fluid within air cells in the petrous apex are diagnosed as abscess or more significant disease. The variations caused by all of these factors are myriad. Before any operative procedure on the temporal bone is undertaken on the basis of relatively subtle MRI findings, a careful CT study of the region of proposed abnormality is in order. Both studies must be interpreted by a person highly skilled in temporal bone analysis and, therefore, aware of the potential diagnostic pitfalls (Fig. 2–36). This helps avoid ill-advised exploratory surgical procedures.

Patients with malignant otitis externa should be initially evaluated with CT study (Fig. 2–22). This helps show the extent of bone and soft tissue disease. If there is evidence of extensive soft tissue involvement or osteomyelitis, it is probably best to obtain a SPECT gallium study as a baseline for following the progress of medical therapy (Fig. 2–22). It has been reported that the SPECT gallium study may return to normal before the infection has been completely eradicated; however, it accurately reflects the progress of therapy in the vast majority of patients. In selected cases, medical therapy may be continued for a period of time beyond the return of the gallium SPECT study to normal. The only reason for use of supplemental MRI in patients with malignant otitis externa may be to identify otherwise undetectable intracranial complications.

Other inflammatory and noninfective inflammatory conditions such as the histiocytoses are usually best handled by imaging in a manner similar to that described for malignant otitis externa. Patients with suspected obliterative labyrinthitis are best studied with CT; this situation most often arises in patients who are possible cochlear implant candidates. A combination of CT and MRI might be necessary to look for extension of an acute or subacute disease process into the bony labyrinth in an immunosuppressed host. A role for contrast-enhanced MRI is to be anticipated in the diagnosis of acute and subacute labyrinthitis when ultrahigh-resolution studies become available.

Infectious and noninfectious inflammatory disease involving the seventh and eighth nerves should be evaluated with contrast-enhanced MRI. This includes patients with known or suspected diseases such as intracranial tuberculosis and sarcoidosis (Fig. 2–21). In the 1970s and 1980s, various authors described an inflammatory process that tends to affect the dura and leptomeninges in the cerebellopontine angle. Its cause is unknown, and some call it idiopathic pachymeningitis; it may mimic other inflammatory conditions (e.g., syphilis, sarcoidosis) or neoplasms such as acoustic schwannoma, meningioma, or metastatic disease, among others.

Trauma

Plain films are of relatively little value in the evaluation of temporal bone trauma. In a critically injured patient, a CT study of the temporal bone in the axial plane is probably sufficient for general diagnostic purposes. This should be done with 1.5- to 2-mm thick sections. Reformatted coronal and sagittal images may be substituted for direct coronal views if the patient is unable to cooperate for direct coronal views. In the acute setting, these examinations are usually done to evaluate the status of the facial nerve canal. Secondary indications might include confirmation of fracture through the bony labyrinth in patients with a nonfunctional ear, or confirmation of ossicular disruption in patients with maximal air bone gaps. Evidence of intracranial injury, such as epidural hematoma and pneumocephalus, is an additional indication.

Outside of the acute setting, imaging investigation of patients who have suffered temporal bone trauma is usually done for chronic cerebrospinal fluid otorrhea or infection. It may also be used to evaluate the status of the ossicles. In cases of cerebrospinal fluid leak, CT is the preferred examination for showing areas of bone dehiscence, which may represent sites of leakage. In the author's experience, this does not require the use of intrathecal injection of contrast. If associated encephalocele is suspected, MRI may be done for confirmation. Such encephaloceles and bony defects are usually seen in the roof of the middle ear or mastoid. Three-dimensional reconstruction of CT data may be used to help anticipate the site and size of the defect (Fig. 2–33).

Angiography plays a role in evaluating the trauma patient if a posttraumatic arteriovenous malformation or aneurysm is suspected on the basis of other imaging studies or clinical symptoms. MRA may be used to help anticipate such a lesion in selected cases; however, definitive diagnosis still probably requires conventional angiography. Endovascular techniques may be used to treat such complications.

Tumors

Benign and malignant tumors that arise primarily in the temporal bone are unusual. Metastases to the temporal bone are relatively rare. Secondary involvement of the temporal bone from tumors arising in adjacent structures is a far more common situation in the author's clinical practice. Plain films are of relatively little value in evaluating tumors in the region of the temporal bone. Evaluation usually begins with CT and often an adjunctive focused MRI study, which may be done with or without paramagnetic contrast enhancement, depending on the questions that need to be answered.

The temporal bone is frequently secondarily involved by squamous carcinoma or basal cell carcinoma arising on or around the pinna. Most patients with skin cancer in this region do not require diagnostic imaging. Those with very advanced primary tumors or deeply infiltrating recurrences do require imaging (Fig. 2–19). In this setting, it is important to study the course of the facial nerve through the temporal bone (Fig. 2–37). The parotid and neck nodes should also be studied.

A variety of benign tumors may involve the external canal, middle ear, and mastoid. These are studied primarily by CT with focused MRI studies as necessary.

Tumors potentially affecting the facial nerve are usually studied with a combination of MRI and CT (Table 2–7; Fig. 2–30). MRI with contrast enhancement may be the only study that is required because the entire nerve can be studied from its root entry zone through its distal ramifications within and beyond the parotid gland. Occasionally, supplemental CT may be used to study the course of the nerve through the temporal bone and help distinguish primary processes involving the temporal bone from disease processes such as acquired cholesteatoma that may be secondarily involving the nerve.

Tumors involving the petrous apex and region of the jugular fossa present considerable therapeutic and, at times, diagnostic challenges. In general, these patients frequently undergo CT and MRI evaluation, and a significant percentage undergo diagnostic angiography; the actual number requiring diagnostic arteriography may be reduced by the use of MRA (Fig. 2–5). A fairly large percentage of this group is made up of patients with the glomus jugulare type of paraganglioma. In some institutions, these lesions are embolized before surgery.

Metabolic Disease and Osteodystrophies

CT is used to evaluate patients with suspected otosclerosis. It may also be used to confirm the diagnosis of more rare diseases such as osteogenesis imperfecta, Paget's disease, fibrous dysplasia, and osteopetrosis that may involve the temporal bones. If CT

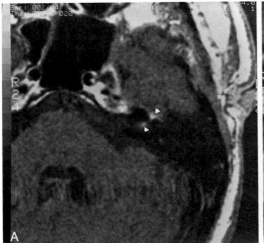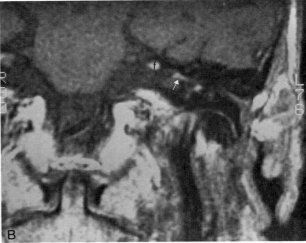

Figure 2–37. Patient with recurrent carcinoma of the pinna and facial nerve paralysis—two views from a contrast-enhanced MR study. *A.* Axial view shows subtle enhancement of the facial nerve at the anterior genu, labyrinthine segment, and fundus of internal auditory canal just adjacent to Bill's bar (arrowheads). *B.* Coronal section confirms nerve enhancement (arrow), not to be confused with petrous apex fat (f). Surgery confirmed gross cancer spread in the facial nerve to a point corresponding to MR findings; microscopic disease extended to the root entry zone of the facial nerve at the brain stem.

is available, other imaging studies play little or no role in the evaluation of these diseases.

Nasopharynx, Parapharyngeal Space, Central Skull Base, Cranial Nerves V and IX to XII, and Cervical Sympathetics

General Indications

Patients with symptoms referable to these areas and structures are now ordinarily evaluated primarily with MRI (Table 2–5). The evaluation may begin with CT, and supplemental MRI may be done when necessary. There is no real routine role for the use of plain radiography. Plain films may be done retrospectively if indicated by the more definitive MRI and CT studies. Conventional tomography should be done only if CT is not available. Contrast nasopharyngography, never a very popular study in the United States, certainly should no longer be done; this study was largely supplanted by improvements in endoscopic equipment. Radionuclide studies play a limited but definite role in evaluating certain inflammatory conditions. Ultrasonography has virtually no role in this subregion of the head and neck. Angiography is a very useful adjunctive study; however, it is virtually always preceded by CT or MRI, except in highly selected circumstances. Fluoroscopic examination, with or without contrast, is used only to evaluate velopharyngeal competence during swallowing and speech. On the basis of this overview, the following sections emphasize the relative role of CT and MRI and imaging problems in this anatomic subregion of the head and neck. These two studies are integrated with angiography and, less commonly, with radionuclide studies as necessary in these specific problem areas.

In general, MRI is chosen as the primary examination in most instances because of its superior soft tissue contrast, multiplanar capabilities, and more direct visualization of the course of the cranial nerves and their intracranial origins. Also, flow-related information on MRI may prove useful in characterizing the vascularity of a lesion. In fact, MRA may replace conventional angiography as a confirmatory diagnostic method in a limited number of these cases (Figs. 2–4, 2–5, 2–20). CT is often used as a supplement for looking for evidence of erosion of the skull base (Fig. 2–17). Whereas CT is more sensitive for detecting bone erosion, MRI is somewhat more accurate at showing the extent of infiltration of the marrow space of the skull base. Still, the evaluation of the skull base with MRI is fraught with interpretive difficulties owing to normal variations in its marrow content, aeration of the petrous bones, and flow-related artifacts (Figs. 2–19, 2–36). This is discussed in detail in the temporal bone section.

Developmental Abnormalities

Few developmental abnormalities involve this area. The most common of these are cysts that occur near the roof of the nasopharynx. The most well known of these is Tornwaldt's cyst. MRI can usually determine whether these predominantly cystic masses have components that extend intracranially. In younger patients, it is always difficult to be sure whether submucosal masses within the nasopharynx represent neoplasms, developmental cysts, or possibly meningoencephaloceles (Fig. 2–23). MRI is the study best suited to differentiation of these possibilities. If MRI is not available, CT may be done; very complex cases might even require CT in combination with the intrathecal injection of contrast agent.

Infectious and Noninfectious Inflammatory Conditions

Acute and subacute adenoiditis usually do not come to imaging unless there is a critical complication suggesting the need for surgical intervention. This might include poor feeding in an infant or airway obstruction. The presence of a large submucosal mass in this setting often leads to imaging because of a suspected retropharyngeal or parapharyngeal abscess. At the University of Florida, the practice is to use CT for evaluating primary inflammatory conditions of the extracranial head and neck. MRI certainly could be used and should be done with paramagnetic contrast agents. Both studies are particularly well suited to separating simple adenoiditis from suppurative retropharyngeal adenitis and true abscesses in the parapharyngeal and retropharyngeal spaces (Fig. 2–38). Studies at the University of Florida have shown that most cases of "retropharyngeal abscess" are, in fact, enlarged suppurative

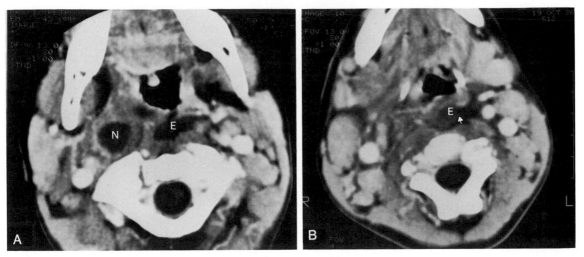

Figure 2–38. Two pediatric patients with suppurative retropharyngeal adenitis, often called retropharyngeal abscess; one case resolved on medical therapy alone, and the other was drained. *A.* Suppurative lateral retropharyngeal node (N) and retropharyngeal edema (E). *B.* Wider window at lower level shows edematous retropharyngeal space (E) with hint of thickened alar fascia (arrow). Findings in *A* and *B* were confirmed at surgery, but this patient could have been cured medically.

retropharyngeal lymph nodes, which usually respond completely to medical therapy. True abscesses in the retropharyngeal space are unusual and most often occur as the result of perforation rather than as a complication of suppurative adenitis.

Invasive fungal disease is becoming more common because of the large population of immunosuppressed patients. The evaluation of these patients should begin with CT because it is important to look for evidence of osteomyelitis involving the skull base. Supplemental MRI may be done, especially if there is a need to detect early intracranial extension of the process and more fully evaluate its extent. Both studies should probably be done in any patient for whom surgery is the primary mode of therapy. If the patient is not a surgical candidate, CT alone is probably sufficient for diagnosing and confirming the extent of the disease. A SPECT gallium study should then be obtained and be used to follow the course of therapy (Fig. 2–22).

Noninfective inflammatory conditions such as sarcoidosis and noninfectious granulomatous processes are usually studied initially with a combination of CT and MRI. MRI may be particularly useful for suggesting an etiologic factor for the finding because these disease processes, in particular, often result in very diminished signal on T2-weighted images, which is suggestive of a fibrous reactive component. This tendency to diminish signal intensity of the disease processes, however, is not specific and may also be seen in invasive fungal disease and occasionally in tumors that incite an intense inflammatory response.

Tumors

In general, tumors in this location fall into one of two broad categories. The benign lesions are usually mucosa-covered and arise primarily within the parapharyngeal space, the adjacent infratemporal fossa, or the masticator space. Occasional malignant tumors mimic this presentation. The other broad category is cancers. These, for the most part, are either keratinizing or nonkeratinizing (lymphoepithelioma) carcinomas and occasionally lymphoma. Rhabdomyosarcomas make up a significant percentage of this group in the pediatric age range. A third group of patients presenting for imaging in this region are those with signs and symptoms suggestive of tumors in this location. These findings are usually related to cranial nerve dysfunction, possible eustachian tube obstruction, or various pain patterns suggesting a deep-seated lesion. If it is available, MRI should be done initially in virtually all of these patients. This can usually be done with fairly standard techniques and usually does not require the injection of paramagnetic contrast agents. Alternatively, CT may

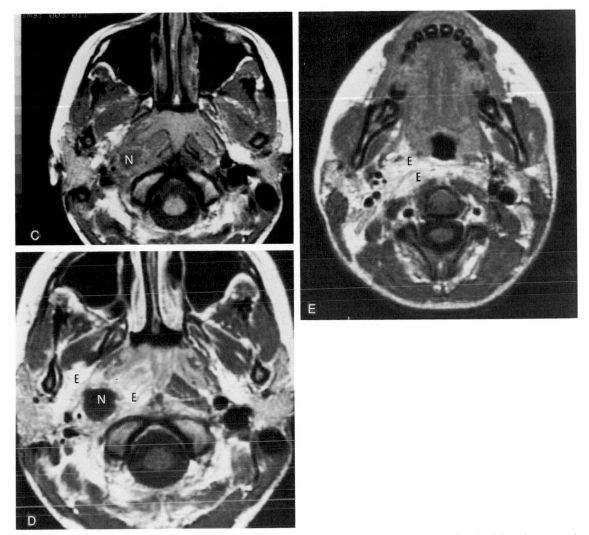

Figure 2–38 *Continued C.* Noncontrast T1-weighted MR shows suppurative retropharyngeal node (N) and surrounding edema. *D.* Contrast-enhanced MR helps distinguish suppurative node (N) from inflamed, edematous tissues (E). *E.* Lower section shows parapharyngeal and retropharyngeal edema (E) and inflammation on right side but no abscess in either space. Correlate this MR view with CT image in *B* for appreciation of the difference in morphologic character between abscess and phlegmon.

be done. Use of angiography is based on CT and MRI findings; angiography is almost never a primary study in these patients. The generalizations just presented may be applied in more specific tumor-related problems as follows.

Parapharyngeal Tumors

Tumors of the parapharyngeal space should be separated into those arising in the prestyloid and poststyloid components of the space. Those arising in the prestyloid parapharyngeal space are almost always benign mixed tumors and may uncommonly represent malignant neoplasms of salivary gland

origin. Those in the poststyloid parapharyngeal space are most usually either paragangliomas or schwannomas (Figs. 2–5, 2–39). Paragangliomas may be either the glomus vagale variety or an inferior extension of a glomus jugulare tumor. Occasionally, enlarged retropharyngeal lymph nodes mimic a mass lesion of the poststyloid parapharyngeal space (Fig. 2–38). The full extent of this lesion is usually best appreciated on MRI because of its multiplanar technique. Supplemental CT may be used if additional information is necessary for treatment planning. Once CT and MRI have been done, it is

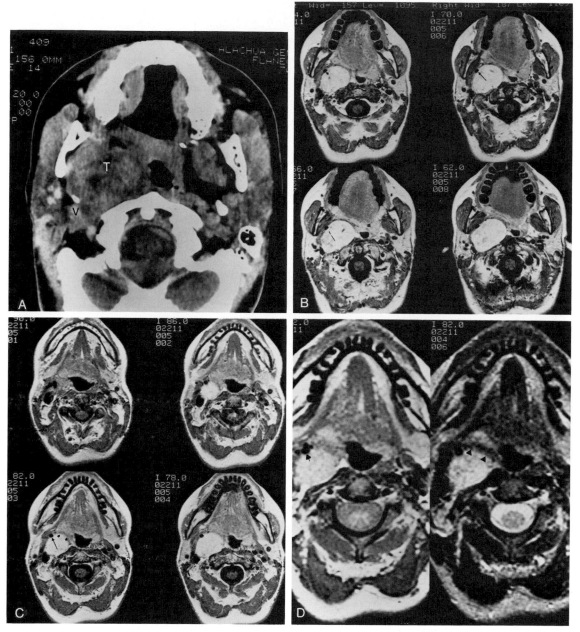

Figure 2–39. A 40-year-old female presenting with a submucosal oropharyngeal mass noticed by her dentist. *A.* Contrast-enhanced CT identifies the tumor (T) but does not clearly demonstrate vector of displacement of carotid artery; the jugular vein (V) is pushed posterolaterally. *B* and *C.* A series of eight contrast-enhanced MR sections. The mass enhances and displaces the carotid artery (arrows) and styloid musculature (arrowheads) anterolaterally; therefore, this is a poststyloid parapharyngeal mass.

usually clear whether angiography is necessary. Angiography is usually done for confirmation that a lesion is, in fact, a paraganglioma. MRI produces such a clear depiction of vascular displacement that angiography is not necessary for confirmation of the position of major vessels (Figs. 2–5, 2–39). MRI or CT

usually clearly shows whether the lesion represents an aneurysm. If this is in question, it may be another indication for diagnostic angiography. In some institutions, therapeutic angiography is used to devascularize a lesion before surgical resection. These same principles can be applied to tumors involving the

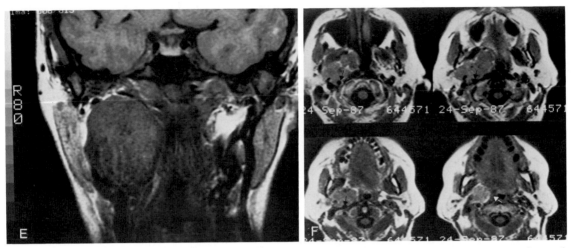

Figure 2–39 *Continued D.* Close-up T2-weighted MR shows the lesion to be bright. Stylopharyngeal muscle (arrowheads) and carotid artery (arrow) are pushed anteriorly. No flow voids or other signs of hypervascularity were seen on any image. *E.* Coronal view shows the relationship of the mass to the skull base. Imaging diagnosis was schwannoma of the poststyloid parapharyngeal space. No angiogram was done. Surgery revealed schwannoma of vagal origin. *F.* A different patient to contrast with the case presented in *A* to *E.* Four axial views from T1-weighted MR show a benign mixed tumor in the *prestyloid* parapharyngeal space displacing the carotid artery posterolaterally (black arrows) and the stylopharyngeal muscle medially (white arrow, lower right).

infratemporal fossa and masticator space regions, although the pathologic spectrum of these lesions differs somewhat from that of those arising in the parapharyngeal space.

Nasopharyngeal Cancer

Most nasopharyngeal carcinomas are obvious mucosal lesions to an experienced examiner. Imaging is done to determine the extent of the lesion after biopsy. MRI is best suited to evaluating a nasopharyngeal carcinoma. Supplemental CT is occasionally used in tumors when MRI shows a lesion immediately adjacent to the skull base but no definite evidence of bone erosion. In these cases, it is best to do a limited, direct coronal CT examination to be sure that the skull base is truly free of tumor involvement (Fig. 2–17). MRI is also ideally suited to the study of nasopharyngeal cancer because the imaging evaluation of cervical and retropharyngeal nodes is not as critical for care as it is in other upper aerodigestive tract primary sites. The neck nodes in patients with nasopharyngeal cancer are usually controlled with radiotherapy. Both sides of the neck are treated routinely. Detection of subtle metastatic disease or early capsular penetration does not seem to be as critical in helping to make the treatment decisions required for control of the neck disease in these patients as it does in patients with cancers at other primary sites.

Juvenile Angiofibroma

The clinical situation is usually fairly obvious in patients suspected of having juvenile angiofibroma. If this lesion is a likely diagnostic possibility, then noninvasive imaging should be the primary method of evaluation before biopsy. MRI or CT may be used (Fig. 2–4). MRI is probably preferable because a careful MRI study can produce most of the morphologic information that suggests the correct diagnosis. The key here is usually to distinguish among simple nasal polyps, fibroangiomatous polyps, and a juvenile angiofibroma. This can often be accomplished by looking at the spread pattern of the lesion (almost all juvenile angiofibromas extend into the pterygopalatine fossa) in combination with the signs of hypervascularity. In larger lesions, the signs of hypervascularity are more obvious on MRI than on CT. On CT images, an enhanced lesion with a typical spread pattern is strongly indicative of the diagnosis; however, strongly enhanced lesions may be ones with large vessels or merely ones that accumulate and hold onto the contrast material. On MRI, if it is properly done, the actual vessels may be visible within the tumor mass (Fig. 2–4). MRA or simply the use of flow-sensitive techniques, augments the capability of MRI to demonstrate the pathologic vascularity of the tumor (Fig. 2–5). MRI, which shows the actual tumor extent versus the secondary obstructive changes in the paranasal sinuses and nasal cavity (Fig. 2–17), is also superior to CT. Once imaging confirms that the lesion is likely to be an angiofibroma, diagnostic angiographic studies are carried out in a high percentage of patients. A combination of typical imaging findings, typical clinical situation, and typical appearing angiographic pattern is essentially as diagnostic as a biopsy. If the spread pattern of the lesion or its appearance on imaging examination and angiography is atypical, then one *must* suspect a lesion other than juvenile angiofibroma and obtain a histologic confirmation of the diagnosis (Fig. 2–40).

Once a diagnosis is firmly established, lesions are usually treated surgically. Devascularization by embolization is an extremely useful adjunct to surgical therapy and is a very safe and effective procedure in these lesions (Fig. 2–40). If there is extensive intracranial spread, surgery may not be possible, and a simple confirmatory diagnostic angiogram may be done. If the patients are irradiated, MRI is a simple and effective means of follow-up (Fig. 2–4).

Other Considerations

Certain other situations exist in which the nasopharynx and parapharyngeal space must be studied in detail in patients who may have tumors. Patients presenting with cervical metastases of uncertain etiology usually undergo fine-needle aspiration of the node (Fig. 2–7). If the node reveals squamous cell carcinoma, imaging may become part of the evaluation before endoscopy. The nasopharynx should be studied in detail, as should the tonsil, tongue base, posterior pharyngeal wall, and pyriform sinuses. Such careful study with imaging before endoscopy may reveal definite evidence of a submucosal mass responsible for the cervical adenopathy or may help identify regions suspicious for pathologic change.

Any patient with a submucosal mass should be imaged before biopsy. This can help avoid damage to a major vascular structure or excessive bleeding from a highly vascular lesion. It can also help avoid transmucosal biopsy of a benign mixed tumor with possible seeding of mucosa that is due to rupture of the tumor pseudocapsule.

Patients with deficits of cranial nerves V and IX to XII and the cervical sympathetics should be evaluated by imaging. This is discussed in detail in the next section.

Cranial Nerves V and IX to XII and Cervical Sympathetics

A wide variety of pathologic processes may involve the cranial nerves. MRI is best suited to the evaluation of the cranial nerves and cervical sympathetics. MRI is capable of studying the central origin of these nerves as

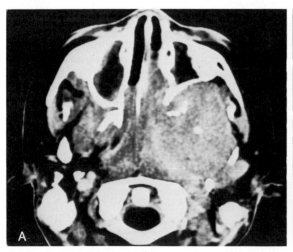
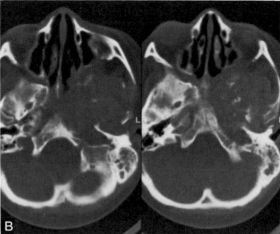

Figure 2–40. A 14-year-old male with nosebleeds and a nasopharyngeal mass. Clinical diagnosis was juvenile angiofibroma. *A.* Although at first glance the findings appear similar to those of juvenile angiofibroma, the involvement of the *entire* infratemporal fossa and poststyloid parapharyngeal space is atypical. *B.* Two views for bone detail show aggressive bone erosion and clival destruction, which again is atypical of angiofibroma. Biopsy or angiography is a reasonable next step. Biopsy was suggested because angiofibroma was considered *very* unlikely. Biopsy confirmed nonkeratinizing squamous cell carcinoma.

TABLE 2–8. Trigeminal Nerve—Clinical Triage

High-Yield	Low-Yield
Atypical facial pain	Typical trigeminal
Progressive history	neuralgia*
All divisions of cranial	Stable complaints
nerve V involved	Strictly subjective
"Hard" supportive	complaints with vague
neurologic findings	localization
Prior history of cancer	Otherwise negative past
(e.g., skin of face,	medical history
remote sites)	Likely myofacial, TMJ, or
	tension headache
	patient†

From Mancuso A: Workbook for MRI and CT of the Head and Neck, 2nd ed. Baltimore: Williams & Wilkins, 1989.

*Even though of low yield, patients with typical tic douloureux should be studied, especially if rhizotomy is planned.

†It is often difficult to decide if this group of patients warrants imaging; a stable versus progressive history is usually the best determinant.

TABLE 2–10. Horner's Syndrome (Oculosympathetic Paresis)—Clinical Triage*

High-Yield	Low-Yield
Complete Horner's triad	Anisocoria only
or at least ptosis and	Pharmacologic pupillary
miosis	testing negative
Pharmacologic	Lack of associated
confirmation of	neurologic findings or
pupillary dysfunction	complaints
and good pre- versus	Negative past medical
postganglionic	history (e.g., for
localization	malignancy)
Associated neurologic	
deficits, cranial nerves	
or others	
History of treated	
malignancy	

From Mancuso A: Workbook for MRI and CT of the Head and Neck, 2nd ed. Baltimore: Williams & Wilkins, 1989.

*True Horner's syndrome alone is an indication for imaging; it has a very high association with structural lesion.

well as their entire course from their root entry zones to the distal sites of innervation. It is absolutely essential that the entire course of the cranial nerve in question be studied. It has been a common fault of diagnostic imagers to study only a portion of the course of the cranial nerve: usually that portion from its origin to some point just at or below the skull base. It has also been a common fault for clinicians to accept such inadequate studies. Because the course of many of these

TABLE 2–9. Cranial Nerves IX, X, XI, and XII—Clinical Triage

High-Yield	Low-Yield
More than one nerve	Otalgia that is stable or
affected	indistinguishable from
"Hard" neurologic	myofacial pain, TMJ
findings	syndromes
Progressive history	Isolated vocal cord
Past history of treated	paresis*
malignancy	Lack of associated
Progressive otalgia with	findings
other symptoms (e.g.,	Complaints stable (i.e.,
dysphagia) or smoking,	not progressive over
ethanol abuse	months or years)
Deep headaches localized	Negative past medical
near the craniocervical	history
junction	
Vocal cord paresis with	
associated findings	
(e.g., brachial	
plexopathy, other	
cranial nerve deficits)	

From Mancuso A: Workbook for MRI and CT of the Head and Neck, 2nd ed. Baltimore: Williams & Wilkins, 1989.

*Although isolated vocal cord paresis is usually idiopathic, imaging demonstrates causative lesions in enough patients to justify the cost of its use.

nerves is highly complex, it is essential for the diagnostic imager to be given complete clinical information about the deficits. Good clinical triage (Tables 2–8 to 2–10) and good communication with the diagnostic imager should lead to highly detailed, efficient studies, which will exclude or confirm a structural lesion as an explanation for the cranial nerve deficit with a very high degree of confidence. It is important that the diagnostic imager have at hand algorithms for tailoring such studies. These are presented in Figures 2–41 to 2–44 for the individual cranial nerves and specific clinical questions at hand. Certainly these algorithms are meant only to serve as a framework for tailoring studies to individual patients. Depending on different institutional and personal biases, somewhat different approaches may be used. It is not really important what specific approach is employed; however, it is essential to have a basic plan of action so that important steps in the process of evaluation are not omitted. The algorithms presented here are meant as a framework for these individualized approaches to evaluating patients with cranial nerve deficits.

Trauma

The evaluation of skull base trauma is usually primarily by CT. This provides a reasonable survey for the extent of bone injury and any intracranial complications. The evaluation of cerebrospinal fluid leaks was discussed in

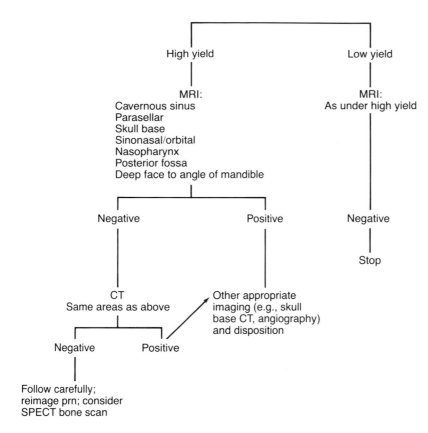

Figure 2–41. Imaging for trigeminal neuralgia after clinical triage. (From Mancuso A: Workbook for MRI and CT of the Head and Neck, 2nd ed. Baltimore: Williams & Wilkins, 1989.)

*High- and low-yield criteria are outlined in Table 2–8.

the sections on sinonasal and temporal bones. In general, sites of possible leak may be identified by careful search for bone defects. It is only in unusual circumstances that this search is aided by the injection of intrathecal contrast. One should be aware of the fact that a significant percentage of spontaneous cerebrospinal fluid leaks occur by dehiscences at the interface between the middle cranial fossa and large lateral recesses of the sphenoid sinus. Such dehiscences are best detected by thin-section, high-resolution CT done in a direct coronal plane. Associated encephaloceles or meningoceles may be detected by supplemental MRI (Fig. 2–33). Again, this search is usually not much aided by injection of intrathecal contrast, although this is frequently done adjunctively. Radionuclide studies may be of value in confirming that cerebrospinal fluid leakage is present; however, their localizing value is limited. In general, a positive result of a radionuclide study leads to an investigation of all possible sites of leak, including the ethmoids, sphenoid, and, if necessary, temporal bone regions. If posttraumatic encephalocele or meningocele is a primary diagnostic consideration, MRI is extremely useful as an adjunctive study in the posttrauma patient. Such patients usually present with cerebrospinal fluid leak, recurrent infections, or possibly poorly controlled or new onset of seizures.

Skull base trauma may lead to posttraumatic arteriovenous malformations or posttraumatic aneurysms. These may present with pulsatile tinnitus or cranial nerve deficits (Fig. 2–35). A dissection, in particular, may cause the acute onset of cranial nerve deficits. If vascular injury is suspected, the diagnostic evaluation may begin with MRI or CT. These studies frequently either make the diagnosis or strongly suggest some manifestation if an injury is present. Angiography is done for confirmation or in light of a negative imaging study along with strong clinical suspicion of vascular injury. Arteriography may also serve as a map for possible endovascular correction of the abnormality.

Figure 2–42. Imaging of cranial nerves IX, X, XI, and XII after clinical triage. (From Mancuso A: Workbook for MRI and CT of the Head and Neck, 2nd ed. Baltimore: Williams & Wilkins, 1989.)

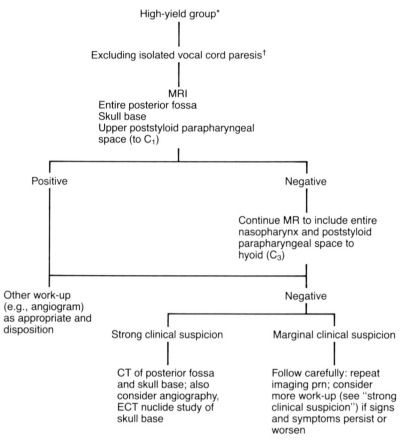

High-yield group*

Excluding isolated vocal cord paresis†

MRI
Entire posterior fossa
Skull base
Upper poststyloid parapharyngeal space (to C_1)

Positive   Negative

Continue MR to include entire nasopharynx and poststyloid parapharyngeal space to hyoid (C_3)

Other work-up (e.g., angiogram) as appropriate and disposition

Negative

Strong clinical suspicion   Marginal clinical suspicion

CT of posterior fossa and skull base; also consider angiography, ECT nuclide study of skull base

Follow carefully: repeat imaging prn; consider more work-up (see "strong clinical suspicion") if signs and symptoms persist or worsen

*See Table 2–9 for triage to high– and low–yield groups.
†See Figure 2–43.

The Parotid and Submandibular Glands

General Indications

Plain films have little, if any, role in evaluating diseases of the major salivary glands. Plain films may be used to look for calcified stones in the submandibular gland or duct. The chances of finding calcified stones involving the parotid ductal system are small and do not justify routine use of plain radiography over other imaging methods. In general, if the ductal systems of the parotid or submandibular glands need to be studied, sialography is the examination of choice (Table 2–5; Fig. 2–3). Mass lesions are generally studied by MRI or CT (Figs. 2–6, 2–7; Table 2–5). Some clinicians have used ultrasonography to study various pathologic processes affecting the parotid gland, including inflammatory disease, ductal disease, and mass lesions. In the author's practice, ultrasonog-

raphy has proved to be cost additive and nondefinitive in most circumstances; however, skilled users can, at times, obviate other diagnostic studies by careful and appropriate application of diagnostic ultrasonography. The patterns of triage of patients to sialography or CT and MRI are outlined in Figures 2–6 and 2–7. Angiography is a rarely used adjunctive study, and radionuclide studies are potentially useful in highly selected patients for studying salivary gland function or confirming the presence of Warthin's tumors.

Developmental Abnormalities

The most common of these to involve the parotid region is the first branchial cleft cyst, tract, or fistula. These frequently do not require any imaging for definitive management. Some clinicians would use ultrasonography to confirm the cystic nature of a mass. Others might use CT or MRI to define the

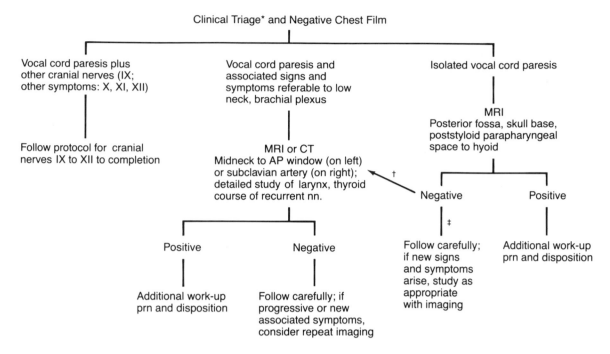

Clinical Triage* and Negative Chest Film

Vocal cord paresis plus other cranial nerves (IX; other symptoms: X, XI, XII)

Follow protocol for cranial nerves IX to XII to completion

Vocal cord paresis and associated signs and symptoms referable to low neck, brachial plexus

MRI or CT
Midneck to AP window (on left) or subclavian artery (on right); detailed study of larynx, thyroid course of recurrent nn.

Positive

Additional work-up prn and disposition

Negative

Follow carefully; if progressive or new associated symptoms, consider repeat imaging

Isolated vocal cord paresis

MRI
Posterior fossa, skull base, poststyloid parapharyngeal space to hyoid

†

Negative

‡

Follow carefully; if new signs and symptoms arise, study as appropriate with imaging

Positive

Additional work-up prn and disposition

*See Table 2–9; this procedure also assumes that complete cranial nerve examination and indirect laryngoscopy have been performed by competent observers.

†Isolated "idiopathic" vocal cord paresis is imagined to be potentially a low-yield situation; this part of pathway is optional and must be evaluated on a cost/benefit basis for individual patients. CT in general will produce a better quality image of the larynx than will MR for most patients.

‡This pathway requires that follow-up include periodic direct visualization of the larynx by an expert observer.

Figure 2–43. Imaging patients with vocal cord paresis of uncertain etiology. (From Mancuso A: Workbook for MRI and CT of the Head and Neck, 2nd ed. Baltimore: Williams & Wilkins, 1989.)

anatomic limits of lesions that are believed to be deeply situated or, for some other reason, a diagnostic dilemma. Sometimes differential diagnosis of a hemangioma or lymphangioma affecting the parotid region versus a branchial cleft cyst is uncertain. MRI or CT is usually definitive and shows the full extent of the lesion, including parotid and extraparotid involvement. MRI is excellent for showing the full extent of hemangiomas and lymphangiomas; however, CT is slightly more effective at demonstrating lesions with a vascular component. In questionable cases, radionuclide blood pool studies could be used to confirm the presence of a hemangioma.

Infectious and Noninfectious Inflammatory Conditions

The only possible role for plain films is perhaps in the identification of calcified stones in the submandibular ductal system or gland. Sialography should be avoided in any patient with evidence of acute sialadenitis. This was

discussed fully in the section on special contrast studies at the beginning of this chapter. In patients *without* evidence of acute infection, sialography is useful for identifying strictures in the ductal system, stones, and evidence of chronic sialadenitis. Ductal changes typical of chronic recurrent sialadenitis of childhood may be present in patients of the appropriate age group, and sialography may prove critical for making the decision of whether to treat the patient medically or surgically. Sialography may also be used to identify the pattern of chronic punctate sialadenitis. Although nonspecific, this pattern of ductal and parenchymal abnormality is strongly suggestive of autoimmune disease within the salivary gland system and can be used to confirm such a condition, if necessary. Sialography is of relatively little value in specifically diagnosing other diffuse parenchymal diseases, but some ductal patterns can suggest that an infiltrating process, such as sarcoidosis, is present.

Multiple masses in the parotid and periparotid region may be due to enlarged lymph

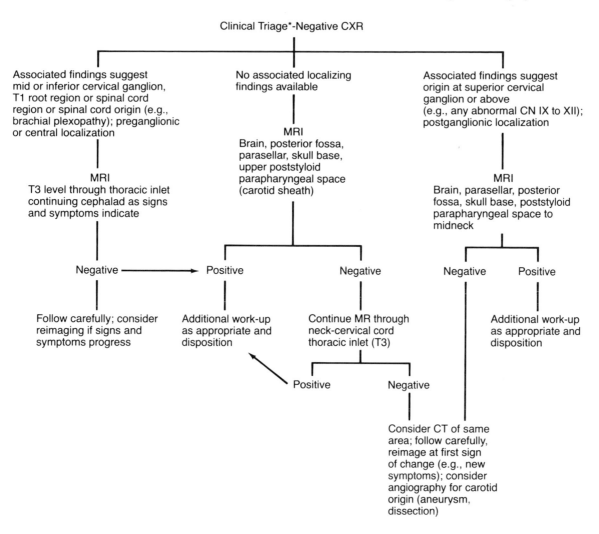

Clinical Triage*-Negative CXR

Associated findings suggest mid or inferior cervical ganglion, T1 root region or spinal cord region or spinal cord origin (e.g., brachial plexopathy); preganglionic or central localization

No associated localizing findings available

Associated findings suggest origin at superior cervical ganglion or above (e.g., any abnormal CN IX to XII); postganglionic localization

MRI
T3 level through thoracic inlet continuing cephalad as signs and symptoms indicate

MRI
Brain, posterior fossa, parasellar, skull base, upper poststyloid parapharyngeal space (carotid sheath)

MRI
Brain, parasellar, posterior fossa, skull base, poststyloid parapharyngeal space to midneck

Negative → Positive

Negative

Negative   Positive

Follow carefully; consider reimaging if signs and symptoms progress

Additional work-up as appropriate and disposition

Continue MR through neck-cervical cord thoracic inlet (T3)

Additional work-up as appropriate and disposition

Positive   Negative

Consider CT of same area; follow carefully, reimage at first sign of change (e.g., new symptoms); consider angiography for carotid origin (aneurysm, dissection)

*See Table 2–44 for triage to high- and low-yield groups; pharmacologic pupillary testing (e.g., cocaine instillation) and localization (Paredrine test) should be done *before* imaging.

Figure 2–44. Imaging patients with Horner's syndrome. (From Mancuso A: Workbook for MRI and CT of the Head and Neck, 2nd ed. Baltimore: Williams & Wilkins, 1989.)

nodes. It is usually unnecessary to image these patients unless there is a clinically compelling reason to do so. Patients with human immunodeficiency virus (HIV) infection may develop multiple masses in the parotid gland. If this situation occurs, one should consider lymphadenitis (possibly related to tuberculosis), lymphoma, metastases from Kaposi's sarcoma, and—the most common etiologic factor—multiple benign lymphoepitheliomatous lesions. Imaging adds little specific information over the clinical evaluation of these patients and is probably unnecessary in most. Imaging is usually done when a clinician thinks that one mass is present and the imaging study, be it MRI or CT,

shows that multiple lesions are, in fact, present.

Tumor

The imaging evaluation of mass lesions in the parotid or periparotid region needs to be integrated with needle biopsy and surgical approaches to such lesions (Figs. 2–6, 2–7). As a general rule, imaging is done before needle biopsy or superficial parotidectomy if the clinician cannot comfortably palpate all margins of the lesion. A superficial, freely movable mass, whether it is high or in the tail of a gland, certainly can be handled by a combination of fine-needle aspiration biopsy and superficial parotidectomy, if necessary. Imaging may be by either CT or MRI. The bias at the University of Florida is to use CT if there is any suggestion of an inflammatory component of the history (Fig. 2–6). This is because sometimes a "mass" actually turns out to be a manifestation of inflammatory disease, and CT is somewhat better than is MRI in identifying stones and ductal dilation (Fig. 2–45). In the author's clinical practice, ultrasonography is not definitive in a sufficient number of cases for justifying its cost. Other groups find more value in the routine use of ultrasonography for parotid mass lesions. In patients with no inflammatory component in the history, MRI or CT might be used. MRI is excellent, and perhaps preferable to CT, because of the ability to manipulate tissue contrast and, therefore, see subtle lesions with more clarity (Fig. 2–46). On the other hand, CT is much less expensive and, if properly done, rarely fails to visualize a parotid mass lesion.

The main aim of imaging in a parotid mass lesion is to determine whether the lesion is intrinsic or extrinsic to the parotid gland (Fig. 2–46). If the lesion is intrinsic, its plane in relation to the facial nerve is described. In the past, such descriptions have been limited to whether the mass was predominantly deep or superficial in relation to the facial nerve. These descriptions were refined in the late 1980s at the University of Florida, and it has been possible to describe not only whether the mass is superficial, or deep to the nerve, but whether it lies in the plane below the main trunk of the facial nerve. Also, success has been achieved in describing the position of intraparotid masses to more peripheral major divisions of the facial nerve. This description is based not on visualizing the main trunk of the nerve or its branches but on merely understanding the approximate position of these branches within the gland (Fig. 2–47). Excellent quality images and highly refined diagnostic skills can greatly aid the surgeon in planning the approach to parotid mass lesions and, most important, anticipating possible facial nerve injury (Fig. 2–47). The third purpose of the study is to determine whether the mass appears to be aggressive or nonaggressive. At the University of Florida, it is the policy to suggest biopsy of lesions that appear grossly

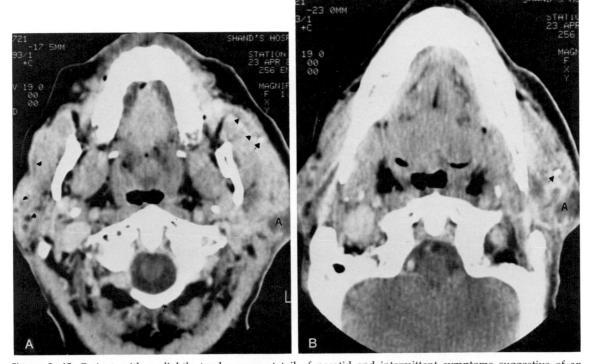

Figure 2–45. Patient with a slightly tender mass at tail of parotid and intermittent symptoms suggestive of an inflammatory condition. The contrast-enhanced CT showed a parotid tail abscess (A), stones in the left parotid ductal system (arrows), and dilation of the left main parotid duct as well as sialectasia on the right (arrowheads).

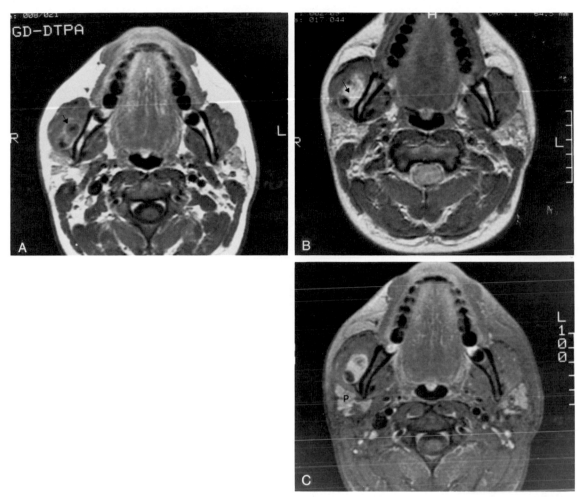

Figure 2–46. Patient presenting with a "parotid" mass. T1-weighted noncontrast *(A)* and contrast-enhanced *(B)* MR show an enhancing mass in the masseter muscle (arrow). C. Fat-suppressed, gadolinium-enhanced MR image shows the mass with the greatest clarity. Rounded calcifications (phleboliths) in the mass are visible on all images. Also note the excellent visualization of the normal parotid (P). The "parotid mass" was in fact a masseteric hemangioma. (Courtesy of Drs. Dan Williams and Alan Elster, Bowman Gray University School of Medicine.)

aggressive before removal. This can help anticipate the presence of malignancy and possibly alter the surgical approach to the lesion. Of course, imaging is not tissue specific, and even well-circumscribed lesions may turn out to be malignant; however, one may anticipate no problem in removal of a well-circumscribed, sharply defined lesion limited to the gland or immediate paraglandular region whether it is benign or malignant.

Over the years, the integration of imaging with clinical evaluation of parotid mass lesions has led to much more informed and safer care of these patients. Imaging occasionally drastically alters the management of the patient but more often serves to increase confidence in the planned surgical management and provides data that can help the clinician more fully inform the patient about the possible risks and benefits of the surgical procedure.

Mass lesions in the submandibular space pose no particular threat to the facial nerve or other vital neurovascular structure. Most often, one is trying to decide whether the mass lesion arises in the submandibular gland or in a lymph node adjacent to the submandibular gland. More rarely, plunging ramulus, dermoids, neuromas, and other benign mass lesions may present in this location. Either MRI or CT may be used to evaluate such lesions. These studies are extremely useful in both differential diagnosis and planning the surgical approach to abnor-

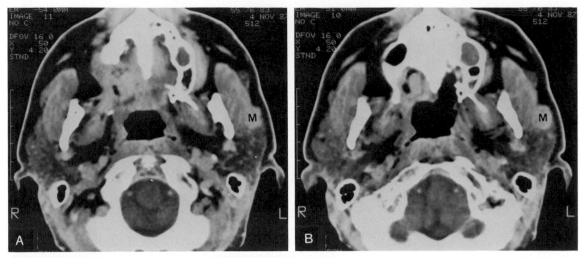

Figure 2–47. A 40-year-old male with a parotid region mass and normal facial nerve function. *A* and *B* show the mass (M) to be intrinsic. It is obviously superficial and distal to the pes anserinus. Branches at risk are the buccal and perhaps zygomatic. Note that there is little normal parotid around the mass. One might anticipate more than the usual challenge of removing the mass with a "cuff" of normal parotid tissue. The patient can be forewarned of increased risk to individual facial nerve branches on the basis of imaging studies done and interpreted as illustrated here.

malities of the submandibular space. In patients previously treated for head and neck cancers, especially those of the oral cavity and floor of the mouth, imaging with CT or MRI can be very useful for differentiating between recurrent disease and metastases to the submandibular lymph nodes and enlargement of the submandibular gland itself, due either to obstruction or to radiation-induced or other sialadenitis. If a tumor mass arises in the submandibular gland itself, imaging can help determine whether the mass is confined to the gland or has an aggressive extraglandular spread pattern.

Trauma

Traumatic lesions to the parotid and submandibular glands usually do not require imaging. Interruption or stricture of the ducts may be identified with sialography. Occasionally a posttraumatic sialocele presents as a parotid mass and come to imaging.

Oropharynx, Oral Cavity, and Floor of the Mouth (Excluding the Mandible)

General Indications

Plain radiography, conventional tomography, and fluoroscopy (with or without bar-

ium) may be used to investigate this area. Sialography was occasionally used to study the submandibular gland as a possible source of disease in this region; these studies now play a very limited role in evaluating oropharyngeal and oral cavity pathologic processes. A major exception is the use of standard plain film and dental radiographic techniques in evaluating the mandible; this was discussed in a previous section on the mandible and TMJ and is discussed in this section mainly as it relates to evaluating cancers. Fluoroscopic studies of this area are still done to evaluate velopharyngeal competence and the swallowing mechanism. These are basically functional, not anatomic, studies and are no longer appropriate for evaluating mass lesions and inflammatory conditions. Ultrasonography may be used to study abscesses, benign masses, and cancers that affect the oral tongue and floor of the mouth, but experience with this technique is limited, and its role in relation to CT and MRI needs to be defined before it is suggested as a routine adjunctive study (Table 2–5). CT and MRI are the primary studies used to evaluate inflammatory conditions, benign masses, and cancers in this region. Radionuclide studies and angiography are infrequently used adjunctive studies; their specific application is usually guided by the results of other imaging examinations (Table 2–5).

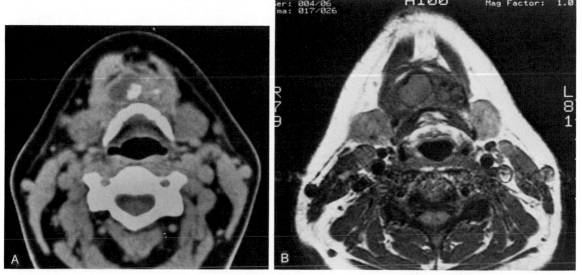

Figure 2–48. A 35-year-old female with a mass in the floor of the mouth–suprahyoid neck region; prior surgery revealed "no tumor," and only fibrous reactive tissue and muscle were seen in the specimen. The patient presented to the author's institution with a postoperative CT and complaints of a persistent mass. *A.* CT without contrast shows partially calcified, partially cystic mass in the suprahyoid neck anterior to the hyoid. *B.* Correlating noncontrast T1-weighted axial MR image.

Developmental Abnormalities

In general, the developmental abnormalities in this region present as submucosal or neck masses. The imaging approach to lesions such as lymphomas or dermoid tumors, which might rightfully be considered developmental, is considered in the following section on mass lesions.

The developmental lesions that most commonly affect this area are those of the branchial apparatus and those related to the development of the thyroid gland. Branchial apparatus abnormalities are evaluated by the techniques described in the previous section on the parotid gland and in a later section on the neck. The diagnosis of the lingual thyroid gland may be suspected in patients with a submucosal mass of the tongue base. This diagnosis is probably best confirmed by a radionuclide examination. In these patients, it is essential to be sure that functioning thyroid tissue is present in the low neck before the lingual thyroid tissue is resected. Often the diagnosis is not suspected, and CT or MRI is done. CT is fairly characteristic in that the soft tissue mass is very avid in its uptake of the iodinated contrast, which strongly suggests the diagnosis. MRI is less specific in its appearance. Thyroglossal duct cysts may extend through or around the hyoid bone and into the tongue base. The full extent of a thyroglossal duct cyst is best evaluated by either MRI or CT. Both studies are adequate. Ultrasonography is of little value because it cannot show the full extent of the anatomic area that needs to be studied. It could be argued that no imaging is necessary in patients with thyroglossal duct cysts if the surgical procedure is, as it should be, the classic Sistrunk approach. Over the years, however, the author has found it useful to be able to fully inform the surgeon about what will be encountered at surgery. This is especially true when there are very large cystic remnants in and about the hyoid region and extending into the tongue base (Fig. 2–48).

The evaluation of craniofacial abnormalities and dental abnormalities related to the lower craniofacial region is discussed in detail in the preceding sections on the orbits, facial bones, and mandible.

Infectious and Noninfectious Inflammatory Lesions

The overwhelming majority of nondental infectious diseases involving the oropharynx, oral cavity, and floor of the mouth do not require any imaging. Nonsuppurative infection of the lingual or faucial tonsils mimics a mass lesion or leads to the suspicion of a

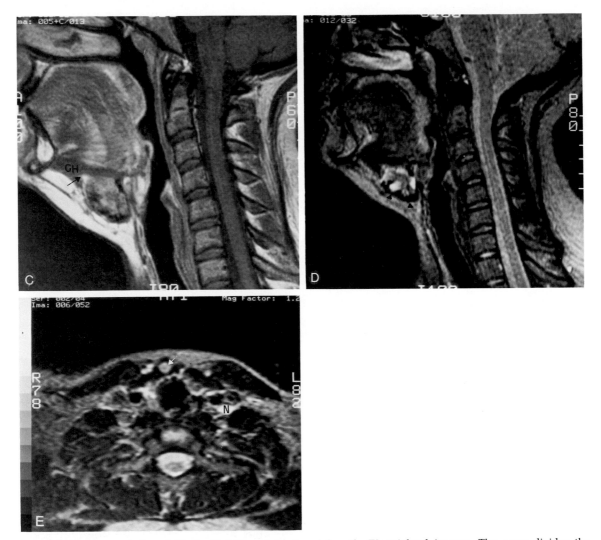

Figure 2–48 *Continued* C *and* D. Sagittal T1-weighted and heavily T2-weighted images. The mass divides the geniohyoid muscle (GH) or separates it from the anterior belly of the digastric muscle (arrow). Dense fibrosis rings the tumor inferiorly (arrowheads), which probably accounts for the negative findings of surgical exploration at the outside institution. The mass does not extend into the tongue base. *E.* Thyroglossal duct tract (arrow) was followed back to isthmus of the thyroid gland, which was in normal position. Low neck node on the left (N) and others not seen were considered suspicious. Because of the mixed appearance of the mass and suspicious nodes, papillary cancer in a thyroglossal duct cyst was considered likely. This was confirmed surgically, and several nodes were positive.

deeper abscess and occasionally causes simple pharyngitis-tonsillitis to come to imaging, which is usually by CT or MRI. Pyogenic infections involving tonsils can progress to tonsillar and peritonsillar abscess, occasionally with extension into the parapharyngeal space and rarely the retropharyngeal space. These conditions more commonly lead to suppurative retropharyngeal lymphadenitis, a condition that is commonly misdiagnosed as an abscess in the retropharyngeal space (Fig. 2–38). Soft tissue lateral views of the

neck are commonly used as a screening examination for patients suspected of having "retropharyngeal abscess." In the adult, this is not an unreasonable step in the work-up; however, a negative examination does not necessarily exclude the possibility of a deep neck or parapharyngeal abscess. In the pediatric age group, it is much less useful because of the tremendous variations in the appearance of the retropharyngeal soft tissues caused by variations in respiration and in positioning of the patient. Still, plain films are not an unreasonable starting point in patients with suspected abscesses if the limitations just described are anticipated. Also, these views can help anticipate the presence of epiglottitis or other gross airway abnormalities. If an abscess in one of the deep spaces of the face and neck is suspected, CT or MRI should be done. The author's preference is CT examination, for reasons stated in the sections on CT and MRI technique. MRI is a reasonable choice, if preferred (Fig. 2–38). Ultrasonography really plays no role in evaluating these abnormalities. CT should also be done in patients suspected of abscesses in the sublingual, masticator, or submandibular spaces. CT is extremely reliable in differentiation of cellulitis from drainable collections of pus. CT examination in these settings should be considered first as a diagnostic tool and second as a map for help in anticipating appropriate drainage pathways. At times, it is difficult to decide from the clinical findings whether the inflammatory lesion is arising predominantly in deep spaces or in adjacent salivary glands. CT is very useful for sorting out whether the origin of disease is due to lymphadenitis, cellulitis, sialadenitis, deep space abscess, or a combination of any of these abnormalities. It may also suggest an alternative diagnosis, in some cases.

Fungal infections are unusual in this location. One should also keep in mind the possibility of infection with actinomycosis. In the immunosuppressed population, multiple necrotic-appearing inflammatory nodes should raise the possibility of tuberculous adenitis. In combination with multiple lesions within the parotid gland, these nodes may also suggest the presence of infectious disease or neoplasm superimposed on HIV infection.

A plunging or diving ranula may present as an inflammatory or noninflammatory mass in the floor of the mouth and submandibular space. The definitive diagnosis may be made with MRI or CT. Ultrasonography merely confirms the cystic nature of the mass but usually is not definitive. These plunging or diving ranulas are usually not infected, and contusion with abscess is unlikely.

Tumors

Benign masses in this region outside of those due to lymph node enlargement are unusual.

After proper clinical screening and, if necessary, a dental radiographic work-up, one should proceed directly to CT or MRI for evaluating a benign or malignant mass. For benign masses, either MRI or CT may be used. The author's preference is CT if the mass is believed to be related to the mandible. If it is strictly soft tissue and most likely nonmalignant, MRI is an equivalent or perhaps better choice.

At the University of Florida, squamous cell carcinomas of this region are evaluated primarily with CT. CT is superior to MRI in its depiction of the lingual and buccal surfaces of the mandible as well as in its ability to evaluate the presence and extent of cervical lymph node disease. The staging of lymph nodes is discussed in the neck section. Adjunctive studies of cancer in this region include dental type radiographs of the mandible if involvement of the alveolar ridge or of lower borders of the mandibular body is suspected. CT is excellent for evaluating the lingual and buccal surfaces of the mandible, and despite some reports suggesting superiority of MRI over CT for the detection of mandibular involvement, the author's colleagues and others have found the approach of combining high-resolution CT and traditional dental radiographs to be highly accurate if done with care. There is some value in using MRI adjunctively to evaluate spread of cancer within the marrow space of the mandible in highly selected cases. After the CT evaluation of patients with cancers in this location, MRI is used occasionally (in no more than 10% to 15% of patients) to evaluate the local extent of the primary tumor. This is done only if the CT evaluation suggests that there is a reasonable chance of yield of information that would alter the therapy or prognosis of the patient. The supplementary MRI examinations are usually confined to relatively small anatomic regions of interest and focused in a way to answer the questions that might alter management.

Larynx and Hypopharynx

General Indications

Numerous radiographic techniques have been employed to evaluate conditions that affect the larynx and hypopharynx. Plain films and conventional tomography have little, if any, role when modern imaging equipment is available. With advances in modern endoscopic techniques, laryngography and pharyngography are basically obsolete studies. Pharyngography may still be used as part of a functional analysis of the upper pharynx but is not indicated for the evaluation of mass lesions. There is still a reasonable role for plain radiography in evaluating the general status of the airway and looking for radiodense foreign bodies. Ultrasonography plays no useful role in evaluating the larynx in the author's clinical practice, although it has been used by some groups to look for cartilage invasion by cancer. Radionuclide studies and angiography are applied only rarely to this anatomic location. CT and MR are the mainstays of imaging at this anatomic site (Table 2–5).

Developmental Abnormalities

The most commonly encountered developmental abnormalities of the larynx and pharynx are laryngoceles and pharyngoceles. It is reasonable to evaluate a patient suspected of having a pharyngocele (such as Zenker's diverticulum) with barium studies. Laryngoceles are most frequently encountered as asymptomatic, minimal dilations of the laryngeal saccule during routine CT studies. The next most common presentation is as a neck mass or submucosal mass in a lesion. These lesions are almost always studied with CT and, more recently, MR before they come to surgery. Any imaging study of a laryngocele must include careful sections through the level of the laryngeal ventricle and false cord for ensuring that there is no obstructing tumor. Occasionally, a laryngopyocele mimics a deep neck infection in its clinical presentation.

There are rare congenital clefts of the larynx that may be imaged, if desired. Again, this is probably best done with CT or MRI.

Infectious and Noninfectious Inflammatory Lesions

Aside from the laryngopyocele, it is unusual for an inflammatory lesion of the larynx or hypopharynx to come to imaging. Occasionally, an inflammatory of inflammatory-like process such as tuberculosis or amyloidosis mimics a neoplasm and is imaged. In this circumstance, it is very important for the imager to be sensitive to findings that may suggest an inflammatory rather than a neoplastic lesion, such as the presence of atypical patterns of cartilage destruction leaving behind sequestra, or excessive enhancement of the laryngeal or pharyngeal lesion. Rare instances of laryngeal and paralaryngeal origin infections, presenting as visceral space abscesses, have been encountered. Clinically, these are difficult to differentiate before imaging from other deep neck infectious processes. CT is preferred to MRI in this setting.

Chondritis and chondronecrosis are usually the result of radiotherapy. CT is preferred for the diagnosis and follow-up of these patients. If infectious perichondritis and chondronecrosis are likely, a gallium study might be useful for following therapy.

Tumor

If patients with benign tumors or malignancies of the larynx and hypopharynx require imaging, CT is the preferred examination at the University of Florida. MRI is done as a supplemental study when necessary. This is mainly because a large proportion (10% to 20% at least) of the MRI studies are of low quality because of motion artifacts (Fig. 2–49). Other specifics involved in this choice are discussed subsequently. There is virtually no role for conventional tomography, laryngography, or plain films in evaluating tumors when CT and MRI are available. Plain films may be done retrospectively if they seem likely to yield useful information as judged from a preceding CT or MRI.

Benign masses of the larynx are unusual. These usually present as submucosal masses, and it is uncertain whether they represent predominantly submucosal cancer or one of the more rare benign lesions that affect the larynx (Fig. 2–50). CT is preferred in evaluating these patients because they often are found to have carcinoma, and CT is preferable for evaluating cervical nodes as well as for its depiction of cartilage detail. A focused, adjunctive MRI study may be done if additional diagnostic information is necessary for therapy. Angiography is rarely used but may confirm a paraganglioma if this is suspected on other studies.

Carcinoma of the larynx and pharynx should be imaged only when it is likely that the imaging findings will alter therapy. Clearly, early T1 lesions of the membranous portion of the true cord do not require im-

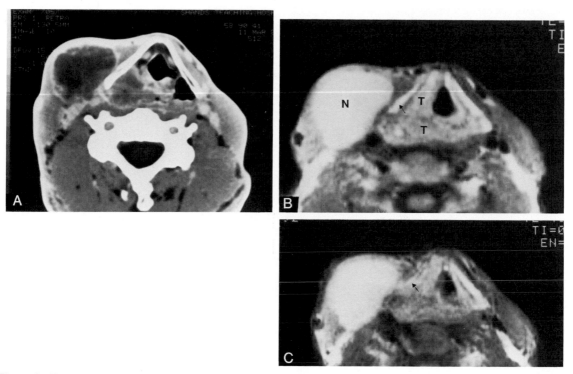

Figure 2–49. Patient with piriform sinus carcinoma. All sections of the CT study were the same as or better quality than that seen in *A. B.* Excellent quality MRI image from the first acquisition shows the primary tumor (T), excellent thyroid cartilage detail (arrow), and an enlarged node (N). *C.* During the second acquisition, the patient coughed several times. The image is only grossly informative compared with *B.* Note the cartilages are not even visible on the right (arrow). Additional acquisitions were equally nondiagnostic, and the study was terminated.

aging. Any tumor that is suspected of deep infiltration, from the history or endoscopic findings, should be studied with CT. Most advanced lesions should also be studied. Some argue that imaging findings do not alter the approach to treating very advanced lesions; however, the following listing of the value of CT and MRI in staging cancers of this region contain some rationale for the imaging even of more advanced lesions. To cite one example, high-volume submucosal spread in the subglottic region may lead to preoperative planning of a tracheostomy site that is lower than usual. Sometimes this degree of subglottic spread cannot be anticipated from the endoscopic study. This certainly does not prevent the patient's loss of the larynx, but such preoperative planning may lower the risk of stomal recurrence. Similar information is available in hypopharyngeal cancer, in which CT or MRI evidence of submucosal spread in the postcricoid region well beyond the apex of the pyriform sinus may indicate that a flap reconstruction or gastric pull-up, rather than primary clo-

sure of the pharynx, is necessary. This certainly does not preserve the patient's larynx or alter the basic operative approach, but it might help avoid failure at the primary site.

The role of CT and MRI imaging in laryngeal and hypopharyngeal cancer is as follows.

1. *Tongue base invasion.* Supraglottic cancers may penetrate the tongue base by cephalad growth from the pre-epiglottic space; this occasionally occurs without obvious mucosal disease in the vallecula or a palpable mass at the tongue base.

2. *Pre-epiglottic space spread.* This is a clinically silent area, and CT and MRI are by far the most accurate means for identifying such spread. From the pre-epiglottic space, very aggressive lesions may involve the attachment of the thyrohyoid membrane to the top of the thyroid cartilage.

3. *Paralaryngeal space spread.* Occult, submucosal spread via the paralaryngeal space is a conduit for the cephalocaudal spread of all laryngeal and hypopharyngeal cancer. The presence of such submucosal disease can

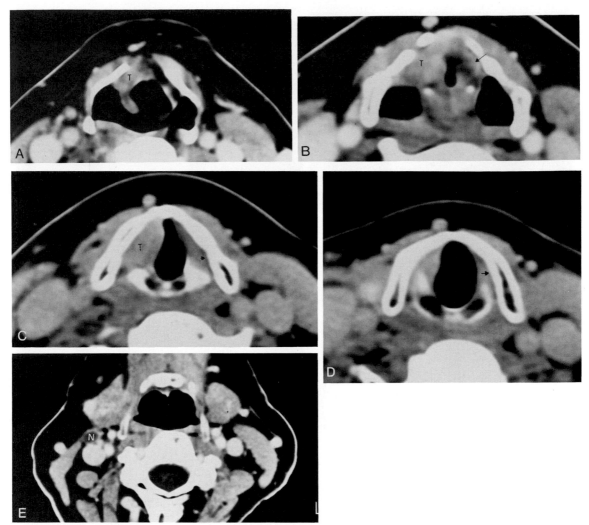

Figure 2–50. Patient with "right true vocal cord paralysis" and no mucosal abnormality seen at two direct laryngoscopic examinations. *A.* CT in low supraglottis shows tumor (T) in paraglottic space. *B.* Tumor (T) crossing the laryngeal ventricle and in the paraglottic space. Note the obliteration of the fat and lack of visualization of the lateral thyroarytenoid muscle (at arrow on normal side). *C.* Tumor (T) at the true cord level obliterates the paraglottic space (arrow on the normal side) and widens the true cord's contour. *D.* Minimal subglottic spread just beneath the undersurface of the true cord. Note the continued obliteration of the paraglottic space (arrow on normal side). *E.* Metastatic node (N) was present at the junction of the upper and middle internal jugular groups. After this CT study, repeat DL revealed no mucosal abnormality. Wedge biopsy at the right false vocal cord–ventricular level revealed squamous cell carcinoma.

greatly alter the surgical approach to lesions. Large volumes of submucosal spread may be predictive of a poor likelihood of control of the primary site with radiotherapy. This information is preliminary but has been reported by two groups (see Suggested Readings).

4. *Subglottic spread.* This is perhaps one of the most critical contributions of CT and clearly has impact on planning of hemilaryngectomy versus total or near-total laryngectomy.

5. *Postcricoid spread.* Spread to this locale occurs mainly in primary hypopharyngeal cancers. CT and MRI may reveal submucosal spread to the postcricoid region or beyond the apex of the piriform sinus. This is useful adjunctive information in evaluating the extent of deep spread of tumor in relation to the esophageal verge (Fig. 2–51). MRI might prove particularly valuable in showing subtle submucosal spread in these regions because of its improved tissue contrast abilities.

6. *Cartilage invasion.* The optimal study for

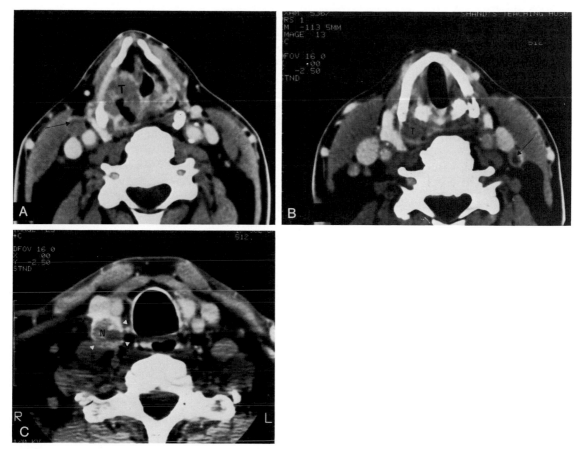

Figure 2–51. Patient with clinical Stage III N0 piriform sinus carcinoma. The neck was negative to multiple examinations by highly experienced clinicians. *A.* Primary tumor (T) shows spread pattern typical of piriform sinus cancer. Focal metastasis (arrow) is present in a 10-mm right neck node. *B.* A positive 1-cm node (arrow) is present on the left; the lucency in the center is either necrosis, the metastasis, or both. Primary tumor involves the apex (T) but does not significantly involve the postcricoid region; such data can help plan the method of neopharyngeal construction. *C.* A 20-mm low neck (scalene) node (N) was also present with possible early capsular penetration (arrowheads). The patient was classified as T4 (cartilage invasion not shown) N3B; right neck N2B, left neck N1 by CT—a staging.

detecting subtle cartilage invasion still does not exist. CT and MRI are good, but the variation and ossification of all the cartilages sometimes makes interpretation difficult. Experienced observers who understand the natural history of cancers can do an excellent job of excluding the presence of cartilage invasion, except for that which might be microscopic or very subtle. This requires careful attention to image quality as well as interpretation. Neither CT nor MRI nor any other imaging study is 100% accurate at predicting cartilage invasion, and none is likely to be that accurate in the near future.

7. *Exolaryngeal spread.* Such spread patterns may critically alter management and prognosis. CT is used as the primary exami-

nation of the larynx, but MRI is very useful in cases in which early exolaryngeal spread is suspected and confirmation is required in order to properly plan therapy. In this setting, MRI can be focused on the area of suspicion, and a relatively quick and efficient study can be planned in order to answer the question of whether early exolaryngeal spread is present. Adjunctive MRI is similarly used in detecting early cartilage invasion.

The evaluation of cervical nodes is often critical, depending on the primary site and extent. CT is preferred for evaluating cervical nodes for reasons discussed in the next section.

CT or MRI may be used to study patients suspected of recurrent cancer. MRI is somewhat better than is CT for differentiating recurrent tumor from end-stage scarring (Figs. 2–48, 2–52); however, CT is still preferred as the initial imaging examination of choice because of its superiority in detecting positive lymph nodes and because it is a reasonable and usually conclusive method for evaluating the neopharynx. MRI is used as a focused examination when the findings on CT are equivocal. In suspicious areas, a supplemental MRI examination might also aid in suggesting a site for imaging-directed biopsy (Fig. 2–15).

Trauma

Plain films or fluoroscopy with barium swallow may be used in evaluating patients suspected of having a foreign body within the larynx or hypopharynx. Supplemental CT may also be used to locate a foreign body if it is suspected of having penetrated through the mucosa into the deep neck. If perforation or infection is suspected, water-soluble contrast should be used. Trauma that may have resulted in penetration or perforation of the airway or pharynx may be imaged in the same way. Certainly, preliminary plain films are helpful for anticipating whether there may be a mucosal tear if air is present in the soft tissues.

If imaging is required in blunt laryngeal trauma, this should be done by CT study. CT clearly shows the status of the airway and surrounding soft tissues, and whether significantly displaced fractures of any of the cartilaginous structures are present. If necessary, reformatting with three-dimensional studies can be done. The lateral digital radiograph, obtained during the CT study, can be substituted for a plain film of the airway if desired. Plain films or xeroradiography can

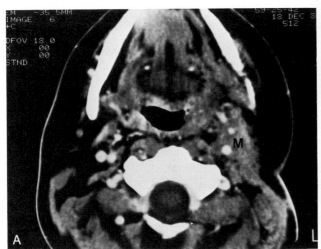
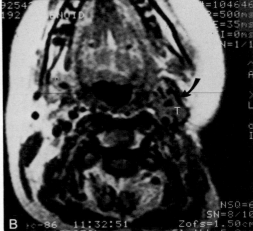
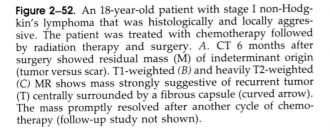
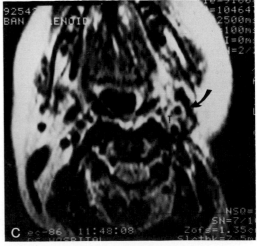

Figure 2–52. An 18-year-old patient with stage I non-Hodgkin's lymphoma that was histologically and locally aggressive. The patient was treated with chemotherapy followed by radiation therapy and surgery. *A.* CT 6 months after surgery showed residual mass (M) of indeterminant origin (tumor versus scar). T1-weighted *(B)* and heavily T2-weighted *(C)* MR shows mass strongly suggestive of recurrent tumor (T) centrally surrounded by a fibrous capsule (curved arrow). The mass promptly resolved after another cycle of chemotherapy (follow-up study not shown).

be done if desired as well, but these do not usually add significant information for the care of the patient. If CT is available, conventional tomography is an obsolete study for evaluating laryngeal trauma. Water-soluble contrast swallow can be used to look for false passages, although these studies tend to be of relatively poor quality in the acutely injured patient.

Neck and Cervical and Retropharyngeal Lymph Nodes

General Indications

The neck is most commonly studied because of the presence of a palpable mass lesion (Table 2–5). At the University of Florida, it is commonly included as part of the evaluation of patients with carcinoma arising in the upper aerodigestive tract. CT is used for the majority of these studies. Plain films are occasionally done as part of the work-up for suspected retropharyngeal abscesses, foreign bodies, or abnormalities involving the airway, but these are rarely definitive, and additional imaging is performed in most patients. For evaluating masses, CT and MRI are integrated with the clinical findings and results of needle biopsy of mass lesions, when appropriate (Fig. 2–7). Ultrasonography is used sparingly because it is rarely definitive and, therefore, is most often cost additive if it is used indiscriminately. Ultrasonography is used mainly to determine whether a mass is vascular or its relationship to vessels before biopsy or definitive management (Fig. 2–7). Angiography is used much less often for similar purposes. Fluoroscopy, with or without contrast, is occasionally used to study the status of the airway and pharynx; this was discussed in previous sections. The use of imaging of the thyroid gland, of the parathyroid glands, and of pathologic changes at the thoracic inlet is discussed in the following sections (Table 2–5).

Developmental Abnormalities

The most common developmental abnormality to involve the neck is a cyst, fistula, or sinus tract deriving from the branchial apparatus. This diagnosis is usually suspected clinically. Imaging is usually done to confirm the diagnosis and evaluate the extent of lesion before surgical treatment. If a fistulous tract is open to the skin, it may be studied by injection. Either CT or MRI may be used to study the extent of branchial apparatus cysts. Ultrasonography is potentially useful for confirming the cystic nature of the lesion but is usually not definitive at showing its extent and, therefore, adds no incremental clinical data. CT or MRI is used to evaluate patients with known or suspected thyroglossal duct cysts. This was discussed in detail in the section on the oral cavity and tongue base (Fig. 2–48).

Infectious and Noninfectious Inflammatory Lesions

Deep neck abscess, jugular thrombophlebitis, infected branchial cleft cyst, and suppurative or malignant adenopathy are the most common considerations entering into the differential diagnosis of inflammatory neck mass. In general, the most efficient pathway to imaging diagnosis is with CT. Ultrasonography may prove useful in a small number of cases; however, it is usually not definitive and only delays the time to diagnosis and adds cost. Also, in patients with inflammatory neck masses, the area of interest is often very tender and, therefore, difficult to examine with the ultrasonographic transducer, even if only gentle pressure is applied to the skin over the infected area. MRI may be used in a manner similar to CT, but unless it is done with and without contrast, or at least with fat suppression techniques and contrast enhancement, studies may not prove as definitive as CT. As in other locations, CT and MRI are extremely useful for mapping the extent of a deep neck abscess before drainage. The examination should be carried into the mediastinum whenever an accumulation of pus is found in the low neck. The basic pathophysiologic mechanism of and suggested imaging evaluation for retropharyngeal abscess were discussed in the section on the oral cavity and oropharynx (Fig. 2–38). Plain films may be part of this evaluation. Occasionally, plain films are warranted and may be supplemented by water-soluble contrast swallow and fluoroscopy; however, evaluation of an inflammatory neck mass can begin and end with a *properly done* CT scan in the majority of patients.

Tumor

Cervical and Retropharyngeal Metastatic Disease

At the University of Florida, CT is the primary imaging study for evaluating cervical and retropharyngeal lymph nodes. It is a safe, efficient study and highly informative when done with proper technique. In general, many studies of the neck region performed with CT are still done with suboptimal technique. Images should routinely appear as those shown in Figure 2–51 and elsewhere in this chapter. If images do not look like these, the fault usually lies in the techniques used, rather than in the patient or imaging equipment. With images of such quality, metastatic foci in nodes under 1 cm are routinely visible, and one can detect early extranodal spread of tumor with a very high degree of confidence. All nodal groups are visible, including the retropharyngeal, scalene (deep low neck), and tracheoesophageal groove nodes, which are difficult to evaluate by palpation (Figs. 2–18, 2–38, 2–51).

CT is preferred as the primary examination to MRI and ultrasonography for several reasons. Ultrasonography is highly user-dependent and does not visualize retropharyngeal nodes and some of the more inferior tracheoesophageal nodes. Ultrasonography may detect gross capsular penetration but is limited in evaluating extranodal spread of tumor; it has some predictive role in evaluating patients for carotid fixation (Fig. 2–8). MRI can visualize all of the nodal groups but is currently unable to consistently demonstrate metastases in nodes smaller than 1 cm with the same clarity as well-done CT scans (Fig. 2–51). It is also more expensive than is CT. Over the 1990s, MRI is bound to improve technically with the application of newer coils, faster imaging techniques, fat suppression, and paramagnetic contrast enhancement. It may be that MRI will prove to be as good as or superior to CT for evaluating cervical metastatic disease by 1995; however, there are insufficient data to make this conclusion at this time. The relative value of CT, ultrasonography, and MRI in evaluating cervical metastatic disease is currently under study by the radiologic-diagnostic oncology group under the auspices of the National Institutes of Health. These coordinated studies may help shed some light on these issues within the next 3 to 5 years. All imaging studies are limited in their ability to show fixation to the carotid artery and deeper neck structures. At times, CT, ultrasonography, and MRI might all be required to help decide whether the carotid artery is fixed. If removal of the carotid artery during surgery is anticipated, a balloon occlusion study, probably supplemented with xenon CT or other method of evaluating brain perfusion, should be done.

Masses of Uncertain Etiology

Patients frequently present with mid- to upper-neck masses of uncertain etiology. Imaging evaluation must be integrated with the clinical situation and results of needle biopsy. A basic decision-making algorithm is suggested in Figure 2–7. At the University of Florida, CT is the primary imaging modality used because of the superiority in evaluating cervical metastatic disease just discussed. Also, it is fast, efficient, and of moderate cost. Ultrasonography is used only when a vascular mass, or a mass arising from a blood vessel, is suspected as the etiologic factor (Figs. 2–7, 2–8). Ultrasonography is also used as a primary study in patients with low neck and thoracic inlet masses if they are believed to be of thyroid or vascular origin. MRI may be substituted for CT. The reasons for the author's using CT rather than MRI have been discussed in the previous section on cervical metastatic disease and in the sections on MRI and CT earlier in the chapter. If a mass is believed to be arising from or involving the spine or neural axis, MRI certainly should be the primary study. This particularly applies in the low neck because of the proximity of the brachial plexus. MRI may also be preferred in the low neck because of the availability of coronal and sagittal images, and for certain other reasons discussed in conjunction with thyroid and parathyroid disease.

Sometimes the cause of a neck mass is known. This is probably most often true in patients with lymphangiomas and cystic hygromas. The main aim in examining these patients is to map the extent of the lesion. MRI demonstrates a fairly classic appearance of these lesions and graphically depicts their relationship to all important structures in the neck. MRI may certainly be substituted for CT in cases in which the cause of a benign neck mass is known and the surgeon requires merely such a preoperative map.

Trauma

There are several mechanisms of trauma to the neck. Ingested foreign bodies may lodge in the airway or pharynx or perforate these structures. The evaluation of these was discussed in a preceding section on the larynx and hypopharynx. Blunt trauma may result in injury to the larynx, hypopharynx, trachea, or esophagus, and this was also discussed in the section on the larynx and hypopharynx. Whenever there is penetrating trauma to the neck, the possibility of vascular injury must be considered. If an acute injury is suspected, it is usually best to proceed to angiography. If a delayed complication is suspected, beginning with a noninvasive technique such as ultrasonography, MRI, or CT may be appropriate; however, a definitive diagnosis usually also requires arteriography.

Cervical spine trauma often occurs in patients suffering craniofacial trauma. The ENT surgeon must be aware of this situation and do appropriate screening and perhaps more advanced imaging studies whenever cervical spine injury is suspected. This is especially true when mandibular fracture is present. One must take great care not to flex or extend the neck to extremes in attempting to study the craniofacial injuries of a patient before the cervical spine has been "cleared" either clinically or by appropriate imaging studies.

Thyroid Gland

General Indications

Diagnostic imaging has traditionally played a major role in the evaluation of both functional and anatomic disease involving the thyroid gland. The approach to imaging of the thyroid gland is anything but straightforward. Radionuclide studies and ultrasonography play primary diagnostic roles (Table 2–5). MRI and CT play only minor, secondary roles. Because of the extreme variations in the clinical approach to thyroid disorders, the imaging approach is probably best driven by the needs of the referring clinician. Basically, the imaging study should make some difference in the approach to the patient. This underlying philosophy is reflected in the triage and imaging approaches suggested in Tables 2–1 and 2–2.

Developmental Abnormalities

The most common developmental abnormality requiring imaging is the thyroglossal duct cyst. This is best evaluated by CT or MRI. These studies are required because they show the full extent of the lesion, especially the course of the cyst in relation to the hyoid bone and tongue base (Fig. 2–48). The diagnosis of a lingual thyroid may be confirmed by radionuclide study or CT. This was discussed in a previous section on the oropharynx. The same studies may be done to look for functioning thyroid tissue in the low neck before removal of lingual thyroid tissue. True absence of the thyroid gland is rare. Any search for functioning thyroid tissue should include the tongue base, low neck, and mediastinum.

Infectious and Noninfectious Inflammatory Disease

Most patients with thyroiditis or paraglandular inflammatory conditions do not require imaging. The diagnosis is made on the basis of thyroid function studies, clinical situation, and physical examination. If the differential diagnosis between a thyroid inflammation and other low-neck inflammatory disease, such as jugular thrombophlebitis or deep-neck abscess, cannot be made on the basis of these studies, imaging with CT, MRI, or ultrasonography may be indicated as discussed in the section on the neck. Frank abscess in the thyroid gland is unusual and could be related to an infected fourth branchial cleft cyst. This, again, would be best evaluated by CT or perhaps MRI. Sometimes ultrasonography is used to confirm diffuse texture abnormality in patients with thyroiditis. Radionuclide studies are sometimes used in the same patients. These are usually not pivotal pieces of information in diagnosis or management.

Tumor

Imaging must be integrated with the clinical approach and results of needle biopsy in the evaluation of low-neck and possible thyroid masses. This basic approach is outlined in Figure 2–7. Ultrasonography is a reasonable starting point in some situations. In others, radionuclide study may be a logical first choice. CT and MRI are reserved for special clinical circumstances; either technique may be used to evaluate the extent of a goiter before surgical removal. The use of radionuclide studies in this setting is unnecessarily redundant and underinformative. What the surgeon basically needs is a map of the extent of the goiter and its relationship to the airway, as well as a full depiction of its extent in the neck and mediastinum. The simplest approach is to use MRI. CT is certainly a reasonable substitute for MRI in this situation. Moreover, if the mass is found to be something other than thyroid-related, MRI is quite useful for showing the relationship of the mass to the brachial plexus, trachea, esophagus, neural axis, and mediastinum in multiple planes. This can prove very useful in differential diagnosis as well as in surgical planning.

If the diagnosis of thyroid cancer is known, imaging is useful in planning overall management. If penetration of the thyroid gland capsule is likely, on the basis of clinical or ultrasonographic findings, MRI is a superior study for showing the local extent of the tumor. MRI is particularly good for detecting early tracheal invasion or involvement of the cervical esophagus (Fig. 2–53). CT is not as well suited to the detection of early tracheal invasion or esophageal invasion but is superior for evaluating cervical nodes. Ultrasonography is limited in its ability to show extraglandular spread but may also be used to evaluate cervical nodes. Radionuclide studies may be used to show residual disease in the neck or body after complete removal of normal, functioning thyroid tissue. MRI is clearly superior to any other imaging study for showing local recurrence of nonfunctioning thyroid cancers (Fig. 2–53). Because the relative contributions of all of these imaging studies are different, their specific use must be tailored to clinical needs in each individual case. Sometimes, more than one study is necessary.

Parathyroid Glands

Imaging of parathyroid glands is basically limited to evaluating patients with hyperparathyroidism. The need for imaging in preoperative localization of parathyroid adenomas is controversial. Some studies have shown that preoperative localization is cost efficient in that it can help limit the operation to one side of the neck, which reduces the time and, therefore, the cost of surgery. This also has the potential of reducing operative morbidity. Others argue that routine exploration of all four glands is curative in 90% of patients with parathyroid adenomas, and therefore preoperative localization is unnecessarily cost additive. Any imaging should be preceded by confirmation of elevated parathyroid hormone. In the patients who have not been previously operated on for hyperparathyroidism, ultrasonography or radionuclide studies (technetium-thallium subtraction studies) may be done. In experienced hands, ultrasonography will correctly

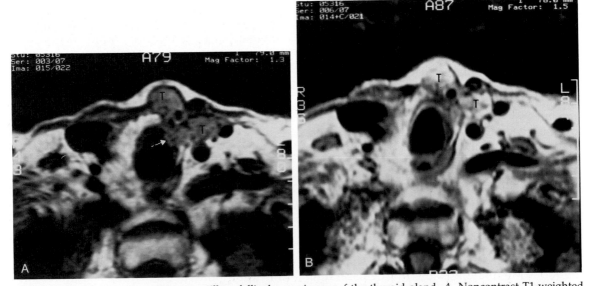

Figure 2–53. Patient with recurrent papillary-follicular carcinoma of the thyroid gland. *A.* Noncontrast T1-weighted image shows multilobulated recurrent tumor (T) with tracheal wall invasion (arrow). *B.* Contrast-enhanced MR shows tumor enhancement (T); tracheal wall invasion is slightly less evident.

localize an adenoma in 65% to 75% of previously nonoperated patients (Fig. 2–54). Radionuclide studies vary in quality, depending on the experience of the center. In the best hands, preoperative localization of parathyroid adenomas is estimated to be between 80% and 90% with these techniques.

For patients who have undergone surgery for recurrent hyperparathyroidism, virtually all surgeons request diagnostic imaging. Ultrasonography is usually not fruitful as an initial test. In this setting, it is probably best to start with technetium-thallium subtraction radionuclide studies. Alternatively, MRI may be done. MRI is probably superior to CT for evaluating patients with recurrent hyperparathyroidism. Ultrasonography may be used to confirm suspicious findings on radionuclide, MRI, or CT studies. Arteriography or venous sampling may also be used for confirmation. In very experienced hands, ablation of recurrent parathyroid adenomas may be attempted through an endovascular or percutaneous approach.

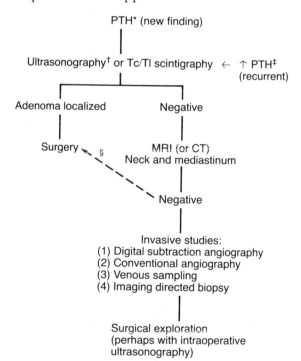

* Parathyroid hormone.

† Ultrasonography preferred for cost and convenience.

‡ Move down algorithm until two studies are positive *and* correlate anatomically. Tc/Tl preferred initially in recurrent cases.

§ Option in *non*recurrent cases.

Figure 2–54. Imaging options for patients with suspected parathyroid adenoma. (From Mancuso A: Workbook for MRI and CT of the Head and Neck, 2nd ed. Baltimore: Williams & Wilkins, 1989.)

Thoracic Inlet and Brachial Plexus

The low neck and thoracic inlet represents an area of crossover in clinical practice between various specialty and subspecialty interests, including the otolaryngologist, the head and neck surgeon, the thoracic surgeon, the neurologist, and the neurosurgeon, among others. Imaging is often pivotal in deciding which groups need to constitute the team that deals with the pathologic process at hand. Whenever abnormalities in the low neck are present, one must consider the thyroid as a source of origin. If the thyroid is likely to be the site of primary pathologic change, suggestions for evaluating the thyroid region in the earlier section on the thyroid gland should be reviewed and applied. Once the thyroid gland is excluded as a site of pathologic change, the imaging examination depends on the physical examination and other clinical factors.

If a mass at the thoracic inlet is suspected of being an abnormal or merely tortuous vessel, ultrasonography is the best starting point and may be the only study necessary. In most circumstances, MRI is probably the next best study for this region, with the possible exception of inflammatory masses. The reasons for the preference of CT to MRI in patients with inflammatory lesions were discussed in preceding sections on the neck, oropharynx, and larynx and hypopharynx. These reasons are, in general, related to morphologic features of the disease. Many of these patients are acutely uncomfortable and better suited to the faster CT examination as well.

If MRI examination can be done, it is perhaps the best study for evaluating lesions at the thoracic inlet. Numerous vascular structures are present, and flow-sensitive imaging techniques, including MRA, can show whether the pathologic process is arising from vessels or the effect of the pathologic process on the major brachial cephalic vessels in the region. The ability to image in multiple planes, especially coronally, is extremely valuable at the thoracic inlet. Also, pathologic change at the thoracic inlet may arise from, or secondarily involve, the brachial plexus or more proximal neural axis; MRI is clearly superior for showing the extent of pathologic change in relation to the central nervous system. Angiography should be used whenever imaging studies or the clinical situation suggests the need. Adjunctive radionuclide studies are sometimes useful in suspected thyroid and parathyroid disease; this was discussed in earlier sections. Gallium SPECT studies might be useful in patients with vertebral osteomyelitis or soft tissue inflammatory disease for both diagnosis and as a means of following medical therapy. Fluoroscopic examination, with either barium swallow or water-soluble contrast swallow, may prove useful in selected circumstances. If perforation of the esophagus is suspected, water-soluble contrast should be used. Plain films and conventional tomography rarely add any additional information; however, subtle observations made on the basis of plain films are often the clues that lead to further investigation with advanced imaging examinations.

SUGGESTED READINGS

Ballantyne AJ: Routines of spread. *In* Fletcher GH, McComb WS (eds): Radiation Therapy in the Management of Cancers of the Oral Cavity and Oropharynx. Springfield, IL: Charles C Thomas, 1962.

Ballantyne AJ: Significance of retropharyngeal nodes in cancer of the head and neck. Am J Surg 108:500, 1964.

Berland LL: Practical CT. Technology and Techniques. New York: Raven Press, 1987.

Brant-Zawadzki M, Normal D: Magnetic Resonance Imaging of the Central Nervous System. Section I, Basic Principles (pp 1–114). New York: Raven Press, 1987.

Friedman M, Shelton VK, Mafee M, et al: Metastatic neck disease: evaluation of computed tomography. Arch Otolaryngol 110:443–447, 1984.

Harnsberger HR (ed): Cranial nerve imaging. Semin Ultrasound CT MR 8(3):163–312, 1987.

Harnsberger HR, Mancuso AA, Muraki AS: The upper aerodigestive tract and neck: CT evaluation of recurrent tumors. Radiology 149:503–509, 1983.

Lederman M: Cancer of the Nasopharynx: Its Natural History and Treatment. Springfield, IL: Charles C Thomas, 1961.

Lederman M: Cancer of the oral cavity: observations on classification and natural history. Int J Radiat Oncol Biol Phys 6:1559–1565, 1980.

Lederman M: Cancer of the oropharynx: classification and natural history. Int J Radiat Oncol Biol Phys 8:1379–1391, 1982.

Mafee MF: Acoustic neuroma and other acoustic nerve disorders: role of CT and MRI: an analysis of 238 cases. Semin Ultrasound CT and MR 8(3):256–283, 1987.

Mancuso AA: MRI and CT of the Head and Neck. Baltimore: Williams & Wilkins, 1989.

Mancuso AA, Hanafee WN: Computed tomography of the injured larynx. Radiology 133:139–144, 1979.

Mancuso AA, Hanafee WN: Elusive head and neck cancer beneath intact mucosa. Laryngoscope 93:133–139, 1983.

Mancuso AA, Hanafee WN: Computed Tomography and Magnetic Resonance Imaging of the Head and Neck, 2nd ed. Baltimore: Williams & Wilkins, 1985.

Mancuso AA, Harnsberger HR, Muraki AS, Stevens MH: Computed tomography of cervical and retropharyngeal lymph nodes: normal anatomy, variants of normal and applications in staging head and neck. Part II. Pathology. Radiology 148:715–723, 1983.

Miller DL, Doppman JL, Shwaker TH, et al: Localization of parathyroid adenomas in patients who have undergone surgery. Parts I and II. Radiology 162:137–141, 1987.

Muraki AS, Mancuso AA, Harnsberger HR: CT of the oropharynx, tongue base and floor of the mouth: normal variations and applications in staging carcinoma. Radiology 148:725–731, 1983.

Muraki AS, Mancuso AA, Harnsberger HR: Metastatic cervical adenopathy from tumors of unknown origin: the role of CT. Radiology 152:749–754, 1984.

Newton TH, Potts DG (eds): Technical Aspects of Computed Tomography, vol 5. Radiology of the Skull and Brain. St. Louis: CV Mosby, 1981.

Oloffsson J, van Nostrand AWP: Growth and spread of laryngeal and hypopharyngeal carcinoma with reflections on the effect of preoperative irradiation; 139 cases studied by whole organ serial sectioning. Acta Otolaryngol 308(Suppl):1–84, 1973.

Peck WW, Higgins CB, Fisher MR, et al: Hyperparathyroidism: comparison of MR imaging with radionuclide scanning. Radiology 162:143–146, 1987.

Rouvier H: Anatomy of the Human Lymphatic System (pp 1–82). Ann Arbor, MI: Edwards Brothers, 1938.

Schaefer SD, Marbel M, Diehl I, et al: Computed tomographic assessment of squamous cell carcinoma of oral and pharyngeal cavities. Arch Otolaryngol 108:688–692, 1982.

Som PM, Bergeron RT: Head and Neck Imaging. St. Louis: CV Mosby, 1991.

Som PM, Braun IF, Shapiro MD, et al: Tumors of the parapharyngeal space and upper neck: MR imaging characteristics. Radiology 164:823–829, 1987.

Swartz J: Imaging of the Temporal Bone. Stuttgart: Thieme Medical Publishers, 1986.

Tucker GF: The anatomy of laryngeal cancer. Can J Otolaryngol 3:417–427, 1974.

Vignaud J, Jardin C, Rosen L: The Ear. Diagnostic Imaging. Paris: Masson Publishing, 1986.

CHAPTER 3

Headache and Facial Pain

Frank E. Lucente, MD, FACS   Jeffrey E. Goldberg, MD

Pain in the head and neck region is a ubiquitous phenomenon that is a constant source of aggravation to millions of patients, as well as a constant diagnostic and therapeutic challenge to physicians and other health care workers in numerous specialties. Approximately 45 million Americans annually have headaches that are sufficiently severe or frequent to prompt them to seek medical attention. Half of those who seek help consider the pain to be a major disruptive force in their daily lives. The economic impact of headache is also significant in that approximately 140 million work days are lost each year, and it is estimated that a loss of $8 billion in productivity and expenditures for health care and medications occurs as a result of headaches.

For some patients headaches are a simple annoyance, whereas for others they become an incapacitating disability. The experience of pain itself is an unpleasant sensation and is often accompanied by the psychologic distress of knowing that this sensation is occurring in a region of many important structures whose functions include communication, cognitive perception, and maintenance of physical appearance. Because of this dual physical and psychologic impact, facial pain and headache necessitate prompt diagnosis and efficient treatment.

It is important to attempt to understand the dual nature of the experience of pain. The perception of pain results from the activation of nociceptive afferent sensory fibers and transmission of impulses along known neuroanatomic pathways. The analysis and processing of these painful impulses are anatomically localized in the brain. For most persons, the mental state or emotion that is the basis for the unpleasant experience is elusive. It is not clear why the same stimulus for two individuals or the same stimulus for a single individual on different occasions produces vastly different emotional responses.

The current understanding of headache and facial pain has evolved over centuries during which physicians, scientists, and medical practitioners of various sorts, including priests and barbers, have studied the uncomfortable phenomena occurring in the head and neck. In ancient civilizations, including the Babylonian society, the source of pain was thought to be external and to result from an intrusion of a magical force or an insidious evil spirit into the body. In some societies, pain was viewed as a punishment for wrongdoing.

Perhaps the first advance in elevating disease above the mystical level was found in ancient Europe. The Edwin Smith papyrus is a document that was copied by scribes of the 16th century B.C. from earlier medical writings ascribed to the era of Imhotep of the third Egyptian dynasty. The papyrus contains classifications of diseases and recommendations for specific therapy. This document represents the first rational approach to treatment beyond previously existing folk remedies. Interestingly, the Egyptian civilization did not prohibit human dissections, and extensive studies were therefore performed on mummies. This was the source of some of the early information regarding nasal, sinus, and cranial anatomy.

The pharmacologic treatment of pain and of other physical complaints began in India; there are records, dating as far back as 4000 B.C., of hundreds of pain remedies derived from mineral, plant, and animal sources. The ancient Chinese viewed the human situation as representative of a harmonious universe with a balance between yin and yang, two primitive forces. Pain was thought to result from disturbance of the balance between these forces, such as what might occur in emotional extremes. The relief of pain came when the balance between yin and yang was re-established.

With the development of civilization in the Greco-Roman world, there was an attempt to understand human phenomena according to rational natural laws. Hippocrates of Cos (c. 460–360 B.C.) was greatly concerned about the causes and relief of pain and focused on the thought that pain was a manifestation of some derangement within the body. However, it remained for the Alexandrian physicians and scientists, such as Herophilus (315–280 B.C.), to perform extensive anatomic dissections to facilitate the identification of the brain as the seat of motor and sensory function. In Rome, Galen (131–201 A.D.) determined that pain was the most primitive form of conscious sensation and was caused by disruption in tissues.

In subsequent centuries, there was great interest in neuroanatomy (with special attention to afferent pain pathways), neurophysiology, and, more recently, neuroendocrinology (including the role of endorphins).

Interestingly, all of the various theories and discoveries led to the current understanding of the anatomic basis of the various painful sensations that originate in the head and neck as being stimuli that originate at peripheral nociceptive sites and are conducted along nerve fibers and across synapses to areas where recognition and interpretation occur.

In this chapter, some of the causes of headache and facial pain according to medical subspecialty are considered. However, it is important to remember that each occurrence of pain should be understood in the comprehensive psychobiologic perspective (mind-body interaction), which influences diagnosis and treatment.

SOURCES OF PAIN IN THE NASAL AND PARANASAL SINUSES

The origins of rhinologic disease are discussed in Chapters 21 to 26 and are not covered in depth here. However, the importance of the nose and paranasal sinuses as a source of primary and referred pain in the head and neck is pertinent to the discussion. The paranasal sinuses share a close anatomic relationship with several neural and vascular structures: the carotid artery, the trigeminal nerve, the optic nerve, the cavernous sinus and pharyngopalatine fossas and their contents, the olfactory nerve, and the sympathetic plexus. These structures are common sites of headache and facial pain. The nose and paranasal sinuses adjoin the orbit, or the cranial fossa, and the oral cavity.

The nose and sinuses are lined with respiratory mucosa, which is susceptible to metabolic, inflammatory, neoplastic, traumatic, developmental, and idiopathic pathologic processes causing pain. A working knowledge of the sensory innervation of the nose and sinuses allows interpretation of pain and patterns of pain referral in this region.

The paranasal sinuses are innervated at their ostia and throughout their mucosal lining. Frontal sinus pain is usually localized above the eyes over the involved sinus but may be sensed over the temporal region or the occiput. The pain of acute inflammation is a persistent aching with pressure. Frontal sinus barotrauma should be suspected if the onset of symptoms occurs after an airplane flight, diving, or use of a high-speed, high-rise elevator; the other sinuses are rarely affected.

Ethmoid sinus pain may be experienced in the medial orbit region, the eye, or the vertex of the head. Ethmoid sinusitis in adults is usually part of a pansinusitis. Solitary ethmoiditis can, however, occur in children, particularly those with cystic fibrosis.

Sphenoid sinus pain is often referred to the vertex and may radiate to the temporal region, the occiput, or the canine tooth. This pain-referral pattern can be explained by a common innervation of the sinus and intracranial structures, such as blood vessels and dura and the first and second branches of the trigeminal nerve. When head pain is dull, diffuse, poorly localized, and unresponsive to therapy, the sphenoid sinus should be evaluated radiographically.

Ethmoid pain may occasionally radiate to the upper cervical region or cause referred pain in the shoulder. This referral pattern may be caused by overlap of the nucleus and spinal tract of the trigeminal nerve with the dorsal horn of the cervical spinal cord. When such overlap occurs after efferent stimulation of the sympathetic neurons, pain receptors are stimulated at the corresponding thoracic levels.

Maxillary sinus pain is perceived over the involved sinus and in the roots of the second premolar and first and second molars. These teeth insert into the sinus, and inflammation may result in lancinating pain. Antral pain is described as a sensation of pressure or burning. Polyps cause pain only if they are situated near a nerve or cause inflammation by ostial obstruction.

It has been suggested that contact of the inferior turbinate with the nasal septum may be responsible for headache that is reported by some patients with septal deviation. Septoplasty may occasionally relieve this pain when other therapies have failed.

HEADACHE AND FACIAL PAIN CAUSED BY OCULAR ABNORMALITIES

Pain and headache of ocular origin are inconsistently accompanied by easily discernible signs on physical examination and merit ophthalmologic evaluation.

Asthenopia refers to a specific group of disorders of the eye that result from strain and subsequent fatigue of the muscles associated with accommodation and convergence. Patients may complain of orbital or periorbital pain, episodic blurring of vision, pulling, retrobulbar pressure, deep pain within the skull, vertigo, and even nausea and vomiting.

Accommodative asthenopia may be due to hyperopia, presbyopia, astigmatism, or paresis of accommodative muscles secondary to pharmacologic mydriasis or intrinsic ophthalmoplegia. Treatment, through corrective lenses, is aimed at eliminating the need for sustained accommodative effort. Symptoms gradually resolve.

Muscular asthenopia results in similar symptoms and is due to muscle fatigue secondary to strabismus correction to allow fu-

sion of images. Surgery may sometimes be necessary to correct the alignment of the eyes. The muscle imbalance may be congenital or acquired secondary to tumor or cerebrovascular accident and should be investigated.

Herpes zoster may cause severe pain of the skin surrounding the eyes. Diagnosis is difficult before presentation of lesions in the distribution of the ophthalmic division of the trigeminal nerve.

Hutchinson's sign or pain involving the tip of the nose suggests intraocular involvement of the nasociliary ganglion.

Blepharitis is inflammation of the eyelid margins that is usually caused by staphylococcal infection. Disruption of normal corneal moisturization can result in irregularity of the corneal epithelium and diffraction of light, which leads to asthenopic symptoms. The patient also complains of eyelid discomfort and puffiness with crusting and irregularity of eyelash alignment. Treatment includes cleansing with warm water and application of a broad-spectrum ophthalmic ointment.

Abnormal eyelid position such as entropion and ectropion can also lead to asthenopic symptoms as a result of direct corneal irritation or tear film abnormalities. Artificial tears may help to avoid corneal ulcerations and ensuing pain. Surgical repair is indicated in severe cases.

Inflammation of the conjunctiva can cause orbital pain and pruritus. Chronic inflammation may compromise mucin production, which is crucial to corneal health. Ocular decongestants are suggested for acute viral conjunctivitis and wide-spectrum antibiotic ointment for bacterial infection. If complaints are severe, with conjunctival scarring, an autoimmune process should be suspected, and ophthalmologic consultation is recommended.

Ulceration and foreign bodies on the cornea can cause sudden severe ocular pain with hyperemia of the conjunctiva. Degeneration of the cornea, the most powerful accommodative structure in the eye, causes asthenopic symptoms.

Glaucoma may cause pain if onset is sudden. This is especially true in acute angle-closure glaucoma. Primary open-angle glaucoma is generally not painful. Acute angle-closure glaucoma presents with sudden, boring eye pain and decrease in visual acuity. Conjunctival hyperemia and dulled corneal reflexes with poor pupillary light reflex are seen. Treatment with timolol maleate drops and acetazolamide is indicated. Laser surgery may be curative. Occasionally, some tumors of the orbit can cause pain associated with glaucoma. Choroid sarcomas and gliomas of the retina classically present with the throbbing pain and signs of glaucoma.

Uveitis, or inflammation of the uvea within the eye, may be of idiopathic, autoimmune, or infectious origin. Patients complain of dull ocular pain with photophobia. Erythema of the sclera surrounding the cornea is often present. Treatment is dictated by cause. Steroids should be withheld until the diagnosis is established because their inappropriate administration in the presence of a bacterial infection may allow the infection to worsen.

Symptoms of optic neuritis include decreased or blurred vision in association with a sharp, boring pain behind the eye. Pain is exacerbated by eye movement. Physical examination usually reveals loss of visual acuity, elevation of the optic disks, and a Marcus Gunn pupil.

Dacryocystitis is an inflammation of the lacrimal gland secondary to impedance of outflow of tears. This obstruction usually occurs at or distal to the origin of the nasolacrimal duct. Rhinitis is a common cause of this disorder. Acute dacryocystitis manifests with fever, excruciating pain, local erythema, and swelling. The diagnosis of acute dacryocystitis should be considered for any patient with nasal mucosal inflammation presenting with the aforementioned symptoms.

HEADACHE AND THE NEURALGIAS

Many causes of headache or facial pain stem from or coincide with neurologic disorders. Early suspicion of these diagnoses allows proper medical therapies and avoids unnecessary search for elusive otolaryngologic causes of pain. Headache is caused by irritation of any of four general pain-sensitive structures in the head: (1) the scalp and attached muscles, (2) intracranial and extracranial blood vessels, (3) the skull and periosteum, and (4) the meninges.

Muscle contraction headaches typically present as dull and aching. Pain may be localized to the frontal, occipital, nuctral, or vertex region. Pain usually begins in the morning and progressively worsens throughout the day, peaking in the late afternoon. These headaches generally respond to the patient's recumbency and to common analgesics; if they do not, intracranial disease should be suspected.

Headaches of vascular origin are often pulsatile and exacerbated by head movement and physical exertion. Pain generally becomes more severe over a period of minutes and may last for hours to days. The patient may also complain of photophobia or sonophobia, nausea, and vomiting.

Headaches caused by expanding intracranial lesions typically worsen in the recumbent position and may awaken the sleeping patient. Focal neurologic signs, as well as nausea and vomiting, may be present.

The migraine headache is a hemicranial vascular headache that reflects a local vascular change in a branch of the external carotid system. Local vasoconstriction precedes vasodilation; release of pain produces polypeptides, kallikreinogens, and prostaglandins. These recurring headaches occur first in childhood or in adolescence. There is often a strong family history of migraine headaches. They are more common in women than in men and are closely associated with menstruation.

The "classic" migraine presents with a prodrome, usually a visual disturbance, although other sensory disturbances as well as aphasia, hemiplegia, and hemianopsia may occur. The prodrome fades within an hour and is followed by typical migraine symptoms. The prodrome actually occurs in less than 10% of migraine headaches. The characteristics of migraine headache are throbbing, hemicranial, and usually frontotemporal pain, which may be accompanied by nausea and vomiting. Sleeping in a dark room may help to relieve symptoms.

Cluster headaches, also called histamine headaches, typically cause unilateral temporal or retrobulbar pain that is described as boring or stabbing. These headaches occur in temporal clusters frequently for weeks to months and are followed by periods of quiescence. There is a preponderance of episodes in spring and fall. Males are more commonly affected than females. Unlike migraine headaches, cluster headaches are never associated with nausea or vomiting. Episodes of cluster headaches often occur at night and are associated with lacrimation and unilateral nasal congestion and rhinorrhea.

Primary therapy includes ergotamines and avoidance of alcohol. Methysergide and prednisone may also be effective in some cases.

Headache may occur secondary to hypertension and result from both vascular dilation and secondary muscle contraction. Its onset typically is gradual with amelioration as the day progresses. Hypertension is rarely the cause of headache in patients whose systolic blood pressure is less than 150 mm Hg. Severity of pain does not correlate with severity of hypertension.

Giant cell arteritis, also termed temporal arteritis, is an idiopathic vasculitis that most commonly affects the ophthalmic, retinal, or temporal arteries of the elderly population, more commonly women. Patients complain of a deep throbbing headache with a burning component and frequently of hyperalgesia of the scalp. Pain is frequently retro-orbital but may be localized to the scalp, the jaws, the tongue, or the neck. On physical examination, the region over the temporal artery is usually exquisitely tender and erythematous. One should suspect temporal arteritis when the erythrocyte sedimentation rate is greater than 40 mm/min. Diagnosis is made from results of temporal artery biopsy. Treatment of choice is steroid administration.

Classic neuralgias include both trigeminal and vagoglossopharyngeal neuralgia and are defined by the following criteria:

1. A stabbing or searing paranasal pain that occurs in the known distribution of a cranial or peripheral nerve. This marked dysthetic sensation generally lasts for seconds to minutes. Patients often report a residual persistent ache.

2. Episodes may be brought on by stimulation of trigger zones within the area of innervation.

3. There is no objective sensory or motor loss in the distribution of the involved nerve.

Perhaps the best-known neuralgia of the head and neck is *trigeminal neuralgia,* also termed *tic douloureux.* This entity may be associated with one of several pathologic conditions. Vascular compromise was reported to be responsible for up to 90% of all cases in one study. In other studies, up to 40% of cases have been reported to be idiopathic. Other associated conditions include multiple sclerosis, intracranial tumors, arachnoiditis, and congenital anomalies. Twenty-five percent of patients with multiple sclerosis have trigeminal neuralgia.

Trigeminal neuralgia has a right-sided preponderance and occurs more commonly in women. Approximately 90% of patients are over 40 years of age. Typically, patients report recurrent episodes of sudden sharp pain that may be described as similar to a bolt of lightning and unbearable. Each episode lasts up to 1 minute. The region innervated by the second and third divisions of the trigeminal nerve is affected in 95% of cases.

The aforementioned trigger zones are typically 2 to 4 mm in size and are usually in the caudal region of the nose, the perioral region, or the gingival regions. Pain may be brought on by the application or the withdrawal of pressure as well as by vibratory stimuli, which affect everyday activities such as brushing teeth, speaking, and chewing and make trigeminal neuralgia a particularly debilitating condition.

In general, medical therapy is tried first in an attempt to control pain. Carbamazepine (Tegretol) is the drug of choice for primary therapy. It has been shown to alleviate symptoms in 70% to 75% of patients. Neurosurgical therapy is aimed at selective lysis of pain fibers of the trigeminal ganglion and relief of vascular compression, if present, through a variety of intranasal approaches. The pain may recur in up to 30% of patients after surgery, and in rare instances patients may suffer from a severe, chronic facial postoperative pain syndrome.

Vagoglossopharyngeal neuralgia is a recurrent lancinating pain that occurs in the somatosensory distribution of the vagus and glossopharyngeal nerves. It usually begins in the throat or the ears and radiates to the tonsillar region, the posterior third of the tongue, the eustachian tube, the external auditory canal, and the larynx. Pain is most commonly triggered by swallowing but may follow coughing, eating spicy food, or even touching the tragus. The cause is often not identified but may be due to cranial nerve compression by vertebral or posterior inferior cerebellar arteries or by metastatic laryngeal cancer.

Vagoglossopharyngeal neuralgia is a rare entity; it occurs only 1% as frequently as trigeminal neuralgia. As with trigeminal neuralgia, 90% of patients with vagoglossopharyngeal neuralgia are 40 years of age or older. However, of vagoglossopharyngeal neuralgia cases a preponderance occur on the left side, and incidences are equal in both sexes. Pain frequently occurs at night.

Diagnosis of this condition is often made after a thorough history and a physical examination. Application of 10% cocaine solution to the trigger zones can aid in eliminating pain. Medical therapy is less effective for vagoglossopharyngeal neuralgia than for trigeminal neuralgia. Carbamazepine is the drug of choice. Surgical approaches include glossopharyngeal rhizotomy, upper vagal root sectioning, microvascular decompression, and radiofrequency coagulation of the petrous ganglion.

Post-herpetic neuralgia occurs most commonly in patients older than 60 years, and patients in this age bracket constitute 90% of all cases. Up to 10% of patients over 70 years of age suffer from post-herpetic neuralgia after a herpes zoster infection. When the trigeminal nerve and its ganglion are involved, the ophthalmic division alone is affected in 80% of patients. The uncommon involvement of the geniculate ganglion (Ramsay Hunt syndrome) is characterized by the presence of an external auditory canal eruption and ipsilateral facial weakness. Pain may precede the cutaneous manifestations by as much as 2 weeks, but vesicular eruptions eventually appear.

Medical therapy for the post-herpetic pain syndrome consists of psychotropic drugs. Amitriptyline hydrochloride is the current drug of choice. Early steroid therapy or administration of acyclovir (Zovirax) during herpes zoster infections may reduce the incidence of subsequent neuralgia.

Raeder's syndrome is characterized by a throbbing, often persistent headache in the distribution of the ophthalmic and upper maxillary divisions of the trigeminal nerve, as well as by ipsilateral Horner's syndrome with preservation of the mechanism for perspiration. Two patient populations have been identified. Group I patients often have presellar cranial nerve involvement. Symptoms may be associated with metastases to the middle cranial fossa, calcification of the internal carotid artery, infections of or trauma to the petrous apex, and meningioma of the gasserian ganglion. Group II patients do not have postsellar cranial nerve involvement. Causes of group II Raeder's syndrome and associated conditions include upper respiratory infection, chronic sinusitis, dental abscesses, hypertension, migraine headache, and aneurysm of the supracavernous portion of the internal carotid artery. Most patients are male. There is a predominance of left-sided occurrences. Treatment of group I patients is directed at the underlying diseases. Group II disease often has a self-limited course. Amitriptyline has proved beneficial for relief of pain in some instances.

Occipital neuralgia can be divided into primary and secondary types. Primary occipital neuralgia is a true neuralgia characterized by lancinating unilateral pain in the distribution of the occipital nerve with identifiable trigger zones. Secondary occipital neuralgia is accompanied by nuchal spasm and may be associated with cervical spondylosis, craniocervical malformations, syringomyelia, and Arnold-Chiari malformation. The pain in this latter group of patients is a more persistent, dull ache that may be bilateral. Treatment of secondary neuralgia depends on the underlying disease. The primary type often responds to amitriptyline or phenytoin (Dilantin). Local blockade of the occipital nerve may be successful when medical therapy fails. Surgery is reserved for unresponsive cases.

Eagle's syndrome is characterized by intense, persistent unilateral facial and parapharyngeal pain, headache, dysphagia, odynophagia, and progressive trismus. Symptoms may mimic those of vagoglossopharyngeal neuralgia but are caused by elongation and calcification of the styloid process and the styloid ligament, which are proximal to cranial nerves V, VII, IX, and X. Diagnosis is made by intraoral palpation of the styloid process and is confirmed by radiograph. Treatment is resection of the styloid process.

Sluder's syndrome is a neuralgia of the sphenopalatine ganglion and is associated with vasomotor abnormalities of lacrimation, rhinorrhea, and salivation. Patients describe a lancinating pain centered on the orbit and radiating laterally and inferiorly to the nose, the palate, the maxillary teeth, the temple, and the zygoma. Relief of symptoms by anesthetic infiltration of the sphenopalatine ganglion confirms diagnosis. Treatment is controversial, but sphenopalatine ganglion neurectomy may offer symptomatic relief.

Causalgia, or reflux sympathetic dystrophy of the face, should be suspected in patients who present with persistent burning facial pain after facial trauma or difficult dental or maxillofacial surgery. Discomfort may be exacerbated by tactile or thermal stimulation and by emotional stress. Successful treatment with sympathetic blockade of the stellate ganglion has been reported. Sympathectomy is reserved for patients who receive only temporary relief from blockade.

TEMPOROMANDIBULAR JOINT PAIN AND MYOFASCIAL PAIN DYSFUNCTION

Three functional and anatomic abnormalities related to jaw movement and mastication can alone or concomitantly produce myofascial pain and headache: (1) functional abnormalities of the muscles of mastication, (2) intrinsic disease of the temporomandibular joint, and (3) static and dynamic abnormalities of dental occlusion. In general, abnormal function of the muscles of mastication, if present, is addressed first.

Myofascial pain dysfunction syndrome is caused by an intrinsic abnormality of the muscles of mastication. This muscle group includes the masseter, the temporalis, and the medial and lateral pterygoids. Spasm secondary to chronic fatigue or injury can cause abnormal function of one or more of these muscles, preventing smooth dynamic action of the functional masticatory unit. Berges (1973) described four signs that are helpful in the diagnosis of myofascial pain syndrome:

1. The jump sign: the patient jumps in response to finger palpation of the involved muscle.
2. The rope muscle sign: muscle fascicles feel like ropes lying next to one another.
3. Dermographia: blanching and hyperemia in response to stroking over the affected muscle.
4. Elimination of pain by local anesthesia administered to trigger zones. Patients frequently give a history of a recent dental or surgical procedure involving intubation or a history of habits such as tooth grinding or chronic gum chewing.

Other common causes include adaptive posturing secondary either to nasal obstruction and mouth breathing or to abnormal dental occlusion, and stress alone may cause myofacial pain dysfunction in these predisposed persons. Symptoms may include muscle tenderness and swelling, trismus, malocclusion, and clicking of the meniscus.

Symptoms related to intrinsic joint disease include preauricular pain, limitation of mandibular movement, swelling, tenderness, crepitus, and changes in dental occlusal relationships. The temporomandibular joint is a highly innervated region. The articular surfaces of the joints are not highly innervated; destruction of these surfaces, however, exposes innervated bone below the fibrous joint capsule and other regional connective tissue that is also innervated and elicits pain. Inflammation of the joint may be secondary to acute or chronic trauma. Patients with a loose joint capsule are predisposed to repeated trauma and subsequent inflammation. Inflammation may be secondary to degenerative osteoarthritis or infection within the joint. The temporomandibular joint is also frequently involved in rheumatoid arthritis. Other causes of temporomandibular joint pain include systemic lupus erythematosus, polyarteritis nodosa, Reiter's syndrome, and psoriasis.

Primary dental occlusive abnormalities may cause facial pain and headache that initially result from spasm of the muscles of mastication and later from intrinsic disease of the temporomandibular joint. Diagnosis requires a careful dental examination because minor malocclusions can be responsible for muscle spasm.

The primary therapy for these associated disorders is aimed at reducing inflammation and, consequently, pain. Nonsteroidal anti-inflammatory medications such as ibuprofen along with warm compresses and a soft diet are helpful. Treatment of neuromuscular dysfunction is addressed first, because its successful therapy may obviate any need for treating joint disease or occlusal abnormalities.

One such treatment is transcutaneous electrical neural stimulation (TENS) therapy. This form of therapy effectively relaxes muscles, which allows attainment of resting occlusal posture. TENS therapy may also cause endogenous analgesia through release of endorphins.

Occlusal adjustment is another effective treatment for many patients with myofascial pain disorders. Orthotics allow for reversible adjustment of occlusion, and coronoplasty offers permanent bite modification. Both allow for a better resting occlusal posture.

DENTAL CAUSES OF FACIAL PAIN

Pain originating in the teeth, like pain of sinus origin, may be localized to the diseased tooth or referred to other regions of the head and neck without any apparent primary site for the pain. Odontogenic pain is usually secondary to dental caries or chronic periodontal disease. Other hard tissue diseases of the oral cavity such as posterior molar eruption, occult tooth, retained roots, odontogenic cysts and tumors, and osseous fractures may be responsible for facial pain or headache. Mandibular molars may cause temporal, auricular, or preauricular pain. Maxillary teeth can be responsible for orbital, retro-orbital, or parietal pain. Peripheral nerve block may help differentiate between primary and referred pain sources.

The pain of dental caries is usually sharp and throbbing and may be triggered by thermal changes or application of irritating substances (including sweets) early in the disease process. Periodontal disease may cause similar symptoms if a periodontal abscess is present. Analgesic therapy and expedient dental consultation are recommended for patients who present with these problems.

PSYCHIATRIC ISSUES IN FACIAL PAIN

The psychiatric contribution to headache or facial pain and the patient's perception of the pain must not be overlooked in the evaluation of such patients. Failure to recognize and provide appropriate treatment for the psychologic aspect of the experience of pain may prevent the success of any proposed program of therapy.

It is important to recognize the strong psychologic investment of most people with regard to the condition of head and neck structures. For example, pain involving the organs of speech and hearing may be interpreted by the patient as a threat to the ability to communicate. Conversely, throat pain and laryngitis may reflect a psychologic conflict concerning communication. Patients may also exhibit almost incredible denial of their illness or of the possible causes of the disease.

The examining physician may have developed attitudes toward pain that influence his or her response to a patient's complaints. These attitudes should not be allowed to interfere with appropriate therapy for the patient.

Recognition of certain descriptive patterns of patients may alert the physician to the psychologic contribution to headache and facial pain. Engel (1951) described a syndrome of "atypical facial pain" that he noted among patients whom he described as a "uniformly unhappy, and unsatisfied group of people." Evidence of psychologic difficulty was consistently present among these patients, all of whom had poor marital, work, and social relationships.

In Engel's description, atypical facial pain is usually aching, poorly localized, and diffuse without neuritic character or correspondence to known neuroanatomy. The pain lasts for hours, days, or months and is variable in intensity and duration. There are no trigger zones or provocative factors. Depression and neurotic (obsessive-compulsive) traits are important factors in causation. Hysterical features are common, as are insomnia, fatigue, mood changes, and weeping spells. The pain is frequently associated with gastrointestinal complaints, dizziness, fainting, and obviously hysterical sensory and motor deficits. Relief has been obtained with antidepressants in a large percentage of patients in controlled studies.

Hacket (1978) developed the seven-item Madison Scale to help evaluate the relative significance of psychogenic factors in a patient's complaint of pain. Each characteristic of pain is evaluated on a scale of 0 to 4. A total score of 15 or above suggests the need for further psychiatric interventions. The Madison scale items are Multiplicity (pain occurs in more than one place or in more than one variety); Authenticity (the patient very much wants the physician to believe that the pain is real); Denial (the patient denies the presence of any emotional problems); Interpersonal relationships (the patient shows evidence of disturbance at the mention of the name of someone who may have something directly and indirectly, or symbolically, to do with him or her); Singularity (the patient stresses that he or she has a singular and unusual pain that distinguishes him or her from all other patients); "Only you" (the patient emphasizes that "only you can help me, doctor"); and Nothing helps (the patient stresses that nothing has worked in his previous therapy).

Patients with certain character disorders

may have syndromes of headache or facial pain as part of their clinical picture. The hysterical personality or compensation neurosis patient may present with intractable pain. Clinical presentation often involves nausea, fatigue, depression, and anxiety.

The patient with a masochistic personality disorder frequently presents with pain and suffering and unconsciously pursues this suffering. The disorder is frustrating to treat because psychiatric therapy is often no more effective than other therapies.

Depression may be a cause or a consequence of chronic pain. Patients with generalized anxiety or depression with stress phenomena, such as jaw clenching, may present with temporomandibular joint pain and myofacial pain disorder. Conversely, a stressful major life event, such as loss of a loved one or divorce, may initiate a facial pain or headache syndrome. Patients with chronic unalleviated pain often exhibit features of a major depressive disorder, including disturbances of appetite or sleep, social withdrawal, and suicidal ideation.

The diagnosis of malingering is a consideration for some patients with chronic pain. Potential secondary gain should be explored. Chronic pain and associated behavior may be reinforced by sympathetic attention, avoidance of conflict by peers and family, and avoidance of work. The diagnosis should be approached carefully when malingering is suspected.

Regardless of the causes of headache and facial pain, it is important for the otolaryngologist to recognize the need for psychiatric consultation when pain is present. Tact, encouragement, and empathy are key ingredients to successful referral, which should be portrayed as an adjunct to the patient's current therapy rather than as a last resort.

In summary, there are numerous causes for headache and facial pain. Formulating a correct diagnosis and initiating a proper therapeutic plan are predicated on the performance of a comprehensive clinical evaluation and the use of consultations as needed. This is one of the most complex aspects of otolaryngology, and the need for interdisciplinary communication is paramount.

SUGGESTED READINGS

Adams R, Victor M: Principles of Neurology, 3rd ed. New York: McGraw-Hill, 1985.

Berges PU: Myofascial pain syndrome. Postgrad Med 53:161–168, 1973.

Cooper BC: Craniomandibular disorders. *In* Cooper BC, Lucente FE (eds): Management of Facial, Head and Neck Pain (pp. 153–254). Philadelphia: WB Saunders, 1989.

Cooper BC, Lucente FE (eds): Management of Facial, Head and Neck Pain. Philadelphia: WB Saunders, 1989.

Dalessio D (ed): Wolff's Headache and Other Head Pain, 5th ed. New York: Oxford University Press, 1985.

Engel GL: Primary atypical facial neuralgia: an hysterical conversion symptom. Psychosom Med 13:375–396, 1951.

Glazer MA: Atypical facial pain diagnosis, cause and treatment. Arch Intern Med 65:340–367, 1940.

Greenidge KD, Dweck M: Head pain associated with the eye. *In* Cooper BC, Lucente FE (eds): Management of Facial, Head and Neck Pain (pp. 77–98). Philadelphia: WB Saunders, 1989.

Hackett TP: The pain patient, the evaluation and treatment. *In* Hackett TP, Cassem NH (eds): MGH Handbook of General Hospital Psychiatry. St. Louis: CV Mosby, 1978.

Kessler JT: Neurological causes of head and face pain. *In* Cooper BC, Lucente FE (eds): Management of Facial, Head and Neck Pain (pp. 23–51). Philadelphia: WB Saunders, 1989.

Kimmelman CP: Rhinologic causes of facial pain. *In* Cooper BC, Lucente FE (eds): Management of Facial, Head and Neck Pain (pp. 99–114). Philadelphia: WB Saunders, 1989.

Lipton JA, Varoscak JA, Lund P, et al: Considerations when diagnosing and treating facial pain patients. N Y State Dent J 49:286–288, 1983.

Lucente FE: Psychiatric problems in otolaryngology. Ann Otol Rhinol Laryngol 82:340–346, 1973.

Lucente FE, Sobol SM: Essentials of Otolaryngology. New York: Raven Press, 1983.

CHAPTER 4

Speech Pathology: Evaluation and Treatment of Speech, Language, Cognitive, and Swallowing Disorders

Daniel Kempler, PhD

Speech pathologists evaluate and treat disorders of voice, articulation, resonance, language, cognition, and swallowing. This chapter provides an overview of the field and is organized as follows. The first section is a review of normal and abnormal speech production, including production of voice at the level of the vocal cords, articulation of sounds by movement of the oral structures, and control of oral and nasal resonance by velopharyngeal valving. The second section concerns the evaluation and treatment of swallowing disorders (dysphagia). The third section is a description of normal and disordered language. The fourth section addresses issues of development and developmental deficits. The fifth and final section addresses the issue of cognitive impairment.

SPEECH PRODUCTION: VOICE, ARTICULATION, AND RESONANCE

Movement of air causes sound, and any sound can be used for communication. Clapping, for instance, is frequently used to com-municate approval. *Speech* refers to the limited number of communicative sounds produced within the *vocal tract*. Speech sounds can be produced in a variety of ways: Zulu speakers, for instance, trap air between the tongue and the hard palate and create a popping sound from the vacuum release when the tongue is lowered. English speakers, however, use egressive pulmonic air passing through the *vocal folds* as the sole basis for speech. This pulmonic air stream is the energy *source* that serves as the basis for sound waves. The vocal tract, which consists of the oral, pharyngeal, and nasal passages, then functions as a *filter*, which shapes this energy into recognizable speech sounds. Speech production can be divided into the three components of *voice*, *articulation*, and *resonance*, and each component has characteristic pathologic conditions and treatment considerations.

Voice

Normal Voice Production

There are two primary settings of the vocal cords during speech: adducted (closed) and abducted (open). When air flow sets adducted vocal cords into vibration, *voiced* speech sounds such as [v] and [z]* can be produced. The production of voiced sounds by vibration of the vocal cords is also referred to as *phonation*. When air flows undisturbed through abducted vocal cords, *voiceless* speech sounds such as [f] and [s] can be produced. In the case of voiceless sounds, air flows through the space between the vocal folds (the *glottis*), and sound is produced by a constriction at some other point in the vocal tract. Many sounds are identical except for the state of the vocal cords: [s] and [z] are both produced with the same articulatory setting (air hitting the back of the top teeth), but the vocal cords are held apart for production of [s] and are brought together and vibrate for [z]. There are other, less common settings of the vocal cords such as *breathy* voice (i.e., the prototypical sexy or secretive voice) in which the vocal cords are vibrating with incomplete closure during each cycle. Figure 4–1 illustrates the vocal cord posture during production of voiced and voiceless speech sounds.

The predominant acoustic and vocal properties of speech arise from the vibrating or voiced portion of the signal. Parameters of vocal cord vibration determine vocal *quality*, *pitch*, and *loudness*.

Vocal Quality. During normal voice production, the vocal cords vibrate symmetrically and evenly; both vocal cords move toward or away from the midline at the same rate. Each cycle is similar to preceding and

---

*Symbols that indicate speech sounds are enclosed in brackets to distinguish them from the letters of the alphabet. See Table 4–3 and the discussion in the section on articulation.

following cycles in duration and extent of movement. Anatomic and physiologic differences between larynges create a vast range of normal vocal qualities. Different phonatory settings can be effectively manipulated to produce various vocal qualities, which are used in English to communicate paralinguistic information such as secrecy (conveyed by whispered voice) and intimacy (by breathy voice). If the symmetry or mechanics of vibration are disturbed, as by incomplete closure of the vocal folds, hyperadduction, or variable rate over adjacent cycles, the voice is perceived as abnormal: rough, harsh, breathy, or hoarse, depending on the specific cause. The exact contribution of each abnormal vibratory characteristic to perceptual abnormality is not known. The terms used to describe abnormal vocal quality (e.g., rough, hoarse, breathy) and the modifiers attached to them (e.g., mild, moderate, and severe) are used subjectively.

Pitch. The rate of vocal cord vibration determines *pitch*. Rate of vocal cord vibration goes by several different names, including fundamental frequency (f_o), cycles per second (CPS), and Hertz (Hz). Large vocal cords vibrate more slowly and produce a voice of lower pitch than small vocal cords; smaller vocal cords vibrate more quickly because they have less mass and produce a higher pitched voice (see Tables 4–1 and 4–2 for normal pitch data). Regardless of the size of their vocal cords, individuals can alter their pitch by specific vocal cord manipulations. For instance, pitch is raised when the vocal cords are lengthened by contraction of the cricothyroid muscles. Changes in pitch furnish much of the intonation contours or melody in voice,

Figure 4–1. Photographs of the vocal cord positions: brought together during production of voice and vibrating (left) and held apart for production of voiceless sounds (right). (From Ladefoged P: A Course in Phonetics. New York: Harcourt Brace Jovanovich, 1975.)

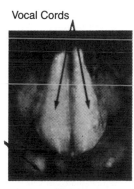

Vocal Cords

Arytenoid Cartilages

Voice

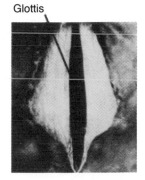

Glottis

Voiceless

TABLE 4–1. Mean Fundamental Frequencies

Age Range	Mean f_o	
	(Males Reading)	*(Females Reading)*
7	294	281
8	297	288
10/11	227	238
19	117	217
20s	120	224
30s	112	196
40s	107	189
60s	112	200
>70	132	202
>80	146	200

Note: Summarized and adapted from information presented in Colton RH, Casper JK: Understanding Voice Problems. Baltimore: Williams & Wilkins, 1990.

also referred to as *prosody*.* Normal prosodic variation signals the speaker's gender and age, as well as emotional and grammatical information (sadness versus surprise; statement versus question intonation). Abnormal pitch is created by abnormality such as vocal fold edema or nodules that, by adding mass and increasing stiffness, can decrease the rate of vibration and therefore lower the perceived pitch. These mass changes also reduce the ability to vary vibratory rate and thereby decrease the dynamic pitch range. The inability to continuously change pitch (which results in a monotone voice) is an abnormality that is also seen in diseases that impair muscular control over the larynx, such as Parkinson's disease, pseudobulbar palsy, and amyotrophic lateral sclerosis (ALS). *Aprosodia* and *dysprosodia* are terms used to refer to an impairment in production and interpretation of prosodic variation.

Loudness. Perceived loudness or vocal in-

---

*Prosody is achieved by alterations in the three parameters of frequency, intensity, and duration. For instance, stress on a word or a syllable generally involves a perceived rise in pitch, increase in loudness, and longer vowel duration.

tensity is achieved by a combination of increased air flow and increased medial adductive force on the vocal cords during phonation. This combination elevates subglottic pressure and vocal cord excursion from midline during each cycle and has the perceptual effect of an increase in loudness. Common abnormalities of loudness include reduced loudness and monoloudness, which are caused by decreased air flow and decreased control over medial adductive force of the vocal folds. Disorders of loudness are common in neurologic diseases, such as Huntington's chorea or Parkinson's disease; in anatomic changes, such as partial laryngectomy; and in physiologic alterations, such as unilateral vocal cord paralysis.

Evaluation of Voice Disorders

Dysphonia refers to any impairment of voice; *aphonia* is used to describe a loss of voice. Although normal voice is difficult to define, aphonia and dysphonia affect vocal quality, pitch, or loudness and are usually easy to identify: they draw attention to themselves, interfere with communication, and bother the speaker. A person may have what appears to the clinician to be a "strange" voice, but it may not be associated with a pathologic disorder, may not represent a change, and may not bother the speaker; the strangeness, therefore, is not a voice disorder. Evaluation of voice disorders requires a detailed history, physical examination, and perceptual evaluation and can involve documentation and quantification of laryngeal function. Important information about the onset, the duration, and changes of the dysphonia (or aphonia), as well as the patient's vocal use patterns, should be obtained. In physical examination, an otolaryngologist or a speech pathologist visualizes the vocal cords through indirect laryngoscopy, fiberoptic laryngoscopy, or stroboscopy. Viewing the vocal

TABLE 4–2. Frequency Range

Age	Males		Females	
	Low Frequency	*High Frequency*	*Low Frequency*	*High Frequency*
<40	80	675	140	1122
35–70s	80	260	136	803
>65	85	394	134	571

Note: Summarized and adapted from information presented in Colton RH, Casper JK: Understanding Voice Problems. Baltimore: Williams & Wilkins, 1990.

Figure 4–2. A pair of vocal fold nodules (left) and a single vocal fold polyp (right). (From Colton RH, Casper JK: Understanding Voice Problems. Baltimore: Williams & Wilkins, 1990.)

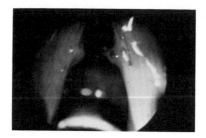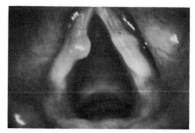

cords with a fixed light source (indirect or fiberoptic) reveals *structural* abnormalities that might affect vocal production. Stroboscopy, the use of an intermittent light source that presents an apparent slow-motion image of the vocal cords, allows more detailed observation of *physiologic* abnormalities in vocal cord vibration, showing symmetry of vocal fold movement, glottal closure, and the presence and the size of the mucosal wave.

Some simple techniques require no instrumentation and yield helpful information. For instance, *maximum phonation duration*—the maximum time that a person can sustain a tone on one continuous expiratory breath—can be used to estimate phonatory control and respiratory support. However, it must be noted that there is a tremendous amount of individual variation with such a measure (the duration for normal adults typically ranges from about 15 to 33 seconds), and the values are affected by age (shorter times for children and the aged), gender, and the general condition of the respiratory system. This technique also provides an ideal opportunity to perform a perceptual evaluation of the patient's voice. Subjective perceptual evaluation of the voice, as mentioned earlier, results in a description of vocal quality and an estimation of severity and, when possible, should be supplemented by instrumental acoustic analyses.

Acoustic analyses can provide objective measurement of the dysphonic voice, which is useful in documentation of the disorder, guiding therapy, and demonstrating efficacy of treatment. Although the speech acoustics armamentarium was greatly developed over the 1980s, few of the instruments are widely or routinely used. Ideally, the clinician makes several measurements of fundamental frequency, including mean f_o and its range. Measures of intensity and measures of *perturbation*—jitter (the cycle-to-cycle variation in frequency) and shimmer (the cycle-to-cycle variation in intensity)—are also collected.

Many commercially produced machines and computer programs are now available to make these measurements, including the Kay Elemetrics Visipitch, the Interactive Laboratory System (ILS), CSpeech, and the PM Pitch Analyzer. Other aspects of vocal cord function can be measured, including formant* and noise components of the acoustic record through sound spectrograms and measures of vocal cord contact and glottal area through electroglottography and photoglottography. Measures of laryngeal aerodynamics including air flow and estimated subglottic pressure can be used to measure vocal tract resistance and are combined with intensity measurements to yield an estimation of vocal efficiency. Measurement of muscle innervation with electromyography can also be helpful in describing the dysfunctional voice.

In the following section, several disorders are discussed in more detail to provide an idea of specific treatment approaches to common phonatory disorders.

Vocal Nodules and Polyps. Vocal nodules are the most frequent cause of hoarseness. Vocal cord nodules are usually bilateral and generally sit at the junction of the anterior and middle thirds of the true vocal cords. The appearance of vocal nodules varies throughout their development. They can appear as a small red, hemorrhagic area (edema) in the early stages or as a white, fibrotic mass later on (Fig. 4–2). The increased mass and stiffness of the vocal cords that result from the nodule disturb the symmetric movement of the cords, prevent full closure during the closed phase of the vibratory cycle, and thereby allow excess air to

---

*Formants consist of a group of overtones or harmonics (particular multiples of the fundamental frequency) that correspond to a resonating frequency of the air in the vocal tract. Vowels are characterized by three formants.

escape throughout the phonation. Vocal cord vibration is aperiodic, with higher-than-normal frequency and amplitude perturbation (i.e., increased jitter and shimmer). The voice sounds hoarse. The patient may appear short of breath, and the voice is low in pitch and limited in pitch range. The speech pathologist may use perceptual observations and acoustic measurements of voice to evaluate the problem. For instance, with the use of commonly available instruments, one can now measure jitter (typically under 1% in a normal voice), which contributes to perceived hoarseness. Videostroboscopy can also be used to record a visual image of the abnormal vocal cord function. Both of these techniques not only provide documentation for the clinician to use in follow-up but also provide objective measures of pathology that can help to formulate goals for the patient during treatment: for example, to reduce jitter by a certain percentage; to increase pitch range by a certain number of cycles per second; and to reduce the size of the nodule visible on the video image.

Although repeated frictional trauma is believed to be the direct cause of vocal nodules, many underlying variables create the right circumstances for the development of nodules. Examples include speaking habits (speaking too loudly, using too high or too low a pitch), drying the vocal cord mucosa (exposure to smoke, alcohol, and strong fumes), coughing, throat clearing, hard glottal attack, and increased muscular tension. Although some nodules, particularly in children, may resolve spontaneously, most nodules can be effectively eliminated with voice therapy. The only treatment for vocal nodules is to eliminate the patterns of vocal abuse that caused the condition. Identification of vocally abusive behaviors, subsequent education, and change of habits form the basis of voice therapy for vocal cord nodules. Specific methods vary with the patient's characteristics (such as age) and the clinician's preferred approach. Although traditionally many clinicians requested that patients begin treatment with strict voice rest (no talking) for 2 weeks in order to reduce edema, this approach is generally unrealistic in terms of patients' compliance and not necessarily helpful in rehabilitation. A more realistic, less stressful "modified voice rest" is preferable, wherein the focus of treatment from the outset is to replace poor vocal habits with good vocal habits. Once the cause is identi-

fied and eliminated, vocal nodules shrink in size, and their effect on vocal cord vibration and voice is reduced. Surgical removal of nodules should be limited to patients for whom voice therapy has failed. Surgical intervention without behavioral change is doomed to failure.

The clinical and histologic distinctions between vocal polyps and vocal nodules are not always clear. Both are caused by vocal abuse, and both create hoarseness. Some descriptions state that vocal polyps are more often unilateral and tend to be larger, more vascular, more edematous, and more inflammatory than are nodules, and some authors explicitly state that the two differ only in degree (see Fig. 4–2).

Vocal Cord Paralysis. Vocal cord paralysis or paresis is a frequent sequela of damage to cranial nerve X, secondary to vascular, traumatic, congenital, degenerative, or metabolic disorders and surgery. Although superior, recurrent, and mixed laryngeal nerve damage are all associated with specific vocal disorders, unilateral damage to the recurrent laryngeal nerve during thyroid or cardiac surgery is probably the most common cause of laryngeal paralyses and is the focus of this discussion. The typical manifestation of recurrent nerve damage is fixation of one arytenoid and one vocal cord, on the same side as the lesion, in a paramedian (abducted) position. In addition to this change in position of the vocal fold, chronic paralysis of the muscle also results in eventual atrophy of the vocalis muscle. The changes in position and mass of the vocal fold are responsible for the resulting vocal dysfunction. Although the remaining intact vocal cord may still vibrate as air flows through the glottis, contact between the cords is limited and results in inability to build up subglottic pressure, which produces a decrease in loudness. The vocal quality is breathy because of the increased air escape through the glottis during phonation. A secondary result of extensive air escape during speech is a limit on phrase length.

In most cases of unilateral vocal cord paralysis, patients recover spontaneously within 6 to 12 months of injury. If in spontaneous recovery the voice does not return to near normal, both surgical intervention and voice therapy are often helpful. Voice therapy is aimed at (1) reducing poor and damaging compensatory vocal habits, such as shouting, and (2) instructing the patient in exercises that can strengthen vocal cord function to compensate for the weak or paralyzed cord. Exercises to achieve vocal compensation generally involve controlled and effortful exertion. Although it has been assumed that improvement of voice from such therapy results from enabling the mobile cord to cross the midline, there is little evidence that this actually occurs. Improvement in voice probably results instead from reduction in the glottal gap and from maintenance of vocal fold stiffness, which allow an increase in vibration of the mobile cord but not necessarily across the midline. Surgical intervention for this type of problem has been varied and successful. Three types of procedures are considered, each aimed at improving the position or the mass, or both, of the paralyzed vocal cord. First, intrafold augmentation by injection of polytef (teflon) or silicone lateral to the fixed cord has the effect of filling in the glottal space sufficiently to allow the mobile cord to meet the fixed cord. Second, reinnervation of the nerve through nerve anastomosis effects an improvement in voice, at least in part by maintaining vocal fold mass. Third, medialization surgery can improve vocal cord position by implanting material lateral to the paralyzed vocal cord or by rotating the arytenoid cartilage and medializing the tip of the vocal process. The range of procedures used for altering the shape and function of the larynx (phonosurgery) is a fast-growing and promising field for this and many other vocal cord problems. Other uses of phonosurgery include life-saving procedures, such as lateralization when both vocal folds are paralyzed medially, which causes dyspnea, and more cosmetic procedures, such as cricothyroid approximation to raise habitually low pitch.

Laryngectomy. The loss of voice altogether from a total laryngectomy presents a different sort of problem for the speech pathologist. Obviously, without a larynx, a voice in the traditional sense cannot be produced. Rehabilitation for communication after a laryngectomy proceeds in several stages; it begins with a preoperative conference that ideally involves the patient, the caregivers, the speech pathologist, the surgeon, and the social worker. A preoperative conference with the speech pathologist is crucial for providing information about the effect of the

surgery on communication and often facilitates a rapid and motivated postoperative recovery. Postoperative voice rehabilitation, depending on the extent of surgery and rate of recovery, can begin soon after the operation. The patient can immediately communicate through writing and gesture. As soon as it is surgically safe (e.g., no risk of exacerbating fistulas), a hand-held electrolarynx can be provided. Electrolarynges are battery-operated tone generators that create a buzz to replace the tone created by the vocal cords. The tone is then introduced into the oral cavity either through a plastic tube (intraoral devices) or through the submandibular skin (under-the-neck devices). The intraoral devices can usually be used soon after surgery and are particularly useful for patients who have significant neck wounds (for example, before removal of staples or sutures) or fibrosis from previous radiation treatment. Many varieties of electronic devices are available and range in price from about $100 to $500. The inexpensive models are plastic and have limited tone capabilities, whereas the expensive models come with rechargeable batteries and include features such as variable pitch capability. The advantages of using an electrolarynx are clear: the device enables patients to communicate easily in face-to-face interaction with family, friends, and medical personnel; it is quicker and less frustrating than writing; it is more intelligible than mouthing words; and most patients can learn to use the machines within a few brief instructional sessions. The disadvantages include the cost of purchase and of batteries; less than perfect intelligibility, particularly in non–face-to-face interaction (such as on the telephone); the negative attention of other people and the patient's self-consciousness associated with use; and the requirement of some manual dexterity and learning, which precludes use by less dextrous and some cognitively impaired patients. Although some patients successfully use an electrolarynx as their long-term primary means of communication, patients are given the option to pursue other, sometimes more appropriate and effective alaryngeal voices through either esophageal speech training or the use of a tracheoesophageal prosthesis.

Esophageal speech has long been considered the gold standard of alaryngeal voice. It can sound indistinguishable from a somewhat low volume and slightly hoarse laryngeal voice. It is estimated that approximately

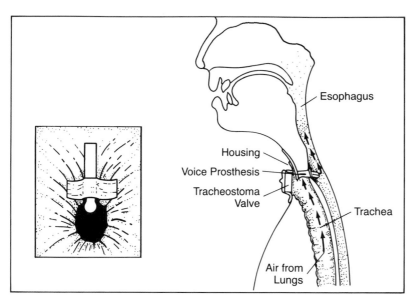

Figure 4–3. The Blom-Singer tracheoesophageal prosthesis. Either a finger or the tracheostoma valve (and housing) is used to occlude the stoma during speech. Inset shows the prosthesis taped in place at the top of the stoma. (From First Steps: Helping Words for the Laryngectomee. Courtesy of the American Cancer Society.)

40% to 70% of patients who enroll in esophageal speech training, and who devote a substantial amount of time to practice, can achieve intelligible esophageal speech within 9 to 12 months. In esophageal speech, the patient is taught to swallow and release air in a controlled manner; as the air returns, it sets the pharyngoesophageal segment into vibration, as when one belches. The advantages of esophageal speech are its naturalness and the lack of any appliance. The primary disadvantages are the amounts of the time and dedication required to master the technique and the relatively high failure rate. Failure to learn esophageal speech is often attributed to psychologic factors (such as poor motivation, poor practice habits) or physiologic limitations, including pouches or diverticula in the pharyngoesophageal segment, radiation fibrosis, and esophageal stenosis. The amount and shape of muscle left in the pharyngoesophageal segment is also a crucial variable.

There have been many attempts over the years to develop voice prostheses, and surgeries to achieve good quality alaryngeal voice. Currently, the most successful surgical/prosthetic technique, often called the Blom-Singer or tracheoesophageal puncture (TEP), requires the surgical creation of a tracheoesophageal fistula, either at the time of the primary surgery or in subsequent surgery, and the use of a one-way valve that allows air to enter the esophagus but does not permit aspiration. This achieves esophageal "voice" with pulmonic rather than esophageal air. To operate the valve, the patient inhales, covers the stoma with a finger, and exhales air through the tracheoesophageal prosthesis; when the pharyngoesophageal segment vibrates, the patient articulates normally over the voice (Fig. 4–3). The quality of voice produced by these patients tends to be slightly stronger than that produced by esophageal speech simply because the power source is the patient's own pulmonic air supply. The advantages of this procedure include the ability to speak with a relatively natural sounding voice and the ability to learn the technique rather quickly (usually only a few sessions are needed to fit the prosthesis and train the patient to produce a voice), and the TEPs have the distinct advantage of allowing longer and more continuous speech than can be produced by the traditional esophageal method. It is estimated that about 80% of TEP patients develop conversational speech. The disadvantages of this approach include the need for an additional operation if the fistula is not created at the time of the primary surgery; the need to use a hand to occlude the stoma when talking, although self-occluding valves can be used with limited success to free the hand; and the need to maintain the prosthesis (changing and cleaning), which makes this procedure a poor option for patients with poor dexterity, cognitive limitations, or poor self-care habits. Complications include temporary loss of voice (for up to 6 months) during and immediately after radiation treatment, and oral-to-tracheal leakage around the prosthesis, which can usually be controlled by cleaning or replacing the prosthesis. Contraindications for TEPs include any of the physical limitations that preclude production of esophageal speech and social and psychologic factors that would preclude maintenance of the puncture site and prosthesis. Speech pathologists are centrally involved in selecting suitable TEP candidates and directing postoperative prosthesis fitting and training.

Many other voice problems present themselves to the practicing otolaryngologist, and although full descriptions are beyond the scope of this chapter, several additional general points can be made. First, hoarseness is the most common vocal symptom. It is associated with a wide range of pathologic conditions and is nonspecific. It is important to recognize, but it gives little information about causes or treatment. Second, laryngeal hyperfunction can produce a harsh or strained or strangled-sounding voice, which is distinct from hoarseness. Although neuromuscular (such as brain stem) and emotional pathologic disorders can produce this type of laryngeal hyperfunction, the most controversial disorder associated with vocal hyperfunction is *spasmodic dysphonia*, a type of laryngeal spasm, which consists of a harsh voice with episodic spasms. This disorder is not well understood and typically runs an irregular course, including periods of normal voice, but no spontaneous remission has been reported. More than most voice disorders, spasmodic dysphonia has been followed by controversy in terms of differential diagnosis, classification (there are several types, including adductor and abductor), causes (organic versus psychogenic), and treatment. Unilateral recurrent laryngeal nerve sectioning, botulinum toxin injection into the vocalis muscle, and traditional voice therapy have all met with some success. Botulinum injections in conjunction with voice therapy is currently the most successful approach to the problem. The variability in the disorder and the inconsistency in responses to treatment indicate that there may be more than one pathologic condition involved. The third and final general point to make about voice disorders is that a great many voice disorders of adulthood appear to be primarily functional in nature and therefore require a broader involvement of health care personnel, including not only the otolaryngologist and the speech pathologist but also the psychotherapist.

The size and the shape of the vocal cords largely determine vocal quality and pitch, and subglottic pressure determines loudness. It is the supraglottic vocal tract that allows people to amplify and shape that basic sound into many other acoustic variations. These supraglottic modifications of the sound wave are referred to as *articulation* and *resonance*.

Articulation

Normal Articulation

Articulation is the shaping of sound within the mouth. Consonants are produced by narrowing or stopping the air flow somewhere between the glottis and the lips by approximating articulators (tongue, palate, lips, teeth). Consonants are described by the manner of articulation, the place of articulation, and the status of the vocal cords with regard to voicing. *Manner of articulation* refers to whether the air flow is completely stopped in the mouth by two articulators actually touching (as in [p,b,t,d,k,g], which are called *stops*), whether the air is funneled through a narrow opening to create friction (as in [f,v,s,z], which are called *fricatives*), a combination of stopping the air and releasing it with friction (as in [tʃ], called *affricates*), or whether the air is just funneled along a specific tongue shape (as in [l,r,w], called *approximants*). *Place of articulation* refers to the point of closest approximation, whether it is at the lips [p,b], the alveolar ridge [t,d,s,z], the hard palate [k,g], or even the glottis (as in "uh-uh"). The description of vowels is a little less straightforward and centers on the shape of the mouth created by lip rounding (rounded as in [u], unrounded as in [i]) and on whether the body of the tongue is front or back and high or low. Traditional writing systems are generally not used to refer to sounds because they do not have a one-to-one correspondence between sounds and symbols. For example, one sound may be represented by many different letters and letter combinations in English, as the sound "e" in *he*, *believe*, *Caesar*, *see*, *people*, *seize*, *sea*, *silly*, *amoeba*, *key*, and *machine*. Other letters are associated with no sound in particular words, such as m*nemonic*, p*terodactyl*,

TABLE 4–3. International Phonetic Alphabet (IPA) Symbols for Transcribing English Sounds

Consonants		Vowels	
Symbol	*Example*	*Symbol*	*Example*
p	p̲ie	I	b̲it
t	t̲ie	e	b̲ait
k	k̲ey	ɛ	b̲et
b	b̲ye	æ	p̲an
d	d̲ye	u	b̲oot
g	g̲uy	U	p̲ut
m	m̲y	ʌ	b̲ut
n	n̲o	o	b̲oat
ŋ	ra̲ng	ɔ	bou̲ght
f	f̲ee	a	p̲ot
v	v̲ie	ə	sofa̲
θ	t̲high	ay	b̲ite
ð	t̲hy	aw	b̲rown
s	s̲igh	ɔy	bo̲y̲
z	z̲oo		
ʃ	s̲hy		
ʒ	vis̲ion		
l	l̲ie		
w	w̲hy		
r	r̲ye		
j	y̲e		
h	h̲e		
tʃ	c̲hime		
dʒ	j̲ive		

in square brackets to distinguish them from standard orthography. Table 4–3 shows IPA correspondences, and Figure 4–4 displays the manner and place of articulation for English consonants.

Pathologic Conditions of Articulation

There are many types and causes of articulation disorders. For the purposes of this discussion, they are divided into apraxia and dysarthria.

Apraxia is the disruption of volitional movement. As limb apraxia is the inability to carry out volitional movement with an arm (e.g., wave goodbye), *oral-motor apraxia* and *apraxia of speech* refer to the inability to perform volitional movements with the articulators. The cause of apraxia is typically a cortical lesion in the left inferior frontal region, the area in and around the left motor strip devoted to the mouth. The symptoms of apraxia are (1) better production of more automatic (less volitional) speech such as cursing, counting, and familiar songs, (2) articulation errors consisting primarily of sound substitutions, additions, repetitions, and prolongations; (3) inconsistent articulation errors (at one point the patient can say "cookie," and at the next the patient cannot say the same word or the same sounds in a different word), (4) good recognition of errors, which inspires self-correction and multiple attempts to produce the target, and (5) intact language comprehension and formulation—that is, no aphasia. An example of

and *debt,* and the same letter may be associated with many different sounds, such as "a" in *dame, dad, father, village,* and *many.* To avoid confusion in referring to sounds, technical discussion of sounds (*phonetics*) is conducted with the *International Phonetic Alphabet* (IPA), in which each sound is associated with only one symbol. IPA symbols are enclosed

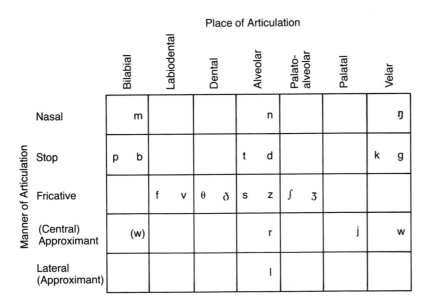

Place of Articulation

Figure 4–4. A chart of the English consonants. Whenever there are two symbols within a cell, the one on the left represents a voiceless sound. All other symbols represent voiced sounds. Note also the consonant [h], which is not on this chart, and the affricates [tʃ,dʒ], which are sequences of symbols on the chart. (From Ladefoged P: A Course in Phonetics. New York: Harcourt Brace Jovanovich, 1975.)

apraxic speech is included here to illustrate the typical features of apraxia (the first four just given). This particular transcript is taken from a recording of an apraxic patient's verbal description of a picture that shows a boy falling from a stool while trying to steal some cookies from a cookie jar on one side of the kitchen, and his mother is washing dishes at the sink on the other side:

OK, the boy is trying to steal some stuky coves, k-k-kopies, ki-ki-kippies, cuppie, kippie. He's ch-chaving, chaving, klip, kli- off the cholbie. That's awful. Stum, stool, stool. OK. He's falling it, off of it. It's tooping over. All right. The mother is cha-chulving the wish-shoving, shov-shov- The letter, la-ladeh-

Dysarthria is the impairment of speech as a result of muscle weakness, incoordination, or other movement limitation and is often associated with neurologic damage. General signs of dysarthria are impaired speech intelligibility and lack of speech naturalness. Dysarthria differs from apraxia in that the symptoms are more consistent across each sound production. If the dysarthric patient suffers from tongue weakness and limited range of lingual motion, he or she may have difficulty articulating [k]. The articulation will likely be distorted in a similar manner in most contexts, unlike that of an apraxic patient whose articulation of even one sound will vary extensively from trial to trial. Dysarthric articulation errors most often consist of imprecise consonant production, and the disorder generally affects many phonemes (i.e., many different speech sounds). Dysarthric speech generally sounds slurred. Distorted rate of speech (either slow or fast), hypernasality, and dysphonia often accompany dysarthria.

Classifications of dysarthria are sometimes based on physiologically descriptive parameters (hypokinetic, hyperkinetic, flaccid, spastic, and ataxic cerebellar) and sometimes on the lesion location (lower motor neuron or upper motor neuron). There is a lack of clarity in most discussions of the dysarthric subtypes, and symptoms often overlap; this situation frequently yields a diagnosis of "mixed dysarthria." The most common dysarthrias result from neurologic impairment of the basal ganglia. Classic hypokinetic dysarthria is typified by parkinsonism and manifests with both dysphonic features (monopitch, monoloudness, reduced pitch, breathiness) and articulation impairments

(imprecise consonants and short rushes of speech). Other dysarthrias such as the hyperkinetic type associated with Huntington's chorea, as well as that seen in various dystonias and voice tremors, also manifest with dysphonic features (irregular pitch fluctuation and voice arrests, harshness, monopitch, monoloudness) and the common dysarthric symptom of imprecise consonant articulation. Ataxic (cerebellar) dysarthria is characterized by irregular breakdown in both phonation and articulation. Imprecise consonant articulation is typical of most dysarthrias and does not distinguish between them.

Dysarthrias also occur as side effects of many medications. The most notable are the side effects produced by the phenothiazine group of tranquilizers used to treat psychoses (e.g., fluphenazine hydrochloride, chlorpromazine hydrochloride, and trifluoperazine hydrochloride). Approximately 40% of patients receiving long-term antipsychotic medication develop tardive dyskinesia with an associated dysarthria. These symptoms may persist for months or years after medication is stopped and in some cases may be permanent. A parkinsonian syndrome may also be produced by these medications, but it usually improves rapidly after medication is ceased.

Although structural modifications of the tongue, the lips, the jaw, and the palate often create speech intelligibility problems similar to the dysarthrias, the term *dysarthria* is generally restricted to speech deficits resulting from peripheral or central nervous system damage. Naturally, the articulation deficit after oropharyngeal surgery is proportional to the amount of tissue excised. However, postsurgical patients, who are otherwise neurologically intact, are remarkably able to compensate for changed anatomy and physiology to produce intelligible speech. Patients who have undergone less extensive surgery have excellent prognoses for recovery of intelligible and natural speech.

Evaluation of Articulation

An evaluation of articulation describes how much of the patient's speech is intelligible and how many and what type of articulation errors are made. Although this evaluation may be accomplished informally in conversation, informal evaluation is inconsistent since clinicians often apply subjective criteria and terms to describe speech. In addition, conversational speech is a relatively uncontrolled context and may not reveal the patient's range of articulation problems and abilities. For these reasons, tests have been developed to assess articulation of sounds in specific contexts that often affect their production: the position of the sound in a word (beginning, middle, or end); mode of production (spontaneous speech, reading, imitation); and whether the sounds are produced in isolated syllables, single words, single sentences, or conversations. Objective assessment of intelligibility can be accomplished by having an independent rater or raters attempt to identify tape-recorded utterances. This method yields a measure of intelligibility in which the articulation of the sounds is the only cue to intelligibility because conversational context and pragmatic cues such as facial expression, eye gaze, and lip reading are eliminated.

Treatment of Articulation Problems

After adverse and unavoidable reactions to drugs have been accounted for and corrected when possible, speech therapy is usually the primary means of improving intelligibility of apraxic and dysarthric speech. Education about articulation and specific advice (e.g., slow down, use shorter sentences, extend the jaw motion, exaggerate articulatory movements) can be combined with oral-motor exercises to improve control over articulators. Severe and untreatable disorders may be compensated for by use of other modalities, including writing and use of augmentative communication devices ranging from a simple pointing board to a computerized speech synthesizer.

Resonance

Normal Resonance

Resonance technically refers to the amplification and shaping of the glottal tone and is used commonly to refer to whether air is allowed to vibrate in the oral cavity or in the coupled oral and nasal cavities. The gateway between the oral and nasal cavities, the velopharyngeal port, is manipulated by control of the soft palate and sphincteric action of the posterior and lateral pharyngeal walls to allow air to enter the nasal passages. In normal articulation, most speech sounds are produced with primarily oral resonance, in which air vibrates in the pharynx and oral cavity but not in the nasal cavity. This method of sound production may have evolutionary roots in speech perception, inasmuch as speech sounds are much less distinct from one another when nasal resonance is superimposed on oral resonance.

Although nasal resonance is probably less important than oral resonance (e.g., in English only three consonants—[m], [n], and [ŋ]—require nasal resonance), a balance between oral and nasal resonance is usually maintained, and any deviation affects speech either in the direction of hypernasality or hyponasality. Hyponasality, or a denasal resonance, is characteristic of speech with congested sinuses or structural blockage of the nasal tract and is generally not the focus of speech therapy. On the other hand, velopharyngeal incompetence (VPI) and resulting hypernasality are created by many pathologic conditions and are frequently the focus of speech treatment.

Disorders of Resonance

Velopharyngeal incompetence can be caused by obvious structural defects associated with a cleft palate or with palatal resection for cancer. It is important to remember that less obvious and nonstructural problems can also cause disorders of resonance. Velopharyngeal incompetence can be caused by neurologic damage that interferes with muscle tone or coordination and can be associated with nerve resections, with chemical/myoneuronal junction disorders such as myasthenia gravis, with stroke, or with degenerative basal ganglia diseases such as Parkinson's or Huntington's. Last, hypernasal resonance may be the result of improper learning. People who are hard of hearing or deaf tend to be hypernasal. This is not the result of any structural or neurologic problem that precludes velopharyngeal competence but rather is attributable to the fact that these individuals cannot hear the oral-nasal contrast. Different pathologic conditions have distinct patterns of nasal resonance. For instance, a gradual rise of nasal resonance through the course of speaking is suggestive of muscle weakening, as from myasthenia gravis; constant nasal resonance suggests obstruction of the nasal tract; and unpredictable variability of nasal resonance is typical of sensory impairment, as in the hearing-impaired population.

Evaluation of Resonance

Evaluation of hypernasal resonance is accomplished by perceptual, radiologic, and physical examinations (e.g., nasal endoscopy with a flexible scope reveals the extent of the defect) and can be augmented by objective measurement of nasal air flow. Various instruments can compare the air flow from the mouth versus the nares during production of sounds. Most of the air flow should come from the mouth during the production of oral sounds, as in isolated English vowels. Manometers can be used to measure oral air flow both with nares occluded and with nares unoccluded; with good velopharyngeal competence, these measurements should be the same. Newer instruments such as the Kay Elemetrics Nasometer directly compare oral and nasal air flow and provide objective measurements of nasal resonance ("nasalence"), which are useful for identifying patterns of nasal resonance associated with specific disorders and for documenting severity of dysfunction and progress in therapy. This instrument also provides a visual display of nasalence that can be used for direct feedback to the patient and is useful for gaining volitional control over nasal resonance.

Treatment of Resonance Problems

Treatment of resonance problems makes use of three modalities: surgery, by construction of a skin flap to reduce the size of the velopharyngeal port; prosthodontics, by construction of a bulb to occlude the velopharyngeal port; and compensation through speech therapy. Surgical and prosthodontic intervention have the best results when combined with speech therapy. Speech therapy focuses on eliminating nonfunctional valving habits, such as using the tongue base to compensate for velopharyngeal incompetence, and on training in the use of volitional velopharyngeal valving, which requires improving sensory monitoring and muscular control.

SWALLOWING AND DYSPHAGIA

Nature is a miser: she builds new functions on old structures. When articulate speech evolved in homo sapiens, it was jury-rigged on top of the swallowing mechanism. The swallowing mechanism compensated, and the end result is that modern human beings can both talk and swallow but always run the risk of aspirating: a small but potentially deadly price to pay for the power of speech.

Normal Swallowing

Normal swallowing function can be broken down into four stages: (1) oral preparation, (2) oral transit, (3) pharyngeal, and (4) esophageal. Oral preparation consists of masticating or forming food and liquid into a cohesive bolus. This requires strong and coordinated tongue and jaw movement, anterior pulling of the soft palate, and adequate facial muscle tone to keep food from accumulating in the lateral sulci between the cheek and the teeth. The oral transit stage takes about 1 second and involves manipulating the bolus into the central, grooved portion of the tongue and propelling it back to the area of the faucial arches, where the pharyngeal stage is initiated. The pharyngeal stage of swallowing is referred to as the swallow "response." The mechanism for initiating the swallow response is not fully understood, but it appears to be partially under reflexive control and partially under voluntary control, mediated by the reticular formation of the brain stem (medulla). The pharyngeal stage also lasts about 1 second and includes (1) tongue retraction, (2) velopharyngeal closure, (3) pharyngeal contraction, (4) closing of the larynx at the three levels of the true vocal folds, false vocal folds, and epiglottis-aryepiglottic folds, and (5) elevation and anteriorization of the larynx. The pharyngeal phase ends with relaxation of the cricopharyngeal region (upper esophageal sphincter, pharyngoesophageal segment) and entry of food or liquid into the esophagus. The bolus is then carried through the esophagus and into the stomach through peristaltic action.

Disorders of Swallowing (Dysphagia)

It is estimated that 6 to 10 million Americans regularly have difficulty swallowing. Because swallowing is controlled at several levels of the nervous system from the neocortex to the peripheral nervous system, a large variety of neurologic conditions are associated with dysphagia. These include stroke (cortical and subcortical), closed-head trauma, and degenerative diseases (e.g., multiple sclerosis, amyotrophic lateral sclerosis, Parkinson's disease, myasthenia gravis, and cerebellar degeneration).

Surgery for cancer of the head and neck is also associated with dysphagia. The surgical procedure that creates the largest risk of aspiration is partial (lateral or supraglottic) laryngectomy. Removal of any portion of the hypopharyngeal and laryngeal valving mechanism, from the vocal folds up to the epiglottis, leaves the airway potentially vulnerable to penetration during the swallow. Although other surgical procedures are thought to run less risk of creating dysphagia, there is significant risk, even, for instance, with a total laryngectomy; this risk, from stenosis and fistulas, is estimated to be between 10% and 50%. Tracheostomy, once thought to reduce risk of aspiration, may actually increase it by decreasing laryngeal elevation, desensitizing the larynx by diminishing protective reflexes (e.g., cough), and discoordinating laryngeal closure. Any other surgery that creates lingual, velopharyngeal, or laryngeal incompetence also carries a risk of dysphagia.

In general, swallowing evaluation is requested, not in the case of any particular diagnosis or procedure, but rather after observation or patient complaint. Swallowing evaluation is generally appropriate for patients who (1) have recurrent aspiration pneumonias, (2) experience unexplained weight loss, (3) cough or choke during or after eating or drinking, (4) have a persistent wet vocal quality, particularly after eating or drinking, (5) have increased mucus production, (6) have an elevated basal body temperature, (7) have a sensation of food sticking in the throat, or (8) complain of pain on swallowing (odynophagia).

Evaluation of Swallowing

As a result of their expertise in the anatomy and physiology of the oral, pharyngeal, and laryngeal structures, speech pathologists serve as a primary resource in the treatment of swallowing disorders. In conjunction with departments of radiology and occupational and physical therapy, speech pathologists evaluate and treat persons with dysphagia. The goals of the evaluation and treatment

are to identify the causes of aspiration, reduce the risk of aspiration, and guide the patient in safe oral intake to maintain adequate nutrition and hydration. Diagnosis and treatment of swallowing disorders improve the patients' chances of leaving the hospital quickly, avoiding pneumonia, living independently, and consuming liquids and solids safely.

The initial evaluation of swallowing disorders begins with a complete medical and swallowing history. Evaluation of swallowing function can then be accomplished by (1) indirect or bedside procedures and (2) a videofluoroscopic examination called a *modified barium swallow*. The indirect bedside evaluation should include testing of oral function (the range of movement and the strength of oral structures) and observation of swallowing behavior. Oral reflexes (palatal and gag reflexes) are documented; however, their role in swallowing is unclear. Control of oral secretions yields some evidence of oral sensitivity. In addition, an oral sensory examination should be performed. These procedures and observations help to identify problems in oral preparation and oral movement. The pharyngeal stage is minimally evaluated at bedside through observation of a dry swallow, a voluntary cough, and trials of food and liquid swallows. The dry swallow allows observation of laryngeal elevation, which is one component of airway protection. Coughing during or after a swallow and a wet voice after drinking water are indications of pharyngeal stage dysfunction.

The obvious disadvantage of the bedside evaluation is that the clinician cannot see the extent of the problem or objectively evaluate the effect and safety of modifications in posture, bolus size, or bolus consistency. The videofluoroscopic modified barium swallow procedure has been developed to allow objective and complete observation of the swallowing mechanism and trial therapeutic intervention. The modified barium swallow allows the clinician to view the patient's oral cavity, pharynx, larynx, and esophagus during swallows of barium mixed with various amounts of liquid, pureed food, and solid food. Both anteroposterior and lateral views are usually obtained. During the procedure, change in bolus size and consistency, postural adaptations, and specific voluntary maneuvers (e.g., supraglottic protective swallow and repeat dry swallows) are tested for efficacy in attaining safe swallowing. If all therapeutic manipulations cannot reduce the risk of aspiration, nonoral feeding or dietary restrictions can be recommended.

Treatment of Dysphagia

Treatment of dysphagia is determined largely by the results of the modified barium swallow procedure. There is no safe amount of aspiration. Although a young, healthy patient may be able to tolerate a minimal amount of aspiration, caution is mandated when any swallowing incompetence is present. Every postural and food consistency manipulation attempted during the modified barium swallow procedure furnishes valuable information regarding the most effective and the safest way for the patient to eat. Follow-up treatment is often required for education and to reinforce use of postures and new eating habits. Standard precautions that are often recommended include restricted food consistencies, slow eating, repeat swallows, and maintaining upright posture while eating and for 30 minutes after eating. Direct therapeutic intervention in the form of thermal stimulation (placing cold instruments in the area of the faucial arches) has been shown to improve pharyngeal motility in some patients. If oral feeding is not safe for nutrition and hydration, non-oral feeding should be recommended. Nasogastric tubes are typically recommended for non-oral feeding, which is expected to be temporary (less than 6 weeks), and gastrostomy tubes are recommended when non-oral feeding is expected to continue over a longer period.

Of particular interest to otolaryngologists is the surgical management of aspiration. Depending on the cause of the dysphagia, there are numerous surgical approaches, all designed to prevent airway penetration by food and liquids. For instance, aspiration can occur with unilateral vocal cord paralysis, which may necessitate a vocal cord augmentation procedure to reduce aspiration. In cases of permanent tracheotomy, a glottic closure procedure may be attempted to separate the tracheal and esophageal passages. Laryngeal diversion (a potentially reversible operation) and laryngectomy are also used to eliminate chronic aspiration.

LANGUAGE

Language is a conceptual symbolic system by which meaning is conveyed (semantics). It is distinct from the ability to speak: people can understand the meaning of words and know whether a sentence is grammatical even if they have no speech capability at all. Language can be subdivided into a system of elements (lexical items or words), rules for combining these elements into grammatical sentences (syntax), and rules for constructing larger units of conversation and narratives (discourse). In addition, there are culture-specific rules of appropriate language use for each context (pragmatics).

Language is discussed in two sections: (1) words and syntax and disorders in this area (aphasia), and (2) normal and disordered discourse and pragmatics.

Words and Syntax

Normal Lexical and Grammatical Abilities

Knowledge of a particular word encompasses its meaning, its pronunciation, its relationship to other words, and its role in sentence structure. For example, people know that the word *computer* should be stressed on the second syllable, not the third; and although the sentence "The tree is frightened" is perfectly grammatical, people know that it does not make any sense because there is something about the meaning of the word *tree* that prevents it from being *frightened*. Knowledge of syntax allows one to tell whether a sentence is grammatical (e.g., "Boy apple the ate the" may convey some meaning, but it is ungrammatical) and to compute the relationship between words in a sentence. For instance, the sentences "The boy gave the girl a disease" and "The girl gave the boy a disease" mean very different things, although the individual words are the same. Syntactic knowledge allows people to determine the aspects of sentence meaning that cannot be determined by the meaning of the individual words.

Disorders of Language: Aphasia

Aphasia is the disruption of formulation and/or comprehension of linguistic symbols. Many forms of aphasia exist, but two predominant varieties are consistently identified. First, damage to the anterior portions of the left cerebral hemisphere is associated with impoverished, often agrammatic output

TABLE 4–4. Age of Acquisition for the Consonants of English

Sound	Age*
m	before 2
n	before 2
p	before 2
h	before 2
w	before 2
b	before 2
d	2
t	2
k	2
g	2
ŋ (sing)	2
f	2.5
j	2.5
r	3
l	3
s	3
z	3.5
tʃ (chew)	3.5
ʃ (shoe)	3.5
dʒ (judge)	4
v	4
θ (thin)	4.5
ð (the)	5
ʒ (leisure)	6

*Age at which 51% of children said sound correctly in more than 50% of test items.

Adapted from Sander E: When are speech sounds learned? J Speech Hear Dis 37:55–63, 1972.

munication system. This developmental process is guided by both innate mechanisms and learning. One of the most striking facts about the child's acquisition of language is the regularity in timing and sequence of language developments despite differences in intelligence, social and cultural environment, amount of language exposure, and the language spoken by parents (Tables 4–4 and 4–5). This regularity of timing and sequence is often taken as evidence of a maturationally based, innate language acquisition system.

Although there is a biologically determined readiness to learn language, this program must be triggered and guided by environmental exposure to language. It is of great theoretical and practical interest to determine the timing, the type, and the amount of environmental stimulation that are necessary for normal development of language.

Information about the timing of language exposure is addressed by the notion of a critical period for language development. This period is a time during which the child is biologically ready to learn language and after which he or she is no longer able to learn the system, regardless of stimulation. Evidence gathered from individuals who were deprived of the opportunity to learn a first language until puberty, for instance, indicates that grammar cannot be natively acquired if exposure and learning begin after this critical period. These data support the notion of a biologically based language acquisition capacity that must be stimulated before puberty (and possibly earlier) if language is to be acquired normally.

Research on the critical period has indicated that environmental stimulation must occur at a particular time in development, but it does not address the nature or amount of exposure required. Is exposure to television sufficient? Or does the input to the child have to be tailored to his or her interests and

TABLE 4–5. Language Acquisition Milestones

0 to 8 weeks	Crying
8 to 20 weeks	Cooing and laughing
20 to 30 weeks	Vocal play (repetitions of sounds)
6 to 12 months	Babbling
9 to 18 months	Melodic utterances
9 to 10 months	Gestures (pointing, reaching, waving)
9 to 12 months	First word comprehension
11 to 16 months	First spoken words
	Pretending to talk (e.g., on a phone, read a book)
16 to 18 months	Surge in vocabulary growth
18 to 24 months	Multiword combinations (two-word sentences)
	50-word vocabulary often by 24 months
24 months	Three- and four-word sentences common
36 months	Grammaticization (e.g., basic sentence structure, word endings)
3 to 7 years	Complex (conjoined and embedded sentences)
6 to 10 years	Complex and discourse-based grammar (e.g., telling stories)
7 to 11 years	Appreciation of jokes

Note: Adapted from Crystal D: Listen to Your Child: A Parent's Guide to Children's Language. Harmondsworth, England: Penguin, 1986.

capacities? Children who have little or no verbal interaction but do have the opportunity to "absorb" language from television do not develop language normally. This and other research suggest that to master the language system, children may need to (1) hear a particular type of simplified and socially relevant language (sometimes called *motherese*), and (2) actively participate in verbal interaction. Barring unethical social deprivation experiments, it is difficult to further establish how much of what type of verbal interaction is sufficient to ensure the normal development of language.

To summarize, there exists an innate biologic language capacity that needs a particular type of environmental stimulation at a particular point in development for normal language development to proceed. Insufficient environmental stimulation or disruption of the underlying neurologic foundation for language creates abnormal patterns of language development.

Disorders of Speech and Language Development

Between 5% and 15% of children have speech or language problems. These problems are among the most common disorders of childhood. Delayed or deviant early communication can negatively affect social, mental, and academic development. Therefore, it is important to identify and remediate speech and language deficits as early as possible.

Neurologic, cognitive, and emotional factors can cause abnormal development of speech and language abilities. For instance, severe mental retardation, such as that seen in children with Down's syndrome, disrupts speech and language development. Children who are abused have been noted to develop atypical language patterns, and children with neurologic impairment, whether it is from vascular lesions, seizure disorders, part of pervasive developmental delays, or associated with maternal drug use, frequently present with deviant communication development.

Several types of developmental problems are particularly common and are described here: developmental disorders of articulation, language, and fluency and the multiple communication disorders associated with hearing impairment.

Developmental Articulation Disorder. About 10% of children under 8 years of age (the ratio of males to females is 2 to 1) have difficulty learning to pronounce one or more sounds, especially the later acquired consonant sounds [r,ʃ,θ,f,z,l]. In the mild cases, errors consist of simple omissions, distortions, or substitutions of a particular sound (e.g., [w] for [r] substitution) or a class of sounds (distortion of [w,r,l]). In the more severe cases, speech can be largely unintelligible and may be the manifestation of a massively disordered sound system. Children with a developmental articulation disorder often have normal language development. Although there appears to be a strong familial pattern, the cause is unclear. Some articulation difficulties are caused by known organic factors (insufficient anatomic structures, neurologic impairment), but most such problems have no known organic cause and are therefore called *functional* articulation disorders. Many children, particularly those with simpler articulation problems, outgrow articulation difficulties without speech therapy. However, for both the mild and severe cases, early therapeutic intervention can have the advantage of eliminating speech disorders before error articulation patterns are overlearned and before significant social stigma can be attached. Standardized tests and observation can reveal the severity of disorder in terms of the degree of delay and degree of handicap (intelligibility). On this basis, a decision can be reached regarding enrollment in speech therapy.

Developmental Language Disorder. Children with developmental language disorder (also called specific language impairment, developmental dysphasia, and language delay) present with a clinical picture of delayed or abnormal first language acquisition that is not associated with mental retardation, hearing impairment, infantile autism, or pervasive developmental disorder. Spelling, reading, and motor skills are also often impaired. The cause is unknown, but it appears to be more common in families with other developmental speech and language disorders. The cause is presumed to be neurologically based because it is frequently associated with memory and motor problems; however, no concrete evidence of neurologic impairment has been found. This disorder is estimated to affect between 5% and 15% of all preschool children. The disorder is often subdivided

TABLE 4–6. Normal Sequence of Oral Motor Development and Eating

Age (Months)	Skill
0 to 4	Strong oral reflexes (sucking-swallowing, rooting, gagging)
	Incomplete lip closure, especially at corner of lips
	Unable to release nipple voluntarily
1 to 2	Better lip closure
	Tongue moves with jaw
	Tongue moves up and down, in and out with sucking
3	Mouth opens or tongue protrudes in anticipation of feeding
4	Recognizes bottle
	Sucking strength increases, tongue starts to raise and lower
	More variety of tongue movements and less reflex movement
	Loses liquids from sides of mouth during sucking
	Cup drinking introduced; messy; tongue may thrust with cup
	Appetite may be erratic
5	Mouth opens for spoon
	Thrusts tongue involuntarily when spoon is removed; ejects food
6	Munches; jaw moves up and down. Biting lacks rotary chewing
	Tongue lateralization (uses tongue to move food from side to side)
	True sucking, stable jaw, tongue moves up and down
	Upper lip comes down well on spoon
	Finger feeding begins (6 to 8 months)
8	Tongue elevation with stable jaw; can handle liquids
	Transfers food well from center of mouth to sides
	Rotary chewing begins; retains some vertical motions
	Holds own bottle
	Makes sounds while eating
12	Controlled bite through food
	Chews adequately with rotary chew
	Plays with tongue; sticks it out experimentally
	More choosy about food, very independent
15 to 18	Begins spoon feeding, may spill
	Drinks well from cup; stabilizes muscle around jaw
	Licks lower lip
21 to 24	Holds small glass with one hand
	Inserts spoon without inverting it
	Food preference stems from taste, form, consistency, or color

Note: Adapted from Hall S, Cicirello N, Reed P, Hylton J: Considerations for Feeding Children Who Have a Neuromuscular Disorder (pp 14–15). Portland: Oregon Health Sciences University, Crippled Children's Division, 1987; Bailey D, Wolery M: Assessing Infants and Preschoolers with Handicaps (p 469). Columbus OH: Merrill Publishing, 1989.

into predominantly expressive problems and predominantly receptive (comprehension) problems. Expressive deficits include, for example, limited vocabulary, difficulty in learning new words, and use of only sentences that are short and grammatically simple in comparison with developmental norms. Receptive dysfunction includes difficulty understanding particular word types (e.g., spatial terms) or grammatically complex sentences. These disorders are usually apparent by 3 or 4 years of age, although mild forms may not be identified until adolescence. When identified in the preschool years, more than half of these children appear to catch up and reach normal language proficiency. The other 30% to 50% of these children manifest persistent language processing problems in adulthood, which are often most apparent in reading difficulty (dyslexia).

Evaluation and Treatment of Developmental Articulation and Language Disorders. Because the rate and sequence of speech and language development are relatively constant in the normally developing child, reliable testing instruments to judge the developmental achievements of children can identify disorders or delays. Tables 4–4, 4–5, and 4–6 show normal developmental sequences in articulation, language, and oral-motor (swallowing) function.

The type and amount of treatment for early childhood articulation and language disorders are determined by the age of the child and the nature and severity of the problem. For instance, the younger and more mildly delayed children (those who have less than a 6-month lag in development) may not be enrolled in direct speech therapy. For these very young children, parental counseling and sufficient exposure to appropriate input (e.g., socially appropriate conversation rather than television; placement in preschool programs in which age-appropriate communication opportunities are frequent) are generally used to facilitate speech and language development. Re-evaluation every 6 months may be recommended to monitor progress during these crucial early years. Older and more severely impaired children require direct therapeutic intervention. Public schools offer individual and group therapy, as well as aphasia classrooms and special programs for children with multiple handicaps.

There exist many formal tests with developmental norms for vocabulary, grammar, and nonverbal communication. Assessment measures yield an age-equivalent score for determining the degree of delay in expressive and receptive language. A 6-month delay should alert the parents and the clinician to a possible problem. A delay of 1 year or more on any portion of a standardized language test generally warrants enrollment in a therapy program. A full audiometric evaluation is essential for all children suspected of having speech or language problems in order to identify hearing impairments that may contribute to the language delay; the evaluation results may possibly indicate the need for amplification and aural rehabilitation as part of the therapy program.

Stuttering. Stuttering (or stammering), an impairment of speech fluency, usually consists of frequent repetitions or prolongations of sounds and syllables. Most cases of stuttering appear in the language acquisition years. Approximately 80% of stutterers recover by adolescence, either spontaneously or with intervention. Young stutterers generally are not aware of the problem until others notice the dysfluency and react to it. The stutterer invariably develops awareness of the problem and a fear of speaking. Situational variables typically exacerbate the problem; certain situations elicit more fear and dysfluency than others. Talking on the telephone and talking with authority figures are commonly reported to cause difficulty. Some stutterers also develop what are called secondary characteristics, which include eye blinking, head jerking, and limb movements that accompany the dysfluent episodes. These are considered to be epiphenomena,

initially used by the speaker to end a dysfluent block, but they generally are ineffective and become habitual. There is no known cause or cure for stuttering. Both neurogenic and psychogenic causes have been proposed. The ratio of male to female stutterers is 4 to 1, and there is a significant familial component. Treatment is usually aimed at reducing the stuttering behavior either directly through behavior modification or indirectly through a psychological approach that focuses on reducing the fear of speaking. Eliminating the secondary characteristics can also be accomplished in therapy.

Hearing Impairment and Language Development. Children with persistent middle ear disease or sensorineural hearing loss (congenital or acquired during language development) constitute two populations of special interest to the otolaryngologist.

The effects of chronic middle ear disease (serous otitis media/otitis media with effusion) on development of speech and language are not clear. Although effect of middle ear disease on hearing is fairly predictable, hearing impairment does not have a uniform effect on language development; language development patterns cannot be predicted on the basis of audiograms. This is because many other factors, in addition to hearing, affect language development, including cognitive development, socialization, and opportunities for learning. Although researchers have found that recurrent early middle ear disease has a negative effect on speech and language development, it has not been clear whether these effects constitute significant delays or persist beyond an initial period of language development.

Severe and persistent (e.g., sensorineural) hearing loss has a very definite and long-lasting effect on speech and language development. Hearing-impaired children typically have poor control over voice and vocal volume, poor articulation, language delay, and, in cases of profound hearing loss, severe limitations on the development of oral language. Although there is an undeniable relationship between the severity of hearing impairment and the ability to acquire auditory-verbal language, there is a significant amount of variability within the population. This variability in the oral language skills of hearing-impaired children has led researchers to conclude that the ability of hearing-impaired children to learn oral language appears to depend on an ill-defined ability to use residual hearing—a cognitive ability that there is currently no way to assess or predict. Two children with objectively similar hearing impairments do not necessarily develop the same proficiency with oral language. This inability to predict oral language skills, along with the political issues surrounding the education of the deaf (oral versus sign language philosophies of education), places the otolaryngologist, the audiologist, and the speech pathologist in an important and yet delicate position regarding educational recommendations for hearing-impaired children. It is helpful to remember that the decisions regarding oral and manual (or simultaneous oral and manual) training are ultimately the responsibility of the patient's caregiver and not of the health professionals. However, it is the responsibility of the health professionals to inform caregivers about (1) alternative methods of communication, including American Sign Language, Signed English, and Total Communication; (2) the importance of being exposed to a natural language (e.g., spoken English or American Sign Language) relatively early in development, because research indicates that people who learn a native language late in development may never develop true nativelike competence; and (3) the positive effects of multiple modality intervention, including amplification through hearing aids, aural rehabilitation, speech therapy, and counseling.

Swallowing Disorders in Children. Swallowing disorders in children are less common than communication disorders. They are generally associated with neurologic and motor disabilities (e.g., cerebral palsy, Down's syndrome) and, of course, can interfere with nutrition and basic health. Table 4–6 outlines normal sequences of oral-motor development and eating. Full evaluations completed by occupational or speech therapists can help identify specific problems and recommend strategies for feeding.

Lifespan Development

Normal Aging

From Table 4–5, it appears that language is basically mastered by about 3 years of age, and even the fine points of syntax and pragmatics are mastered by 10 years of age. It has been largely assumed that no significant changes in speech or language, other than an indefinite increase in vocabulary size, occur after childhood. However, the growing literature on gerontology has identified changes in speech and language throughout the lifespan. It is essential to be aware of these normal speech and language changes in order to accurately diagnose pathologic conditions in the elderly.

The effects of normal aging on communication are subtle but pervasive. Voice is known to change over the course of adulthood, probably from reduction of respiratory support, calcification and atrophy of the vocal folds and larynx, lowering of the larynx, and reduced elasticity of the pharyngeal walls. Routine and accurate identification of a speaker's age over the telephone confirms that there are acoustic correlates of the aging vocal mechanism. Fundamental frequency appears to increase for males and to decrease or stay the same for females (see Tables 4–1 and 4–2). Many older voices are also said to be mildly hoarse, which possibly reflects the increased jitter that has been shown to accompany age. Resonance and articulation appear to remain relatively unchanged during normal aging.

Normal reduction in brain weight, atrophy of dendritic elaboration, neurotransmitter reduction, and loss of myelin are all natural occurrences in the aging brain. There are concomitant changes in older adults' cortically mediated language behavior: older adults produce a more limited array of words and sentence structures than do younger adults and have some difficulty understanding complex sentences. Some of these problems may be attributed to declines in nonlinguistic cognition, such as attention and memory, and to age-related declines in hearing (presbycusis).

Diagnostic Considerations With the Elderly

Differential diagnosis is often harder with an aging population than with a younger group. Several factors must be considered when diagnoses are made for elderly patients. First, normal age-related changes and indications of pathologic conditions can overlap. Some patients complain that they have trouble coming up with words now and again. Is that an age-aggravation of the normal "tip of the tongue" phenomenon, or is it the early stage of dementia? Some patients may complain that their voice is becoming weak or mildly hoarse. Is that an effect of a normally aging larynx, the first symptom of laryngeal cancer, or a degenerative neurologic disorder?

Second, the incidences of certain diseases increase dramatically with age. Approximately 75% of strokes occur in people over 65; Alzheimer's disease occurs almost exclusively in the elderly; Parkinson's disease and cancer also occur much more frequently with age. Clinicians must have an awareness of the relative likelihood of certain diseases in each age group.

Other complicating factors in evaluating and diagnosing deficits in an elderly patient include the following:

1. Elderly patients often present with multiple changes such as hearing loss, cataracts, and dementia, which make symptoms complex and a single diagnosis unlikely.

2. Reactions to drugs may be more pronounced in the elderly, and the elderly are more likely to be taking multiple prescriptions, other people's prescriptions, and nonprescription drugs.

3. Elderly patients do not always have the same reactions to disease as younger people do; for example, mental disturbance such as confusion in the elderly is likely to result from a physical illness or a fall, whereas confusion in a younger patient is more likely to indicate an underlying organic brain syndrome.

4. Elderly patients are more likely than younger patients to underreport illness; they may accept deafness, dementia, or motor problems as part of inevitable aging and do not consider them important symptoms of potentially reversible pathologic changes.

Evaluation and Treatment of the Elderly

Evaluation of the elderly does differ in significant ways from that of the younger population. Some of the considerations are simple, such as allowing more time for an evaluation of an older person, compensating for known sensory deficits in hearing and vision with hearing aids and eye glasses, and asking for confirmation of medical history from a reliable source. Treatment considera-

tions and prognoses are also sometimes different for an elderly patient. For instance, in counseling patients about recovery from aphasia, clinicians must consider the fact that older patients typically recover more slowly and less completely. There are also more likely to be certain mitigating circumstances not found for younger patients, such as reduced opportunity for verbal interaction and progressive hearing loss.

Cognitive Disorders and Cognitive Rehabilitation: The Bigger Picture

Normal communication and other daily activities rely heavily on a range of nonlinguistic cognitive abilities, including memory, attention, calculation, judgment, inference, problem solving, and orientation to time and place. Disorders in these areas may interfere with communication and create other significant disabilities. In these cases, cognitive rehabilitation to recover functional skills is crucial if the patient is to return to work and independent living. Whether these cognitive disorders appear in association with language disorders or in isolation, they are frequently identified, evaluated, and treated by speech pathologists. When these disorders impinge on communication abilities, speech pathologists are essential participants in the rehabilitation effort.

Pathologic Conditions of Cognition

Organic brain syndromes and *neurobehavioral disorders* are terms used to describe a wide range of cognitive deficits ranging from basic impairment in arousal that is seen in acute confusional states (delirium) to high-level impairment in problem solving or abstract thought. These disorders result from insult or injury to the central nervous system, including closed-head trauma, focal cortical and subcortical lesions (e.g., strokes), exposure to toxic substances (e.g., drugs, carbon monoxide), infections (e.g., syphilis, meningitis), epilepsy, neoplasms, degenerative neurologic diseases (e.g., Alzheimer's and Parkinson's), and affective disorders.

Cognitive disorders can be described either as focal or as part of a dementia syndrome. Focal deficits are often associated with circumscribed lesions caused by stroke, neurosurgery, or central nervous system infection. The deficits are focal in that they affect one aspect of cognition more than any other. For instance, specific amnesias may be among the unavoidable side effects of neurosurgery to control temporal lobe epilepsy, or they may be the permanent sequelae of herpes encephalitis. Another example of a focal cognitive deficit occurs in some patients who suffer a right-hemisphere stroke and who recover well except for a persistent left-space neglect. In contrast, dementia syndromes are caused by more widespread pathologic processes and are associated with deficits in multiple areas of mental activity. Some dementias are potentially reversible, such as those caused by hydrocephalus, metabolic disorders (e.g., hypothyroidism), vitamin deficiencies (e.g., B_{12} deficiency), and brain tumors. However, approximately half of all dementias are attributed to Alzheimer's disease, which is degenerative, irreversible, and of unknown origin. Other disease processes that affect primarily subcortical regions have also been associated with dementia syndromes, including Parkinson's disease, progressive supranuclear palsy, and Huntington's chorea. Although the specific deficits vary across dementia syndromes, they all create significant impairment in several spheres of mental function.

Closed-head trauma, because of its prevalence, deserves independent mention as a cause of cognitive disorders. It is currently the third leading cause of death in the United States; it is estimated that 500,000 new cases of serious head injury occur every year. At least 50,000 of these patients are chronically disabled. The most common neuropsychologic effects associated with head trauma include personality changes that are characteristic of frontal lobe damage (apathy, euphoria, irritability, and inappropriate behavior), cognitive disturbance (conceptual disorganization, disconnected thought processes, posttraumatic amnesia), aphasia, and depression.

Evaluation and Treatment of Cognitive Disabilities

Cognitive disorders can be evaluated by many members of the rehabilitation team, including the neurologist, psychiatrist, neuropsychologist, occupational therapist, and speech pathologist. The most common tool for estimating the range and severity of cognitive dysfunction is the mental status examination. Although many specific mental status instruments exist, they all cover a similar range of basic cognitive functions, including emotional status, level of consciousness, attention, language, memory, constructional ability, and what are called *higher cognitive processes*, which usually include interpretation of proverbs and problem solving.

As with all rehabilitation efforts, the goal of the speech pathologist is to help the patient compensate for lost function and, if possible, return to an independent and meaningful life within the community. Specific treatment programs for cognitive disorders vary as much as the symptoms. In some cases, compensation for lost ability is accomplished by direct teaching. For instance, for severe memory dysfunction, a patient can often be trained to use a memory book that is constructed and organized according to the patient's need and is used to accomplish specific tasks. Patients can be successfully taught to look up information that they have difficulty remembering, including personal and family history, new acquaintances, and daily schedules. In other cognitive disorders, such as the dementia associated with Alzheimer's disease, the severity and progressive nature of the cognitive limitations preclude teaching patients new strategies to compensate for their deficits. Nonetheless, programs can be developed to improve communication and function at various stages of the disease by training caregivers to compensate for the memory problems of the patient. For instance, because early memory deficits in Alzheimer's disease can impair the patient's ability to follow instructions, the use of short sentences and written cues by the caregiver can help improve the patient's communication and performance of daily activities. In addition, because many of these cognitive impairments affect the interaction of the patient with the social support system, extensive family counseling by the speech pathologist is part of any cognitive rehabilitation program. Naturally, prognosis varies with severity of the deficit and is largely determined by whether the impairment is reversible, degenerative, or stable.

SUMMARY AND CONCLUSIONS

Speech pathologists are responsible for the evaluation and the treatment of a wide range of disorders, ranging from the hoarse voice to life-threatening dysphagia, to the rehabilitation of cognition after head injury. Considering the wealth of expertise within the field, speech pathology is, by any estimation, an underused resource in both acute care and rehabilitation. The goal of this chapter was to introduce the practicing physician to the range of services that the speech pathologist can provide. It will have achieved its goal if the reader makes a single appropriate referral that would otherwise not have been made.

Acknowledgments

I gratefully acknowledge comments made by several colleagues on early drafts of this chapter, including Barbara Cone-Wesson, Shaun Brayton-Gerratt, Bruce Gerratt, Patricia Gomeztrejo, Peter Persic, and Steven Peskind.

SUGGESTED READINGS

Speech and Voice

Aronson AE: Clinical Voice Disorders. New York: Thieme-Stratton, 1980.

Baker RJ: Clinical Measurement of Speech and Voice. Boston: Little, Brown, 1987.

Colton RH, Casper JK: Understanding Voice Problems. Baltimore: Williams & Wilkins, 1990.

Darley FL, Aronson AE, Brown JR: Motor Speech Disorders. Philadelphia: WB Saunders, 1975.

Fry DB: The Physics of Speech. Cambridge, England: Cambridge University Press, 1979.

Hirano M: Clinical Examination of Voice. New York: Springer-Verlag, 1981.

Keith RL, Darley FL (eds): Laryngectomee Rehabilitation. San Diego: College Hill Press, 1986.

Ladefoged P: Elements of Acoustic Phonetics. Chicago: University of Chicago Press, 1962.

Ladefoged P: A Course in Phonetics. New York: Harcourt Brace Jovanovich, 1975.

Perkins WH, Kent RD: Functional Anatomy of Speech, Language, and Hearing. San Diego: College Hill Press, 1986.

Swallowing

Aspiration and swallowing disorders. Otolaryngol Clin North Am 21(4)595–788, 1988.

Logemann J: Evaluation and Treatment of Swallowing Disorders. San Diego: College Hill Press, 1983.

Language and Cognition

Berko Gleason J: The Development of Language. Columbus, OH: Merrill, 1989.

Goodglass H, Kaplan E: The Assessment of Aphasia and Related Disorders. Philadelphia: Lea & Febiger, 1983.

Holland A: Language Disorders in Children. San Diego: College Hill Press, 1984.

Kolb B, Whishaw IQ: Fundamentals of Human Neuropsychology. New York: WH Freeman, 1985.

Lezak M: Neuropsychological Assessment. New York: Oxford University Press, 1983.

Sarno MT: Acquired Aphasia. New York: Academic Press, 1981.

Sohlberg MM, Mateer CA: Introduction to Cognitive Rehabilitation: Theory and Practice. New York: Guilford Press, 1989.

Strub RL, Black RW: Neurobehavioral Disorders. Philadelphia: FA Davis, 1988.

General

Lass NJ, McReynolds LV, Northern JL, Yoder DE: Handbook of Speech-Language Pathology and Audiology. Toronto: BC Decker, 1988.

CHAPTER 5

Geriatric Otolaryngology

Charles F. Koopmann, Jr., MD   Bradford S. Patt, MD   William L. Meyerhoff, MD, PhD

The demographic alteration of age characteristics within the United States population makes it imperative that otolaryngologists understand specific problems as they relate to the elderly patient. Since 1945, 4 years have been added to the average life expectancy of a 65-year-old male (from 78 years in 1945 to 82 years in 1990). By the year 2000, 20% of the American population will be 65 years of age or older, and by 2030, people age 65 or older will outnumber people between the ages of 18 and 34 in the United States. By 2005, the number of Americans 85 years of age or older will double. As this group of patients increases in number, so too do the demands on the health care system and expectations that the patients' problems will be understood and solved. It is because of this data that this chapter addresses voice changes, swallowing difficulties, hearing loss and balance disorders, cutaneous problems, the loss of senses of smell and taste, and other aspects of aging.

WOUND HEALING

Factors involved in manifestations of the aging process in connective tissue include the type of tissue evaluated, mechanical and sexual differences, and nutritional, vascular, and neurogenic factors. Nutrition and endocrinologic changes markedly affect the amounts of soluble and insoluble collagen, collagen synthesis, and the multiplication and growth rate of fibroblasts and their connective tissue. Soluble collagen content decreases with age, whereas insoluble collagen increases. Blood vessels and skin show a decrease in the elastic fibers, although the absolute amount of elastin may increase. Thus although the amount of collagen in tissues increases as a person ages, the older connective tissue contracts because of lower binding ability of fluid.

Nutrition, especially vitamins, is essential to adequate wound healing. Vitamin E (a free radical scavenger) inhibits inflammation. Deficiencies of thiamine cause a reduction of tensile strength. Vitamin C is essential to collagen synthesis, and a deficiency causes marked problems in wound healing. Vitamin A deficiency causes a decreased rate of collagen synthesis and reduction in epithelial coverage. Finally, a zinc deficiency causes problems with tensile strength of the wound as well as a loss of macrophages and polymorphonuclear leukocytes.

Endocrinologic disorders may significantly affect wound healing. The most important of these is diabetes mellitus. Patients with diabetes mellitus exhibit decreased tensile strength and a reduction of new collagen. Ingrowth of blood vessels in new fibroblasts is markedly reduced. Many aged persons take nonsteroidal anti-inflammatory drugs, which affect contractile strength and wound healing. Liver disease, or other chronic disease states, may lead to low serum albumin levels and increase protein metabolism, which cause a marked reduction in the ability to heal wounds.

Thus satisfactory wound-healing ability in the aging patient can potentially be reduced for many reasons.

RHINOLOGIC, OLFACTORY, AND TASTE FUNCTIONS

The nasal cavity, the olfactory system, and the sense of taste all show significant changes with aging. Hormonal changes, especially in the female, lead to a reduction of internal moisture as well as in size of the inferior turbinates, which thus predisposes the patient to atrophic rhinitis. The previously mentioned changes in connective tissue lead to atrophy of the collagen, absorption of fatty tissue, and increased fragility of the blood vessels. The third aspect, when combined with arteriosclerosis, makes the intranasal vessels highly subject to significant bleeding. The treatment of epistaxis in the elderly follows the same principles as that for other age groups. Specifically, the physician should attempt to identify the site of bleeding before the initiation of therapy. Elderly patients are more likely than younger patients to have renal problems, to be taking medication such as nonsteroidal anti-inflammatory agents, aspirin, or anticoagulants, or to have high blood pressure; therefore, a complete medical history should be obtained if time permits. Anterior epistaxis can be treated either by applying pressure or by cauterizing the affected vessel (thermally or chemically). Intranasal humidification and increased moisture, maintained with either propylene glycol or saline solution, are important. If this conservative approach fails, light packing of the nostrils with any type of gauze pack or hemostatic agent (such as oxidized cellulose [Oxycel]) may be used. Posterior epistaxis may either require anterior or posterior nasal packing or arterial ligation. If posterior nasal packing is necessary, the elderly patient should be hospitalized to minimize the risks of hypoxia, arterial oxygen desaturation, sleep apnea, and potential cardiac oxygen compromise. Occasionally, arterial ligation of either the ethmoidal arteries or the internal maxillary arteries is warranted. If surgical risks to the patient are too high, arterial embolization could be considered.

The cartilaginous and osseous structures of the nose are also affected by the aging process. The cartilaginous structures show separation and fragmentation of the lower lateral, upper lateral, and nasal septal cartilages, as well as a loss of fibrous tissue supporting the nasal tip, which results from absorption of the fat pad and weakening of the collagenous support. The nasal tip loses additional support when the feet of the medial crura of the lower lateral cartilage spread laterally and retract posteriorly. The result of these changes is a shortened retracted columella with both a downward rotation of the lobule and a reduction of nasal air flow. There is also a reduction in body fluid; this reduction increases the nasal mucus viscosity. When these changes are combined with atrophy of the mucus-secreting glands, the patient complains of postnasal drip and a feeling of nasal obstruction.

The olfactory neuroepithelium (located along the cribriform plate and superior aspects of the nasal septum and lateral nasal walls) shows significant degeneration in the elderly population. This process begins at approximately age 20 and continues throughout life.

The clinical sequelae of the aging process include changes in odor detection, odor identification, odor discrimination, and odor hedonic. Odor detection testing reveals impairment in the ability to detect low concentrations of odors and in chemical perceptions as a person ages. Specifically, for an elderly person to perceive the same odor intensity perceived by a younger person, a tenfold increase in the odor's concentration may be required. Nasal receptors for irritation are innervated by the trigeminal nerve. Often the same substances stimulate both the chemical and the olfactory receptors. The chemical stimulation may cause mucus reduction, cough, sneezing, or tearing.

Use of the University of Pennsylvania Smell Identification Test (UPSIT) has led to the discovery that odor identification is most accurate between the ages of 30 to 50, and impairment is significant after the age of 65. Finally, odor hedonics (measurements of good versus bad sensation) are significantly affected. This may result in the failure of the elderly to derive the same degree of pleasure from food that is blended or that may have a slightly bitter taste. Also, the nasal mucosa is affected by diuretics, antihypertensives, and antidepressants. The change in odor hedonics has been postulated to be one reason why many elderly people complain of a reduction in pleasures of taste. This problem may be ameliorated by use of food additives that may stimulate the chemical as well as the taste or small receptors.

The therapy for nasal obstruction resulting

from the retraction of the columella and drooping tip includes surgical procedures to shorten the nose by rotation of the upper tip. This is accompanied by removal of the cephalic third of the lower lateral cartilage and trimming of the caudal end of the nasal septum. Also, nasal tip support is improved by cartilaginous grafts placed anterior to the nasal spine. Tip elevation may also be increased by undermining the nasal dorsum and allowing it to redrape in combination with conservative removal of the dorsal hump. Antihistamines should be avoided in the treatment of the complaint of postnasal drip because they may cause lethargy, oversedation, or increased dryness of the mucosa. Decongestants may increase hypertension, may cause urinary retention, or may worsen cardiac problems. Nasal dryness may be treated with increased humidity, nasal saline drops, or topical water-soluble ointments. Oily preparations must be used with extreme caution because of the risk of lipoid pneumonia.

LARYNX AND VOICE

Phonation is a function of three factors: (1) pulmonary function, (2) laryngeal function, and (3) oral, anatomic, and physiologic functions. The pulmonary system of the elderly patient shows loss of compliance, reduction of vital capacity, limitation of expiratory force used for phonation, and reduction in the maintenance of intraoral breath pressure in vowel sounds. The larynx shows changes in ossification and in endocrinologic and neuromuscular functions. The false vocal cords show squamous metaplasia, decreased mucous production, and parakeratosis. The muscle mass in the thyroarytenoid cartilage is decreased and the cricoarytenoid joint may show either fixation or relaxation with poor arytenoid approximation. The latter leads to a significantly hoarse voice. The vocal folds show varying changes, depending on the sex of the patient: in males the folds show atrophy, which leads to a thin, reedy voice with increased pitch and a higher fundamental frequency; in women, the vocal cords show edema, which produces a lower fundamental frequency of the voice and light hoarseness. In an attempt to compensate for these changes, men frequently attempt to lower their pitch, which results in a gravely,

breathy, glottal voice. This type of voice fatigues easily. Women attempt to raise their pitch, which results in a strained, squeezed sound and a very effortful voice. Both sexes may show varying degrees of "senile bowing" of the vocal cords that results from connective tissue changes. Vocal tremor may result from hoarse qualities that are combined with higher pitch and reduced strength of amplification. This must be differentiated from the changes associated with spastic dysphonia or parkinsonism. Spastic dysphonic patients show excessive approximation of the true vocal cords without tremor. Patients with dysarthria may improve with either medical therapy or active speech intervention, and L-dopa administered for Parkinson's disease reduces dysarthria. Another cause of dysphonia in the elderly is gastroesophageal reflux resulting from the direct action of acid on the supraglottic larynx. Symptoms include a globus sensation, paroxysmal cough, dysphagia, pharyngeal clearing, a feeling of heartburn, and possibly otalgia and cervical pain. The findings on physical examination are arytenoid edema or granulomas and possibly point tenderness over one superior laryngeal nerve. Therapy is aimed at reduction of the reflux or neutralization of the acid.

Laryngeal framework surgery may provide the otolaryngologist with an important therapeutic tool to assist in the treatment of vocal problems in the elderly. The procedure has some limitations in the elderly patient because of significant relaxation of the tissue. The theory behind this surgery is anterior displacement of the anterior commissure with placement of a tantalum sheeting implant to displace the midline cartilage and anterior commissure anteriorly. The resultant anterior displacement of the attachment of the vocal ligament results in a higher pitch and decreased breathiness. However, it is difficult to predict which elderly patients will derive long-term benefit from this procedure.

ORAL CAVITY

Some of the more common complaints of the elderly patient relate to the physiologic or pathophysiologic changes in the oral cavity. The elderly patient may have an increased incidence of problems with dentition, inasmuch as 50 to 75% of patients over 70 years of age are completely edentulous. Contributing factors to these problems are dental caries, many years of bruxism, chronic periodontal disease, and reduction of salivary flow. Also, there is a progressive loss of both mandibular and maxillary alveolar bone. Xerostomia results from a combination of atrophy or fibrosis of the salivary glands (which creates a sensation of burning of the mouth or tongue), increase in dental caries, and alteration in the sensation of taste. Xerostomia should be treated with increased fluid intake, the use of artificial saliva, and stimulation of the remaining salivary flow with sialogogues. The oral epithelium also changes because of alterations in the epithelium and underlying connective tissue. The epithelium becomes thinner, and the prickle cell layer shows the most changes. In areas of chronic irritation secondary to denture use or other irritants, parakeratosis and hyperkeratosis can be found. The oral mucosa is more susceptible to injury, and traumatic wounds take longer to repair because of the thinning of the epithelium and the reduction of vascular supply.

Nicotinic stomatitis has been seen in up to 10% of the elderly population; it is heavily predominant among males. The area most often affected is the palatal mucosa. The lesions usually resolve with the cessation of use of the irritant (most commonly tobacco). If no improvement occurs, a biopsy may be necessary to rule out carcinoma. Angular cheilitis is seen at the oral commissure, either unilaterally or bilaterally, and most commonly manifests with erythema or cracking of the skin with surrounding maceration. A multitude of factors contribute to angular cheilitis, including redundant facial skin folds, ill-fitting dentures, pooling of saliva, chronic monilial infection, systemic disorders such as pernicious anemia or vitamin B complex deficiency, and the loss of osseous support. Treatment should be directed at the underlying nutritional or vitamin deficiency and should include thorough cleansing of the area, refitting of dentures when indicated, and the application of topical antifungal ointments. Occasionally when angular cheilitis is associated with glossodynia, the patient may be found to have vitamin B_{12}, iron, or folic acid deficiencies or diabetes mellitus.

Lichen planus is a chronic disease of the oral cavity that occasionally is confused with carcinoma but is most commonly a result of physical or emotional stress or the intake of numerous types of medication. This is a benign condition that may have two forms: nonerosive and erosive (or bullous). Nonerosive lichen planus is usually asymptomatic; the majority of the lesions occur on the buccal mucosa (in 80% of cases), although the tongue, lips, or hard palate may also be affected. These lesions are usually reticular or lacy in appearance and are white or gray. Erosive bullous or lichen planus is painful and in the earliest stages may be mistaken for herpetic lesions. The erosive form of lichen planus must be differentiated from syphilis, nutritional deficiency, benign pemphigoid, or erythema multiforme. Treatment involves reassurance and relief of pain, most often with 0.5% dyclonine hydrochloride or topical lidocaine.

Hyperkeratotic lesions are frequently seen in the elderly and are a cause of concern because of the fear of carcinoma. These lesions may include leukoplakia, verruciform hyperkeratosis, frictional hyperkeratosis carcinoma in situ, or invasive squamous cell carcinoma. When frictional keratosis is seen, some type of irritant must be suspected, usually denture, trauma from the teeth, or occasional pipe smoking. This disorder can be compared with callus formation, and the treatment is removal of the causative agent. When this treatment is unsuccessful, an incisional biopsy is warranted.

Actinic cheilitis (or keratosis) can be found along the vermilion border of the lower lip in patients who have had chronic sun exposure. Any areas that show ulceration should be biopsied to rule out early invasive squamous cell carcinoma. If the cutaneous lesion is entirely actinic keratosis, then a lip shave is performed, and the remaining mucosa is advanced to the vermilion cutaneous border. The patient is postoperatively counseled in the use of sunscreen preparations and wide-brim hats or caps to protect the involved areas from ultraviolet rays.

Erythroplasia is seen in one of three forms: interspersed with leukoplakia, multifocal, or homogeneous. The lesions are usually red and appear inflamed. The incidence of carcinoma or severe dysplasia has been reported to be up to 90% in these lesions. When the areas localize, an attempt to excise the area can be made.

Carcinomas of the lip, the tongue, and the floor of the mouth are discussed in Chapter 32.

CUTANEOUS PROBLEMS OF THE HEAD AND NECK

Chronic exposure to ultraviolet light from the sun can cause damage to the epidermis, especially to cells involved in the production of melanin and keratin. Clinical manifestations are wrinkling of the skin along with capillary fragility, easy bruisability, and telangiectasia. Seborrheic dermatitis is often seen in the elderly, especially in debilitated patients. The lesions are characterized by scaling red lesions along the scalp margin, the eyebrow glabella, the nasolabial folds, and the postauricular regions. These lesions must be differentiated from those of psoriasis. Treatment includes a medicated shampoo such as Neutrogena (benzoyl peroxide), T-Gel (coal tar), Sebulex (salicylic acid and sulfur), or Selsun (selenium sulfide). If the lesion becomes inflamed, one could use a topical fluorinated steroid cream such as betamethasone valerate (Valisone).

Seborrheic keratosis is distinguishable by its flat, sharply marginated edges and the brown to tan color. Differential diagnosis includes cutaneous warts or actinic keratosis. Although most of these lesions require no treatment, they occasionally can be cosmetically disturbing, and they can be removed with cryosurgery, a shave excision, or, in rare instances, a surgical excision.

Lentigo maligna can occur anywhere in the head and neck but is usually seen over the anterior face and along the nasolabial crease. The lesions have a distinct black pigmentation surrounded by a brown to tan area and must be considered melanoma in situ. Consequently, they must be entirely removed surgically and often require regional advancement flaps for wound closure. Keratoacanthomas are lesions that are considered benign, although they can be closely associated with squamous cell carcinoma. Keratoacanthomas usually grow rapidly and are characterized by central depression, which is most commonly filled with keratin. The lesions should be totally excised so that the base can be examined microscopically because in many areas that appear to be benign, invasive squamous cell carcinoma is in the base. Basal and squamous cell carcinomas of the skin are discussed in Chapter 46.

HEAD AND NECK ONCOLOGIC DISORDERS

Too often, medical and surgical colleagues have felt that head and neck malignancies in the elderly should be treated in a markedly different fashion than those in younger patients because of a mistaken impression that elderly patients are intolerant of head and neck surgery. Studies to date fail to substantiate this philosophy. Johnson and coworkers (1977) demonstrated that a composite resection is a procedure well tolerated by the elderly patient. They found that the elderly experienced major and minor wound complications with a frequency similar to that in younger patients. It is true that the elderly are more likely to have medical problems related to the surgery, but surgical morbidities such as wound infection, flap necrosis, carotid artery rupture, hematoma formation, or orocutaneous fistulas do not increase in the aged patient. Associated medical complications such as pulmonary difficulties, cardiac arrhythmias, and gastrointestinal hemorrhage are slightly increased in the elderly. However, composite resection offers not only a chance for a cure but also an effective method of palliation with an acceptable complication rate in this age group.

Tucker (1977) and associates reviewed their experiences with conservation laryngeal surgery in the elderly and found that the total complication rate approached 11%. Among patients who underwent vertical hemilaryngectomy and most candidates for supraglottic laryngectomy, there were no major surgical difficulties, minimal pulmonary complications, and no surgical mortalities. These data showed that the complication rate was totally acceptable, and so the argument for withholding the conservation procedure in the elderly because high morbidity and mortality were anticipated does not seem to be appropriate. Again, a patient with carcinoma of the larynx should be viewed as an individual, irrespective of age, and if the patient's cardiac status and pulmonary status are acceptable, then conservation laryngeal surgery is warranted. John and Vaughn (1980) found that elderly patients tolerate total laryngectomy well, and Gall and coworkers (1977) found that laryngopharyngeal surgical complications had no relation to age and sex. Thus, again, if the patient does require total laryngectomy, age should not be a contraindication. Finally, McGuirt and coauthors (1977) reviewed complications of major head and neck procedures in the elderly over a 10-year period. Their findings showed that the incidence of surgical complications was no different than that in younger groups, although medical complication were 8% higher in elderly patients. Consequently, in all the studies just mentioned, the evidence is clear that if a patient's pulmonary status and cardiovascular status are reasonably acceptable, age should not be a deterrent for major surgical extirpation of head and neck malignancies.

AUDITORY AND VESTIBULAR SYSTEMS

External Auditory Canal: Anatomy

Two kinds of hair grow within the external auditory canal. Minute vellus hairs cover almost all of the ear canal; the larger tragi hairs are laterally situated in the external canal and are found only in adult males. These tragi are a secondary sex characteristic and become coarser, larger, and more noticeable in the third and fourth decades of life. These larger hairs are also found on the tragus, the antitragus, and the helix.

Cerumen glands are actually modified apocrine sweat glands. In the ear canals, they are responsible for the distinctive odor of cerumen. Cerumen glands open onto the skin or more frequently into hair follicles just external to the opening of the sebaceous gland ducts. In the hair follicle, sebum, apocrine secretions, and desquamated epithelial cells combine to form wet or dry cerumen, which are two genetically controlled phenotypes. Cerumen glands atrophy in the ear canals of the elderly. Because of this reduction in the number of glands, cerumen has the tendency to become drier in older persons, and this tendency may be partially responsible for more frequent cerumen impactions.

Cerumen impaction tends to occur more frequently in the elderly male because of the large tragi in the ear canal, which become entangled with the drier wax and prevent the natural dislodgment of cerumen. Impaction may be removed in several ways. If the

wax is relatively soft, gentle irrigation of the ear canal with water at body temperature may be attempted. Firmly impacted cerumen often resists removal even with vigorous irrigation and must therefore be manually extracted by the use of a curet and an otoscope. It is important to avoid trauma to the skin of the canal, especially the medial portion, which is quite sensitive and easily injured during cerumen removal. Dry wax may be softened with ceruminolytic agents for 24 to 48 hours, after which the softened wax may be removed by irrigation from the ear canal. A tympanic membrane perforation precludes the use of irrigation or ceruminolytic agents to clean the ear canal.

Itching within the external auditory canal results from anatomic and biochemical changes related to aging that leave the skin atrophic. Pruritus of the skin is usually related to dryness, but it may be a major complaint even when no apparent abnormality exists. The problem may be exacerbated by efforts to remove accumulated dry wax with cotton-tipped applicators and other foreign objects.

Frequently, chronic pruritus of the ear canal is not a sign of chronic otitis externa or serious dermatologic problems but merely an itch-scratch-itch cycle initiated by the skin dryness that results from atrophy of the epithelium and epidermal sebaceous glands. Efforts must be directed toward breaking the cycle by avoiding moisture, trauma, and defatting agents (alcohol-vinegar mixtures) in the external canal and occasionally by using an emollient, which acts as an epidermal seal and slows the loss of moisture from the skin. Several drops of glycerin or mineral oil instilled in the ear canal daily decrease the dryness and preclude the need for alcohol irrigations after bathing and swimming. A steroid ointment may be applied to the outside of the external ear canal to help resolve chronic pruritus. If alcohol douches are used, they should be followed by the instillation of glycerin or other emollients.

Aging is *not* associated with a higher incidence of infections in the ear canal. Otitis externa is manifested by otalgia and tenderness of the external canal. The infection may be manifested by aural discharge, hearing loss, increasing tenderness, fever, and periauricular erythema and swelling. Treatment should include thorough cleaning of the ear canal and avoidance of the entry of water into the canal. Antibiotic steroid drops are prescribed three times daily for 7 to 10 days, and if periauricular erythema and tenderness are marked, oral antibiotics may be prescribed. The presence of continued infection of the canal despite local measures and oral antibiotics may in rare instances require the use of intravenous antibiotics. Pain may be severe, especially at night, and may require narcotic or nonsteroidal anti-inflammatory medications. Malignant (necrotizing) otitis externa is an osteitis and osteomyelitis of the temporal bone caused by *Pseudomonas aeruginosa*. It is most commonly seen in elderly diabetics and may present as a persistent external otitis. Malignant otitis externa is most likely related to a compromised vasculature and immunologic system rather than to the age of the patient, inasmuch as the disease has also been seen in children.

Tumors involving the external canal include squamous cell carcinoma, basal cell carcinoma, and ceruminoma. These growths are most commonly seen in patients from 50 to 61 years old, although they can occur in both younger and older patients. Tumors of the external canal, although more prevalent in the elderly, are not manifestations of the aging process. These tumors should be suspected in all patients complaining of chronic otalgia (with or without otorrhea), hearing loss, vertigo, or facial nerve paralysis. Abnormal tissue seen in the external canal should undergo biopsy for pathologic examination.

Middle Ear

The normal middle ear undergoes age-related changes that most commonly involve the ossicular joints. Arthritic changes within the joint capsule may range from mild to severe and can occasionally lead to narrowing of the joint space. Severe changes may lead to calcification of the joint capsule, diffuse calcification of the articular cartilages and disk, and fusion or obliteration of portions or all of the joint space. Two-thirds of people 30 to 70 years old have mild to severe arthritic changes in middle ear joints; furthermore, all persons over 70 years of age show moderate to severe arthritic changes, which are symmetric in both ears and most severe in the incudomalleal joint. Arthritic changes have been evaluated audiometrically, and even complete obliteration of the joint space has no identifiable effect on sound transmission through the middle ear. Aging alone does not result in conductive hearing loss. Osteitis deformans has been linked to sensorineural hearing loss in the elderly, although the pathophysiologic process of the hearing loss has not been clearly elucidated.

Tumors

Middle ear tumors are rare and occur in the same age range as do tumors of the external canal, and they therefore are not considered manifestations of aging. The most common middle ear tumors found in aging patients are adenocarcinoma and nonchromaffin paragangliomas. An objective finding of pulsatile tinnitus in a patient with an abnormal-looking tympanic membrane may represent the presence of a middle ear tumor. Other symptoms of middle ear masses are similar to those seen with external ear tumors.

Inner Ear

Dizziness, disequilibrium, and vertigo are common complaints by the elderly. A National Health Interview Surgery Supplement on Aging (Havilik, 1986) found that 34% of people between 65 and 74 years of age were restricted in their everyday actions by dizziness. An estimated 12.5 million persons over the age of 65 in the United States are thought to be significantly affected by dizziness or balance disturbance.

Furthermore, falls are a significant cause of morbidity in the elderly population. They are the precipitating cause of more than 200,000 hip fractures and various other fractures that occur annually in Americans over 65. The reported incidence of falls increases with age and disability, being 0.2 to 0.6 per person per year in the healthy elderly community and 0.6 to 3.6 among institutionalized patients. Multiple factors have been linked to falls, including general health status, change in vision, impairment of activities of daily living, cardiac and cerebrovascular disease, environmental hazards, medication use, muscle weakness, and gait disorders. Whether vestibular dysfunction is a significant factor in falls has not been proved. Vertigo seldom directly accompanies falls, being associated with only 7.2% of falls documented by one study and 6.4% in another study.

Balance, or the sensation of equilibrium,

is regulated by inner ear vestibular function, vision, and projections from the skeletal muscles in the neck, the trunk, and the extremities. Balance disorders contribute to severe deficits in ambulation that may impair a person's ability to carry out the activities of daily living. In evaluation of the cause of disequilibrium or dizziness in the elderly, etiologic factors other than those involving the vestibular system must be considered. Thus visual disturbances, musculoskeletal disorders, neurologic dysfunctions, and metabolic causes of dizziness as well as cardiovascular disorders must be considered for the elderly patient complaining of a balance disturbance (Table 5–1). Studies show that significant structural and physiologic changes in the vestibular system occur with age. However, vestibular function shows increased variability in the elderly, which makes definitive conclusions on the effect of aging alone on balance disorders difficult.

TABLE 5–1. Disorders Associated With Dizziness

Peripheral Vestibular System
Meniere's disease
Chronic otitis media
Vestibular neuronitis
Luetic (neurosyphilis)
Iatrogenic (otologic surgery)
Head trauma
Cupulolithiasis
Ototoxic drugs
Otosclerotic inner ear syndrome
Alternobaric vertigo
Primary tumors of temporal bone (congenital
    cholesteatoma, glomus tumor, facial nerve neuroma,
    squamous cell carcinoma)
Metastatic tumors of temporal bone (prostate, breast,
    kidney, lung)
Cerebellopontine angle tumors (acoustic neuroma,
    cholesteatoma, meningioma)

Central Nervous System
Demyelinating diseases (multiple sclerosis, diffuse
    sclerosis, acute disseminated encephalitis)
Localized encephalitis
Metastatic tumors of the brain stem
Posterior fossa tumors
Seizures (temporal lobe epilepsy)
Orthostatic hypotension
Vascular lesions or disease (thrombotic and embolic)

Systemic and Metabolic
Hypoglycemia
Hypothyroidism
Anemia
Drug intoxication
Allergic inner ear syndrome

Cervical
Cervical vertigo

The peripheral vestibular system has been studied to determine the effect of aging on hair cells, peripheral vestibular neurons, and supporting elements of the vestibular end organ. An age-related progressive loss has been found in the sensory epithelia and components of the labyrinth.

Progressive hair cell reduction begins at about 40 years of age. Paralleling the loss of hair cells are similar reductions in peripheral vestibular neurons and a decrease in the caliber of remaining peripheral myelinated nerve fibers. There is almost a 40% decrease in the number of myelinated vestibule nerve fibers in persons over 74 years of age in comparison with those under 35 years of age.

Vestibular Function Testing

Vestibular function tests are attempts to quantify the degree to which a person is affected by disequilibrium and dizziness, and they may help identify the source of the problem. Unfortunately, these tests show great variability, especially in the elderly population. Tests of vestibular function encompass portions of the neurologic examination as well as certain quantitative laboratory procedures. Quantitative testing includes caloric stimulation, rotational testing, and posturography.

Caloric responses measured by electronystagmography have been found to increase until middle age, to peak at ages 50 to 70 years, and to then decline modestly. Although age-related effects on caloric responses exist, there appear to be only minor differences between age groups.

Rotational testing has yielded no conclusive data to determine whether age-related changes occur in the elderly. Some studies have shown decreased responses to rotational testing in persons older than 70 years of age.

Posturography is a relatively new quantitative procedure to investigate postural control capabilities. The integration of visual, vestibular, and proprioceptive cues (sensory integration) with motor response output and of coordination of the lower limbs is tested by posturography. In posturography, test conditions are used to evaluate balance disorders and sensory organization (Fig. 5–1). Although posturography is a new procedure in testing balance disorders, especially in the elderly, it represents a systematic investiga-

Sensory Organization Test

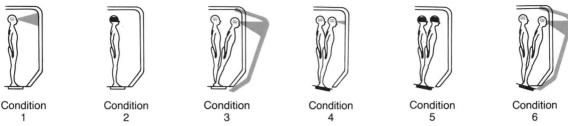

| Condition 1 | Condition 2 | Condition 3 | Condition 4 | Condition 5 | Condition 6 |

Figure 5–1. Six testing conditions used in posturography to evaluate dizziness.

tion of balance disorders that provides a new dimension that has been lacking in the routine work-up of the patient with dizziness. Further studies are needed to document reliability.

Conditions of Dizziness and Disequilibrium

Although there is a general decrease in vestibular sensitivity with aging, this decrease generally leads to only a modest decline in function. Clinicians should not dismiss dizziness or disequilibrium as a symptom of normal aging or multiple sensory deficits without a careful evaluation for specific disease processes. Although a tremendous variety of disorders are associated with dizziness (see Table 5–1), a specific cause can be identified in 85% of patients.

Four clinically documented age-related conditions of disequilibrium found in the elderly are (1) benign positional vertigo, (2) ampullary disequilibrium, (3) macular disequilibrium, and (4) vestibular ataxia of aging.

Benign Positional Vertigo. Cupulolithiasis, or benign positional vertigo, is characterized by sudden severe episodes of vertigo precipitated by a particular head position. Benign positional vertigo may result from head injury, ear surgery, otitis media, or inner ear vascular occlusion, or it may occur spontaneously in persons over 40 years of age. The elderly, therefore, have been shown to suffer an increased incidence of benign positional vertigo. When cupulolithiasis does occur in older patients, it tends to persist indefinitely. If vestibular suppressant medication is ineffective or if patients are unable to adapt to this disability, surgical section of

the vestibular nerve is effective in alleviating benign positional vertigo.

Ampullary Disequilibrium. Turning the head quickly to the right or left or extension or flexion of the head may precipitate vertigo. The causes of this problem are not known, and treatment is to avoid the precipitating movement.

Macular Disequilibrium. Macular disequilibrium of aging is characterized by vertigo precipitated by a change of head position in relation to the direction of gravitational force after the head has been maintained in a given position for some time. For example, on attempting to rise from the bed, the patient may have such pronounced vertigo that sitting up may have to be accomplished in stages. Orthostatic hypotension may cause similar symptoms but it is usually accompanied by other signs of intracranial ischemia as well as changes in blood pressure. As with ampullary disequilibrium, the treatment is to avoid movements that elicit these symptoms.

Vestibular Ataxia. Vestibular ataxia of aging is characterized by a constant feeling of imbalance with ambulation. Walking is hesitant, with frequent side steps and a fixed head position to gain optimal advantage of visual points of reference. Also, the fixed head position may lead to recurrent headaches. The cause of this disease entity may be loss of vestibular control over the lower limbs.

Rehabilitation

It is clear that vertigo and disequilibrium are important clinical problems in the elderly. Although adaptation may occur over time, the elderly patient tends to have greater problems with balance than does the younger patient. Medical and surgical treatment can often ease the symptoms of disequilibrium, but a significant proportion of patients continue to have some balance disturbances. Rehabilitation of the patient with dizziness is aimed at enhancing adaptation of the vestibular system and substituting alternative strategies to replace lost vestibular function. A vestibular exercise program that was originally introduced by Cawthorne in the 1940s is directed at improving visual following when the head is stationary, gaze stability during head movements, visual-vestibular interactions during head movement, and balance in stance and during ambulation (Cawthorne, 1964). Alternative strategies to replace lost vestibular function emphasize the substitution of visual and proprioceptive information to stabilize the visual world and to maintain posture stability.

AUDITORY DYSFUNCTION

Types of Hearing Loss

Hearing impairment is classified as conductive, sensorineural, or mixed. *Conductive* hearing loss may be caused by anything that precludes the normal transmission of sound energy through the external auditory canal, the tympanic membrane, or the middle ear. Various conditions that frequently result in conductive hearing loss include impacted cerumen, tympanic membrane perforation, otitis media, and discontinuity of fixation of the ossicles (e.g., otosclerosis). *Sensorineural* hearing loss results when the inner ear, the auditory nerve (cranial nerve VIII), the brain stem, or the cortical auditory pathways are not functioning properly. A *mixed* hearing loss is a conductive hearing loss superimposed on a sensorineural hearing loss.

Presbycusis

Presbycusis, a sensorineural form of hearing loss, represents the most common form of hearing loss in the elderly. Studies have indicated that approximately 25% of people between 65 and 74 years of age and 50% of people 75 years of age or older experience hearing difficulties.

The cause of presbycusis remains unclear. Researchers have attempted to link effects of diet, metabolism, arteriosclerosis, noise,

stress, and heredity on hearing without clear correlation. Presbycusis remains a diagnosis of exclusion and requires that other causes of bilateral progressive sensorineural hearing loss be ruled out before the diagnosis is made (Table 5–2). In some research, long exposure to environmental noise has been correlated with presbycusis, but it would be overly simplistic to assume that noise is the only etiologic factor.

Schuknecht (1974) classified four types of presbycusis:

1. The most common type, sensory presbycusis, is characterized by changes at the basal end of the organ of Corti. Audiometrically, these changes caused high-tome hearing loss. Speech discrimination remains fairly good.

2. Neural presbycusis results from loss of cochlear neurons. Audiometrically, loss of speech discrimination is greater than lowering of pure-tone hearing thresholds.

3. Metabolic presbycusis has been connected with atrophy of the stria vascularis. The audiometric changes consist of a flat sensorineural hearing loss and relatively good speech discrimination.

4. Inner ear (cochlear) conductive presbycusis is thought to be caused by the stiffening of the basilar membrane. Audiometrically, a gradual downsloping curve is seen with speech discrimination more or less in the range that would be expected from the level of pure-tone hearing threshold (Fig. 5–2).

Because more than one area of degeneration is usually present in a given ear, the diagnosis of one of the four types of presbycusis is not frequently made.

In a more recent classification, presbycusis is categorized into three types: primarily peripheral (cochlear and cochlear neuron), central (central auditory processing problems), or mixed peripheral and central. More research is needed before the extent to which central auditory factors are involved in hearing loss in the elderly is known.

Characteristics. Most patients with presbycusis experience a slowly progressive type of hearing loss with a fairly consistent pattern of pure-tone hearing loss (represented by the curve of an audiogram). An additional documented auditory handicap in the elderly is a decrease in word intelligibility. It is com-

TABLE 5–2. Causes of Bilaterally Symmetric Sensorineural Hearing Loss

Disorder	Characteristics	Diagnosis	Treatment
Meniere's disease	Episodic attacks of fluctuant SNHL, vertigo, tinnitus, aural fullness or pressure; bilateral in 20%–30% of cases	History of typical attacks with symptom-free intervals; hearing loss involves low tones initially and later all frequencies; rule out neurosyphilis	Medical: Diuretic and low-salt diet Surgical: Decompression or shunt of endolymphatic sac; section of vestibular nerve
Luetic hearing loss (late acquired syphilis)	Frequently bilateral SNHL with no characteristic audiometric pattern; speech discrimination score often worse than would be predicted on basis of pure-tone thresholds; often associated with vestibular symptoms; may mimic Meniere's disease	Positive FTA-ABS test, with or without clinical history of syphilis	Penicillin and oral steroids
Osteitis deformans	Slowly progressive SNHL and CHL; SNHL worse for high frequencies; maximum CHL of 20–30 db at 500 Hz	Skeletal deformities of skull and long bones of extremities; elevated levels of serum alkaline phosphatase and urinary hydroxyproline	Calcitonin
Hypothyroidism	Slowly progressive SNHL affecting all frequencies equally	Usual clinical stigmata of hypothyroidism; decreased levels of serum T_4	Desiccated thyroid or synthetic mixture of T_4 and T_3
Ototoxic drugs	Hearing loss with or without vestibular dysfunction after treatment with known ototoxic drug	History	None
Hereditary progressive SNHL	Progressive SNHL beginning at earlier age than expected for presbycusis; possible family history	Family history	None
Noise-induced hearing loss	History of prolonged exposure to loud continuous noise or brief exposure to loud impulse noise	History; characteristic audiogram with maximal hearing loss at 4000 Hz; may not be distinguishable from presbycusis	None; use of ear protectors may prevent further loss from noise exposure
Head trauma	Severe head injury often resulting in loss of consciousness and bilateral temporal bone fractures	History	None
Cochlear otosclerosis and far advanced clinical otosclerosis	Far advanced clinical otosclerosis (stapedial fixation) and cochlear otosclerosis (SNHL) may appear on audiogram as severe to profound SNHL; good speech modulation (in contrast to profound SNHL) and wearing of a bone conduction hearing aid; possibly a family history for otosclerosis	History is suggestive but surgical exploration of stapes footplate is diagnostic and therapeutic; poststapedectomy patient may be able to wear ear-level hearing aid with good results	Stapedectomy, sodium fluoride

Note: The hearing loss from any of these diseases may be improved with hearing aids unless it is of such a degree that hearing aids are inadequate or unsatisfactory. Persons with bilateral profound SNHL may be candidates for a cochlear implant and should be evaluated by an otologist to determine their suitability for such a device.

Abbreviations: SNHL = sensorineural hearing loss; FTA-ABS test = fluorescent treponemal antibody test; CHL = conductive hearing loss; T_3 = triiodothyronine; T_4 = thyroxine.

Figure 5–2. Cross-section of cochlea, showing cochlear neurons, organ of Corti, and stria vascularis.

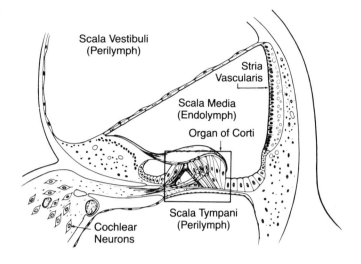

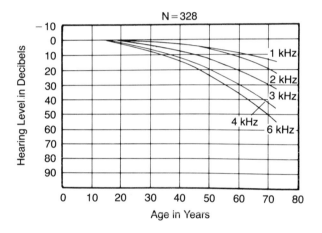

mon for an older person to hear people talking but be unable to understand the words being said. At a given level of hearing, many elderly persons have a significantly poorer speech discrimination than does a younger person with the same hearing level. Some research has linked poor word intelligibility to changes in the central auditory system. It is thought that presbycusis may be caused by an interaction of changes in the auditory periphery and central nervous system.

Additional auditory problems in the elderly are related to directional hearing. Elderly people complain that it is much more difficult to hear when more than one person is talking or when there is background noise. Loss of directional hearing has also been linked to deficits in central auditory processing and leads to further deterioration of word intelligibility.

Obviously, presbycusis is not a simple entity but rather a complex disorder involving a wide range of problems from loss of speech processing to decreased word intelligibility. The elderly require careful explanations of the problem to help prevent the isolation or the frustration that may result from progressive hearing loss. Auditory rehabilitation plays an important role in keeping the older person with a hearing deficit from withdrawing from society.

Audiometric Evaluation

Hearing sensitivity is measured in units of sound that are known as decibels (db). A decibel is not a fixed value of sound but represents a logarithmic ratio based on a standard reference level of acoustic pressure. In standardized hearing tests, discrete frequencies of sound from 250 to 8999 Hz (cycles per second) are presented in a prescribed manner until the listener responds to the stimulus being presented, at which point the threshold of hearing sensitivity is established. The more decibels of sound that are required for a person to hear, the poorer the hearing is. Although an average hearing threshold of 30 db or less in speech frequencies (500 to 3000 Hz) is satisfactory for routine listening needs, amplification may be indicated if psychosocial needs or work-related requirements demand better hearing.

Although pure-tone hearing tests provide significant information regarding auditory function, another important consideration involves the ability to understand speech. *Speech discrimination,* or word intelligibility, is determined by use of a standardized list of monosyllabic words, which are presented to the patient at a comfortably loud listening level. Results are calculated in percentages that are based on the number of words that the patient correctly repeats, 100% being a perfect discrimination score. Thus the higher the discrimination is, the better is the ability to understand speech. In general, persons whose speech discrimination is less than 70% to 80% have noticeable problems understanding speech.

AUDITORY REHABILITATION

Factors Determining Candidacy for Hearing Aid

The use of a hearing aid should be considered once a complete otologic examination and audiologic evaluation have confirmed bilateral sensorineural and medically untreatable hearing loss. The success of auditory rehabilitation depends on the person's auditory capabilities as well as physical capabilities, including manual dexterity and mobility, level of social activity, motivation, and adaptability.

Physical Aspects of Hearing Aids

A hearing aid is a miniature amplifier of acoustic energy and is designed specifically to improve hearing. Its primary function is to increase the intensity of sound and to deliver it to the ear with as little distortion as possible. Every hearing aid contains four basic components: a *microphone* that receives sound and converts it into an electrical signal;

an *amplifier* that increases the amplitude of the electrical signal; a *power source,* which is a small battery, that provides energy to the amplifier; and a miniature loudspeaker, called an *earphone* or a receiver, that converts the electrical energy back to sound.

Hearing aids are available in different styles, all of which function in basically the same fashion. The selection of a particular style of hearing aid depends on the type and degree of hearing loss and on the patient's cosmetic desires, personal preference, and manual dexterity for inserting the aid and adjusting the controls (Fig. 5–3). The post-auricular (behind-the-ear) aid is currently the most popular because of its small, neat appearance, wide application, and versatility of fitting. The body aid is appropriate for patients who may have difficulty manipulating the smaller hearing aid control on the ear-level models. The all-in-the-ear aid has gained increasingly wide acceptance and is able to provide adequate power for patients with a variety of hearing losses.

A certified audiologist should help determine the appropriate hearing aid needed as well as the proper ear mold, the style of the aid, and whether one or both ears should be aided. It is particularly important, especially for the elderly patient, that he or she actually experiences hearing aid use before purchasing an aid. Many elderly people deny auditory difficulties and may refuse to wear a hearing aid. They are difficult to fit because of acquired poor listening habits, unwillingness to make changes in their lives, poor word intelligibility, and often decreased tolerance to loud sounds.

Once a hearing aid is selected, a carefully planned rehabilitation program is followed to maximize the efficiency of the hearing aid. Although a hearing aid can help the elderly overcome the handicap of hearing loss, it cannot return hearing to normal. The patient and family members must be counseled with regard to the limitations of a hearing aid and in this way avoid unrealistic expectations and future frustration for the hearing aid user.

Other Rehabilitative Programs

Aural rehabilitation is an attempt to minimize the handicap of hearing impairment. Although a hearing aid plays an integral part in achieving the goal of hearing rehabilitation, the procedures—including speech read-

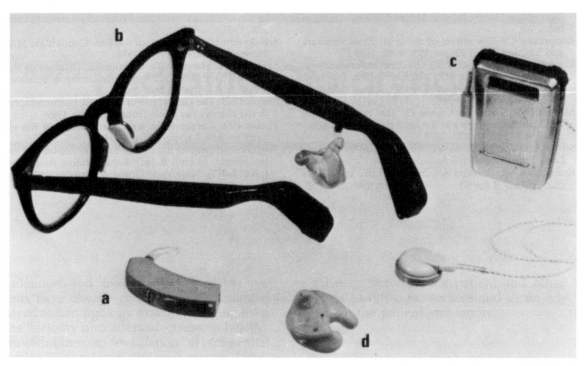

Figure 5–3. Commonly used hearing aids. *A.* Postauricular (behind-the-ear) aid. *B.* Eyeglass hearing aid. *C.* Body aid. *D.* All-in-the-ear hearing aid.

ing training, auditory or listening training, speech hearing training, and lip-reading instruction—all play an important role in helping the elderly overcome severe hearing loss. Each patient requires an individualized approach tailored to his or her audiologic, mental, and physical deficits. The ultimate goal of an aural rehabilitation program is to enable the patient to perform in society with the least hearing handicap possible.

CONCLUSION

It is clear that the otolaryngologist of today must be cognizant of the specific problems affecting the elderly population. Evaluation and treatment of elderly patients require an understanding of their particular disease states. The diseases affecting the elderly are varied, and appropriate treatment should not be deferred on the basis of age alone. If the physician treating the aged can understand their problems, a better relationship will develop, and good medical care will result. By being aware of the particular medical problems affecting the elderly, physicians can help them lead more active and happier lives.

SUGGESTED READINGS

Baloh RW, Sakala SM, Yee RD, et al: Quantitative vestibular testing. Otolaryngol Head Neck Surg 92:145, 1985.

Boucek RJ: Factors affecting wound healing. Otolaryngol Clin North Am 17(2):243–264, 1984.

Cawthorne T: Otological aspects in the differential diagnosis of vertigo. *In* Fields W, Alford B (eds): Neurological Aspects of Auditory and Vestibular Disorders (pp 271–282). Springfield, IL: Charles C Thomas, 1964.

Goldstein JC, Kashima HK, Koopman CF: Geriatric Otolaryngology. Toronto: BC Decker, 1989.

Gacek RR, Ham R: A clinical approach to the management of geriatric disequilibrium. Ear Nose Throat J 68:958, 1989.

Gall AM, Sessions DG, Ogura JH: Complications following surgery for cancer of the larynx and hypopharynx. Cancer 39:624–631, 1977.

Havilik RJ: Aging in the 80's: Impaired Senses for Sound and Light in Persons Age 65 and Older. [Preliminary data from the Supplemental on Aging to the National Health Interview Survey, United States, January–June 1984. Advance data from Vital and Health Statistics No. 125, DHHS Publication O(PHS) 86–1250.] Hyattsville, MD: Public Health Survey, 1986.

John AC, Vaughn SD: Laryngeal resection in patients of seventy years and over. J Laryngol Otol 94:629–635, 1980.

Johnson JT, Rabrizzi D, Tucker H: Composite resection in the elderly: A well tolerated procedure. Laryngoscope 87:1509–1515, 1977.

Koopmann CF: Otolaryngologic surgery in the elderly. *In* Katlic MR (ed): Geriatric Surgery: Comprehensive

CHAPTER 7

Anatomy and Embryology of the Ear

H. Alexander Arts, MD   Larry G. Duckert, MD, PhD

The peripheral auditory system can be divided both functionally and anatomically into three distinct parts. The *external ear* consists of the auricle, the external auditory canal, and the lateral surface of the tympanic membrane. It serves both as a passive acoustic resonator, which increases the sound pressure of certain frequencies at the tympanic membrane, and as a passive acoustic filter that aids in detecting the direction of sound. The *middle ear* consists of the tympanic cavity, the ossicles, and the middle ear muscles, and it couples sound energy from the external ear to the inner ear. It functions as an acoustic transformer that matches the acoustic impedance of the external ear canal to the much higher impedance of the cochlear fluids. The middle ear muscles provide a degree of protection from excessive sound pressure. The *inner ear* consists of the bony and membranous labyrinths and serves as an electromechanical transducer that converts acoustic energy into neural impulses. In addition, the inner ear serves as an accelerometer, generating neural signals that indicate head position and acceleration. In this chapter the anatomy of the temporal bone and the anatomy of each portion of the auditory apparatus are described. The development of the ear is then briefly reviewed.

TEMPORAL BONE

The auditory apparatus is contained within the temporal bone, which makes up a major portion of the lateral aspect and the base of the skull. The temporal bone can be divided into four parts: the squamous portion, the tympanic portion, the mastoid portion, and the petrous portion (Fig. 7–1).

Squamous Portion

The large superior squamous portion articulates with the occipital bone, the parietal bone, and the greater wing of the sphenoid bone. It forms the lateral boundary of the middle cranial fossa. On its medial aspect a sulcus for the middle meningeal artery exits from the foramen spinosum. It articulates anteriorly with the petrous bone at the petrosquamous suture or fissure. The zygomatic process originates anteriorly and laterally from the squamous portion of the temporal bone. Posteriorly, on the lateral surface, a curved crest called the temporal line marks the inferior attachment of the temporalis muscle. Inferiorly, the squamous portion articulates with the tympanic bone at the tympanosquamous suture. A hiatus between the tympanic and squamous portions superiorly is termed the notch of Rivinus. Anterior to the external auditory meatus and inferior to the posterior buttress of the zygoma lies the glenoid fossa, where the mandible articulates with the squamous portion of the temporal bone. The medial part of the glenoid fossa is separated from the tympanic bone by the tympanosquamous fissure. Medially, a plate of bone, a portion of the

Figure 7–1. Right temporal bone. *A.* Dry temporal bone viewed from the lateral aspect. *B.* Medial aspect. *C.* Inferior view. (From Anson BJ, Donaldson JA: Surgical Anatomy of the Temporal Bone, 3rd ed. Philadelphia: WB Saunders, 1981.)

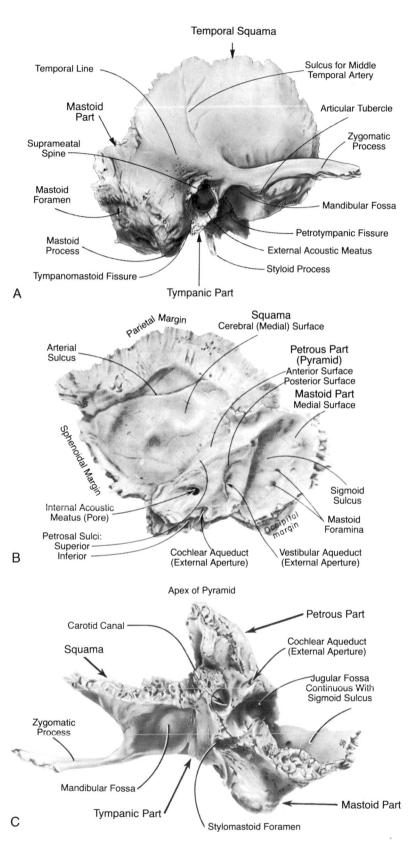

petrous bone, is inserted into this fissure. This formation creates the petrotympanic plate medially. The petrotympanic fissure leads into the tympanic cavity and is called the canal of Huguier. The chorda tympani nerve passes through this canal as it travels anteriorly.

Mastoid Portion

The mastoid portion forms the posteriormost aspect of the temporal bone. It is actually a postnatal development of the petrous portion. Its lateral surface is roughened by attachments of the sternocleidomastoid and occipitalis muscles. Just inferior to the temporal line and posterior to the external auditory meatus is a depression called the cribriform area, or the suprameatal triangle. This surgical landmark is important because the mastoid antrum lies immediately medial to this area. Just anterior to the cribriform area lies the suprameatal spine of Henle. On the posterior aspect of the mastoid bone, a foramen usually exists for a mastoid emissary vein that connects the sigmoid sinus to the occipital veins. There may also be an indentation for the occipital artery and a foramen for a meningeal branch of the occipital artery. Inferiorly and medially, a groove for the posterior belly of the digastric muscle is present. The stylomastoid foramen, which contains the facial nerve, lies immediately anterior and medial to this groove.

The interior of the mastoid is variably pneumatized. It may be divided into medial and lateral components by a thin plate of bone called Körner's septum, which is a remnant of the petrosquamous suture. The mastoid air cells communicate with the middle ear through the mastoid antrum. The tegmen tympani is the bone underlying the middle cranial fossa dura and limits the interior of the mastoid superiorly. Posteriorly, the interior is limited by a large indentation for the sigmoid sinus. Inferiorly, the digastric ridge corresponds to the digastric groove and marks the location of the facial canal just anterior to it. The interior of the mastoid is limited anteriorly by the posterior wall of the external auditory canal and the mastoid portion of the facial nerve. The mastoid portion is limited medially by the labyrinth and the bone overlying the posterior fossa dura.

Petrous Portion

The petrous portion of the temporal bone is wedged between the occipital bone and the greater wing of the sphenoid bone. It is shaped like a quadrilateral pyramid, with its apex directed anteromedially and slightly superiorly. In addition to a base and an apex, it has a superior, a lateral, a medial, and an inferior aspect. The apex is blunt and irregular and articulates with the posterior border of the greater wing of the sphenoid bone and the basilar part of the occipital bone. Through it passes the carotid canal and the eustachian tube. The apex forms the posterolateral border of the foramen lacerum. The base corresponds to the petrosquamosal junction, the remnant of which is thought to be Körner's septum. The base may be more practically assumed to be the mastoid antrum. The lateral aspect of the petrous portion defines the medial wall of the middle ear. It is discussed in detail in the section on the middle ear.

The superior surface of the petrous portion forms part of the floor of the middle cranial fossa. Anteriorly, there is a depression for the trigeminal ganglion. The arcuate eminence lies approximately half of the way back on the superior surface, and the superior semicircular canal lies underneath it. Lateral to this canal is the tegmen tympani, which is a thin plate of bone separating the middle cranial fossa from the mastoid air cells posteriorly and from the middle ear cleft anteriorly. The petrous portion joins the squamous portion laterally at the petrosquamous suture line, where the petrous bone turns inferiorly to form the lateral aspect of the pyramid. Between the arcuate eminence and the trigeminal depression is the facial hiatus, from which a small groove runs anteriorly; this hiatus transmits the greater petrosal nerve (sometimes called the greater superficial petrosal nerve), which arises from the geniculate ganglion. Slightly lateral to this is a second hiatus for the lesser petrosal nerve, which arises from the tympanic plexus. Medially, the superior surface is limited by a groove for the superior petrosal sinus.

The medial aspect of the petrous bone forms the anterolateral wall of the posterior cranial fossa. Near the center of the medial aspect is the internal auditory canal, through which cranial nerves VII and VIII and the internal auditory artery run. The canal is limited laterally by a bony plate that is the medial wall of the cochlea and the vestibule. At its lateral end, the canal is divided into superior and inferior parts by a small ridge of bone called the transverse, or falciform, crest. In the superior compartment the facial nerve lies anteriorly and the superior vestibular nerve lies posteriorly. These two nerves are separated by Bill's bar, a small vertical ridge of bone. Inferior to the transverse crest, the cochlear nerve lies in an anterior position, whereas the inferior vestibular nerve lies posteriorly. Posterior to the internal auditory meatus and midway between it and the sigmoid sinus is a small slit in the bone that leads to the vestibular aqueduct. The vestibular aqueduct transmits the endolymphatic duct and sac. Slightly superior and lateral to the internal auditory meatus is a small depression called the subarcuate fossa. The medial surface is limited posteriorly by a large groove for the sigmoid sinus. The superior petrosal sinus can be seen to join the sigmoid sinus superiorly.

The inferior aspect of the temporal bone forms a portion of the base of the skull. Most anteriorly is an area for the attachment of the levator veli palatini. Posterior to this is a large oval opening to the carotid canal. From here the canal courses in a cephalad direction and then turns anteriorly to leave the temporal bone at the foramen lacerum. Immediately posterior to the carotid foramen is the jugular foramen, which is formed by the temporal bone anteriorly and the occipital bone posteriorly. The carotid and jugular foramina are separated by a small ridge of bone called the carotid crest. The lateral part of the jugular foramen transmits the jugular vein as it becomes the sigmoid sinus, whereas the medial part transmits the glossopharyngeal, the vagus, and the accessory nerves as well as the inferior petrosal sinus. Just posterior to the carotid ridge is a large depression for the jugular bulb; this depression underlies the hypotympanic floor. The cochlear aqueduct has a funnel-shaped opening medial to the jugular fossa and inferior to the internal auditory meatus. Along the carotid ridge lies a small canaliculus that transmits the tympanic, or Jacobson's, nerve. Just lateral to the jugular bulb is the styloid process and the stylomastoid foramen, which transmits the facial nerve.

Tympanic Portion

The tympanic part of the temporal bone is a C-shaped curved plate that lies below the squamous part and in front of the mastoid process. Medially, it is fused with the petrous portion. It is separated anteriorly from the glenoid fossa of the squamous portion by the tympanosquamous suture and posteriorly from the mastoid by the tympanomastoid suture. The tympanomastoid suture is important as a surgical landmark because the stylomastoid foramen lies immediately medial to it. The open portion of the "C" is directed superiorly and forms the notch of Rivinus. In the adult, the inner aspect of the tympanic ring is grooved to accept the annulus of the tympanic membrane. The annulus lies free in the region of the notch of Rivinus. The inferior border of the tympanic ring is sharp and splits to surround the root of the styloid process. The lateral part of this split is called the vaginal process.

EXTERNAL EAR

The external ear consists of the cartilaginous auricle, the cartilaginous and bony portions of the external auditory canal, and the lateral surface of the tympanic membrane.

Auricle

The auricle, or pinna, consists of a single cartilaginous framework covered by perichondrium and skin (Fig. 7–2). The auricular cartilage is part of the cartilaginous external ear canal and is attached to the tympanic bone medially. The auricular cartilage is also attached to the temporal bone by several minor intrinsic muscles. The skin overlying the posterior aspect of the auricle is more loosely attached than the skin overlying the anterior aspect. Posterior to the external auditory meatus is a large convexity in the auricle called the concha. Anterior to the meatus is a projection of the same cartilage called the tragus. The superior border of the auricle is a rim of cartilage called the helix. The helix is directed anteriorly and inferiorly toward the center of the concha, where it is called the crus of the helix. The conchal bowl is limited laterally by another rim of cartilage termed the antihelix. The antihelical rim bifurcates at the superior limit of the conchal bowl. This bifurcation is called the crus of the antihelix. Between the helix and the antihelix is a flat region of cartilage called the scaphoid fossa. At the inferior end of the antihelix is a prominence called the antitragus. The antitragus is separated from the

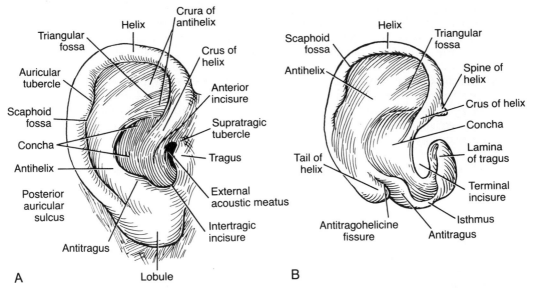

Figure 7–2. External ear *(A)* and auricular cartilage *(B)*. Lateral surface. (From Duckert LG: Anatomy of the skull base, temporal bone, external ear, and middle ear. *In* Cummings CW, Harker LA [eds]: Otolaryngology—Head and Neck Surgery, vol 4. St. Louis: CV Mosby, 1986.)

tragus by the intertragic incisure. The non-cartilaginous inferior appendage of the auricle is called the lobule.

External Auditory Canal

The external auditory canal is a tunnel into the temporal bone extending from the concha to the tympanic membrane. It has a slight S shape and courses in an anterior and slightly inferior direction. The temporomandibular joint lies anterior to the canal, and the mastoid process is posterior. The outer third is cartilaginous, and the inner two thirds are osseous. The cartilaginous portion is contiguous with the cartilage of the auricle, which is attached to the osseous canal by fibrous tissue. The skin overlying the cartilagenous portion is thicker than that over the osseous portion and contains hair follicles, sebaceous glands, and ceruminous glands. The medial ear canal skin is very thin and tightly adherent to the underlying bone, the only subcutaneous tissue being the periosteum of the temporal bone. This portion of the ear canal is highly sensitive to touch. The bony portion of the ear canal is formed primarily by the C-shaped tympanic ring. Superiorly, it is formed by the squamous and petrous portions of the temporal bone.

Blood Supply and Innervation

The blood supply to the auricle and external auditory canal is from the superficial tem-poral and posterior auricular arteries, both of which are branches of the external carotid artery. Venous drainage is supplied by the corresponding veins as well as by the mastoid emissary vein. Lymphatic drainage is to the anterior auricular nodes and then to the superficial parotid nodes anteriorly, or to the retroauricular nodes or superficial cervical nodes, and from there to the upper deep cervical nodes posteriorly or inferiorly.

The external ear receives sensory innervation from cranial nerves V, VII, and X as well as the third cervical nerve through the greater auricular nerve. The greater auricular nerve supplies the lateral and medial aspects of the auricle and the skin overlying the mastoid process. The auriculotemporal branch of the trigeminal nerve supplies the anterior part of the auricle and the superior and anterior portions of the bony and cartilaginous ear canal. The auricular branch of cranial nerve X (Arnold's nerve) supplies a small portion of the auricle and the floor and posterior wall of the external auditory canal. A branch of the facial nerve may supply the posterosuperior ear canal and small areas of the auricle.

Tympanic Membrane

The tympanic membrane is a thin, semitransparent membrane that lies at the medial end of the external auditory canal and separates

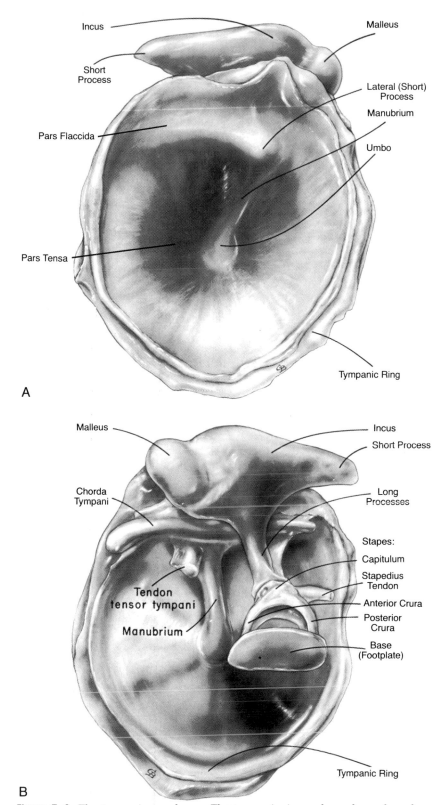

Incus

Malleus

Short
Process

Lateral (Short)
Process

Manubrium

Pars Flaccida

Umbo

Pars Tensa

Tympanic Ring

A

Malleus

Incus

Short Process

Chorda
Tympani

Long
Processes

Stapes:

Capitulum

Stapedius
Tendon

Tendon
tensor tympani

Anterior Crura

Posterior
Crura

Manubrium

Base
(Footplate)

Tympanic Ring

B

Figure 7–3. The tympanic membrane. The tympanic ring and membrane have been excised in one piece with the auditory ossicles. *A.* Lateral aspect. *B.* Medial aspect. (From Anson BJ, Donaldson JA: Surgical Anatomy of the Temporal Bone, 3rd ed. Philadelphia: WB Saunders, 1981.)

it from the middle ear (Fig. 7–3). It is in an oblique position in relation to the ear canal and forms an angle of about 55° with the floor of the ear canal and a similar angle with the anterior canal wall. It is oval in shape: its vertical diameter is approximately 9 to 10 mm, and its horizontal diameter is 8 to 9 mm. The membrane's average thickness is 0.074 mm.

The tympanic membrane is made up of three distinct layers: (1) an outer layer of keratinizing stratified squamous epithelium that is contiguous with the skin of the external ear canal, (2) a middle lamina propria, and (3) a medial mucosal layer that is contiguous with the mucosa of the tympanic cavity. The lamina propria consists of connective tissue fibers arranged in two layers: an outer layer of radially directed fibers and an inner layer of circularly oriented fibers. Centrally, the fibers are attached to the manubrium of the malleus.

The greater part of the circumference of the tympanic membrane is thickened into a fibrocartilaginous ring that is inserted into the annular sulcus of the tympanic bone. This sulcus is absent superiorly at the notch of Rivinus. From the ends of the notch, two bands, called the anterior and posterior malleolar folds, extend toward the short process of the malleus. The portion of the tympanic membrane superior to these folds is called the pars flaccida, and the portion inferior to the folds is called the pars tensa. The tympanic membrane is concave, the most depressed point being the umbo, which is where the tip of the manubrium of the malleus is attached. The manubrium, or handle, of the malleus is attached to the tympanic membrane along its length from the umbo to the short process.

The tympanic membrane is innervated laterally by the auriculotemporal nerve and the auricular branch of the vagus. The medial surface of the membrane is supplied by the tympanic branch of the glossopharyngeal nerve (Jacobson's nerve). The blood supply of the tympanic membrane is from the deep auricular, the anterior tympanic, and the stylomastoid arteries. The deep auricular and anterior tympanic arteries are both branches of the internal maxillary artery. The stylomastoid artery is a branch of the posterior auricular artery and passes through the stylomastoid foramen. The deep auricular artery is thought to supply the lateral aspect of the membrane; the anterior tympanic and stylomastoid arteries are thought to supply the mucosal aspect.

MIDDLE EAR

The middle ear or tympanic cavity is an air-filled space between the tympanic membrane laterally and the osseous labyrinth medially (Fig. 7–4). It is lined with mucous membrane and can be divided into several subspaces. The tympanic cavity proper is the space immediately medial to the tympanic membrane. Superior to the superior border of the tympanic membrane is a space called the epitympanic recess, or "attic," and caudal to the inferior border of the tympanic membrane is the hypotympanic recess. Posteriorly is the tympanic antrum with the mastoid air cells.

Walls of the Tympanic Cavity

The tympanic cavity is best thought of as a rectangular, box-shaped space. The roof, or tegmen tympani, separates the middle ear cleft from the middle cranial fossa. The floor separates the hypotympanic area, which contains numerous air cells, from the jugular bulb posteriorly and the carotid artery anteroinferiorly. The floor may sometimes be incompletely formed, and thus the jugular bulb may be exposed. The jugular bulb is variable in position and may, on occasion, rise as high as the tympanic cavity proper. The anterior wall of the box is made up by the opening of the eustachian tube. The superior portion of the posterior wall consists of the mastoid antrum, which is the opening to the mastoid air cell system (Fig. 7–5). Further inferiorly, at the level of the stapes, is the pyramidal eminence where the stapedius tendon leaves its canal to attach to the neck of the stapes. Lateral to the pyramidal eminence lies a depression in the posterior wall called the facial recess, and lateral to this is the canal for the chorda tympani nerve. Medial to the pyramidal eminence is a cavity called the sinus tympani, which is bounded medially by the posterior rim of the oval window. The vertical portion of the facial nerve separates the facial recess from the sinus tympani. Much of the lateral wall is composed of the medial aspect of the tympanic membrane. Superior to the tympanic membrane, the lateral wall consists of the

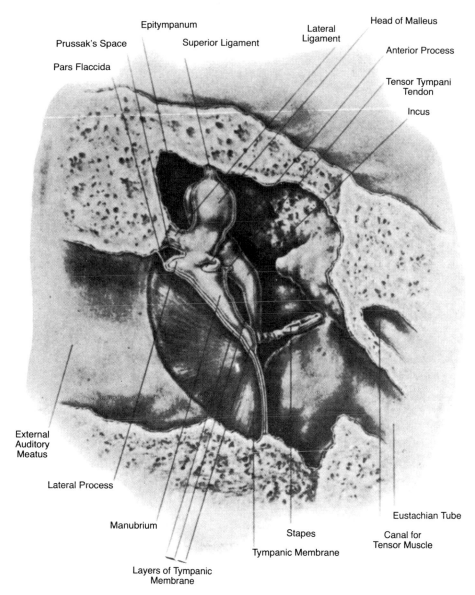

Epitympanum

Prussak's Space

Pars Flaccida

Superior Ligament

Lateral Ligament

Head of Malleus

Anterior Process

Tensor Tympani Tendon

Incus

External Auditory Meatus

Lateral Process

Manubrium

Stapes

Tympanic Membrane

Eustachian Tube

Canal for Tensor Muscle

Layers of Tympanic Membrane

Figure 7–4. The middle ear. This view illustrates the suspension of the ossicles within the middle ear cavity. Note the attachment of the manubrium of the malleus to the tympanic membrane and the insertion of the stapes into the vestibular fenestra. (From Deaver JB: Surgical Anatomy of the Human Body. Philadelphia: Blakiston, 1926.)

scutum, which is the portion of the squamosa adjacent to the notch of Rivinus.

The majority of the medial wall of the middle ear is made up of the promontory, which is the bone that overlies the basal turn of the cochlea (Fig. 7–6). The promontory is limited posteriorly by the round window niche; underneath the niche lies the round window proper. Over the midportion of the promontory is a vertical groove for the tympanic branch of the glossopharyngeal nerve (Jacobson's nerve). Posterior to the promon-

tory, the round window is separated superiorly from the anterior portion of the sinus tympani by a ridge of bone called the subiculum. The sinus tympani is then separated from the oval window superiorly by another ridge of bone, the ponticulus. Above the oval window is the posterior limit of the horizontal segment of the facial, or fallopian, canal. The anterior limit of the horizontal facial canal is marked by the cochleariform process, where the tensor tympani tendon turns laterally to insert onto the malleus near its neck.

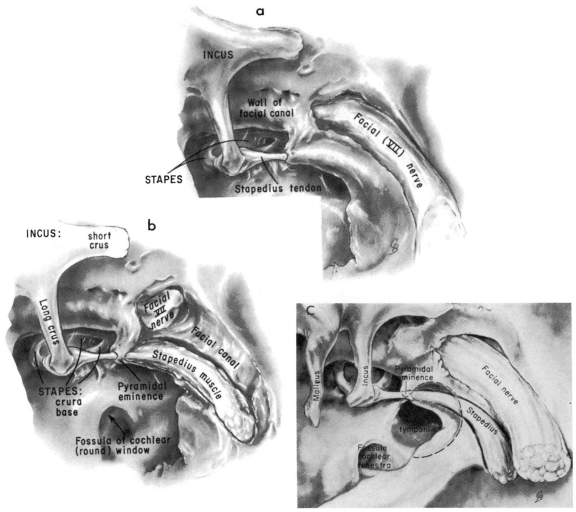

Figure 7–5. Posterior tympanum. Dissected unembalmed temporal bone. *A.* The facial nerve has been uncovered as it finishes the horizontal course and curves gently toward its vertical course. The relationship of the intact facial nerve to the prominence of the stapedius muscle and its tendon can be seen. *B.* The facial nerve has been removed from the facial canal and the stapedius muscle uncovered. The compartment housing the stapedius muscle may be entirely separate from the facial canal, the two may communicate in part, or the two may be housed in a common compartment. *C.* In another specimen, the facial nerve and the stapedius muscle have been uncapped. The dashed line indicates the extent of the sinus tympani in this specimen.

At this point the facial canal turns medially to become the labyrinthine segment. Anterior to the cochleariform process, the medial wall is made up of the canal for the tensor tympani muscle superiorly and the internal carotid artery inferiorly as it turns from its vertical portion to its horizontal portion through the temporal bone. These two structures continue farther anteriorly to become the medial and superior walls of the eustachian tube.

Ossicles

The three auditory ossicles are small bones that bridge the tympanic space from the tympanic membrane to the oval window and provide for the transmission of sound between these structures (Fig. 7–7). The lateral ossicle is the malleus, which consists of a manubrium (or "handle") and the head. The manubrium is attached to the tympanic membrane along its length, and the tip of the manubrium corresponds with the umbo. The head of the malleus lies in the epitympanum, where it is suspended from the walls of the middle ear by the superior, anterior, and lateral ligaments of the malleus. The head of the malleus is connected to the manubrium by a narrow neck, and just below the neck

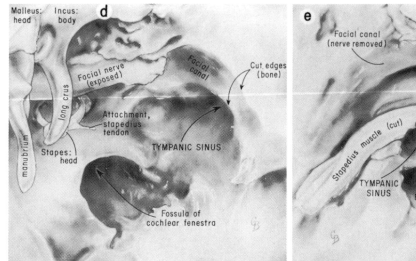

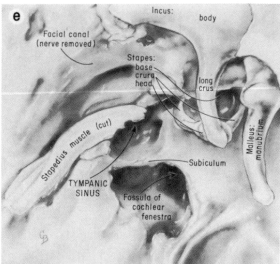

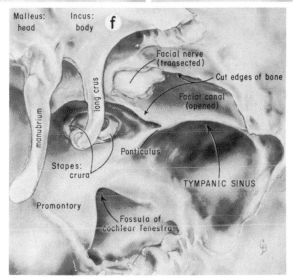

Figure 7–5 *Continued D.* The sinus tympani has been exposed. It almost reaches the posterior margin of the vertical portion of the facial nerve. *E.* The sinus has been exposed as in *D.* It is quite small and could have been adequately exposed and cleaned without damaging the facial nerve. The subiculum bounds the sinus inferiorly. *F.* The sinus has been exposed by removing its lateral wall, demonstrating the relation of the ponticulus to the sinus. (*A, B* from Paparella MM, Shumrick DA: Otolaryngology [2nd ed, vol 1]. Philadelphia: WB Saunders, 1980. *C* from Donaldson JA, Anson BJ, Warpeha RL, Resnik MJ: The perils of the sinus tympani. Trans Pacific Coast Oto-Ophthalmol Soc, 49:101, 1968. *D, E, F* from Anson BJ, Donaldson JA: Surgical Anatomy of the Temporal Bone, 3rd ed. Philadelphia: WB Saunders, 1981.)

the tensor tympani tendon inserts onto the manubrium. Opposite this insertion, on the lateral aspect of the malleus, the lateral, or short, process of the malleus can be seen. The head of the malleus articulates posteriorly, through a true synovial joint, with the body of the incus.

The incus is composed of a globular body, out of which a short process and a long process extend. At the tip of the long process,

the bone turns a right angle to form the lenticular process. The body of the incus is supported anteriorly by its articular ligaments to the malleus and posteriorly by the posterior ligament of the incus to the wall of the tympanic cavity. The short process lies in the fossa incudis lateral to the mastoid antrum, where its tip is attached by a ligament to the posterior wall of the tympanic cavity. The long process is directed inferiorly,

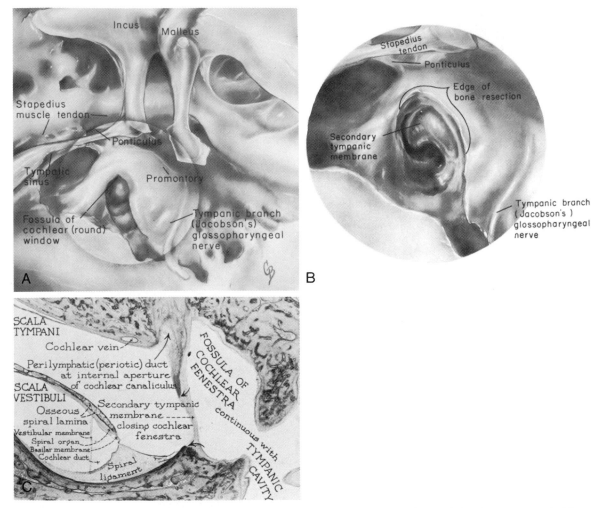

Figure 7–6. Anatomy of the medial wall of the tympanic cavity. Dissection of unembalmed specimen. *A.* The tympanic membrane and external acoustic meatus have been removed, exposing the medial wall of the tympanum. The ossicles remain in situ. Note the ponticulus extending from the promontory to the pyramidal eminence. The encircled area contains the external aperture of the fossula of the cochlear fenestra. *B.* The area encircled in *A* is shown after the anterior and posterior margins of the external aperture have been pared away, until the edge of the secondary tympanic membrane can be seen. *C.* Horizontal section through the temporal bone, again showing the relationship of the orifice of the fossula to the secondary tympanic membrane. (*A* and *B* from Donaldson J: Fossula of the cochlear fenestra. Arch Otolaryngol 88:124–130, Fig. 2, 1968. *C:* source unknown.)

and at its tip the lenticular process articulates with the capitulum of the stapes, again through a synovial joint.

The stapes is shaped like a stirrup, with a footplate, an anterior and a posterior crus, a neck, and a head (or capitulum). The footplate of the stapes is attached circumferentially to the rim of the oval window by the annular ligament. The stapedius tendon inserts onto the neck of the stapes.

Tympanic Mucous Membrane

The mucosa of the middle ear cavity is continuous with that of the nasopharynx through the eustachian tube. It consists of ciliated columnar (respiratory) epithelium and a flatter, nonciliated epithelium. The mucosa that lines the mastoid air cells is cuboidal and nonciliated. There is considerable variation in the distribution of ciliated mucosa. The mucosa creates a number of folds where it invests various middle ear structures. Some of these folds create saclike pouches important in the progression of retraction cholesteatoma. One pouch, termed the superior recess of the tympanic membrane, or Prussak's space, lies between the neck of the malleus and the pars flaccida.

Figure 7–7. The auditory ossicles from the right ear, shown separately, five times natural size. (From Wever EG, Lawrence M: Physiological Acoustics, 2nd ed. Princeton, NJ: Princeton University Press, 1954.)

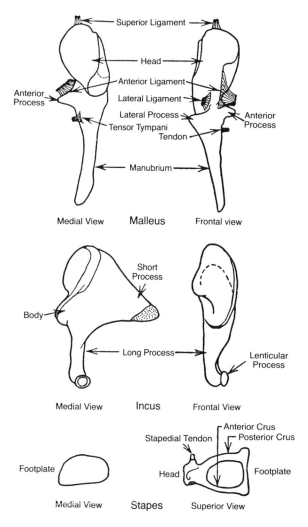

Two other recesses, termed the anterior and posterior recesses of the tympanic membrane, or the anterior and posterior pouches of von Tröltsche, are limited by the tympanic membrane laterally, by the manubrium of the malleus posteriorly or anteriorly, and by the anterior or the posterior mallear fold, respectively.

The Mastoid Air Cells

The mastoid air cells are a series of intercommunicating, mucous-membrane–lined, air-filled spaces within the mastoid portion of the temporal bone. The size and the number of air cells vary considerably, and they may extend into the petrous portion, the root of the zygoma, the occipital bone, or the parietal bone. In some cases the mastoid process consists of dense bone with minimal pneumatization. Körner's septum, a

residual of the petrosquamous suture, sometimes separates lateral mastoid cells from medial mastoid cells and from cells extending into the petrous portion. Anterosuperior in the mastoid cavity and medial to the cribriform area lies the mastoid antrum, which connects the mastoid cells to the tympanic cavity.

Eustachian Tube

The eustachian tube is directed anteriorly, medially, and inferiorly from the anterior wall of the tympanic cavity. The bony portion within the temporal bone connects laterally with a cartilaginous portion medially. The bony portion is approximately 12 mm long, and the entire tube is about 37 mm long in the adult. In the neonate, the tube is about half as long and is more horizontally directed. The cartilaginous portion of the tube is fixed to the base of the skull in a groove between the petrous bone and the greater wing of the sphenoid bone. The bony portion of the tube is lined with ciliated columnar epithelium, whereas the cartilaginous portion is lined with pseudostratified columnar cells and has many mucus-secreting goblet cells. At the pharyngeal orifice there is an abundance of lymphoid tissue called the tubal tonsil of Gerlach.

Vessels and Nerves of the Middle Ear

The inner surface of the tympanic membrane and the anterior portion of the tympanic cavity are supplied principally by the anterior tympanic artery, a branch of the internal maxillary artery that passes through the petrotympanic fissure to arrive in the tympanic cavity. The posterior half of the tympanic cavity, as well as the mastoid air cells, is supplied primarily by the stylomastoid artery, a branch of the posterior auricular artery or the occipital artery. The stylomastoid artery enters the tympanic cavity through the stylomastoid foramen. Other smaller arteries derived from the external carotid artery provide additional blood supply. Two branches of the internal carotid artery also supply the middle ear: the caroticotympanic branch and the subarcuate artery. Venous return corresponds roughly to the arterial supply and terminates in the pterygoid plexus and the superior petrosal sinus.

The primary nerve supply to the tympanic cavity is through the tympanic branch of the glossopharyngeal nerve (Jacobson's nerve). This accounts for the frequent clinical finding of pharyngeal pain that is referred to the ear. Additional innervation is from the inferior and superior caroticotympanic nerves from the internal carotid plexus (sympathetic) and the lesser petrosal nerve. Branches of the tympanic plexus supply the lesser petrosal nerve, which ultimately supplies the parotid gland. The chorda tympani passes through the middle ear on its way to the tongue. The tensor tympani muscle is innervated by a branch of the mandibular division of the trigeminal nerve through the otic ganglion. The stapedius muscle is innervated by the nearby facial nerve.

FACIAL NERVE

The facial nerve deserves special comment because of its importance and its complicated route through the temporal bone. The facial nerve is composed of a motor root and a sensory root (also called the nervus intermedius). The two roots exit the brain stem at the caudal border of the pons in the cerebellopontine angle. The nervus intermedius is usually within the substance of the vestibular nerve and passes from cranial nerve VIII to cranial nerve VII as it approaches the internal auditory canal. In many cases, it may not be a separate nerve until it reaches the internal auditory meatus. The motor root supplies the muscles of the face, the scalp, and the auricle as well as the buccinator, the stapedius, the platysma, the stylohyoid, and the posterior belly of the digastric muscle. The sensory root consists of afferent taste fibers from the chorda tympani and the greater petrosal nerve as well as of preganglionic parasympathetic fibers to the salivary and lacrimal glands.

Within the internal auditory canal the facial nerve is superior to the cochlear nerve and anterior to the superior vestibular nerve (Fig. 7–8). At the lateral end of the internal auditory canal, the nerve passes superior to a ridge of bone called the transverse, or falciform, crest and anterior to a vertical wedge of bone called Bill's bar. Lateral to this, the labyrinthine segment of the facial nerve begins. Here the nerve travels slightly anteriorly between the basal turn of the cochlea and the ampulla of the superior semicircular canal. The geniculate ganglion lies at the lateral end of the labyrinthine segment. Here the nerve turns posteriorly to become the horizontal, or tympanic, segment. The greater petrosal nerve exits the geniculate ganglion anteriorly and leaves the temporal bone through the facial hiatus. The tympanic segment passes along the medial wall of the tympanic cavity superior to the oval window. The nerve curves around the oval window niche and then travels in an inferior direction as the vertical or mastoid segment. This bend around the oval window is frequently termed the second genu, the first genu being located at the geniculate ganglion. The bony canal for the tympanic and mastoid portions of the nerve is called the fallopian canal. The nerve to the stapedius muscle is the first branch of the mastoid segment, followed by the chorda tympani. The facial nerve then exits the temporal bone through the stylomastoid foramen.

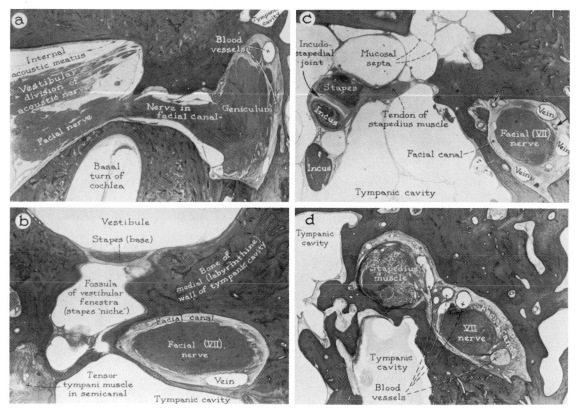

Figure 7–8. Facial canal—the contents, course, and related anatomy. *A.* The nerve passes from the fundus of the internal acoustic meatus into the facial canal. *B.* After bending sharply, the nerve passes posteriorly and laterally. The canal courses medial to the vestibular window. Note the prominent blood vessels within the canal. *C.* Assuming its vertical course, the nerve descends to the stylomastoid foramen. *D.* Near the lower limit of the stapedius muscle, the canal for the facial nerve and that for the stapedius muscle are continuous. (From Paparella MM, Shumrick DA: Otolaryngology, 2nd ed, vol I. Philadelphia: WB Saunders, 1980.)

INNER EAR

The inner ear is composed of two parts: the bony labyrinth, a system of cavities within the petrous portion of the temporal bone, and the membranous labyrinth, a system of ducts and sacs within the bony labyrinth.

Bony Labyrinth

The bony labyrinth houses the sense organs of hearing and balance and is located within the dense bone of the otic capsule in the petrous pyramid. It can be divided into five parts: the vestibule (housing the saccule and utricle), the cochlea, the semicircular canals, the vestibular aqueduct, and the cochlear aqueduct (Figs. 7–9, 7–10).

The vestibule is an ovoid cavity just medial to the tympanic cavity. It is connected to the tympanic cavity through the oval window, which is occupied by the footplate of the stapes. Its inner surface is notable for two recesses: the spherical recess on the medial wall and the elliptical recess on the roof and medial wall. The spherical recess contains the saccule, and the elliptical recess contains the utricle. In the anterior wall there is an elliptical opening into the scala vestibuli of the cochlea. Posteriorly are the five openings of the semicircular canals into the vestibule. Just inferior to the elliptical recess lies the opening to the vestibular aqueduct.

The cochlea is anterior to the vestibule and is a snail-shell–shaped canal within which lies the membranous cochlear duct. The apex of the cochlea is directed anteriorly and laterally. The cochlea makes two and one-half turns about a central structure called the modiolus, through which the cochlear vessels and nerves pass. A shelf of bone, termed the spiral lamina, protrudes into the osseous cochlear canal from the modiolus. The spiral lamina partially divides the cochlear canal

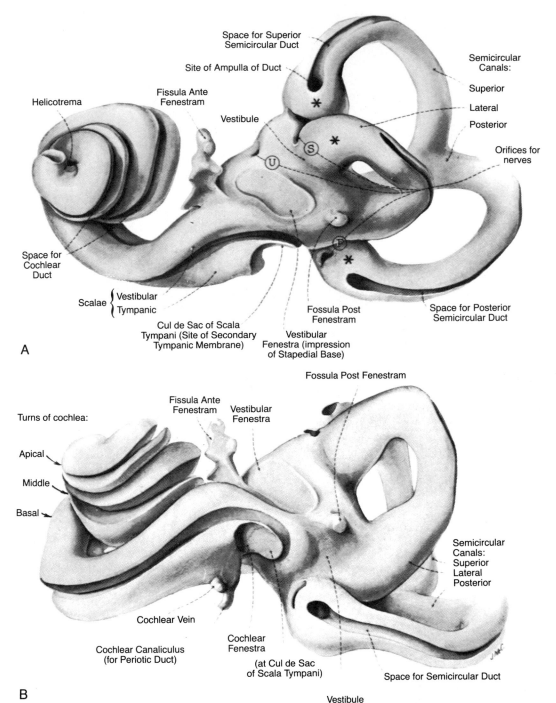

Figure 7–9. Reconstruction of osseous labyrinth, demonstrating form of perilymphatic space proper and its continuity with fossula ante fenestram, fossula post fenestram, and cochlear canaliculus (310 mm. fetus). *A.* Anterior-lateral view. Note form of labyrinthine system for perilymph comprising scali, vestibule, semicircular canals, and perilymphatic appendages; spaces (represented by sulci) of cochlear and semicircular ducts; points of entry of the utricular part of the acoustic nerve at *u*, of saccular part at *s*, and of nerve to ampulla on lateral semicircular duct at *p*; extension of tympanic scala as a cul de sac related in fresh state to a corresponding prolongation (cecum) of the cochlear duct. Asterisk indicates ampulla. *B.* Inferior-lateral view with reconstruction rotated on its long axis through approximately one eighth of a turn, demonstrating: relation of two windows (vestibular and cochlear fenestrae) to each other, and their relation, in turn, to perilymphatic appendages; proximity of cochlear canaliculus to channel for cochlear vein; form of saucer-shaped cul de sac of tympanic scala (produced by shape of secondary tympanic membrane); relatively great capacity of osseous labyrinth, in comparison with that of a membranous labyrinth. (From Paperella MM, Shumrick DA: Otolaryngology, 2nd ed, vol I. Philadelphia: WB Saunders, 1980.)

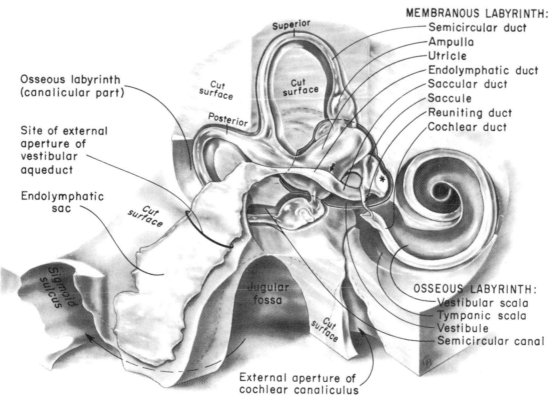

Osseous labyrinth
(canalicular part)

Site of external
aperture of
vestibular
aqueduct

Endolymphatic
sac

Cut
surface

Sigmoid
sulcus

Superior

Cut
surface

Cut
surface

Posterior

MEMBRANOUS LABYRINTH:
—Semicircular duct
—Ampulla
—Utricle
—Endolymphatic duct
—Saccular duct
—Saccule
—Reuniting duct
—Cochlear duct

Jugular
fossa

Cut
surface

OSSEOUS LABYRINTH:
—Vestibular scala
—Tympanic scala
—Vestibule
—Semicircular canal

External aperture of
cochlear canaliculus

Figure 7–10. Membranous and osseous labyrinth. Reconstruction prepared by the Born method. Adult, 69 years of age. (Wisconsin Collection.) This demonstrates especially the relations between the membranous and bony labyrinths, but in particular, the form, size, and relations of the endolymphatic sac. The saccus extends for a considerable distance beyond the external aperture of the vestibular aqueduct into the posterior cranial fossa. In the latter position it occupies a foveate impression on the posterior surface of the petrous pyramid where it may be prolonged inferiorly to the level of the sulcus for the sigmoid venous sinus. The unlabeled arrow points to the utriculoendolymphatic duct; the asterisk is on the saccule. (From Paparella MM, Shumrick DA: Otolaryngology, 2nd ed, vol I. Philadelphia: WB Saunders, 1980.)

into the scala tympani below and the scala vestibuli above; the division is completed by the basilar membrane of the cochlear duct. The two compartments join at the helicotrema, located at the apex of the cochlea. Fibers of the cochlear nerve fan out in the spiral lamina to reach the sensory cells in the cochlear duct. There are three openings into the cochlear canal: (1) the fenestra vestibuli, which connects the scala vestibuli with the vestibule; (2) the round window, which connects the scala tympani with the tympanic cavity; and (3) the cochlear aqueduct. The round window is located at the termination of the scala tympani and is sealed from the tympanic cavity by the secondary tympanic membrane. The cochlear aqueduct is also located at the termination of the scala tympani and runs inferior to the internal auditory canal to open into the subarachnoid space. It provides a variable degree of communication

between the perilymphatic space and the subarachnoid space.

The three semicircular canals lie posterosuperior to the vestibule and are termed the horizontal, the posterior, and the superior semicircular canals. Each canal forms about two thirds of a circle and communicates at each end with the vestibule. Each canal lies at right angles to the others. The posterior limb of the superior canal joins the superior limb of the posterior canal to form the common crus, which enters the vestibule as a single opening. The sensory cells of the semicircular canal system are located in dilated portions of each canal that are termed the ampullae. The ampullae of the superior and horizontal semicircular canals are located at the junction of the canals and the vestibule on the anterosuperior aspect of the vestibule. The ampulla of the posterior semicircular canal is located at the junction of the canal

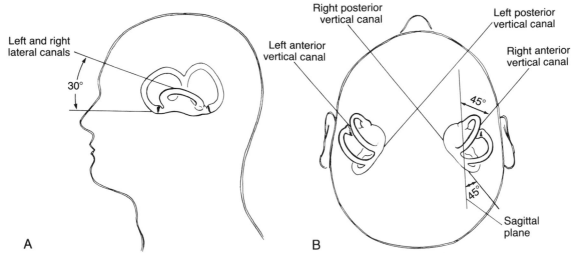

Figure 7–11. Planes of semicircular canals. *A.* Left and right lateral canals. *B.* Anterior and posterior canals. Size of canals is greatly exaggerated. (From Ryu JH: Anatomy of the vestibular end organ and neural pathways. *In* Cummings CW, Harker LA [ed]: Otolaryngology—Head and Neck Surgery, vol 4. St. Louis: CV Mosby, 1986.)

with the vestibule on its posteroinferior and lateral aspects. The second genu of the facial nerve lies immediately adjacent to the ampullated end of the horizontal semicircular canal. The superior canal on one side of the head is roughly parallel to the posterior canal on the opposite side, and vice versa. The superior canals are located in a vertical plane roughly 45° from the sagittal plane, and the posterior canals are in a vertical plane perpendicular to the superior canals (Fig. 7–11). The horizontal canal on each side is in a plane 30° off the axial plane.

Blood Supply of the Labyrinth

The internal auditory artery (or labyrinthine artery) supplies the entire inner ear. It originates as a branch of either the anterior inferior cerebellar artery or the basilar artery. It then travels laterally in the internal auditory canal, where it eventually divides into the vestibular artery, the vestibulocochlear artery, and the cochlear artery. The vestibular artery supplies the vestibular nerve and parts of the saccule, the utricle, and the semicircular ducts. The vestibulocochlear artery supplies the basal turn of the cochlea, as well as the saccule, the utricle, and the semicircular canals. The cochlear artery enters the modiolus and gives rise to the spiral arteries, which supply most of the cochlea. According to some authors, the labyrinth also derives some blood supply from the stylomastoid

artery. Three vessels supply venous drainage from the labyrinth: the internal auditory vein, the vein of the cochlear aqueduct, and the vein of the vestibular aqueduct.

Membranous Labyrinth

The membranous labyrinth consists of a system of epithelium-lined tubes and spaces that are contained within the bony labyrinth and that contain endolymph (Figs. 7–10, 7–12). The membranous labyrinth is surrounded by a fluid of different composition called perilymph, which is contained within the bony labyrinth. The membranous labyrinth is divided into five major portions: the endolymphatic duct and sac, the saccule, the utricle, the semicircular ducts, and the cochlear duct.

Cochlear Duct

The cochlear duct lies within the bony cochlear canal and follows the canal's spiral shape. It begins at the vestibule and ends at the apex of the cochlea, the cupular cecum. At its vestibular end it is connected by a small duct, the ductus reuniens, to the saccule.

The cochlear duct is triangular in cross-section. The floor of the duct is formed by the basilar membrane, which is attached to the spiral lamina medially and to the spiral ligament laterally. The lateral wall of the duct is lined by a very vascular epithelium called

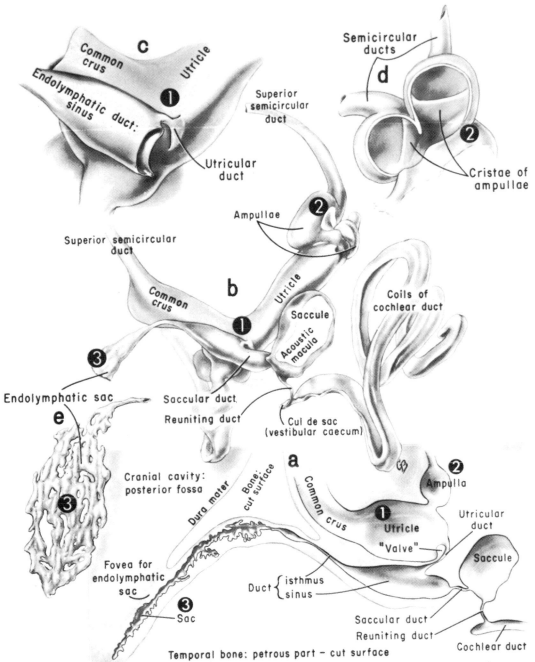

Figure 7–12. Membranous labyrinth. Based upon a reconstruction by David G. Harper, MD. Infant of 6 months. (Wisconsin Collection, series 121.) *A.* This shows schematically the form of the labyrinth in the area of the endolymphatic duct, the utricle, and the interconnecting utricular (or utriculo-endolymphatic) duct. The numeral designations correspond throughout the succeeding figures. The utricle *(1)* communicates widely with the common crus and with the semicircular ducts *(2)*. Differing from this relationship, the utricle opens into the endolymphatic duct beneath a valvelike form, formed by their epithelial walls and the intervening connective tissue. The endolymphatic duct expands proximally, where it communicates with the utricle. The sinuslike enlargement continues into a narrowed segment, the isthmus. Although it is wide at the sinus, the endolymphatic duct narrows at the isthmus to widen again in the plicated sac. *B.* The utricle (at one end) and the common crus together form a V-shaped common chamber. The utricle communicates widely with the ampullae *(2)*. *C* and *D.* Toward the cochlear side *(c)* the connection of the utricle with the sinuslike expansion of the endolymphatic duct is through an aperture, which has a spatulate form (compare value in *A*). It is to be likened to a chink. Comparably, the space at the free surface of the cupula of each crista is also narrow (less than at *2* in *C*, shrinkage having resulted in widening of the opening). *E.* The termination expansion of the endolymphatic duct is characterized by multiple folds *(3)*. As this "cast" of the lumen demonstrates, the facing epithelial surfaces meet, dividing the entire space into intercommunicating chambers.

Illustration continued on following page

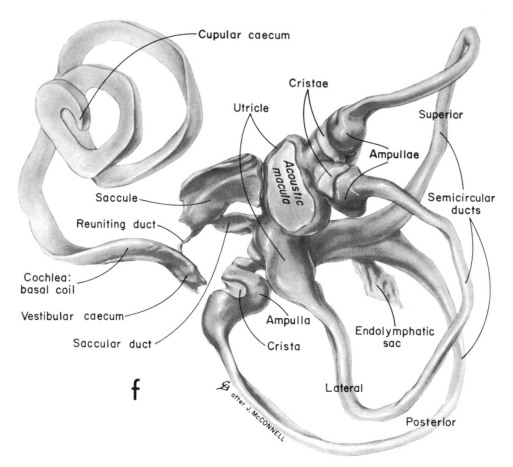

Figure 7–12 *Continued F.* Reconstruction of the entire membranous labyrinth as viewed from the lateral aspect to bring into perspective all the details depicted in *A* through *E*. (From Paparella MM, Shumrick DA: Otolaryngology, 2nd ed, vol I. Philadelphia: WB Saunders, 1980.)

the stria vascularis. The third wall of the triangular duct is made up by the vestibular, or Reissner's, membrane. Thus the basilar membrane and Reissner's membrane divide the cochlear canal into three spaces: the scala vestibuli above Reissner's membrane, the scala tympani below the basilar membrane, and the scala media within the cochlear duct itself. The scala media contains endolymph, and the scala tympani and the scala vestibuli contain perilymph. The scala tympani and the scala vestibuli are connected at the apex by a space called the helicotrema.

Organ of Corti

The sense organ responsive to acoustic energy is located on the basilar membrane and is called the organ of Corti. The organ of Corti is best examined in a transverse cross-section of the cochlear duct (Fig. 7–13). A detailed description of the organ is beyond the scope of this chapter, but a brief outline follows. The organ is located on the endolymphatic aspect of the basilar membrane. The sensory cells are columnar cells surmounted by 50 to 100 hairlike stereocilia and are called hair cells. There are three rows of outer hair cells and one row of inner hair cells; each row is aligned with the length of the cochlear duct. There are approximately 3500 inner hair cells and 12,000 outer hair cells. A number of supporting cells surround the hair cells and provide rigidity to the organ. The stereocilia and the apical end of the hair cells are located in the endolymphatic space, and the lateral and basal aspects of the hair cells are surrounded by perilymph. The differences between inner and outer hair cells are diagrammed in Figure 7–14.

The organ of Corti is covered by a gelatinous flap called the tectorial membrane. The tectorial membrane is attached only on its inner edge to the spiral limbus. Laterally, the

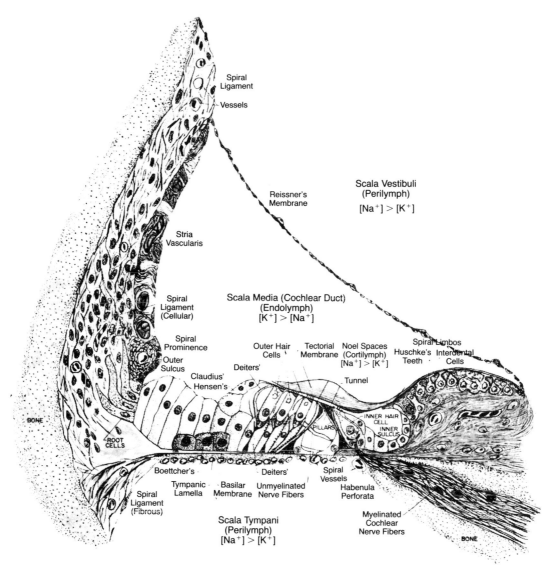

Spiral
Ligament

Vessels

Reissner's
Membrane

Scala Vestibuli
(Perilymph)

$[Na^+] > [K^+]$

Stria
Vascularis

Spiral
Ligament
(Cellular)

Scala Media (Cochlear Duct)
(Endolymph)
$[K^+] > [Na^+]$

Spiral
Prominence

Outer Hair
Cells

Tectorial
Membrane

Noel Spaces
(Cortilymph)
$[Na^+] > [K^+]$

Spiral Limbos
Huschke's Interdental
Teeth Cells

Outer
Sulcus

Deiters'

Claudius'
Hensen's

Tunnel

BONE

INNER HAIR
CELL

INNER
SULCUS

PILLARS

ROOT
CELLS

Boettcher's

Deiters'

Spiral
Vessels

Tympanic
Lamella

Basilar
Membrane

Unmyelinated
Nerve Fibers

Habenula
Perforata

Spiral
Ligament
(Fibrous)

Scala Tympani
(Perilymph)
$[Na^+] > [K^+]$

Myelinated
Cochlear
Nerve Fibers

BONE

Figure 7–13. Diagram of transverse (midmodiolar view of cochlear duct). See text. (From Hawkins JE Jr: Hearing: Anatomy and acoustics. *In* Best CH, Taylor NB [eds]: The Physiological Basis of Medical Practice, 8th ed. Baltimore: Williams & Wilkins, 1966.)

stereocilia of the outer hair cells are firmly embedded within the tectorial membrane. The stereocilia of the inner hair cells are not firmly embedded but rest in a groove on the undersurface of the tectorial membrane called Hensen's stripe. The arrangement of the basilar membrane, the organ of Corti, and the tectorial membrane is such that a deflection of the basilar membrane would result in a shearing movement between the hair cells and the tectorial membrane, which in turn would result in lateral or medial deflection of the stereocilia. This bending movement of the stereocilia initiates the

transduction of acoustic energy into neural signals.

Auditory neurons synapse with the basal portions of both inner and outer hair cells. Approximately 90% to 95% of the afferent neurons connect directly with inner hair cells; each inner hair cell receives about 20 fibers. The remaining afferent fibers synapse with the outer hair cells, each fiber synapsing with about 10 hair cells. Auditory efferent fibers synapse with outer hair cells directly and terminate on the dendrites of afferent fibers that innervate the inner hair cells. Inner and outer hair cells therefore have entirely differ-

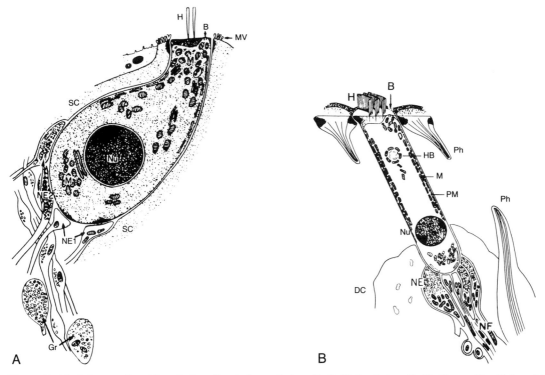

Figure 7–14. Schema of cochlear hair cells. *A.* Inner hair cell. *B.* Outer hair cell. *H*, Stereocilia; *B*, basal body of kinocilium; *MV*, microvilli on supporting cell; *NE₁*, afferent nerve ending (agranulated); *NE₂*, efferent nerve ending (granulated); *M*, mitochondrion; *Ph*, phalangeal process. (From Hawkins JE Jr: Hearing: Anatomy and acoustics. *In* Best CH, Taylor NB [eds]: The Physiological Basis of Medical Practice, 8th ed. Baltimore: Williams & Wilkins, 1966.)

ent patterns of innervation and appear to play completely different functional roles in auditory perception.

Utricle and Saccule

The saccule is a small spherical sac in the membranous labyrinth connected to the cochlear duct by the ductus reuniens and to the utricle by the utriculosaccular duct. It is located in the spherical recess of the vestibule. The utricle is a similar sac but is larger and more flattened than the saccule and lies in the elliptical recess of the vestibule. Posteriorly, the semicircular ducts are connected to the utricle.

The maculae of the saccule and the utricle are sensory organs responsive to changes in position. The macula of the utricle is a thickened area of the utricular wall in the axial plane. The macula of the saccule is a similar thickened area in the medial saccular wall and lies in a vertical plane, perpendicular to the macula of the utricle. The maculae are innervated by the saccular and utricular

branches of the inferior and superior vestibular nerves, respectively.

The two maculae are anatomically similar. As in the cochlea, the primary receptor cells are hair cells. There are two morphologic types of hair cells: type I cells are chalice-shaped, and type II cells are more test-tube–shaped (Fig. 7–15). On the upper surface of these cells are a number of stereocilia and a single kinocilium. Each hair cell is surrounded and supported by a number of supporting cells. The cilia project into an otolithic membrane that lies atop each macula. Within the otolithic membrane, a number of calcium carbonate crystals called otoconia are embedded. The location of the kinocilium in relation to the stereocilia determines the polarity of the hair cell. The primary afferent discharge rate of the hair cell is increased when its stereocilia are deflected away from the kinocilium and is decreased when its stereocilia are deflected toward the kinocilium. Throughout each macula the hair cells are distributed with systematically different polarities (Fig. 7–16). The mass of the otolithic membrane with its otoconia and the different

Figure 7–15. Diagrammatic representation of Types I and II vestibular hair cells. The flask-shaped Type I cell *(HC I)* is surrounded by a nerve calyx *(NC)*, which makes contact on its outer surface with granulated (presumably efferent) nerve endings *(NE 2)*. Unmyelinated fibers *(UMN)* are extensions of myelinated fibers *(MN)* which lose their myelin sheaths as they pass through basement membrane. Type II sensory cell *(HC II)* is roughly cylindrical and is supplied by two types of nerve endings *(NE 1* and *NE 2)* which can be seen at its basal end. Several groups of mitochondria *(M₁-M₅)* are found in the sensory cells and neural elements. Two kinds of hairs project from the surfaces of sensory cells, stereocilia *(H)* and kinocilium *(KC)*, single kinocilium always being the longest on each cell. Supporting cells are easily distinguished from sensory cells by virtue of their numerous population of rather uniformly distributed granules *(Gr)*. (From Ades HW, Engstrom H: Form and innervation of the vestibular epithelia. *In* Graybiell A: The Role of the Vestibular Organs in Space. Washington, DC: National Aeronautics and Space Administration, 1965. NASA Publication No. SP-77.)

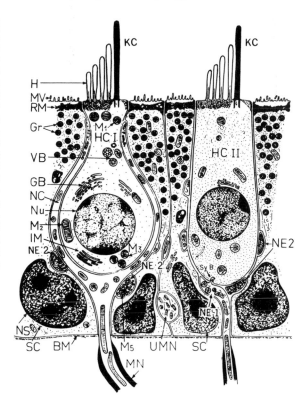

polarizations of the hair cells in relation to the head create different vestibular signals with variation in head position and linear acceleration.

Semicircular Canals

Like the osseous semicircular canals, the semicircular duct portion of the membranous labyrinth takes on a tubular shape. The membranous ducts, however, take up only one fourth of the diameter of the bony canals and, like the remainder of the membranous labyrinth, are surrounded by perilymph. At one end of each duct is a dilated portion called the ampulla. The ampullated ends of each duct open directly onto the utricle. The nonampullated end of the horizontal semicir-

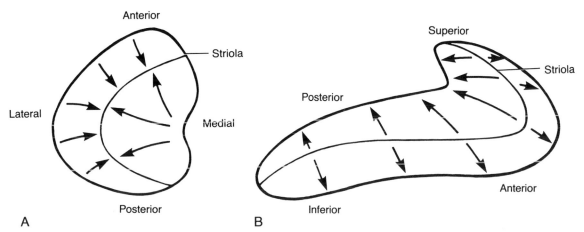

Figure 7–16. Polarization of sensory hairs in macula utriculi *(A)* and macula sacculi *(B)*. Arrows indicate direction of polarization. (From Ryu JH: Anatomy of the vestibular end organ and neural pathways. *In* Cummings CW, Harker LA [eds]: Otolaryngology—Head and Neck Surgery, vol 4. St. Louis: CV Mosby, 1986.)

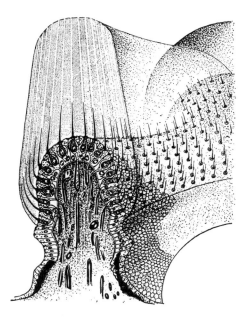

Figure 7–17. Diagrammatic representation of section through ridge of crista ampullaris. The organization of hair cells along the surface of the crista may be seen. Moreover, the insertion of the cilia into the cupula is shown. (From Wersall J, Lundquist PG: Morphological polarization of the mechanoreceptors of the vestibular and acoustic systems. *In* Graybiel A: Second Symposium on the Role of the Vestibular Organs in Space Exploration. Washington, DC: National Aeronautics and Space Administration, 1966. NASA Publication No. SP-115.)

cular duct also opens directly onto the utricle. The nonampullated ends of the superior and posterior ducts join to form a common crus that subsequently opens into the utricle.

The ampulla of each duct contains a ridge of sensory epithelium and supporting cells called the crista ampullaris (Fig. 7–17). In microscopic views, the crista ampullaris is very similar to the maculae of the saccule and utricle. Both type I and type II hair cells are found, but, unlike hair cells in the maculae, they are all polarized in the same direction. In the horizontal duct, the kinocilium is located on the utricular side of the cell, and in the superior and posterior ducts, the kinocilia are located on the side of the cell away from the utricle. The cilia insert into a gelatinous cupula that extends from the surface of the crista to the roof of the ampulla. Movement of the endolymphatic fluid within the semicircular duct deflects the cupula, which subsequently deflects the cilia and causes excitation or inhibition of the hair cell.

Endolymphatic Duct and Sac

The endolymphatic sac typically lies partly within the vestibular aqueduct and partly on the posterior surface of the petrous portion of the temporal bone between layers of posterior fossa dura. The sac is connected to the rest of the endolymphatic system by the endolymphatic duct and the utriculosaccular duct. The size, the shape, and the location

of the endolymphatic sac are quite variable. Surgically, the canal is found by removal of mastoid cells between the posterior semicircular canal and the sigmoid sinus. The cephalad border of the sac usually lies at or below a line through the horizontal semicircular canal (Donaldson's line).

EMBRYOLOGY OF THE EAR

Inner Ear

The inner ear is first evident at about 3 weeks of gestational development as a thickened area of the surface ectoderm called the otic placode (Fig. 7–18). Shortly thereafter these placodes invaginate and sink through the ectoderm into the underlying mesoderm to form the otic vesicles or otocysts. The otocyst eventually becomes the membranous labyrinth.

At about the 5th week of development, after the otocyst loses its connection with the surface epithelium, a diverticulum grows from the otocyst and elongates to form the endolymphatic duct and sac. The otocyst then divides into two parts: (1) a ventral portion, which gives rise to the saccule and cochlear duct, and (2) a dorsal portion, which develops into the utricle, the semicircular ducts, and the endolymphatic duct (Fig. 7–19). The dorsal portion corresponds to what is sometimes called the pars superior, and

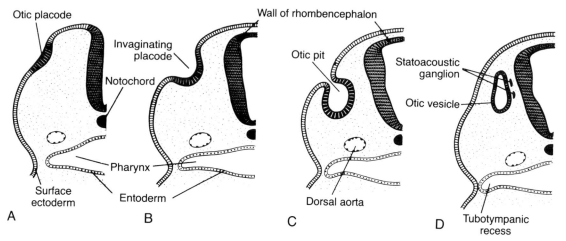

Figure 7–18. Schematic transverse sections through the region of the rhombencephalon at various stages of development, showing the formation of the otic vesicles. *A.* At 22 days. *B.* At 24 days. *C.* At 27 days. *D.* At 4.5 weeks. Note the appearance of the statoacoustic ganglion. (From Langman J: Medical Embryology, 3rd ed. Baltimore: Williams & Wilkins, 1975.)

the ventral portion corresponds to the pars inferior.

From the dorsal portion, three disklike diverticula appear and form the semicircular ducts (Fig. 7–20). A tubular diverticulum grows from the ventral portion and coils to form the cochlear duct. The connection between the cochlear duct and the saccule becomes narrower and develops into the ductus reuniens.

The membranous labyrinth is initially surrounded by mesoderm that becomes cartilaginous and finally ossifies to become the bony labyrinth. As the membranous labyrinth develops, vacuoles appear in the cartilaginous otic capsule and form the perilymphatic space.

During formation of the otocyst, a small group of epithelial cells breaks away from its wall and forms the statoacoustic ganglion. This ganglion subsequently splits into cochlear and vestibular portions and eventually innervates the sensory cells of the membranous labyrinth.

Middle Ear

The tympanic cavity and the eustachian tube are derived primarily from the first branchial pouch, an endodermal outpocketing of the pharynx (Fig. 7–21). The pouch appears at about 4 weeks of intrauterine development and grows laterally to meet the inwardly developing first branchial cleft, which gives

rise to the external auditory canal. The proximal portion of the pouch forms the eustachian tube, and the distal portion forms the tubotympanic recess, which later forms the primitive tympanic cavity. Further expansion of the tympanic cavity in the latter stages of fetal development creates the mastoid antrum. Pneumatization of the mastoid region develops after birth. By 2 years of age the mastoid cells are well developed.

The tympanic membrane is derived from the ectodermal lining of the first branchial cleft and from the endodermal lining of the first branchial pouch. Between the ectodermal and the endodermal layers is a thin layer of connective tissue.

Situated above the primitive tympanic cavity at the 7th week of intrauterine development are several condensations of mesenchyme derived from the dorsal ends of the first and second branchial arches (Fig. 7–22). These condensations ultimately develop into the auditory ossicles. The malleus and incus are derived from the cartilage of the first branchial arch (Meckel's cartilage), and the superstructure of the stapes is thought to develop from the cartilage of the second arch (Reichert's cartilage). The footplate of the stapes may be derived from the otic capsule rather than from the second branchial arch cartilage.

As the endodermal tympanic cavity expands, it envelops the ossicles, their tendons and ligaments, and the chorda tympani

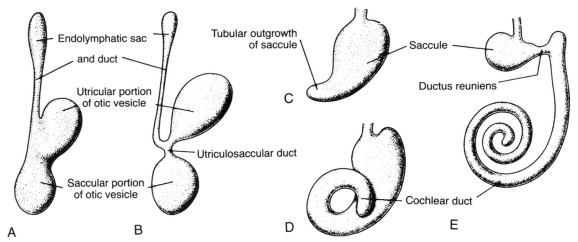

Figure 7–19. *A* and *B.* Further development of the otocyst during the 5th week of development, showing a dorsal utricular portion with the endolymphatic duct, and a ventral saccular portion. *C, D,* and *E.* Development of the cochlear duct shown at 6, 7, and 8 weeks, respectively. Note the formation of the ductus reuniens and the utriculosaccular duct. (From Langman J: Medical Embryology, 3rd ed. Baltimore: Williams & Wilkins, 1975.)

nerve. This development creates the various mesentery-like mucosal folds and pouches within the middle ear space.

Because the malleus is a first arch derivative, its associated muscle, the tensor tympani, obtains its innervation from the cranial nerve of the first arch, the trigeminal nerve. The facial nerve is associated with second arch structures and therefore innervates the stapedius muscle.

External Ear

The external auditory canal is derived from the first branchial cleft, which grows inward as a funnel-shaped tube until it meets the

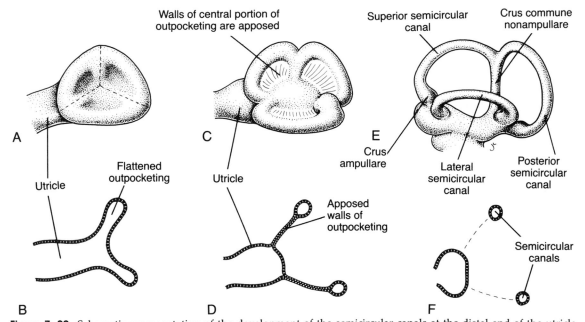

Figure 7–20. Schematic representation of the development of the semicircular canals at the distal end of the utricle. *A.* At 5 weeks. *C.* At 6 weeks. *E.* At 8 weeks. *B, D,* and *F* show diagrammatically the apposition, fusion, and disappearance of the central portions of the walls of the semicircular outpocketings. Note the ampullae in the semicircular canals. (From Langman J: Medical Embryology, 3rd ed. Baltimore: Williams & Wilkins, 1975.)

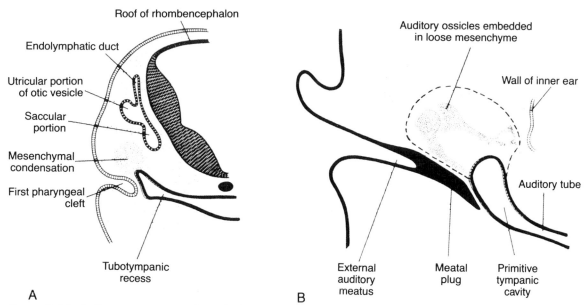

Figure 7–21. *A.* Transverse section through the cephalic end of a 7-week embryo in the region of the rhomben-cephalon, showing the utricular and saccular portions of the otic vesicle, the tubotympanic recess, the first pharyngeal cleft, and the mesenchymal condensation between the otic vesicle and the primitive tympanic cavity, foreshadowing the development of the ossicles. *B.* Schematic representation of the middle ear, showing the cartilaginous precursors of the auditory ossicles embedded in loose connective tissue. Broken line indicates future expansion of the primitive tympanic cavity. Note the meatal plug extending from the primitive auditory meatus to the future tympanic cavity. (From Langman J: Medical Embryology, 3rd ed. Baltimore: Williams & Wilkins, 1975.)

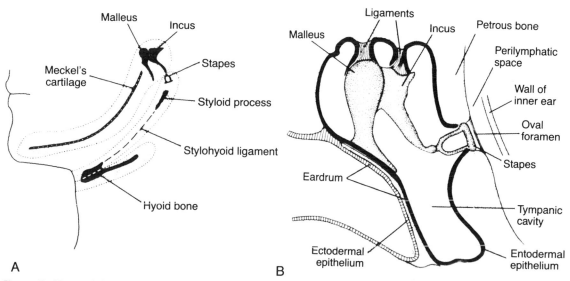

Figure 7–22. *A.* Schematic representation of the derivatives of the cartilaginous components of the first three branchial arches. Note the malleus and incus at the dorsal tip of the first arch and the stapes at that of the second arch. *B.* Schematic representation of the middle ear, showing the handle of the malleus in contact with the eardrum. The stapes establish contact with the membrane in the oval window. The wall of the expanded tympanic cavity is covered with epithelium of entodermal origin. (From Langman J: Medical Embryology, 3rd ed. Baltimore: Williams & Wilkins, 1975.)

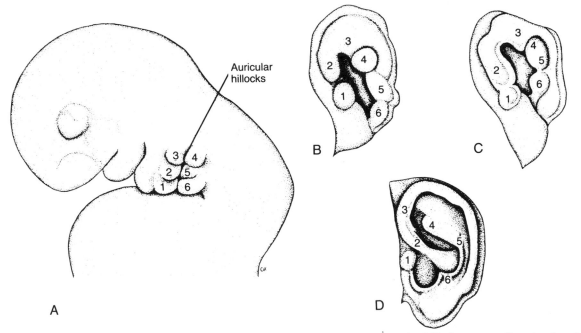

Figure 7–23. *A*. Lateral view of the head of an embryo, showing the six auricular hillocks surrounding the dorsal end of the first pharyngeal cleft. *B, C,* and *D* show the fusion and progressive development of the hillocks into the adult auricle. (From Langman J: Medical Embryology, 3rd ed. Baltimore: Williams & Wilkins, 1975.)

endodermal lining of the first branchial pouch, which develops into the tympanic cavity (Fig. 7–21). At the beginning of the 3rd month of gestation, the ectodermal cells at the bottom of the canal proliferate to form a solid epithelial plate called the meatal plug. During the 7th month this plug breaks down and becomes the lateral surface of the tympanic membrane.

The auricle develops from six mesenchymal proliferations located at the dorsal end of the first and second branchial arches and surrounding the dorsal limit of the first branchial cleft (Fig. 7–23). These swellings, or hillocks, appear during the 6th week of development and later fuse to form the auricle.

Abnormalities of this fusion result in auricular anomalies.

SUGGESTED READINGS

Anson BJ, Donaldson JA: Surgical Anatomy of the Temporal Bone, 3rd ed. Philadelphia: WB Saunders, 1981.

Gulya AJ: Developmental anatomy of the ear. *In* Glasscock ME, Shambaugh GE: Surgery of the Ear, 4th ed (pp. 5–33). Philadelphia: WB Saunders, 1990.

Pickles, JO: An Introduction to the Physiology of Hearing, 2nd ed. London: Academic Press, 1988.

Schuknecht HF, Gulya AJ: Anatomy of the Temporal Bone with Surgical Implications. Philadelphia: Lea & Febiger, 1986.

Sadler TW: Langman's Medical Embryology, 6th ed. Baltimore: Williams & Wilkins, 1990.

CHAPTER 8

Peripheral Auditory Physiology

Harold C. Pillsbury III, MD   Adam S. Wilson, MD

THE NATURE OF SOUND

Study of the mechanisms of hearing requires some background in the physics of sound production and propagation. Sound energy is a mechanical disturbance propagated through an elastic medium and is brought about when a structure within that elastic medium (gaseous liquid or solid) vibrates sufficiently to impart kinetic energy to the particles of the medium. The vibrations of the sound-producing body (or sound source) cause vibrations of the particles about their mean positions with alternating increases (condensation) and decreases (rarefaction) in the particle density (or pressure) adjacent to the sound-producing body. This induces vibrations in progressively more distant particles, and the sound wave is propagated through the medium.

Simple Harmonic Vibrations

The simplest type of sound wave is a sine wave, or a pure tone. Such a wave is characterized by a smooth change in particle pressure around the ambient value as a function of time, and it is in the form displayed in Figure 8–1.

A pure tone is defined by the parameters of peak amplitude and frequency. Peak amplitude is the maximal pressure fluctuation from mean atmospheric pressure. Frequency is the number of cycles per second and is given in units of hertz. One cycle is completed when a particle has gone through the points of maximal displacement in the positive and negative directions and has returned to the initial position. Changes in frequency are perceived as changes in pitch. Changes in amplitude (or intensity) are perceived as changes in loudness.

The wavelength (λ) of a sound wave is the distance between equivalent points on two successive waves and is related to the sound frequency (f) and the propagation velocity (c) by the equation

$$c = f * \lambda.$$

The propagation velocity is a physical constant characteristic of the medium.

Particular points in the cycle of a pure tone may be specified on a time axis or a distance axis; however, it is often convenient to use the measure of phase angle. Phase angle is specified in degrees (360° = one cycle) or in radians (2π radians = one cycle). The beginning, the middle, and the end of a cycle are specified by 0°, 180°, and 360°, respectively. The positive and negative points of maximal amplitude are specified by 90° and 270°, respectively, when the wave begins at a zero crossing (Fig. 8–1).

Phase angle is useful in comparisons of two or more different tones. For example, the simultaneous outputs of two sound sources with the same frequency combine to form a single waveform of the same frequency that depends on the relative amplitude and phase of the two source compo-

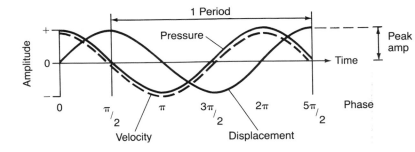

Figure 8–1. The variation of the pressure, the velocity, and the displacement of the particles of the medium in a sinusoidal sound wave, measured at one point, are plotted as a function of time. (Redrawn from Pickles JO: An Introduction to the Physiology of Hearing. London: Academic Press, 1988.)

nents. When the two components are in phase, *reinforcement* occurs, and the amplitude of the resultant waveform is the sum of the amplitudes of the components. When the two waveforms have equal amplitudes and are exactly 180° out of phase, *cancellation* occurs, and the amplitude of the resultant waveform is zero.

Complex Vibrations

Pure tones are the simplest acoustic signals but are rarely encountered in natural settings. Complex tones have nonsinusoidal waveforms. The simplest complex waveforms have a regularly repeating pattern that

represents the sum of two or more pure tones of different frequencies (Fig. 8–2). Any complex, periodic waveform of frequency f can be analyzed as a set of component sine waves with frequencies equal to whole number multiples of f. This analysis is known as Fourier transformation and produces a unique result that specifies the frequencies, the relative amplitudes, and the phase relationships of the components. In many instances, phase has little effect on the resultant wave, and so the Fourier transformation may be summarized in a Fourier *spectrum* that contains the amplitude of each frequency component.

Figures 8–3A and 8–3B show examples of Fourier transformation of various signals. In

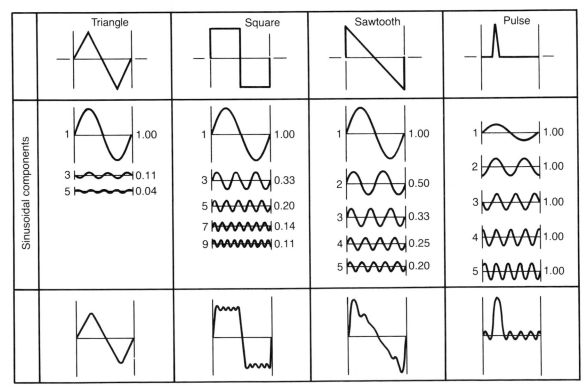

Figure 8–2. The synthesis of various waveforms from their constituent sinusoids is shown. (Adapted from Berg RE, Stork DG: The Physics of Sound. Englewood Cliffs, NJ: Prentice-Hall, 1982.)

Figure 8–3. Analyses of various types of sound stimuli into their Fourier spectra are shown. *A.* Sine wave. *B.* Square wave. *C* Ramped sine wave. *D.* Gated sine wave. *E.* Click. *F.* White noise. (Redrawn from Pickles JO: An Introduction to the Physiology of Hearing, p. 9. London: Academic Press, 1988.)

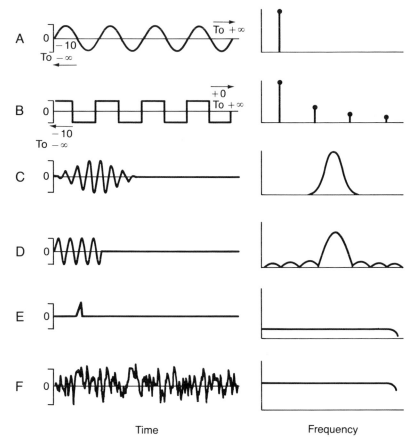

Time   Frequency

the case of the sine wave and the square wave, the durations of which are infinite, the Fourier spectra show discrete lines that represent the frequencies of the components. The shorter duration signals (Figs. 8–3C, 8–3D) result in continuous spectra with frequency bands rather than lines. The relationship between duration ($\Delta\tau$) and frequency band (Δf) is given by

$$(\Delta\tau \times \Delta f \sim 1).$$

Thus for a signal of infinitely short duration, the spectrum is infinitely broad. In Figure 8–3E the signal does have a finite duration and thus has an upper limit to its frequency spectrum. Another signal that has a similarly broad frequency content is *white noise,* which has a large number of components that include random phases and frequencies across a wide band width.

Intensity

As with any form of physical energy, a measure of the magnitude of sound is needed.

Pressure is the most convenient parameter for measurement. Intensity is a measure of the average rate of energy flow through a unit area and is directly related to the square of the pressure.

The mean sound pressure of sine waves is equal to the mean atmospheric pressure because the fluctuations of pressure caused by condensations are canceled by those caused by rarefactions. Measuring sound intensity in terms of the root mean square (RMS) pressure avoids this problem. The RMS pressure is found by squaring the value of the pressure measurements and finding the square root of the mean of these values. Furthermore, RMS pressure allows comparison of the energy transfer of dissimilar sound waves, whereas the peak pressure does not. For sinusoidal waveforms, the peak pressure is related to the RMS pressure by the following formula:

$$RMS = p/1.414,$$

where p = the peak pressure.

RMS pressure may be expressed directly in terms of newtons/m² (pascals) or dynes/cm². This scale is somewhat unwieldy because the range of sound pressures from absolute threshold to the threshold of pain is about 10 million. A more convenient scale, therefore, is the decibel. The decibel (db) is a dimensionless unit expressing the relative difference in intensity of two sounds. Given two sounds, of intensities I′ and I″ (W/cm²), the formula for I′ in decibels in relation to I″ is

$$db = 10 * \log(I'/I'').$$

Because intensity varies as the square of the sound pressure, the formula for determining decibels with pressure is

$$db = 10 * \log(p'/p'')^2$$
$$db = 20 * \log(p'/p'').$$

To express intensity or sound pressure in absolute terms, reference standards have been adopted. For pressure the reference standard is $2 * 10^{-5}$ newtons/m², which is the threshold for detection by the normal human ear of a 1000-Hz tone. Sound pressures given in decibels in relation to this level are known as *sound pressure levels* (SPLs).

Inverse Square Law

The simplest theoretical (hypothetical) sound source is a pulsating sphere of negligible volume. In an unbounded space, the leading condensation, or wavefront, is a sphere advancing concentrically outward from the sound source at the center. The surface area of the sphere varies with the square of its radius. If the energy transferred by the advancing wavefront is constant, the intensity of the sound varies inversely with the square of the distance from the sound source.

Linearity

A concept important to the discussion of auditory physiology is that of linearity. In a linear system, the ratio of the input and output amplitudes is constant. Similarly, the output of two simultaneous inputs equals the sum of outputs resulting from individual inputs. The output of a linear system contains only frequency components that are present in the input. Each of these criteria

must be met for a system to be considered linear.

OUTER AND MIDDLE EARS

The human auditory system is most conveniently treated as a series of individual stages, each responsible for some steps in translating the information contained in acoustic waveforms into perceptions of speech, music, and environmental sound. The outer and middle ears transfer acoustic energy to the cochlea, where acoustic filtering and transduction into neural action potentials occur.

Outer Ear

The outer ear is composed of the auricle (or pinna), the external auditory meatus, and the tympanic membrane. The outer ear alters the sound pressure at the tympanic membrane in relation to that in the free field and provides clues for the localization of sound sources.

Pressure Gain of Outer Ear

The individual structures of the external ear, as well as of the head, the neck, and the torso, each result in acoustic pressure changes at the tympanic membrane in relation to the free field that vary as a function of the frequency and angle of incidence of the sound. Figure 8–4 shows the sound pressure gain contributed by individual structural elements of the external ear. The head presents an obstacle to sound propagation and thus causes reflection and diffraction. The reflected and incident waves combine to increase sound pressure near the head in relation to the free field for some frequencies (the *baffle effect*). Conversely, the head casts a *sound shadow* for short wavelengths (short in relation to the size of the head), which results in reduced sound pressure at the far ear. Reflection of sound by the auricle toward the meatus also depends on the angle of incidence of sound waves. The external auditory meatus is essentially a tube that is closed at one end and, with the concha, acts as an acoustic resonator. The meatus should have a resonant wavelength equal to four times its length, or about 10 cm (2.6 kHz). Both the tympanic membrane and the walls of the meatus are pliant; this pliancy causes

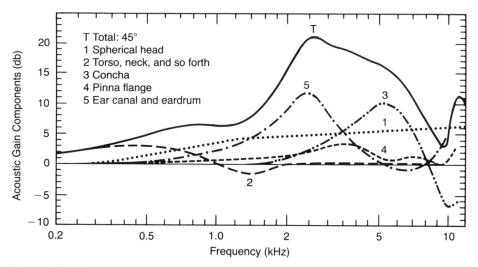

Figure 8–4. The average pressure gains contributed by various components of the external ear are shown. (Redrawn from Shaw EAG: The external ear. *In* Keidel WD, Neff WD [eds]: Handbook of Sensory Physiology, vol. 5/1 [pp 455–490]. Berlin: Springer, 1974.)

some energy absorption and results in a broadly tuned resonance peak that extends for almost three octaves.

The pressure gain at the tympanic membrane is the sum of pressure gains contributed by the separate elements; this sum results in a broad peak between 2 and 5 kHz of 15 to 20 db.

Sound Localization

The ability of the auditory system to localize sound-producing bodies in space is based on the ability to detect differences in intensity, phase, and timing of sound that reaches the ears from sources located off the medial-sagittal plane. The reduction in intensity is greater for high than for low frequencies because of increasing shadowing of short wavelength sounds by the head. The *duplex theory* holds that for sinusoidal stimuli, temporal cues are used for localization of low-frequency tones, and intensity cues are used for localization of high-frequency tones. In natural settings the process of localization is much more involved than the duplex theory suggests. Natural sounds are complex and often transient. There is now evidence that the auditory system can use temporal information contained in the envelope of amplitudes or in frequency-modulated waveforms for localization cues.

Sounds from sources located in the medial-sagittal plane lack interaural differences,

which would otherwise provide localization cues. Judgments of localization in this plane are based on the acoustic filtering properties of the auricle and concha. The convolutions of the auricle and concha may modulate the spectra of incoming sound, especially for shorter wavelengths. The changes in the spectrum are dependent on the location of the sound in relation to the auricle and thus provide cues for distinguishing back from front and above from below. When unfamiliar sounds are encountered, slight exploratory movements of the head can provide the context for making localization judgments.

Middle Ear

The middle ear mechanically couples sound energy striking the tympanic membrane with the oval window of the cochlea. The vibrations of the stapes footplate in turn set the cochlear fluids into motion; the motion results in movement of the organ of Corti, where transduction of hydromechanical energy into neural action potentials occurs.

The efficient transmission of mechanical energy to the cochlea depends on the impedance-matching function of the middle ear. Impedance is a concept applied to acoustic, electrical, and mechanical systems relating the motive force (sound pressure, RMS voltage, or force) to the response of the system (particle velocity, current, or velocity of displacement). Different media respond differently to sound pressure; for example, a given pressure produces a much higher particle velocity in air than in water. The impedance of a large, unbounded medium is called the *specific impedance* (Z) and is defined by the equation

$$Z = \rho * c,$$

where ρ is the density of the medium and c is the propagation velocity. When sound traveling in one medium (impedance = Z_1) encounters a boundary with another medium (Z_2) the proportion of incident power transmitted (T) is given by the equation

$$T = 4r/(r + 1)^2,$$

where r is the ratio of the two impedances.

Where the impedances of the two media are equivalent, $T = 1$. The specific impedance of water is approximately 4000 times that of air. Thus at an air-water interface, only 0.1% of the incident sound is transmitted, an attenuation of about 30 db.

The transformer action of the middle ear minimizes the impedance mismatch between the external air and the cochlear fluids by increasing the pressure acting on the oval window. Impedance transformation by the middle ear is determined by three factors (Fig. 8–5). The first factor is the relative areas of the tympanic membrane and the stapes footplate. The force acting on the tympanic membrane equals the sound pressure multiplied by its area. This force is then applied over the smaller area of the stapes footplate and results in a pressure gain equal to the ratio of the areas. This *hydraulic action* makes the greatest contribution to impedance matching by the middle ear.

The second factor is the lever action of the ossicular chain. The malleus and the incus move as a unit; the manubrium and the long process of the incus serve as the arms, and the head of the malleus serves as the fulcrum of a simple lever system. The manubrium is longer than the long process of the incus and thereby increases the force and decreases the velocity at the stapes.

The third factor is the movement of the tympanic membrane. The tympanic membrane does not move as a rigid cone; rather, it has areas that vibrate with different displacements. The points of maximal displacement lie to either side of the manubrium.

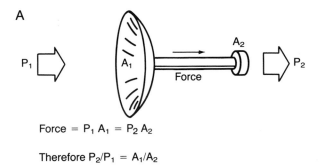

Force = $P_1 A_1 = P_2 A_2$

Therefore $P_2/P_1 = A_1/A_2$

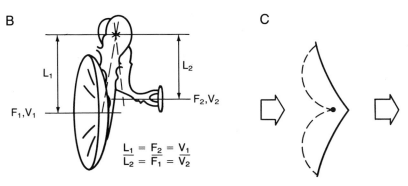

$$\frac{L_1}{L_2} = \frac{F_2}{F_1} = \frac{V_1}{V_2}$$

Figure 8–5. The components of the middle ear transformer ratio. *A.* The ratio of the areas of the tympanic membrane and the stapedial footplate results in the greatest increase in mechanical advantage. *B.* The greater length of the manubrium in relation to the malleus results in an increase in the force and a decrease in the velocity of the stapedial footplate motion. *C.* Buckling of the tympanic membrane also increases the force and decreases the velocity of stapedial footplate motion. A, area; F, force; L, length; P, pressure; V, velocity. (Redrawn from Pickles JO: An Introduction to the Physiology of Hearing. London: Academic Press, 1988.)

This has the effect of reducing the velocity and increasing the pressure applied to the manubrium.

By multiplying the three factors, it should be easy to calculate the final transformer ratio. However, the situation is not nearly as simple as this description suggests. A number of additional factors contribute to a frequency-dependent loss of efficiency. As mentioned previously, the pattern of vibration of the tympanic membrane changes with frequency. The effective area of the tympanic membrane is progressively reduced with increasing frequencies above 2 kHz until it becomes equal to the area of the manubrium itself. Furthermore, the center of effort of the tympanic membrane changes as a function of frequency and is not centered at the tip of the manubrium. Thus the form of the tympanic membrane is transmitted through a lever arm shorter than the actual length of the manubrium. The ossicular chain also has mass and elastic and frictional forces that reduce efficiency of transmission in a frequency-dependent manner. The peak velocity of displacement in response to a given sound pressure is independent of frequency. However, accelerational forces are directly proportional to frequency. Thus inertia is more likely to reduce the efficiency of transmission for high-frequency stimuli. The peak displacement is inversely proportional to frequency. Elastic forces exhibited by the joints of the ossicular chain and the compression and expansion of air in the closed space of the middle ear cavity are directly proportional to the displacement of the system; it therefore follows that these forces have their greatest effect at lower frequencies.

To accurately characterize the transmission of sound over a range of frequencies, it is necessary to plot a *transfer function*, which is a plot of the ratio of input and output pressures of the middle ear as a function of frequency (Fig. 8–6).

Middle Ear Muscles

The middle ear muscles (the stapedius and the tensor tympani) are activated by acoustic signals with sound pressure about 80 db above absolute threshold, as well as by vocalization or movement of the head. The middle ear muscles have several possible functions. It has been suggested that they serve to maintain the ossicular chain in

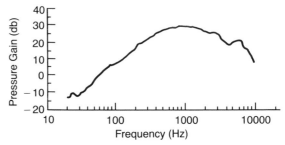

Figure 8–6. The transfer function of the middle ear (expressed as the pressure gain in the cochlea over that at the tympanic membrane) as a function of frequency. (Redrawn from Nedzelnitsky V: Sound pressures in the basal turn of the cat cochlea. J Acoust Soc Am 68:1676–1689, 1980.)

proper position. Because the muscles contract in response to loud stimuli, they have also been thought to protect the inner ear from noise damage. Patients with unilateral paralysis of the stapedius muscle show much greater auditory fatigue in response to intense low-frequency sounds than do people with intact stapedial reflexes. However, because of the long latency between sound onset and muscle contraction, the reflex is ineffective protection against intense noise with a sudden onset. Contraction stiffens the ossicular chain, resulting in selective attenuation of lower frequencies. This provides a means for gaining control of intense low-frequency sounds, which can mask higher frequency sounds. The attenuation of these low-frequency components by the middle ear reflex may serve to enhance the intelligibility of speech at high sound levels.

COCHLEA

The two main functions of the cochlea are acoustic filtering of the sound waves transmitted to the oval window by the middle ear and transduction of the sound waves into neural action potentials. This section provides a brief description of the principles underlying cochlear mechanics and transduction.

Cochlear Mechanics

Traveling Wave

Understanding of the mechanism of acoustic filtering was greatly advanced by von Békésy with his description of the traveling wave

distance from the base as a result of decreasing stiffness. Conversely, the mass-limiting effect on amplitude increases toward the apex. For a given stimulus frequency, there is a point on the longitudinal axis of the basilar membrane where the stiffness-limiting and mass-limiting effects are equal but 180° out of phase, and so they cancel each other. This is the point of maximal displacement. Earlier, in the description of the middle ear transfer function, it was noted that stiffness is a greater impediment to low-frequency vibration than is mass, whereas inertia (mass) is a greater impediment to high-frequency vibration than is mass. Therefore, the place of maximal displacement for low-frequency stimuli is toward the less stiff apex, whereas the place for high-frequency stimuli is toward the base, which has less mass. As the stiffness gradient is exponential, the places are arranged on the membrane as a function of *log frequency*.

The independence of the direction of propagation of the traveling wave on the location of the stimulus is also related to the gradients of stiffness and mass just described. A stiffness-limited system responds earlier than a mass-limited system; therefore, the traveling wave begins at the base and travels apically regardless of whether the base or the apex is stimulated.

The stiffness gradient is also responsible for the difference in phase of different loci along the basilar membrane. The velocity of the traveling wave is related to the stiffness of the membrane. At the stiffer (basal) end of the cochlea, the propagation velocity of the traveling wave is high, and the wavefront passes through different loci in rapid succession. The phase differences between these loci are therefore relatively small. As stiffness decreases, the velocity of the wavefront decreases as well, and the time interval between passage of the wavefront through various loci increases, with a corresponding increase in the phase difference in these loci.

These physical properties account for why the older experimental data showed a broadly tuned peak. Contemporary models that successfully account for the sharp tuning such as that shown in Figure 8–8 include an active mechanical process that amplifies the traveling wave in such a way that the tuning of the basilar membrane is sharpened. An active process would account for the dependence of basilar membrane tuning on the physiologic state of the cochlea. On the basis of a number of intriguing lines of evidence, the structure that most likely plays an active role in tuning is the outer hair cell. The first direct evidence of an active source of energy in the cochlea came from the discovery of measurable acoustic emissions in the ear canals of humans and experimental animals, either spontaneously or after acoustic stimulation. Acoustic emissions have also been generated by delivering a.c. current to the scala media. The deterioration of neural tuning with destruction of outer hair cells provides direct evidence of their role. Outer hair cells have both fast and slow motile responses and lengthen or shorten in response to hyperpolarizing or depolarizing currents, respectively. Apparently, the energy for the motile responses of the outer hair cells is derived from the endocochlear potential, described in the next section.

It is believed that the energy from the motile responses of the outer hair cells is added only on the basal slope of the traveling wave. As the wave passes through the region of maximal displacement, the outer hair cells are in some way stimulated and deliver energy to the traveling wave, which results in increased displacement. This in turn results in more feedback, which makes the wave grow more and more steeply. After passing through the active region, the amplitude of the wave declines rapidly.

Fluid Spaces of the Cochlea

The scala media are bounded above by Reissner's membrane, laterally by the stria vascularis, and below by the reticular lamina of the organ of Corti and Claudius cells of the basilar membrane, and they contain endolymph. There is some controversy as to the actual boundaries of the endolymphatic space because of some evidence that the lower boundary is formed by the tectorial membrane rather than by the reticular lamina. Endolymph closely resembles intracellular fluid in its ionic composition, with a K^+ concentration of 140 mM and an Na^+ concentration of 2 mM. The perilymph in the scala vestibuli and the scala tympani is similar to extracellular fluids. Table 8–1 provides a comparison of the ionic composition of the cochlear fluids in the various cochlear compartments.

The resting electric potential in the scala media is 80 mV in relation to the scala tym-

TABLE 8-1. Cochlear Fluids Composition

Composition	ST Perilymph	Endolymph	SV Perilymph	CSF
Na$^+$ (mM)	147	1	141	145
K$^+$ (mM)	3.4	158	6.7	2.7
Ca^{2+} (mM)	0.68	0.023	0.64	—
Mg^{2+} (mM)	—	0.011	—	—
pH	7.28	7.37	7.26	7.28
Cl$^-$ (mM)	129	136	130	131
HCO$_3^-$ (mM)	19	21	18	19
Osmolarity (mOsm/kg H$_2$O)	293	304	294	—
Electrical potential (mV)	0	90	5	0

ST, scala tympani; SV, scala vestibuli; CSF, cerebrospinal fluid.
From Jahn AF, Santos-Sacchi J (eds): Physiology of the Ear. New York: Raven Press, 1988.

pani. The endocochlear potential is thought to be the energy source for hair cell transduction and the active mechanical response of the basilar membrane. Endolymph is believed to be secreted by the stria vascularis. The source of both the high concentration of K$^+$ and the endocochlear potential is felt to be active ion transport pumps in the stria vascularis. Anoxia results in a concomitant decline in the endocochlear potential and strial adenosine triphosphate content, which is normally 12 times higher than in any other site in the cochlea. The most positive resting potentials are recorded in the marginal cells of the stria. After disruption of Reissner's membrane to allow mixing of perilymph and endolymph, the only site that continued to show a positive potential was the stria vascularis. Na$^+$/K$^+$ transport inhibitors such as ouabain also cause a decline in the endocochlear potential, which becomes negative within minutes. The mechanism underlying maintenance of the endocochlear potential seems to be secretion of K$^+$ into endolymph. Perfusion of the scala media with low K$^+$ fluid results in a decline in the endocochlear potential; the recovery of the endocochlear potential and the normal concentration of K$^+$ are closely correlated. The cellular mechanisms underlying endolymphatic secretion of K$^+$ are not known. The source of K$^+$ appears to be perilymph: perfusion of the cochlear vasculature with K$^+$ free blood has no effect on the endocochlear potential, whereas replacement of the perilymph with K$^+$ free solution causes a very rapid decline in the endocochlear potential. Once produced, the endolymph flows through the ductus reuniens to the endolymphatic duct and then on to the endolymphatic sac, where it is resorbed.

The resting potentials in the perilymph of the scala vestibuli and the scala tympani are approximately those of plasma: $+5$ mV in the scala vestibuli and $+7$ mV in the scala tympani. Whereas the cochlear aqueduct connects the perilymphatic space with the cerebrospinal fluid, perilymph is thought to be produced by local mechanisms in the cochlea, including passive diffusion, facilitated diffusion, and active transport of solutes. Exchange is thought to occur across a barrier that is composed of pericytes, fibrocytes, and endothelial cells associated with the capillaries of the spiral ligament.

The fluid in the spaces of the organ of Corti has the same ionic composition as perilymph but possibly has a higher protein content, which leads some investigators to refer to it as *cortilymph*. The fluid in these spaces has a resting potential of approximately 0 mV. The cells in the organ of Corti have negative resting potentials that vary with the cell type. Supporting cells have potentials ranging from -70 mV to -100 mV. Outer hair cell potentials are approximately -70 mV, a value similar to that of most nerve cells. The resting potential of inner hair cells is approximately -45 mV.

Transduction

Most of the afferent cochlear neurons come from the inner hair cells, and so it is believed that the inner hair cells are the proximal sensory receptors and are responsible for the transduction of basilar membrane movement into neural action potentials. The endocochlear potential and the negative intracellular resting potential in the inner hair cells result in a large transmembrane potential (125 mV) across the apical membrane of the hair cell.

Deflection of the stereocilia of the hair cell that results from basilar membrane motion opens ion channels in the stereocilia, allowing diffusion of ions down the potential gradient and thereby causing intracellular voltage fluctuations. This depolarization causes the release of neurotransmitter at the synaptic cleft between the hair cell and the afferent cochlear nerve fiber.

Mechanism of Hair Cell Deflection

The means by which stereocilia are deflected in response to basilar membrane motion are still not clear. The stereocilia of the outer hair cells are attached to the undersurface of the tectorial membrane; this attachment led many investigators to believe that radial shear between the organ of Corti and the tectorial membrane during basilar membrane displacement was responsible for deflection of the stereocilia. However, data show that the tectorial membrane is much less stiff than the stereocilia, which indicates that the tectorial membrane acts on outer hair cell stereocilia through its inertia. The inner hair cells are not embedded in the tectorial membrane; therefore, deflection of inner hair cell stereocilia is thought to result from viscous drag of the fluids in the subtectorial region.

Inner Hair Cell Responses. Deflection of hair cell stereocilia modulates the inward flow of current and changes the membrane potential. The modulation of the inward current is thought to result from the action of ion transduction channels at the tips of the stereocilia. The current is presumed to be carried by K^+, which has a high concentration both in the endolymph and in the hair cells. The inward flow of K^+ is driven by the high potential between the endolymph and the interior of the cell.

Deflection of the stereociliary bundle toward the tallest stereocilium increases the flow of K^+ into the cell, with a depolarization of the intracellular potential. Deflection in the opposite direction decreases the inward flow of K^+, with a hyperpolarization of the intracellular potential. The transduction channels are presumed to be operated mechanically by links between the tips of stereocilia in different rows. Deflection of the stereocilia in one direction (toward the stria vascularis) stretches the links and opens the ion channels, whereas deflection in the op-

posite direction (toward the modiolus) compresses the links and closes the channels. The hair cell receptor potential depends on the magnitude of the deflection of the stereocilia. However, the response is not symmetric; the magnitude of depolarization for a given deflection in the positive direction is greater than the magnitude of the hyperpolarization for the same degree of deflection in the negative direction (Fig. 8–10).

Receptor potentials recorded from inner hair cells show both alternating current (a.c.) and direct current (d.c.) responses (Fig. 8–11). The a.c. response represents a distorted version of the stimulus waveform, whereas the d.c. response results from the hair cell deflection-response asymmetry. The a.c. response becomes progressively attenuated with increasing stimulus frequency because of the electrical capacitance of the hair cell

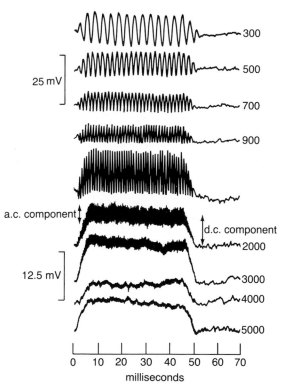

Figure 8–10. Input-output functions: the instantaneous value of the intracellular voltage change (vertical axis) is plotted against the instantaneous value of the stimulus pressure during sinusoidal stimulation (horizontal axis). Voltage changes in the depolarizing direction (upwards) are greater than those in the hyperpolarizing direction (downwards). The stimulus frequency is 600 Hz. (Redrawn from Cody AR, Russell IJ: The responses of hair cells in the basal turn of the guinea-pig cochlea to tones. J Physiol [Lond] 383:551–569, 1987.)

Figure 8–11. The relative size of the a.c. component of intracellular voltage changes in an inner hair cell declines at higher stimulus frequencies (numbers on right of curves). (Redrawn from Palmer AR, Russell IJ: Phase-locking in the cochlear nerve of the guinea-pig and its relation to the receptor potential of inner hair-cells. Hear Res 24:1–15, 1986.)

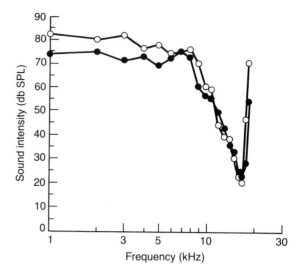

membrane, which limits the cell's ability to follow changes in transmembrane current. The higher the frequency of stimulation is, the greater is the attenuation of the a.c. response, so that at high frequencies, the a.c. response is quite small in relation to the d.c. response.

Depolarization of inner hair cells results in release of neurotransmitter at the base of the hair cell, which produces action potentials in the afferent neurons of the cochlear nerve.

To construct *tuning curves*, the response of the system in question is kept constant by varying the stimulus intensity while the frequency is varied. Figure 8–8 shows tuning curves for inner and outer hair cells. The two curves show a high degree of correspondence. All frequencies show a low-threshold, sharply tuned tip at the characteristic frequency. The lower frequencies show a high-threshold, broadly tuned tail. This indicates that hair cell tuning is based on the tuning of the basilar membrane response.

Outer Hair Cell Responses. As mentioned earlier, the resting potential of outer hair cells (about −70 mV) is more negative than that of inner hair cells. The hair cells show both a.c. and d.c. responses; however, their magnitudes are about one half to one third the size of the responses.

Outer hair cell responses differ in the apical and basal regions of the cochlea. In the apical (low-frequency) region, there is a depolarizing d.c. component of the response around the CF, but below the CF the d.c. component is hyperpolarizing, given that the

stimulus intensity is low (Fig. 8–12). If the stimulus intensity is high, the d.c. potentials are depolarizing at all frequencies.

The situation is a bit more complex for basal (high-frequency) outer hair cells. These cells show attenuated a.c. responses at the CF, whereas stimulation at a lower frequency produces a greater response. There is no d.c. response at the CF, but there is a measurable response with lower frequency stimulation. The low-frequency d.c. response is hyperpolarizing at moderate stimulus intensities, but it becomes depolarizing at high intensities.

Gross Evoked Potentials

Electrodes in or near the cochlea can record gross stimulus-evoked responses that represent the average of the responses of large numbers of the individual receptor and nerve cells.

The cochlear microphonic is generated by the hair cells. The inward flow of current into the hair cells during transduction causes fluctuations of the endocochlear potential, which are 180° out of phase with the voltage fluctuations of the hair cells. The cochlear microphonic is greatly reduced with selective destruction of the outer hair cells, which indicates that they are the source of the cochlear microphonic. The cochlear microphonic shows frequency localization that reflects localization of the traveling wave; at low frequencies it is found at the apex, and at high frequencies it is found at the base.

The d.c. shift in the baseline of the signal

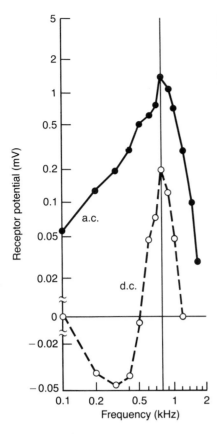

Figure 8–12. The a.c. and d.c. responses of an apical (low-frequency) outer hair cell. Stimuli near the best frequency (800 Hz) cause a d.c. depolarization, whereas stimuli below the best frequency (500 Hz) cause a d.c. hyperpolarization. The stimulus intensity is 30 db. (Redrawn from Dallos P: Response characteristics of mammalian cochlear hair cells. J Neurosci 5:1591–1608, 1985.)

seen in Figure 8–13 is referred to as the summating potential. The summating potential is not well understood, but it is probably derived directly from the d.c. receptor potentials of outer hair cells in the same way that the cochlear microphonic is derived from the a.c. receptor potentials. When the asymmetry of the hair cell response results in intracellular d.c. hyperpolarization, the endocochlear potential (and hence the summating potential) tends to become more positive. Intracellular d.c. depolarization results in a negative summating potential. Figure 8–14 shows the frequency response of both the summating potential and the cochlear me-

chanic. The frequency response is very similar to that of outer hair cells shown in Figure 8–12.

THE COCHLEAR NERVE

The cochlear nerve in humans comprises about 30,000 afferent neurons that synapse with the hair cells. Although the outer hair cells are more numerous than the inner hair cells, they synapse with only 5% to 10% of the cochlear nerve fibers; the rest of the fibers synapse with the inner hair cells. The pattern of innervation is also different. Each inner

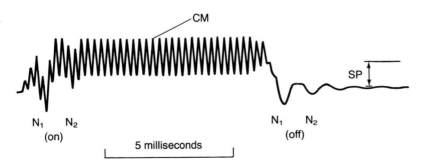

Figure 8–13. Typical response to a tone burst, recorded with gross electrodes, showing the cochlear microphonic (CM), preceded and followed by the gross action potentials N_1 and N_2, and the d.c. shift from baseline, or summating potential (SP). (Redrawn from Pickles JO: An Introduction to the Physiology of Hearing. London: Academic Press, 1988.)

Figure 8–14. The cochlear microphonic (CM) and summating potential as a function of stimulus frequency. The potentials were recorded with gross electrodes and expressed as the difference between the scala. (Modified from Dallos P, Schoeny ZG, Cheatham MA: Cochlear summating potentials: descriptive aspects. Acta Otolaryngol [Suppl 302]:1–46, 1982.)

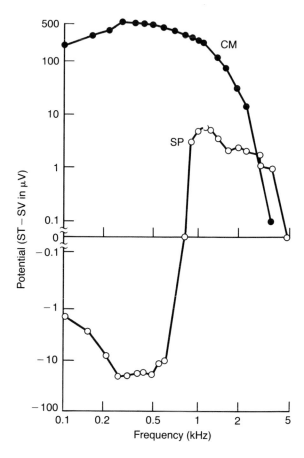

hair cell synapses with about 20 afferent neurons, each of which connects with one and only one hair cell. Outer hair cells synapse only 5 or so afferent neurons, each of which branches and innervates about 10 other hair cells. Innervation of the inner hair cells is described as convergent, whereas innervation of the outer hair cells is described as divergent. The cell bodies of the afferent neurons are in the spiral ganglion of the cochlea. There are no synapses with afferent neurons from their origin in the cochlea to their termination in the cochlear nucleus.

The afferent neurons of the cochlear nerve are organized spatially in an orderly cochleotopic (or tonotopic) arrangement, so that adjacent neurons in the cochlear nerve have adjacent sites of origin in the cochlea.

Single Unit Recordings

The first single unit recordings were made by Tasaki in 1954. Most recordings are made at the level of the internal auditory meatus, which is approached through the posterior fossa. Some researchers record from the cell bodies in the spiral ganglion. Experimental animals are anesthetized, and so their middle ear reflexes and efferent input to the cochlea are minimal or absent. It is assumed that most, if not all, recordings are from fibers innervating inner hair cells.

Many afferent neurons from inner hair cells show random spontaneous activity. The distribution of mean discharge rates is bimodal. About 25% of the fibers discharge at less than 20 spikes per second; of those, most have rates of less than 0.5 spikes per second. The other 75% have a mean discharge rate of about 60 spikes per second. The threshold is related to the spontaneous discharge rate; the most sensitive neurons have the highest spontaneous rates. The spontaneous activity is the result of random release of neurotransmitter into the synaptic cleft between the hair cells and the afferent neurons.

Acoustic stimulation modulates the receptor potentials in hair cells, which in turn modulates the release of neurotransmitter. This, in turn, results in the depolarization of the afferent neurons with propagation of an action potential toward the cochlear nucleus.

Response to Pure Tones

Single pure tones are always excitatory; that is, they elicit an increase in the mean discharge rate of afferent neurons. There is no neural inhibition at the cochlear nerve because there are no inhibitory neurons or synapses to mediate such an effect. Responses are quantified and analyzed in the form of poststimulus- (or peristimulus-) time histograms (PSTH). A PSTH is constructed by presenting a stimulus many times and recording the action potentials in bins corresponding to the time after the beginning of the stimulus. Figure 8–15 shows a PSTH in response to a tone burst. There is a high rate of discharge at the onset, which is followed by a rapid decline for 10 to 20 milliseconds and then a more gradual decline. When the tone burst terminates, the spontaneous discharge rate is initially lower than the prestimulus rate and then gradually returns to the prestimulus level. The time required to return to the prestimulus level depends on the length and the intensity of the preceding test tone. This effect is termed *adaptation* and is apparently related to depletion of neurotransmitters in the presynaptic hair cell.

Cochlear neurons are characterized by the relationship of the stimulus parameters of frequency and intensity to the discharge rate evoked by the stimulus. Plotting the threshold intensity of a tone burst that results in a criterion increase in the mean discharge rate, as a function of frequency, produces a frequency threshold curve, or tuning curve, that is very similar to those constructed for hair cell receptor potentials (Fig. 8–16). The CF is the frequency with the lowest threshold and represents the "tip" of the tuning curve. Thresholds rise quickly with change in stimulus frequency. Neurons with CF below 1 kHz show symmetric tuning curves when plotted on a log-frequency scale. Neurons with CFs above 1 kHz have asymmetric tuning curves, with steep slopes on the high-frequency side and shallower slopes on the low-frequency side. Single cochlear neurons therefore behave as band-pass filters with an asymmetric filter shape. The CF of cochlear neurons appears to be based on the location of their origin on the organ of Corti, and so it is probably derived from the frequency selectivity of the basilar membrane and hair cell responses.

The distribution of fiber thresholds at the CF encompasses a range of 60 to 80 db when units with low spontaneous rates and high thresholds are taken into account. However, as mentioned, most fibers have relatively high spontaneous discharge rates and correspondingly low thresholds. Therefore, the majority (80%) of fibers have thresholds within the lowest 20 db of the entire range.

The frequency selectivity can be quantified by the slope of the tuning above and below the CF. The tuning curve slopes are a function of the neuron's CF; the steepest slopes are found with CFs around 10 kHz. The low frequency slopes become shallower, whereas

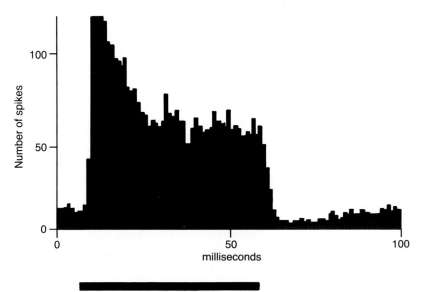

Figure 8–15. A peristimulus histogram constructed from the response of a single auditory nerve fiber to repeated presentations of a tone burst. (Redrawn from Kiang NYS, Watanabe T, Thomas EC, Clark LF: Discharge Patterns of Single Fibers in the Cat's Auditory Nerve. Cambridge, MA: MIT Press, 1965.)

Figure 8–16. Tuning curves of cat auditory nerve fibers recorded from six frequency regions. (Redrawn from Liberman MC, Kiang NY-S: Single neuron labeling and chronic cochlear pathology. IV: Stereocilia damage and alterations in rate- and phase-level functions. Hear Res 16:75–90, 1984.)

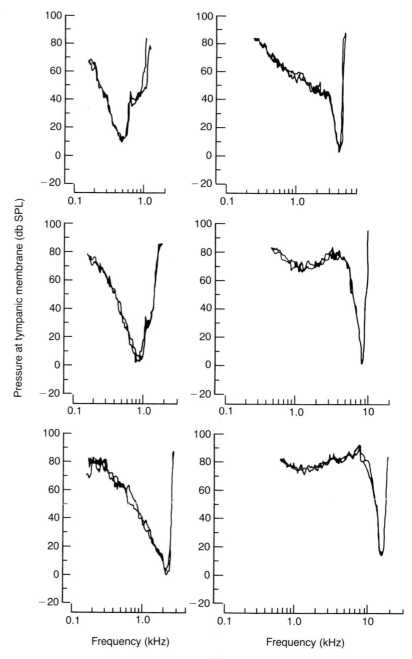

the high-frequency slopes become steeper, as the stimulus frequency is moved away from the CF.

Frequency selectivity can also be quantified by measuring the band width of the filter at an intensity set some increment over the threshold at CF. The most common formula is to divide the CF by the band width of the tuning curve 10 db above the best threshold. The higher this value is, the narrower is the band width and the greater is the frequency resolution of that neuron.

Once the threshold response of a neuron has been obtained, the suprathreshold responses may be expressed as *isorate contours*, in which the intensity necessary to achieve a criterion discharge rate is plotted as a function of frequency (Fig. 8–17). This figure shows that the frequency selectivity is greater for higher criterion rates but begins to dete-

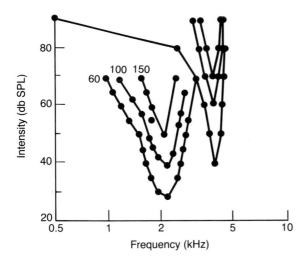

Figure 8–17. Isorate curves constructed by plotting the stimulus intensity necessary to evoke a criterion firing rate (numbers on the curves) as a function of frequency. (Redrawn from Evans EF: Cochlear nerve and cochlear nucleus. *In* Keidel WD, Neff WD [eds]: Handbook of Sensory Physiology, vol 5/2 [pp 1–108]. Berlin: Springer, 1975.)

riorate as the discharge rate saturates. *Isointensity contours* are constructed by plotting the rate of discharge for a fixed intensity stimulus as a function of frequency (Fig. 8–18). These contours show that at low stimulus levels, the highest rate is evoked near the CF. As the stimulus intensity is raised, the highest rate is evoked by stimulus frequencies above the CF for fibers with CFs below 1 kHz and by stimulus frequencies below the CF for fibers with CFs above 1 kHz. *Rate-intensity functions* are constructed by plotting the discharge rate as a function of intensity for a fixed frequency stimulus (Fig. 8–19). These figures show a sigmoidal shape, with the discharge rate saturating at levels 20-50 db above threshold. Different stimulus frequencies evoke different maximal firing rates. Frequencies below the CF of the neuron evoke higher firing rates than do frequencies above the CF.

Intensity Coding

The dynamic range over which people can perceive a change in stimulus intensity as a change in loudness is greater than 100 db. The dynamic range of single cochlear neurons is at most 50 db. This discrepancy raises the issue of how intensity information is encoded to produce the much larger perceptual dynamic range. It appears that different neurons code smaller overlapping segments of the perceptual dynamic range.

Temporal Relationships

Stimulus frequencies below 3 to 5 kHz tend to evoke responses in cochlear neurons at a

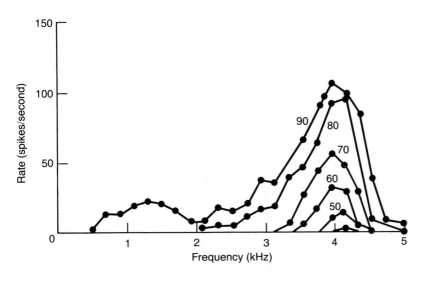

Figure 8–18. Isointensity functions show that at the lower intensities, the greatest response is produced by tones near the CF; at higher intensities the most effective frequencies move toward 1 kHz. Numbers on curves represent intensity in decibels' sound pressure level. (Redrawn from Rose JE, Kind JE, Anderson DJ, Brugge JF: Some effects of stimulus intensity on response of auditory nerve fibers in the squirrel monkey. J Neurophysiol 34:685–699, 1971.)

Figure 8–19. Rate-intensity functions for one auditory nerve fiber plotted with different stimuli frequencies (numbers on the curve). The fiber goes from threshold to saturation in about 40 db when stimulated at the CF. Stimulus frequencies below the CF produce higher firing rates than stimulus frequencies above the CF. (Redrawn from Pickles JO: The neurophysiological basis of frequency selectivity. *In* Moore BCJ [ed]: Frequency Selectivity [pp 51–121]. London: Academic Press, 1986.)

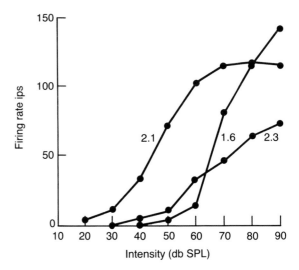

particular phase in relation to the stimulus. This may be revealed by a PSTH that is synchronized to a particular phase of the stimulus waveform (repeated-period histogram; Fig. 8–20). The discharges do not necessarily occur in each cycle, but when they do occur, it is at the same point on the stimulus waveform. The intervals between spikes tend to be integer multiples of the stimulus period. Phase-locking occurs in hair cells with a pronounced a.c. receptor potential. Deflection of the stereocilia in one direction depolarizes the hair cell and effects the release of neurotransmitter at the hair cell synapse. The a.c. receptor potential has a constant phase relationship to the stimulus and is directly responsible for release of neurotransmitter at the hair cell synapse. Therefore, neuron discharges also occur in a constant phase relationship to the stimulus waveform. As the stimulus frequency is increased, the a.c. response is progressively attenuated by the capacitance of the hair cell membrane, and neuron discharges are in response to the d.c. receptor potential. Phase locking declines in direct proportion to the decline in the inner hair cell's a.c./d.c. ratio.

The degree of phase-locking is expressed as the number of discharges occurring in the most effective half-cycle as a percentage of the total number of discharges (*coefficient of synchronization*).

Figure 8–20. With low-frequency stimuli, nerve fiber spikes appear to occur in only half of the cycle. The number of spikes increases little above 70 db SPL, which indicates that even though the firing is saturated, phase-locking of nerve fiber activity to the stimulus waveform is maintained. (Redrawn from Rose JE, Kind JE, Anderson DJ, Brugge JF: Some effects of stimulus intensity on response of auditory nerve fibers in the squirrel monkey. J Neurophysiol 34:685–699, 1971.)

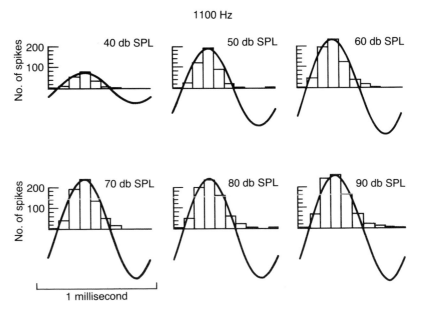

Phase-locking can occur with no change in the mean firing rate. This allows the construction of tuning curves at levels 20 db below the mean threshold. Phase-locking is preserved as the stimulus intensity increases, even though the number of spikes does not increase above 70 db SPL. With the neuron well into saturation, the repeated-period histogram still follows the waveform of the stimulus.

Response to Clicks

The response of cochlear neurons to clicks depends on the filtering characteristics of the basilar membrane at the neuron's place of origin. A click has a short duration but also a broad frequency range. Figure 8–21 shows the PSTHs of a number of neurons with different CFs. The histograms from low-frequency fibers show decaying peaks, with interspike intervals that are the reciprocal of the neuron's CF. The response appears to be produced by decaying oscillations or "ringing" of the cochlear filter. Because basilar membrane motion in only one direction effectively elicits neuron action potentials, the PSTH represents a half-wave rectified version

of the oscillations of the filter (Figs. 8–22A, 8–22B). It appears that motion of the basilar membrane toward the scala vestibuli is the effective direction, because an intense rarefaction click produces the earliest response (Fig. 8–22B). By inverting a PSTH from a rarefaction click and placing it underneath a PSTH from a condensation click, a *compound histogram* is created and provides a representation of the "ringing" of the basilar membrane (Fig. 8–22C). In fibers with CFs above about 5 kHz, there is no periodic discharge seen, apparently because of the lack of a significant a.c. receptor potential.

For pure tones of long duration, the temporal characteristics of a particular neuron's discharge are related to the frequency of the stimulus. For click stimuli, the temporal characteristics are related to the filtering characteristics of the neuron. For stimuli with intermediate durations, the temporal response characteristics are related both to the frequency of the stimulus and to the filtering characteristics of the basilar membrane.

Response to Noise Stimuli

Another way to investigate the frequency selectivity of the cochlear afferent neurons

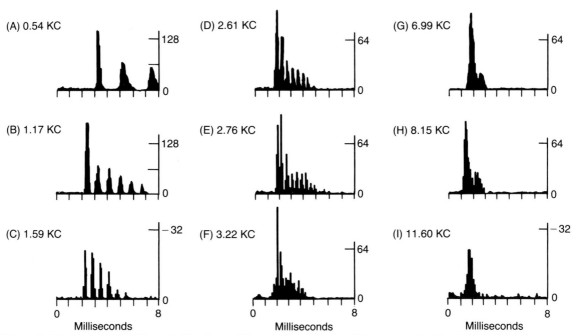

Figure 8–21. Fibers with different CFs show different responses to clicks as revealed by PSTHs. Low-frequency fibers "ring" (*A* to *F*), whereas high-frequency fibers do not (*G* to *I*). High-frequency fibers also show a later phase of activation (*F* to *H*). (Redrawn from Kiang NY-S, Watanabe T, Thomas EC, Clark LF: Discharge Patterns of Single Fibers in the Cat's Auditory Nerve. Cambridge, MA: MIT Press, 1965.)

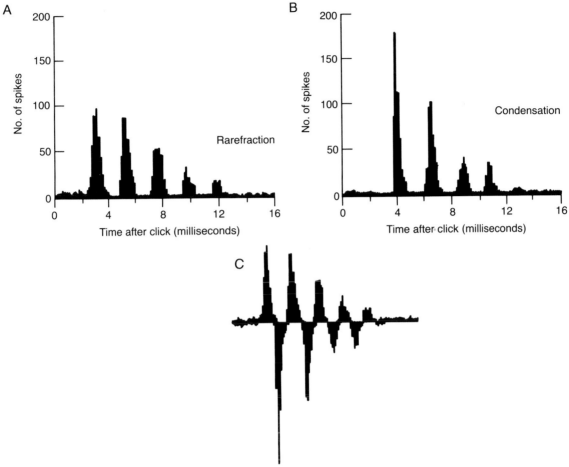

Figure 8–22. PSTHs constructed from responses to rarefaction *(A)* and condensation clicks *(B)*. A compound histogram is formed by inverting the histogram of responses to condensation clicks under that of responses to rarefaction clicks *(C)*. The fiber CF is 450 Hz. (Redrawn from Kiang NY-S, Watanabe T, Thomas EC, Clark LF: Discharge Patterns of Single Fibers in the Cat's Auditory Nerve. Cambridge, MA: MIT Press, 1965.)

involves correlating the firing pattern with stimulation by broad-band noise. Broad-band noise contains components of different frequency and phase. Only components that are passed by the basilar membrane filter and that have sufficient intensity result in neuronal discharge. For neurons whose CF is below 4 to 5 kHz, the action potentials are phase-locked to the stimulating component. By sampling only those segments of the noise immediately preceding action potentials, and by averaging many such samples, a waveform representing the impulse response of the system responsible for initiating action potentials is obtained. This waveform can then undergo a Fourier transformation to reveal the frequency response of that fiber. Tuning curves obtained through the reverse correlation technique show close agreement with pure-tone tuning curves.

Two-Tone Suppression

The response of a cochlear neuron to a single tone is always excitatory. However, the simultaneous presentation of a second tone of the proper intensity and frequency suppresses the normal increase in firing rate elicited by presentation of the first (probe) tone alone. Figure 8–23 shows the tuning curve of a cochlear fiber with a CF of 8 kHz, along with the intensity and frequencies of tones (shaded areas) that reduce the firing of a probe tone by 20% or more. The suppressive areas lie almost entirely outside of the normal excitatory areas.

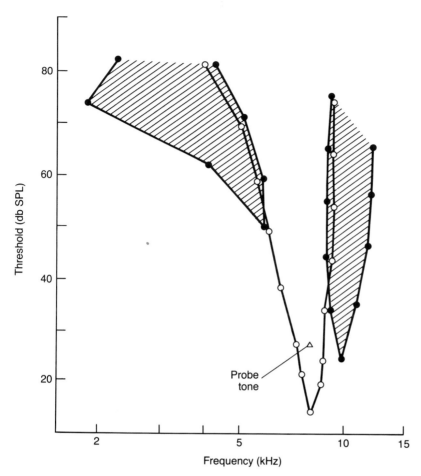

Figure 8–23. Suppression areas of an auditory nerve fiber (shaded) flank the excitatory tuning curve (open circles). Stimuli in the suppression areas reduce the mean firing rate evoked by the probe alone by 20% or more. (Redrawn from Arthur RM, Pfeiffer RR, Suga N: Properties of "two-tone inhibition" in primary auditory neurones. J Physiol 212:593–609, 1976.)

In addition to suppressing the firing rate of the neuron in response to a tone, the presence of a suppressor tone also interferes with phase-locking, an effect termed *synchrony suppression*. The area for synchrony suppression extends throughout the area of excitation, with maximal effect near the CF.

Two-tone and synchrony suppression is believed to be based on the mechanical response of the cochlea. The latency of the response is too short to be based on neural inhibition; furthermore, there is no neuroanatomic basis for such inhibition.

Noise Masking

The simultaneous presentation of background noise with tone or click stimuli reduces or abolishes the response of a cochlear neuron; this process is known as *masking*. An incremental increase in the noise level results in the same incremental increase in the threshold at CF but also elevates the threshold in the tail of the tuning curve much less.

There are two possible mechanisms for masking. The first is that underlying two-tone suppression. The second is known as the *line-busy effect*: simply stated, if one stimulus produces a given response, a second, less intense stimulus causes little or no increase in the overall response. Figure 8–24 shows a rate-intensity function for a tone presented alone and in the presence of broadband noise of constant intensity. The firing rate produced by the noise and the tone is not increased until the intensity of the tone exceeds about 50 db. This is the result of the line-busy effect. When the tone is above 50 db, its response in the presence of the noise is less than the response of the tone presented alone. This is the result of a process similar to two-tone masking.

Combination Tones

When stimulated with two simultaneous tones, combination tones that are not physically present may be heard. The most com-

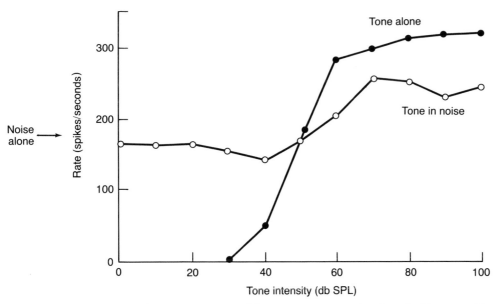

Figure 8–24. Rate-intensity functions constructed from a tone presented with and without masking noise. The tone frequency is 2.9 kHz (CF of the fiber); the noise band is 2.5 to 4 kHz. (Adapted from Rhode WS: Some observations of cochlear mechanics. J Acoust Soc Am 64:1218–1231, 1978.)

mon combination tones are the difference tone of frequency $f_2 - f_1$, and the cubic distortion tone $2f_1 - f_2$, where f_1 and f_2 represent the frequencies of the stimuli and $f_2 > f_1$. It is believed that they result from nonlinearities in basilar membrane mechanics. For example, if $f_1 = 1000$ Hz and $f_2 = 1300$ Hz, then the cubic difference tone is 700 Hz. A fiber with a CF of 700 does not respond to either of the two primaries presented alone, but it does respond to both tones presented together. The tuning curves produced by cochlear neurons with the cubic difference tone is as sharp as those produced with pure tones. Furthermore, the firing of the neurons shows phase-locking to the cubic

difference tone, provided that its frequency is below 3 to 5 kHz.

SUGGESTED READINGS

Green DM: An Introduction to Hearing. New York: Lawrence Erlbaum, 1976.

Gulick WL, Gescheider GA, Frisina RD: Hearing. Oxford, England: Oxford University Press, 1989.

Jahn AF, Santos-Sacchi J. (eds): Philosophy of the Ear. New York: Raven Press, 1988.

Moore BCJ: An Introduction to the Psychology of Hearing. London: Academic Press, 1982.

Pickles O: An Introduction to the Physiology of Hearing. London: Academic Press, 1988.

von Békésy G: Experiments in Hearing. New York: McGraw Hill, 1960.

CHAPTER 9

Central Auditory Physiology

George M. Gerken, PhD

Audition involves large portions of the human brain, either directly through the classic ascending pathway from cochlea to cortex or indirectly through neurons that are within one or two synapses of the primary system. The objective of this chapter is to consider aspects of central auditory function that are relevant to the electrophysiologic measures of hearing that are used in the clinic. To provide a frame of reference, the chapter begins with a brief introduction to central auditory anatomy. Then the neurophysiology of the central system is described to the extent needed to provide an interpretation of clinically relevant measures of central auditory function. A discussion of auditory evoked potentials builds on neuronal behavior, and the dipole is introduced as a useful explanatory concept. Then the fundamental principles of electrical measurements, including near-field and far-field evoked potentials and evoked potential averaging, are described. Finally, a broad view of topographic mapping of event-related electrical potentials and magnetic fields is presented. Throughout the chapter the emphasis is on the relation of basic physiologic phenomena to useful indexes of audition.

The pressure variations in the sounds that have been collected by the ear provide information about the environment in which the organism finds itself. It is the purpose of the central mechanism to extract portions of this information and supply them to the remainder of the brain in a form useful for the direction of behavior. In humans, of course,

this information includes speech and language as well as a description of the surrounding acoustic space. Different species have different needs for auditory information. Nevertheless, auditory systems across mammalian species exhibit numerous common capabilities that seem to be mediated by similar neural processes. This is fortunate because only few data about human auditory physiology are available. The data that are available, however, are quite compatible with corresponding animal findings.

CENTRAL AUDITORY ANATOMY

The entry of cranial nerve VIII into the brain stem (Fig. 9–1) marks the functional beginning of the central auditory system. Some components of the system are partly visible as elevations on the surface of the brain stem. The other nuclei and tracts lie deep within the brain stem. The ascending auditory system is conventionally represented by a stick-and-ball type of model (Fig. 9–2). Nuclei in the system that are not indicated in Figure 9–1 are shown in Figure 9–2 with light shading. Neural input from the cochleas progresses upward through the nuclei shown. The target of the brain stem auditory system is generally represented as auditory cortex; however, it is usually accepted that the coding and processing carried on in the lower levels of the auditory system are prerequisites for the more complex analyses mediated

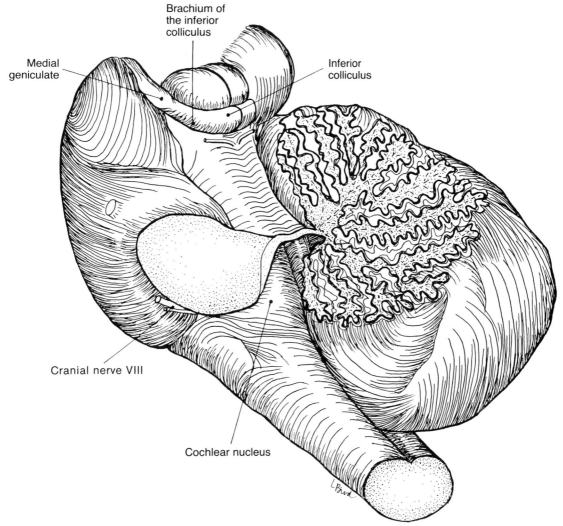

Medial geniculate

Brachium of the inferior colliculus

Inferior colliculus

Cranial nerve VIII

Cochlear nucleus

Figure 9–1. Diagram of the human brain stem, showing the portions of the auditory system located on or near the surface. (Drawing by Laura Bird.)

by the auditory cortex. Although this may be so, birds generate and discriminate remarkably involved acoustic stimuli by using only the equivalent of the human inferior colliculus. Figure 9–2 is a simplified model in which important divisions within each of the nuclei shown or within the auditory cortex are not recognized; a number of smaller pathways and nuclei have also been omitted.

Even a simple diagram such as Figure 9–2 raises the questions of why there are multiple pathways and which auditory functions are mediated by these pathways. Presumably, there are well-established criteria within the auditory system for distributing information to the various nuclear subdivisions, but the identification of the functions me-

diated by a given pathway has proved to be a difficult task. Some firm conclusions have been reached, however. For example, the medial portion of the superior olivary complex (the medial superior olivary nucleus) processes timing differences between the ears for low-frequency sounds, whereas the lateral portion of the complex (the lateral superior olivary nucleus) processes intensity disparities between the ears for high-frequency sounds. Analyses of this sort are needed for the extraction of information from the acoustic signal concerning the spatial location of the sound source.

The fibers from the bipolar neurons of the cochlea that form the auditory branch of cranial nerve VIII number about 30,000 per

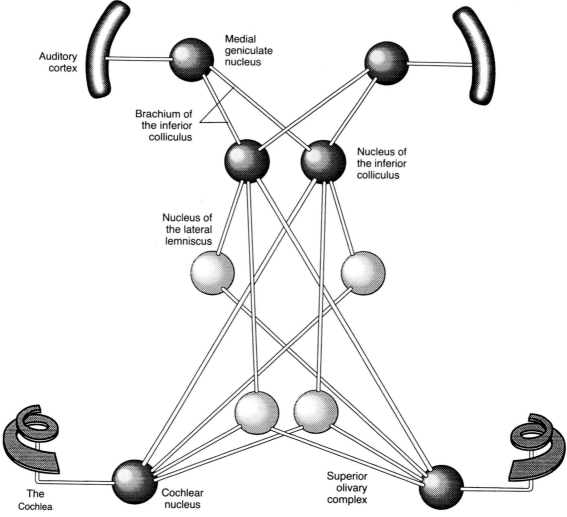

Figure 9–2. Model of the human auditory system showing the principal nuclei and pathways. The darker spheres correspond to the structures visible in Figure 9–1.

ear. These fibers enter the brain stem and synapse in the cochlear nucleus with each fiber dividing so that it is represented in at least the three major divisions of the nucleus: anteroventral, posteroventral, and dorsal cochlear nucleus (not shown in Fig. 9–2). Pathways continue from the cochlear nucleus, as schematically indicated in Figure 9–1, to the superior olivary complex or to the inferior colliculus. Again, each nucleus has several subdivisions that not only are morphologically distinct but also receive and originate specific pathways. The multiple tracts and nuclei that collectively form the main afferent pathway continue to the medial geniculate nucleus and the auditory cortex. Thus a number of parallel pathways convey

auditory information from the cochlea to the cortex. In addition, there are outputs to non-auditory brain areas. Each of these multiple pathways and multiple outputs may represent a class of functions that constitutes one part of hearing. Thus an output from the inferior colliculus acts to initiate turning of the eyes in the direction of a sound. Another output from the brain stem is critical for middle ear muscle action. Neural activity that reaches the cortex through the multiple afferent pathways is received in multiple subdivisions of the auditory cortex. Presumably identification of the person speaking is mediated by a cortical mechanism different from that used for localizing a sound source in space. Hearing is therefore not a unitary function. It may be divided into subfunctions, each of which is supported by a set of neurons (which possibly overlaps other sets) within the auditory system.

A diagram complementary to Figure 9–2 that would describe the descending system is not included. Perhaps it can be visualized, however, because the descending system runs parallel to, and is interconnected with, the ascending portion. It consists of a distinct set of pathways and nuclei within or near the nuclei of the ascending system. The descending system conveys signals in the opposite direction and ultimately ends within the cochleas. Thus the ascending and descending branches form a closed loop. In a closed loop, input influences output, and vice versa, so that the contribution of any specific portion of the system is difficult to determine. At a minimum, the central auditory system comprises the cochlear nucleus, the superior olivary complex, the nucleus of the trapezoid body (not shown in Fig. 9–2), the nuclei of the lateral lemniscus, the inferior colliculus (and its brachium), the medial geniculate nucleus, the auditory cortex, and the corresponding components in the descending system.

The location of the primary auditory cortex in humans is in Heschl's gyrus in the temporal lobe within the infolding of cortex in the lateral fissure. Because of its buried location, the human auditory cortex is particularly difficult to access. Much less is known about the organization of the auditory cortex in humans than about that in monkeys or cats. It may be assumed, however, that the human cortex is at least as diverse and complex as that of the monkey. In the monkey, there are a dozen or more subdivisions of the auditory cortex. Each subdivision has different physiologic properties. Furthermore, a given subdivision has anatomic connections with contralateral and other ipsilateral subdivisions of the auditory cortex and with lower levels of the auditory system. An auditory cortex subdivided into numerous functional regions forms a logical end-station for the numerous parallel pathways in the brain stem. It would be pleasant to report that another brain area has been found in which the outputs from the several subdivisions of auditory cortex are integrated into the sense modality termed *hearing*. No such area has been located, but the search is an active one, and some positive findings have been obtained (e.g., the late evoked potentials that correlate with some cognitive functions). Alternatively, it may be that the known interconnections of auditory cortex are sufficient to support the level of integration required to generate auditory perceptual experience. This possibility is compatible with clinical observations that no single higher brain region is essential for all aspects of auditory experience. In this view, hearing is truly a system function based on the orchestrated participation of the multiple cortical subdivisions.

PHYSIOLOGY OF AUDITORY NEURONS

What Figures 9–1 and 9–2 do not reveal is the greater part of the story; namely, what functions are performed as a result of the anatomic interconnections. It is necessary to further explore the role in audition of the fundamental unit of the nervous system, the neuron (also called a *single unit* in physiologic studies). A basic question is how individual neurons in the auditory system are affected by sound delivered to the ear. *Neuronal coding* is the term used to describe the complex manner in which an acoustic stimulus is represented as a pattern of neural impulses at any given point within the auditory system. Within the central auditory system, a neuron is typically two or more synapses removed from the hair cells of the cochlea. Thus the description of neural coding for that neuron includes the cumulative effects of all the synaptically related neurons interspersed on the paths that can be traced back to the hair cells of the cochlea.

With respect to neural coding, perhaps the most obvious physical dimension of sound is frequency. Neurons in the auditory system typically respond very selectively to stimulus frequency: that is, they are *tonotopically organized* on the basis of the cochlear region from which they are activated. The frequency analysis performed by the cochlea is preserved in the tonotopic stratification in the central auditory system. Thus the answer to the question of how auditory neurons in different parts of the system respond to acoustic stimuli presented to the ear usually involves stimulus frequency (or frequency spectrum) as an important parameter. Stimulus intensity is equally important. Before neuronal coding is discussed further, however, a brief

offset; it may fire at the onset, stop, and then start again; it may tend to fire only with the cycles of the stimulus (this can be seen in Figure 9–3B). In spite of the tremendous possible variability in response patterns, it has been found experimentally that they can be combined into perhaps six major groups. Thus at the neuronal level of analysis, the auditory system seems to use a finite number of response patterns to code the information contained in an acoustic stimulus.

Spontaneous Neural Activity. Several spikes occur in Figure 9–3B at times when the stimulus is not present. Such firing in the absence of an obvious stimulus is called *spontaneous activity* and is another example of seemingly random neuronal behavior. Figure 9–4 also indicates the level of spontaneous activity for the neuron in question. The time interval before the presentation of the stimulus is particularly useful in this regard because with proper experimental technique it may be assumed that spikes in this interval are not caused by the stimulus. There seems to be a reduction in spontaneous activity after the cessation of the stimulus. If spontaneous activity occurred at a rate higher than that shown in Figure 9–3B, the presence of a signal could also be unequivocally indicated by a reduction of spontaneous activity even if there were no increase in firing rate during the stimulus. Response patterns of this type have been observed.

Spontaneous activity is found throughout the nervous system, and the obvious question is, Why is it there? Does spontaneous activity represent a failure of the nervous system to exclude randomly generated activity within itself? If so, the level of spontaneous activity would place a central nervous system limitation on the detection of weak signals. With regard to weak signals, it is more likely that there is noise in the transduction process that must be separated from the sensory signal. But then why brain regions far removed from sensory inputs still show significant levels of spontaneous activity remains a puzzle. Alternatively, spontaneous activity could represent other neural signals (e.g., control signals) multiplexed into what is regarded as the afferent signal channel. If this is the case, then to fully separate control signals from informational signals, it would be necessary to access or to know the multiplexing strategies that are present in the auditory system. The usual approach, however, is simply to consider spontaneous activity to be neural noise.

At a far less abstract level, it is clear that in Figures 9–3A and 9–3B, the firing rates of the neuron increased immediately after and during the stimulus, respectively. In general, regardless of the nature of spontaneous activity, it will always be a practical statistical issue for the neurophysiologist to decide whether the response to the stimulus is significantly greater than the spontaneous activity. In Figure 9–3 it is apparent that the answer is affirmative even without formal statistical analysis.

Other Aspects of Neuronal Coding. Again with regard to the neuronal coding concept, several straightforward relations with stimulus parameters deserve mention. A given neuron generally responds most readily to a narrow range of frequencies called the *best frequency*, or the *characteristic frequency*, of that neuron. The intensity of a stimulus at the best frequency can be reduced further than at any other frequency, and the stimulus will still activate the neuron. The neuron responds less vigorously at frequencies above and below the best frequency, and at these other frequencies, a more intense stimulus must be used to yield a given firing rate. Thus a neuron has a V-shaped frequency-intensity function that is minimal for the best frequency. This selective responsiveness based on stimulus frequency is the hallmark of the tonotopic organization of the auditory system.

Neurons within the auditory system are grouped on the basis of responsiveness to stimulus frequency. Thus low frequencies are represented at a place in a nucleus or a fiber bundle that is anatomically different from the placements of middle or high frequencies. However, although a neuron typically responds best when the stimulus is at the best frequency, the neuron also responds to a considerable range of other frequencies. Neurons higher in the auditory system than the neuron in question do not necessarily "know" what the stimulus frequency is. Thus their input, which is a train of spike responses, could have been produced by many combinations of frequency and intensity. This trading relation among stimulus parameters (in this case, frequency and intensity) is very much a part of the concept of neuronal coding, and care must therefore be taken in interpreting the role of stimulus frequency. One interpretation is that the tonotopic organization of the auditory system provides an organizational framework that supports a number of analytic processes. As a classification scheme, tonotopic organization is most prevalent at the lower and middle levels of the system. At the level of the auditory cortex, some of the cortical subdivisions are clearly tonotopically organized, whereas others are not.

The effect of stimulus intensity is, in general, that more intense sounds produce higher firing rates (more nerve impulses per second). A plot of the relation between stimulus intensity and firing rate is called the *response rate function*. This function expresses an important aspect of neuronal coding and is usually determined through the use of a stimulus at the best frequency of the neuron. For very low-stimulus intensities (i.e., below threshold), the firing rate is the spontaneous rate for the neuron in question. At stimulus intensities above threshold, the neuron typically responds to the stimulus by firing at higher rates as the intensity is increased. Finally, the neuron saturates, and no further increases in response rate are obtained. In fact, the curve may roll over and actually decrease at still higher intensities. One puzzle in the coding of stimulus intensity is that a given neuron may have only a 20- to 40-db range from threshold to saturation. Thus elaborate explanations involving a number of neurons are necessary to relate perceived loudness to the full range (100 db or more) of stimulus intensities handled by the auditory system.

It was previously noted that the spikes in response to the tone burst can occur within the same portion of a stimulus cycle. This synchronized firing is called *phase locking,* and it occurs only in a minority of neurons that are usually located lower in the system. It also tends to occur for lower frequency stimuli because timing is not as critical at low frequencies. The neuron in Figure 9–3B demonstrates phase locking, whereas the neuron in Figure 9–3A does not show phase locking because the response follows the end of the stimulus. Phase-locked firing in neurons driven by one or the other ear makes possible temporal comparisons within about 12 microseconds between the ears. These comparisons are critical for the localization of sound sources.

Processing of Complex Sounds. Sinusoidal tone bursts are convenient for the researcher, but such single-frequency tone bursts are the exception rather than the rule in real life. Real stimuli are usually more complicated and contain more than one frequency. The acoustic domain that consists of sounds with two or more frequency components is large indeed, and it is in this domain that the auditory system normally operates. Thus the barking of a dog is a sound with many frequency components. These components can be separated mathematically by *Fourier analysis* and can be physically separated by electronic equipment designed for this task. The frequency components in a complex sound really do exist. An interesting question that arises is whether the complex sound is one sound or many. Is the dog's bark one sound or many? The answer of the auditory system is that a single bark is a single sound, because the various frequency components are tightly linked in time. However, the various frequencies in the bark come from many regions of the cochlea in the same way that a word spoken by a friend also activates many regions of the cochlea. The bark and the word are perceived as single sounds. If they overlap in time, they share the activation of many common neural elements in the auditory system, but the perceptions are still kept separate. To deal with barks and words simultaneously, the coding strategies in the lower levels of the auditory system must clearly feed into far more sophisticated coding and processing strategies in the upper portions of the system.

In the bark and word example, these sounds are composed of acoustic components that relate to one another in ways that are not in the least intuitively obvious. In the visual domain, a house built of toy blocks is an example in which the blocks are physically related to one another in obvious ways. Although each block exists in itself, the house is perceived as an entity: a visual object. Thus barks and words are auditory objects with relations among the acoustic components that are also physically specifiable. The discussion has now gone beyond simple sounds (single-frequency sinusoids) to the realm of complex sounds that constitute the auditory objects of real life. These sounds are perceived and discriminated, but how, specifically, does the central auditory mechanism process complex sounds? At present, the question has been approached experimentally, but much more work is needed before satisfactory answers are available.

Two important aspects of hearing are the abilities of the auditory system (1) to resolve two or more sounds (simple or complex) as distinct entities, and (2) to identify (name) one sound as opposed to other similar sounds. An example of the first ability is hearing a coin hit the floor even though a radio is playing. Failure to hear the coin under these circumstances would be called *masking*. An example of the second ability is that the coin can be identified as a quarter, dime, and so forth. This is called *identification*. *Discrimination* is the term used if the sound of one coin can be distinguished from the sound of another even though neither coin can be specifically identified. As suggested later, some measures at the neuronal level can be related to the auditory function of discrimination.

Masking. Masking is interference in the detection of one stimulus that is caused by the presence of another stimulus. The stimuli can be simple, complex, or one of each. Masking is thus a failure of resolution: the first stimulus cannot be separated from the second. Physiologic responses such as single unit firing or evoked potentials (to be described) can be used as measures of masking. At the single unit level, if two stimuli are individually capable of increasing the firing rate of a given neuron, a masking experiment can be performed by noting the firing rate produced in the neuron by stimulus 1. If stimulus 2 is also presented at very low intensity every time that stimulus 1 is presented, there is no incremental increase in firing rate resulting from stimulus 2. Stimulus 2 is said to be masked by stimulus 1. Increasing the intensity of stimulus 2 step by step ultimately results in a firing rate in the presence of both stimuli that is greater than that produced by stimulus 1. Stimulus 2 is no longer masked (according to physiologic measurements). The failure to detect one stimulus in the presence of a second of different frequency depends, in part, on the resolving power of the inner ear. But masking also depends on the analytic capabilities of the central auditory system. There is a match between the peripheral and central mechanisms: neither is analytically overdesigned in relation to the other.

Masking can be obtained not only with neuronal responses but also with other, more clinically applicable measures. Evoked potentials (to be described) can be used to demonstrate masking, as can behavioral procedures during audiometric evaluations. The audiogram indicates the sensitivity of an ear to different pure-tone stimuli. The information that can be provided by masking goes beyond the audiogram in that it invokes the use of acoustic sensitivity with regard to the resolution (or nonresolution) of stimuli.

Active Interactions of Two Stimuli. The same two stimuli that were used to measure masking physiologically can be used under slightly different experimental conditions to yield results that relate to discrimination. The simultaneous presence of the two acoustic stimuli provides opportunities throughout the auditory system for nonocclusive types of interactions between the neural populations activated by the two stimuli. Such interactions occur and have been studied in detail. Even in the cochlear nucleus, the inhibitory effects of one stimulus on the neural responses elicited by the second stimulus are both present and extremely important. At higher levels of the system, the interactions become more complicated and include excitatory processes as well. The complexity is increased by the fact that the two stimuli do not have to occur simultaneously to produce interactive effects. Sequential stimulation can also yield interaction.

As an example of the effects of two stimuli, consider a neuron, in the inferior colliculus, that is activated by one stimulus but not by another. It may be that the frequency of the first stimulus is in the vicinity of the best frequency of the neuron, whereas the second stimulus is somewhat removed in frequency and is not sufficiently intense to activate the neuron. On the other hand, it may be that the second stimulus does influence the response of the neuron to the first stimulus. Why is this not some aspect of masking? It is not masking because the second stimulus was by itself ineffective in activating the neuron. When the effects of the two stimuli on the firing rate of the neuron are studied further, it often turns out that the mapping of firing rate in relation to the frequencies and intensities of the two stimuli yields a remarkably involved plot. The stimuli interact, as measured by this one neuron, in well-specified ways that may include either inhibitory or excitatory effects. This interaction goes beyond masking and is an active processing strategy of the sort that would be expected to underlie auditory discrimination.

As a second example, a neuron in the superior olivary complex may be excited (an E response) by an ipsilateral stimulus (which is applied to the ear on the same side of the head as the neuron) and inhibited (an I response) by a contralateral stimulus. A response rate function that relates the intensities of the two stimuli with neuronal firing rate can be experimentally measured: a formal playing of excitation against inhibition. Often, the neuron responds if the ipsilateral stimulus is more intense. If the contralateral stimulus is more intense, the neuron is inhibited and does not fire. This type of neuron (EI) is thought to be involved in the localization of sound. A sound source in a forest, for example, would not stimulate both ears equally because of numerous acoustic factors. The cues provided by these factors, in conjunction with other time and frequency cues, can be used to estimate the position of the sound source in three-dimensional space, as in locating a bird after it is heard singing.

In Figure 9–5, a prototypical listener is shown listening to a prototypical bird. The sound path to the right ear (R) is longer than that to the left ear (L). Sound attenuates with distance, and so the right ear receives a sound that is slightly weaker than the sound received by the left. In addition, it also takes a little longer, as little as 10 or 20 microseconds, for the sound to reach the right ear. These slight differences in intensity and time are processed by the interaction of excitatory and inhibitory processes in the auditory system to locate the sound source to the right or the left of midline. The calculation of the elevation of the sound source cannot be described so simply. It is known, however, that the frequency filtering and waveform processing of the auricle is necessary for accurate elevation judgments. In the examples just given of neurons in the inferior colliculus and the superior olivary complex, inhibition and excitation processes were activated in the former case by frequency differences in one ear and in the latter case by time and intensity differences between the two ears.

Functions of the Descending System. The anatomy of the descending system reveals that it parallels and interconnects with the ascending system from the cortex down to the cochlea. This arrangement suggests a system that modifies, modulates, or emphasizes activity within the ascending system on the basis of conclusions reached at the higher levels of the auditory system. Thus selective attention, facilitated discrimination, and

Figure 9–5. A sound source is slightly above the horizontal plane and to the left of the listener. Location in the environment can be determined on the basis of the acoustic signals reaching the two ears. (Drawing by A. Craig Lockhart.)

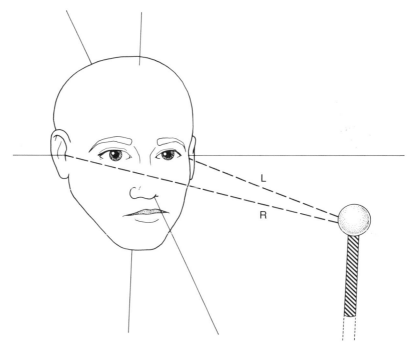

switching between listening modes are possible functions. Some support for facilitated discrimination under difficult (noisy) listening conditions has been obtained in studies of animals. The experiments are clearly important and difficult to perform, and more of them are needed.

Overview of Auditory Physiology. The auditory neuron is the basic building block in the auditory system, and neuronal responses to a wide variety of acoustic stimuli have been studied extensively. Frequency, intensity, and other stimulus parameters are demonstrably of paramount importance for neuronal coding. The neurons exhibit a diversity of response patterns, however, which suggests that more involved processing strategies exist. Although these strategies have been described, it is not currently understood how sound is thereby analyzed and processed to yield acoustic objects.

A great deal is known about the neuronal coding of sound as expressed in patterned neuronal activity; however, the relation between neuronal responses and ordinary auditory experience remains elusive. This is a fact of neurophysiologic life. It is proving difficult to analyze neuronal behavior with a reductionistic neuronal approach and then to return to the perceptual/experiential level.

Beyond investigations of the neuron, little work has been done on the *relative* firing patterns in groups of neurons. Even simple systems of several neurons can exhibit amazingly complex collective response patterns. The number of possible states within a neural system of as few as 15 or 20 neurons rapidly becomes astronomic. There is virtually no mathematical framework for describing neural networks, although the area is one of intense current research. Hence in observing a neuron in the inferior colliculus, researchers may be *not* seeing much more than they do see.

In regard to the manner in which two or more neurons respond to a single stimulus, these response patterns can quickly become of immense complexity, as noted earlier. However, there is a measure, the evoked potential, that does provide an indication of the activities of a multitude of neurons. By its nature, the evoked potential avoids the subtleties and complexities of neuronal interaction and emphasizes instead the modal response patterns in large groups of neurons.

AUDITORY EVOKED POTENTIALS

As a generic term, *auditory evoked potential* has many meanings. Each is associated with a different set of recording procedures, and each provides a different type of information concerning auditory processing. The approach taken herein is to describe this continuum of evoked potentials, starting with those closest to neuronal activity and building progressively toward more global measures.

As described earlier, the behavior of an auditory neuron can be recorded and summarized statistically by a poststimulus-time histogram such as that in Figure 9–4. However, because of the tonotopic organization of the auditory system, there may be hundreds or even thousands of neurons that respond as a group when a tonal stimulus is used. Because of neuronal coding, a diversity of response patterns can be expected from this neuronal group. The diversity, however, is finite because of the small number of basic coding patterns. Even so, this diversity can lead to rather complex neuronal group behavior. The auditory evoked potential is another statistical summary of neuronal activity, and the critical question is, What types of neuronal activities are included in this statistical measure? To record an evoked potential, the electrical data are gathered by an electrode that is larger than the microelectrode previously discussed. What does this electrode detect in the way of neuronal activity? A technical digression is needed.

Electrodes. The electrodes used in evoked potential work range from small wires (e.g., 50 μm in diameter) of stainless steel or platinum to disks a centimeter in diameter. What the electrode detects in the brain depends upon two factors: (1) electrode size and (2) the proximity of the electrode to the source of neural activity. Small electrodes can record from relatively small populations of neurons but only if they are quite close to the active neurons. Large electrodes are usually positioned on the scalp and hence are always at some distance from the target neural population. In practice, the difference between large and small electrodes is like the difference in perspective between the expansive views from the mountaintop and the detailed views of small groups of flowers and trees from the valley floor.

An electrode not designed to function as

a microelectrode is generally called a *gross electrode*. Clearly, even the smallest gross electrode cannot be in contact with each neuron, and large gross electrodes may not be in contact with any neurons. Gross electrodes thus provide a statistical summary of neuronal activity without identifying individual neurons. It is simpler to record with gross electrodes because they are intrinsically less specialized than microelectrodes. The smaller gross electrodes may be used invasively in both animals and humans, however, to record from specific neural populations. When electrodes are introduced into brain tissue, they produce some damage that can alter the potentials to be recorded. If the electrodes can be left in place for a period of days, some of the transient damage effects subside. It is always important to know about the effects of the intrusion of the measuring instrument—in this case, the electrodes—on the phenomenon under consideration.

What does the gross electrode detect? Small electrodes (which are wires insulated everywhere except at the tips) may under optimal conditions record the aggregate of all the spike potentials. However, spike potentials are hard to pick up, for reasons to be discussed, unless the electrode is extremely close to the active axons. A class of slower neural events, the postsynaptic potentials, is more visible electrically. To relate these neuronal potentials with evoked potentials, several terms and concepts are needed.

It is useful to distinguish between *near-field potentials* and *far-field potentials*. The recording situation is described as near-field when the recording electrode is in the immediate vicinity of a number of auditory neurons that are activated by an acoustic stimulus. The situation is considered far-field when the distance between the recording electrode and the source of the recorded potentials is at least several times the diameter of the source of voltage. Other terms relevant to the process of recording the electrical activity of neurons must also be described at this time.

The Dipole. The *dipole* is a concept of sufficient importance to merit its own section and it is fundamental to an explanation of evoked potentials. Ideally a dipole is considered to be a voltage and current source, much like a miniature battery, with a positive pole on one end and a negative pole on the other.

Dipoles can be described by (1) the magnitude of the voltage difference between the positive and negative poles, (2) the physical separation of the two poles, and (3) the orientation of the dipole in space. A fourth property that goes beyond the miniature battery image is the manner in which the dipole voltage changes over time. A battery immersed in an electrically conducting medium such as cerebrospinal fluid or intracellular fluid gives rise to the flow of electrical current. Such current flow can be rigorously associated (through Ohm's law) with voltage differences. A dipole is usually considered to be composed of equal and opposite charges separated in space. The voltage difference in the dipole is due to these separated charges, and placing the charges in a conducting medium results in a current. Thus charge, voltage, and current are all interrelated. If the charge were not replenished (as in a battery or a neuron), the energy available in the dipole would dissipate in the conducting medium and the dipole would cease to exist. Although the interrelatedness of charge, voltage, and current rests on firm physical principles, the battery model of the dipole is not a bad approximation. Because the electrical current and voltage are external to the "battery" and exist in the conducting medium, it is possible to record the electrical activity of the nervous system.

The battery is the neuron. Alternatively, on a smaller scale, it may be just a part of a neuron; on a larger scale, it may be a group of neurons. On the small scale, a neuronal membrane is highly polarized, with the negative charges on the inside of the cell. Now the required mental exercise is to regard the cell membrane as being composed of a sheet of tiny batteries all standing side by side and all oriented in the same way with the negative poles toward the inside of the cell. How can this view be reconciled with the fact that the dipole model apparently requires the outside of the neuron to have a positive voltage, as opposed to the apparent zero voltage of the rest of the body? First, one end of a battery does not have a voltage: the battery voltage is the difference between the two ends. Second, if the positive ends of all the batteries are connected together, as are the outer sides of all the cell membranes in the body through the body fluids, the positive ends of the billions of batteries become a reference that can be treated as a zero voltage. In relation to the bodily reference, the interior of the cell is then negative.

Exactly how do dipoles relate to neurons? In the preceding paragraph, the cell membrane was modeled as a sheet of dipoles. The full description of a single neuron in this manner could keep a large computer busy for a long time. The dipole model is supposed to aid description, not hinder it. The method in relating dipoles to neurons is to choose an *equivalent dipole* that models the particular neural phenomenon of interest, whether it is the active region of an axon, the overall effect of a neuron, or the collective potential produced by thousands of neurons. As an example, consider 500 dipoles oriented vertically but tilted 20° to the right and an equal number of dipoles tilted equally to the left. All 1000 dipoles can be represented by one equivalent dipole that is oriented vertically but produces a voltage somewhat less than that produced by 1000 individual dipoles oriented vertically. Why somewhat less voltage? The question can be answered by a brief mental exercise: if the two groups of 500 were oriented completely in opposition, the net voltage difference would be zero. Partial opposition, as with the tilted dipoles, moves the voltage toward zero (mathematically, this is a vector operation).

There is more to the question of how dipoles relate to actual neurons. While a neuron is quiescent, the polarization within the cell produces only a minor flow of current in the surrounding tissue. It is true that the cell membrane is polarized and thus resembles a sheet of dipoles, but it is also true that the membrane is a poor conductor of electricity in relation to the surrounding tissue. The net result is that the quiescent neuron is virtually invisible electrically. This is not the case, however, when the neuron generates a spike response. Membrane conductivity alters radically in the active region, and the transmembrane voltage interacts much more effectively with the adjacent tissue; this interaction results in marked external current flow during the spike. The movement of the spike along an axon is considered to consist of a series of equivalent dipoles activated sequentially in time; thus this sequential activation mimics the movement of the spike. Alternatively, the sequentially activated series of equivalent dipoles could be replaced with a single moving dipole. In either case, considerable computational effort is required to model an axon.

Other neural elements such as synapses can also be modeled by using dipoles. In fact, the postsynaptic membrane is the best candidate for accounting for the potentials recorded by gross electrodes. When presynaptic activity reaches a neuron, the transmitter substance released at the synapse acts to either incrementally depolarize (excite) or incrementally hyperpolarize (inhibit) the neuron. Activity at one synapse is of no consequence: typically hundreds or thousands of synapses are required to fire the neuron or, alternatively, to prevent it from firing. Incoming activity is spatially summed in this manner across the dendrites to determine the behavior of the cell. Because the depolarization or hyperpolarization effects persist for tens of milliseconds or more before decaying to zero, the input to the neuron is also summed across time as well. These changes in polarization tend to affect the entire neuron, and because at least some neurons are relatively long physically, an easily recordable potential results. The temporal persistence of the postsynaptic potentials also favors electrical visibility. Finally, if a number of neurons are simultaneously generating postsynaptic membrane potentials, the resulting equivalent dipole can be quite robust.

The equivalent dipole can be used to model neural activity and is an excellent explanatory concept. In practice, the modeling process can be extremely complex. It is a major blessing that only some evoked potential work requires actual calculation of equivalent dipoles.

Evoked Potentials and the Dipole. Several mental exercises illustrate some of the properties of equivalent dipoles as they relate to the auditory system. Begin by imagining 10 dipoles all oriented the same way, all having the same voltage, and all suspended in a beaker of saline solution. Then introduce two recording electrodes, because it is always a voltage *difference* that is recorded from brains (and beakers). One of the electrodes, the "hot," or active, electrode, is positioned in the vicinity of the dipoles. Moving this electrode from one spot to another in the beaker produces voltage readings that depend on the location of the electrode in relation to the dipoles. The second electrode is the "ground," or "indifferent" or "reference," electrode and is usually treated as if it were at a considerable distance from the dipoles.

(Locating the reference electrode well away from the active neural tissue is a matter of great importance in the recording of evoked potentials.) Presumably, the reference electrode is suitably placed, but obviously there are limits to how remotely it can be located in a small beaker. If this were a real experiment, this reference electrode would cause real problems. When the active electrode is near the positive ends of the dipoles, a positive voltage difference is recorded. The voltage is greatest when the electrode touches the positive ends of the dipoles and gradually decreases to zero as the electrode is pulled farther and farther away (now the size of the beaker must be increased). The same changes in voltage occur for the negative ends of the dipoles. If, however, the active electrode is located halfway between the positive and negative ends of the pack of dipoles (i.e., in the plane perpendicular to the lines connecting the positive and negative ends of the dipoles), the voltage difference recorded is zero. This is because the positive and negative contributions cancel out, in spite of the fact that the active electrode may be relatively close to the ends of the dipoles. This geometric factor is of great importance in the understanding of the electrical potentials produced by dipoles.

As a second experiment, imagine two dipoles suspended side by side in the beaker, with the polarity of one dipole reversed with respect to the other. In this configuration, the dipoles almost completely cancel each other so that the voltage differences recorded are essentially zero; that is, the effects produced by the opposing dipoles cancel. If a number of dipoles were present but were randomly oriented, no net voltage difference between active and reference electrodes would again be recorded, and the equivalent dipole would be of zero magnitude.

As a third experiment, mentally compare voltages recorded in the beaker by using a short dipole (positive and negative poles are close together) with those recorded by using a longer dipole (the poles are more separated). A hint is in order: from any point in the beaker, the recording electrode has a harder time detecting the short dipole than it does the long dipole. This is analogous to being able to see large, widely spaced pickets in a fence more easily than narrow, closely spaced pickets. The phrase "recording a voltage difference" is now truncated to "recording a voltage"; the latter form is in common

use, and it seems to indicate that a voltage was recorded from a given electrode without specifically involving another (reference) electrode. The phraseology is jargon: two electrodes are always needed because only voltage differences can be recorded. Evoked potentials are recorded only as voltage differences between two electrodes. It is essential to keep this in mind when laboratory or clinical data are interpreted.

As a final experiment, consider the effects of varying the dipole voltage. Imagine that the active electrode is properly located in the beaker so that a voltage is recorded. If the dipole voltage is increased, the recorded voltage increases proportionally. If the dipoles were modeling a time-varying voltage such as the spike potential, the electrode in the beaker would record a voltage proportional to the spike. This example shows that a time-varying neural generator can be recorded by a properly positioned electrode. However, the sheets of dipoles (arranged in a cylindric form to mimic the axonal membrane) that are used to model the axon are composed of very small dipoles. Small dipoles in a small circular configuration (modeling the axon) are hard to detect; hence the spike potential is hard to record except when a small recording electrode is extremely close to the axon. Synaptic circuits, however, are modeled by much larger dipoles, and these can be detected by a recording electrode at a much greater distance from the neuron.

Superposition. Superposition resembles ordinary addition. If event 1 occurs along with event 2, the net result is the sum of the effects of events 1 and 2. Given that the two events do not interact and that the order of addition does not affect the outcome, then the process is described as linear. If the two events are voltages produced by two dipoles, it is convenient to have a linear system. Although the principle is straightforward, the calculation is not. For one thing, the correct measures to add are generally currents, not voltages. For example, superposition of the effects of two dipoles is not simply the sum of their individual voltages. The currents produced by the dipoles in a small region of the beaker (or the brain) must be summed before the resultant voltage can be calculated. This disclaimer is particularly critical when tens of thousands of dipoles must be used to model a neural event (one does not obtain 1000-V evoked potentials). Superposition does, however, hold within the brain for all of the neuronally produced currents, and the resultant current yields the voltage difference termed the *evoked potential*. With far-field sources, however, superposition can be used in an intuitive way with voltage to account for the effects of multiple generators on evoked potentials.

A Typical Evoked Potential. An auditory evoked potential is a time-varying electrical potential that occurs after the presentation of an acoustic stimulus and that is usually recorded from a gross electrode. In principle, an evoked potential can be thought of as being generated by a time-varying equivalent dipole. This single equivalent-dipole model, however, is unquestionably too simple. Typically, multiple equivalent dipoles are needed to account for any evoked potential.

Given that evoked potentials are complicated, one can nevertheless continue with the train of thought concerning neurons and dipoles. There is an abundance of neuronal activity in the auditory system after even a simple acoustic stimulus such as a click or a brief tone. The question is how large-scale neuronal behavior relates to auditory evoked potentials. The neuronal firing patterns in Figures 9–3A and 9–3B and the poststimulus-time histogram in Figure 9–4 suggest that an evoked potential may simply be the sum of the neuronal spike activity in the vicinity of a gross electrode. Spike potentials, as mentioned earlier, may not be easily detected by gross electrodes, but the spatially more ex-

tensive postsynaptic potentials can be recorded more easily. The varied patterns of the neuronal activity and the associated slower synaptic potentials generate a diverse series of potentials that may cancel or reinforce one another by superposition. Cancellation and reinforcement can occur within a neuronal population (i.e., within a neural generator) or between neuronal populations.

It is at the onset of the stimulus, however, that the responses of the various neural populations generally reinforce one another so that the auditory evoked potential is, in essence, an onset potential. Because evoked potentials reflect the neural responses to only a limited portion of the stimulus, they are of limited use as indicators of the complexities of processing throughout the stimulus. Under certain conditions, an evoked potential related to stimulus offset can also be seen, because this is a second period of time during which neural activity tends to be synchronized.

The evoked potential shown in Figure 9–6 is a simulation of an evoked potential obtained from an electrode in the human inferior colliculus. This potential would be obtained from an indwelling electrode (no doubt from the central nucleus of the inferior colliculus), so that the evoked potential is recorded near-field. Once again the 1-kHz tone burst is used as a stimulus. S marks the time of arrival of the tone burst at the tympanic membrane. The interval between S and A is the *onset latency*, which is the time required for the stimulus to pass through the middle ear and the inner ear, to be trans-

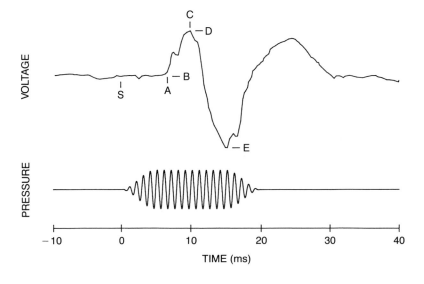

Figure 9–6. An evoked potential from the inferior colliculus. S corresponds to the arrival of the tone burst at the tympanic membrane; A through E are measures used to describe the evoked potential.

duced, and to progressively activate neural elements between the cochlea and the recording electrode. At A the neural generators in the vicinity of the electrode are activated. If positive recorded voltage is assumed to produce an upward deflection (in practice, this is known from the calibration of the recording equipment), the potential that peaks at C represents the net effect by superposition of all the generators involved. The time interval between S and C is the *peak latency*. Subsequently the potential becomes negative and then positive before returning to baseline. The difference in voltage between the mean *baseline* (B) and the *peak amplitude* at D is the *baseline-to-peak amplitude*. The voltage difference between D and E is the *peak-to-peak amplitude* of the first series of deflections. Similar latency and amplitude measures could also be used with the later, unlabeled peaks of the evoked potential.

The evoked potential in Figure 9–6 is a near-field recording. Yet it cannot be assumed that all components of the potential are attributable to neurons in the inferior colliculus. Some far-field contributions from large generators external to the colliculus may also be included. It is most important to realize that the evoked potential is the result of superposition of contributions from numerous equivalent dipoles. Recall that some neuronal configurations (e.g., random orientations) cannot be detected even by near-field electrodes, whereas neurons that lie parallel with each other and that are spatially extensive may be detected over considerable distances. Success in recording from a given source depends jointly on neuronal configuration, the orientation of the neurons (dipole orientation), and the magnitude of the voltage that the neurons generate. Furthermore, some multiple equivalent dipoles will cancel or partially cancel each other simply because they happen to be of opposing polarities. Finally, as the electrode location is changed, most of these factors will vary, with the result that the evoked potential will also vary in latency, magnitude, and waveform.

Electrode location may be changed by switching between electrodes or by physically moving the electrode. This latter case might occur in animal research or in human patients during invasive surgical procedures. Small changes in electrode position tend not to affect the far-field contributions to the evoked potential. The same changes in position, however, may produce marked changes in the contribution to the evoked potential from near-field generators. For example, at one location there may be neuronal activity representing a given tonotopic channel, whereas at an adjacent location the neurons may be associated with another channel and are not activated. Or the electrode may move across a subdivision boundary within the nucleus and thus encounter quite different neuronal response patterns. Both components and latencies may change with electrode location. Neural generators that make essentially no contribution at one electrode location can make a prominent contribution at another electrode location. None of these factors are directly related to the message the neurons are carrying. Furthermore, no series of deflections categorically is *the* evoked potential for the inferior colliculus. Figure 9–6 would, however, be a member of the set of evoked potentials obtained from the inferior colliculus.

Of what use, then, is the evoked potential if there is such uncertainty as to its meaning? The amount and type of information concerning auditory processing that the evoked potential can convey are limited. A vast volume of careful previous and ongoing research has delimited the contributions of the various recordable auditory evoked potentials, and numerous research and clinical applications have been developed. For humans, the most important usage in the field of hearing has been to obtain indications of central auditory activity from noninvasive scalp electrodes. The evoked potentials generated in the auditory system, with rare exception, cannot be seen in the scalp-recorded electroencephalogram. As is discussed in the next section, a special procedure involving several presentations of an acoustic stimulus (and hence repeated production of an evoked potential) and summation of the appropriate window of electroencephalographic (EEG) activity permits an auditory evoked potential to be seen, whereas otherwise it would be invisible.

EVOKED POTENTIAL AVERAGING

In practice, it may or may not be possible to record the evoked potential from the inferior colliculus by using a far-field electrode placement because of the various factors related to equivalent dipoles, as just described. In a more flexible approach to the situation, however, it is possible to obtain potentials from the auditory system by the process of *evoked potential averaging*. Whereas researchers may or may not succeed in recording inferior colliculus evoked potentials per se, they certainly will succeed in obtaining a large amount of auditory system activity, some of which may well include potentials from the inferior colliculus.

There is, however, a new factor of great importance in the far-field recording configuration. That factor, which is related to the spontaneous spikes described previously, is the normal ongoing EEG activity that exists throughout the brain. The EEG activity is large-amplitude electrical activity that must be considered disruptive noise in attempts to record auditory evoked potentials. Evoked potential averaging is the means to circumvent this noise.

In the mathematical operation of averaging, entries are summed, and the total is divided by the number of entries (N). Entries that are randomly sometimes positive and sometimes negative tend to sum to zero. Entries that are small but tend, for example, to be positive yield a small positive average. In evoked potential averaging there are two types of entries that, because of superposition, can be treated independently. First, there is large EEG activity that at any given time may be randomly positive or negative but that for large N tends to sum to zero. Second, there is the small, but consistently present, far-field evoked potential activity from the auditory system. This latter activity becomes visible during evoked potential averaging because of the reduction in the EEG noise that ordinarily obscures the evoked potential.

In evoked potential averaging, time is of critical importance. The auditory evoked potential is spread over a specific interval of time that immediately follows the acoustic stimulus; the auditory evoked potential is said to be time-locked to the stimulus. Thus if an interval of EEG activity that extends 10 milliseconds beyond each presentation of the acoustic stimulus is selected to be averaged, each of the entries contains a sample of large EEG activity plus a tiny contribution that is the evoked potential.

To actually compute the average evoked potential, the 10-millisecond window must be divided into a series of briefer time intervals, and whatever voltage appears in each of these time intervals must be averaged separately. Thus the 10-millisecond window may be broken into 200 time slots, which yield a 0.05-millisecond ($10/200 = 0.05$) temporal resolution of the averaged evoked potential. Each time the stimulus is presented, the next 10-millisecond window is divided into 200 time slots, and whatever voltage appears in each time slot is the entry for that slot. Thus the average evoked potential is, in this case, really 200 separate averages, each representing what happened at some specific time after the stimulus. These 200 averages, when plotted in sequence, form what appears to be a continuous line (if all calculations have been performed correctly), which is the averaged evoked potential.

The Auditory Brain Stem Response. With brief acoustic stimulation (such as a click) and a far-field recording configuration, what one records and averages is called the *auditory brain stem response* (ABR). (The term *brain stem electrical response* is also used.) For a given configuration of the active and reference electrodes, the ABR is the composite of the evoked potentials from all of the brain stem sources activated by acoustic stimuli. By consensus among the workers in the field, the ABR is considered to be complete within 10 milliseconds after presentation of a click stimulus. The ABR is widely used because it is easy to record from far-field electrodes and because it gives much useful information about the neural signals in the early stages of the auditory system. Because of the computerized averaging process, the effects of EEG noise are greatly reduced, and a waveform that is as uncluttered as that shown in Figure 9–6 is obtained. Accomplishing this, however, requires a moderately intense stimulus that is presented 1000 or 2000 times.

Because the EEG activity, which may be 25 μV in amplitude, is essentially random in relation to the presentation of the tone burst, the average of the EEG activity over many stimulus presentations (say, 1000) approaches, but does not equal, zero. The far-field evoked potential from the auditory system is quite small (0.1 to 0.5 μV) when measured at the scalp. Because the noise does not go to zero, the averaged far-field evoked potential is intrinsically not as accurate a description of the neural generator activity as the near-field potential. The non-invasive nature of the ABR recording process, however, overrides most other considerations.

Typically, the human ABR is recorded in a clinical setting for the purpose of objectively evaluating the ear and the brain stem portion of the auditory system. The active electrode is on the middle of the head (the vertex) and the reference electrode is on the mastoid or the earlobe of the ear that receives the acoustic stimulus. Usually clicks instead of tone bursts are used. The tones also produce evoked potentials, but because of the gradual rise used with tones, the latencies are different from latencies for clicks. Also, because of the tonotopic organization of the auditory system, the frequency of the tonal stimulus is important, and this introduces another dimension that is usually not welcome in a clinical situation. An example of a human ABR to a click stimulus is shown in Figure 9–7. The ABR consists of several surface positive waves labeled I to VII. The latencies and relative amplitudes of these waves have been studied extensively, as described in Chapter 10.

The concepts presented in the earlier sections of this chapter can be used to account in principle for the waveform shown in Figure 9–7. In Figure 9–2, imagine an active electrode positioned at the top of the figure (i.e., at the vertex) that will pick up the far-field potentials from equivalent dipole sources throughout the head. The neural activity induced by a click stimulus begins in cranial nerve VIII and progresses sequentially through the nuclei and pathways of the auditory system. The neural generators can be modeled by dipole arrays that are correspondingly turned on and off as the neural activity passes by. How well the vertex electrode can detect a given generator depends on the same factors described previously:

1. The pattern of neuronal-level activity and synaptic potentials in the generator: activity that occurs in a bunch is more visible than activity distributed over time, and an abundance of neural activity is more visible than a paucity of neural activity.

2. The physical extent of the neural generator: spatially larger generators are more visible.

3. The orientation of the neural generator with respect to the axis defined by the active and indifferent electrodes: a 90° difference in orientation can make the difference between electrically visible and electrically invisible.

4. The superposition of generator potentials: in the same manner that vectors can be added or subtracted, the generator potentials can add to or diminish each other.

5. The timing of the neural activity: the net result of superposition depends on how the neural activity is distributed in time.

It follows from these points that even minor differences in procedure such as location of the electrodes or parameters of the acoustic stimulus (e.g., rate of presentation of the clicks) can produce marked differences in the averaged evoked potentials recorded. Thus for effective use of the ABR in the clinic, clinicians must employ a rigorous set of procedures that exactly specifies all aspects of electrode positioning, stimulus parameters, gain and bandwidth settings on the amplifiers, computer operations used in averaging, the manner in which the data are to be analyzed, and the norms against which the results are to be compared.

At one time it was thought that each of the peaks in the ABR represented activity in a different nucleus; thus the inferior colliculus evoked potential would be one of the waves such as V. Unfortunately this view proved to be too simple. Activity in a given

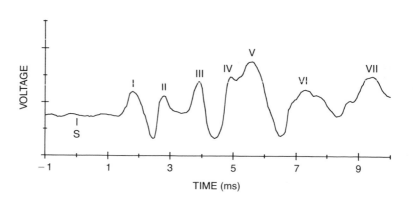

Figure 9–7. A human auditory brain stem response (ABR) recorded from vertex to the mastoid of the ear ipsilateral to the stimulus. The arrival of the stimulus, a click, at the tympanic membrane is indicated by S.

auditory nucleus does not occur in a brief burst after the arrival of an input volley. Rather, it occurs over an interval of time that, as a rule, is several times larger than the latency of the initial response of the nucleus. Furthermore, the activity in this interval does not form a single wave but instead must be represented as multiple waves (as in Fig. 9–6). Apparently this reflects the complex internal connections of the nucleus or even the arrival at the nucleus of neural volleys from several sources. A few multiple pathways are shown in Figure 9–2. The worst-case situation would be that the seven waves of the ABR may each be composed of activity from a number of nuclei in the auditory system, so that what looks like a real wave of the ABR (i.e., any of the seven waves) is simply a statistical accident.

In a more positive vein, waves I and II seem to be identified with auditory nerve activity. As cranial nerve VIII passes through its canal in the temporal bone, wave I apparently arises from the lateral side of the canal, whereas wave II arises from the medial side. Wave III is associated with the cochlear nucleus, and wave V has been attributed principally to the nuclei of the lateral lemniscus. Wave IV is presumably associated with structures between the cochlear nucleus and the nuclei of the lateral lemniscus. The remaining waves, VI and VII, may then represent the upper levels of the brain stem auditory system. These assignments of waves to nuclei do not at all negate previous concerns of overlapping waves and multiple sources. Through the extensive ongoing research on the ABR, the specific details of the origins of the waves are emerging, as are methods of extracting useful information from them.

Cortical Evoked Potentials. If the time base used to obtain the ABR is extended to 50 or even 500 milliseconds and the averaging process is carried out, a new series of positive and negative waves is obtained on the new time scale. On the longer time base, the ABR is compressed into insignificance, whereas new and slower waves dominate the average evoked potential. Waves in the 10- to 50-millisecond range are termed *middle-latency evoked potentials*. From 50 to 500 milliseconds they are termed *long-latency*, or *late*, *evoked potentials*. Collectively, these waveforms may also be termed the *auditory evoked potential* or the *auditory evoked response*. In obtaining the

middle- or long-latency potentials, attention must be paid to numerous recording technicalities, but no new principles are required to explain the results. The slower time scale, however, does permit observation of much slower or prolonged neural events than of those that constitute the ABR.

The middle-latency auditory evoked potential (also called *middle-latency response*) consists at the vertex primarily of a triphasic waveform composed of negative (Na), positive (Pa), and negative (Nb) peaks. The corresponding peak latencies are roughly 20, 30, and 40 milliseconds. Other preceding waves (No and Po) and following waves (Pb, Nc, and Pc) can sometimes be recorded as well. (The P and the N designations refer to positive and negative deflections, respectively.) The amplitude of the triphasic group is on the order of 1 to 2 μV, which makes the group easier to record than the ABR: fewer stimulus presentations are needed to extract an acceptable waveform from the EEG ongoing activity. On the other hand, there are some scalp muscles that twitch reflexively to moderately intense acoustic stimuli and that have response latencies in the same range as the middle-latency response. Thus interpretation of the average evoked potentials is sometimes difficult. The bulk of the evidence indicates that the middle-latency response originates in the auditory cortex in the vicinity of Heschl's gyrus, but some data indicate that other brain areas are responsible for these potentials. Although the interpretation may be somewhat uncertain, the middle-latency response can be used to measure audiometric threshold, test the integrity of the ascending system, and evaluate central auditory function.

The late evoked potentials consist of two sets of positive and negative waves, designated P1, N1, P2, and N2, that are spaced over the interval from approximately 60 to 220 milliseconds. These waves are typically recorded by means of a vertex electrode placement (with, of course, a second electrode located on the neck or lower side of the head). Although the ABR is a stable series of potentials that are relatively unaffected by attention, by sleep, and by many medications, the late potentials are extremely labile. The most extreme case is a still later potential, the P3 (or P300, so designated in recognition of its roughly 300-millisecond latency), that appears when an infrequent or an unexpected acoustic event occurs. In fact, the P300 can also occur in the *absence* of an expected acoustic event. The difficulty in accounting for a potential evoked by the absence of a stimulus has given rise to the more general term *event-related potentials*. The late components are still easier to record than the ABR or the middle-latency potentials because amplitudes may be up to 10 μV so that an acceptable waveform can be obtained after 25 to 50 stimulus presentations. In general, the subject's state of mind is a critical variable that affects the recording of the late potentials. Although this may be considered a disadvantage in that variability is increased, it is actually an advantage because these potentials provide a view of the operation of higher level mental processes.

The dipole model is effective in accounting for the cortical potentials evoked by acoustic stimuli. All of the factors given for the ABR are relevant to the understanding of cortical potentials as well. The cortex, however, is physically more extensive than the brain stem nuclei, and so the potentials generated tend to be larger and hence easier to record. Although cortical potentials can be obtained from simple stimuli such as clicks or tone bursts, these stimuli hardly engage the analytic mechanisms of the cortex. Hence with simple stimuli, cortical evoked potentials principally indicate no more than the presence of basic physiologic function in the areas in question. More complex stimuli are required to gather evidence of the higher level functions of cortex. It is in experiments with such stimuli that the term *event-related potentials* must be used to recognize the more complex conditions that give rise to these potentials.

The late evoked potentials are thought to arise from more than one generator because they are differentially affected by the subject's state (e.g., sleep), by drugs, and by brain lesions. Furthermore, visual or somesthetic stimuli as well as acoustic stimuli can give rise to a P300 potential, whereas this is not true for the P1-N2 components. Much work has been done to locate the generators of the late potentials, and it seems that some of them may not even be cortical potentials. It is hypothesized that cortical outflow has activated subcortical areas.

The large areas of the cortex devoted to audition are organized in the orderly manner typical of neocortex. However, the auditory cortex is buried in the lateral fissure, and it consists of multiple subdivisions innervated by multiple ascending pathways. On the basis of what has been said thus far, a complex series of evoked potentials might be expected from these subdivisions. On the other hand, these multiple potentials most likely cannot be separately resolved with scalp electrodes. Thus the middle and late evoked potentials recorded from the vertex are probably produced by a number of cortical generators. With the ABR, there is uncertainty as to which nuclei or tracts contribute to a given wave, but the brain stem auditory system is compact and well defined. With the middle and late potentials, the difficulties are compounded: the auditory portions of the cortex that contribute to evoked potentials are not well defined, there are numerous subdivisions of auditory cortex whose functions are at best poorly understood, the cortex is both extensive and convoluted, subcortical areas may participate as well, and there may be multisensory contributions to an evoked potential. This all suggests that a larger framework is needed for the presentation and analysis of middle and late potentials from the auditory system; a framework of this sort is provided by topographic mapping of event-related potentials.

TOPOGRAPHIC MAPPING

Computed tomography and magnetic resonance imaging have dramatically increased the ability to visualize the structural aspects of the central nervous system. Positron emission tomography scans of blood flow have shown that cortical areas differentially increase demand for blood in a manner that relates to the task that the subject is required to perform. Thus there is a difference in blood flow to the auditory cortex that depends on whether the subject is, for example, listening to speech or to music. This technique may ultimately help specify the functions of the numerous subdivisions of auditory cortex, although at present the relatively coarse resolution of the technique is a limiting factor.

Electrical Measures

Given the present technology, recordings can be made not from just several electrodes but from several dozen electrodes simultaneously. An array of, say, 30 electrodes can generate immense amounts of data in short order. In essence, one can observe over time the distribution of the EEG across the surface of the scalp, and this distribution forms a research area of its own. Through this method, the so-called noise of the EEG can be examined in temporal and spatial detail. As might be expected, the voltage obtained from a given electrode differs from the voltages at neighboring electrodes, although there is some correlation. Of relevance to this chapter, however, is the fact that average evoked potentials can be obtained from any and all of the electrodes in the array. Great care must be taken, however, to ensure that all recording amplifiers are functioning in exactly the same manner (e.g., same gain, same frequency response).

The approach thus far to evoked potentials has been to plot the potentials as a function of time while commenting on the changes that might be observed if a differently located recording electrode had been used. Now it is necessary to think in terms of spatial distributions as well. In the previous plots of voltage against time (Figs. 9–6 and 9–7), spatial location was held constant; that is, the data were obtained from one electrode. In a plot of voltage versus spatial location, time is held constant; that is, the plot describes the voltage distribution on the head at one instant in time.

Topographic mapping is one way of handling the large volumes of information that are produced by large arrays of electrodes. The familiar topographic map used by hikers describes the elevation of the land by a series of isoelevation contours. By locating oneself on the map, one can then decide whether the land rises or falls in any given direction. A topographic map of voltage of the scalp plots isovoltage contours at some given instant in time. If average evoked potentials or event-related potentials are recorded from large arrays of electrodes on the scalp, it is possible to compute the distribution of voltage contours on the head for any instant of time. This process is termed *topographic mapping*. Figure 9–8 shows a simple voltage distribution on the scalp that would result from a dipole within the brain. The positive end of the dipole would be closest to the top of the head and would be located in the right hemisphere. The contours in Figure 9–8 are extrapolations of the voltages between the electrodes. If greater spatial resolution is re-

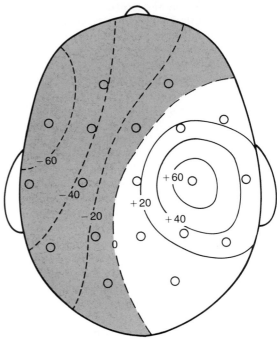

Figure 9–8. Topographic distribution of voltage across the scalp. This distribution represents one instant in time. More electrodes could be used to provide better spatial resolution.

quired, more electrodes would have to be used.

A variation on this theme relates the diagram in Figure 9–8 to evoked potentials. As a mental exercise, imagine a picture of a head with 30 average evoked potentials displayed on the scalp, each evoked potential being associated with one electrode. The amount of information in such a display is extremely large, and although differences among the evoked potentials may be obvious, there is the problem of organizing an approach to all this information. To continue with the exercise, take the voltage from each evoked potential that occurred at some specific time (e.g., 54.5 milliseconds) after the presentation of the stimulus. On the basis of these 30 voltages, draw isopotential contours like those in Figure 9–8. Using the equivalent dipole approach, one can analyze this plot to determine (or attempt to determine) the location of the neural generators. Mathematically, the problem is quite difficult.

This exercise in drawing isopotential contours was performed at one particular instant in time. Each instant after the stimulus gives rise to a related isopotential plot. If these successive plots were made into a motion picture, the spatial distribution of voltage across the scalp would be experienced as varying with time. Some commercially available topographic mapping equipment has sufficient computer capacity to present such a motion picture on its monitor. With the successive frames in this motion picture (played in slow motion), one can see the waxing and waning of voltage distributions moving across the scalp. It is a dynamic picture indeed.

The computerized display of isopotential contours is interesting and attractive, but, more important, the method permits intra-subject statistical comparisons between brain hemispheres and intersubject comparisons within hemispheres. Thus through existing data bases, an individual with a suspected neuropathologic disorder can be compared with normal persons. As a research tool, topographic mapping frequently permits useful estimates of the location of the neural sources underlying the potential maps.

Evoked Magnetic Fields

Any time an electrical current flows, a magnetic field (a magnetic dipole) is also produced. Superconducting detectors immersed in liquid helium are sensitive enough to detect the magnetic fields produced by the neural activity in the cerebral cortex. One magnetic detector is sufficient to obtain the magnetic equivalent of an average auditory evoked potential. Such evoked magnetic fields have properties that resemble electrical evoked potentials. As an example, the tonotopic organization of the auditory cortex in humans has been demonstrated with evoked magnetic fields.

The waveform of the average evoked magnetic field as a function of time resembles that obtained with electrical measures in that a series of increases and decreases in field strength are obtained. Magnetic fields, however, have one extremely important advantage. The electrical fields used in far-field recordings are distorted by conductivity differences between the brain and the skull or between intracellular fluid and myelin. The most serious distortion, however, is produced by the boundary between the scalp and air. Magnetic fields are unaffected by conductivity differences and thus may be used to locate active neural tissue with far more accuracy. The limitation of magnetic evoked responses is limited sensitivity. Under ordinary recording conditions, neural activity that occurs more than a few centimeters below the scalp cannot be detected. The use of heavily shielded rooms makes it possible to record brain stem magnetic activity, but successful recording by this method is still considered a tour de force.

With improvements in technology, the original single-detector systems were replaced by systems with 7 or 14 detectors. Systems with several dozen superconducting detectors have become available, and even larger systems are planned. Multiple detectors make possible the simultaneous recordings needed to produce topographic maps of magnetic field strength. These maps can be used to derive the equivalent magnetic dipoles associated with neural activity in the auditory system. The independence of the magnetic fields from the medium in which they originate is extremely important for deriving the magnetic dipoles. With magnetic fields, the mathematical calculations are merely extremely difficult as opposed to virtually impossible for electrical field calculations. In conjunction with other noninvasive measures, evoked magnetic fields offer fascinating possibilities for viewing the workings of the auditory system in the conscious human brain.

CONCLUSION

The purpose of this chapter was to survey the aspects of central auditory physiologic processes that are most relevant to clinically important aspects of hearing. The auditory system can be thought of as being organized on a number of levels. The discussion began with neurons (and portions of neurons) and progressed to near-field potentials obtained from aggregates of hundreds or thousands of neurons within nuclei or cortical subdivisions. Finally, the more global far-field and topographic measures were discussed.

With each change in level of analysis, there are also changes in the rules that govern the responses obtained. For example, the neuronal coding strategies at the neuron level cannot be used to derive in any simple manner the evoked potentials recorded with near-field electrodes. More parametric measures of synaptic potentials are needed to accomplish this task. Near-field evoked potentials are different from far-field potentials for reasons that are explainable in terms of equivalent dipoles, but the mathematical transforms are quite complex. Each of these measures has a place in research on audition from the extremely detailed neuronal level response to the global results obtained with topographic mapping. In addition to a role in research, the measures described provide the foundation for the interpretation of electrical and magnetic data obtained from the auditory system in a clinical setting. The development of the increasingly sophisticated, noninvasive indices of hearing is an ongoing process.

SUGGESTED READINGS

Aitkin L: The Auditory Midbrain. Clifton, NJ: Humana, 1986.

Duffy FH: Topographic Mapping of Brain Electrical Activity. Boston: Butterworth's, 1986.

Gevins AS, Rémond A (eds): Methods of Analysis of Brain Electrical and Magnetic Signals. Amsterdam: Elsevier, 1987.

Hood LJ, Berlin CI: Auditory Evoked Potentials. Austin, TX: Pro-Ed, 1986.

Kaas JH: The organization of neocortex in mammals: Implications for theories of brain function. Ann Rev Psychol 38:129–151, 1987.

Moller AR, Jannetta PJ: Comparison between intracranially recorded potentials from the human auditory nerve and scalp recorded auditory brainstem responses (ABR). Scand Audiol 11:33–40, 1982.

Moller AR, Jannetta PJ: Evoked potentials from the inferior colliculus in man. Electroenceph Clin Neurophysiol 53:612–620, 1982.

Moore EJ (ed): Bases of Auditory Brain-Stem Evoked Responses. New York: Grune & Stratton, 1983.

Musiek FE: Neuroanatomy, neurophysiology, and central auditory assessment. Part II: The cerebrum. Ear Hear 7:283–294, 1986.

Musiek FE: Neuroanatomy, neurophysiology, and central auditory assessment. Part III: Corpus callosum and efferent pathways. Ear Hear 7:349–358, 1986.

Pickles JO: An Introduction to the Physiology of Hearing. London: Academic Press, 1988.

Regan D: Human Brain Electrophysiology. New York: Elsevier, 1989.

Schlag J: Generation of brain evoked potentials. In Thompson RF, Patterson MM (eds): Bioelectric Recording Techniques. Part A (pp 273–316). New York: Academic Press, 1973.

Vaughan HG Jr, Weinberg H, Lehmann D, Okada Y: Approaches to defining the intracranial generators of event-related electrical and magnetic fields. In McCallum WC, Zappoli R, Denoth F (eds): Cerebral Psychophysiology: Studies in Event-Related Potentials (pp 505–544). New York: Elsevier, 1986.

Yost WA, Nielsen DW: Fundamentals of Hearing: An Introduction. New York: Holt, Rinehart & Winston, 1985.

CHAPTER 10

Auditory System Tests

Barbara Cone-Wesson, PhD

The practice of audiology encompasses the identification, diagnosis, description, and rehabilitation of hearing disorders. Hearing and its disorders are assayed by a combination of tests that are based on psychophysical and physiologic principles; the purpose of this chapter is to describe their clinical application and interpretation. A brief review of the physics of sound, sound measurement, and psychophysical principles is included at the outset of this chapter, which together with George M. Gerken's chapter on auditory physiology (Chapter 9) provides an orientation to the rationale and methods of clinical tests of hearing. Many important aspects of audiology are excluded from this chapter in order to maintain the focus on specific auditory tests. Pure-tone, speech audiometry, psychophysical site-of-lesion, acoustic immittance, auditory evoked potential, central auditory dysfunction, pseudohyperacusis, and pediatric and otoacoustic emission test procedures are reviewed.

Audiology textbooks and monographs in the suggested reading list offer exhaustive review of the history and development of auditory testing. The reader is encouraged to consult these sources for a historical perspective as well as an in-depth description of procedures.

SUMMARY OF HEARING SCIENCE AND PSYCHOACOUSTICS

Auditory tests are based on principles of hearing science and psychoacoustics. The following section introduces the basics of acoustics and perception relevant to clinical tests of audition. The discussion includes (1) mathematical formulas for describing sound waves; (2) the physical aspects of sound including frequency, level (amplitude), spectrum, and phase; and (3) the perceptual aspects of sound including pitch, loudness, tonality, adaptation, localization, and masking.

The Sound Wave

Frequency

A sound wave travels through air in a longitudinal fashion, and air molecules are alternatively *compressed* (pushed together) and *rarefacted* (drawn apart) by the wave motion. This can be visualized by considering the air particle movement that takes place as a result of a loudspeaker (or earphone diaphragm) movement (Fig. 10–1). If the movement of one air molecule is followed, it appears to oscillate back and forth about a point in space. This type of pendular motion, when plotted as a function of time, describes a *sinusoidal* wave. The interval that it takes for one particle to be compressed and rarefacted is the *period* of the sound. The number of cycles of motion completed in 1 second is the *frequency* of the signal. Frequency (in hertz, Hz) and period are related by the formula

$$Hz = 1/P,$$

where P is the period in seconds (Fig. 10–2). The distance between two successive rarefactions or condensations is the *wavelength* (λ). The relationship between frequency and wavelength is formulated as

$$\lambda = C/F,$$

where C equals the velocity of sound, or C equals 343 m/second in air at a temperature of 20°C.

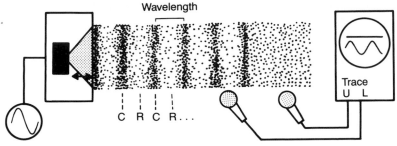

Figure 10–1. Propagation of a sound wave (an example of longitudinal propagation) generated via a speaker driven (electrically) by a sine wave generator. The sound pressure is being monitored by microphones connected to the upper (U) and lower (L) channels of a dual-trace oscilloscope. Peaks of condensation (C) and rarefaction (R) phases are indicated. (From Durrant JD, Lovrinic JH: Bases of Hearing Science, 2nd ed. Baltimore: Williams & Wilkins, 1986.)

Level (Amplitude)

Decibel. The level of sound can be measured as power (that is, how much work is done by sound), expressed in W/cm², or as pressure, expressed in dynes/cm², or pascals (Pa). The loudest tolerable sound is 10,000,000 times greater in amplitude than a signal that is barely detectable. A logarithmic scale is used to express this wide range. The decibel sound pressure level (db SPL) scale expresses sound level with reference to a *minimum audible pressure* of 2×10^{-5} Pa,

$$db\ SPL = 20 \times \log P_1/P_0,$$

where P_1 is sound pressure in Pa, and P_0 is the reference value 2×10^{-5} Pa.

Because the sound pressure of a sinusoidal signal is constantly changing, its level cannot be described at one instantaneous point in time. The level of a sinusoidal wave is expressed as the root mean square (RMS) of the peak-to-trough amplitude (Fig. 10–2), or

$$A_{RMS} = 0.354\ \text{peak-to-trough amplitude}$$

Phase

For a periodic signal (that is, a sound wave that repeats regularly, such as a sine wave), it is also possible to specify its phase. The phase is the portion of the cycle through which the periodic signal has advanced in relation to a fixed point in time. There are clinical auditory tests based on detectability

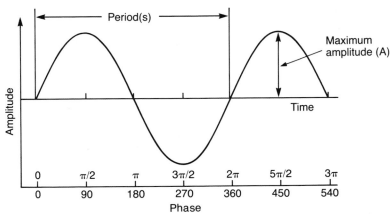

Figure 10–2. The waveform of a sine wave or sinusoidal vibration. Only 1.5 cycles are shown, although the waveform should be pictured as repeating indefinitely. The instantaneous amplitude is given by the expression $A \cdot \sin(2\pi ft)$, where t = time, f = frequency, and A = maximum amplitude. Phase is indicated along the bottom, where the first zero-crossing of the wave is used as a reference point. Phase may be measured in degrees or in radians. One complete cycle corresponds to 360° or 2π radians. (Redrawn from Moore BCJ: An Introduction to the Psychology of Hearing, 3rd ed. Orlando, FL: Academic Press, 1989.)

of phase differences that exist between the ears. Signal phase is also important for some electrophysiologic tests in which signal-onset phase influences test results.

Spectra: How to Describe Simple and Complex Sound Waves

Complex signals are those that have more than one frequency component. Most environmental sounds are complex signals, and speech is a prime example of a complex signal. Other complex signals used in auditory testing are narrow-band noise, white noise, warbled tones, frequency and amplitude modulated tones, tone bursts, and clicks. A sound wave can be analyzed to show its component frequencies and their amplitudes, a process known as *Fourier analysis* (Fig. 10–3). The spectrum of a complex signal is a graphic representation of each frequency component and its amplitudes. Spectra for various signals are shown in Figure 10–4. The *fundamental frequency* of a complex signal, F_0, is the component with the lowest frequency. The components of a spectrum that are integral multiples of F_0 are called *harmonics*.

Psychophysics

Psychophysics attempts to quantify perception. The perception of an acoustic signal is determined by its level, frequency, phase, and spectral complexity. Psychophysics tells us how the perception of threshold, pitch, loudness, adaptation, tonality, localization, and masking relate to the physical parameters of the signal. Clinical auditory tests involve the use of these psychophysical relationships.

The relationship between signal and response is often described by a *psychometric function*. Psychometric functions relate listener performance to sound dimension. For example, Figure 10–5 shows percentage signal detection plotted as a function of signal level. It illustrates that there is a range of levels over which the listener responds. The minimum signal detection level can be described by a point on the function—for example, the level at which the listener achieves 50% detectability. The 50% point is an arbitrary definition of minimum signal detectability; any value on the ordinate could be used as an operational definition of this listener's minimum signal detection level.

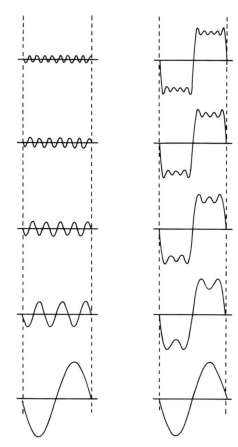

Figure 10–3. An example of how a complex waveform (a square wave) can be built up from a series of sinusoidal components. The square wave is composed of odd harmonics only, and the 1st, 3rd, 5th, 7th, and 9th harmonics are shown on the left. The series on the right shows progressive changes from a simple sine wave as each component is added. If enough additional harmonics, with appropriate amplitudes and phases, were added, the composite wave would approach a perfectly square shape. (Redrawn from Moore BCJ: An Introduction to the Psychology of Hearing, 3rd ed. Orlando, FL: Academic Press, 1989.)

Clinical auditory test findings, including *threshold*, are often best described by psychometric functions, and later sections of this chapter highlight their applications.

Threshold. The concept of threshold is basic to clinical auditory testing. Threshold is the minimal detectable level of a stimulus required for a response. *Absolute threshold* is the threshold for a signal in the absence of all other stimuli; but threshold is not "absolute" in the literal sense because it can vary with the measurement method, the listener's criteria for threshold, the listener's motivation, and even the instruments used to deliver the signal to the ear.

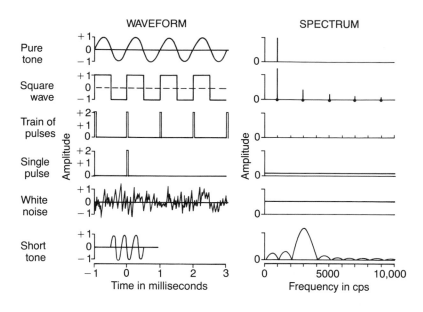

Figure 10–4. Left: the waveforms of some common auditory stimuli. Right: the corresponding spectra. The periodic stimuli (pure tone, square wave, and train of pulses) have line spectra, whereas the nonperiodic stimuli (single pulse, white noise, and short tone burst) have continuous spectra. (Redrawn from Moore BCJ: An Introduction to the Psychology of Hearing, 3rd ed. Orlando, FL: Academic Press, 1989.)

Psychophysicists use precise methods for determining threshold, and these methods have been adapted for clinical auditory testing. Three psychoacoustic methods for determining threshold are

1. *Method of limits:* The tester controls the stimulus, systematically increasing or decreasing one stimulus parameter (such as level). The listener reports when the stimulus is detected.

2. *Method of adjustment:* The listener controls the stimulus and varies it until the stimulus is detected.

3. *Method of constant stimuli:* The tester presents stimuli varied on a continuum (such as level) in random order. The listener responds to each trial: yes, stimulus detected; no, stimulus not detected.

Because the testing method affects threshold, it is important that test methods are standardized within and across clinics. The method of limits is used for clinical pure-tone threshold evaluation; a criterion of 50% detectability for four signal trials is common.

Sensitivity as a Function of Frequency. The ear is not equally sensitive at all frequencies. When sensitivity is measured as the least intense signal detectable, or threshold, the human ear is most sensitive in the range from 125 to 8000 Hz (Fig. 10–6), and this is the range of frequencies tested in the clinic. The graph of sensitivity as a function of frequency (with level in db SPL) is called the *minimum audible pressure* (MAP) curve (Fig. 10–6).

Pitch. Signal frequency is perceived as pitch. Pitch has been defined as "that attribute of auditory sensation in terms of which sound may be ordered on a musical scale" (American Standards Association, 1960). For a pure tone, the pitch corresponds to frequency; for a complex periodic sound, the pitch corresponds to F_0. Pitch judgments are influenced by other signal parameters such as signal level and duration. For example, for signals below 2000 Hz, pitch decreases with increasing level, and for signals above 4000 Hz, pitch increases with increasing level. Pitch judgments are also influenced by signal duration and the spectral complexity

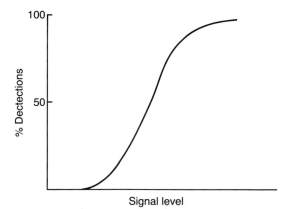

Figure 10–5. A typical psychometric function showing how the percentage of times a signal is detected varies with signal level. (Redrawn from Moore BCJ: An Introduction to the Psychology of Hearing, 3rd ed. Orlando, FL: Academic Press, 1989.)

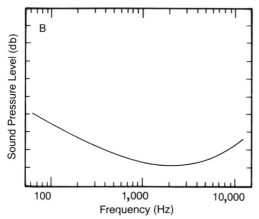

Figure 10–6. Minimum audible pressure (threshold) for normal adults is shown as a function of frequency. (From Humes L: Psychoacoustic foundations of clinical audiology. *In* Katz J [ed]: Handbook of Clinical Audiology, 3rd ed. Baltimore: Williams & Wilkins, 1985.)

of the signal. Clinical pitch-matching tests have been used to evaluate patients suffering from tinnitus. Pitch perception tests also may be used as part of test batteries for determining candidacy for cochlear implantation.

Loudness. The psychologic percept of sound level is loudness. A signal can be ordered on a scale from soft to loud, or alternatively, one signal can be compared with a standard for determination of a loudness judgment. Loudness judgments are used in clinical auditory testing for determining tolerance for amplification (hearing aids), for tinnitus evaluation, and for tests of recruitment.

Tonality (Timbre). The perceived tonality, or timbre, of a sound is dependent on its spectrum. The auditory system is, to some extent, able to detect individual components of a complex periodic signal. The relative magnitude of spectral components and their harmonic relationships influence perception of sound quality. In the clinic, patients are asked to make judgments of sound quality when, for example, evaluating the difference between hearing aids.

Adaptation. All sensory systems undergo adaptation to ongoing stimulation. *Adaptation* refers to a change in the perception of stimulus magnitude that takes place during stimulation or immediately after stimulation. Auditory adaptation takes place even for signals of low level and short duration. *Auditory fatigue* is not equivalent to adaptation, however; the term is used to refer to the change

in auditory sensation that occurs when high-level signals are used. Adaptation is discussed further in the site-of-lesion and acoustic immittance test sections.

Localization. The auditory system uses two cues for localizing sound in space: interaural time and level differences. Consider a sound source in the same plane as that of the two ears. Unless the sound source is directly in front of the head, or directly behind it, the sound first reaches the ear closer to the source, and it is more intense in comparison to the ear farther from the source. The auditory system is able to detect small differences in timing or level between the two ears. The auditory system uses interaural time differences for localization of low-frequency signals and interaural level differences for localization of high-frequency signals. Localization of sound in space is a crucial benefit of binaural hearing, although some localization can take place monaurally. Binaural cues are also used to discriminate speech in noise, and patients with unilateral hearing loss or other problems affecting binaural hearing often have difficulty with this type of discrimination.

Signals played through earphones are not localized to a point in space but, rather, *lateralized*, which means that the sound is perceived at a certain point (in the lateral plane) within the head. Interaural time differences and level differences have been exploited in clinical hearing tests such as the Stenger and the Masking Level Difference tests.

Masking. Masking is the amount (or process) by which the threshold for one sound is raised by the presence of another (masking) sound. Masking is used to study fundamental properties of hearing such as frequency and temporal resolution. Masking is also used to eliminate the possibility of response from the nontest ear when ear-specific tests are given. Although the mechanisms of masking are beyond the scope of this discussion, the general principle that presentation of one signal influences the response to another signal is crucial to the understanding of many auditory system tests.

PURE-TONE THRESHOLD TESTS

Pure-tone threshold tests describe a patient's hearing sensitivity for frequency. Sensitivity is the number of decibels above or below the minimum audible pressure (MAP) curve at which threshold is defined. The frequency range usually tested in the clinic is 125 to 8000 Hz, at octave (doubling of frequency) intervals.

Hearing impairment is defined by the number of decibels above the MAP curve needed to reach the patient's threshold and is measured as decibels hearing level (db HL). Minimum audible pressure has been determined for a large group of normal adult listeners and is the basis for audiometer calibration. Audiometer output (in db SPL) at 0 db HL varies as a function of frequency to correct for normal threshold differences on the MAP curve. The relationship between MAP and audiometric threshold is shown in Figure 10–7. Table 10–1 contains the American National Standards Institute (ANSI) db SPL values for audiometric 0 at each test frequency as delivered through a standard (TDH–39) earphone.

Procedure for Testing Threshold

The modified *Hughson-Westlake* procedure is recommended for clinical threshold tests. First, the patient is alerted to listen for a tone that is presented at a level above threshold. Subsequent test trials are presented at 20-db decrements until the patient no longer responds; then the level is increased in 5-db steps until another response is obtained. Thereafter, the signal is successively decreased 10 db for each signal detection and raised 5 db for each miss. Threshold is deter-

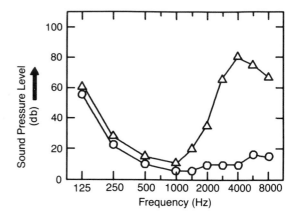

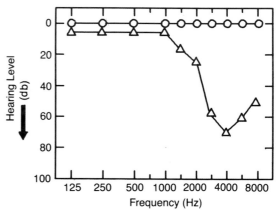

Figure 10–7. The relationship between the decibel hearing level (db HL) scale and the decibel sound pressure level (db SPL) scale of sound level is shown. *Upper panel:* circles indicate thresholds of normal hearing young adults; triangles indicate thresholds of an individual with high-frequency hearing loss. Increasing hearing loss is indicated by higher sound pressure levels at threshold. The difference between normal threshold at 4000 Hz (10 db SPL) and the patient's threshold (80 db SPL) is 70 db. *Lower panel:* data have been replotted on the db HL scale. Normal hearing threshold = 0 db HL at all frequencies. Increasing sound level is shown in a downward direction on the audiogram. Note that threshold for the hearing-impaired subject at 4000 Hz is 70 db HL. (From Bess FH, Humes LE: Audiology: The Fundamentals. Baltimore: Williams & Wilkins, 1990.)

TABLE 10–1. ANSI (1969) Standards for Audiometric Zero: Sound Pressure Level at the Earphone

When the Audiometer Dial Reads	And the Frequency Is	The Actual SPL* Is
0	125	45.0
0	250	25.5
0	500	11.5
0	1000	7.0
0	1500	6.5
0	2000	9.0
0	3000	10.0
0	4000	9.5
0	6000	15.5
0	8000	13.0

*Norms for TDH–39 earphones.
From Hodgson W: Basic Audiologic Evaluation, p. 23. Baltimore: Williams & Wilkins, 1980.

mined on the level-ascending trials and is the lowest level at which the patient responds for 50% of the trials.

The patient is given simple, clear instructions about the test, including an explanation of the signal and the desired response—for example, raising the hand or pushing a signal button. It is often necessary to emphasize that the patient must respond even when the signals are very faint.

Air Conduction Pure-Tone Thresholds

Signals for air conduction threshold tests are presented through supra-aural, circumaural, or insert phones (Fig. 10–8). Earphone placement for supra-aural phones may affect the results of pure-tone tests, especially for patients who have collapsing ear canals. Circumaural phones reduce the probability of ear canal collapse, and insert phones eliminate this problem. Insert phones also reduce the amount of low-frequency sound leakage that occurs when the earphone and the ear are not well coupled. Interaural attenuation is an important consideration in choice of earphones for audiometric tests. Interaural attenuation is the amount of attenuation created by the skull for a signal played in one ear, in relation to the contralateral ear. That is, the skull and its contents can be considered as "sound-proofing material" between the two ears, but signals of sufficient intensity to one ear will permeate ("cross over") the barrier and stimulate the opposite cochlea. Interaural attenuation of air-conducted signals is on the order of 70 db for insert phones, in comparison to 40 to 50 db for supra-aural or circumaural phones. Although insert phones offer clear advantages for air conduction testing, the use of supra-aural phones is widespread in clinical testing.

Masking of the nontest ear is essential when the possibility of "cross-over" hearing exists—that is, when the signal levels exceed the interaural attenuation. Masking noise must be presented to the nontest ear at levels that mask any signal that crosses over. Interaural attenuation ranges for air-conducted signals through supra-aural phones are shown in Table 10–2. Narrow-band noise signals are the most effective maskers for pure-tone threshold tests. The determination of the amount of masking to use must take into account the effectiveness of the masker (i.e., how much noise is required to mask a signal at a given level), the interaural attenuation for both the signal and the masker, the cochlear sensitivity of the nontest ear, and conductive loss for the nontest ear.

Bone Conduction Pure-Tone Thresholds

Pure-tone thresholds are also tested by use of bone conducted signals. Three simultaneous transmission routes for bone conduction must be considered in order to interpret the

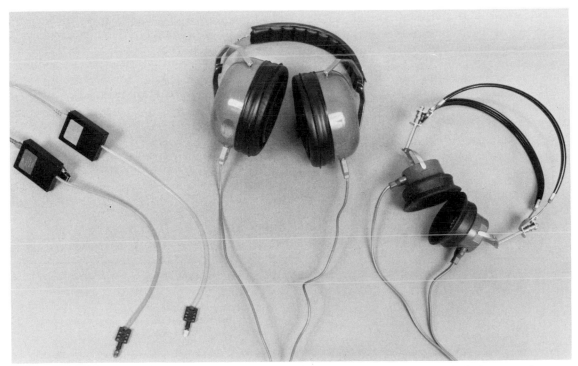

Figure 10–8. Earphones used for air conduction tests. *Left:* insert phones; *center:* circumaural phones; *right:* supra-aural phones.

TABLE 10–2. Range of Interaural Attenuation Values for Air-Conducted Signals

Study	Frequency (Hz)						
	125	*250*	*500*	*1000*	*2000*	*4000*	*8000*
Coles and Priede (1968)		50–80	45–80	40–80	45–75	50–85	
Liden et al. (1959)	40–75	45–75	50–70	45–70	45–75	45–75	45–80
Chaiklin (1967)	32–45	44–58	54–65	57–66	55–72	61–85	51–69

From Goldstein BA, Newman CW: Clinical masking: a decision making process. *In* Katz J (ed): Handbook of Clinical Audiology, 3rd ed. Baltimore: Williams & Wilkins, 1985.

test results. First, signals are transmitted through the skull through the *compression* mode: the skull is set into vibration by the bone conduction oscillator placed on either the mastoid prominence or the forehead. The bone conducted oscillation radiates to the cochlea, resulting in a neural response; that is, the basilar membrane displacement that causes hair cell stimulation is identical to that for air conducted signals. Second, signals may also be transmitted via the *inertial* mode of bone conduction. The vibration of the bone conduction oscillator against the skull causes the ossicles to vibrate. The ossicles vibrate out of phase with the temporal bone from which they are suspended because their mass is much less than that of the temporal bone. The difference in vibration between the ossicles (including stapes footplate) and temporal bone (including oval window) results in movement of the stapes footplate in and out of the oval window, thereby stimulating the cochlea. Third, the *osseous* (or *osseotympanic*) mode refers to the sound energy radiated to the ear canal by the vibration of the oscillator on the skull. The bone and cartilage surrounding the ear canal transmit this vibration to the standing air column in the external auditory meatus, which in turn causes tympanic membrane and ossicular vibration, resulting in cochlear stimulation.

Bone conduction through the compressional mode does not depend on middle ear integrity; however, it is not possible to isolate completely the external and middle ear from participating in bone conduction transmission. The thresholds determined by bone conduction are therefore a best estimate rather than a direct measurement of cochlear hearing sensitivity. Middle ear pathology can result in abnormal bone conduction thresholds, even when the cochlea is normal, because of disruption of the osseous and inertial bone conduction transmission modes.

Masking for the nontest ear is essential in bone conduction testing because the intra-aural attenuation for bone conducted signals is close to 0 db. The determination of effective masking levels for bone conduction testing follows the same principles as for air conduction testing.

Test Interpretation

Comparison of thresholds for air and bone conducted signals is the foundation of pure-tone test interpretation. First, the threshold levels are considered. The thresholds are described by a range of hearing levels from normal to profound hearing impairment (Fig. 10–9). There is some variability in the literature regarding the decibel range for each category. Despite the lack of consensus for each category, this scale helps to characterize the patient's hearing handicap for conversational speech. In addition, thresholds for 500, 1000, and 2000 Hz (sometimes 3000 Hz is included) are averaged for each ear to yield the pure-tone average that in most cases has a high correlation with the patient's threshold for speech signals. Conversion of threshold values to percentage scores is sometimes used (Table 10–3).

Air conduction thresholds are then compared with bone conduction levels. For patients with normal hearing, the air and bone conduction thresholds agree ±10 db, and all thresholds are in the normal range (0 to 25 db HL). Patients with conductive hearing

TABLE 10–3. Conversion of Pure-Tone Thresholds to "Percentage" of Hearing Impairment

Determine the pure-tone threshold average (PTA) for 500, 1000, 2000, and 3000 Hz for each ear, air conduction only
Subtract 25 db from the PTA
Multiply the result by 1.5% to find the percentage of hearing impairment for each ear
Multiply the smaller of the two percentages by 5
Add the percentage impairment for the poorer ear
Divide by 6 to find the combined "percentage of hearing handicap"

Figure 10–9. Classification of hearing impairment in relation to handicap for speech recognition. (From Bess FH, Humes LE: Audiology: The Fundamentals. Baltimore: Williams & Wilkins, 1990.)

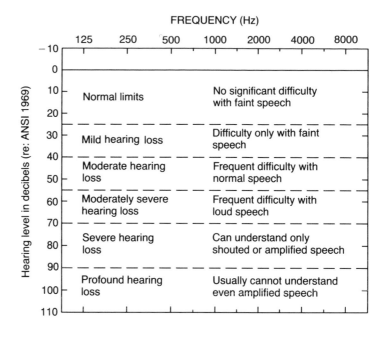

impairment have bone conduction thresholds that are within normal range and air conduction thresholds that are at least 10 db poorer than the air conduction thresholds. Sensorineural impairments result in abnormal thresholds for both air and bone conduction; however, the air and bone thresholds agree ±10 db. Finally, for mixed-type impairments, the bone conduction thresholds are poorer than normal, and air conduction thresholds are at least 10 db poorer than the bone conduction thresholds. The difference between air and bone conduction thresholds is sometimes referred to as the *air-bone gap*, and its size is used to indicate the extent of conductive impairment.

Conventions for Plotting Data

Certain conventions are used for audiogram construction and data presentation. The dimensions of the frequency versus threshold level grids are standardized; frequency is represented on a log scale, and amplitude is represented on a linear scale. The aspect ratio is one octave interval to 20 db on the ordinate scale of hearing level (Fig. 10–10). Symbols for unmasked, masked, and sound field thresholds are shown in Figure 10–10. Traditionally, right ear thresholds are plotted in red and left ear thresholds in blue. The use of separate audiograms for each ear results

in a clearer presentation of the data, particularly when unmasked and masked air and bone thresholds for each ear are plotted.

Pitfalls. Pure-tone threshold tests help define the site-of-lesion (conductive versus sensorineural), but in general, the audiogram does not define the etiology of the impairment. For example, otitis media can cause a conductive hearing impairment of mild to moderate degree, as can cholesteatoma or otosclerosis. Mass-increasing conductive pathologies reduce high-frequency transmission to the cochlea. Stiffness-increasing conductive pathologies decrease low-frequency transmission, and increased friction (resistance) attenuates transmission of all frequencies (Fig. 10–11). (The transmission of sound through the middle ear is determined by the principles of acoustic impedance that are addressed in the acoustic immittance section of this chapter.) For many middle ear disorders, mass, stiffness, and friction are concomitantly affected, and audiogram shape does not contribute to an understanding of the underlying disease. Similarly, an audiogram indicating high-frequency sensorineural impairment does not generally offer etiologic clues. When combined with case history and other audiometric and medical tests, however, the audiogram is a critical piece of the diagnostic puzzle.

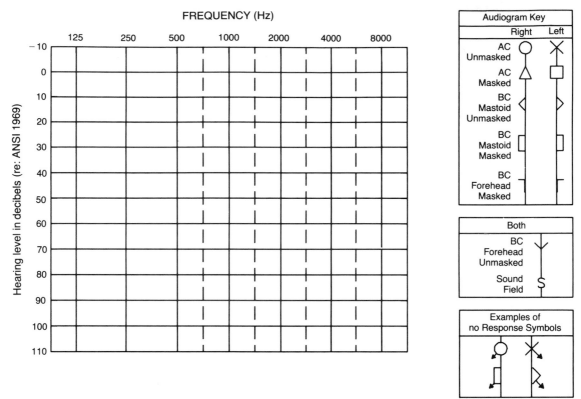

Figure 10–10. *Left:* audiogram used for plotting pure tone air and bone conduction threshold. *Right:* audiogram key displays the symbols commonly used on audiograms. AC, air conduction; BC, bone conduction. (From Bess FH, Humes LE: Audiology: The Fundamentals. Baltimore: Williams & Wilkins, 1990.)

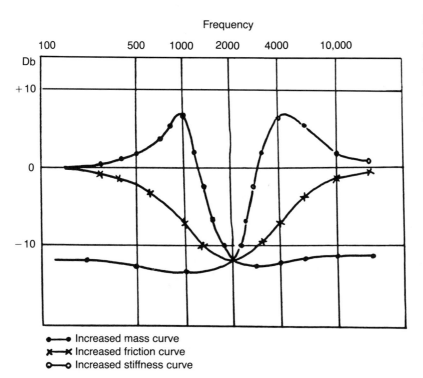

●—● Increased mass curve
✗—✗ Increased friction curve
○—○ Increased stiffness curve

Figure 10–11. Graphic display of expected audiometric patterns in conductive pathologies by their influence on middle ear impedance. Note that increased mass affects high-frequency transmission; increased stiffness impairs transmission of low frequencies, and increased friction affects transmission of all frequencies. (From Shambaugh GE: Surgery of the Ear, 2nd ed. Philadelphia: WB Saunders, 1967.)

Ultra-High Frequency Audiometry

The conventional pure-tone threshold test is given for frequencies in the 125 to 8000 Hz range. Pure-tone threshold testing above 8000 Hz offers special benefits and challenges. The major benefit is that cochlear pathology, resulting from ototoxicity or noise trauma for instance, may first be evident in threshold changes above 8000 Hz. A clinical test for the ultra-high frequency thresholds would be more sensitive to this pathology, thereby increasing the probability of early detection and treatment. The major problem for ultra-high frequency pure-tone tests is signal calibration. The length of the ear canal is greater than the wavelength of signals above 8000 Hz. Standing waves may be present in the ear canal when signals of exceedingly short wavelength (ultra-high frequencies) are used. Standing waves can reverberate and be additive or cancel one another, depending on the dimensions of the canal. Definition of the minimum audible pressure (at the eardrum) is quite variable from subject to subject; an audiometer calibration standard for frequencies above 8000 Hz is not yet available. The standard audiometric earphone, furthermore, is not suitable for testing at frequencies above 8000 Hz. Although earphones capable of transducing frequencies above 8000 Hz are commercially available, it is necessary for each testing facility to develop normative data.

Automatic Tests: Békésy Audiometry

It is possible to test pure-tone thresholds with use of a method of adjustment so that the patient has control over signal level. The procedure, called automatic or Békésy audiometry (after Georg von Békésy, a Nobel Prize–winning scientist in audition), utilizes an instrument that sweeps through the 125 to 8000 Hz frequency range at a rate of one octave per minute. The attenuator is controlled by the patient, who is instructed to depress a switch while the signal is audible and to release it when the signal is inaudible. The depressed switch increases signal attenuation, and switch release raises the level. The patient's threshold is traced automatically by a plotter controlled by the attenuator switch.

Békésy audiometry declined in popularity in recent years. Pure-tone tests given manually are more rapid and yield reliable threshold values, and so there is no advantage to automatic audiometry procedures for finding thresholds.

Pure-Tone Threshold Tests—Summary

The threshold of hearing plotted as a function of frequency, the audiogram, is a simple and elegant tool for defining auditory sensitivity or impairment. Many diagnostic and rehabilitative decisions can be based on the audiogram. Pure-tone air and bone conduction threshold data define conductive versus sensorineural loss and indicate the degree of impairment. At the very least, the audiogram aids in determining the need for other diagnostic tests.

SPEECH AUDIOMETRY

Hearing-impaired persons often describe their problem in terms of difficulty understanding speech. The patient's deficit for perceiving and understanding speech must be described in order to proceed with treatment or rehabilitation. Speech audiometry can help to quantify this problem.

There are two basic tests in the *speech audiometry battery*, the speech recognition threshold (traditionally called the *speech reception threshold*, SRT) and the word recognition test (also called the *speech discrimination test*, SDT). The speech recognition threshold defines the lowest level at which a patient can recognize a spoken word. The word recognition test measures the *accuracy* of word recognition for speech presented at suprathreshold levels. Materials and procedures for each test have been standardized.

Speech Recognition Threshold

To measure the SRT, the patient is first familiarized with a list of test items. *Spondaic* words, two-syllable words with equal stress on both syllables (Table 10–4), are used for defining SRT. The words are presented through a microphone-attenuator circuit of the audiometer (monitored live voice), or, preferably, recorded stimuli (tape or compact disk format) can be used. The patient is instructed to repeat the words as they are heard. The lowest signal level at which 50% of the words are correctly repeated is the

TABLE 10–4. CID Auditory Test W–1, List A

1. greyhound	10. duckpond	19. baseball	28. oatmeal
2. schoolboy	11. sidewalk	20. stairway	29. toothbrush
3. inkwell	12. hotdog	21. cowboy	30. farewell
4. whitewash	13. padlock	22. iceberg	31. grandson
5. pancake	14. mushroom	23. northwest	32. drawbridge
6. mousetrap	15. eardrum	24. railroad	33. doormat
7. eardrum	16. workshop	25. playground	34. hothouse
8. headlight	17. horseshoe	26. airplane	35. daybreak
9. birthday	18. armchair	27. woodwork	36. sunset

speech recognition threshold. The SRT and the pure-tone average (PTA) should be nearly equal (± 7 db), and discrepancies between the two measures suggest that the patient should be reinstructed and re-evaluated for both tests. The SRT may be considered the minimum sound level required by the patient for hearing and understanding speech.

Word Recognition Test

Estimates of a patient's ability to hear speech clearly are made on the basis of word recognition tests. The test items are chosen to evaluate the patient's ability to recognize speech sounds typical in normal conversation. The most widely used tests are composed of "phonemically balanced" words—that is, word lists constructed to contain speech sounds (phonemes) in relatively equal proportion to that found in a corpus of familiar words. The phonemic balancing is supposed to ensure that the word list is comparable to the speech sounds in normal conversation. The words are familiar, are monosyllabic, and have a consonant-vowel-consonant structure (Table 10–5). There are normally 50 items per list. The most commonly used word lists are the CID W–22, NU–6, Maryland–50, and PAL–50.

The percentage of words correctly recognized as a function of sensation level differs for subjects with normal hearing or conductive, sensorineural, and retrocochlear impairments. Psychometric functions relating word recognition score and signal level for these groups of patients are shown in Figure 10–12. (These functions are sometimes referred to as *PI-PB functions*, the performance versus intensity function for phonetically balanced words.) Patients with sensorineural or retrocochlear disorders have scores that are lower than those for normal-hearing or conductively impaired patients, even when signal

TABLE 10–5. NU–6 Word Lists

List 1A	List 2A	List 3A	List 4A
1. laud	1. pick	1. base	1. pass
2. boat	2. room	2. mess	2. doll
3. pool	3. nice	3. cause	3. back
4. nag	4. said	4. mop	4. red
5. limb	5. fail	5. good	5. wash
6. shout	6. south	6. luck	6. sour
7. sub	7. white	7. walk	7. bone
8. vine	8. keep	8. youth	8. get
9. dime	9. dead	9. pain	9. wheat
10. goose	10. loaf	10. date	10. thumb
11. whip	11. dab	11. pearl	11. sail
12. tough	12. numb	12. search	12. yearn
13. puff	13. juice	13. ditch	13. wife
14. keen	14. chief	14. talk	14. such
15. death	15. merge	15. ring	15. neat
16. sell	16. wag	16. germ	16. peg
17. take	17. rain	17. life	17. mob
18. fall	18. witch	18. team	18. gas
19. raise	19. soap	19. lid	19. check
20. third	20. young	20. pole	20. join
21. gap	21. ton	21. road	21. lease
22. fat	22. keg	22. shall	22. long
23. met	23. calm	23. late	23. chain
24. jar	24. tool	24. cheek	24. kill
25. door	25. pike	25. beg	25. hole
26. love	26. mill	26. gun	26. lean
27. sure	27. hush	27. jug	27. tape
28. knock	28. shack	28. sheep	28. tire
29. choice	29. read	29. five	29. dip
30. hash	30. rot	30. rush	30. rose
31. lot	31. hate	31. rat	31. came
32. raid	32. live	32. void	32. fit
33. hurl	33. book	33. wire	33. make
34. moon	34. voice	34. half	34. vote
35. page	35. gaze	35. note	35. judge
36. yes	36. pad	36. when	36. food
37. reach	37. thought	37. name	37. ripe
38. king	38. bought	38. thin	38. have
39. home	39. turn	39. tell	39. rough
40. rag	40. chair	40. bar	40. kick
41. which	41. lore	41. mouse	41. lose
42. week	42. bite	42. hire	42. near
43. size	43. haze	43. cab	43. perch
44. mode	44. match	44. hit	44. shirt
45. bean	45. learn	45. chat	45. bath
46. tip	46. shawl	46. phone	46. time
47. chalk	47. deep	47. soup	47. hall
48. jail	48. gin	48. dodge	48. mood
49. burn	49. goal	49. seize	49. dog
50. kite	50. far	50. cool	50. should

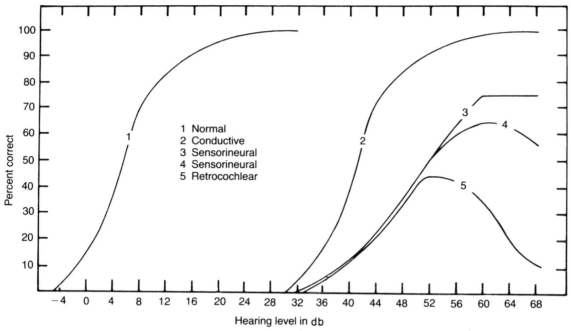

Figure 10–12. Illustrative examples of performance-intensity functions seen with normal hearing, conductive hearing losses, sensorineural impairments and retrocochlear lesions. (From Bess FH: Basic hearing measurement. *In* Lass NJ, McReynolds LV, Northern JL, Yoder D [eds]: Handbook of Speech-Language Pathology and Audiology. Philadelphia: BC Decker, 1988.)

presentation levels are markedly increased. Also, patients with retrocochlear disorders may show poorer recognition scores as signal level is increased. This finding, known as *roll-over*, describes the shape of the psychometric function in this case (Fig. 10–12).

Test items for word recognition tests are presented via monitored live voice or, preferably, with a recorded format, and the patient is asked to repeat the words as they are heard. Signal presentation level (SL) is usually based on the patient's SRT or pure-tone average; 25 db SL above SRT (i.e., SRT + 25 db) is used initially. The percentage of words correctly repeated is measured. If the score is less than 92%, the signal level is increased by 15 db, and another trial (of 50 words) is given. This procedure is repeated until a score of 92% is obtained, or until the patient's loudness tolerance is reached. The highest score achieved (PB-Max) and minimum score (PB-Min) can be used for calculating the roll-over ratio:

$$\text{Roll-over ratio} = (\text{PB-Max} - \text{PB-Min})/\text{PB-Max}.$$

Word recognition scores are used to characterize the patient's hearing handicap for speech understanding. A PB-Max score of 88% or better is considered good or normal, 72% to 86% is fair, and below 72% is poor. Roll-over ratios have been used for site-of-lesion determination; ratios of 0.45 or greater are associated with neural rather than cochlear impairment. The PI-PB function is also used for fitting hearing aids and other amplification devices.

Other Word Recognition Tests

The California Consonant Test (CCT), the Speech Perception in Noise (SPIN) test, and the Synthetic Sentence Identification (SSI) test are also tests of word recognition. Each test has a strategy somewhat different from the standard phonetically balanced word tests just described.

The CCT is a multiple-choice test of consonant recognition. The CCT is more difficult a test than is the NU–6; however, it also appears to differentiate more patients with word recognition problems. The SPIN test evaluates recognition abilities as a function of background noise and is also designed to evaluate the role of phonemic or contextual cues. The results of the test indicate how well the patient can recognize words in or out of linguistic context, with or without competing noise. This test simulates more accurately the challenge of the hearing-impaired listener in everyday life.

The SSI test items are "synthetic sentences"; these sentences do not make sense semantically, but they follow syntactic rules for construction (e.g., "Forward march said the boy had a"; "Small boat with a picture has become"). The patient's task is to identify the sentence, as it is spoken, from a written list of 10 alternative items. A competing message (a speaker reading a passage from a book) is presented simultaneously with the test items. SSI has been used to show differences in performance as a function of hearing loss type or to show an individual's difference in performance with different hearing aids.

Pitfalls. The ability to hear and understand conversational speech is very different from the ability to hear and understand single words presented in a quiet environment. Even tests with competing noise may not adequately characterize the handicap that the patient experiences outside the audiometric test booth. Thus the traditional word recognition tests do not predict hearing handicap and only grossly estimate the difficulties the hearing-impaired patient may have in realistic listening situations. The number of items that must be presented to show statistically significant differences in performance (e.g., when the patient is tested with different hearing aids) is large; therefore, the tests can be time consuming. Tests with competing messages or noise are also somewhat more difficult for the patient to perform, and motivation may wane, compromising validity and reliability.

Most Comfortable Listening Level; Uncomfortable Listening Level

Speech signals are often used to determine the most comfortable listening level (MCL) and the uncomfortable listening level (ULL), or the loudness discomfort level (LDL). The MCL is the signal level that the patient judges to be most comfortable for listening to conversational speech. The ULL is the signal level that is judged to be intolerable to the patient.

Test Interpretation. The MCL and the ULL help to determine the patient's dynamic range of hearing, which in turn can be used to aid in differential diagnosis or to plan rehabilitation. A reduced dynamic range— that is, small differences (in decibels) between the patient's threshold, MCL, and ULL—suggests a recruiting type of hearing loss and cochlear disease (see next section for an explanation of recruitment). This finding also indicates that the patient should use amplification designed to compensate for a limited dynamic range.

Pitfalls. Intrasubject variability limits the diagnostic use of these measures. Similarly, test reliability is limited as a result of nonstandardized test methods. Conversion of MCL and ULL levels to values for the electroacoustic specifications of hearing aids is fraught with problems in calibration. Despite this fuzziness, many audiologists determine MCL and ULL levels as part of a hearing aid evaluation.

SITE-OF-LESION TESTS

Several tests, developed in the 1950s before the widespread use of computed tomographic scans, magnetic resonance imaging, and electrophysiologic assessment, have been used to distinguish between sensorineural and retrocochlear impairment. Two underlying principles determine test method. First, the impaired cochlea demonstrates *loudness recruitment*; second, the impaired eighth nerve demonstrates *abnormal adaptation*.

Recruitment. According to the classic definition, recruitment is an abnormally rapid growth of loudness with an increase in level. Loudness growth is tested by comparing the loudness of suprathreshold signals between an impaired ear and an unimpaired ear. Figure 10–13 illustrates loudness growth functions by a plot of equal loudness (loudness balance) as a function of hearing level. The illustration demonstrates that loudness sensation for the impaired ear *at suprathreshold levels* is equal to that of the unimpaired ear. It is only the *reduced dynamic range* between threshold and the perceived loudness of a suprathreshold signal that is abnormal.

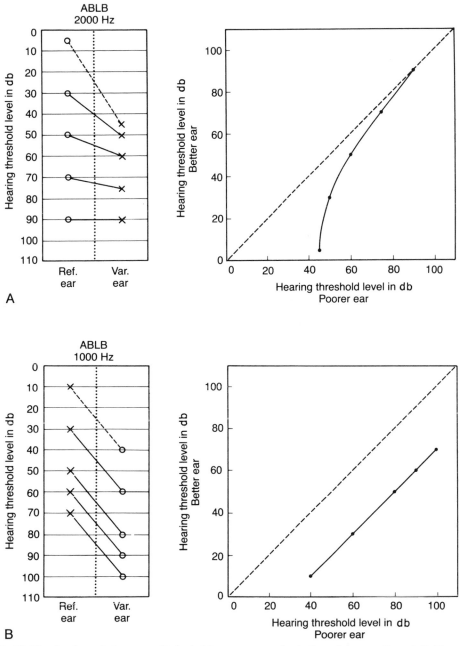

Figure 10–13. Plotting loudness balance results by laddergram or graph. *A.* Complete recruitment. *B.* No recruitment. (From Brent ME: Bekesy audiometry and loudness balance testing. *In* Katz J [ed]: Handbook of Clinical Audiology, 3rd ed. Baltimore: Williams & Wilkins, 1985.)

The sensation of loudness balance between the ears is reached at equal sensation levels (an equal number of decibels above threshold) for the normal ear, for a nonrecruiting ear, or for a conductive hearing impairment. An example of this is illustrated in Figure 10–13A. The left ear threshold at 1000 Hz is 10 db HL; the right ear threshold is 40 db HL. A signal presented at 100 db HL (100 − 40 = 60 db SL) to the right ear is judged to be as equally loud as a 70 db HL (70 − 10 = 60 db SL) signal to the left ear. On the other hand, an equal loudness judgment with a *decreased sensation level* to the impaired ear indicates abnormal loudness growth and cochlear dysfunction. In the example in Figure 10–13B, a signal presented to the impaired ear at 45 db SL is judged to be as equally loud as a signal at 85 db SL for the normal ear. Loudness balance test results are interpreted by use of three categories:

1. *No recruitment:* equal loudness achieved at *equal sensation levels* (±10 db) (Fig. 10–12A).
2. *Total recruitment:* equal loudness achieved at *equal hearing threshold levels* (±10 db) (Fig. 10–12B).
3. *Partial recruitment:* equal loudness achieved at sensation levels between those for no recruitment and total recruitment (Fig. 10–12C).

Loudness Balance Tests. Recruitment is a symptom of cochlear pathology associated with hair cell damage, particularly to outer hair cells. Loudness balance tests can be given to evaluate this phenomenon. Loudness balance can be compared between the two ears by use of the normal ear as a reference (*alternate binaural loudness balance test,* ABLB). Alternatively, comparisons can be made between two different frequencies for one ear if one frequency lies in the range of normal hearing (*monaural bifrequency loudness balance,* MBLB).

Pitfalls. Loudness balance tests cannot be used for every hearing-impaired patient because the constraint of normal hearing for one ear (for ABLB) or one frequency (for MBLB) is not met. Some patients, moreover, have difficulty performing reliable loudness balances, requiring tedious training trials in order to yield valid measures. The use of loudness balance tests to distinguish between cochlear and cranial nerve VIII lesions has been eclipsed by imaging and electrophysiologic techniques. The measurement of recruitment, however, may provide useful information about the patient's dynamic hearing range, which in turn can guide amplification strategies.

Abnormal Adaptation

Adaptation, the change in sensation that results from prolonged stimulation, is a normal phenomenon in all sensory systems. The impaired ear, however, may show abnormal or pathologic adaptation. Abnormal metabolic processes in the cochlea or auditory nerve may result in a very rapid decrease in the neural response and lead to a significant decrease or change in sensation. Although some adaptation may be evident with cochlear impairment, tests of adaptation, or *tone decay,* are used to differentiate retrocochlear from cochlear lesions.

Adaptation is tested with relatively simple procedures. The patient is asked to listen for a pure tone and to indicate when the tone fades away or changes in loudness. A puretone signal is presented at 5 db SL, and a timer is activated. The length of time (in seconds) between tone onset and the patient's report of adaptation is measured. If no adaptation is reported within 60 seconds, the test is normal. If adaptation takes place within 60 seconds, the signal level is raised 5 db, and the timer is reset. This procedure is repeated until a signal level is reached at which the patient has no measurable adaptation within a 60-second interval.

Test Interpretation and Pitfalls. Adaptation in the 5- to 20-db SL range is consistent with cochlear impairment. Adaptation that exceeds 20 db SL is associated with neural or retrocochlear impairment. The test is easily and quickly administered and requires no special instrumentation beyond that of a pure-tone audiometer and a watch. However, another test of adaptation, the acoustic reflex decay test, can be used in its place with more accuracy. The acoustic reflex decay test relies not on the patient's perception of adaptation but rather on an electrophysiologic correlate of adaptation. The tone decay test may still be applicable, especially for patients with middle ear disease or cochlear lesion, which precludes the measurement of the acoustic reflex.

Békésy Audiometry Revisited

A description of Békésy audiometry was provided in the pure-tone test section. Békésy threshold traces may indicate abnormal adaptation when thresholds for a continuous tone are compared with those for a pulsed signal. Also, abnormal adaptation may be evident when comfortable listening levels, rather than thresholds, are traced. Békésy audiometry, traditionally part of the audiometric site-of-lesion test battery, has fallen into disuse with the introduction of electrophysiologic tests. Tests of acoustic reflex threshold and acoustic reflex decay and the auditory brain stem response have higher sensitivity and specificity for retrocochlear lesions. Still, Békésy audiometry may be useful for testing patients with losses too severe to be assessed by electrophysiologic methods. Békésy audiometry may also be used for indicating pseudohypacusis, which is considered later in this chapter.

Summary

Recruitment is an indicator of cochlear disorder, whereas adaptation is an indicator of cranial nerve VIII disorder. These signs can be detected and quantified by using tests that rely on the patient's perception. The combination of word recognition, loudness balance, tone decay, and Békésy audiometry test results (the so-called site-of-lesion battery) has dubious efficacy for delineation of cranial nerve VIII disorders from cochlear disorders. These psychophysical site-of-lesion tests, however, retain limited usefulness when electrophysiologic tests are not feasible. Also, the results from the classic test battery may be used to describe and characterize abnormal perception that may not be evident from electrophysiologic tests.

ACOUSTIC IMMITTANCE MEASURES

The external ear and middle ear are a remarkable sound transmission system. The external and middle ear provide "tuning" for the signal reaching the cochlea. The middle ear is an impedance-matching device for the airborne sound wave that must be transmitted to the fluid medium of the cochlea. Sound transmission through the middle ear system can be measured indirectly. Opposition to the flow of sound energy through the middle ear is called *acoustic impedance;* reciprocally, the amount of acoustic energy transfer is called *acoustic admittance;* the measurement of these properties is called, generically, *acoustic immittance.* External and middle ear disease can change the sound transmission properties, as can contraction of the stapedius muscle and changes in external or middle ear pressure. Aural acoustic immittance measurements are made to characterize the effect of pathology or stapedius muscle contraction on the middle ear transmission system.

Introduction to the Physical Principles of Acoustic Immittance

Sound transmission through the external and middle ear is determined by its physical properties. Acoustic impedance is the opposition to the flow of sound energy and is dependent on the friction, elasticity, and mass of the middle ear system. Acoustic admittance, the reciprocal of acoustic impedance, is measured by commercially available acoustic immittance instruments. Formulas describing impedance and admittance and their components, summarized as follows, are helpful in predicting the effect of disease on middle ear sound transmission.

Impedance is the ratio of force and velocity needed to produce energy transfer:

$$\text{impedance} = \text{force/velocity; or}$$
$$Z = F/V.$$

Acoustic impedance can be determined by measuring the sound pressure level of a pure tone in an enclosed volume of air:

$$\text{acoustic impedance} = \text{pressure/volume velocity; or}$$
$$Z_a = P/V_v.$$

Acoustic admittance is the reciprocal of acoustic impedance; it follows that

$$\text{acoustic admittance} = \text{volume velocity/pressure; or}$$
$$Y_a = V_v/P.$$

Resistance (friction), mass, and stiffness (elasticity) combine to impede the flow of energy. These properties are related to impedance by the formula

$$/Z/ = (R^2 + X^2)^{1/2},$$

where R^2 is resistance and X^2 is reactance. The reactance term X^2 is defined as

$$(X_m - X_c)^2,$$

where X_m is mass reactance and X_c is stiffness reactance; and

$$X_m = 2\pi FM,$$
$$X_c = C/2\pi F,$$

where F is frequency, M is mass, and C is stiffness (elasticity).

Similarly, total admittance is determined by the same physical properties of the system. Admittance due to friction is called *conductance (G)*, and mass and elasticity properties contribute *mass susceptance (B_m)*, and *compliant susceptance (B_c)*. These properties are related to admittance by the formula

$$/Y/ = (G^2 + B^2)^{1/2},$$

where G^2 is conductance and B^2 is total susceptance. The susceptance term, B^2, is defined as

$$(B_c + B_m)^2,$$

where B_m is compliant susceptance and B_c is mass susceptance; and

$$B_m = -S^2/2\pi FM,$$
$$B_c = 2\pi FCS^2,$$

where F is frequency, M is mass, C is compliance, and S is the surface on which sound pressure acts.

Resistance is the loss of energy (converted to heat) due to friction. A major source of resistance to acoustic energy is encountered at the tympanic membrane and also at the oval window, the site at which mechanical energy (ossicular vibration) is transformed into hydraulic energy. *Conductance*, the reciprocal of resistance, determines the energy transfer that takes place through elements that provide friction.

Reactance is the storage of energy due to stiffness and mass characteristics. In a stiffness-dominated system, energy is stored rather than returned to the system. Conversely, systems with elasticity store less energy and transfer more energy. The tympanic membrane, ossicular joints, and air of the middle ear cavity all contribute to the stiffness of the conductive mechanism. Energy flow is also affected by mass and its inertia. The mass opposes the flow of energy. The mass of the conductive mechanism is determined by the tympanic membrane, ossicles, mucosa, middle ear muscles and ligaments, and middle ear space.

From the formulas given, it can be seen that reactance has two components, *stiffness reactance* and *mass reactance*. Stiffness reactance varies inversely with the frequency, and mass reactance varies directly with frequency. Stiffness-increasing middle ear lesions result in decreased low-frequency sound transmission, and mass-increasing lesions result in decreased high-frequency sound transmission. The so-called stiffness tilt and mass tilt effects on the pure-tone audiogram are shown in Figure 10–11.

Susceptance is the analog of reactance in the admittance equation. Similarly, total susceptance is composed of *compliant susceptance* and *mass susceptance*. Compliant and mass susceptance are frequency dependent; compliant susceptance varies directly with frequency, and mass susceptance varies inversely with frequency. Thus compliance-reducing middle ear lesions result in decreased low-frequency sound transmission, and mass-increasing lesions result in decreased high-frequency sound transmission (Fig. 10–11).

The formulas assume that resistance, stiffness reactance, and mass reactance can be described as independent of one another, or as pure elements. This is not the case, however, and the phase relationship of the force (sinusoidal pressure wave) and the flow of energy needs to be considered. In a resistance-dominated system, the pressure and the flow are in phase. In a stiffness-dominated system, the flow (energy transfer) is 90° out of phase with the pressure; the flow leads in phase. In a mass-dominated system, the pressure and flow are out of phase; the pressure wave leads the flow of energy by 90°. Because of the phase relationships, impedance is the vector sum of resistance and total reactance; admittance is the vector sum of conductance and susceptance (Fig. 10–14). The phase angle between conductance and total admittance determines the flow of energy in relation to the pressure wave that varies with the compliant and mass susceptance components. When the phase angle is 0, or when the susceptance term is 0, the system is said to be at resonance and is completely conductance dominated.

A summary of immittance terms and units is found in Table 10–6.

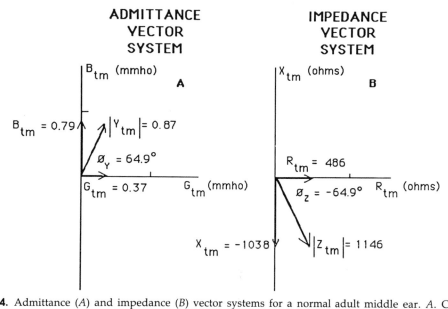

Figure 10–14. Admittance (*A*) and impedance (*B*) vector systems for a normal adult middle ear. *A*. Compensated conductance (G_{tm}) and susceptance (B_{tm}) vectors and the resultant compensated admittance magnitude (Y_{tm}) vector at a normal phase angle (O_y) of 64.9°. *B*. Compensated acoustic resistance (R_{tm}) and reactance (X_{tm}) vectors and the resultant compensated impedance magnitude (Z_{tm}) vector at a normal phase angle (O_z) of −64.9°. (From Margolis RH, Shanks J: Tympanometry: basic principles. *In* WF Rintelmann [ed]: Hearing Assessment, 2nd ed. Austin, TX: Pro-Ed, 1991.)

TABLE 10–6. Terminology for Acoustic Immittance Measurements

Factor	Acoustic Impedance (Z_a) Term, Unit	Acoustic Admittance (Y_a) Term, Unit
Resistance	Acoustic resistance R_a, 10^8 Pa·s/m³ acoustic ohm	Acoustic conductance G_a, 10^{-8} m³/Pa·s acoustic mmho
Reactance	Acoustic reactance X_a, 10^8 Pa·s/m³ acoustic ohm	Acoustic susceptance B_a, 10^{-8} m³/Pa·s acoustic mmho
Stiffness/compliance	Acoustic stiffness K_a, Pa/m³	Acoustic compliance C_a, m³/Pa
Mass	Acoustic mass M_a, Pa·s²/m³	
Volume	Acoustic equivalent volume V_{ea}, m³ or cm³	
Pressure	Pressure Pa or mm H₂O	

Immittance Measurement Principles

A schematic diagram of an immittance-measuring device is shown in Figure 10–15. The probe, hermetically sealed in the ear canal, provides

1. A pure-tone signal of known level directly in the plane of the tympanic membrane (loudspeaker component).
2. Measurement of the signal reflected back from the plane of the tympanic membrane (microphone-analysis component).
3. Variation of pressure in the ear canal and against the tympanic membrane (air pump–manometer component).

The unit of admittance is the *acoustic millimho* (mmho), although acoustic admittance of an equivalent volume of air, in cubic centimeters (cm³) is also frequently used and is popularly although inaccurately referred to as compliance. This measurement is based on the inverse relationship between sound pressure level and cavity size. If the sound source and the sound pressure level within a cavity are known, then the admittance of the cavity can be determined. The analogy for admittance measurements is that the probe tone is a constant sound source in a cavity created between the probe tip and the tympanic membrane. The microphone measures the sound pressure level in that cavity. The sound pressure is converted into an admittance value. For conditions of very high tympanic membrane or middle ear stiffness, very little sound is admitted into this system, and the sound pressure level is thereby raised in the cavity: a small admittance value will be measured. For conditions of high elasticity, such as tympanic neomembrane or ossicular discontinuity, the amount of sound admitted is large. The sound pressure level

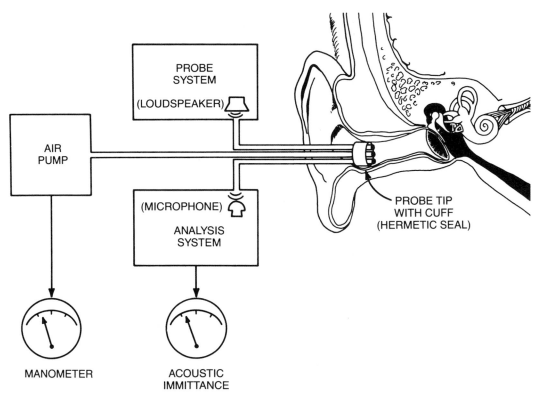

Figure 10–15. Block diagram of an electroacoustic immittance instrument and its coupling. The instrument is coupled to the ear by a probe tip, hermetically sealed in the ear canal by a soft rubber cuff. Probe tip openings are connected to three basic instrument subsystems. The air pump opening is used to introduce air pressure changes in the ear canal. The probe system opening connects the loudspeaker to the ear canal for presentation of probe tones or acoustic reflex-activating signals or both. The analysis system microphone opening allows ear canal sound pressure level monitoring. Acoustic immittance at the tympanic membrane is proportional to the sound pressure level of the probe tone developed in the ear canal. (From Wiley TL, Block MG: Overview and basic principles of acoustic immittance measurements. *In* Katz J [ed]: Handbook of Clinical Audiology, 3rd ed. Baltimore: Williams & Wilkins, 1985.)

in the cavity is low, and a large admittance value is the result. Thus the term *high compliance* is used to describe a system with large admittance values, and *low compliance* describes a very stiff system with small admittance values.

The frequency of the probe tone is a crucial variable for immittance measurements. Probe frequencies at 220 to 226 Hz are well below the resonance frequency of the middle ear, and measurements made at this frequency result in an adequate description of a stiffness-dominated system. Middle ear pathologies can shift the resonance peak of the ear, and higher probe frequencies (i.e., 678 Hz or 1000 Hz) are more sensitive to many abnormalities. The probe frequency must be specified when acoustic immittance measurements are made.

Static Immittance and Tympanometry

Middle ear pathology results in abnormal immittance that can be measured at ambient or atmospheric pressure or under various conditions of applied pressure. *Static acoustic immittance* is the immittance quantity at a specified probe frequency and ear canal pressure (usually a pressure that produces maximum admittance), corrected for the ear canal volume. The range of normal values is shown in Table 10–7.

Tympanometry is the measurement of immittance as a function of applied pressure. The pressure is usually varied over a range of 400 to −400 daPa by the air pump–manometer component of the immittance probe. The findings are plotted as a pressure versus immittance function. Applied pressure causes an increase in the stiffness of the tympanic membrane–middle ear system; thus the immittance varies as a function of applied pressure. Three tympanometric parameters can be quantified: the pressure point at which maximum immittance is found, the peak-compensated immittance (immittance measured at the peak immittance point and corrected for ear canal volume), and the shape of the applied pressure-immittance function. These parameters are used to indicate normal versus abnormal functions, from which diagnostic inferences are made.

Test Interpretation. The normal tympanogram (used with a 220-Hz probe) is distinguished by an immittance peak that falls within ±50 daPa of 0 daPa applied pressure, a peak-compensated immittance that is within the range of normal values, and an essentially symmetric shape around the pressure peak (Fig. 10–16).

Many types of abnormal tympanograms exist, and classification systems for abnormal findings are presented in Figure 10–16. Rather than reliance on a classification system, consideration of tympanometric parameters can be used to indicate the type of abnormality, at least when a single probe tone and single component system are used. In general, pathologic conditions that increase stiffness will reduce overall admittance (acoustic impedance), and the tympanogram shape becomes flatter, with no discernible peak. Pathologic conditions that cause increased elasticity will result in increased admittance with one or more peaks seen in the tympanogram. Changes in middle ear pressure will displace the tympanogram peak, and admittance may also be reduced.

When multiple components of immittance are measured, results may be classified according to the number of extrema (peaks and valleys) that appear in the admittance, susceptance, and conductance tympanograms. A single peak for both the conductance and susceptance tympanograms (1B1G) indicates that reactance is greater than resistance; this is found in normal ears when low-frequency probe tones are used (Fig. 10–17). More complex patterns exist (Fig. 10–17), and the relationship between conductance and susceptance components as a function of probe tone frequency can be determined. This, in

TABLE 10–7. Normal (90% range) 226-Hz Admittance (Y) and Impedance (Z) Values for Two Age Groups and Two Rates of Ear Canal Pressure Change

| Group | | Rate of Pressure Change | | | |
| | | ≤50 daPa/s | | 200 daPa/s | |
		Y	Z	Y	Z
Children	Lower limit	0.35	1100	0.40	970
(3–5 years)	Median	0.53	1900	0.63	1600
	Upper limit	0.90	2900	1.03	2500
	Lower limit	0.50	570	0.57	500
Adults	Median	0.91	1100	1.08	925
	Upper limit	1.75	2000	2.00	1750

From Shanks J, Lilly DJ, Margolis RH, et al: Tympanometry. J Speech Hear Disord 53:354–377, 1988.

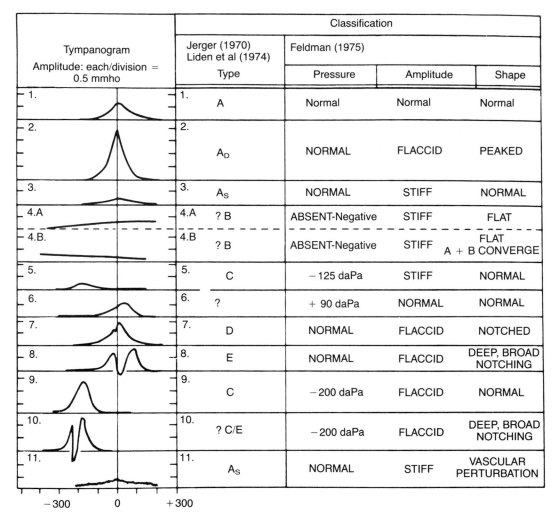

		Classification			
Tympanogram Amplitude: each/division = 0.5 mmho	Jerger (1970) Liden et al (1974) Type	Feldman (1975)			
		Pressure	Amplitude	Shape	
1.	1. A	Normal	Normal	Normal	
2.	2. A_D	NORMAL	FLACCID	PEAKED	
3.	3. A_S	NORMAL	STIFF	NORMAL	
4.A	4.A ? B	ABSENT-Negative	STIFF	FLAT	
4.B.	4.B ? B	ABSENT-Negative	STIFF	FLAT A + B CONVERGE	
5.	5. C	− 125 daPa	STIFF	NORMAL	
6.	6. ?	+ 90 daPa	NORMAL	NORMAL	
7.	7. D	NORMAL	FLACCID	NOTCHED	
8.	8. E	NORMAL	FLACCID	DEEP, BROAD NOTCHING	
9.	9. C	− 200 daPa	FLACCID	NORMAL	
10.	10. ? C/E	− 200 daPa	FLACCID	DEEP, BROAD NOTCHING	
11.	11. A_S	NORMAL	STIFF	VASCULAR PERTURBATION	

−300   0   +300

Pressure (daPa)

Figure 10–16. Tympanogram classification schema. (From Margolis RH, Shanks JE: Tympanometry: basic principles and clinical applications. *In* Katz J [ed]: Handbook of Clinical Audiology, 3rd ed. Baltimore: Williams & Wilkins, 1985.)

turn, offers a more complete description of the effect of middle ear disease on sound transmission. Although clinical use of multicomponent, multiprobe tone tympanometry is not yet widespread, instruments for this are commercially available.

Pitfalls. Static immittance has, in the past, been cited as a weak indicator of middle ear disease. This critique is based on early investigations that showed low correspondence between static immittance values and middle ear pathology. These studies are flawed because they failed to measure immittance in absolute physical units or to consistently compensate for ear canal volume. Although

there is a wide range of normal compensated static immittance values and some overlap with values from pathologic middle ears, compensated static immittance (in physical units) is often helpful in the differential diagnosis of middle ear pathologies.

Procedural variables for tympanometry, including choice of probe tones, immittance components, rate of pressure change, and even the number of consecutive pressure sweeps, can influence test findings. Although tympanometry is very sensitive to tympanic membrane and middle ear pathology, differential diagnosis cannot be based on tympanometric findings alone. Otoscopic and pure-tone threshold data should be con-

Figure 10–17. Four examples (1B1G, 3B1G, 3B3G, 5B3G) of normal tympanogram patterns recorded by using a 660-Hz probe tone. *A.* Relationship between reactance (X) and resistance (R): *B.* Susceptance (B) tympanogram. *C.* Conductance (G) tympanogram. *D.* Admittance (Y) and phase-angle (θ) tympanograms. (From Osguthorpe JD: Effects of tympanic membrane scars on tympanometry: a study in cats. Laryngoscope 96:1366–1377, 1986.)

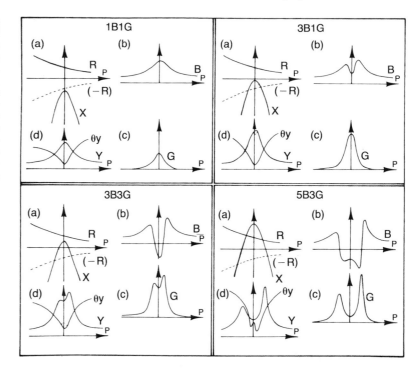

Acoustic Reflex Tests

A stapedius muscle contraction can be elicited with auditory stimulation as well as by other motor maneuvers, such as phonation or chewing. The stapedius muscle contraction changes the transmission properties of the middle ear. Low-frequency signals are attenuated in comparison to high-frequency sounds; that is, signals are high-pass filtered as a result of stapedius muscle contraction.

The neural pathway for stapedius muscle contraction is shown in Figure 10–18, which illustrates the essential feature of bilateral innervation. When the stapedius muscle contracts, the stapes footplate is rocked laterally from the oval window, the ossicular chain is stiffened, and the tympanic membrane may move outward, inward, or diphasically. The stapedius contraction alters transmission properties of the middle ear with a resultant change in acoustic immittance. The stapedius muscle contraction is monitored by observation of acoustic immittance with acoustic stimulus presentation. The abrupt change in immittance in conjunction with the eliciting signal is the basis of clinical acoustic reflex

considered in conjunction with acoustic immittance findings.

ACOUSTIC-REFLEX ARC

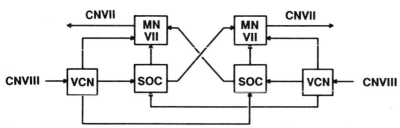

Figure 10–18. A schematic of the acoustic reflex arc. The arc involves input through cranial nerve VIII to the ventral cochlear nucleus (VCN) from which there are neural pathways through the two superior olivary complexes (SOC) to the motor nuclei of cranial nerve VII (motor nerve VII) that innervates the stapedius muscle. (From Wilson RH, Margolis RH Acoustic reflex measurements. *In* Rintelman WF [ed]: Hearing Assessment. 2nd ed. Austin, TX: Pro-Ed, 1991.)

tests, which include determination of acoustic reflex threshold and acoustic reflex decay (adaptation).

Acoustic Reflex Threshold

The threshold, amplitude, and latency of the acoustic reflex can be measured; however, acoustic reflex threshold (ART) as a function of frequency has the most widespread use. The threshold of the acoustic reflex is the lowest stimulus level that produces a detectable change in baseline immittance. Threshold is dependent on the method used for measurement. Most instruments provide some sort of visual display, such as video display, immittance meter needle deflection, or pen movement on a hard-copy plotter. For activator signals in the 250 to 4000 Hz range and an immittance probe frequency of 220 to 226 Hz, the mean ART in normal ears is 80 to 90 db HL, with an upper limit of normal at 95 db HL for 250 to 2000 Hz, and 95 to 105 db HL for 4000 Hz. Figure 10–19 shows the acoustic reflex at threshold and the growth of the acoustic reflex as a function of signal level.

Test Interpretation and Pitfalls. The ART may be altered by a lesion at any level of the afferent pathway, including the external ear, middle ear, cochlea, cranial nerve VIII, and brain stem pathways. The ART must be considered in terms of the type and degree of hearing loss present for the stimulus ear. Conductive hearing losses produce ART elevation that is directly related to the attenuation produced by the conductive lesion. For cochlear lesions, the relationship is more complex (Fig. 10–20). ART levels remain normal for impairments of 40 db or less. The ART level increases at a rate of 0.38 db for each decibel of hearing loss at hearing loss levels above 40 db HL. The incidence of absent reflexes for losses in the 70 db HL to 100 db HL range increases from 40% to over 80%.

The ART profile in patients with cranial nerve VIII disorders is different still from the conductive and cochlear profiles. Even small hearing losses, of 10 db or less, result in a high percentage of absent reflexes (Fig. 10–21). Of patients with retrocochlear losses of 60 db HL or more, 80% have an absence of acoustic reflexes.

Disorders of the efferent portion of the acoustic reflex, including the facial nerve, the stapedius muscle, and the middle ear, result in abnormal test results for the probe ear—that is, the ear in which the acoustic immit-

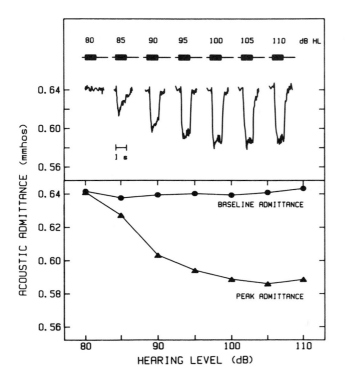

Figure 10–19. *Top:* acoustic reflex responses (in acoustic mmhos) monitored with a 226-Hz probe and corrected for ear canal volume; activator signal was a 1000-Hz tone presented at 80 to 110 db HL for 1 second, with a 5-second interstimulus interval. *Bottom:* acoustic-reflex growth function; baseline admittance (circles) represents the acoustic admittance of the middle 100 milliseconds before presentation of the activator signal (Y_{tm}), and peak admittance (triangles) represents the acoustic admittance during the last 500 milliseconds of the activator signal (Y_r). (From Wilson RH, Margolis RH: Acoustic reflex measurements. *In* Rintelmann WF [ed]: Hearing Assessment, 2nd ed. Austin, TX: Pro-Ed, 1991.)

Figure 10–20. *Top*: mean acoustic reflex thresholds (in db SPL) for 500-, 1000-, and 2000-Hz activators as a function of mean hearing level at 500, 1000, and 2000 Hz (355 ears). Solid line represents a best-fit, third-degree polynomial. *Bottom*: mean acoustic reflex thresholds (in db SPL) for broadband noise activator as a function of mean hearing level at 500, 1000, and 2000 Hz (355 ears). Solid line represents a best-fit, third-degree polynomial. (From Popelka GR: The acoustic reflex in normal and pathologic ears. *In* Popelka GR [ed]: Hearing Assessment With the Acoustic Reflex. New York: Grune & Stratton, 1981, as illustrated by Wilson and Margolis, 1991.)

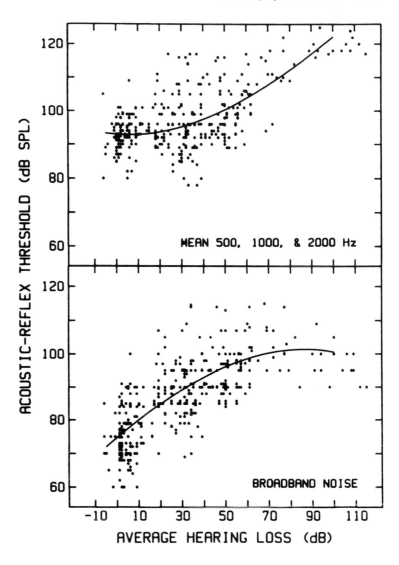

Figure 10–21. The percentage of absent acoustic reflexes in the ear to which reflex-activator signal is presented as a function of hearing threshold (db HL). Dashed line, patients with cranial nerve VIII hearing loss; solid line, conductive hearing loss; dotted line, cochlear hearing loss. (From Jerger J, Clemis J, Harford E, Alford B: The acoustic reflex in eighth nerve disorders. Arch Otolaryngol 99:409–413, 1974.)

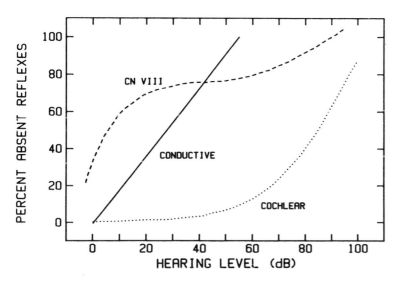

tance change is monitored. Facial nerve lesions such as Bell's palsy result in absent reflexes when the site-of-lesion is proximal to the branching of the stapedius nerve from cranial nerve VII. Middle ear abnormality precludes measurement of acoustic reflexes. For example, otitis media or ossicular discontinuity alters the middle ear transmission characteristics so profoundly that a stapedius contraction does not result in a measurable change in acoustic immittance.

Hearing Loss Prediction. Acoustic reflex thresholds have been used to estimate hearing loss, or at least the presence of an impairment. It has been suggested that the ART is linearly related to the area of excitation on the basilar membrane produced by the reflex activator. Thus comparison of reflex thresholds for high-pass, low-pass, and broad-band noise, as well as for pure tones, can contribute to the prediction of hearing impairment. The variability in the relationship between hearing loss and ART is evident from Figure 10–20, and this is a limiting factor for predicting the amount or degree of hearing loss. The classification of patients into impaired and unimpaired groups, however, is possible when ARTs for tones and noise are considered.

Acoustic Reflex Adaptation

A sustained signal of sufficient level activates a sustained stapedial contraction. The acoustic reflex in response to a continuous signal is measured by observation of the immittance change at signal onset and during continuous stimulation. Relaxation of the stapedial contraction will result in immittance change back to the prestimulus state. Relaxation of acoustic reflex during sustained stimulation is the result of adaptation and is called *acoustic reflex adaptation,* or *acoustic reflex decay.*

Normal Findings. Because adaptation is a characteristic of all sensory systems, it is not surprising that adaptation can be measured by monitoring the acoustic reflex. The amount and rate of adaptation is related to the signal frequency and level. The amount of adaptation is determined by observing the percentage of change in reflex amplitude during the sustained activation (Fig. 10–22). The rate of adaptation can be measured by dividing the percentage change over the signal duration. The 50% adaptation point occurs at well over 10 seconds for 500- and 1000-Hz signals at levels of 10 db above ART. For 2000- and 4000-Hz signals at levels of ART + 10 db, the 50% adaptation point may be reached within 1 second. Clinical acoustic reflex decay tests employ 500- and 1000-Hz activators at levels of ART + 10 db, with a duration of 10 seconds.

Abnormal Findings. Patients with cranial nerve VIII lesions demonstrate a high rate of adaptation in comparison to normal findings. When reflex amplitude declines 50% or more

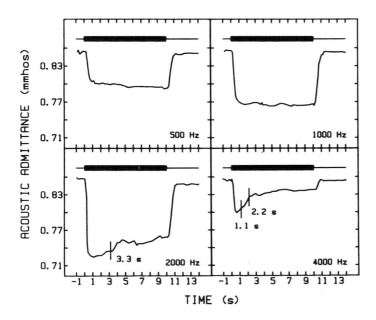

Figure 10–22. Acoustic-reflex adaptation functions elicited from a young adult with normal hearing; 500-, 1000-, 2000-, and 4000-Hz activator signals presented for 10.2 seconds, 10 db above acoustic reflex threshold. (From Wilson RH, Margolis RH: Acoustic reflex measurements. *In* Rintelmann WF [ed]: Hearing Assessment, 2nd ed. Austin, TX: Pro-Ed, 1991.)

within 5 seconds for 500- and 1000-Hz stimuli, the results are positive for retrocochlear disease. Reflex adaptation as a function of type of hearing loss is shown in Figure 10–23. This illustration shows that some patients with cochlear lesions demonstrate adaptation, but the patient with cranial nerve VIII lesion has much more pronounced adaptation. Reflex adaptation appears to decrease with increased signal level for patients with cochlear lesions, whereas it increases with increased signal levels for patients with cranial nerve VIII disorders.

Pitfalls of Acoustic Reflex Tests. The choice of acoustic immittance probe signal (i.e., 220 versus 660 Hz) can influence acoustic reflex threshold results. A 220-Hz probe is typically used, but for the young infant or the neonate, a higher frequency probe tone is needed for accurately detecting an acoustic reflex. The acoustic reflex measurement system is sensitive to artifact from movement of the probe, movement of the tympanic membrane, and interaction between the probe and acoustic reflex–activating signal. The determination of acoustic reflex threshold or adaptation is made from visual detection of immittance changes. Differences in measurement procedures can lead to increased variability in test results. A number of patients cannot be tested with these procedures because the presence of middle ear pathology, although mild, can preclude acoustic reflex measurements.

AUDITORY EVOKED POTENTIALS

Auditory evoked potentials, changes in nervous system electrical activity resulting from stimulation, have an important role in clinical auditory testing. Auditory evoked potential tests yield results from which hearing thresh-

Figure 10–23. Acoustic reflex adaptation from three subject groups; squares, normal hearing; circles, Meniere's disease; triangles, cranial nerve VIII disorders. There were 15 subjects in each group. *Top:* 500-Hz reflex-activator signal; *bottom:* 1000-Hz activator signal. (From Cartwright WR, Lilly DJ: A comparison of acoustic-reflex decay patterns for patients with cochlear and VIIIth-nerve disease. ASHA 18:678, 1976.)

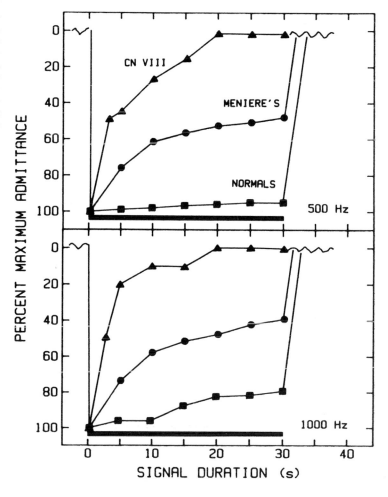

olds can be estimated; cochlear, retrocochlear, and higher brain lesions can be delineated; and cognitive brain processes can be described. The physiology and signal-averaging principles of auditory evoked potentials have been reviewed in Chapter 9. The purpose of the discussion that follows is to describe their clinical application.

Electrocochleography

Electrocochleography (ECochG) is the recording of bioelectrical responses of the cochlea and cranial nerve VIII by means of an electrode placed as close as possible to the cochlea. A transtympanic electrode may be placed on the promontory near the round window, but noninvasive methods of recording, such as recording electrodes placed in the external auditory meatus close to the tympanic membrane or on the tympanic membrane itself, have become more prevalent. ECochG is frequently performed simultaneously with auditory brain stem response recordings (ABR). This is because ECochG yields better definition of summating potential (SP) and cranial nerve VIII action potential (AP) than is evident in ABR recordings, whereas the ABR is crucial for defining auditory pathway integrity above the level of cranial nerve VIII.

Figure 10–24 shows an ECochG recording with each component labeled. *Latency*, the

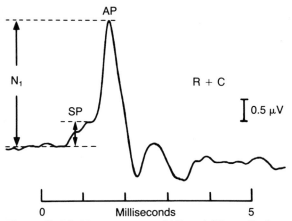

Figure 10–24. Measurements of N1 and SP amplitudes used for clinical assessment of presence or absence of SP enlargement. Waveform shown is sum of responses to rarefaction (R) and condensation (C) clicks presented at 115 db SPL at a rate of 8/second. Both the AP-N1 peak amplitude and the SP amplitude are measured from the prestimulus baseline. (From Coats AC: Electrocochleography: recording techniques and clinical applications. *In* Seminars in Hearing, vol 7, no. 3. New York: Thieme Medical Publishers, 1986. Reprinted by permission.)

time interval (in milliseconds) between signal onset and a resulting component, and *amplitude*, the peak-to-trough size (in microvolts), are the standard response parameters measured. The AP–N1 response latency varies from 1.5 milliseconds for high-level signals to over 3 milliseconds for near-threshold responses. Response amplitude has high intrasubject variability, but ranges from a few tenths of a microvolt up to 4 μV are seen.

The testing strategy for ECochG includes measurement of AP latency and amplitude as a function of signal level. The latency-level and amplitude-level functions are used to estimate threshold and determine the type of hearing loss. Another response parameter, the ratio between the SP and AP amplitude, is used to detect endolymphatic hydrops.

AP Threshold, Latency-Level, and Amplitude-Level Functions. A click stimulus (100 microseconds square wave pulse) is used to elicit the ECochG, and threshold is visualized as the lowest stimulus level at which ECochG is clearly distinct from the background noise. For normal hearing subjects, the AP is identified at levels of 10 to 20 db nHL—that is, within 10 to 20 db of psychophysical threshold for the click stimulus. The AP threshold correlates highly with pure-tone thresholds in the 4000- to 8000-Hz region of the cochlea, from which the most synchronous neural response is generated. Tone burst signals can also be used to elicit AP. Threshold prediction with use of tone burst signals is best for high-frequency thresholds (2000 and 4000 Hz) for patients with less than 60-db impairments in that frequency range. It should be noted, however, that discrepancies of more than 20 db between AP and pure-tone threshold are not uncommon.

The latency of AP–N1 decreases monotonically as level increases, and the amplitude increases monotonically. Of the two functions, the latency versus level function has lower intrasubject and intersubject variability, making it suitable for clinical use. Deviations from the normal latency versus level function can be used to predict hearing loss. For example, elevated thresholds and prolonged latencies are typical of hearing impairment, particularly with a lesion of the conductive mechanism. A latency versus level function showing elevated thresholds and an abnormal slope is characteristic of cochlear impairment.

SP–AP Amplitude Ratio. The SP–AP amplitude ratio can be used to identify endolymphatic hydrops. Endolymphatic hydrops causes an increase in SP amplitude in relation to the AP–N1 amplitude. There is considerable variability in absolute SP and AP–N1 amplitude, variability that increases with stimulus level. Several methods for determining abnormal SP/AP–N1 amplitudes exist. SP enlargement is seen in 55% to 70% of patients with endolymphatic hydrops when hearing is only mildly or moderately impaired (Fig. 10–25). Another application of the SP/AP–N1 ratio is for glycerin challenge tests. The theory is that glycol ingestion reduces fluid accumulation in the cochlea and decreases SP amplitude. Pre– and post–glycol ingestion SP–AP measurements are made, and those patients who experience a reduced SP post–glycol ingestion are considered "positive" for endolymphatic hydrops.

Auditory Brain Stem Response

The auditory brain stem response (ABR) is the auditory evoked response from cranial nerve VIII and ascending auditory pathways of the brain stem. The ABR waveform is composed of up to seven peaks that are conventionally labeled with Roman numerals (Fig. 10–26). Wave I is the far-field recording of AP–N1. The most prominent response peak recorded at the skull vertex, wave V,

has a latency that varies from more than 8 milliseconds for near-threshold signals to less than 6 milliseconds for suprathreshold signals. The ABR, like the ECochG, has variable amplitude that is influenced by recording technique. Amplitude ranges from 100 μV to at least four times that value.

The ABR has been the subject of an enormous amount of basic and clinical investigation in the past 15 to 20 years, and it has become an indispensable diagnostic procedure in audiology, otology, and neurology. This description emphasizes its uses in audiology for predicting hearing impairment and for neuro-otologic diagnosis.

Stimulus Variables

A description of stimulus-response and non-pathologic subject-related variables is needed to understand clinical application of ABR. The ABR is elicited by brief stimuli, such as clicks or tone bursts. ABR threshold and latency characteristics are exquisitely sensitive to changes in level, phase, rate, frequency, and stimulus rise time, making definition of stimulus parameters crucial for response interpretation.

Level. ABR wave V can be recorded at levels as low as 10 db nHL when click (i.e., 100-microsecond square wave pulse) stimuli are used. The ABR threshold for clicks cor-

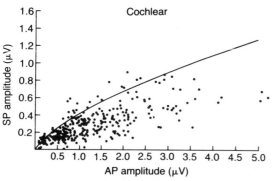

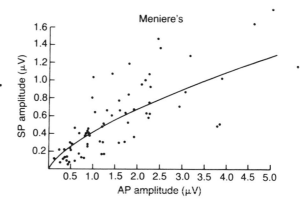

Figure 10–25. Scatterplots of summating potential (SP) versus action potential (AP) amplitudes for normal, cochlear, and Meniere's study groups. The curves represent upper normal limit derived from the normal test group (the upper 95% confidence limit from the log-normalized data replotted on an arithmetic scale). (From Coats AC: The summating potential and Meniere's disease. Am J Otol 5:443–446, 1984.)

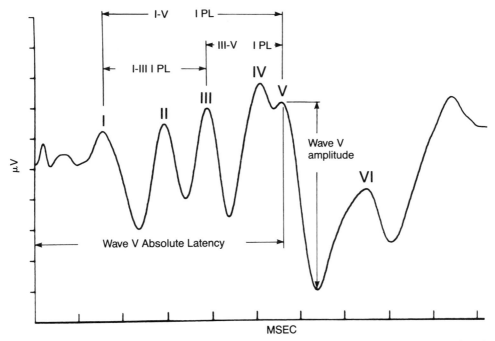

Figure 10–26. Example of a normal auditory brain stem response (ABR) for an adult male. Shown is the Jewett scheme for peak labeling (vertex-positive up) and the measurement of absolute and interpeak latency and peak-to-trough amplitude. (From Schwartz D, Berry GA: Normative aspects of the ABR. *In* Jacobson JT [ed]: The Auditory Brainstem Response. Austin, TX: Pro-Ed, 1985.)

responds to pure-tone thresholds in the 1000- to 4000-Hz frequency range because of the broad-band nature of the stimulus. When brief tonal stimuli are used, such as tone bursts, pure-tone threshold can be estimated from the ABR threshold. The ABR threshold for tone burst signals at 2000 and 4000 Hz appears to be within 10 to 20 db of pure-tone threshold, and for lower signals (at 1000 and 500 Hz) the correspondence is somewhat poorer, in the 20- to 40-db range. The transient nature of the tone burst signal limits the frequency specificity of the ABR response, because responses to brief stimuli, regardless of frequency, cause the basal portion of the cochlea to respond. Some specialized maneuvers, such as shaping the signal onset, selective filtering of the response, or use of band-limiting masking noise, can help to improve the frequency specificity of the response and thus improve correspondence of the ABR and the pure-tone threshold.

The ABR wave V latency versus level function, in conjunction with response threshold, is the basis for determining the presence and, to some extent, the type of hearing impairment. Wave V latency increases with decreasing level (Fig. 10–27). The normal latency values as a function of signal level are plotted on a graph so that deviations from normal can be assessed (Fig. 10–28). A patient with conductive hearing impairment demonstrates elevated thresholds and prolonged latencies, with a latency versus level function that runs parallel to normal. The patient with cochlear impairment shows elevated thresholds, but a latency versus level function with very rapidly decreasing latencies at suprathreshold stimulus levels. Some patients with moderate or severe sensory impairment have elevated ABR thresholds (e.g., at 70 db nHL) and *normal* latencies at threshold and at suprathreshold levels. Patients with retrocochlear disorders cannot usually be distinguished on the basis of response threshold and the latency versus level function alone because their responses may follow a pattern typical of either conductive or sensorineural impairment.

Phase. The polarity of a click stimulus can be positive or negative. These polarities are known as *condensation,* or *rarefaction,* clicks. The click phase affects response latency and

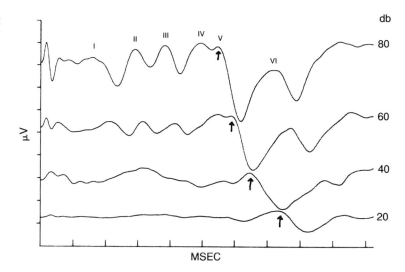

Figure 10–27. Effect of decreasing stimulus intensity on wave V latency, amplitude, and morphology. Time window is 10 milliseconds. (From Schwartz D, Berry GA: Normative aspects of the ABR. *In* Jacobson JT [ed]: The Auditory Brainstem Response. Austin, TX. Pro-Ed, 1985.)

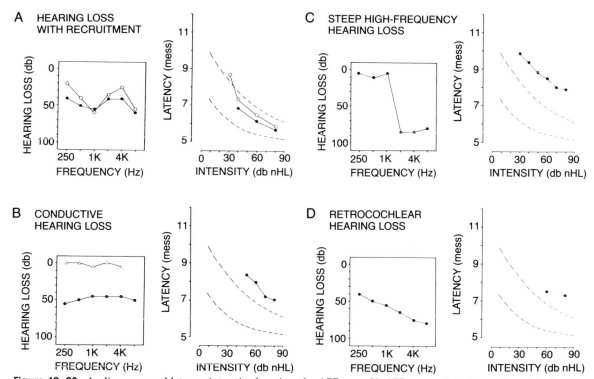

Figure 10–28. Audiograms and latency-intensity functions for ABR wave V. ABRs were elicited by using click signals. Area between dotted lines on the latency-intensity functions indicates normal latency range. *A.* Meniere's disease. *B.* Conductive hearing loss. *C.* Steep, high frequency sensorineural hearing loss. *D.* Retrocochlear hearing loss. (From Stappels D, et al: Frequency specificity in evoked potential audiometry. In Jacobson JT [ed]: The Auditory Brainstem Response. Austin, TX: Pro-Ed, 1985.)

may also affect response morphology. In clinical practice, it is typical to use either one polarity or the other or to alternate polarity and average responses for the alternating stimuli. The phase of the stimulus, however, must be known and specified to aid interpretation of test results.

Rate. Stimulus rate affects ABR wave V latency and amplitude. Latency increases and amplitude decreases with increased stimulus rate as a result of the decreased synchronization of neural elements as they undergo adaptation from rapidly repeated click stimuli. Rate-induced latency change can be predicted by multiplying the change in rate of stimulation (rate of test minus the base rate) by 0.006 milliseconds for rate changes between 10 and 90 per second.

Frequency. ABR latency and amplitude for tone burst signals are dependent on stimulus frequency. ABR wave V latency increases with decreasing frequency, a relationship in part dependent on the cochlear site of generation of the ABR. The more apical the response site, the longer the latency of the response. Tone burst stimuli at high levels do, however, generate a broad excitation pattern in the cochlea regardless of tone burst frequency. There is spectral spread even at low stimulus levels, with reduction of frequency specificity. Tone burst stimuli are shaped with gradual rise times that reduce neural synchrony and result in reduced response amplitudes as well as prolonged latencies. The correspondence between ABR thresholds for tone bursts and psychophysical thresholds for pure tones is determined by these differences in stimulus and response types. Yet, as noted, ABR thresholds for tone burst signals in the 500- to 4000-Hz range have reasonably good correspondence with pure-tone thresholds, and threshold predictions can be based on ABR recordings.

Rise Time. Temporal parameters of the stimulus, including rise time, duration, and shape of the stimulus envelope at onset, affect the ABR latency and amplitude. ABR wave V latency increases and amplitude decreases with increasing rise time, for noise or tone burst signals. This is a result of the decreased synchronization of neural firing at stimulus onset. Duration of the stimulus has little effect, as long as the interstimulus interval is held constant. The gating of the tone burst signal at onset determines the spectral spread of energy beyond the center or nominal frequency of the burst. The spread of spectral energy reduces the frequency specificity of the response, which affects the correspondence of ABR threshold with pure-tone thresholds.

Subject Variables

Nonpathologic subject variables influencing ABR characteristics are age, gender, temperature, and subject state.

Age. A subject's age is the most significant nonpathologic subject variable encountered in clinical application of ABR. The ABR is dependent on neural integrity at peripheral and brain stem levels, and both development and aging have demonstrable effects on the ABR.

Maturational changes in the auditory system are reflected in ABR latencies and amplitudes. ABRs can be recorded from premature infants as young as 28 weeks' gestational age. Responses from premature infants have elevated thresholds, prolonged latencies, and reduced amplitudes in comparison with adult responses. In the neonatal period, ABR threshold appears to be elevated 10 to 20 db, latency is prolonged, and amplitude is lower in relation to adult norms. Wave I latencies reach adult values by 2 months of age, and wave V latencies continue to mature (shorten) through 12 to 18 months of age. The age-dependent latency changes mandate that age-specific latency norms be used for accurate diagnosis of impairment.

There also appear to be age-dependent latency changes for subjects over the age of 50 years, although these effects are confounded by concomitant sensorineural impairment. Subjects over the age of 50 years with normal hearing have a 0.1- to 0.2-millisecond prolongation of wave I, wave III, and wave V latencies in comparison with subjects 20 to 30 years old. More study of ABR aging effects is needed, especially with protocols designed to control for hearing impairment.

Gender. Adult female subjects have shorter wave latencies and larger response amplitudes in comparison with male subjects. This finding suggests that separate sex-specific norms are needed for response interpretation, particularly for neuro-otologic diagnosis. Yet there is considerable overlap between normal values for male and female subjects, making the cost/benefit ratio for developing gender-specific norms unfavorable for clinical use.

Temperature. As core temperature is decreased, absolute and interpeak ABR latencies increase. This is of concern when ABRs are measured from patients with extremely low core temperatures: for example, during certain surgical procedures or during coma. When ABRs are used to monitor neuro-otologic surgical procedures, temperature variables must be borne in mind.

Subject State. The level of a patient's consciousness does not affect the ABR. The ABR is unaffected by most sedatives and anesthetic agents. It is crucial to keep background myogenic and electroencephalographic noise at a minimum for adequate signal averaging to take place, and for that reason, sedatives are often prescribed for subjects who are unable to lie quietly during the test procedures.

Test Interpretation

There are two primary ABR test strategies. The first is to determine abnormalities in ABR threshold and latency versus level function. Evaluation should include the determination of ABR threshold for click or tone burst signals and also sample latency at several suprathreshold levels. The second strategy is to evaluate interpeak latency values and waveform morphology associated with retrocochlear disease. (Interpeak latency is the latency difference that exists between components of the ABR, such as wave I to wave III, wave III to wave V, and wave I to wave V.) Evaluation should employ suprathreshold click stimuli presented at rates that increase or decrease neural synchrony so that the effect on ABR latency and amplitude can be quantified.

Conductive Impairment. When conductive hearing impairment affects the frequency range of the ABR stimulus (e.g., for clicks, 1000 to 4000 Hz), ABR threshold is elevated and latency prolonged. The conductive impairment can be thought of as an "attenuator" to cochlear input; therefore, ABR latency

at a given stimulus level is prolonged in relation to an unimpaired ear. The latency versus level function is displaced from, but runs parallel to, the normal function (Fig. 10–28B). Threshold elevation for air conduction clicks is based on the degree of conductive impairment in the high-frequency range. ABR interpeak latency is unaffected by conductive impairment.

Just as for conventional pure-tone threshold tests, contralateral masking should be employed whenever stimulus levels exceed the crossover value. Interaural attenuation for click stimuli is 70 db. Stimuli may also be presented by bone conduction for estimating the air-bone gap. Stimulus calibration, the frequency-response characteristic of the bone conduction oscillator for transient stimuli, and acoustic and electric artifact from the oscillator must all be accounted for before bone conduction ABR tests are used. Development of a clinic-specific data base for ABR threshold and latency values for bone conducted stimuli is recommended.

Cochlear Impairment. The effects of cochlear impairment on ABR threshold and latency may be considered according to the pure-tone threshold configuration. For flat sensory impairment, ABR threshold is elevated, and latency near-threshold is prolonged. With increasing signal level, latencies reach normal values. This gives a steep appearance to the latency versus level function (Fig. 10–28A). For some patients, ABR threshold may be elevated, yet latency at threshold may be comparable with normal latency at the same signal level (Fig. 10–28A). Patients with precipitously sloping high-frequency losses may have only slightly elevated ABR thresholds for click stimuli, with latencies that are prolonged, but latencies may be closer to normal for low levels in comparison with high levels (Fig. 10–28C). When hearing impairment is greater than 70 db HL at 1000 Hz, the ABR may be absent. Because of this circumstance, it is not possible to distinguish severe from profound impairments on the basis of ABR tests.

Interpeak latency values are normal or even shorter than normal because of differences in AP–N1 latency, amplitude, and morphology encountered in cochlear impairment. Furthermore, ABR wave V may be the only component recorded in some sensory impairments.

There is no consensus for the best way to estimate degree of hearing impairment when tonal stimuli are used for ABR tests. Cochlear impairment would be expected to alter the threshold and the latency of tone burst–evoked responses; however, the correlation between tone burst ABR thresholds and pure-tone thresholds is diminished when cochlear impairment is present. Response filtering, stimulus gating, and band-limited noise masking may improve threshold prediction for tone burst responses, but there are no standardized protocols for these methods.

Retrocochlear Impairment. The most significant ABR finding in retrocochlear impairment is prolonged wave I to wave V interpeak latency for the affected side. Interpeak latency abnormality can be judged on the basis of age-specific norms, and also an interaural comparison can be made. Another abnormality found in retrocochlear impairment is that the ABR wave V latency may show larger than normal shifts as stimulus rate is increased. The amplitude of wave V in relation to wave I may be reduced, but this finding is more common in upper than in lower brain stem lesions.

The presence of hearing loss in an ear with retrocochlear disease is not unusual and may confound the interpretation of wave V latency prolongation, especially when wave I is absent. Latency correction factors for accounting for degree of impairment are based on unproved assumptions about latency delays encountered in sensorineural impairment. For this reason, interaural latency differences for wave V alone must be interpreted cautiously.

Simultaneous ECochG and ABR recording is recommended for identifying the AP–N1 peak so that interpeak latencies can be determined. Recording the AP with an ear canal or transtympanic electrode is advantageous because the AP amplitudes are much larger than those observed in the far-field ABR response. Normal interpeak latency differences are 4 milliseconds plus or minus two standard deviations (usually 0.2 to 0.3 milliseconds). Prolonged interpeak latencies are indicative of retrocochlear disease at the level of cranial nerve VIII or higher.

ABR test sensitivity for detecting acoustic neuroma is quite high (over 90%). The so-called false-positive finding must also be carefully considered: there are retrocochlear lesions other than acoustic neuromas that yield a similar pattern of ABR test results but are considered false-positive when there is no neuroma. For example, prolonged interpeak latencies are found in patients with vertebral basilar disease, vascular disease of the lower brain stem, compression of the arterial loop in the cerebellar-pontine angle, and multiple sclerosis and other demyelinating diseases. The ABR is sensitive to cranial nerve VIII disorders and brain stem disease, but the abnormal test findings cannot be used to specify neoplastic versus vascular versus demyelinating disease.

Pitfalls of ECochG and ABR Tests

ECochG and ABR indicate electrophysiologic integrity of the cochlea, cranial nerve VIII, and brain stem pathways. Some critics observe that these are not tests of "hearing," which implies perception. It is possible, for example, to obtain normal ECochG and ABR results from patients who have no cortical function and are functionally deaf. The limitations for predicting pure-tone threshold are also cited as a drawback. The use of ABR for detecting acoustic neuromas may be superseded by magnetic resonance imaging techniques. Despite these drawbacks, ECochG and ABR are methods of primary importance for estimating the type and degree of hearing impairment in infants and other subjects who are difficult to test as well as for site-of-lesion determination.

Other Auditory Evoked Potentials

Auditory evoked potentials generated at cortical levels have also been used to estimate hearing impairment. These include the *middle latency response;* the *late, cortical,* or *vertex potential;* and various *event-related potentials* (ERPs) such as the P_{300} response. In general, the cortical evoked potentials with latencies longer than 100 milliseconds have high intrasubject and intersubject variability, are affected by subject state, and have proved unsuitable for audiometric tests. The middle latency response can be used to predict pure-tone thresholds, but it may be unsuitable for pediatric evaluations because of its variability as a function of the subject's age, state of consciousness, and susceptibility to sedatives. Event-related potentials are used for testing the cognitive aspects of auditory function. ERP test protocols for determining pure-tone thresholds require a degree of subject cooperation comparable with that for conventional (psychophysical) test methods.

TESTS OF THE CENTRAL AUDITORY NERVOUS SYSTEM

Disorders that affect the central auditory nervous system (CANS) at the brain stem and cortical levels may not be evident from standard audiologic evaluation. For example, stroke, neoplastic disease, and neural degeneration due to presbycusis may result in auditory-perceptual deficits. Tests designed for evaluating these deficits provide limited site-of-lesion identification and, more important, may characterize the CANS disorder.

There are pure-tone and speech tests of the CANS, and one of two strategies is usually apparent. Degraded (filtered, interrupted, time-compressed) speech stimuli are used to evaluate the patient's compensation for the missing information in the speech signal, an ability that is impaired by CANS lesions. A second strategy is to test for binaural integration or discrimination of speech or tonal stimuli, which are also disrupted by CANS impairment.

The application of CANS tests is limited; for that reason, detailed descriptions of various tests are not provided. Hearing impairment severely contaminates all CANS tests, rendering them uninterpretable. Only patients with no more than mild symmetric sensory impairments and excellent speech discrimination are candidates for CANS assessment. This means that a large segment of the target population (for example, the elderly) cannot be tested. It is possible that research on the effect of hearing impairment on CANS test performance may eventually yield a test battery suitable for patients with peripheral lesions.

CANS tests are time intensive and require subject cooperation. CANS test validity for site-of-lesion application is based on very small subject groups who have had surgically or radiographically confirmed lesions. These tests have been recommended for use with school-aged children with learning disabilities even though correlation of test results with definitive neurologic findings is tenuous. An argument for their inclusion in the clinical armamentarium is that they provide a description of CANS function and deficits that would not be possible from conventional pure-tone or speech tests. These descriptions may lead to more directed rehabilitation techniques.

TESTS FOR PSEUDOHYPACUSIS

Some patients with normal hearing feign hearing impairment, and other patients exaggerate an existing hearing impairment. Some patients are simply uncooperative, and others cannot understand instructions for taking hearing tests. There are patients who believe there are tangible rewards for demonstrating poor hearing (e.g., disability compensation). In others, the motivation for malingering may not be apparent.

A patient's behavior may alert the clinician to malingering. There may be a failure to obtain test-retest reliability for pure-tone thresholds. Very often, there is a failure of agreement between the pure-tone threshold average and the speech recognition threshold. Another discrepancy is the failure to obtain a shadow curve in the case of a supposed unilateral impairment: a patient with a true unilateral impairment responds to a signal that is greater than 60 db HL in the poor ear because of crossover hearing to the good ear. The malingerer does not respond to signals at any level in the "dead" ear.

Electrophysiologic tests such as acoustic reflex thresholds and the ABR are used to indicate pseudohypacusis. Patients who feign severe or profound impairment but have normal acoustic reflex thresholds are suspect. ABR threshold measures are extremely useful for detecting the malingerer and predicting true threshold. Furthermore, the sight of a clinician entering the test suite with a long, sharp, needle-like transtympanic recording electrode for ECochG may motivate the patient to perform pure-tone threshold tests more accurately.

There are several psychoacoustic tests that reveal the feigning of hearing loss. Most tests are based on the principle that the patient's test-taking strategy can be disrupted by a competing or confounding signal.

Stenger Test. The Stenger test is used routinely for patients demonstrating unilateral hearing loss. The Stenger test employs pure-tone or speech signals. The test is based on the fact that subjects lateralize a binaural signal to the ear in which the signal is perceived as louder and are unaware of the signal in the other ear. The test is given by presenting signals simultaneously at 10 db SL above the admitted threshold for the better ear and 10 db SL below the admitted threshold for the "poor" ear. A truly hearing-impaired patient responds to the signal because it is heard only in the good ear. The malingerer perceives the signal in the "poor" ear and is unaware of the signal in the "good" ear and does not respond. The Stenger procedure can be used to estimate threshold in the "poor" ear by determining the minimum contralateral interference level, or the level in the "poor" ear at which the patient fails to respond. The Stenger test can also be performed with word stimuli, either spondee or monosyllabic words. The Stenger test is applicable only for cases of unilateral or grossly asymmetric impairments.

Low-Level PB Word Tests. Word recognition tests can be given at levels of 5, 10, and 20 db SL above the admitted threshold. For the patient with a true hearing impairment, scores are below 75% for the 20 db SL level and 50% or poorer for the lower presentation levels. If the patient demonstrates better scores at low levels, it can be assumed that the true threshold is lower than admitted threshold.

Yes-No Test. The patient is asked to say "yes" when a tone is heard and "no" when it is not. Although the strategy of this test is quite obvious, a number of malingerers, especially child malingerers, can be detected by this test when they respond "no" to signals presented below their admitted threshold.

Békésy Ascending-Descending Gap Evaluation (BADGE). The discrepancy between thresholds when the signal level is swept from low-to-high versus high-to-low may indicate pseudohypacusis. The pseudohypacusic patient is unable to maintain a constant response criterion under such conditions, and wide discrepancies (greater than 15 db) between the ascending and descending traces result. This test can also be given by using manual audiometry techniques.

Pitfalls. The Stenger, low-level PB words, yes-no, and BADGE tests can be used routinely to detect the malingerer. ABR and ECochG methods appear to be most sensitive for detecting the malingerer *and* estimating threshold. Other tests for pseudohypacusis have diminished in importance in comparison with electrophysiologic procedures because they do not estimate true threshold.

ASSESSMENT PROCEDURES FOR THE PEDIATRIC POPULATION

Detection of hearing impairment in early infancy is crucially important because unidentified losses can lead to irreversible speech, language, cognitive, educational, social, and vocational handicaps. Technology exists for the performance of sensitive and specific tests of hearing acuity for even the youngest infant. Although the emphasis of this chapter has been on describing specific test procedures, detection and *management* of hearing impairment in early childhood is truly a process rather than a procedure. There is no one test given at a single point in time that can yield a thorough description of auditory impairment in infancy.

The assessment of hearing in infancy and early childhood is based on behavioral, electrophysiologic, and acoustic immittance measures. A distinction should be made at this point between assessment and screening. *Assessment* is the in-depth examination of auditory function by behavioral, electrophysiologic, and acoustic immittance measures to determine the degree, the configuration type, and the symmetry of an auditory impairment, or to determine that the infant does not have hearing impairment that could impede normal communication development. *Screening*, on the other hand, is used to determine which infants, among the population of all infants, have hearing impairment and require assessment. At the present time, the recommended hearing screening procedure for neonates at risk for hearing impairment is the ABR test. Infants at risk are those who demonstrate one or more risk criteria (Table 10–8). There are no published guidelines for screening older infants or toddlers, but common sense suggests that older infants at risk should be evaluated.

Age-specific considerations are needed

TABLE 10–8. Joint Committee on Infant Hearing

A. Risk Criteria: Neonates (Birth to 28 Days)

The risk factors that identify those neonates who are at risk for sensorineural hearing impairment include the following:

1) Family history of congenital or delayed onset childhood sensorineural impairment
2) Congenital infection known or suspected to be associated with sensorineural hearing impairment such as toxoplasmosis syphilis, rubella, cytomegalovirus, and herpes
3) Craniofacial anomalies, including morphologic abnormalities of the pinna and ear canal, absent philtrum, low hairline, etc.
4) Birth weight less than 1500 grams (3.3 lb.)
5) Hyperbilirubinemia at a level exceeding indication for exchange transfusion
6) Ototoxic medications, including but not limited to the aminoglycosides used for more than 5 days (e.g., gentamicin, tobramycin, kanamycin, streptomycin) and loop diuretics used in combination with aminoglycosides
7) Bacterial meningitis
8) Severe depression at birth, which may include infants with Apgar scores of 0–3 at 5 minutes or those who fail to initiate spontaneous respiration by 10 minutes or those with hypotonia persisting to 2 hours of age
9) Prolonged mechanical ventilation for a duration equal to or greater than 10 days (e.g., persistent pulmonary hypertension)
10) Stigmata or other findings associated with a syndrome known to include sensorineural hearing loss (e.g., Waardenburg's or Usher's syndrome)

B. Risk Criteria: Infants (29 Days to 2 Years)

The factors that identify those infants who are at risk for sensorineural hearing impairment include the following:

1) Parent/caregiver concern regarding hearing, speech, language and/or developmental delay
2) Bacterial meningitis
3) Neonatal risk factors that may be associated with progressive sensorineural hearing loss (e.g., cytomegalovirus, prolonged mechanical ventilation, and inherited disorders)
4) Head trauma, especially with either longitudinal or transverse fracture of the temporal bone
5) Stigmata or other findings associated with syndromes known to include sensorineural hearing loss (see item A.10)
6) Ototoxic medications (see item A.6)
7) Children with neurodegenerative disorders such as neurofibromatosis, myoclonic epilepsy, Wernig-Hoffmann disease, Tay-Sachs disease, infantile Gaucher's disease, Niemann-Pick disease, any metachromatic leukodystrophy, or any infantile demyelinating neuropathy
8) Childhood infectious diseases known to be associated with sensorineural hearing loss (e.g., mumps, measles)

Modified from AAO-HNS The Bulletin, March 1991.

when acoustic immittance and ABR tests are used for pediatric patients. Behavioral test methods, including behavioral observation, visual reinforcement audiometry, and other operant conditioning techniques, are also described.

Auditory Brain Stem Response

Age-specific norms for ABR tests are needed because maturational changes at the peripheral and brain stem level throughout the first 18 months of life affect ABR latency and amplitude. In most investigations of the effect of maturation on the ABR, only click stimuli have been used, and less is known about the stimulus-response functions for signals that vary in frequency, rise time, rate, or phase. The evaluation of hearing for a young infant may include both click and tonal stimuli, presented through air and bone conduction. It is important to consider differences between infants and adults in ABR latency, amplitude, and threshold. Use of signals for which only adult norms are available requires cautious interpretation of the infant's test results. Neonatal ABR thresholds for air-conducted click signals are within 10 to 20 db of adult values, and the difference grows smaller with age. It is reasonable to expect that infant ABR thresholds for tonal signals are close to adult values. This has been the basis of using ABR threshold measures to estimate auditory sensitivity in early infancy. This assumption must be kept in mind when ABR is used in early infancy for predicting hearing threshold.

The use of ABR in the pediatric population has facilitated assessment of infants and children once thought to be too young or too neurologically impaired to be evaluated. Sedation is often needed, however, to perform ABR tests for patients who would not otherwise tolerate the procedure. Sedation risks should be weighed against the benefits of the ABR results. For many patients, the benefits far outweigh the risks. The need for sedation discourages the use of serial ABR assessment, for example, in cases of chronic otitis media. Infant ABR test results are often limited to the determination of click threshold for both ears because the mild sedatives used do not always allow lengthier test protocols employing tonal signals. Again, the benefit of ABR results must be weighed against the risk of prolonged or multiple exposures to sedation required for more thorough tests. This author is in favor of using the ABR to its fullest extent to characterize hearing impairment and believes that ABR can be the cornerstone of assessment for infants at risk for hearing impairment.

Acoustic Immittance

Age-specific norms are needed for interpretation of acoustic immittance results. External and middle ear immaturity influences absolute immittance values, and special consideration is also needed for acoustic reflex threshold determination. The neonatal ear canal exhibits distensibility as a function of applied pressure, and this in turn affects determination of immittance values. Highly distensible ear canals and tympanic membranes found in neonates and very young infants may mask middle ear disease when immittance measurements are made. This has discouraged some clinicians from using tympanometry in very young infants. The determination of immittance values in absolute rather than relative units can be used to overcome the dilemmas encountered when only relative immittance changes are measured. More data from neonates with confirmed middle ear pathology are needed to clarify abnormal versus normal findings. For infants older than 4 months of age, ear canal and tympanic membrane stability is sufficient to yield adultlike tympanometric patterns, although absolute immittance values differ from those of older subjects.

The neonate's middle ear resonance frequency is higher than the adult's, and because of this, a higher immittance probe tone frequency is required to measure acoustic reflexes; that is, the use of a probe tone closer to the resonance frequency of the middle ear improves reflex detectability. For neonates, the use of a 660-Hz probe tone yields more consistently detectable reflexes in comparison to a 226-Hz probe tone. For older infants and young children, the 226-Hz probe tone is sufficient for measuring acoustic reflexes.

Behavioral Observation Audiometry

Neonates and infants respond to sound in stereotypical ways. Normal-hearing neonates can be awakened from sleep by a loud sound. A startle response, also called the *cochleopalpebral reflex*, can be elicited, and there are changes in respiration and heart rate that accompany sound presentation. Crying babies may quiet when sound is presented; others may become agitated. Head or eye movement toward the sound source may also be detected in infants as young as 2 months of age. Observation of these behaviors in a controlled environment with signals of known frequency and level is called *behavioral observation audiometry* (BOA). BOA has, in the past, been used for both screening and assessment purposes. BOA validity and reliability are diminished by observer bias and tenuous response criteria that have been used. Threshold determination is not possible with this method; it is not recommended as a screening procedure.

BOA is not recommended for threshold prediction; however, systematic observation of an infant's interaction with the (sound) environment is important for hearing assessment. Behavioral observation can be used to corroborate the parent's or the caretaker's report of the infant's auditory behavior and provide information that may guide further assessment or rehabilitation.

Visual Reinforcement Audiometry

The determination of threshold by employing a strict operant conditioning procedure is called *visual reinforcement audiometry* (VRA), or the *conditioned orienting response* (COR). The infant's response to sound can be shaped by operant conditioning techniques. An auditory signal is used to cue the infant that a reinforcer is available if a correct response is made. The correct response is a head turn toward the direction of the reinforcer. The reinforcer is a pleasing visual display, usually a lighted animated toy or an animated display on a video monitor. The reinforcers are hidden from view until the desired response is made. The behavior is initially shaped by exploiting the infant's localization (head turn) to the sound source or by pairing the auditory signal and the presentation of the reinforcer. Threshold determination is initiated after the head turn behavior has been conditioned. The level of the signal that cues reinforcer availability is decreased for each trial until there is no response. Then, the signal level can be increased until the head turn response is once again emitted. The infant's minimal response level, or threshold, can be bracketed in this way.

VRA procedures can be used with infants aged 5 months or older who have normal neurologic and motor development and unimpaired vision. VRA techniques lose their effectiveness for infants older than 24 months. The signals for VRA can be tonal (warble or pure tones or narrow-band noise) or speech, presented through earphones or a bone conduction oscillator or in the sound field through loudspeakers. Sound field signal presentation prohibits the assessment of each ear separately but is commonly employed when an infant does not accept earphone or bone conduction oscillator placement. Another procedural consideration is determination of the infant's "false-positive" rate of response. Catch trials, during which no signal is presented, must be interspersed with signal trials for determining the reliability and validity of the infant's response. Several test sessions may be necessary to accustom the infant to wearing earphones, to establish the correct conditioned response, and to determine thresholds for frequencies in the 500- to 4000-Hz range.

Thresholds determined with VRA for normal-hearing infants are similar to adults' thresholds. Deviations from normal are generally interpreted by use of the same pure-tone threshold criteria established for adults, indicating mild, moderate, severe, or profound impairment (Fig. 10–9).

VRA can be used with developmentally delayed or neurologically impaired infants, but extensive training for establishing the head turn response is needed. The hearing-impaired infant who has had less experience with sound may also require more test sessions for shaping the operant behavior required for VRA. The clinician must recognize when the infant is too disabled to be conditioned successfully and must then move on to other test strategies.

Visual/Tangible Reinforcement Operant Conditioning Audiometry (VROCA/TROCA)

Older infants can be conditioned to push a button or response bar after a signal is presented. The reinforcer can be a pleasing visual display or something tangible, such as food (cereal, fruit bits, tokens). This technique has been used successfully with older infants, toddlers, and preschoolers aged 2 to 4 years. The same procedural concerns outlined for VRA, including shaping the correct response, determining the reliability and validity of response, and sampling threshold over a range of frequencies, apply to VROCA/TROCA.

Play Audiometry

Toddlers and preschoolers aged 30 months or more can usually be taught to listen for and respond to sound in a consistent fashion when the listening task is made into a game. For example, the child is allowed to throw a block in a bucket each time a sound is detected; the child's task is to fill the bucket with blocks obtained for each correct response. A child can be reinforced for completing the task successfully. Wooden puzzles, block towers, and string beads are among the many play activities that can be used to engage children in listening tasks.

Speech Audiometry

VRA, VROCA/TROCA, and play audiometry can be used to determine the *speech awareness threshold*, the lowest level of response to a speech signal. The speech signal can be a syllable, word, or phrase. Standardized speech recognition threshold and word recognition tests involving a point-to-picture response (rather than oral word repetition) have been created for children as young as 3 years of age. The choice of speech audiometry materials and response mode must take into account the child's receptive and expressive vocabulary. Informal assessment methods include having the child perform simple commands ("Simon says . . .") or object identification.

Pitfalls

Multiple measures, including ABR, VRA, and immittance, that sample different aspects of auditory system integrity are needed for this age group. Procedures for resolving discrepancies between tests, however, are not well established. The clinician must advise the infant's parents or caregivers when discrepancies exist and counsel them about the need for repeated tests. It is unconscionable to "wait and see" when so many tools for diagnosis are available to the clinician.

OTOACOUSTIC EMISSIONS

The cochlea is not a passive organ. Hair cell physiology research has demonstrated that the outer hair cells have electromotile capacity. This motility is thought to contribute to the exquisitely fine frequency tuning that is evident in the response of the auditory nerve fibers. The hair cells make an active contribution to tuning. As a result of this process, the cochlea produces sound in response to sound. The sound produced by the cochlea is called the *otoacoustic emission* (OAE). The emission is detected by placing a miniature microphone in the external ear canal and recording the sound emitted by the cochlea that is transmitted through the middle ear space, ossicles, and tympanic membrane. Amplification and spectral analysis of the sound present in the ear canal is needed to detect the emission.

At the time of this writing, the use of OAEs for auditory assessment is in its initial phase. Reports from research laboratories suggest that various forms of OAEs can be used to test cochlear integrity at the hair cell level.

Some cochleas produce sound spontaneously. The so-called *spontaneous otoacoustic emissions* (SOAEs) are found in about 50% of normal-hearing subjects, and women exhibit SOAEs more often than do men. The frequency of the SOAEs varies little over time for the individual subject; most SOAEs occur in the 500- to 6000-Hz range and rarely exceed 20 db SPL. The use of SOAEs for diagnosis has been focused on patients with tinnitus; however, SOAEs are related to tinnitus in only 6% to 12% of tinnitus sufferers.

Acoustic emissions can also be recorded in response to a click or tone burst signal and are called *transient evoked otoacoustic emissions* (TEOAEs; Fig. 10–29). TEOAEs have been recorded in normal-hearing and hearing-impaired adults as well as from neonates, older infants, and children. TEOAEs are present in over 98% of all normal-hearing subjects, regardless of age or gender. TEOAEs can be detected at stimulus levels below psychophysical threshold, and the relationship between TEOAE threshold and psychophysical threshold is not well defined. TEOAEs are absent in patients with sensorineural hearing losses exceeding the mild range (25 to 40 db HL) and are exceptionally vulnerable to even slight cochlear dysfunc-

tion. The use of TEOAEs in the clinic may be confined to screening for cochlear impairment rather than for estimating pure-tone thresholds.

Otoacoustic emissions can also be recorded as a cochlear distortion product. Distortion in the cochlea is a result of nonlinear properties of the system. Distortion products are measured when two or more frequencies are used and frequencies not present in the input signal are created from intermodulation distortion within the cochlea. The most prominent distortion product in the human ear is found at $2F_1 - F_2$, when F represents stimulus frequency, and F_1 is lower in frequency than is F_2. *Distortion product otoacoustic emissions* (DPOAEs) are present in nearly 100% of all normal-hearing adult subjects. DPOAEs appear to reflect integrity in discrete frequency ranges of the cochlea. The relationship between pure-tone threshold and DPOAE threshold and input-output functions needs further investigation, but it appears to be a promising tool for predicting hearing impairment. This prediction may, however, be limited to the 1000- to 8000-Hz range and only for hearing losses not exceeding 60 db HL because DPOAEs are absent for more severe hearing losses.

Pitfalls. The paucity of clinical research about OAEs at this time limits discussion of the test pitfalls. One problem is that middle ear and external ear status must be nearly normal in order to record an OAE. This means that OAEs may not be useful for testing many young children at risk for hearing impairment resulting from chronic ear disease. That TEOAEs are absent for even mild impairments and that DPOAEs are absent for moderately severe or severe impairments may be limiting factors for describing cochlear dysfunction. In spite of these limitations, the OAEs are a window to cochlear processes in humans.

SUMMARY AND CONCLUSIONS

Psychoacoustic and electrophysiologic tests provide a description of auditory system integrity from the external ear to cortical auditory response areas. Auditory assessment can be provided at any age. The rationale for most tests in the audiologic test battery is to determine the degree of hearing impairment

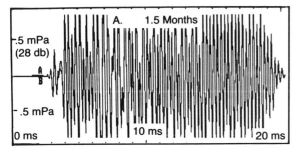

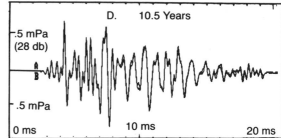

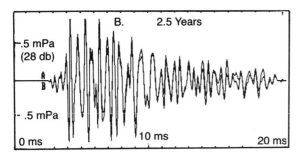

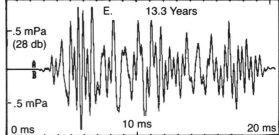

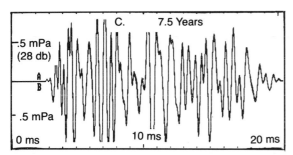

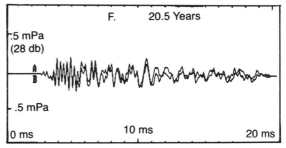

Figure 10–29. Evoked otoacoustic emission (EOAE) waveforms for normal hearing subjects. Ages are (*A*) 1.5 months; (*B*) 2.5 years; (*C*) 7.5 years; (*D*) 10.5 years; (*E*) 13.3 years; (*F*) 20.5 years. (From Norton SJ, Widen JE: Evoked otoacoustic emissions in normal hearing infants and children. Emerging data and issues. Ear Hear 11:121–127, 1990. Reprinted by permission of Williams & Wilkins, Baltimore, MD.)

and define the site-of-lesion. There will no doubt be continued efforts toward creating more sensitive and specific tests for this purpose. Another challenge for scientists and clinicians is to develop tests that determine appropriate treatment and rehabilitation. This should include electrophysiologic and psychoacoustic procedures to guide the design and use of signal-processing devices, both externally worn and implantable, to overcome auditory system impairment.

Acknowledgments

The author is grateful for comments provided by colleagues on early drafts of this chapter, including those of Daniel Kempler, Richard H. Wilson, Cynthia Fowler, and Nancy Cambron.

SUGGESTED READINGS

Hearing Science and Psychoacoustics

American Standards Association: Acoustical Terminology SI, 1-1960. New York: American Standards Association, 1960.

Durrant JD, Lovrinic JH: Bases of Hearing Science, 2nd ed. Baltimore: Williams & Wilkins, 1984.

Moore BCJ: An Introduction to the Psychology of Hearing, 3rd ed. San Diego: Academic Press, 1989.

Audiology

Bess FH, Humes LE: Audiology, The Fundamentals. Baltimore: Williams & Wilkins, 1990.

Hannley M: Basic Principles of Auditory Assessment. San Diego: College Hill Press, 1986.

Katz J (ed): Handbook of Clinical Audiology, 3rd ed. Baltimore: Williams & Wilkins, 1985.

Lass NJ, McReynolds LV, Northern JL, Yoder DE (eds): Handbook of Speech-Language Pathology and Audiology. Philadelphia: BC Decker, 1988.

Rintelmann WF (ed): Hearing Assessment, 2nd ed. Austin: Pro-Ed Publishers, 1988.

Speech Audiometry

Konkle DF, Rintelmann WF (eds): Principles of Speech Audiometry. Baltimore: University Park Press, 1983.

Aural Acoustic Immittance

Shanks JE, Lilly DJ, Margolis RH, et al: Tympanometry. J Speech Hear Disord 53:354–377, 1988.

Van Camp KJ, Margolis RH, Wilson RH, et al (eds): Principles of Tympanometry. Rockville, MD: ASHA Monograph Number 24, 1986.

Auditory Evoked Potentials

Durrant JD, Ferraro RC, Fowler CG, et al: The Short Latency Auditory Evoked Potentials. Rockville, MD: American Speech-Language and Hearing Association, 1988.

Ferraro JA (ed): Electrocochleography. Semin Hearing 7:241–337, 1986.

Jacobson JT (ed): The Auditory Brainstem Response. San Diego: College Hill Press, 1985.

Pediatric Assessment

Bess FH (ed): Hearing Impairment in Children. Parkton, MD: York Press, 1988.

Otoacoustic Emissions

Shimizu H (ed): Otoacoustic Emissions: Clinical Implications. Ear Hear 11:81–166, 1990.

CHAPTER 11

Conductive Hearing Loss: Inflammatory and Noninflammatory Causes

Jeffrey P. Harris, MD, PhD   Roberto A. Cueva, MD

As discussed in Chapter 8, the tympanic membrane and ossicles serve to transmit (conduct) the mechanical energy of sound waves, propagated by the compression and rarefaction of gas molecules in the air, to the fluid environment of the inner ear. In order to prevent the attenuation of sound energy that would normally occur at the interface between gaseous and liquid environments, the tympanic membrane and ossicles amplify the sound energy. This amplification is accomplished by two major factors: (1) the difference in the surface area between the tympanic membrane and the oval window and (2) the lever advantage of the ossicular chain. Another important function of the tympanic membrane is sonic shielding of the round window. Any process that affects the functional efficiency of this sound-conducting mechanism results in a conductive hearing loss.

Conductive hearing losses can have a variety of etiologic factors. In an effort to group related causes, this discussion is organized first by anatomic location and then into inflammatory and noninflammatory causes. The chapter focuses primarily on acquired disorders; congenital problems are addressed in Chapter 14. Under each broad category, specific causes are discussed. The mechanism by which conductive hearing loss is caused by each disorder is covered. Medical and surgical treatment options are reviewed as they pertain to each disorder.

THE EXTERNAL AUDITORY CANAL

The external auditory canal (EAC) serves as a conduit for sound to travel from the external environment to the tympanic membrane.

Inflammatory Causes

Inflammatory diseases of the EAC cause conductive hearing loss by a mechanical obstruction of sound travel by edema or scarring of the skin of the EAC as well as by accumulation of debris in the canal or against the tympanic membrane.

Otitis Externa

An acute episode of otitis externa causes edema of the skin of the EAC. The inflamed skin has a more rapid turnover rate and desquamates an abundance of keratinous debris. This combination of edema and squamous debris may obstruct the canal, effectively attenuating sound travel through the EAC and thus causing a conductive hearing loss. The clinician is led to the correct diagnosis by the common preceding history of water exposure to the involved ear, the sign of tragal/auricular motion tenderness, and the physical appearance of the inflamed EAC and relatively normal tympanic membrane.

Otitis externa is a localized infection of the skin of the EAC. It generally does not require parenteral antibiotics for successful treatment. Topical medication suffices unless there is a clear-cut cellulitis of the auricle or surrounding tissues. Topical medications include acetic acid solutions, Domeboro solution, antibiotic- and steroid-containing drops, and antifungal drops and creams. The physician's choice for treatment is largely dependent on how the physician was trained and personal preference. Cultures need be done only for patients who do not respond rapidly to conventional treatment or for patients with immune compromise such as diabetes. When the EAC is severely swollen, it may be necessary to place a wick for therapeutic success to be achieved.

Chronic Stenosing Otitis Externa

Chronic stenosing otitis externa is an unusual condition characterized by ongoing inflammation of the EAC skin with resultant progressive thickening of the skin that blocks effective clearance of proximal canal skin and cerumen. This accumulation of debris perpetuates the inflammation. Often, in spite of medical treatment, this condition progresses to the point of total EAC stenosis with blocking of sound transmission through the EAC.

Medical therapy for this disease focuses on careful EAC hygiene for the removal of debris. Topical steroids may provide some benefit. Surgical intervention is commonly required in the form of canalplasty. In this procedure, all the skin of the EAC is removed; the squamous covering of the tympanic membrane is left intact. The EAC is then carefully skin-grafted with suitable thin skin harvested from the back of the auricle or from the inner aspect of the upper arm. Once an adequate EAC passage is re-established, hearing should return to normal.

Noninflammatory Causes

Cerumen

Something as simple as an accumulation of cerumen can cause a 20- to 30-db conductive hearing loss. The amount of cerumen need not be excessive; it only needs to form an airtight seal across the lumen of the EAC.

Removal of the cerumen can be accomplished in many ways. Irrigation of the ear should be avoided if there is any question about the presence of a tympanic membrane perforation. During irrigation, care should be taken to prevent high pressures that can produce iatrogenic perforations. Cerumen curets, loops, and suction can be used with and without magnification for removal of cerumen. It is often useful to perform Weber and Rinne tuning fork tests before and after cerumen removal for documenting correction of the conductive loss. If it is not corrected by cerumen removal, another cause may be present.

Foreign Bodies

Foreign bodies of all types are introduced into the EAC both purposely and by accident. Foreign bodies of the EAC are most commonly encountered in the pediatric population. Pebbles, beans, seeds, pieces of plastic, beads, insects (dead and alive), miniature batteries, and many other objects have been described as EAC foreign bodies. It is important to try to ascertain the nature of the foreign body and how long it has been in the EAC. Infection may or may not be present. A perforation may have been caused by introduction of the object into the ear. Conductive hearing loss is caused, again, by a mechanical obstruction to the passage of sound through the EAC or by perforation of the tympanic membrane.

In children, general anesthetic is often necessary for safe removal of the foreign body. This removal should be done under the operating microscope, and the EAC and the tympanic membrane should be carefully inspected for signs of injury or infection. If the ear is painful, adults may be adequately anesthetized with local anesthetic. However, apprehensive adults or mentally incompetent patients may also require general anesthetic for a safe removal and a thorough examination of the ear to be effected. As a special case, live insects may be immobilized by the use of mineral oil before their removal.

Exostoses and Osteomas

Exostoses and osteomas of the EAC are fairly common and generally do not cause conductive hearing loss. Hearing loss may occur when they are large enough to obstruct the

EAC or press against the tympanic membrane or the malleus and thereby impede movement. Exostoses are believed to be caused by exposure of the proximal EAC skin to cold water or air. Cold temperature exposure is thought to create an irritation of the periosteum with stimulation of bone growth. On histologic examination, exostoses have a lamellar growth pattern, which supports the theory of periosteal irritation by cold temperature. Osteomas, on the other hand, arise de novo without any known precipitating cause.

Surgical excision is the only cure for these lesions. However, surgery is necessary only when the lesions are causing symptoms of conductive hearing loss or recurrent otitis externa (as a result of accumulation of debris behind the growths). The operative techniques are described in surgical atlases, but the basic purpose of the operation is to remove the excess bone. Care must be taken to avoid iatrogenic injury of the tympanic membrane, the ossicles, and the facial nerve from misdirected drilling.

TYMPANIC MEMBRANE AND MIDDLE EAR

The tympanic membrane, ossicular chain, and aerated middle ear allow efficient conversion of sound energy traveling by air to the fluid medium of the inner ear. Any alteration of this mechanism that reduces the efficiency of this conversion results in a conductive hearing loss.

Inflammatory Causes

Myringitis

The tympanic membrane can be affected with inflammation or infection without middle ear involvement. This situation is fairly unusual but seen in the case of granular myringitis. In this entity, the patient complains of otalgia, diminished hearing, and often otorrhea. On examination, the eardrum or a portion of it is covered by a velvety layer of granulation tissue. Pneumatoscopy often reveals fair mobility of the tympanic membrane, which suggests an aerated middle ear.

Oral antibiotics and even topical steroid-containing drops mildly ameliorate symptoms. Often conservative cauterization of the granulations with silver nitrate followed by

the application of Mycolog ointment or cream effectively returns the tympanic membrane to a normal appearance. On rare occasions, one must resort to skin-grafting the canal and the drum head after curettage of the granulations has been performed.

Acute Otitis Media

More common is the situation of middle ear and tympanic membrane inflammation in the form of acute otitis media. In acute otitis media, the middle ear mucus membranes are inflamed because of infection. A purulent exudate is usually present in the middle ear, which then dampens tympanic membrane movement and results in a conductive hearing loss. Subacute or chronic infection may lead to the development of hypertrophic middle ear mucosa or granulations, which can add to the conductive hearing loss by hampering ossicular movement. Otitis media is often preceded by an upper respiratory tract infection. The symptoms of otalgia, diminished hearing, and often fever suggest otitis media. On examination, the external auditory canal is often fairly normal in appearance, and there is no auricular/tragal motion tenderness. The tympanic membrane is erythematous, bulging, and sometimes desquamating; pneumatoscopy may elicit pain.

Typically, acute otitis media responds to oral antibiotics that would cover streptococcal pneumonia, *Haemophilus influenzae* infection, and beta-hemolytic streptococcal infections. If no relief of pain or fever is achieved with 24 to 48 hours of therapy, myringotomy or tympanocentesis is indicated for removing pus from the middle ear and obtaining a specimen for culture.

Serous Otitis Media

Once the infection has cleared, a residual sterile middle ear effusion is commonly referred to as serous otitis media. An effusion may remain as long as 1 month after acute otitis media in up to 50% of patients. During this time, hearing may continue to be impaired (approximately 10 to 30 db) because of the vibration-dampening effect of middle ear fluid. Once the effusion resolves, hearing should return to normal.

Whereas serous otitis media commonly follows an episode of acute otitis media, serous otitis media may arise de novo from underlying eustachian tube dysfunction. The suboptimal anatomic relationships of the eustachian tube in childhood, chronic rhinosinusitis of allergic or infectious etiology, and palatal dysmotility that results from cleft palate or other craniofacial abnormalities can all contribute to the formation of serous otitis media. Physical examination may demonstrate an air/fluid level in the middle ear space or the presence of bubbles as an obvious finding. Often the tympanic membrane appears amber colored with no bubbles, but pneumatoscopy reveals no or paradoxical movement of the eardrum.

Commonly recommended treatment consists of a course of antibiotics, with the optional use of decongestants. Bacterial colonization of nonpurulent middle ear effusions has been demonstrated in up to 30% of cultures from ears. If the effusion does not clear with the first trial of antibiotics, up to three courses of different antibiotics may be tried over a 3-month time period. If effusion persists after 90 days, myringotomy with tube placement is generally recommended. Treatment of underlying causes such as allergy or infectious rhinosinusitis is an essential part of therapy.

Chronic Otitis Media

The complications of chronic otitis media often result in conductive hearing loss. This can occur as the result of many mechanisms. The following discussion divides these etiologic mechanisms into those with an intact (but not normal) tympanic membrane and those with tympanic membrane perforation.

Intact Tympanic Membrane

Atelectasis. Tympanic membrane atelectasis is a long-term complication of chronic serous otitis media. The tympanic membrane can become very thinned and retract to such an extreme degree that differentiation between perforation and retraction can be difficult. The middle ear space is filled by a thick mucoid effusion with the consistency of glue; hence the derivation of the term "glue ear." In extreme cases, the tympanic membrane is adherent and draped over the promontory and ossicles, with virtual elimination of the middle ear space. Prolonged contact of the retracted tympanic membrane with the ossicular chain causes erosion of the ossicles, most commonly the incus. Conductive hearing loss is caused by poor tympanic

membrane vibration secondary to effusion, excess tympanic membrane laxity, tympanic membrane retraction, ossicular erosion/discontinuity, and impaired sonic shielding of the round window.

Treatment usually requires surgical intervention. In early cases, the placement of a long-lasting pressure equalization tube may provide some benefit. In advanced cases, the weakened tympanic membrane is resected. In patients who have recovered fairly good eustachian tube function, fascia may be used to graft the membrane. In patients in whom continued eustachian tube dysfunction is anticipated, cartilage with attached perichondrium may be employed as an effective retraction-resistant graft material. It may be necessary to reconstruct the ossicular chain for improvement of hearing in cases in which ossicular erosion or discontinuity has occurred.

Tympanosclerosis. Tympanosclerosis can cause conductive hearing loss through tympanic membrane or ossicular chain involvement. Tympanosclerosis is formed by hyaline deposits (which often calcify) in tissues subjected to the inflammation of repeated bouts of otitis media. It can be found as plaques in the fibrous layer of the tympanic membrane and in submucosal regions of the middle ear, such as along the ossicular chain. If tympanic membrane tympanosclerosis is extensive enough, it can impede membrane vibration or even fix the membrane and the malleus. Tympanosclerosis can involve the ossicular chain in the oval window, causing stapes fixation. The round window may also be diseased, preventing perilymph movement during stapes vibration. It can affect the malleus head and incus in the epitympanum, causing fixation in this location.

Treatment requires surgical removal of involved tissues. This is effectively accomplished in the tympanic membrane during tympanoplasty surgery. Ossicular chain tympanosclerosis is more difficult to eradicate completely and has a tendency to re-form, particularly in the oval window. Removal of tympanosclerosis from the round window is fraught with the hazard of creating a perilymphatic fistula. Involvement of the malleus and the incus in the epitympanum usually requires removal of the malleus head, along with removal and sculpting of the incus as an incus interposition for re-establishing the ossicular chain. Oval window and stapes involvement can be treated by stapedectomy. These cases have a higher incidence of postoperative sensorineural and recurrent conductive hearing loss. In severe cases, removal of tympanosclerotic deposits over the promontory can lead to inadvertent opening of the cochlea with the risk of sensorineural hearing loss.

Ossicular Discontinuity. The tympanic membrane may appear fairly normal, but with a history of repeated bouts of otitis media, ossicular discontinuity must be considered as an etiologic factor for conductive hearing loss. During otitis media, the ossicles are subject to the effects of bacterial toxins and inflammatory mediators, which can cause bone resorption or jeopardize the blood supply to the ossicles. The incus long process is most susceptible to erosion that leads to ossicular discontinuity. Next most frequently affected is the superstructure of the stapes. The malleus is rarely eroded to a significant degree unless cholesteatoma is present.

Once again, treatment is surgical in nature. The general goal of surgery for ossicular discontinuity is re-establishment of an effective sound-conducting connection between the tympanic membrane and the inner ear. The procedure of choice is selected on the basis of the anatomy found at the time of middle ear exploration. There are numerous techniques for ossicular chain reconstruction involving the patient's own ossicles, homograft ossicles, and synthetic materials. Discussion of all these options is not within the scope of this chapter, and the reader is directed to the suggested readings for a more in-depth description of surgical techniques.

Tympanic Membrane Perforation

Tympanic membrane perforation alone can cause conductive hearing loss by essentially two mechanisms. The first is the loss of vibratory surface area for the reception of sound waves. With a smaller surface area, the amplifying properties of the tympanic membrane are compromised. For a significant conductive hearing loss to be achieved by this mechanism alone, the perforation must be fairly large, approaching 50% of the surface area. The second mechanism by which conductive hearing loss may occur with tympanic membrane perforation is the loss of sonic shielding for the round window. The round window serves as the release valve for the perilymphatic fluid displacement generated by stapes movement in the

oval window. To function effectively, the round window membrane must remain sonically shielded; if not, the round window would be subject to the same sound waves being transmitted through the stapes, and phase cancellation of perilymphatic movement would occur. This results in a conductive hearing loss. It is by this mechanism that even small perforations near the area of the round window may cause a greater conductive hearing loss than expected, in accordance with their size.

Treatment is determined by a multitude of factors. The age and size of the perforation and the mechanism of its formation are the two most important factors. Relatively small perforations of traumatic origin commonly heal spontaneously. However, perforations resulting from chronic or recurrent bouts of otitis media generally require a combination of medical and surgical intervention. Any predisposing conditions that may affect eustachian tube function or the likelihood of recurrent infection should be dealt with. Allergic or infectious rhinosinusitis, adenoid hypertrophy, and other conditions require concomitant or antecedent treatment for maximizing the chances of successful tympanic membrane repair. Active otitis media should be treated appropriately. Preferably the ear should be free from recent infection before tympanoplasty surgery. Water precautions and the judicious use of topical and parenteral antibiotics can achieve this goal. Tympanoplasty performed under the proper conditions and by experienced clinicians can achieve a success rate for tympanic membrane closure approaching 90% to 95%. Once again, in-depth descriptions of tympanoplasty techniques are not covered, and the reader is directed to the sources included in the suggested readings.

Cholesteatoma. A complication of tympanic membrane perforation and pars flaccida retraction pockets is cholesteatoma formation. Cholesteatoma can be likened to a skin-lined cyst in which the continuous accumulation of squamous debris allows expansion and destruction of adjacent structures by a combination of pressure and the biochemical effects of its lining matrix. Cholesteatoma is a serious condition and requires surgical removal in all cases with rare exceptions. Left untreated, cholesteatoma can, through its erosive properties, invade the inner ear, causing sensorineural deafness and vertigo; erode the bone, separating the middle ear and intracranial cavity of the middle or posterior fossa with risk of central nervous system infection; compress the facial nerve, leading to paralysis; and, least of all, erode the ossicles, causing a conductive hearing loss. The diagnosis can usually be made on physical examination when an onionskin or cottage cheese–appearing material is seen to exude from a tympanic membrane perforation or pars flaccida retraction. If cholesteatoma is suspected, careful examination of the tympanic membrane should be performed under the operating microscope. What may appear to be a small cholesteatoma by clinical examination can extensively involve temporal bone structures hidden from view. For assessment of the extent of cholesteatoma and for identification of the possible aforementioned complications of cholesteatoma, high-resolution computed tomography (CT) of the temporal bones is recommended.

Treatment, as mentioned, is surgical. Mastoidectomy combined with tympanoplasty is the general procedure of choice. The extent of mastoidectomy and whether the bony external auditory canal is left intact is a judgment made at the time of surgery. The specific technique employed reflects the extent of disease as well as the training and experience of the surgeon. Excellent descriptions of various surgical techniques can be found in the suggested reading material.

Noninflammatory Causes

Atraumatic Etiologies

Otosclerosis. The best-known cause of conductive hearing loss in which the tympanic membrane appears normal is otosclerosis. The reason this entity receives so much attention is the dramatic reversal of conductive hearing loss achieved by stapedectomy. The condition begins as an abnormality of bone metabolism and turnover affecting the bone of the otic capsule. In the oval window, it most commonly affects the anterior portion of the stapes footplate and the fissula ante fenestrum. It begins as an area of exuberant bone turnover that is actually otospongiotic. As these lesions mature, calcium is deposited, and they become densely sclerotic. Stiffening and fixation of the stapes footplate occurs and causes conductive hearing loss. Otosclerotic foci can also occur adjacent to the endosteum of the membranous labyrinth, causing sensorineural hearing loss and occasionally vertigo.

The patient most often complains of a slowly progressive hearing loss. On examination, the tympanic membrane is normal. In unilateral cases, Weber tuning fork testing lateralizes to the affected ear. Rinne testing reveals (if conductive loss is greater than 20 db) that sound through bone conduction is louder than that through air conduction. Audiometric testing discloses a conductive hearing loss. Impedance testing reveals that acoustic reflexes are diminished or absent in the affected ear. A review of the family history often reveals relatives who have been similarly afflicted.

Some controversy exists over the efficacy of medical treatment of otosclerosis with sodium fluoride ingested orally. Controlled clinical studies suggest that this agent protects the inner ear from further deterioration that results from otosclerosis. The surgical treatment of this entity, once frowned upon, was revolutionized by the advent of the binocular operating microscope and improved sterile technique in the early 1950s. The basic principles of stapedectomy are removal or bypassing of the fixed stapes footplate and re-establishing a vibratory connection between the inner ear and the ossicles by means of a prosthesis bridging from the incus long process to the oval window. This procedure, performed under local anesthesia, carries a 90% to 95% success rate for improved hearing. The variety of specific techniques and prostheses available is considerable, and the reader is referred to the suggested readings for detailed descriptions.

Ossicular Fixation. Ossicular fixation may result from acquired or congenital causes. Ear infections causing middle ear scarring and tympanosclerosis can fix the ossicles at any point. Congenital ossicular fixation must be considered in a child presenting with conductive hearing loss, a normal-appearing tympanic membrane, and no history of ear infections. Most commonly, the malleus and incus are fixed in the epitympanum by bony attachment. The conductive hearing loss occurs as a result of limitation of ossicular vibration. Treatment is surgical and involves the removal of the head of the malleus; removal and sculpting of the incus forms an interposition graft from the malleus to the stapes capitulum. Simple mobilization of the ossicles or limited procedures for removing bony points of fixation provide short-term results because refixation is common. Occasionally the stapes may be congenitally fixed in the oval window and requires either mobilization or, a more dependable procedure, a stapedectomy to correct the conductive hearing loss.

Neoplasms. Tumors arising in the middle ear can impede the movement of the ossicles or tympanic membrane, causing a conductive hearing loss. Glomus tumors, adenomas, meningiomas, and malignancies can all manifest in the middle ear with conductive hearing loss. Any middle ear tumor should be suspected to be of vascular origin until proven otherwise. Diagnostic evaluation is primarily accomplished with radiologic tests in the form of high-resolution CT scan, magnetic resonance imaging scan, and possibly arteriography. If a biopsy is undertaken, it should be done only after imaging studies suggest a nonvascular etiologic origin.

Treatment of neoplastic lesions of the middle ear is entirely dependent on their histologic type and extent. The reader is directed to the literature for the treatment of specific tumor types.

Traumatic Etiologies

Tympanic Membrane Perforation. Tympanic membrane perforation of traumatic origin may result in conductive hearing loss for the same reasons as do perforations of nontraumatic origin. However, the clinician must keep in mind the possibility of a coexistent ossicular injury when evaluating a traumatic perforation. A conductive hearing loss out of proportion to the size of perforation, any inner ear symptoms (i.e., sensorineural hearing loss or vertigo), or an injury in the posterosuperior quadrant of the tympanic membrane (location of the ossicles) should alert the clinician to the possibility of ossicular damage.

Treatment varies, depending on the size of the perforation, whether infection is present at the time of presentation, and whether ossicular injury is suspected. In noninfected ears, even sizable traumatic perforations heal spontaneously. Whenever possible, any visible flaps of the torn tympanic membrane should be approximated with the use of cigarette paper or adhesive-backed paper to facilitate healing. If, however, infection is present or likely to develop (i.e., middle ear contamination by water or other material at the time of injury), parenteral and topical antibiotics should be employed to eradicate or prevent infection. Surgical intervention is indicated for perforations that fail to heal spontaneously after 2 to 3 months or for cases in which ossicular or inner ear injury is suspected. The latter cases require prompt surgical exploration for assessment of the status of the ossicles and oval and round windows. Tympanoplasty techniques are employed in the repair of these perforations and are well described in surgical atlases.

Hemotympanum. Barotrauma from flying, underwater diving, forceful nose blowing, and other sources can result in the rupture of blood vessels in the middle ear space. A hemotympanum is thus formed and results in the sensation of aural fullness, often pain, and conductive hearing loss. The presence of fluid in the middle ear dampens tympanic membrane vibration; hence a conductive loss ensues. At the time of examination, the history of the inciting event is usually elicited, and the tympanic membrane appears blue and opaque.

Conservative treatment consists of the use of oral decongestants to promote the evacuation of blood from the middle ear via the eustachian tube. Pain may prompt the physician to perform myringotomy for achieving relief. If the tympanic membrane does not return to normal after treatment, then further work-up is indicated for ruling out a possible vascular tumor of the middle ear.

Ossicular Injuries. Conductive hearing loss may result from an ossicular injury even without tympanic membrane perforation or temporal bone fracture. A concussive blow to the head and a rapid barometric shift in external auditory canal pressure transmitted to the tympanic membrane in the form of a slap injury are examples of the types of forces that may result in isolated ossicular injury. The susceptibility of each ossicle to injury is directly related to its fibrous and bony supports. The malleus long process is well supported by its attachment to the tympanic membrane. In addition, the anterior, posterior, superior, and lateral malleolar ligaments, as well as the tensor tympani tendon, provide further stabilization for the malleus head and neck. The stapes footplate is firmly anchored in the oval window by its annular ligament; the superstructure receives stabilization from the stapedius muscle tendon. The incus, however, is supported only by the incudomalleolar joint, the posterior incudal ligament, and the incudostapedial joint. This relative lack of support renders the incus most vulnerable to traumatic injury.

The most frequent traumatic ossicular lesion is disarticulation of the incudostapedial joint. This is followed by complete dislocation of the incus. Fracture of the stapes crura is next most common and may be associated with perilymph fistula. In spite of its degree of stability, the malleus may be injured. The most frequent lesion is malleus head fixation to the bony wall of the middle ear. A less common but important injury is the malleus handle fracture. The fracture usually occurs in the region of the malleus neck, forms a pseudarthrosis, and may effectively disconnect the tympanic membrane from the rest of the ossicular chain. Close examination of the tympanic membrane under magnification with the use of pneumatoscopy allows identification of the fracture site. The importance of this lesion is that it may be confused with a stapedial crural fracture. Both manifest clinically with a mild conductive hearing loss and hypercompliant tympanic membrane on tympanometry. As mentioned, the correct diagnosis may be made with careful pneumatoscopy. Differentiating between the two types of injury can help the surgeon decide whether surgical exploration of the middle ear is necessary. An unrecognized perilymph fistula, such as may occur with a stapedial fracture, can result in chronic vertigo or permanent deafness; hence middle ear exploration would be indicated in the patient with these clinical features in the absence of a malleus handle fracture.

An ossicular injury is immediately suspected in the patient presenting with complaints of hearing loss after an auricular or a head trauma. If examination is performed soon after the traumatic event, a hemotympanum is often present. Later, if conductive hearing loss persists after the blood has cleared, ossicular injury is very likely. If the lesion is not readily identified (i.e., malleus handle fracture), middle ear exploration is indicated for the purposes of diagnosis and treatment. The decision to explore is tempered by the degree of symptoms. In patients without temporal bone fracture, any symptoms of inner ear dysfunction (vertigo or sensorineural hearing loss) warrant prompt exploration for the diagnosis and treatment of possible perilymphatic fistula.

The successful treatment of traumatic ossicular injuries involves use of the principles of ossicular reconstruction pertinent to ossicular defects found in chronically diseased ears. Care must be taken to assess the integrity and mobility of all three ossicles. Removal of bone from the posterosuperior scutum may be necessary to adequately visualize the stapes and oval window. Interposition grafting or the use of synthetic ossicular implants may be necessary to achieve optimal reconstitution of the ossicular chain. Any area of suspected perilymph fistula (i.e., oval and round windows) must be repaired with a suitable tissue graft.

Temporal Bone Fracture. Substantial trauma to the temporal region or the occiput can result in a temporal bone fracture. These fractures are traditionally divided into transverse and longitudinal varieties. Transverse fractures are less common (20%) but have a higher rate of associated sensorineural hearing loss and facial nerve injury. Longitudinal fractures are more common (80%) and result in visible fracture lines in the EAC as well as conductive hearing loss. A mixed type of temporal bone fracture is not uncommon. In these injuries, a hemotympanum is almost always present and causes a conductive hearing loss.

Once other factors have been resolved (usually closed-head injury associated with the trauma), attention may be directed to assessment of the hearing loss. If conductive hearing loss persists after the hemotympanum has cleared, then ossicular injury is very likely. Audiometric testing should establish whether the hearing loss is solely conductive in nature or whether a sensorineural component is present. Impedance testing provides information regarding tympanic membrane compliance and the presence or absence of stapedial reflexes. Often CT scans have already been obtained as part of the initial trauma evaluation. If not, high-resolution CT scan of the temporal bones is in order for defining the sites of fractures and the involved anatomy.

For conductive hearing loss, middle ear exploration with reconstruction of the ossicular chain is the treatment of choice. A 3- to 4-month period of observation to allow spontaneous resolution of the hearing loss is recommended. In patients without CT scan evidence of a fracture through the labyrinth and with a sensorineural component to their hearing loss, exploration is also warranted for determining whether a perilymphatic fistula is present. If, for medical reasons, the patient is not a good surgical candidate, a hearing aid may be used to rehabilitate hearing. Mastoidectomy may be necessary at the time of ossicular reconstruction for assessing facial nerve integrity or for repairing a source of persistent cerebrospinal fluid leak.

SUMMARY

In this chapter, a variety of clinical situations in which conductive hearing loss may occur have been reviewed. Discussion organized by anatomic location has helped to present related etiologic factors and the mechanisms by which they cause conductive hearing loss. For in-depth study of a specific etiologic factor or surgical technique, the reader is encouraged to refer to the materials in the suggested reading list.

SUGGESTED READINGS

Austin DF: Ossicular reconstruction. Arch Otolaryngol 94:525–535, 1971.

Cummings C (ed): Otolaryngology—Head and Neck Surgery. St. Louis: CV Mosby, 1987.

Glasscock ME, Shambaugh GE: Surgery of the Ear. Philadelphia: WB Saunders, 1990.

Harris JP, Butler D: Recognition of malleus handle fracture in the differential diagnosis of otologic trauma. Laryngoscope 95:665–670, 1985.

Jackson CG, et al: Ossicular reconstruction: the TORP and PORP in chronic ear disease. Laryngoscope 93:981–988, 1983.

Sade J: Pathogenesis of attic cholesteatomas. J Soc Med 71:716–732, 1978.

Schucknecht HF (ed): Pathology of the Ear. Cambridge: Harvard University Press, 1974.

The Otolaryngologic Clinics of North America: Otology—current concepts and technology. Philadelphia: WB Saunders, February 1989.

CHAPTER 12

Sensorineural Hearing Loss: Sudden, Fluctuating, and Gradual

Dennis R. Maceri, MD

Sensorineural hearing loss is immediately characterized in the presenting patient as a unilateral versus a bilateral loss and as to whether it is sudden or fluctuating as opposed to gradual. The emphasis here is on the sudden fluctuating loss because it represents an otologic emergency requiring immediate diagnosis and treatment. The treatment of such losses closely parallels the therapy for Meniere's disease or endolymphatic hydrops.

The myriad congenital and hereditary syndromes that are responsible for sensorineural hearing loss (SNHL) are not discussed here except where pertinent. The focus is also placed on adult problems rather than pediatric SNHL. Of course, some syndromes are common to all ages and are discussed accordingly.

The starting point should be to divide SNHL into cochlear and retrocochlear lesions. In general, bilateral symmetric lesions tend to be cochlear, nonconductive, and gradual in nature. Unilateral losses that are more sudden and fluctuating in nature present a more significant diagnostic challenge to the physician and receive the most attention.

Table 12–1 lists the major cochlear and retrocochlear lesions that account for sudden SNHL (SSNHL). These can present as the more gradual forms or as a fluctuating hearing loss as well.

INCIDENCE

Byl (1984) has estimated that true idiopathic SSHL accounts for up to 20 new cases per 100,000 patients per year. A sudden hearing loss can be a most frightening experience for patients because of the rapid onset and fear of a more severe underlying disease that might progress to total deafness in both ears. The incidence may in fact be quite a bit higher because of a lack of attention by patients and the spontaneous recovery that occurs in many cases.

This in general is a disease that has an increasing incidence with age, being more common for people over 65 years than in children less than 14 years (Mattox and Simmons, 1977).

Mattox and Simmons found the mean overall age for SSHL to be 46 years. In general, the following breakdown of ages applies (Van Canegham, 1958):

Incidence by Age	Rate per 100,000
20–30 years	4.7
50–60 years	15.8
70–80 years	13.0

Sheehy and Shaia (1976) have shown that there is no sex difference in SSHL, men and women being equally affected.

The incidence of bilateral involvement var-

TABLE 12–1. Etiology of Sudden and Fluctuating Sensorineural Hearing Loss

Cochlear Disorders

Congenital lesions
Hereditary syndromes
Acquired losses
Acquired disorders
Inflammatory
Traumatic—includes spontaneous fistula
Vascular
Hematologic
Polycythemia rubra vera
Sickle cell disease
Hypercoagulation states
Leukemia
Immune disorders
Metabolic
Renal failure
Alport's disease
Diabetes mellitus
Hyperlipidemia
Hypothyroidism
Toxic—drug-induced
Antibiotic
Contraceptives
Miscellaneous
Bypass
Vaccinations
Meniere's syndrome
Presbycusis
Cochlear otosclerosis

Retrocochlear Lesions

Multiple sclerosis
Tumors of the cerebellopontine angle
Sarcoidosis
Vogt-Koyanagi-Horada syndrome
Miscellaneous

ies a great deal but is generally believed to be present in less than 10% of the cases.

DEFINITIONS

What is a sudden sensorineural hearing loss? A true definition is hard to find, but otolaryngologists agree that it consists of a rapid-onset loss that occurs within hours or one that is present when the patient awakens. This loss can be progressive over a few hours to a few days, making the time of the initial presentation key (Byl, 1984). Byl found that the speed of onset, severity, and rate of recovery are quite variable. In general, the typical patient presents with a spontaneous, sudden hearing loss that is unilateral and of unknown etiology.

CHARACTERISTICS OF HEARING LOSS

In the work by Byl, the loss generally occurred within 2 hours of or was present upon the patient's awakening and was most commonly seen in the age group in the fourth and fifth decades. The loss audiometrically varies from a mild high-frequency SNHL to a more complete absent reaction to acoustic stimulation. The patterns seen were up-sloping, down-sloping, and flat losses. Byl found that 18% of the patients had a *normal* recovery when the pure-tone threshold was better than 25 db in all test frequencies. Patients were categorized as having a *complete* recovery (27%) when they had a 25-db or better pure-tone average. A *partial recovery* was seen in 24% of the patients and was characterized by a 10-db improvement in pure-tone average from the initial audiogram. Thirty-one percent had no demonstrable improvement (Table 12–2). In terms of recovery, 83% showed improvement if the loss was mild, and, as expected, the rate of improvement was less in the more profound losses. The more severe the initial loss was, the poorer was the recovery. The presence of vertigo was also a negative factor, as was the duration of the loss. In Byl's series, if the loss was seen to improve within 7 days, 56% had a normal or complete recovery. The average age of onset was a factor only in the incidence, not in the rate of recovery.

A 28% recurrence rate was seen in the series by Byl, and up to 11% had continual fluctuations.

TABLE 12–2. Recovery from Sudden Sensorineural Hearing Loss

Percentage Recovery	Definition
18% normal	Pure-tone threshold level better than 25 db in all test frequencies
27% complete	25 db or better pure-tone threshold average
24% partial	10 db improvement in pure-tone threshold average from initial audiogram
31% improvement	

Adapted from Byl FM: Sudden hearing loss: eight years' experience and suggested prognostic table. Laryngoscope 94:647–661, 1984.

COCHLEAR LESIONS

Congenital Cochlear Losses

Congenital losses at birth that result from a SSHL have not been reported. However, there are congenital problems that predispose to SSHL later in life, such as a patent endolymphatic or perilymphatic duct, a narrowed or stenosed internal auditory canal, abnormalities of the oval and round windows, and cochlear anomalies. Goodhill and associates (1980) have postulated implosive or explosive pressure change mechanisms as the cause of labyrinthine window ruptures. Congenital defects in the cochlea could in fact enhance these pressure changes by alterations of endolymphatic flow. Progression of SSHL can occur unilaterally or bilaterally in congenital cochlear deformities such as Mondini's dysplasia, in which there is both a bony defect and a membranous defect in the cochlea. The hearing canal is flat or circular, the cochlear duct is short, and the auditory and vestibular nerve endings are poorly developed (Jackler et al., 1987).

After these causes have been excluded, it is assumed that the loss is a result of an acquired cochlear problem.

Acquired Cochlear Losses

The group of acquired cochlear lesions responsible for SSHL can be divided into three causes (Table 12–1): inflammatory, traumatic, and vascular.

Inflammatory Causes of SSHL

Under the inflammatory causes, the viral illnesses are seen to predominate. These include mumps (with or without clinical parotitis), measles, rubella, herpes zoster oticus, varicella, and mononucleosis. The prototypic viral lesion may be unilateral or bilateral. Mumps is more commonly unilateral whereas measles manifests bilaterally. On histologic examination, there is atrophy of the stria vascularis and the organ of Corti; the hair cells are destroyed; and Reissner's membrane is collapsed because of a viral labyrinthitis (Schuknecht, 1974).

In *herpes zoster* oticus (Ramsay Hunt syndrome), there is tinnitus and a high-frequency SNHL that shows some recovery. Presence of facial paralysis with vesicular lesions in the external canal confirms the diagnosis.

Bacterial causes of a septic labyrinthitis are seen in meningococcal, pneumococcal, and staphylococcal meningitis. The source of meningeal infection is usually a respiratory pathogen, especially in children. The pathologic process is rarely an encephalitis. Syphilis can also cause sudden deafness in the acquired congenital form. Acute syphilitic labyrinthitis may occur with lymphocytic meningitis in secondary syphilis. In the late or latent tertiary stages, the lesion is more commonly a syphilis-induced temporal bone osteitis (Hendershot, 1973).

Traumatic acquired cochlear losses result in sudden hearing loss from temporal bone fractures, high-energy electric shocks, and lightning. Head and neck radiation can produce a secondary serous labyrinthitis with doses above 50 Gy. These are high-frequency losses and may show some fluctuation over the years. Degenerative changes are seen in the spiral and annular ligaments with atrophy of the stria vascularis and degeneration of the organ of Corti (Pfaltz, 1988).

Goodhill and coworkers (1973) have proposed that stress episodes resulting in a Valsalva type maneuver lead to increased cerebrospinal fluid pressure, which can be transmitted to the scala tympani and serve as a source of potential leaks around the oval and round windows in adults.

Perilymphatic Fistula

A fistula is an abnormal communication between the fluids surrounding the membranous labyrinth and the middle ear space. The existence of such an entity has been questioned in many instances but must be considered in the differential diagnosis and management of SSHL or of fluctuating SNHL with or without tinnitus and vertigo.

The decision of when to explore an ear in a patient with fluctuating hearing loss and vertigo is based on a failure of response to conservative medical management. There is no question that patients with a history of rhinorrhea, otorrhea, or trauma, with or without recurrent meningitis, should be explored after a thorough work-up has been done. The work-up should include a high-resolution computed tomographic scan of the temporal bones in order to check for cochlear anomalies or signs of fracture.

What is not clear is the management of the patient who does not have otorrhea or rhinorrhea and has a negative history for head trauma, recurrent meningitis, or barotrauma (sneezing, coughing, straining with a Valsalva type motion), but has fluctuating hearing loss and vertigo. This situation suggests a "spontaneous" perilymphatic fistula that usually arises from the round or oval window. The incidence of such fistulas is difficult to determine because of the number of negative explorations in patients who improve with time after surgery. There is no question that patients improve if they are treated with fat or fascia packing of suspected sights even if no fistula is documented. Some otolaryngologists believe that a problem cannot be found unless it is looked for. Because there is no clear-cut laboratory test that is specific enough to increase the yield at exploration, an absolute recommendation as to when surgery should be done cannot be given.

In the pediatric population, a history of recurrent meningitis of unknown etiology is an indication of a possible fistula. Reilly (1989) studied 244 children with sensorineural hearing loss who had no antecedent history of meningitis prospectively over 3 years and found a fistula rate of 6% (15 of 244 cases).

Shelton and Simmons (1988) explored 66 patients in an adult population with recurrent balance problems in anticipation of finding a perilymphatic leak. The explorations were positive in 51% of the cases. They found that the cure rate with surgery was no higher than the rate of spontaneous recovery in the natural course of the disease. The authors drew attention to the fact that fistula symptoms are quite similar to attacks of Meniere's disease, which creates a serious diagnostic dilemma as to the true etiology. It was believed that the intermittence or fluctuation of a perilymphatic leak may account for the fact that negative explorations, when treated surgically, were seen to improve patients' symptoms. For this reason, all explorations should be done with the technique discussed in the following section, regardless of findings.

Surgical Repair. Most otologists agree that at the time of exploration, a tissue graft of temporalis fascia, perichondrium, or muscle with or without fibrin glue is recommended. The two areas of concern are the annular ligament around the footplate and the round window niche. The mucosa is roughed up before the packing is placed. In fistulas resulting from a traumatic stapedectomy, the oval window membrane is preserved, and a new tissue graft and a prosthesis are applied. If the crura are intact, the mucosa is stripped around the footplate, packed with ear lobule fat, and covered with fascia or perichondrium. The round window is treated in a similar fashion. Again, it is important that *all* explorations are treated regardless of the findings at surgical exploration (Althaus, 1981).

Vascular Etiologies

The most important theories of SSHL encompass the vascular causes despite the fact that such an etiology remains unproved. Most treatment regimens evolve around the philosophy that improvement results from increasing the blood flow to the inner ear. In vascular lesions, the onset is sudden, the recovery is quite good, and there does seem to be a response to the therapy. There is, however, a liability to relapse, and there may be increased triggers related to stress, shock, and other systemic vasoactive influences.

Current research is directed toward the basic sciences of cochlear blood flow. The team at the University of Michigan has published data in animal models on the neurocirculation of the cochlea, specifically, the vasoconstrictor mechanisms and the response to certain vasodilators and hemorrheologic agents such as pentoxifylline (Trental) in the guinea pig (La Rouere et al., 1989). When pentoxifylline is given intravenously, cochlear blood flow increases by 20%. This effect seems to be separate from vasodilation, inasmuch as the flow was increased with use of pentoxifylline despite maximal prior dilation achieved with a nitroprusside infusion (La Rouere et al., 1989).

Hughes has carried out similar experiments with hemorrheologic agents, including pentoxifylline, in patients with sensorineural hearing loss in high-noise environments. Hughes found that pure-tone threshold changes were minimal during the 6-week test period but that a substantial improvement in speech reception thresholds occurred while patients were receiving the drug.

The mechanism of action of pentoxifylline

is to reduce the pathologic rigidity of deformed red cells and decrease the ability of thrombocytes to aggregate. The net effect is to increase the blood's fluidity (decrease viscosity) under pathologic conditions (Hulcrantz, 1988).

Although vascular lesions can produce sudden deafness, hearing loss usually occurs in association with a known systemic vascular disease or in patients with associated cardiac risk factors. Other disorders such as hyperviscosity states, macroglobulinemia, and thrombotic end artery disease have also been implicated. The cause of the hearing loss can be an arterial obstruction, atherosclerotic vascular disease, a microembolic phenomenon, or venous obstruction of labyrinthine veins (Pfaltz, 1988).

Finally, the basilar artery migraine syndrome demonstrates the consequences of acute interruption of basilar artery flow. Specifically, ataxia, vertigo, tinnitus, nausea, and severe headache of the migraine type are seen. The hearing loss fluctuates and is associated with a fullness in the ear (Love, 1978). Intracranial aneurysm as a cause of SSHL is rare; there would be an expected fluctuation with improvement of symptoms once the aneurysm is clipped.

In vascular lesions with tissue ischemia, it would be assumed that autoregulatory mechanisms have maximally dilated capillary beds in the brain. The microcirculation is dilated by local tissue autoregulatory mechanisms in response to hypoxia, elevated carbon dioxide, and metabolic byproducts. This is most important in therapeutic considerations because pharmacologic agents are unable to further dilate these beds. Disease states that cause vascular sludging result from altered or increased red cell mass and hyperviscosity syndromes. The sludging causes capillary engorgement, decreased blood flow, and oxygen deficiency, which leads to hearing loss. This is seen in polycythemia rubra vera, sickle cell disease, and hypercoagulation states. Jaffe (1970) described this and believed that it resulted from possible vascular plugs in the vessels of the spiral ligament or stria vascularis.

Leukemia has also been implicated in SSHL because of leukemic infiltrates, hemorrhage, or infection from altered host immunity resulting as a consequence of the underlying disease.

Treatment Summary. Most forms of ther-apy for sudden deafness are based on less than sound scientific rationale. Whatever the cause, the theory of vascular compromise implies blood vessel narrowing, hypercoagulation and sludging of blood, and possibly thrombosis with subsequent ischemia of the inner ear. The first step is to treat any systemic disorder that may be acting to decrease cochlear blood flow.

In the series of Meyerhoff and Paparella (1980), the treatment in most instances required hospitalization and strict bed rest. After the complete neuro-otologic examination, an audiogram, electronystagmograph, and appropriate laboratory studies are obtained. Specifically, tests for syphilis, thyroid disease, diabetes, cholesterol, and triglycerides and serologic tests for autoimmune disorders are obtained.

Meyerhoff and Paparella (1980) have suggested subcutaneous heparin 5000 to 10,000 units every 12 hours, systemic steroids at 1 mg/kg/day, low-molecular-weight dextran, and papaverine hydrochloride (Pavabid) orally every 12 hours. The duration of treatment is usually given for a minimum of 3 days and up to 1 week.

Some use daily doses of intravenous vasodilators such as histamine for 3 days in conjunction with the oral regimen.

Morimitsu (1977) has reported a 37% patient response to intravenous diatrizoate meglumine (Hypaque) in 60 patients. However, none of these patients had vertigo, and they probably were in a group that would have had a favorable response regardless of treatment.

Immunologic Causes

In 1979, McCabe proposed a form of sensorineural hearing loss thought to be due to an autoimmune mechanism in 18 patients. This proposal was based on a composite representative patient who presented with all the signs and symptoms of SNHL but who failed to fit a known etiologic category.

Harris (1983) has studied both cell-mediated and humoral immunity in patients with suspected autoimmune hearing loss by use of modern immunologic techniques that included lymphocyte transformation and Western Blot analysis. This work has demonstrated that a number of patients show a positive antibody to inner ear antigens, which suggests the possible existence of an organ-specific *autoantibody* similar to that seen in a guinea pig animal model. An antigenic challenge sensitizes the cells and makes them more responsive to second and third challenges with antigen.

In addition, both animal and human studies have shown that perilymph contains immunoglobulins, which demonstrates that the inner ear is not immunologically isolated.

In the study of Harris (1987), animals were immunized with a preparation of heterologous bovine inner ear antigen. Thirty-two percent of the animals developed hearing defects and lesions within the inner ear without direct inoculation or manipulation of the inner ear.

A similar situation has been postulated by Harris for the human autoimmune cochlear hearing loss. In this theory, the antigen of the inner ear is somehow recognized as foreign, and antibodies develop, which leads to local immune deposition and destruction of the entire membranous labyrinth. Furthermore, it is suspected that the immune competent cells that are responsible for the lesions develop outside the ear and migrate to the site of antigen challenge or exposure. One possibility is that the endolymphatic sac acts as the site where antigens are processed. It is believed that some of the immune reactions, especially to viruses such as cytomegalovirus, may protect the ear.

Several clinical entities of autoimmune etiology are associated with inner ear disease. These include polyarteritis nodosa, Behçet's disease, relapsing polychondritis, lupus erythematosus, and rheumatoid arthritis. It is believed that the hearing loss may be either a result of organ-specific disease or the result of a systemic disorder. In support of the latter concept, Veldman (1984) has reported a case in which circulating immune complexes were identified in a patient with systemic vasculitis resulting from systemic juvenile chronic arthritis. In this 14-year-old girl, the inner ear was identified as a target organ in the autoimmune response for circulating immune complexes. This case proved to be responsive to steroids.

It is therefore clear that the cochlea is *not* to be considered a passive end organ in the immune response when it is challenged by antigen or infection or when it is part of a systemic disease.

Treatment. When clear-cut evidence of autoimmune disease exists, the patient should be placed on an immunosuppressive regimen. The individuals are placed on large doses of steroids, 1 to 2 mg/kg/day for 2 to 3 weeks. In more significant nonresponsive cases, cyclophosphamide at doses of 2 to 5 mg/kg/day can be added. With drugs like cyclophosphamide, the peripheral blood count must be monitored for leukopenia on a regular basis. It is helpful to have consultation with rheumatologic specialists in more advanced disease with systemic manifestations. In recalcitrant patients, plasmapheresis can be considered if circulatory immune complexes appear to be at work. Typically these patients are treated daily for 5 days, then at decreasing intervals over the next month for a total of 10 runs (Harris, 1989).

Cases have been seen by the author that require months of steroid therapy and that relapse quickly if attempts are made to taper the drug too soon. In the series by McCabe (1979), a patient was treated with steroids for more than 10 months; an attempt to wean at 3 to 5 months was associated with a rapid drop in hearing.

In summary, autoimmune inner ear disease is a disease whose diagnosis is difficult to prove, and as yet there is no absolute diagnostic test specific enough for the diagnosis to be certain. At times the work-up is equivocal, and the diagnosis is made by a steroid challenge. Tests of lymphocyte status such as lymphocyte transformation, lymphocyte lymphokine assays, macrophage migration inhibitory factor, and leukocyte migration inhibitory factor are specific tests for demonstrating lymphocyte sensitization to previous antigenic challenge. Much more sophisticated tests are done in research settings and are not commonly found in the average clinical laboratory. Serum protein electrophoresis, immunoelectrophoresis, sedimentation rate, cryoglobulins, quantitative immunoglobulins, antinuclear antibody, and LE preparation are commonly available tests. These are often abnormal in many autoimmune disorders. They are sensitive but not very specific. The C1q complement-binding assay provides strong evidence of circulating immune complexes that interact with complement with use of IgG and IgM.

Cochlear Loss of Metabolic Origin
Renal Failure

The nephron has many similarities to the stria vascularis of the inner ear. These include a common epithelial origin, high vascularity and metabolism, and the physiologic function of creating and maintaining steep electric gradients. In addition, both end organs arise from epithelial precursors at relatively the same time and are frequently found to have simultaneous pathologic problems seen in congenital and hereditary syndromes.

These two organs are similarly affected by many ototoxic drugs that poison metabolic activity and therefore prevent maintenance of electrochemical gradients. In the kidney, this translates to an inability to excrete urine of proper osmolality. In the scala media, the metabolic dysfunction alters the endocochlear potential and ultimately prevents mechanoelectric transduction.

The prototypic lesion commonly discussed is Alport's syndrome, also known as familial hematuric nephritis or hereditary nephritis with sensorineural hearing loss. The syndrome includes progressive nephritis, bilateral high-frequency SNHL, a positive family history, and visual problems. The hearing loss may start in early infancy with progression or may present as a rather sudden loss (Winter et al., 1968).

Temporal bone findings in Alport's syndrome show spiral ligament projections that cause partitioning of the scala vestibuli bilaterally, atrophy of the stria vascularis, and decreased spiral ganglion cells in the basal turn (Gussen, 1973).

Diabetes Mellitus

In diabetes, the question is often raised as to whether the hearing loss is due to the diabetes. The hearing loss is similar to that seen in presbycusis—that is, a bilateral high-frequency sloping SNHL—except that it occurs earlier in life. This can also manifest as a sudden SNHL, especially in the younger diabetic, with a variable recovery rate. It is known that diabetes affects the capillaries and small vessels with a type of intimal proliferation and with deposition of lipid. This vascular disease is also seen in the retina and the kidney. In addition, an enhanced form of arteriolosclerosis occurs in these patients throughout the body, and it is characterized by thickening of the intima and endothelial proliferation (Schucknecht, 1974). Makishima and Tanaka (1971) found in human temporal bones a type of microangiopathy as well as direct neural injury with

hemorrhage and exudates that even involved some of the higher central pathways.

Disorders such as hyperlipidemia have also been implicated in fluctuating low-tone SNHL. The losses are seen in both the primary and secondary forms of hyperlipidemia; both the cholesterol and triglycerides are elevated. Hypothyroidism is often listed in the differential diagnosis of SNHL but is not well documented in the literature. The hereditary syndrome of Pendred's disease is an autosomal recessive disorder in which the cochlear hearing loss is bilateral and is associated with a goiter and hypothyroidism. This disorder is responsible for about 7.5% of all congenital deafness with an incidence of 1 in 50,000 (Fraser, 1969). The pathologic change is thought to result from a peroxidase enzyme defect that affects the organification of iodine. The hearing loss does not usually respond to hormonal replacement, and it is believed that the cochlear pathologic process occurs in utero during the first trimester (Illum et al., 1972).

Ototoxicity

Many drugs of varied pharmacologic types act in the inner ear either as therapeutic agents or in the form of ototoxic effects. This section deals with the most common classes of drugs that are known to be ototoxic, the most common of which is the family of aminoglycoside antibiotics followed by the nonsteroidal anti-inflammatory agents, diuretics, and cancer chemotherapy agents. The aminoglycoside antibiotics have their effect on either the auditory or vestibular systems or, in many cases, both. The toxic effects are related to the dose, the route of administration, and the patient's renal function. The site of action is in the hair cell itself, the outer row of hair cells being the most vulnerable in a basal-to-apical progression. In severe forms, the hair cells are replaced by scar tissue with degeneration of cochlear neurons (Hawkins and Johnson, 1981). Several theories as to the mechanism of toxicity have been proposed, including a direct binding of the drug to the phospholipid moiety of the hair cell membrane with subsequent loss of permeability and function. The possibility of an inhibition of calcium uptake by the cells, thereby blocking electric conduction, has also been suggested (Weiner and Schacht, 1981; Wagner et al., 1987). Whatever the cause, the antibiotic therapy must be monitored closely with peak and trough levels of the drug throughout the course of therapy. The doses must be adjusted according to the patient's renal function. This is, of course, complicated by the fact that the aminoglycosides are also nephrotoxic. Whenever possible, baseline and interval audiograms should be obtained. An associated and dangerous interaction exists between the aminoglycosides and loop diuretics, which act synergistically to enhance the ototoxic effect of both drugs (West et al., 1973). The physician must always be concerned with the potential for ototoxic effects when topical preparations that contain neomycin sulfate are used as an irrigation in body cavities with high absorption potential, such as the pleural and peritoneal spaces. Extremely high levels of neomycin sulfate in the blood and tissues can result from this type of irrigation, with complete and total SNHL as a consequence.

Of the nonsteroidal anti-inflammatory agents, salicylates are the most frequent causes of ototoxic effects. High levels of salicylate can cause severe tinnitus and hearing loss, both of which are usually reversible when the drug is stopped. It is believed that the action is a temporary metabolic alteration at the hair cell level, perhaps by an inhibition of some prostaglandin synthesis (Dovek et al., 1983). The other agents in this group, such as ibuprofen, indomethacin, and naproxen, produce a much lower rate of toxicity than does aspirin.

The loop diuretics ethacrynic acid and furosemide act on the ascending loop of Henle in the kidney to block the resorption of sodium and chloride. In animal models, these drugs also have an effect at the level of the stria vascularis for blocking the Na^+/K^+ ATPase activity and thereby abolishing the endocochlear potential. The effect is most severe when the drugs are given intravenously (Prazma, 1981). As mentioned, a synergy exists with the aminoglycosides for potentiating ototoxicity. The mechanism of action of these agents is thought to result from a resultant swelling in the stria vascularis that renders it incapable of metabolic activity (Prasma, 1981). The effects can be temporary or permanent, depending on the duration of the treatment and the renal function.

Antineoplastic drugs such as cisplatin, the nitrogen mustards, and vincristine have a direct effect on the hair cells in the inner ear. They cause both vestibular and auditory lesions that occur first in the hair cells by alteration of the stereocilia in a random unorderly fashion. The effects of cisplatin in the temporal bone include degeneration of the stria vascularis, fusion of the stereocilia, loss of spiral ganglion cells, and loss of fibers in cranial nerve VIII with a resultant high-frequency hearing loss first, followed by a complete progression (Strauss et al., 1983).

Meniere's Disease

The syndrome first described by Prosper Meniere as an inner ear disease remains an enigma to otologists because of its fluctuation and spontaneous recovery. Many medical regimens are available, all of which share about the same degree of success. A full discussion of the syndrome is beyond the scope of this chapter, but a word about the pathologic process and treatment options is appropriate. The symptoms of fluctuating hearing loss, vertigo, and tinnitus are felt to be secondary to endolymphatic hydrops within the membranous labyrinth. Whatever the cause of the hydrops, either too much endolymph is generated or too little is absorbed from the endolymphatic sac. These concepts have led to the various medical and surgical treatments used today. Certainly, the presence of hydrops is not unique to Meniere's disease and is seen in acute labyrinthitis, syphilis, and some leukemic states. The author has personally treated a patient with a petrous ridge meningioma that arose from the endolymphatic sac and presented with a fluctuating hearing loss in the low frequencies, persistent tinnitus, and severe incapacitating episodic vertigo. Initially, the patient even responded to a challenge of steroids. Removal of the tumor stabilized the hearing but did not improve it. The symptoms of vertigo also subsided.

The pharmacotherapy in Meniere's disease is designed to reduce the amount of endolymph produced within the membranous labyrinth or to destroy the vestibular end organs within the temporal bone. Endolymph fluid reduction is achieved by dietary restrictions of salt, by diuretic therapy, and possibly, at the inner ear level, by carbonic anhydrase inhibitors such as acetazolamide, although this has not been proved in humans (Watanabe and Ogawa, 1984).

Streptomycin therapy has also been used

to chemically ablate the vestibular labyrinth in patients unable to have vestibular nerve sections (Graham and Kemink, 1984). This use of streptomycin, although toxic to sensory cells, affects the vestibular function first. The drug is given by intramuscular injections on a daily basis while the hearing is constantly followed for a 2-week period.

Surgical treatment for Meniere's disease is designed for patients who fail medical management. The type of surgical procedure used depends on the status of the hearing in the affected ear.

Endolymphatic Sac Decompression. Endolymphatic sac decompression and shunts drain the sac with some type of valve or Silastic stent into the mastoid cavity. This is designed to relieve the pressure in the membranous labyrinth. This procedure is still employed today in patients with good hearing. Success rates vary from center to center, and some feel that sac operations have no further place in the surgical treatment of hydrops. The cure rates range from 35% to 90% with an average of about 67% (Glasscock et al., 1977; Maddox, 1981; Arenberg and Stahle, 1981). Arenberg and Stahle reported a 90% control of vertigo with Arenberg's special unidirectional shunt. Thomsen and coworkers (1981) evaluated the placebo effect of endolymphatic sac surgery and found that patients who underwent a mastoidectomy alone without any manipulation of the sac recovered just as well as those patients who received shunts of mastoid type. House (1964) initially proposed a shunt procedure that drained the sac into the subarachnoid space. However, most surgeons have abandoned this shunt in favor of the type that drains directly into the mastoid.

Vestibular Nerve Section. In patients with intact hearing, most centers are going directly to a retrolabyrinthine vestibular nerve section. Some otolaryngologists still prefer the middle fossa vestibular nerve section, but the results of vertigo control are higher in the retrolabyrinthine procedure: 97% was reported by Silverstein and colleagues (1985), and 94% was reported in the series by Glasscock and associates (1984). Total hearing loss occurs in about 2% of the cases; more than 75% of the patients are maintained near the preoperative level (McElveen et al., 1988).

Translabyrinthine Vestibular Nerve Sec-

tion. This is the most reliable technique and is the procedure to which all others are compared. It is used only when hearing conservation is not an issue. The surgical procedure incorporates not only a vestibular neurectomy but also a labyrinthectomy and sections the nerves in a preganglionic location. Control of vertigo is as high as 98% (Nelson, 1986).

RETROCOCHLEAR LESIONS

Retrocochlear causes of sudden SNHL or fluctuating hearing loss must be considered in the work-up but occupy a small percentage of the cases.

Multiple Sclerosis

Bilateral sudden deafness in multiple sclerosis is known to occur especially in the more advanced disseminated forms. Rarely, however, does multiple sclerosis present in the initial stages as a hearing loss, but it does so as an isolated vestibular lesion in about 5% of the new cases. The pathologic change is due to demyelinization that occurs in the brain and spinal cord. The brain stem evoked response is abnormal with absent or distorted waveforms and prolonged latencies characteristic of a retrocochlear problem (Pfaltz, 1988).

Tumors of the Cerebellopontine Angle

Lesions of the cerebellopotine angle, in order of frequency, include acoustic neuromas, meningioma, cholesterol granuloma, and facial nerve neuroma. Sudden hearing loss as the sole presenting sign of an acoustic neuroma is unusual, although it has been reported in as high as 10% to 15% of the cases in some series (Pensack, 1985). The cause of the sudden loss in angle tumors, especially acoustic neuromas, is thought to be a rapid change in tumor size due to either hemorrhage within the mass or necrosis with secondary vascular compromise. The more common presentation is a slow, steady unilateral loss of cochlear function and tinnitus.

Miscellaneous

Many other more unusual lesions such as sarcoidosis, cortical encephalitis leading to an auditory aphasia, Vogt-Koyanagi-Horada syndrome, carcinomatous neuropathy, and a Guillain-Barré type syndrome have been reported as causal in sudden SNHL, but they are most infrequent (Pfaltz, 1988).

HEARING AIDS

For the patient who does not respond to the various medical therapies and continues to progress with nerve loss, a hearing aid must be considered. Normally a unilateral loss does not require an aid unless there is an absolute indication, such as the need to function in a binaural environment. The most important aspect of hearing aid fitting is to provide the patient with a device that is used regularly and not one that sits in the drawer.

Hearing aids are worn either in the ear or behind the auricle, depending on power needs and canal anatomy. The behind-the-ear model is more conspicuous, has more power, and can be adjusted more easily by the patient with regard to gain and loudness settings. Most of the hearing aids available today can fit into three major categories: (1) analog hearing aids; (2) hybrid hearing aids; and (3) digital hearing aids.

Analog Hearing Aids

This is the traditional hearing aid that has been around for years with constant modifications and gimmicks for enhancing sales. The acoustic signal is converted to an electric signal by a microphone. This electric signal is then acted on by filters, amplifiers, and an auditory gain control device that modifies the characteristics of the signal. The processed signal is then converted back to an acoustic signal and delivered to the ear. One of the changes that has occurred in both analog and digital devices has been the use of compression circuits. These circuits are analogous to the Dolby noise reduction used in audio recordings. The weaker signals of importance are amplified above the noise on the magnetic tape. The electronic circuit compresses or reduces the dynamic range of the signal to fit the channel being recorded. At the receiver end, the signal is re-expanded to establish the dynamic range without the noise. In hearing aids, compression is used against the overamplification of intense sounds that may be unpleasant. In the older

devices, the power output was limited by transistors that prevented amplification over a preset level. With compression, the hearing aid amplifier can limit its output gracefully and at a level that can be adjusted by the professional fitter. This type of compression has no effect at ordinary speech levels but rather becomes operative at the maximal power output of the device that is chosen to suit the tolerance level of the wearer. The net effect is to reduce amplifier gain as the input level increases. This works to make even low-level speech cues audible without overamplification of the intense sounds and thus make the signal more intelligible and comfortable (Walhauer and Villchur, 1988).

Hybrid Hearing Aids

A hybrid hearing aid processes the sound in the same way that an analog device does. The signal is converted to an electric signal by a microphone, acted on by filters, amplifiers, and the auditory gain control circuit, and converted back to an acoustic signal. The difference is that the operation on the electric signal is accomplished by digital circuits in the hearing aid. The parameters of control are computer generated externally and stored within the device. The parameters are used to set the gain, filter frequencies, and adjust the gain control. The advantage is that many configurations can be generated by computer to work on the electric signal, much as a graphic equalizer does in a stereo system. This allows more independent and precise control of the settings, which are always reprogrammable for different environments. The disadvantages are that these devices are more expensive than analog aids, are more difficult to fit, and require a dedication for programming them.

Digital Hearing Aids

Digital aids process the acoustic signal differently from the analog or hybrid devices. The acoustic signal is converted to an electric signal by the microphone, which is then sampled by an analog to digital converter. This means that the voltage amplitude of the electric signal is measured at fixed intervals of time and assigned a number that corresponds to a given amplitude value. The numbers are then stored in the computer within the aid. The signal no longer represents a physical or electric entity but rather represents a series of numbers that describe the signal. The processing of the signal is then accomplished by mathematical manipulations on the numbers, which generate new numbers that are converted back to an electric signal by a digital to analog converter. The analog signal is changed back to an acoustic signal at the receiver. The signal-processing capabilities are endless and can be reprogrammed to fit the desired needs of the patient. The disadvantages are cost, size, and power consumption, as well as the infinite capabilities of programming, which can serve as a dilemma for the programmer.

Cochlear Implants

Since the 1970s, interest in multichannel cochlear implants has led to many clinical and basic science advances. Today, more than 3000 patients with profound bilateral sensorineural hearing loss have received cochlear implants. This is most gratifying to the physician, who can provide sound to a patient who was previously isolated from the outside world. In June of 1990, the Food and Drug Administration approved the 22-channel cochlear implant, manufactured by the Nucleus Corporation (Englewood, Colorado), for children aged 3 to 18 years. These are post- or perilingual children who have bilateral profound hearing loss with no help from conventional amplification devices. The initial studies in children also included some prelingual recipients, who have a much more involved and rigorous rehabilitation postoperatively.

The device is surgically implanted in the basal turn of the cochlea and advanced about 1.5 cm along the spiral lamina. A standard mastoidectomy is performed with inclusion of a wide opening of the facial recess. The cochleostomy is made just above the round window, with care being taken to verify the true basal turn rather than a hypotympanic air cell tract. The patients are usually kept in the hospital overnight with an indwelling suction drain. Stimulation and programming take place in 4 to 6 weeks. Acceptance by the patients has been high: more than 90% of the recipients use the device more than 12 hours per day. All patients gain sound awareness, more than 90% have improved lip reading skills, and as many as 60% to 75% have open set discrimination.

The characteristic that separates the various available implants is the number of electrodes available and the coding strategy. The Nucleus 22-channel device uses a feature extraction strategy by which the sound is analyzed according to its fundamental frequency F_0, which provides a rate pitch analysis, as well as formants F_1 thru F_5. The formants are mathematically selected energy peaks that describe the acoustic signal. The last three formants have recently been added to the sound processor, which essentially gives three high-pass filters for further characterization of the sound. In this way, the energy from the filters can be assigned to certain electrodes along the 22-channel array, which are programmed to fire in bipolar or bipolar plus N configuration where N is the number of electrodes between the stimulating electrode and the sink electrode. This strategy serves to enhance speech understanding. It is quite clear that as the number of electrodes increases and the maximal number of formants used increases, so does the speech discrimination (Holmes et al., 1987; Walhauer and Villchur, 1988).

What is actually being stimulated in the damaged cochlea is uncertain. Most agree that the recipient of stimulation must be either the spiral ganglion cells or the remaining auditory nerve fibers. Most centers attempt to determine preoperatively the relative number of auditory neurons that have survived the insult. This determination is usually made through a transtympanic electric promontory stimulation. These data are far from precise but give an idea of the future success of the patient.

As cochlear implants gain acceptance worldwide, it becomes more evident that the learning curve with rehabilitation in postlingual adults is virtually open ended. The single-channel device is no longer being manufactured in favor of multiple-channel implants that provide increased speech discrimination capabilities. The product reliability has been quite good for the Nucleus device. A 1% implanted hardware failure rate worldwide is reported. The major drawback at the present time is cost. At present, the average hospital bill for an overnight stay is approximately $35,000. Most insurance companies pay for the implant but balk at the rehabilitation expenses. Medicare covers cochlear implants, but none of the Medicaid type plans underwrite implantation.

The present level of technology has merely

scratched the surface and opened the door for more research and advancements in sound processing and coding strategies. The future certainly looks a lot brighter for the profoundly impaired patient. Being able to offer a patient renewed sound exposure is truly a rewarding part of otology.

SUGGESTED READINGS

References

Althaus SR: Perilymphatic fistulas. Laryngoscope 91:538–562, 1981.

Arenberg IK, Stahle J: Endolymphatic sac operations for Meniere's disease. Am J Otol 2:329–334, 1981.

Byl FM: Sudden hearing loss: eight years' experience and suggested prognostic table. Laryngoscope 94:647–661, 1984.

Dovek EE, Dodson HC, Bunnister HC: The effects of sodium salicylate on the cochlea of the guinea pig. J Laryngol Otol 93:793–797, 1983.

Fraser GR: The genetics of thyroid disease. Prog Med Genet 6:89–115, 1969.

Ganz BJ, Tyler RS: Cochlear implant comparisons. Am J Otol 92 (Suppl):92–95, 1985.

Glasscock ME, Kveton JF, Christiansen SG: Middle fossa vestibular neurectomy: an update. Otolaryngol Head Neck Surg 92:216–220, 1984.

Glasscock ME, Miller GW, Drake FD, et al: Surgical management of Meniere's disease with the endolymphatic subarachnoid shunt. A five year study. Laryngoscope 87:1668–1675, 1977.

Goodhill V: The idiopathic group and the labyrinthine group. Approaches to sudden sensorineural hearing loss. *In* Snow JB (ed): Controversies in Otolaryngology (pp 12–22). Philadelphia: WB Saunders, 1980.

Goodhill V, Harris I, Brockman SJ: Sudden deafness and labyrinthine window rupture. Ann Otol Rhinol Laryngol 82:2–17, 1973.

Graham MD, Kemink JL: Titration streptomycin therapy for Meniere's disease, a progress report. Am J Otol 5:534–535, 1984.

Gussen R: Scala vestibuli partition with deafness and renal disease. Ann Otol Rhinol Laryngol 82:871–875, 1973.

Harris JP: Immunology of the inner ear: response of the inner ear to antigenic challenge. Otolaryngol Head Neck Surg 91:17–23, 1983.

Harris JP: Experimental autoimmune sensorineural hearing loss. Laryngoscope 97:63–76, 1987.

Harris JP: Immunologic Mechanisms in Disorders of the Inner Ear. Course Outline (pp 37–52, personal communication). San Francisco Otology Update, 1989.

Hawkins JE, Johnson LG: Histopathology of cochlear and vestibular ototoxicity in laboratory animals. *In* Lerner JS, et al (eds): Aminoglycoside Ototoxicity (pp 175–214). Boston: Little, Brown, 1981.

Hendershot EL: Luetic deafness. Laryngoscope 83:865–870, 1973.

Holmes AE, Kemker FJ, Merwin GE: The effects of varying the number of cochlear implant electrodes on speech perception. Am J Otol 8:240–247, 1987.

House WF: Subarachnoid shunt for drainage of hydrops:

a report of 63 cases. Arch Otolaryngol 79:338–342, 1964.

Hughes EC, Gott PS, Weinstein RC: Effects of hemorrheologic blood modifiers on speech intelligibility of the sensorineural hearing impaired in high noise. Laryngoscope (submitted for publication).

Hulcrantz E: Clinical treatment of vascular inner ear disease. Am J Otolaryngol 9:317–322, 1988.

Illum P, Kiaer HW, Hvidberg-Hansen J, et al: Fifteen cases of Pendred's syndrome. Arch Otolaryngol 96:297–304, 1972.

Jackler RK, Luxford WM, House WF: Congenital malformations of the inner ear: a classification based upon embryogenesis. Laryngoscope 97:2–14, 1987.

Jaffe BF: Sudden deafness; a local manifestation of systemic disorders: fat emboli, hypercoagulation and infection. Laryngoscope 80:788–801, 1970.

La Rouere MJ, Sillman JS, Nuttall AL, Miller JM: A comparison of laser Doppler and intravital microscopy measurements of cochlear blood flow. Otolaryngol Head Neck Surg 10:373–384, 1989.

Love JT: Basilar artery migraine presenting as a fluctuating hearing loss and vertigo. J Otolaryngol 86:450–455, 1978.

Makishima K, Tanaka K: Pathologic changes of the inner ear and central auditory pathways in diabetes. Ann Otol Rhinol Laryngol 80:218–223, 1971.

Maddox HE: Surgery of the endolymphatic sac. Laryngoscope 91:1058–1062, 1981.

Mattox DE, Simmons FB: Natural history of sudden sensorineural hearing loss. Ann Otol Rhinol Laryngol 86:463–480, 1977.

McCabe BF: Autoimmune sensorineural hearing loss. Ann Otol Rhinol Laryngol 88:585–589, 1979.

McElveen JT, Shelton CL, Hittselberger NE, et al: Retrolabyrinthine vestibular nerve section: a reevaluation. Laryngoscope 98:502–506, 1988.

Meyerhoff WL, Paparella MM: Medical therapy for sudden deafness. *In* Snow JB (ed): Controversy in Otolaryngology (pp 3–11). Philadelphia: WB Saunders, 1980.

Morimitsu T: New theory and therapy of sudden deafness. *In* Shaumbaugh G, Shea J (eds): Proceedings of the Shambaugh 5th International Workshop on Middle Ear Surgery and Fluctuating Hearing Loss (p 10). Huntsville: Strode, 1977.

Nadol JB, Wilson WR: Treatment of sudden hearing loss is illogical. *In* Snow JB (ed): Controversy in Otolaryngology (pp 22–32). Philadelphia: WB Saunders, 1988.

Nelson RA: Surgery for control of vertigo. *In* Wiet RJ, Causse (eds): Complications in Otolaryngology Head and Neck Surgery. Ear and Skull Base, vol 1 (pp 149–159). Philadelphia: BC Decker, 1986.

Pensak M: Sudden hearing loss and cerebellopontine angle tumors. Laryngoscope 95:1188–1193, 1985.

Pfaltz CR: Sudden and fluctuating hearing loss. *In* Alberti PW, Ruben RJ (eds): Otologic Medicine and Surgery, vol II (pp 1577–1603). New York: Churchill Livingstone, 1988.

Prazma J: Ototoxicity of diuretics. *In* Brown, Daingneault (eds): Pharmacology of Hearing (pp 197–229). New York: John Wiley, 1981.

Reilly JS: Congenital perilymphatic fistula: a prospective study in infants and children. Laryngoscope 99:393–397, 1989.

Schuknecht HF: Pathology of the Ear. Cambridge: Harvard University Press, 1974.

Shaia FT, Sheehy JL: Sudden sensorineural hearing impairment (report of 1220 cases). Laryngoscope 86:389–398, 1976.

Shelton CL, Simmons FB: Perilymphatic fistula: the Stanford experience. Ann Otol Rhinol Laryngol 97:105–108, 1988.

Silverstein H, McDaniel A, Wazen J, et al: Retrolabyrinthine vestibular neurectomy with simultaneous monitoring of the eighth nerve and brainstem auditory evoked potentials. Otolaryngol Head Neck Surg 93:736–742, 1985.

Strauss M, Towfighi J, Lord S, et al: Cis-platinum ototoxicity: clinical experience and temporal bone histopathology. Laryngoscope 93:1554–1559, 1983.

Thomsen J, Bretlau P, Tos M, et al: Placebo effect in surgery for Meniere's disease. Arch Otolaryngol 107:221–227, 1981.

Van Canegham D: La sordite subite. Acta Otorhinolaryngol Belg 121:5–17, 1958.

Veldman JE, Roord JJ, O'Conor AF, Shea JJ: Autoimmunity and inner ear disorders: an immune complex mediated sensorineural hearing loss. Laryngoscope 94:501–507, 1984.

Wagner JA, Oliver BM, Snyder SH: Aminoglycoside effects on voltage sensitive calcium channels and neurotoxicity. N Engl J Med 317:1669–1670, 1987.

Walhauer F, Villchur E: Full dynamic range multiband compression in a hearing aid. Hear J Sept: 1–4, 1988.

Watanabe K, Ogawa A: Carbonic anhydrase activity in the stria vascularis and dark cells in the vestibular labyrinth. Ann Otol Rhinol Laryngol 93:262–266, 1984.

Weiner ND, Schacht J: Biochemical model of aminoglycoside induced hearing loss. *In* Lerner et al (eds): Aminoglycoside Ototoxicity (pp 113–121). Boston: Little, Brown, 1981.

West BA, Brummett RE, Himes DL: Interaction of kanamycin and ethacrynic acid. Arch Otolaryngol 98:32–37, 1973.

Winter LW, Cram BM, Banovitz JD: Hearing loss in hereditary renal disease. Arch Otolaryngol 88:238–241, 1968.

CHAPTER 13

Otalgia

William L. Meyerhoff, MD, PhD   Patrick H. Pownell, MD

Otalgia (ear pain) is a symptom that does not always signify primary ear disease; rather, it may represent referred pain from a regional or distant abnormality. For the sake of clarification, otalgia can therefore be divided into that caused by local disease, that caused by regional disease, and that caused by disease at a distant site. Ear pain from local causes originates from pathologic changes in the auricle, the external auditory canal, the tympanic membrane, and the middle ear cleft. Regional ear pain is defined as pain that is experienced in the ear but whose true source is referred from dental-related causes or temporomandibular joint abnormalities. Distant causes of otalgia are those arising from pathologic processes in other areas of the upper aerodigestive tract and, rarely, the cardiovascular system. In the adult population, it is estimated that 50% of patients complaining of ear pain are suffering from local disease, and the remainder are actually experiencing regional or distant disease. For better understanding of the many causes of ear pain, the complex neural pathways from the auricle, the external ear canal, the tympanic membrane, the middle ear, and the surrounding head and neck regions must be understood.

NEUROANATOMY

The sensory and motor distribution of the head and neck region represents the most complex network of neural innervation in humans. Sensory fibers can be divided into general sensory (general somatic afferent), special sensory (special afferent), and visceral sensory (general visceral afferent) neurons. General sensory fibers are afferent neurons responsible for pain, temperature, touch, and proprioception. The general sensory fibers innervating the auricle, the external ear canal, the tympanic membrane, the middle ear, and the remainder of the head and neck involve an intricate system of fibers from cranial nerves V, VII, IX, and X as well as sensory fibers from the second, third, fourth, and fifth cervical roots. Special sensory neurons are defined as those responsible for smell, vision, taste, balance, and hearing and include the olfactory, optic, facial, vestibulocochlear, and glossopharyngeal nerves. Visceral sensory fibers represent information necessary for visceral reflexes such as swallowing and are contained in cranial nerves IX and X.

Motor fibers are subdivided into somatic motor (general somatic efferent), branchial motor (special visceral efferent), and visceral motor (general visceral efferent) neurons. Somatic motor fibers consist of voluntary motor neurons from cranial nerves III, IV, VI, and XII innervating the extraocular muscles and the majority of the intrinsic and extrinsic tongue muscles. Branchial motor fibers are those supplying voluntary muscles from the branchial complexes and include cranial nerves V, VII, IX, and X. Visceral motor fibers are autonomic fibers supplying the head and neck region and include fibers from cranial nerves III, VII, IX, and X.

To begin the understanding of otalgia, the general sensory (general somatic afferent) innervation to the auricle, the external ear canal, the tympanic membrane, and the middle ear is reviewed. The neural distributions are quite variable from individual to individual, but generalities can be described (Fig. 13–1).

Cranial Nerve V. The auriculotemporal branch of the mandibular division of the trigeminal nerve provides general sensory innervation to the skin of the tragus, the anterior half of the external auditory canal, and the anterior half of the tympanic membrane. Sometimes the superior wall of the external auditory canal, the anterior limb of the helix, and a portion of the crus can be supplied by this branch as well. Evidence also exists suggesting that the trigeminal nerve provides some sensory innervation to the middle ear and the eustachian tube.

Cranial Nerve VII. The facial nerve supplies general somatic afferent fibers to variable portions of the external auditory canal, the concha, and the posterior tympanic membrane. At times, a portion of the postauricular skin is also supplied by this branch. Hitzelberger's sign represents hypesthesia of the posterior wall of the external auditory canal believed to be due to early compression of the facial nerve by a cerebellopontine angle lesion.

Cranial Nerve IX. The tympanic branch of the glossopharyngeal nerve joins the superior and inferior caroticotympanic branches of the sympathetic plexus of the internal carotid artery to form the tympanic plexus. This plexus supplies the majority of the general sensory innervation to the middle ear cleft and to the medial surface of the tympanic membrane.

Cranial Nerve X. The auricular branch of the vagus nerve (Arnold's nerve) supplies general somatic afferent innervation to the inferior and posterior walls of the external auditory canal and the remainder of the posterior part of the tympanic membrane.

Cervical Branches. The greater auricular nerves (C2, C3) and the lesser occipital nerve (C2) supply general sensory fibers to the cranial surface and the posterior part of the lateral surface of the auricle.

Regional and Distant Neuroanatomy

Regional and distant disease can manifest as ear pain via referred neural pathways. Referred pain can be defined as that pain experienced in a part of the body distant from its true source. The most commonly accepted explanation for referred otalgia is the complex neural convergences of cranial nerves V,

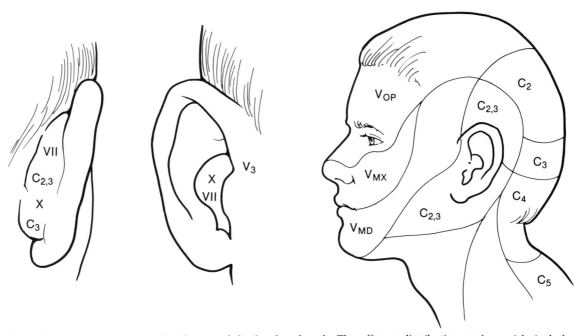

Figure 13–1. General sensory distribution of the head and neck. The afferent distribution to the auricle includes cranial nerves V, VII, and X with second and third cervical root fibers.

VII, IX, and X with the spinal tract nucleus of the trigeminal nerve. This spinal tract descends from the caudal pons and medulla to the level of C2 and C3. This convergence of cranial nerves with the upper cervical nerve along somatic afferents in the brain stem provides a logical explanation for the occurrence of referred pain from the head and neck to the ear.

Any pathologic process in regions that are supplied by the nerves that also innervate the ear may therefore cause referred or secondary otalgia. A review of the sensory and motor fibers of the nerves that provide sensory innervation to the ear will be discussed. Again, these represent generalities because of the great variability that exists between individuals.

Cranial Nerve V. The trigeminal nerve is the largest cranial nerve, and it has the most extensive distribution in the head and neck. This nerve is divided into three major branches: ophthalmic, maxillary, and mandibular. This nerve essentially supplies general sensory fibers to the face and anterior scalp. It also supplies the conjunctiva, the bulb of the eye, the mucous membranes of the paranasal sinuses, the nasal and oral cavities (including tongue and teeth), the temporomandibular joint, the parotid region, and the meninges of the anterior and middle cranial fossae. In addition, the nerve supplies branchial motor fibers to the muscles of mastication and the tensor tympani, the tensor veli palantini, the mylohyoid, and the anterior belly of the digastric muscles.

Cranial Nerve VII. The majority of fibers within cranial nerve VII constitute branchial motor fibers innervating the stapedius muscle, the stylohyoid muscle, and the posterior belly of the digastric muscles. It also supplies the muscles of facial expression and the buccinator, platysma, and occipitalis muscles. The remaining fibers enter the internal auditory canal as a distinctly separate group termed the *nervus intermedius*. Included within this nerve are visceral motor, general sensory, and special sensory branches. Also parasympathetic fibers and visceral motor fibers arise from the superior salivary nucleus and divide into three branches at the geniculate ganglion. One division, the greater petrosal nerve, gains fibers from the deep petrosal nerve to then become the vidian nerve.

This nerve travels with a division of cranial nerve V to supply the lacrimal, palatine, and nasal glands. The second branch joins the fibers from the inferior salivary nucleus of cranial nerve IX to become the lesser petrosal nerve, which innervates the parotid gland. The third division courses with the chorda tympani nerve through the middle ear. It then travels with the lingual branch of the trigeminal nerve and sends parasympathetic fibers to the sublingual and submaxillary glands. Special sensory fibers form the chorda tympani nerve, which supplies taste from the anterior two thirds of the tongue and the hard and soft palates. The general sensory fibers are described earlier.

Cranial Nerve IX. The glossopharyngeal nerve supplies fibers to the oronasopharynx and the superior hypopharynx. Branchial motor fibers supply only the stylopharyngeus muscle. Visceral motor fibers, which constitute Jacobson's nerve, arise from the inferior salivatory nucleus in the brain stem and course through the middle ear with a branch of cranial nerve IX that carries parasympathetic fibers to the parotid gland along with the previously mentioned fibers from cranial nerve VII. Visceral sensory fibers carry information from the carotid body and from the carotid sinus. General sensory pathways constitute those previously mentioned as well as sensation from the posterior third of the tongue. Special sensory fibers innervate taste receptors in the posterior third of the tongue.

Cranial Nerve X. The vagus nerve supplies branchial motor fibers to the striated muscles of the pharynx, the tongue (palatoglossus), and the larynx (except the stylopharyngeus [IX] and the tensor veli palatini [V3]). Visceral motor fibers innervate the smooth muscles and glands of the pharynx, the larynx, and the thoracic and abdominal viscera. Visceral sensory fibers arise from the larynx, the trachea, the esophagus, and the thoracic and abdominal viscera. Fibers also arise from receptors in the walls of the aortic arch and chemoreceptors in the aortic bodies adjacent to the arch. General sensory fibers include Arnold's nerve to the inferior and posterior external auditory canal which innervate the oropharynx, the hypopharynx, and the larynx. The bronchial branch contains general sensory fibers from the trachea and the bronchi. The visceral afferents from the thoracic and abdominal viscera have been reported to be sympathetic neurons, but otalgia from these regions in selected patients has been described.

Cervical Branches. The greater auricular nerve (C2, C3) supplies general sensation from the skin of the face over the parotid gland and the skin over the mastoid process. The lesser occipital nerve (C2) supplies general sensation from the posterior scalp behind the auricle. The spinal accessory nerve (cranial nerve XI) arises from the upper cervical spinal cord and consists of motor fibers to supply the sternocleidomastoid and the trapezius muscles.

EVALUATION OF THE PATIENT WITH EAR PAIN

A careful history is the first step leading to an accurate diagnosis in the cause of ear pain. Knowledge regarding onset, character, attributing factors, and time and frequency of the pain is useful in helping distinguish the source of the pain. Identification of associated medical conditions such as temporomandibular joint disease, significant dental disease, weight loss, and gastrointestinal disorders can be helpful in diagnosis. Past medical history can also be helpful for establishing an association with other medical conditions.

The physical examination begins with a careful evaluation of the auricle and the surrounding skin. Otoscopic and microscopic examination follows in an effort to identify any local causes for the ear pain that arise from the external canal or tympanic membrane. Careful evaluation of the cranial nerves is the essential next step. The remainder of the examination centers on any abnormalities of the oral cavity, the oropharynx, the nasopharynx, the larynx, or any specific area of the head, the neck, or the thorax. These areas are the source of most referred pain caused by regional and distant lesions. Further examination can then be performed as the history directs.

Otalgia can be subdivided into that caused by local factors, that caused by regional factors, and that caused by distant factors. A differential diagnosis of otalgia with concern

to these divisions is presented in the remainder of the text.

Local Ear Pain

Local ear pain originates from the auricle, the external auditory canal, the tympanic membrane, and the middle ear cleft. The pathologic process is usually easily identified with a careful history and physical examination. A microscopic examination, however, should always be included if no apparent source is easily identified. Common causes of primary otalgia are listed in Table 13–1 and can be grouped into general categories of trauma, infection and inflammation, neoplasm, degeneration, and idiopathic causes.

Auricle

Trauma to the auricle is a common source of otalgia. Severe sunburn or chemical burn is quite painful because of the relatively thin skin of the auricle and its firm attachment of the perichondrium. Lacerations of the auricle can of course cause ear pain and require careful reapproximation of the cartilage and the soft tissue components. Blunt trauma to

TABLE 13–1. Local Causes of Otalgia

Auricle
  Trauma
  Perichondritis
  Abscess of the auricle
  Malignant or benign growth
  Radiation-induced chondritis
  Relapsing polychondritis
  Winkler's disease
  Frostbite of the auricle
External Auditory Canal
  Otitis externa
  Furunculosis
  Foreign body
  Impacted cerumen
  Malignant otitis externa
  Herpes zoster oticus
  Malignant or benign growth
  Fungal infections (otomycosis)
  Trauma
Tympanic Membrane or Middle Ear
  Acute otitis media
  Acute mastoiditis
  Acute aero-otitis media (barotrauma)
  Bullous myringitis
  Acute eustachian tube obstruction
  Complications of chronic otitis media
    and cholesteatoma
  Trauma
  Malignant or benign growth

the auricle can cause otalgia, and careful attention must be placed on the possibility of a subperichondrial hematoma. Such lesions require incision and drainage for prevention of a "cauliflower ear" deformity.

Infection or inflammation of the auricle is usually related to previous trauma or burn. A change in the characteristics of a previously injured auricle or an increase in the intensity of pain is the hallmark of the onset of bacterial perichondritis. This infection can quickly destroy the helical and conchal cartilage because of the relatively poor vascularity to the auricle. Careful and meticulous wound care combined with prophylactic antibiotics is the key to preventing this dreaded wound infection. Should perichondritis occur, wound debridement and drainage should be performed as soon as possible, in combination with large doses of intravenous antibiotics.

The auricle is a common site for sun-induced skin malignancies. The most common sites for such malignancies are those receiving the most sun exposure: the helical and antihelical regions. Wide local excision is usually curative, but larger malignant lesions require a superficial parotidectomy for removal of the first level of draining lymphatics. Severe otalgia usually suggests perichondrial invasion, and excision should be performed to include the cartilage.

Patients who have received radiation therapy can suffer from ear pain that is due to radiation-induced chondritis. Careful observation and treatment of radiation burns with acidic solutions is needed for prevention of perichondritis.

Relapsing polychondritis represents an autoimmune connective tissue disorder characterized by recurring episodes of inflammation of the cartilages of the ear, the nose, the larynx, and the joints. Otalgia is accompanied by polyarthralgias, nasal deformity, and often a high-frequency sensorineural hearing loss. Diagnosis is made on the basis of history and nonspecific autoimmune laboratory analysis such as an elevated erythrocyte sedimentation rate. Biopsy of the affected cartilage may be needed for confirmation of the diagnosis. Treatment must be directed toward the autoimmune cause and includes systemic steroids and occasionally cytotoxic agents.

Chondrodermatitis nodularis chronica helicis, or Winkler's disease, is a rare condition of unknown origin that affects the auricle. The lesion is usually noted at the top of the helix in elderly men. Patients may present with complaints of pain when recumbent with the ear on a pillow. On histologic examination, this lesion consists of tiny lesions similar to a glomus lesion. Surgical excision is curative.

External Auditory Canal

The external ear canal is commonly a site for primary otalgia. Otitis externa represents the most common cause of ear pain from the external canal. Trauma from a cotton-tipped applicator or water in the external canal is a frequent predisposing factor in this type of infection. Of note, the pain usually intensifies during the late night or early morning because of edema associated with the supine position. Occasionally, this pain can be quite severe and can incapacitate the patient. The tragus is usually tender on palpation, and an inflamed canal is noted. Bacteriologic cause is usually *Pseudomonas aeruginosa*. Treatment involves careful clearing of debris from the canal and topical otic drugs directed toward the inflammation and infection. In cases in which swelling obstructs the canal, a wick is of benefit to allow better penetration of the otic drops. Furunculosis represents an inflammatory process of a hair follicle inside or surrounding the canal. The responsible microorganism is usually *Staphylococcus aureus*, and simple incision and drainage is curative. A foreign body in the external ear canal may be hidden in a cerumen impaction and involved in the pathogenesis of external otitis. Careful microscopic removal without injuring the canal is necessary. Examination and removal while the patient is anesthetized may be required for pediatric patients.

Malignant otitis externa represents an osteomyelitis of the temporal bone and possibly the skull base. The otalgia is usually described as boring pain that peaks in severity in the early morning hours. Granulation tissue may be present in the posterior external auditory canal at the bone-cartilage juncture, although the physical findings are usually minor in comparison with the pain described by the patient. *P. aeruginosa* is the usual pathogen, and the usual patient is diabetic or immunocompromised and has been suffering from otitis externa for some time. The facial nerve is the cranial nerve most commonly involved, and its involvement worsens the prognosis. Treatment should include a systemic aminoglycoside in combination with a third-generation penicillin effective against *Pseudomonas*. The oral macrolide antibiotics have also shown effectiveness as single-agent coverage with avoidance of long-term hospitalization. Surgical intervention is necessary only in refractory cases. Mortality may approach 20% despite the advances in surgical and antibiotic therapy.

Herpes zoster oticus (Ramsay Hunt syndrome) causes an intense otalgia that is out of proportion to the usual physical findings. In addition, the pain may precede the physical findings by several days. The etiologic organism is the varicella zoster virus that has invaded the geniculate ganglia to remain dormant until reactivation occurs. The physical examination findings include tender vesicles on an erythematous base that involve the auricle, the external auditory canal, and possibly the tympanic membrane. In some cases, the palate may be involved as well. The facial nerve is usually paretic to some degree, and recovery occurs in only approximately 40% of patients in whom complete paralysis occurs.

Malignant and benign growths of the external auditory canal can cause primary otalgia. These lesions are usually easily detected by physical examination, although with an early neoplasm involving the ear canal, the examination may appear normal. In the occult lesion, placement of the ear speculum or gentle instrument palpation may elicit the pain, which suggests that deep biopsy should be performed for identifying these early lesions as soon as possible.

Tympanic Membrane and Middle Ear

Most conditions causing primary otalgia arising from the tympanic membrane, the middle ear, and the mastoid are infectious and should be recognized easily with otoscopic or microscopic evaluation. Acute otitis media is the most common finding, especially in the pediatric population. A history of a recent upper respiratory tract infection can accompany the acute symptoms. Intense otalgia is usually reported, and an inflamed tympanic membrane with decreased mobility is noted. Suppurative perforation of the tympanic membrane usually greatly reduces the pain as a result of the reduction of pressure in the middle ear cleft. Treatment involves oral antibiotics directed toward *Streptococcus pneu-*

moniae, Haemophilus influenzae, group A *Streptococcus*, and *Branhamella catarrhalis*. Of note, chronic otitis media from cholesteatoma or chronic mastoiditis usually does not cause significant ear pain. Should pain occur in this condition, a complication of chronic otitis media, such as abscess formation or petrous apicitis (Gradenigo's syndrome), should be suspected. Computed tomography scan should be obtained for further investigation as soon as possible, and surgery should not be delayed.

Bullous myringitis is a virus-induced inflammation of the tympanic membrane that causes severe otalgia. In adults, the condition is usually associated with a concurrent viral illness. In children, bacteria similar to those causing acute otitis media have also been implicated. On physical examination, the tympanic membrane contains hemorrhages or serous-filled bullae. Treatment involves supportive care and oral antibiotics when indicated.

Barotrauma resulting from diving or flying may cause acute and intense otalgia. The tympanic membrane surface may contain small hemorrhages, or gross hemotympanum may develop because of the injury. Treatment is also supportive, and prophylactic antibiotics are elective.

Eustachian tube dysfunction with relative negative pressure in the middle ear can cause otalgia. This can be a chronic problem or can be associated acutely with an upper respiratory tract infection. Diagnosis is made with pneumatic otoscopy or with impedance testing. Treatment is usually supportive with decongestants and pain control until the eustachian tube function returns to normal.

Regional Ear Pain

Regional ear pain can be defined as pain that is experienced in the ear but whose true source is referred from dental-related causes or temporomandibular joint abnormalities (Table 13–2). This type of pain represents the most common form of referred pain to the ear. For this reason, a careful examination of the oral cavity must follow in the patient who has both otalgia and a normal otologic examination. Dental neuralgias that are due to carious or abscessed teeth of the mandibular molars are referred to the ear via the mandibular branch of the trigeminal nerve. Unerupted or impacted teeth are also a common

TABLE 13–2. Regional Causes of Otalgia

Dental neuralgias
  Dentine exposed, pulp inflamed, or nerves dying
  Unerupted or impacted molars or wisdom teeth
  Traumatic occlusion of teeth, faulty jaw closure, and
    improperly fitting denture
  Teething
Bruxism
Temporomandibular joint disease
Myofacial pain dysfunction syndrome
Malignant or benign growths

cause of otalgia because of local infections surrounding the tooth, causing pain fiber excitation. When indicated, an anesthetic block of the nerve supplying the suspected tooth can be performed for diagnostic relief of the pain.

Bruxism is another cause of referred otalgia. This condition is due to nocturnal or daytime grinding of teeth that is usually related to stress. Many of these patients do not recognize their condition, and family members must witness and report the activity. Otalgia is frequently noted bilaterally, and on physical examination, wear facets are noted on the canine teeth. Treatment consists of bite appliances and behavior conditioning. Medical treatment with tricyclic antidepressants is used only in refractory cases.

Temporomandibular joint disease has long been known as a common cause of otalgia. Many patients with this syndrome report otalgia as their most common or only complaint. Any pathologic change of the joint can be the source of the referred pain. Previous trauma can be a common initiator of the derangement, with accelerated osteoarthritis thereafter involving the joint. A locking, clicking, or crunching sound may be elicited with joint movement. Other symptoms may include retro-orbital headaches, facial pain, tinnitus, and facial paresthesias. Treatment involves anti-inflammatory agents, physiotherapy, variable appliances, and, rarely, surgical interventions on the joint.

A syndrome related to temporomandibular joint disease is the myofascial pain dysfunction syndrome, or Costen's syndrome. The syndrome, first described in 1934, consists of otalgia, temporomandibular joint dysfunction, facial neuralgias, tinnitus, dizziness, headache, trismus, and tenderness of the temporalis muscle, the sternocleidomastoid muscle, and other muscles of mastica-

tion. This syndrome is believed also to be stress related, and it is important to identify the underlying psychologic component for treatment success. The typical patient is a young adult female with complaints of these symptoms over months to years. On physical examination, tenderness of the sternocleidomastoid, masticatory muscles, and posterior neck muscles is noted in the majority of cases. The actual cause of the cochleovestibular findings is to date not fully explained. Treatment involves anti-inflammatory agents, physical therapy, muscle relaxants, and referral for the underlying psychologic cause.

Benign or malignant neoplasms of the mandible or maxilla are uncommon causes of regional otalgia but must be considered when the physical examination directs. Screening radiographic studies can be obtained with plain films or a Panorex view. Computed tomography scanning will better define a mass when present, and biopsy is needed to confirm the diagnosis. Treatment is designed once the malignant or benign nature is determined.

Distant Causes of Otalgia

Distant causes of otalgia are defined as those causes of referred pain arising from pathologic processes in other areas of the upper aerodigestive tract and, rarely, the thoracic cardiovascular system (Table 13–3). The involved areas include those innervated by cranial nerves V, IX, or X and the upper cervical roots (Fig. 13–2).

Lesions involving the nasal cavity and nasopharynx are an uncommon source of otalgia referred via the second division of the trigeminal nerve and the pharyngeal plexus. Inflammation due to sinusitis can cause the usual manifestations of maxillary pain, facial fullness, and headache as well as otalgia. Treatment is antibiotic therapy with aggressive nasal hygiene. Benign or malignant neoplasms of the nasal cavity or the nasopharynx can occasionally cause otalgia as an accompanying symptom. Treatment is directed to the eradication of the neoplasm.

Any inflammatory process, malignant or benign growth, or ulceration involving the oral cavity, the oropharynx, or the hypopharynx can present with otalgia as the only symptom or as part of a symptom complex. The pharyngeal plexus, consisting of cranial nerves IX and X, constitutes the sensory

TABLE 13–3. Distant Causes of Otalgia

Nasal Cavity and Nasopharynx
  Sinusitis
  Malignant or benign growth
Oral Cavity and Pharyngeal Lesions
  Acute glossitis or stomatitis
  Pharyngitis
  Acute tonsillitis (palatine, lingual, pharyngeal)
  Peritonsillar abscess
  Retropharyngeal abscess
  Ulceration
  Post adenoidectomy or tonsillectomy
  Malignant or benign growth (especially tonsil
    or tongue)
Larynx
  Ulceration
  Perichondritis and chondritis
  Arthritis of cricoarytenoid joint
  Malignant or benign growth
Esophagus
  Foreign body
  Hiatal hernia
  Gastroesophageal reflux
  Malignant or benign growth
Lung and Bronchus
  Inflammation or infection
  Malignant or benign growth
Cardiovascular System
  Angina pectoris
  Thoracic or innominate artery aneurysm
Cervical Spine
  Osteoarthritis
  Whiplash injury
  Subluxation of the atlantoaxial joint
  Malignant or benign growth
Idiopathic (Ticlike Pain Confined to the Ear)
  Geniculate complex of cranial nerve VII
  Tympanic branch of cranial nerve IX

afferent fibers in this setting. Tonsillopharyngitis can be a common cause of referred otalgia, especially in the pediatric population. Otalgia is also a common complaint after tonsillectomy or adenoidectomy and is due to this same referred pathway. In the adult population, a complaint of otalgia with a normal otologic examination represents a tonsillar or a base-of-tongue malignancy until proved otherwise. This area of the pharynx represents a common site for occult lesions, and a careful examination is absolutely necessary for identifying these lesions, especially in the high-risk smoking and alcohol-abusing population.

Laryngeal lesions are also an uncommon cause of referred otalgia. The superior laryngeal branch of the vagus nerve allows pain to originate in the larynx and to be referred to the ear. Physical examination in this region requires careful indirect or fiberoptic evaluation. Ulceration from trauma, infection, or

neoplasm usually manifests with symptoms of hoarseness and swallowing complaints, but it may also manifest with associated otalgia. Arthritis of the cricoarytenoid joint may be present in the arthritic patient and may in unusual cases manifest with ear pain. Diagnosis is made on the basis of flexible laryngoscopy and direct palpation of the joint while the patient is under general anesthesia.

The stylohyoid syndrome (Eagle's syndrome) represents an elongation of the styloid process or an ossification of the stylohyoid ligament that manifests as facial or neck pain, dysphagia, restricted movement of the neck, and otalgia. Tenderness of the tonsillar fossa and radiographic findings confirm the diagnosis. Treatment involves anti-inflammatory agents or possible surgical excision of the styloid process or ossified ligament.

Otalgia can be referred from distant visceral organs, usually via the vagus nerve. Esophageal malignancy or inflammation from gastroesophageal reflux can occur with ear pain as a contributing symptom. Lung and bronchial lesions are referred via the bronchial branch of the vagus. Pain from myocardial ischemia has been reported to be referred via sympathetic afferents, but a few cases of isolated otalgia that is due to angina have been reported. A thoracic, an aortic, or an innominate artery aneurysm can also cause ear pain as a result of tension on the vagus nerve.

Cervical spine disease is an uncommon cause of referred otalgia. Any chronic inflammatory process, such as osteoarthritis, can manifest as persistent otalgia in the presence of a normal otologic examination. Cervical trauma, such as "whiplash," may cause referred ear pain. A condition seen in the pediatric population, Grisel's syndrome, is due to subluxation of the atlantoaxial joint that usually follows an upper respiratory tract infection or an adenoidectomy. These patients present with stiff neck, palpable cervical dislocation, and otalgia. Malignant or benign growth of the cervical spine is also an uncommon cause of ear pain. Cervical radiographic films or computed tomography scans usually confirm the suspected diagnosis.

Idiopathic ticlike pain is a rare condition originating from cranial nerves VII or IX that can cause referred otalgia. Primary medical management with an antiepileptic agent such as carbamazepine should be the first line of

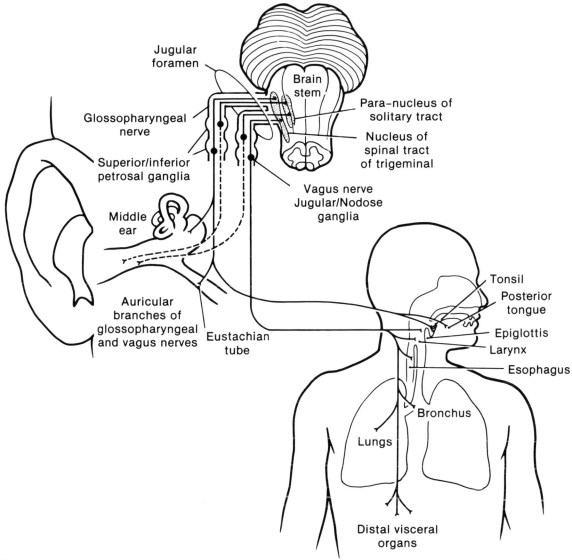

Figure 13–2. Local and distant origins of otalgia from cranial nerves IX and X.

therapy once neoplastic, vascular, and inflammatory causes have been ruled out. Surgical decompression of the nerve may be necessary if medical therapy fails.

OTALGIA IN THE PEDIATRIC POPULATION

The causes of otalgia in children are similar to those in adults, although the usual cause of ear pain is some form of local otalgia in approximately 80% of the patients. The physical examination in children can be difficult because of the small canal, cerumen occlusion, and the uncooperative status of some children. Because approximately one in five children with otalgia has ear pain from another source, a prudent examination is warranted in all children. Teething in the early years can cause otalgia and fever that, in combination, simulate acute otitis media; this scenario again emphasizes the need for a careful physical examination. Ear drops and antibiotics by mouth are not the treatment of choice in all children with the complaint of otalgia.

CONCLUSION

Otalgia can be due to local, regional, or distant causes. Understanding of the complex neuroanatomy of the head and neck is needed for a complete evaluation of the patient with ear complaints. Local lesions are the cause of otalgia in approximately 50% of adults and 80% of children. In the patient with a normal otologic examination, a careful history and physical examination of the head and neck is always necessary to uncover the etiologic basis of this symptom. Treatment can then be directed to the local or referred cause.

SUGGESTED READINGS

Al-Sheikhle AR: Pain in the ear—with special reference to referred pain. J Laryngol Otol 94:1433–1440, 1980.

Blake DN, et al: Temporomandibular joint dysfunction in children presenting as otalgia. Clin Otolaryngol 7:237–244, 1982.

Brookes GB: Costen's syndrome—correlation or coincidence. Clin Otolaryngol 5:23–36, 1980.

Bryhn M: Ear pain due to myocardial ischemia (letter). Am Heart J 107:186–187, 1984.

Correll RW, Wescott WB: Eagle's syndrome diagnosed after history of headache, dysphagia, otalgia, and limited neck movement. J Am Dent Assoc 104:491–492, 1982.

Curtis AW: Myofascial pain-dysfunction syndrome: the role of nonmasticatory muscles in 91 patients. Otolaryngol Head Neck Surg 88:361–367, 1980.

Ingvarsson L: Acute otalgia in children—findings and diagnosis. Acta Paediatr Scand 71:705–710, 1982.

Kreisberg MK, Turner J: Dental causes of referred otalgia. Ear Nose Throat J 66:398–408, 1987.

Messer EJ, et al: The stylohyoid syndrome. J Oral Surg 33:664–667, 1975.

Nelms RC, Paparella MM: Otalgia. Minn Med 10:955–958, 1969.

Paparella MM, Shumrick DA: Otalgia. In Otolaryngology. Philadelphia: WB Saunders, 1980.

Wilson-Pauwels L, et al: Cranial Nerves. Philadelphia: BC Decker, 1988.

CHAPTER 14

Congenital Aural Atresia and Microtia

Robert O. Ruder, MD   Dennis R. Maceri, MD   Dennis M. Crockett, MD

The term *congenital aural atresia* usually refers to abnormal or lack of development of the external auditory canal and the meatus, the tympanic membrane, and the middle ear cleft; the term *microtia*, although imprecise, refers to hypoplastic development of the auricle (or pinna). Any degree of severity of congenital aural atresia may be associated with any degree of severity of microtia; however, the degree of microtia generally correlates with that of the middle ear abnormalities.

The purpose of this chapter is to discuss the embryology, normal and abnormal anatomy, and the assessment and management of congenital aural atresia and microtia. Within the specialty of otolaryngology–head and neck surgery, the evaluation and surgical correction of congenital aural atresia are undertaken by the otologic surgeon, whereas the assessment and reconstruction of the microtic auricle are accomplished by the facial plastic surgeon. Often a social worker, an audiologist, and a psychologist work together with the surgeon. Each group of subspecialists must coordinate a common treatment philosophy and communicate to the patient and his or her family what functional and cosmetic expectations are attainable.

CONGENITAL AURAL ATRESIA

Congenital ear malformations exist within a spectrum of related malformations of the auricle (microtia), the external auditory canal, the tympanic membrane, and the contents of the middle ear. The surgical repair of canal atresia can be a most satisfying, as well as frustrating, experience.

Timing of surgery, parental counseling, evaluation of the patient, and surgical technique are discussed in this chapter. In general, microtia repairs are first undertaken when the patient is around 5 or 6 years of age. In cases of bilateral atresia, repair immediately follows healing. In cases of unilateral atresia, repair is usually delayed until the late teens or adulthood unless chronic infection or risk for cholesteatoma is present. For all cases, the authors urge craniofacial evaluation by a team that consists of pediatricians, geneticists, otologists, reconstructive surgeons, psychiatrists, social workers, audiologists, and speech and language specialists. Such a team helps the parents deal with the myriad problems associated with craniofacial anomalies and facilitates the appointment process for the multiple specialists.

Embryology

All three germ layers participate in the formation of the auricle and the external ear canal, the tympanic membrane, the middle ear structures, and the labyrinth (Table 14–1). The external ear develops at about the sixth week of uterine life from six knoblike hillocks situated around the primitive meatus.

TABLE 14–1. Embryologic Derivatives of the Ear

Ectodermal Derivatives
Auricle (six hillocks)
External canal
Tympanic membrane
Otocyst (future inner ear)
Mesenchymal Derivatives
First branchial arch (Meckel's cartilage)
   Malleus
   Incus body
   Tensor tympani
Second branchial arch (Reichert's cartilage)
   Long process of incus
   Stapes superstructure
   Stapedius muscle
Endodermal Derivatives
Auditory (eustachian tube)
Mucosa of middle ear cavity

The tissue destined to become the external ear canal migrates inward as a solid core of epithelium from the future auricle toward the first branchial pouch during the second month of gestation (Fig. 14–1). At the junction of the inward and outward migrations, a plate or a bar of tissue known as the presumptive meatal plate, which ultimately becomes the tympanic membrane, forms. The external auditory canal starts to recanalize during the sixth intrauterine month. Concurrently, the malleus and incus are forming from the first and second branchial arch cartilages. Formation is complete by the end of

the seventh or eighth month of gestation. The fully formed ossicles are covered with mucous membrane derived from the endoderm of the first branchial pouch.

Two key steps are required in the formation of a normal ear canal: (1) recanalization of the external canal and (2) posteroinferior migration of the mastoid, which allows for the development of the tympanic ring and the canal from a mass of tympanic bone. The tympanic bone recanalizes into a cylinder and separates the glenoid fossa from the mastoid. As the mastoid moves posteriorly, it carries the facial nerve to its ultimate location. This posterior migration may be arrested at any point from the beginning of the tympanic bone development, deep over the middle ear space in complete atresia (Fig. 14–2), to a stage at which canalization is complete at the lateral end of the external ear canal but remains stenotic (Fig. 14–3). The time of developmental arrest varies and accounts for the spectrum of types of atresia seen.

Types of Atresias

Meatal atresias can be divided into minor, moderate, and severe, as described by Colman (1971). Severe atresias entail complete or nearly complete absence of the tympanic bone and, therefore, of the external canal (Fig. 14–2). The middle ear cavity sits anterior

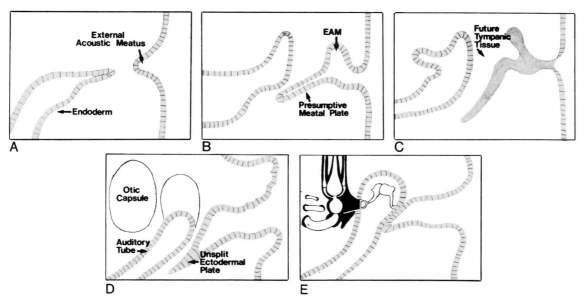

Figure 14–1. *A.* Embryology. *B.* Migration of tissue inward to form the presumptive meatal plate. *C.* Note future tympanic tissue that gives rise to the ossicles. *D.* The ectoderm of the external canal begins to recanalize. *E.* By the eighth month, endoderm surrounds the ossicles in the tympanic cavity.

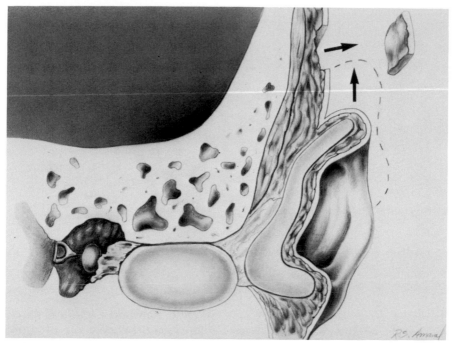

Figure 14–2. Left ear tympanic bone has failed to recanalize; all that is left is a solid core of bone. The glenoid fossa remains lateral to the tympanic cavity because the mastoid migration posteriorly has been arrested. The tegmen is identified.

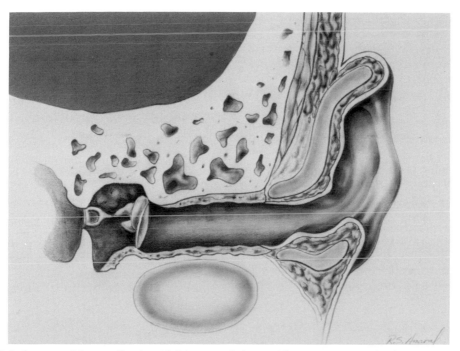

Figure 14–3. Left ear partial recanalization of the tympanic bone with more posterior displacement of the mastoid bone. This results in a more anteriorly placed glenoid fossa. The canal remains stenotic.

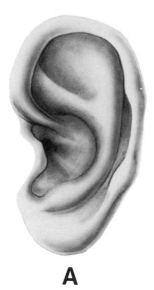

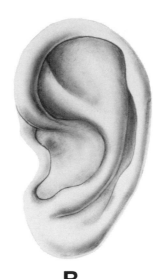

Figure 14–4. *A.* A slitlike or conical meatus, which usually ends in a blind pouch or a fistula, is depicted. *B.* A flat thumbprint depression exists with a false meatus. See text for details.

A

B

and medial to any tympanic bone remnant and to the condyle of the mandible. The malleus and incus exist as a globular mass of ill-defined bone that may or may not articulate with the stapes. The auricle is usually severely deformed and consists of cartilage nubs. The only signs of an external meatus may be a flat depression over the condyle. The examining surgeon must look for a poorly pneumatized mastoid and for possible cochlear anomalies as well. A thorough work-up for associated malformations is indicated.

Minor aplasias involve some tympanic bone development and partial recanalization of the ear canal. The canal eardrums are smaller than normal. This type of atresia may go unnoticed until a conductive hearing loss is eventually identified and evaluated. The auricle is frequently normal or only slightly deformed (Fig. 14–3). In the moderate aplasias, the major problem is incomplete recanalization of the tympanic bone. The auricle varies in shape but usually has a slitlike meatus or looks like a fistula. The bony canal is severely narrowed and ends in a blind pouch. The middle ear space is again anterior and medially placed, behind the tympanic bone remnant and condyle. Alternatively, the meatus is a flat depression with no visible canal.

Preoperative Evaluation

Sufficient time must be set aside in the initial consultation to answer parents' questions, to provide assurances of future surgical success, and to plan the steps for aural rehabilitation. Counseling the parents with regard to the potential outcome, the timing of the surgery, and the risks is vital. The patient's history must be thorough and must include pregnancy and family histories. No detail is to be overlooked. The craniofacial team concept is important with regard to genetic counseling, especially when a family has a history of genetic anomalies.

The physical examination should focus on uncovering other craniofacial anomalies such as Treacher Collins syndrome, hemifacial microsomia, and facial paralysis. The size, the shape, and the position of the auricle are important. The relationship of the auricle to the temporomandibular joint is important for surgical planning. The type of meatus (flat or slitlike) is defined. A slitlike opening may indicate a partially developed tympanic bone, whereas a flat depression usually implies absence of the tympanic bone (Figs. 14–4*A*, 14–4*B*). A well-developed mastoid tip usually indicates a well-pneumatized mastoid cavity. The temporomandibular joint is palpated, and its location in relation to the mastoid tip is determined; this also may provide a clue about the degree of tympanic bone development. The authors find drawings and structural models helpful in explaining the problem to parents.

Audiology

An accurate and early audiologic evaluation is critical. This usually requires two well-trained pediatric audiologists who work as a team to obtain meaningful results. In difficult cases of bilateral atresia, a brain stem evoked response is elicited in order to try to sort out a masking dilemma; however, it is not always possible to sort it out. In cases of unilateral atresia, earphones can be used for checking both ears to determine the presence of one good, normal hearing ear. In cases of bilateral atresia, the most common finding is a maximal conductive loss, with a normal bone line and a 50- to 60-db air bone gap. At times, an early computed tomographic (CT) scan of the temporal bones is performed; this procedure requires sedation in order to assess morphologic characteristics of the cochlea. The appearance of a normal cochlea can be extrapolated to mean an intact auditory nerve. The most important part of this analysis is to reassure the parents that normal inner ear function exists and that with early amplification and aural rehabilitation, speech and language will develop.

Early auditory stimulation is provided with bone conduction aids at age 4 to 6 months. Implantation of bone conduction devices should be delayed until the child reaches the age of 2.5 to 3 years. At that time, skull thickness is adequate to accommodate the implant.

Radiographic Evaluation

Radiographic imaging of the temporal bone is essential in the evaluation of atresia patients. Timing is of concern because an infant or a young child will require sedation. The technique used is high-resolution CT scanning in the coronal and axial planes. These scans show the anatomic structure of the cochlea, the middle ear, and the external ear canal. In cases of bilateral atresia, CT scanning is performed before the first surgery at age 5. In cases in which there is concern about congenital abnormalities of the cochlea and possible sensorineural hearing loss resulting from an elevated conduction threshold, scanning is performed at a much earlier age. In cases of unilateral atresia, without suspicion of cochlear anomalies, CT scanning is performed before any surgical procedure. Three-dimensional CT algorithms, magnetic resonance imaging, or conventional plain films contribute little to the preoperative work-up.

The radiographic study is used to help plan the surgical procedure and to predict the outcome of surgery. Cole and Jahrsdoerfer (1990) stated that one absolute requirement for operating on an atretic ear is the presence of a functioning normal inner ear. They suggested that a good-quality CT scan should depict a normal-appearing inner ear, the presence of stapes, patency of the oval and round windows, and a reasonably normal facial nerve course that will not hamper ossicular reconstruction. Other factors that influence the course of surgery include the extent of the tympanic bone development and its degree of canalization. Without a tympanic bone, there is nothing but soft tissue around the temporomandibular joint adjacent to the middle ear space. In addition, the degree of mastoid pneumatization, the location of the sigmoid sinus, and the position of the middle fossa plate are important. The triangle formed by the tegmen, the sigmoid sinus, and the condyle of the mandible determines the angle of approach to the middle ear and the position of the external canal and the meatus.

Aguilar and Jahrsdoerfer (1988) developed a rating system of radiologic analysis that serves as a predictor of surgical outcome in atresia (Table 14–2). In this system, nine key radiographic findings are weighted equally, except for the stapes, which receives two points. Ten points is a perfect score, and a score of eight or above implies that the patient is a good surgical candidate; a score of five or below implies that the patient is a poor candidate for surgery.

Final Recommendations to the Patient's Family

With all information at hand, the surgeon operates on a patient with bilateral atresia

TABLE 14–2. Congenital Atresia Preoperative Rating System

Anatomic Finding	Point Value
Intact stapes	2
Open oval window	1
Adequate middle ear space	1
Normal facial nerve course	1
Malleus/incus complex	1
Well-pneumatized mastoid	1
Incus/stapes articulation	1
Good appearance of the external ear	1
Ear canal stenosis with malleus bar	1

Data compiled from Aguilar EA, Jahrsdoerfer RA: The surgical repair of congenital microtia and atresia. Otolaryngol Head Neck Surg 98:600–606, 1988.

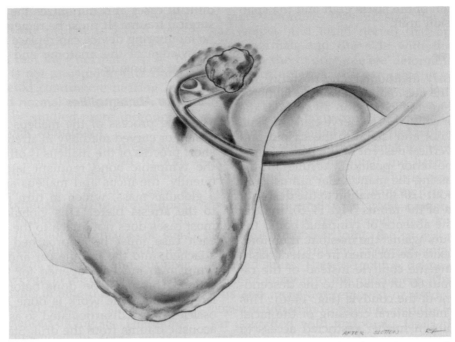

Figure 14–6. Complete developmental arrest. The course of the facial nerve is altered, turning more abruptly across the condyle of the mandible. A remnant of tympanic bone can be seen.

Surgical Technique

The authors advocate a curved postauricular incision well away from the glenoid fossa and mastoid tip. When the repair of microtia has preceded repair of atresia, the entire cartilage framework can be elevated with the soft tissue flap to expose the mastoid cortex. A cortical mastoidectomy staying high and posterior is begun. The sigmoid sinus is not skeletonized, so that some bone may be saved for the new posterior canal wall. The middle fossa plate is followed anteriorly and medially until the fossa incudus is reached. Here the horizontal canal and the ossicular mass are encountered. Again, care is taken to avoid trauma to the ossicles with the burr. The facial nerve is identified, and the incudostapedial joint is separated.

At this point, the remaining bone over the temporomandibular joint is removed; this removal exposes the tympanic or atretic plate, which lies over the ossicles. The middle ear is smaller than normal and medial to the condyle of the joint. Bone removal, commonly in the posterior part only, is maximized to facilitate ossicular reconstruction and grafting. The existing ossicular chain is rarely of value and is removed for grafting later. An annular ledge is fashioned ante-riorly above the eustachian tube orifice with the drill in order to hold the new tympanic membrane graft. The ossicles are reconstructed from the previously removed bone or autologous cartilage.

At times, the use of tissue glues is helpful at this stage to facilitate the reconstruction. The temporalis fascia is used for grafting and is placed on the surgically created annular ledge described earlier. The graft is carried posteriorly and covers the facial nerve and the horizontal canal. The new meatus will be located in a posterior superior position; therefore, the auricle must be rotated up and back from its original location, whether it is the natural cartilage or the fabricated rib cartilage framework. The skin over the cartilage framework, in either case, is incised and elevated as an anteriorly based flap, exposing the cartilage framework. The cartilage is cut and removed; this procedure creates a large meatus. The anterior skin flap is then dunked into the new meatus against the bone of the anterior canal wall. In some cases, this skin comes to rest against the soft tissues of the temporomandibular joint. A large split-thickness graft is harvested from the anterior abdominal wall or from medial upper arm skin. The graft is sutured to the posterior margin of the meatus and lines the canal and the mastoid cavity. A free graft is placed anteriorly and overlaps the fascia along the surgically created annulus. A template of polymeric silicone (Silastic) can be used lateral to the skin graft and the fascia graft in order to help the skin conform to the fascia and to minimize blunting. The canal is then filled with an absorbable gelatin sponge (Gelfoam) soaked in antibiotic solution in the standard fashion.

At the lateral end of the meatus, a petroleum jelly (Vaseline) gauze strip ½ inch thick is rolled into a stent and placed into the newly created meatus. The stent remains for 10 to 14 days, and administration of ear drops is started in 3 weeks. The Silastic template is removed in the physician's office.

Complications

The most common problems in repair of atresia are infection, recurrence of stenosis, neural hearing loss, and injury to the facial nerve. Postoperative infections cause graft failures. Fortunately, such infections are rare, but when present, they are treated locally with topical drops, curettage, and packing with antibiotic ointment. Occasionally, spot skin grafting is necessary, especially when infectious granulation tissue is a chronic problem.

Recurrence of stenosis is a feared complication that is best treated by prevention. Techniques include a wide meatoplasty with removal of as much soft tissue as possible. The posterosuperior repositioning of the auricle aids in preventing scar contracture, because of the direction of the force vectors. Bony stenosis is also possible, especially in the small, poorly pneumatized mastoid. Any technique that minimizes postoperative infection is advised. Patients who are known to form keloids receive injections of local steroids.

Hearing loss of the neural type can be of the temporary threshold shift type, can result from drill trauma, or can be a permanent result of direct drill injury to the ossicles, the oval window, or the balance canals. Late-developing conductive losses may imply a middle ear effusion or a failure in the reconstructive process that results from prosthesis migration or fixation. Blunting, or lateralization of the graft, and of course recurrence of stenosis must be looked for.

Injury to the facial nerve is best avoided by early identification and preservation of the nerve. For this purpose, the facial nerve monitor serves as a useful adjunct to thorough anatomic knowledge and meticulous surgical technique. Rerouting the nerve should be avoided because of the trauma that results from disruption of vascularity to the nerve sheath.

Hearing Results

Treatment of most minor atresias yields good hearing results within 20 to 25 db of the cochlear reserve in 80% to 90% of patients. In more severe atresias, good long-term hearing results are seen in 60% to 75% of patients. Reversal rates run about 30% in most series, mainly because of recurrence of stenosis, graft failure, or a failure to achieve the deserved hearing result. However, poor hearing with a patent, clean, dry canal is also correctable with a hearing aid. This is especially true in cases of severe atresia with extensive abnormalities of the middle ear. In these cases it may not be physically possible to reconstruct the ossicular chain in any fashion that maximizes sound transmission to the footplate.

Summary

Surgical treatment of congenital bilateral atresia is advised when the patient is around 5 years old. The repair of atresia follows the repair of microtia whenever possible. In some cases, the underlying craniofacial anomaly prevents successful reconstruction of the middle ear conducting system. In such cases, an implantable bone conduction device may serve the patient well and with better frequency responses than do conventional bone conduction hearing aids. Most unilateral atresias with normal hearing in the contralateral ear are not surgically treated until the late teens or early adulthood. The authors believe that the decision should be left to the individual patient whenever possible. Most important, early sound amplification and aural rehabilitation must begin as soon as possible to ensure appropriate speech and language development.

MICROTIA

Embryologic Considerations

The auricular anlage is first recognizable by the fourth week of gestation and is composed of ectoderm and mesoderm in the form of six external swellings, or hillocks. The first three hillocks (1, 2, and 3) are derived from the first pharyngeal (mandibular) arch and give rise to the tragus, the root of the helix, and the superior portion of the helix. The second three hillocks (4, 5, and 6) are derived from the second pharyngeal (hyoid) arch and give rise to the antihelix, the superior crus, the inferior crus, the antitragus, and, probably, the lobule (Fig. 14–7). During the second month of gestation, as the mandible and facial structures grow and develop, the developing auricle migrates from an inferior medial position to a superior lateral position opposite the developing external auditory canal and inner ear structures. By the 20th week of development, the auricle has attained adult configuration, although it is smaller and more interiorly positioned than the neonatal ear.

During the first trimester, even the most subtle adverse genetic or environmental factors may severely interfere with the rapid sequence of developmental changes and may cause catastrophic auricular anomalies. Because of the temporal and anatomic proximity of the developing auricle to other organ systems, a malformed auricle often occurs concomitantly with developmental anomalies of the first and second branchial arches derivatives, the heart, and the kidneys. The high incidence of auricular malformations with preauricular appendages, maxillary and mandibular hypoplasia, facial nerve paresis and paralysis, and cervical vertebral anomalies necessitates a close working relationship of the otologist with other members of a craniofacial team. Consultation with experts in pediatrics, plastic surgery, genetics, dentistry, orthodontics, prosthodontics, nursing, audiology, speech pathology, psychiatry, and social work is often essential to effectively assist the patient and his or her family.

After all elements of the auricle have developed, other forces in the second and final trimesters may cause dysmorphic anomalies. Abnormal intrauterine positioning or cervical masses may displace the developing auricle and cause a lop ear, a cup ear, or a prominent ear. At birth, the ear is approximately two thirds of the size of an adult ear and reaches almost adult size by age 6 years. Hence it is generally accepted that the minimal age to begin auricular reconstruction is 6 years.

Anatomic Considerations

When evaluating any patient with an auricular anomaly (especially microtia), the facial plastic surgeon must have a thorough understanding of normal position, contour, and form (Fig. 14–8). The range of normalcy must be studied, with the understanding that no two auricles are exactly the same, even on the same patient. The normal adult auricle is approximately 60% as wide as it is long and has a vertical height of almost 6 cm. The superior level of the ear approximates that of the tail of the eyebrow, and the inferior aspect reaches the level of the nostril and the upper lip. The auricle is not vertical but is inclined posteriorly, closely paralleling the dorsum of the nose. The distance from the root of the helix to the lateral orbital rim is approximately one ear length, or 6 cm (Fig. 14–9). An ear that is delicately and carefully sculptured but poorly positioned on the head is less attractive than a poorly sculptured ear that is properly positioned.

The auricle must have the essential elements of (1) a multicontoured flaplike structure, (2) a slightly distorted oval shape, (3) proper placement and positioning in relation to other facial structures, and (4) some protrusion from the skull. In three dimensions,

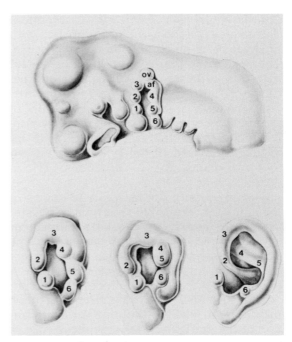

Figure 14–7. Derivation of the six hillocks from the pharyngeal arches to form the parts of the external ear.

Figure 14–8. The normal position for the auricle is depicted in *A*.

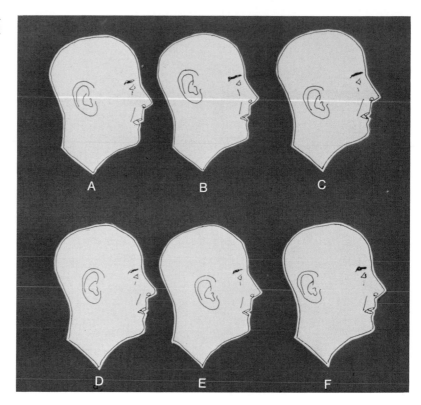

the ear may be conceptualized as a three-layered structure of cartilage (Fig. 14–10). The concha is the most medial or interior tier and surrounds the ear canal. The scapha is the second layer and is the main structural support of the auricle. When deficient or weak, the scapha appears to fall upon itself, furrowing like a window shade, and loses

Figure 14–9. Distance from the root of the helix to the lateral orbital rim, depicted as one ear length.

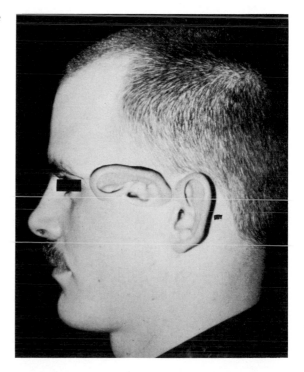

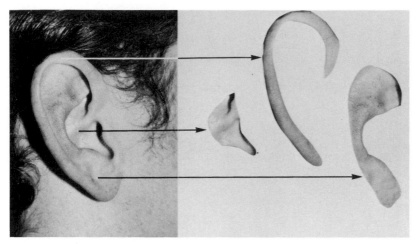

Figure 14–10. Conceptualization of the ear as a three-layered structure of cartilage.

vertical height, as seen in a lop ear (Fig. 14–11). The superior and most lateral layer is the helix, which delineates the delicate periphery and silhouettes the auricle.

Anomalies of the auricle have been classified, typed, grouped, and graded in numerous articles. Then they have been further subcategorized into such descriptive terms as prominent, protruded, cupped, lop, hooded, lidded, cryptotic, macrotic, and microtic. The authors have used a grading system of three levels of severity. Grade I anomalies include ears in which all anatomic subunits are present but are misshapen (Fig. 14–12). This includes the prominent or protruding ear,

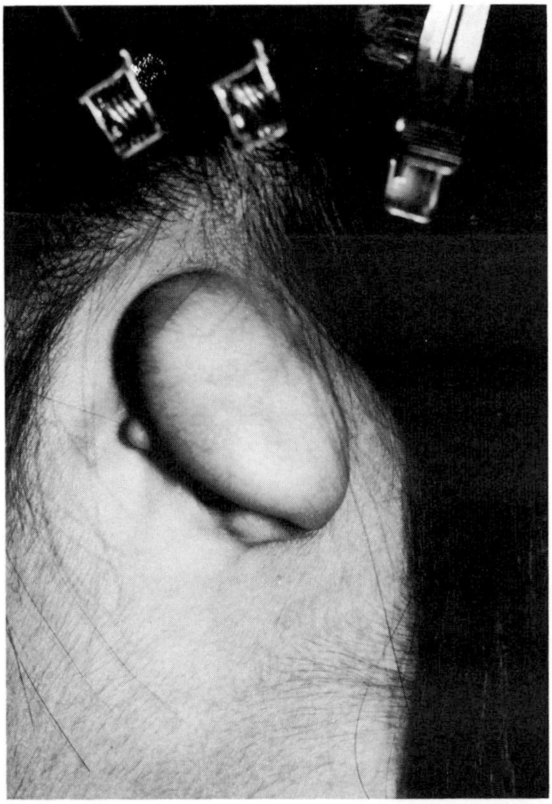

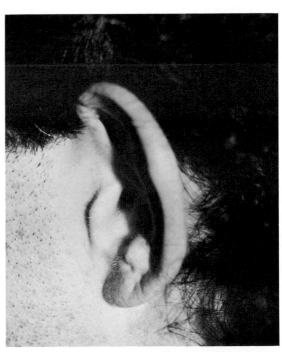

Figure 14–11. Lop ear, caused by a weak or deficient scapha.

Figure 14–12. Example of a grade I anomaly, in which all anatomic subunits are present but misshapen.

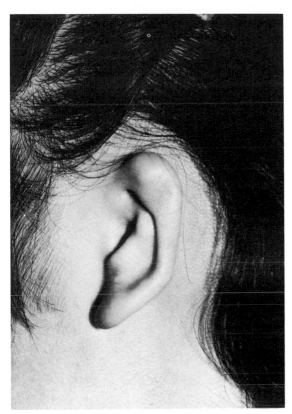

Figure 14–13. Example of a grade II anomaly, in which some anatomic subunits are missing.

with its unfurled antihelical fold, and cup ears, with their excessively deepened, angulated conchae. These anomalies need only to be resculptured by standard otoplastic techniques and do not require cutaneous or cartilage grafts.

Grade II deformities include auricles that lack some anatomic subunits (Fig. 14–13). The cryptotic, lidded, and severely constricted ears result from deficient development of the scapha supporting layer, which causes the superior aspect of the ear to fold over on itself. The fossa triangularis is usually absent, the helical arch is flattened and foreshortened, and the height of the ear is inadequate. Reconstruction usually requires repositioning of the existing vestige and the addition of chondrocutaneous composite grafts from the opposite auricle.

Grade III anomalies include the most severe deformities, in which few or no normal auricular remnants exist (depicted later in Fig. 14–27A). The classic microtic ear consists of a vertically oriented rudimentary fold of misshapen skin and cartilage superiorly and

a fibroadipose remnant of lobular tissue interiorly. Correction of grade III deformities requires harvesting rib cartilage and sculpting it into a delicately shaped auricle.

Classic Microtia

The classic form of microtia is described as a peanut-shaped appendage consisting of hypoplastic cartilage superiorly and a lobular remnant below. The superior nubbin of cartilage can often be unfolded, after dissection, into a rudimentary scapha, a helix, and a concha. The inferior portion of fibroadipose tissue is the most constant and best-developed subunit. It represents a lobule that often lies at a level different from that of the normal ear in cases of unilateral microtia (Fig. 14–14). The superior nubbin is too small and misshapen to be useful for reconstruction and is usually discarded. If the entire microtic vestige fails to migrate, it may lie anywhere along the path of migration and lie anteriorly and interiorly, even beneath the mandible (Fig. 14–15).

Sequence and Timing of Operation

Reconstruction usually involves four staged operations spaced at 3-month intervals: (1) implantation of the autogenous sculptured rib graft; (2) posterior positioning of the fibroadipose remnant into a lobule; (3) con-

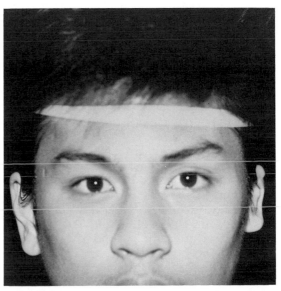

Figure 14–14. The normal auricle is on the patient's right.

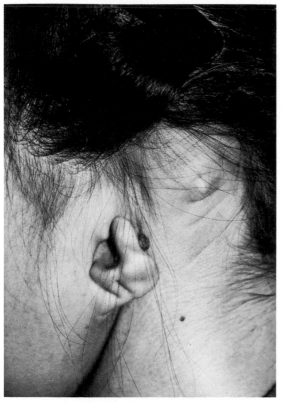

Figure 14–15. Anomalous position of a microtic auricle, a result of failure of the microtic vestige to migrate.

years, the rib cage is adequately large to permit harvesting enough costal cartilage without deforming the chest wall.

Studies have suggested that by the age of 5 years, children become extremely sensitive to their body image and can emotionally suffer from their heightened awareness and from ridicule by peers. Therefore, by age 6, most of the authors' patients are psychologically ready to begin reconstruction. Children with bilateral microtia have compound problems. Their hearing loss must be improved as early as possible. If external bone conduction amplification is inadequate, unilateral atresia repair should begin by age 4 years, before auricular surgery. The team must understand the full spectrum of this deformity. It is a developmental anomaly of the first and second branchial arch structures. The auricle is one part of this multifaceted problem. If the team approach is not coordinated, the reconstructed auricle and the canal may be on different levels (Fig. 14–16).

Preoperative Consultation

Both the parents and the child are present during the initial consultation. The four-stage

struction of the tragus and neointroitus for the external canal; and (4) elevation of the helix from the mastoid. Some patients neither need nor want a postauricular sulcus for glasses or hearing aid to rest on, and therefore elevation is not performed.

Three important factors must be considered in deciding on the ideal age to begin reconstruction in the child with unilateral microtia: (1) growth of the normal auricle; (2) the size and conformation of the chest wall, which may enable the harvesting of a sufficiently sized rib graft; and (3) the psychologic maturity of the child. In general, reconstruction of unilateral microtia should precede repair of canal atresia. The sculptured rib graft must be placed in an unscarred and well-vascularized skin pocket for the optimal aesthetic outcome. Although some teams repair atresia after the second stage (lobular transposition), the authors have delayed temporal bone surgery until the patients have reached adulthood in cases of unilateral microtia. By age 6 years, the auricles of most children are 85% of adult size. Also by age 6

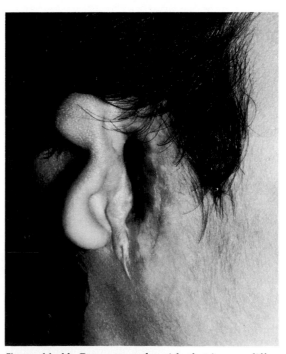

Figure 14–16. Reconstructed auricle that is on a different level than the canal. This is a result of an uncoordinated approach to reconstruction by the surgical team.

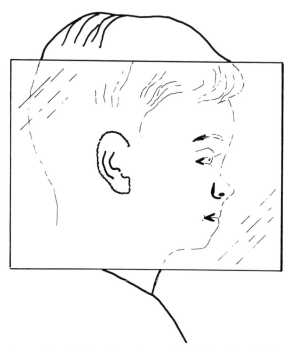

Figure 14–17. Template of normal facial landmarks for repair of microtia.

reconstructive procedure can be performed at 3-month intervals and completed in 1 year. A nurturing relationship must be initiated with the patient to allay his or her anxieties and to establish an environment of confidence and cooperation for better postoperative care.

Reconstruction of auricular defects with more than 15 mm disparity in vertical height between the normal and abnormal side requires augmentation with skin, cartilage, or pedicle grafts. If a rib graft is needed, the patient's chest wall is evaluated for adequate size and shape. The parents are shown the area where the incision is made and the grafts are taken. Exposed clear x-ray film is used as a template. Normal facial landmarks from the normal side are drawn on the x-ray film (Fig. 14–17). Distances from the normal ear to the eyebrow, the nostril, and the corner of the mouth are marked to ensure proper positioning, size, and configuration of the reconstruction. The pattern is then reversed and tattooed to the microtic side. A second x-ray template slightly smaller than the normal auricle is traced to allow for thickness of the skin (Fig. 14–18).

Operative Technique

Several materials have been used with varying success for the auricular skeleton. The authors use rib cartilage grafts because of their superior durability and resistance to absorption and infection. Grafts are taken from the chest wall on the side of the normal auricle because the natural curvature of the cartilage more closely simulates the configuration of the normal auricle. An incision is made 2 cm above and parallel to the inferior border of the rib cage. Dissection extends through the skin, the fascia, and the rectus sheath and muscle until the underlying ribs are exposed. The previously contoured x-ray template is placed over the cartilaginous portion of the ribs to delineate the amount of donor cartilage necessary. Careful dissection of the seventh, eighth, and ninth ribs is vital to avoid perforation of the closely adherent underlying pleura. After a block of seventh and eighth rib cartilage is taken, an additional part of the ninth rib cartilage is necessary to create a helical rim (Fig. 14–19).

It is essential to leave intact as much perichondrium as possible to prevent postoperative absorption and infection. A three-layered auricle is sculpted to simulate a concha, a scapha, and a helical rim. Each subunit of the auricle must be carved into the donor cartilage and be slightly exaggerated in

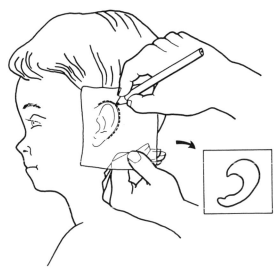

Figure 14–18. Template of the normal ear, drawn slightly smaller than the actual ear in order to allow for skin thickness.

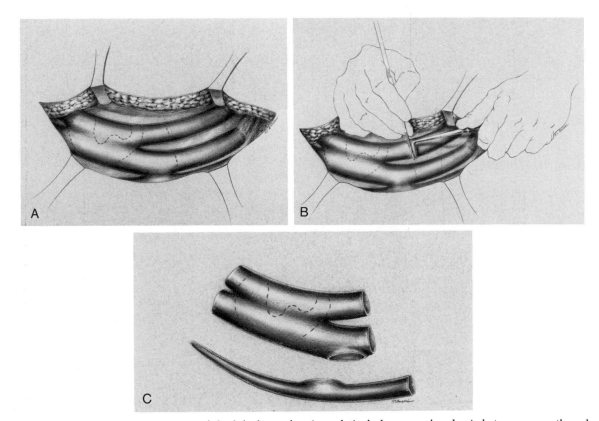

Figure 14–19. *A.* Surgical exposure of the left chest, showing relatively large synchondrosis between seventh and eighth cartilaginous ribs. *B.* Harvesting cartilage. *C.* Harvested seventh and eighth costal cartilage with synchondrosis intact as well as the ninth costal cartilage.

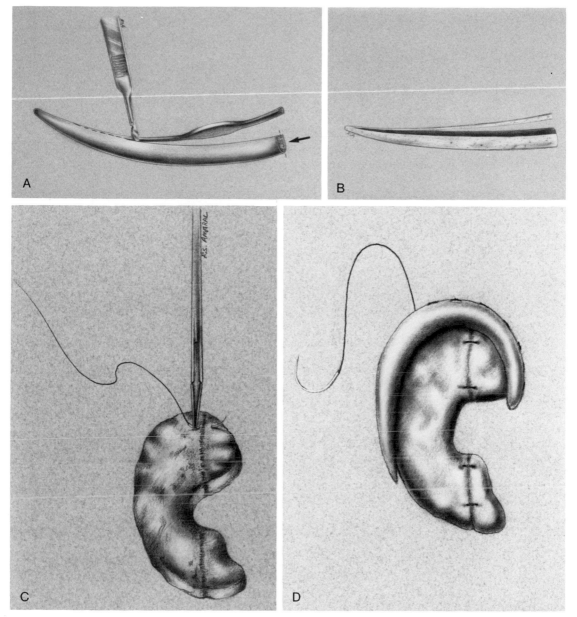

Figure 14–20. *A.* Cut along superior surface of ninth costal cartilage. *B.* Cut along posterior surface of ninth costal cartilage to facilitate bending of the graft into a curve. *C.* Stabilizing wire sutures to synchondrosis of sculpted base plate. *D.* Securing the helix to base plate with wire sutures.

Illustration continued on following page

height and depth to allow for the thickness of the mastoid skin. The shape and length of the ninth rib are ideal for the helical rim. This rib is thinned on its convex surface to create a gently curving helix while enough height is maintained to exaggerate the helical ridge. After the helix is secured to the sculpted base plate with 4–0 and 5–0-wire sutures, the fossa triangularis and the scapha are sculpted with carving tools. This three-layered technique, created by Tanzer and refined by Brent (1980a, 1980b), is far superior to the previously utilized expansile and monoblock cartilage frameworks, which tend to flatten and lose definition with time (Fig. 14–20).

The previously made x-ray template of the normal side is placed over the microtic side.

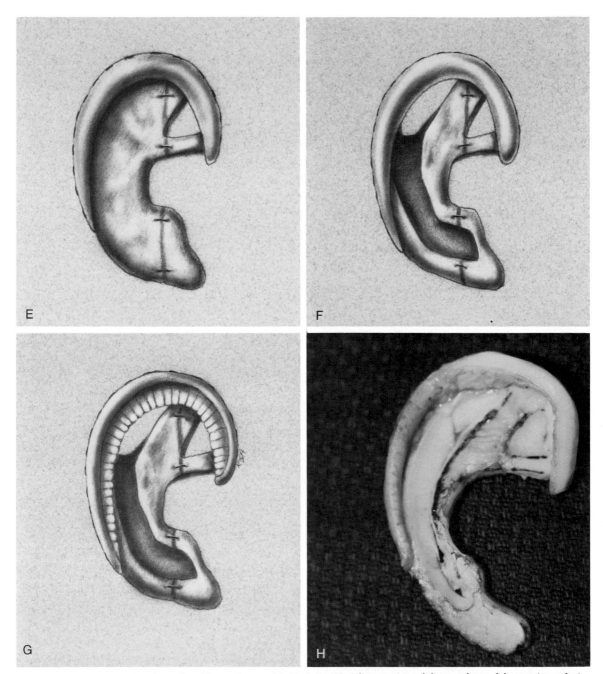

Figure 14–20 *Continued E.* Completed base plate and helical rim. *F.* After carving of the scapha and fossa triangularis. *G.* Horizontal grooves may be carved in the convex (posterior) surface of the graft to facilitate bending into a curve. *H.* Completed base plate and helical rim.

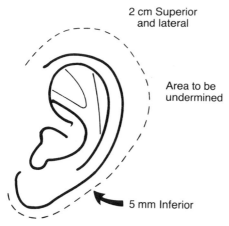

Figure 14–21. Subdermal skin pocket created 2 cm superiorly and 5 mm interiorly beyond the tattooed outline.

Its periphery is tattooed on the skin with methylene blue and 18-gauge needles to ensure proper positioning. An incision is made anterior to the microtia remnant, and all cartilage in the vestige is dissected and removed. This gains skin pliability and allows better coaption of the skin to the cartilage graft. A delicate subdermal skin pocket, 2 to 3 mm thick, is created 2 cm superiorly and 5 mm interiorly beyond the tattooed outline to gain enough skin laxity to adequately conform to the contours of the sculpted rib graft (Fig. 14–21). Any excessive skin tension may cause necrosis and exposure of the underlying cartilage. The graft is inserted into the pocket (Fig. 14–22) and rotated into the proper position. Better coaption of skin to cartilage is accomplished by two drainage tubes attached to continuous wall suction at 80 mm Hg, which avoids bolsters and mattress sutures. The anterior incision is closed, and the newly created sulci are packed with petroleum-saturated gauze and covered with mastoid dressings. Continuous wall suction is maintained for 3 days, and antibiotics are given for 1 week, at the end of which the dressings and sutures are removed.

Lobular Transposition

Three months later, the fibroadipose lobule is transposed to form the inferior third of the auricle (Fig. 14–23). An interiorly based flap encompassing the fibroadipose tissue is sculpted and rotated along the inferior surface of the neoauricle to continue the gentle curvature of the helix and create a lobule. It is unnecessary to have internal support in this ear lobe to maintain its form. However, the flap must be sutured without tension to avoid disappearance of the lobe by shrinkage. Any redundant skin in the superior remnant is excised.

Tragal Reconstruction

The third reconstructive stage consists of constructing a tragus and deepening of the conchal bowl (Fig. 14–24). A composite chondrocutaneous graft is harvested from the anterior aspect of the cavum concha of the normal ear. A full-thickness postauricular skin graft, 2 cm in diameter, is taken, and the donor sites are closed. A J-shaped incision is made in the microtic ear in the proposed area of the tragus. The skin is elevated anteriorly, and the crescent-shaped chondrocutaneous graft is sutured to the skin. Interiorly, the graft bends onto the previously sculpted cartilage graft to simulate an incisura between the tragus and the antitragus. Skin over the conchal area is also elevated posteriorly, and the underlying soft tissue is excised to the level of the mastoid periosteum. The full-thickness skin graft is sutured to the posterior aspect of the composite graft anteriorly and to the skin of the excavated conchal bowl posteriorly (Fig. 14–25).

These three sutures (anterior skin, composite chondrocutaneous graft, and full-thickness skin graft) are folded like an accordion to create a tragus and a deepened, widened conchal bowl. This firm tragal supporting structure avoids the shrinkage of other amorphous soft tissue advancement flaps. The newly excavated conchal bowl and

Text continued on page 348

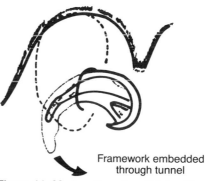

Framework embedded through tunnel

Figure 14–22. Insertion of graft into skin pocket.

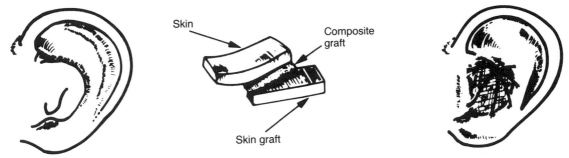

Figure 14–25. The full-thickness skin graft is sutured to the posterior aspect of the composite graft anteriorly and to the skin of the excavated conchal bowl posteriorly.

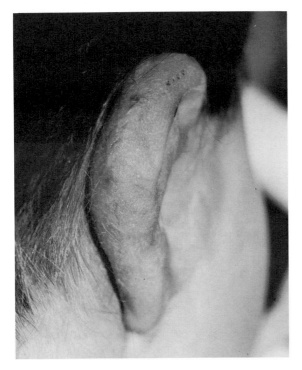

Figure 14–26. Additional protrusion of ear, obtained through elevation and scalp advancement.

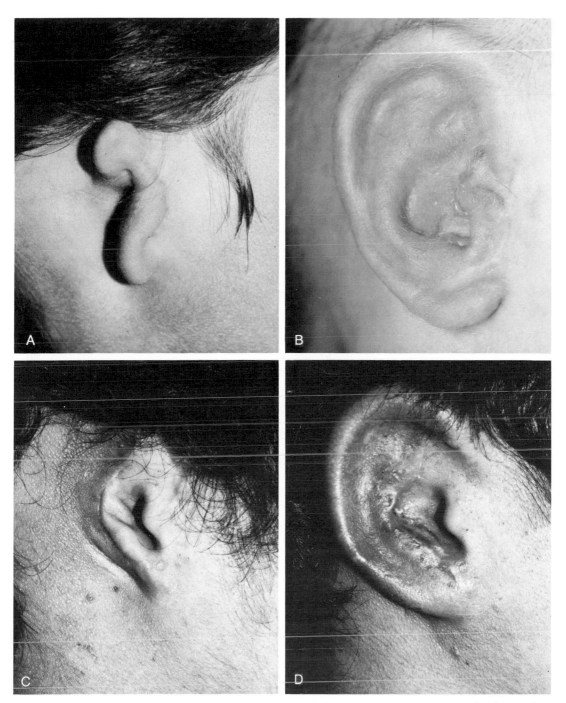

Figure 14–27. *A.* Preoperative microtia. *B.* Postoperative result from *A. C.* Preoperative microtia that has undergone previous atresia repair. *D.* Postoperative result from *C.*

Illustration continued on following page

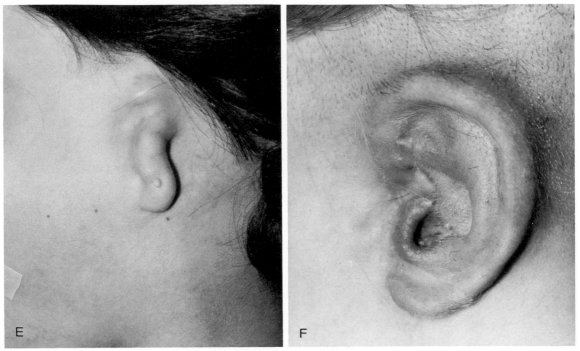

Figure 14–27 *Continued E.* Preoperative microtia. *F.* Postoperative result from *E.*

the entrance of the external canal are packed with bismuth tribromophenate (Xeroform) to prevent blunting of their depth and detail.

Elevation of the Helix

After tragal reconstruction, the auricle should have a pleasing contour but may still lack adequate projection. The patient has an appendage for glasses or a hearing aid at this point but may need a postauricular groove or sulcus to anchor these appliances. If no hypertrophic scarring from the previous stages has occurred, the helix can be elevated simultaneously as the otologic surgeon constructs an external canal and a middle ear. A curvilinear incision is made 5 mm posterior and parallel to the helix. The scalp is elevated in a subgaleal plane 6 to 7 cm posteriorly. The cartilage framework is dissected from the periosteum; the surgeon must take extreme care to avoid exposing the bare cartilage. If the framework is denuded of its soft tissue covering, it must be recovered with soft tissue. If a large section of cartilage is exposed, the procedure must be terminated because no skin graft will adhere to it directly. The framework should be dissected and elevated to the level of the concha.

Excessive elevation causes the superior pole to fall anteriorly and displace the framework. The periosteum is dissected separately by the otologist, and the bony canal is subsequently constructed.

A postauricular sulcus is developed as the undermined scalp is advanced anteriorly and secured to the periosteum beneath the auricle. The denuded posterior surface of the auricle is covered with a full-thickness skin graft from the groin. The sulcus is packed with bismuth tribromophenate gauze and tied over with sutures for 10 days. This elevation and scalp advancement gain additional protrusion and create better harmony with the opposite side (Figs. 14–26, 14–27).

ATYPICAL MICROTIA

Patients who have previously undergone ear surgery or who have a low-lying hairline present additional problems. Excessive scarring with extensive fibrosis makes dissection of a thin subdermal pocket quite difficult. Thick, nonelastic scar tissue does not conform to the delicately sculptured cartilage framework. This type of skin must be re-

Figure 14–28. Cartilage framework placed over the pocket and removal of nonusable, scarred, wrinkled skin.

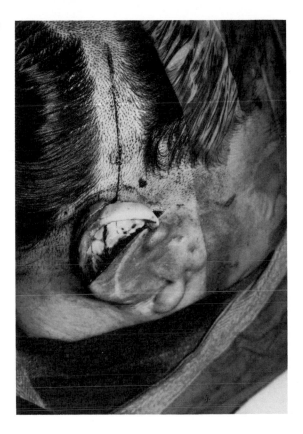

moved and replaced with a skin graft. Well-vascularized tissue must be placed between the cartilage and the skin. The proximity of the temporalis fascia, with its branches of the superficial temporal artery, makes this tissue excellent coverage to nourish the skin graft.

An attempt is made to create a subdermal pocket and any remnants of microtic cartilage are removed. The cartilage framework is placed over the pocket, and nonusable, scarred, wrinkled skin is removed (Fig. 14–28). The temporal vessels are outlined on the parietal skin with a Doppler ultrasonographic flowmeter. No epinephrine is injected into the scalp or fascia, so that vascularity can be better evaluated and necrosis of the most distal margins of the flap can be avoided. A vertical incision 12-cm long is made above the pocket. Scalp flaps are elevated anteriorly and posteriorly just beneath the hair follicles.

When enough length is dissected to cover the exposed framework, a horizontal incision 6 cm long is made through the temporal fascia. A fascial flap is elevated and rotated interiorly to cover the framework. A closed suction drain is inserted, and the fascia is sutured to the undersurface of the skin

pocket (Fig. 14–29). An 0.4-mm skin graft is harvested and sutured over the fascia to the skin. To have any definition, the contours of the framework must have been even more exaggerated to allow for the additional thickness of these two layers of tissue. Continuous suction drainage is used for 3 days to enhance coaption of the fascial flap and skin graft with the cartilage (Fig. 14–30). Additional stages are continued in the same sequence as with classic microtia construction.

SUMMARY

Re-creation of the absent or deformed auricle requires a thorough analysis of each specific deformity and the methods of repair. The ear should be a flaplike structure, bordered by a gently sloping helical rim placed in a proper axis, at a proper inclination, and in a proper position. There is little agreement as to what constitutes an ideal ear. Perhaps a "normal" auricle can best be described as one that calls little attention to itself.

Reconstruction of the microtic ear should be started as early in life as possible to help avoid many psychologic problems often

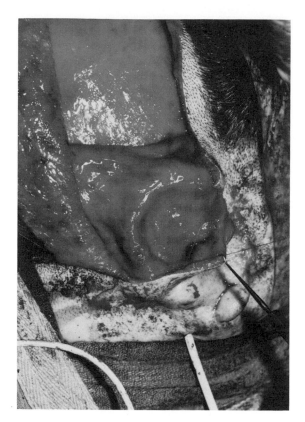

Figure 14–29. Insertion of closed suction drain and suturing of fascia to the undersurface of the skin pocket.

Figure 14–30. Continuous suction drainage, used for 3 days, to enhance coaption of the fascial flap and skin graft with the cartilage.

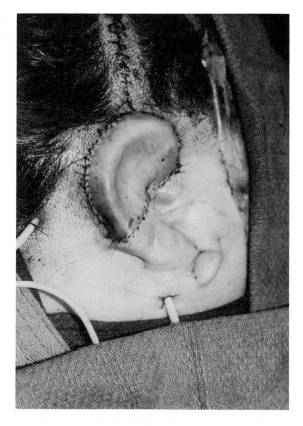

caused by the deformity. When microtia is unilateral, the auriculoplasty must first be completed before any temporal bone surgery is begun, so that a pocket for the costal cartilage graft will be well vascularized and nonscarred. Elements of the sculptured graft must be exaggerated so that height and definition are adequate. A well-structured, communicative team approach with the facial plastic surgeons and the otologic surgeons is essential to maximize the aesthetic and functional results.

SUGGESTED READINGS

Aguilar EA, Jahrsdoerfer RA: The surgical repair of congenital microtia and atresia. Otolaryngol Head Neck Surg 98:600–606, 1988.

Brent B: The correction of microtia with autogenous cartilage grafts: I. The classical deformity. Plast Reconstr Surg 66:1–12, 1980a.

Brent B: The correction of microtia with autogenous cartilage grafts: II. Atypical and complex deformities. Plast Reconstr Surg 66:13–21, 1980b.

Cole RR, Jahrsdoerfer RA: Congenital aural atresia. Clin Plast Surg 17:367–371, 1990.

Colman BH: Congenital atresia: aspects of surgical care. Acta Otorhinolaryngol Belg 25:929–935, 1971.

Cosman B: The constricted ear. Clin Plast Surg 5:389–394, 1988.

Crabtree JA: Congenital atresia: case selection, complications, and prevention. Otolaryngol Clin North Amer 15:755–762, 1982.

Crabtree JA: The facial nerve in congenital ear surgery. *In* Graham MD, House WF (eds): Disorders of the Facial Nerve. New York: Raven Press, 1982.

Farkas LG: Anthropometry of the normal and defective ear. Clin Plast Surg 17:213–217, 1990.

Gill NW: Congenital atresia of the ear: A review of the surgical findings in 83 cases. J Laryngol 83:551–587, 1969.

MacGregor FC: Ear deformities: social and psychological implications. Clin Plast Surg 5:347–350, 1978.

Roush J, Rauch SD: Clinical application of implantable bone conduction hearing device. Laryngoscope 100:281–285, 1990.

Ruder RO: New concepts in microtia repair. Arch Otolaryngol Head Neck Surg 114:1016–1019, 1988.

Tolleth H: A hierarchy of values in the design and construction of the ear. Clin Plast Surg 17:193–197, 1990.

CHAPTER 15

Acquired Lesions of the Auricle and Ear

Vincent G. Caruso, MD

THE EXTERNAL EAR CANAL

Otitis Externa

Otitis externa is one of the most common diseases encountered by the otolaryngologist. The treatment of otitis externa is usually simple and easily accomplished in one or more office visits. However, it may be protracted and frustrating and have a fatal outcome. Successful treatment depends on a thorough understanding of the pathophysiologic mechanism in each patient, a proper diagnosis, and treatment tailored to the individual case.

Pathophysiology. The external auditory canal is designed to be protected from the entrance of foreign bodies and from infections. The tragus helps shield the orifice of the canal from foreign bodies. The anterior direction of the canal from lateral to medial, the hairs of the lateral third of the canal, and the narrow isthmus protect the canal from foreign bodies. The sebaceous and apocrine glands of the outer third of the ear canal that empty into the hair follicles and produce cerumen also protect the external auditory canal. The cerumen covering the squamous epithelial lining has an acid reaction that inhibits the growth of bacteria and fungi. It collects in the outer third of the ear canal, providing a chemical barrier to infection and an additional obstruction to the entrance of foreign bodies. Its lipid content tends to prevent moisture within the external canal

from entering the pilosebaceous units, thereby preventing maceration of the squamous epithelium of the external auditory canal.

Many local factors may interfere with the normal defenses against infection. Fastidious persons who feel that the presence of cerumen in the ear canal is a sign of uncleanliness carefully clean cerumen from their own and their children's external auditory canals. Removing the cerumen eliminates an important barrier to infection. Recurrent douching of the external auditory canal with water, which occurs with swimming or scuba diving, also tends to remove the cerumen from the ear canal and dissolve some of its more water-soluble elements. This increases the possibility of penetration by bacteria. The heat and humidity and increased swimming in warmer climates tends to increase the moisture within the external auditory canal, which leads to increased colonization with bacteria and fungi. Washing the ear canal with soapy water leaves a film of alkali along the canal wall. This also predisposes the patient to otitis externa. A narrow canal or excessive cerumen may permit the accumulation of water within the external canal during swimming and lead to recurrent otitis externa. Cleaning the external auditory canal, whether performed with cotton-tipped swabs, bobby pins, fingernails, or the tip of a pen or pencil, may cause abrasion of the epithelial barrier and permit the entrance of organisms into the tissue. Many patients, in times of emotional stress, have a habit of scratching their ears with fingernails or other objects. The feeling of fullness caused by serous otitis media may cause a patient to scratch and dig at the ears, and this may lead to otitis externa. The mild inflammation caused by scratching produces itching that leads to further scratching; this cycle continues until the skin becomes infected.

Many systemic conditions, such as anemia, vitamin deficiency, endocrine disorders, and various forms of dermatitis, lower host resistance to infection. Seborrheic dermatitis is a systemic disease that may predispose a patient to otitis externa. It usually manifests with a history of infantile eczema, severe dandruff, and seborrhea corporis. Characteristic findings in patients with seborrheic dermatitis involving the external auditory canal are retroauricular eczema (Fig. 15–1) and scaling within the outer third of the canal that may extend into the cavum conchae. Psoriasis may be present in the external auditory canal and must be considered as a possible predisposing cause of otitis externa. Circumscribed neurodermatitis, which is occasionally present in the external auditory canal, produces spasmodic itching associated with anxiety. Contact dermatitis involving the auricle and the external auditory canal is very common. It may be caused by the use of hair sprays or chemicals leached from the earpieces of eyeglasses or from the earmolds of hearing aids. Contact dermatitis commonly occurs after drugs are instilled into the external canal. Neomycin is probably the most common sensitizing drug used in the ears. Allergies to bacteria may play a role in external otitis when, as in the case of chronic otitis media, the external auditory canal is subjected to constant purulent drainage. In these cases, the organisms and their metabolites elicit an allergic response in the skin of the external canal.

The normal ear canal is sterile in some persons. In others, *Staphylococcus albus* is cultered alone or in combination with other organisms, usually diphtheroids. *Staphylococcus aureus* and *Pseudomonas pyocyanea* species, the most common pathogens in otitis externa, are rarely cultured from normal ears. In cases of otitis externa, bacteriologic cultures most commonly show a mixed flora, with *Pseudomonas* species predominating. The most common fungus isolated in both normal and infected ears is *Aspergillus*. Except in very grossly contaminated water, the water quality, as measured by bacterial counts, is not usually related to the incidence of otitis externa in swimmers.

Diagnosis. In general, the diagnosis of otitis externa is not a problem to the experienced otolaryngologist. The patient usually presents with a characteristic picture. This includes pain, discharge from the external auditory canal, tenderness on movement of the tragus and the auricle, and occasionally fever and celulitis. The tenderness of the auricle, the tragus, and the canal wall and the redness and swelling of the canal wall skin help in distinguishing otitis externa from suppurative otitis media. However, the predominant symptoms may be itching, hearing loss, a feeling of fullness, or aural discharge. The symptoms and the physical findings are helpful in determining the specific factors that play an etiologic role in each case of otitis externa. Dry, scaly skin associated with an itchy external canal suggests the presence of a seborrheic dermatitis, especially in the presence of severe dandruff or other signs of seborrhea. Itching may also be characteristic of a superficial fungal infection of the ear canal, contact dermatitis or eczema, or a sensitivity (dermatophytid) reaction to a distant fungal infection such as tinea pedis or monilial vaginitis. The weeping, crusting, and itching associated with eczematous otitis externa is diagnosed by examining the ear and by noting the related dermatoses elsewhere on the skin. Neurodermatitis, which

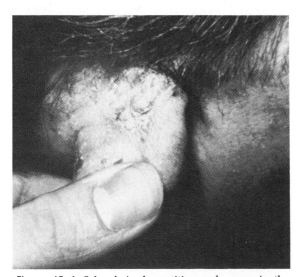

Figure 15–1. Seborrheic dermatitis can be seen in the retroauricular crease.

is presumably caused by chronic rubbing or scratching of the skin, is usually diagnosed from the anxiety that the patient exhibits, from the thickened skin of the external auditory canal, and from other patches of neurodermatitis on the body. A feeling of fullness with itching in the ear may represent otomycosis in the external auditory canal. In the usual case of *Aspergillus niger* infection, examination reveals the characteristic grayish membranes.

Treatment. No single therapeutic approach can cure all cases of otitis externa. The principles of therapy for otitis externa are as follows: (1) relief of pain or discomfort; (2) elimination or control of predisposing causes; (3) thorough cleansing of the aural canal; (4) acidification of the external auditory canal; and (5) judicious, limited use of specific medication. The need for the relief of pain seems obvious but is often overlooked in the rush to apply medications to the external auditory canal. Otitis externa can be a severely painful and debilitating condition, requiring the use of codeine or meperidine hydrochloride for a short time while the disease is being controlled. Successful treatment of otitis externa must begin with an understanding of the causes of the particular case at hand. Systemic conditions, including anemia, hypovitaminosis, endocrine disturbances, and dermatologic conditions, are treated. It is often necessary to control severe dandruff of the scalp before a refractory external otitis responds to local treatment. Persistent trauma to the ear canal must be controlled before other therapy can be effective. On rare occasions, patients are allergic to methyl methacrylate in their hearing mold. Patch tests may be used to confirm the diagnosis. The mold may be coated with polyvinyl chloride or made from vulcanite, silicone rubber, or gold, which are less allergenic.

The most important factor in the treatment of most cases of otitis externa is the thorough and repeated cleansing of the external auditory canal. Medications placed in the canal in the form of drops are unlikely to reach the surface epithelium unless the canal is thoroughly cleansed of desquamated epithelium, pus, and cerumen. Repeated, thorough cleansing of the ear canal in the physician's office with irrigation and suction is usually necessary until the infection is controlled. Because the canal is extremely painful and tender, it is preferable to flush the canal with a solution such as Burow's solution. In particularly refractory cases, the patient is given a 60-mL syringe and a prescription for Burow's powders or tablets. The patient is instructed to dissolve two tablets in a pint of boiling water at home and allow the solution to cool to room temperature. This is the stock solution. A portion of it is warmed to body temperature by diluting it in half with very warm tap water before each instillation. About 60 mL is used for each irrigation three or four times daily. The patient can tell when the ear is being irrigated adequately because it feels similar to the irrigation performed in the office by the physician. A member of the family can usually perform this maneuver for the patient over the sink. Although this procedure is messy and inconvenient, it is usually acceptable to the patient if the physician explains the necessity for its use. Alternatively, after thorough cleaning in the office, the patient may be given any one of a number of proprietary preparations to place in the ear canal three times daily. These preparations should have an acid pH and be in a nonsensitizing base such as propylene glycol. Whichever agent is selected must be applied in sufficient quantity to cover the whole surface of the external auditory canal. Therefore, the patient should be instructed to place from three drops to a whole dropperful in the ear canal, with the head kept to the side to allow the drops to remain in the ear canal and coat the surface before the head is straightened and the excess medication is allowed to run out. Culturing of the ear canal is usually not necessary. It may be performed on the second or third visit if the otitis externa appears to be an infectious process and is not responding to therapy.

If the external auditory canal is infected and there is no accumulation of pus or debris in the ear canal, one of the many proprietary ear drops containing a combination of antibiotics effective against *Staphylococcus* and gram-negative organisms with a topical steroid and an acid pH may be prescribed. This therapy is easier to implement than is irrigation. However, the physician must be constantly alert to the development of hypersensitivity to one of the antibiotics, particularly neomycin. This reaction may be partially masked by the steroid that is usually included in such preparations. This sensitivity reaction may appear to the untrained eye to be a worsening of the original infection. In severe infections, the skin and the subcutaneous tissue of the external auditory canal are swollen to such a degree that medication cannot be instilled into the ear canal. Debris has collected and is trapped within the canal. In these cases, a cotton wick soaked with ear drops is gently placed into the canal. Medication placed on the wick is carried medially by capillary attraction. After 1 or 2 days, the canal is usually open, and cleaning and instillation of the medication is permitted without the wick.

Fungal infection of the external auditory canal is usually secondary to colonization with *Aspergillus niger*. This infection may be recognized by the velvety grayish membranes that line the medial two thirds of the external auditory canal and frequently fill the canal. Suction removal of the membranes reveals an inflamed epithelial lining of the canal. The canal must be thoroughly cleansed by suction and irrigation and then treated with a fungicidal drug. Castellani's paint is usually effective topically but has the disadvantage of staining the tissues of the cavum conchae and sometimes the patient's clothes. It may be applied in the physician's office after thorough cleansing of the ear canal. Proprietary ear drops are prescribed. In particularly refractory cases of fungal external otitis, clotrimazole (Lotrimin) drops instilled three times daily with weekly or biweekly cleansing of the ear canal in the physician's office has been successful. When the ear canal is healed and the infection cleared, therapy should be terminated. If the symptoms recur, the patient should return to the physician rather than begin self-treatment with a prescription from a previous infection.

Systemic antibiotics with a broad spectrum of bactericidal effect are helpful when there is a surrounding cellulitis, cervical lymphadenopathy, or signs of systemic infection. Amoxicillin is effective in most instances. Cefoperazone may be particularly effective because of its activity against *Staphylococcus* and *Pseudomonas*. Because of the nature of the mixed flora cultured in cases of otitis externa, the systemic antibiotic is usually not selected on the basis of a culture.

Furuncles may form in the outer third of the external auditory canal. These are staphylococcal infections of the pilosebaceous units and manifest with the symptoms previously described for otitis externa. Although they are usually treated with analgesics, systemic antibiotics, local heat, and topical antibiotic solutions, incision and drainage may be necessary.

In rare instances, chronic, irreversible changes occur within the skin and subcutaneous tissue of the external auditory canal. These changes may render the canal susceptible to persistent, chronic otitis externa. In these cases, the skin is markedly thickened. The pilosebaceous units are usually nonfunctioning, and the cerumen and acid mantle are not present to aid in the prevention of infection. In instances of chronic, intractable otitis externa, excision of all infected skin with a meatoplasty, with or without skin grafting, has been successful.

Prevention. Prevention of recurrent otitis externa may be accomplished only by strict attention to the predisposing causes. Seborrheic dermatitis, psoriasis, eczema, and contact dermatitis must all be treated adequately. Trauma to the external canal must be avoided. Patients with a history of recurrent attacks of otitis externa after swimming are given directions for prophylactic use of acidic alcohol drops in their ears before and after exposure to water. A 10-mL bottle is filled with rubbing alcohol (70%) and four drops of vinegar (4%). Alternatively, alcohol drops may be purchased. This solution is somewhat less effective, but more patients comply with its regimen because it can be bought at the local pharmacy. A dropperful of the solution is placed in each ear before and after the day's swimming. Divers exposed to water regularly and for long periods of time find this particularly helpful in preventing otitis externa.

Malignant Otitis Externa

Malignant otitis externa is a progressive, debilitating, often fatal infection of the external auditory canal, the surrounding tissue, and the base of the skull. Although uncommon, it is seen perhaps once or twice yearly in a busy otolaryngology practice. It is an uncommon infection caused by *Pseudomonas aeruginosa* in patients with low resistance to infection.

Pathophysiology. The disease typically occurs in elderly diabetics. The vasculitis of diabetes enhances the vasculitis produced by *Pseudomonas*. Other predisposing conditions include arteriosclerosis, immunosuppression by chemotherapy, steroid administration, hypogammaglobulinemia, neutropenia with decreased neutrophil chemotactic activity, and other disorders of cellular immunity. *Pseudomonas* is cultured from the external auditory canal in pure or mixed culture. This organism produces exotoxins, including a neurotoxin, and contains enzymes, including lecithinase, hemolysin, lipase, esterase, and a variety of proteases. These enzymes cause a necrotizing vasculitis that aids the organism in destroying local tissues and resisting phagocytosis. Leukocidin and hemolytic toxin, also produced by *Pseudomonas*, destroy white blood cells and inhibit their phagocytic chemotactic activity. The infection begins in the external auditory canal, probably as a mixed infection, and later becomes a pure *Pseudomonas* infection. The disease may spread from the external auditory canal through Santorini's fissures in the conchal cartilage to invade the periauricular tissue, including the parotid gland, the temporomandibular joint, and the soft tissue at the base of the skull. From there, the infection ordinarily progresses along the base of the skull, causing paralysis of cranial nerve VII at the stylomastoid foramen; cranial nerves IX, X, and XI at the jugular foramen; and the hypoglossal nerve at the hypoglossal canal. The jugular vein may become thrombosed, and progression to a lateral sinus thrombosis may occur. Alternatively, the infection may progress from the external auditory canal through the tympanic membrane into the middle ear and throughout the mastoid air cell system. From here it has access to the petrous apex, the intracranial structures, and the brain stem. The infection may progress into the mastoid air cell system by producing an osteitis in the bony external auditory canal wall. The progressive cranial polyneuropathy is indicative of a very poor prognosis, with impending meningitis and lateral sinus and cavernous sinus thromboses.

Diagnosis. The diagnosis is based on a history of refractory, progressive otitis externa in an elderly diabetic or an immunosuppressed patient. Invariably, there is granulation tissue at the junction of the cartilaginous and bony external auditory canal; bare or necrotic cartilage and bone occasionally can be seen at this site. The tympanic membrane is usually intact. Culture reveals *Pseudomonas aeruginosa*. The severe pain produced by this infection is monitored in following the progress of treatment. Recurrent pain after apparent control of the infection is an ominous sign and warrants aggressive management. Although the diagnosis of malignant external otitis is usually made by use of clinical criteria, the extent of the disease is difficult to determine. Additional information regarding the exact extent of infection in the soft tissue and bone at the base of the skull is needed. Conventional radiographs and computed tomography are insensitive to the presence or extent of cellulitis or early osteomyelitis. In contrast, both technetium 99 and gallium 67 scans are very sensitive and accurate in the early diagnosis of malignant otitis externa. Gallium 67 is picked up by granulocytes and technetium 99 by osteoblasts. These scans are usually normal in patients with benign otitis externa. Although technetium 99 scans remain positive long after the osteomyelitis has cleared, gallium 67 scans become negative as the infection clears. Thus gallium 67 scans offer a means for following the progression of disease or recovery (Fig. 15–2). Because uncertainty about the extent of the disease results in undertreatment with increased morbidity and mortality, these scans provide an important contribution to successful treatment. Magnetic resonance imaging is helpful in evaluating the anatomic extent of the soft tissue changes, although abnormalities on imaging resolve more slowly than does the condition itself.

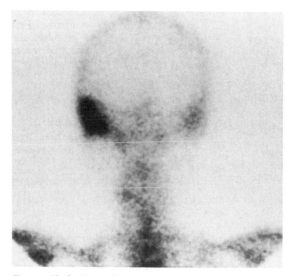

Figure 15–2. Area of intense uptake can be seen on a gallium scan of a patient with malignant otitis externa.

Treatment. The principles of successful treatment include control of the diabetes, administration of antibiotics, and aggressive local wound care, usually with limited surgical debridement. The standard antibiotic treatment has included the combination of a semisynthetic antipseudomonal penicillin such as carbenicillin and an aminoglycoside such as gentamicin. They act synergistically to delay the development of resistance by *Pseudomonas.* These drugs must be administered parenterally, and each has potentially serious side effects. The aminoglycosides are nephrotoxic and ototoxic; patients' blood aminoglycoside levels and renal and cochlear function must be monitored during therapy. Antipseudomonal cephalosporins, such as ceftazidime, and ciprofloxacin, a fluoroquinolone, have been used successfully either alone or in combination. They have less renal toxicity and no known ototoxicity. Ciprofloxacin may be administered orally. Hyperbaric oxygen may be considered as adjuvant therapy when a hyperbaric pressure chamber is available and may add significantly to the treatment protocol. Local wound care often includes limited debridement of the infected tissue; however, it may include bone, cartilage, and the parotid gland. Each case should be treated individually, and a mastoidectomy should be avoided if the mastoid air cell system is not involved. After debridement, topical wound care may be accomplished with use of antibiotics effective against *Pseudomonas* (e.g., colistin, polymyxin B, and neomycin). Four percent acetic acid soaks are also effective. Patients who have had this disease must be followed closely, and close cooperation between the internist and the otolaryngologist is necessary.

Trauma

Abrasions and Lacerations. Abrasions and lacerations of the external auditory canal are common and may be caused by the patient or by the physician. In most instances, these injuries heal spontaneously unless they are grossly contaminated. The status of the tympanic membrane and facial nerve should be recorded, and the patient should be followed closely for signs of infection. Proprietary ear drops containing antibiotics are usually effective in treating infected superficial lacerations and abrasions of the external auditory canal. Deeper lacerations or avulsion of skin may require packing the external auditory canal with petrolatum gauze covered with neomycin-containing ointment. This allows lacerations to heal without infection or stenosis. Partial avulsion of the skin usually does not require grafting because the remaining skin of the external auditory canal regenerates quickly if there is no infection.

Temporal Bone Fractures. Temporal bone fractures may follow head trauma and may be of the transverse, the longitudinal, or the mixed variety. The transverse fracture is usually produced by a blow to the occiput. It runs translabyrinthine, traverses the internal auditory canal and cochlea, and ends in the foramen lacerum or spinosum. It may also run posterolaterally across the whole labyrinth and fallopian canal and end in the middle ear. In transverse fractures, the external auditory canal is usually spared. Sensorineural hearing loss, facial nerve paralysis, nystagmus, and hemotympanum are the usual findings. In the longitudinal variety, however, the fracture runs through the bone that surrounds the carotid artery, passes through the middle ear and thus causes a tear in the tympanic membrane, and terminates as a fracture in the roof of the exernal auditory canal. Patients with a longitudinal fracture usually manifest conductive hearing loss as a result of ossicular and tympanic membrane injury and bloody otorrhea (occasionally mixed with cerebrospinal fluid). Facial nerve paralysis is present in approximately 25% of the cases. The mixed type of temporal bone fracture may include any combination of these findings. Treatment of temporal bone fractures is usually conservative, with systemic antibiotics and careful cleansing of the external auditory canal when otorrhea is present. Facial nerve paralysis of immediate onset may require exploration.

Temporal bone fractures may result in aural meningoceles or in meningoencephaloceles. Surgical correction is performed through a mastoidectomy approach if the patient has not had previous mastoid surgery. If a radical mastoidectomy has been performed previously, repair is done through a middle cranial fossa approach.

Foreign Bodies. Foreign bodies in the external auditory canal are a challenge for the otolaryngologist, who usually has an operating microscope and several microsurgical instruments including metal suctions, ring curets, wire loops, and hooks of various sizes. Inanimate objects that are lateral to the isthmus of the canal are usually removed easily. Objects medial to the isthmus of the canal are more difficult to remove because they must be brought through the isthmus, where the canal wall skin is thin and quite sensitive. Often, hematomas and maceration are produced in the skin of the inner two thirds of the external auditory canal by minimal trauma. Care must be taken for avoidance of injuries to the tympanic membrane and the ossicles when larger objects medial to the isthmus are being removed. Several drops of oil are useful for killing insects before their removal. Compressed air may be used to flush the ear canal with Burow's solution or hydrogen peroxide when smaller objects are removed from the ear canal. This procedure causes little discomfort to the patient. Irrigations should not be used to flush out vegetable seeds and beans because they may expand in a position medial to the isthmus and this expansion makes their extraction more difficult. Older children and adults may be anesthetized locally before a difficult extraction. In young children or in cases of difficult extractions in adults, it is best to begin the attempted extraction under general anesthesia in the operating room. One or two drops of blood, some maceration of the canal wall skin, and some pain may make the procedure very difficult and uncomfortable for the patient.

Exostoses. Exostoses of the external auditory canal are caused by repeated cooling of the bone of the external auditory canal. This cooling is produced by swimming repeatedly in cold water. It is uncommon in warm climates unless the patient has lived previously in northern climates. Exostoses may be large enough to prevent water from exiting from the sulcus lateral to the tympanic membrane after swimming. Patients with this condition may have recurrent external otitis and a collection of epithelial debris medial to the exostoses. In these cases, the exostoses should be removed surgically.

THE AURICLE

Trauma

Sharp Trauma. A detailed review of the reconstructive techniques employed for re-

pairing the injured auricle is beyond the scope of this chapter, but reviews on this subject are available.

As in other soft tissue trauma, injuries to the auricle must be carefully treated in the emergency room for obtaining the best possible long-term cosmetic result. The blood supply in this area is plentiful, and debridement should be judicious and minimal. Every effort is made to preserve perichondrium because cartilage that is devoid of perichondrium is subject to necrosis. Local flaps and skin grafts have been used to cover exposed cartilage and perichondrium. Incomplete avulsion injuries to the ear are treated conservatively to preserve tissue. Free composite grafts of auricular tissue that is not too heavily contaminated will probably survive repair. Large pieces of auricular cartilage that are devoid of perichondrium may be buried under postauricular skin for later use in a reconstruction, with a pedicled flap. Complete avulsion of the auricle has been treated successfully by immediate reanastomosis by use of microsurgical techniques. However, the successful reattachment of totally amputated ears is still rare because of the small diameter of the vessels to be anastomosed (0.3 to 0.7 mm), avulsion of the vessels, and venous thrombosis. Iced saline has been used to decrease the metabolic needs of the composite graft, and dextran, heparin, and antibiotics have been used to prevent intravascular coagulation and infection in the flap.

Although keloids usually occur in black persons, they may occur in white people. Commonly found on the lobule of the ear, they may be a result of ear piercing. They usually respond to intralesional injection of triamcinolone at weekly intervals. For prevention of recurrence, large keloids may require excision followed by triamcinolone injection and low-dose irradiation. Earrings worn on pierced ears may be pulled through the earlobe (Fig. 15–3). This often occurs when women are holding children who pull on large, attractive earrings and in patients who wear unusually heavy earrings. There are a variety of methods for repair of a defect that results from earlobe keloid removal or repair of an earlobe that has been cleft as a result of pierced earrings.

Blunt Trauma. The most common complication of blunt trauma to the ear is the formation of hematomas (Fig. 15–4). When

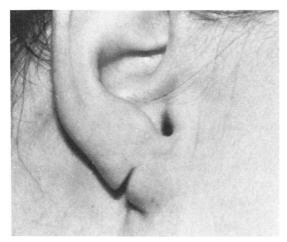

Figure 15–3. Typical lesion created by forceful extraction of a pierced earring can be identified in the lobule.

hematomas form below the perichondrium, they must be evacuated for prevention of infection or "cauliflower ear" deformity. Aspiration and application of pressure are often successful but may have to be repeated. If a hematoma recurs, incision and drainage are performed and followed by application of a pressure dressing. The "cauliflower ear" deformity is a thickening of cartilage in the location of an earlier hematoma. It is repaired by thinning the cartilage under a skin-perichondrial flap.

Burns. Burns of the auricle are common in patients presenting with extensive facial burns. Of these patients, about 25% develop suppurative chondritis. Burns may be caused by fire, hot liquids, sun exposure, or electric current. Most important in treating the burned auricle is avoidance of pressure. First-degree burns are treated conservatively with pain medications. Second- and third-degree burns may be treated with silver sulfadiazine, mafenide acetate, or silver nitrate and Surgifix mesh dressing. Full-thickness auricular burns may lead to demarcation and autoamputation of the affected portion of the auricle. Third-degree burns may be extensively debrided and grafted or closed. However, more conservative management usually leads to less tissue loss and may carry no higher incidence of suppurative chondritis. In conservative management, granulation tissue is allowed to form over the full-thickness burned area, and split-thickness grafts are used for cover. Chemical burns are treated by flushing the surface with saline, half-strength vinegar (2% acetic acid), or a mild alkali (1 teaspoonful of baking soda in a 12-oz glass of water), depending on whether the burn is chemical, alkaline, or acidic.

Frostbite. Frostbite is a condition in which tissue is frozen. Temperatures below 10°C block sensory nerve input and thereby deprive the patient of advanced warning of impending danger. Once the temperature falls below freezing, the frostbite injury begins. Initially, vasoconstriction produces a pallor. Ice formation occurs in extracellular fluid, resulting in a hypertonic state in the remaining fluid and intracellular dehydration. As the affected area thaws, subcutaneous edema resulting from extravasated fluid causes bullae to form (Fig. 15–5). Later, erythema occurs around the demarcating tissue, which is distinguishable over a period of weeks or months. Treatment consists of rapidly rewarming the frostbitten area with moist cotton pledgets at a temperature of 38°C to 42°C. Silver nitrate (0.5%) soaks are applied to superficial infections only. Ordi-

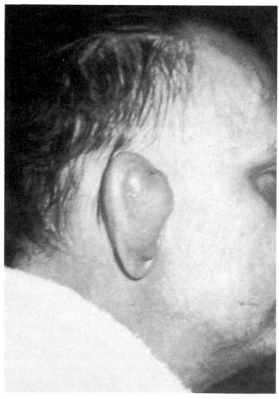

Figure 15–4. Extensive auricular hematoma after blunt trauma.

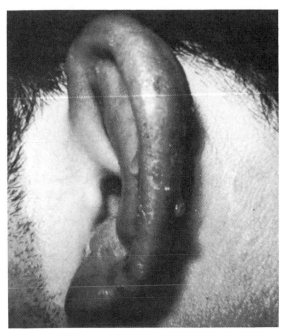

Figure 15–5. Typical frostbite injury to the auricle, showing weeping of fluid and bullae formation.

narily, the auricle is kept sterile, but no dressings are used. The use of sympathectomy, hyperbaric oxygen, and low-molecular-weight dextran remain controversial. Rubbing with snow or exposure to radiant heat is contraindicated.

Inflammation

Cellulitis and Perichondritis. Cellulitis of the auricle is usually secondary to otitis externa. It is managed with mild, local heat and systemic antibiotics. Perichondritis is an inflammation of perichondrium that complicates burns or trauma to the auricle. It usually occurs 3 to 5 weeks after a burn and manifests initially with severe pain. This is followed within several hours by redness, swelling, tenderness, and elevated temperature in the affected area. Prevention of perichondritis begins with general supportive care in the burn patient, strict avoidance of pressure on the injured ear, and topical antimicrobial chemotherapy. Polyurethane foam doughnuts are used to prevent injury from pressure. Perichondritis and chondritis are usually caused by infection with *Pseudomonas aeruginosa* and *Staphylococcus* species. Mild cases may be treated by debridement and drainage and topical and systemic antimicrobial agents. Severe cases may require debridement by the bivalve technique. Diabetes may be a predisposing factor in patients with perichondritis of the auricle, especially when there is no history of burns.

Relapsing Polychondritis. Relapsing polychondritis is an episodic, inflammatory disease of the connective tissue and various cartilages in the head and neck and the upper respiratory tract. The etiologic factor is probably an autoimmune reaction. It manifests most commonly as an acute inflammation of the cartilage of the ears, the larynx, and the nasal septum but may affect the trachea, causing respiratory obstruction. The "saddle nose" and "cauliflower ear" deformities are late signs commonly seen in the disease. Fever is the most common clinical symptom but is nonspecific. Auricular manifestations occur in about half of the cases. Steroids are used to control the acute attacks and suppress recurrence. A high index of suspicion is necessary for early diagnosis of this disease.

Varicella–Herpes Zoster. The varicella–herpes zoster virus may affect the auricle. It has two primary clinical forms. The varicella form has an incubation period of 14 to 17 days, followed by prodromal malaise and fever for 1 to 2 days and a subsequent maculopapular cutaneous eruption. Pneumonia, encephalitis, neuritis, and myelitis occur in rare instances. In the zoster form of the disease, the incubation period is unknown. The cutaneous eruption is usually unilateral and confined to one or more dermatomes corresponding to the distribution of the extramedullary cranial nerve ganglia. The cutaneous lesion is painful but self-limiting, and local treatment is usually unnecessary. Facial nerve paralysis and vertigo may occur in Ramsay Hunt syndrome when cranial nerves VII and VIII are involved.

SUGGESTED READINGS

Kraus D, Rehm S, Kinney S: The evolving treatment of necrotizing external otitis. Laryngoscope 98:934–939, 1988.

Locher A, Blitzer A: The traumatized auricle—care, salvage, and reconstruction. Otol Clin North Am 15:225–239, 1982.

Mills D, et al: Suppurative chondritis: its incidence prevention, and treatment in burn patients. Plast Reconstr Surg 82:267–276, 1988.

Mutimer K, Banis J, Upton J: Microsurgical reattachment of totally amputated ears. Plast Reconstr Surg 79:535–541, 1987.

Quaba A: Reconstruction of a posttraumatic ear defect using tissue expansion: 30 years after Newmann. Plast Reconstr Surg 82:521–524, 1988.

Rubin J, et al: Malignant external otitis: vitality of CT in diagnosis and follow up. Radiology 174:391–394, 1990.

Rubin J, Yu V: Malignant external otitis: insights into pathogenesis, clinical manifestations, diagnosis, and therapy. Am J Med 85:391–398, 1988.

Sessions D, et al: Frostbite of the ear. Laryngoscope 81:1223–1232, 1971.

Shupak A, et al: Hyperbaric oxygenation for necrotizing (malignant) otitis externa. Arch Otolaryngol 115:1470–1475, 1989.

Noninflammatory Lesions of the Ear and Skull Base

Peter S. Roland, MD

A wide variety of both malignant and benign lesions may involve the temporal bone. Selection of the appropriate therapeutic modality depends not only on accurate identification of the type of neoplasm but also on precise mapping of the tumor. The temporal bone is a structure of such complexity that tumor extension of a few millimeters in one direction or another may make a critical difference in whether the tumor can be successfully resected. The temporal bone surgeon must use all available diagnostic modalities to ascertain with as much precision as possible the precise limits of tumor involvement.

BENIGN TUMORS

Acoustic Neuroma

"Acoustic neuroma" is a misnomer because it suggests that this neoplasm arises from neural elements in the statoacoustic nerve. In actuality, the tumor usually arises from the investing Schwann cell of the superior or the inferior vestibular nerve. Therefore, "benign vestibular schwannoma" is a more accurate term. The term acoustic neuroma is, however, irrevocably enshrined in the medical literature as the accepted name for this tumor.

The surgical outcome for patients with acoustic neuroma has altered dramatically since 1950. During the late 1940s and the early 1950s, the surgical mortality for removal of acoustic neuroma averaged 40% in the United States. Most tumors were diagnosed when relatively large. Facial nerve paralysis and deafness were regular and expected sequelae of these dangerous operations.

Advances in anesthesia, the introduction of the operating microscope, improved diagnostic audiometry, innovations in diagnostic imaging, and the pioneering work of William House and William Hitzelberger have reduced surgical mortality to 1% or 2%. The facial nerve is now regularly salvaged, and with smaller tumors, conservation of hearing is a realistic goal in selected patients.

Although as many as 5% of patients with acoustic neuroma may have normal preoperative auditory function, unilateral hearing loss is the diagnostic hallmark of acoustic tumors. Hearing loss most commonly starts with loss of ability to hear the high frequencies and slowly progresses to involve lower octaves. As many as 20% of patients, however, may experience the loss as a sudden event. Complete or partial recovery of hearing after such sudden losses is common and does not eliminate the possibility of a neoplastic cause. A similar percentage may experience fluctuating hearing losses. Tinnitus is a regular accompaniment of the hearing loss induced by acoustic neuroma and is often present even when hearing loss is not. Unilateral aural pressure and a feeling of fullness may also occur.

Few patients volunteer complaints of vertigo or dysequilibrium. However, if carefully questioned, many patients reveal that they have experienced vertigo, dysequilibrium, or ataxia at some time before diagnosis. Occasional patients present with the classic Meniere's triad of fluctuating hearing loss accompanied with tinnitus and severe rotational vertigo. Because tinnitus, hearing loss, aural fullness, or vertigo may occur alone as the earliest manifestation of acoustic neuroma, an axiom of good otologic practice is that all unilateral otologic symptoms require some evaluation to rule out acoustic neuroma.

Neurologic signs or symptoms are late findings and occur with large tumors. Hitzelberger's sign, which is hypoesthesia of the posterior-superior external auditory canal, may be an early sign of facial nerve compression, but weakness or paralysis of cranial nerve VII is uncommon; this is surprising, given the amount of stretching and attenuation that these nerves have been subjected to by tumor growth. In fact, cranial nerve V dysfunction is a more common preoperative finding than is motor dysfunction of cranial nerve VII. Facial paralysis caused by a small to medium-sized tumor (<2.5 cm) should lead one to question the diagnosis of acoustic neuroma. Extremely large tumors may result in cerebellar ataxia because of displacement of midline cerebellar structures. Eventually, large tumors distort the brain stem sufficiently to obstruct the ventricular aqueduct and produce hydrocephalus. Severe headache with rapid obtundation may then occur.

Evaluation. After a careful neurotologic examination, the evaluation of a person suspected of having acoustic neuroma should begin with routine audiometry. The characteristic audiometric finding of an acoustic neuroma is unilateral hearing loss with a speech discrimination score reduced out of proportion to the pure-tone hearing loss. Thus a patient with a pure-tone threshold average of 30 db might have a speech discrimination score of 8% or 12%. Of all patients with acoustic neuroma, 75% have a speech discrimination score below 60%. Some patients have "roll-over," in which the ability to understand words diminishes at higher loudness levels. Ninety-five percent of patients with acoustic neuromas have abnormalities of stapedius reflex (the reflex may be absent or may decay), and 98% have abnormal audiometric auditory brain stem responses (ABRs). The ABR may be entirely absent, or there may be a marked delay in the appearance of wave V. Waves I to V interpeak latency differences of more than 0.2 milliseconds should arouse suspicion of retrocochlear disease. Stapedius reflex testing and ABR audiometric evaluation are good screening tests to rule out the presence of cranial nerve VIII lesions. Patients who have normal stapedius reflex test and ABR results are unlikely to have an acoustic neuroma. It is reasonable to follow patients in whom these studies are normal with repeated audiometric evaluation every 6 to 12 months (Fig. 16–1).

Although 80% of patients with acoustic neuroma have abnormal electronystagmographic (ENG) results, this test has a limited role in the diagnosis because both stapedius reflexes and ABRs have higher sensitivities and specificities. ENG testing retains some utility in the evaluation of patients for hearing conservation operations. Because electronystagmography tests the horizontal semicircular canal, which is innervated by the superior vestibular nerve, patients with acoustic neuroma who have normal ENG

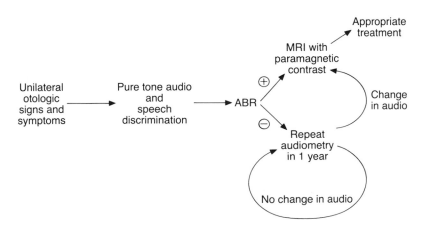

Figure 16–1. Patients with unilateral otologic signs and symptoms should always be evaluated for acoustic tumors. Even if the ABR is negative, audiometry should be repeated regularly.

results are likely to have an acoustic tumor arising from the inferior vestibular nerve. When the tumor arises from the inferior portion of the vestibular nerve, it is more likely that the cochlear nerve and the blood vessels supplying the cochlea are involved by the tumor. Therefore, patients with normal ENG results are *less* likely to experience successful hearing conservation operations.

Diagnostic imaging for acoustic neuroma has gone through many changes. In the 1940s and the 1950s, arteriography was the only neuroradiologic modality available. Only relatively large tumors were detected by this method. Plain film evaluation, hypocycloidal tomography, iophendylate (Pantopaque) posterior fossa cisternography, contrast-enhanced computed tomography (CT) scanning, and air-contrast CT posterior fossa cisternography have been some of the steps leading to the present reliance on gadolinium-enhanced magnetic resonance imaging (MRI) (Fig. 16–2). MRI without injection of paramagnetic contrast agents can enable visualization of the cranial nerve VIII bundle as it passes from the pons across the cerebellopontine

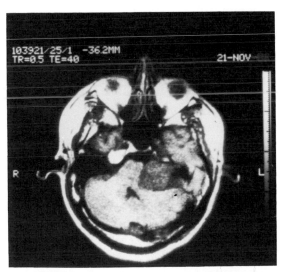

Figure 16–2. MRI scanning with paramagnetic contrast is the definitive radiologic study. A large 4-cm acoustic neuroma is seen in the left cerebellopontine angle. This tumor was removed through a translabyrinthine technique. Although the facial nerve was anatomically intact at the end of the procedure, a portion of it was quite thin and attenuated. At 1.5 years postoperatively, the patient had regained approximately 75% of her facial function. Although she had symmetry at rest and good corneal protection, marked asymmetry was noticeable when she smiled. The high-signal area in the right petrous apex represents fat in the nonpneumatized narrow space and is not pathologic.

angle and through the internal auditory canal. A small star-shaped signal that represents the fluid-filled membranous labyrinth can be seen in the large void space produced by the temporal bone. If the statoacoustic and facial nerves are well visualized without paramagnetic contrast and are symmetric, an unenhanced study may be sufficient. Mild asymmetry or thickening of the cranial nerve VIII bundles may still leave a question as to the presence or absence of tumor. The use of paramagnetic contrast agents produces dramatic enhancement of even small acoustic tumors. Tumors 2 to 3 mm in diameter can be detected through this technique. For detection of acoustic neuromas, evaluation of their size, and assessment of the relationships of the tumor to the surrounding brain structures, gadolinium-enhanced MRI is the definitive radiographic study.

Each scan should be carefully scrutinized to determine whether the internal auditory canal is enlarged on the side of the tumor mass. If the internal auditory canal is normal, or if the mass is placed eccentrically over the porus acousticus, the lesion should be suspected of being a meningioma and not an acoustic neuroma. The amount of anterior extension should be determined, and whether there is impingement on, or displacement of, either vertebral or basilar arteries should be noted. Every scan should be inspected to ascertain the superior level of involvement and associated distortion of the tentorium. When the inferior extent of tumor growth is assessed, thought should be given as to whether cranial nerves IX to XII are involved. The MRI scan should be evaluated to determine whether the tumor impinges on the brain stem and, if so, how much brain stem distortion or displacement has occurred. The presence or absence of hydrocephalus should be noted and its extent evaluated. In patients who have significant preoperative hydrocephalus, consideration should be given to perioperative placement of a ventriculostomy.

Because MRI shows no bony detail, there is a continuing, although restricted, role for CT. In some cases, knowing the details of bony anatomy is helpful in preoperative planning. When a large tumor is seen in a patient with good hearing, meningioma should be suspected. If fine-cut CT shows no evidence of expansion or involvement of the internal auditory canal, the chances that the tumor is a meningioma are higher. When a meningioma is suspected, the surgeon may elect a hearing conservation procedure, even for large tumors. The chance for successful conservation of hearing when the lesion is a meningioma is significantly higher than it would be with a large acoustic neuroma. When hearing conservation surgery is selected, knowledge of the precise anatomy of the internal auditory canal is helpful. Preoperative CT scans can be used to measure precisely the distance between the most medial portion of the labyrinth (either the vestibule or the posterior semicircular canal) from the posterior lip of the porus acousticus. Such information can be quite helpful when the posterior lip of the porus acousticus is removed during a hearing conservation operation. Occasionally more needs to be known about the relationship of the sigmoid sinus, the jugular bulb, and the internal auditory canal than can be obtained from MRI scanning. In all these situations, fine-cut CT is a useful adjunct to MRI scanning.

Eighty percent of tumors involving the cerebellopontine angle are acoustic neuromas. Another 15% are meningiomas. Of the remaining 5%, the majority are lipomas, cholesteatomas, cholesterol granulomas, hemangiomas, or arachnoid cysts. The preoperative diagnosis of lipoma and arachnoid cyst is now possible through MRI scanning. However, the distinction between acoustic neuroma and meningioma cannot be made reliably before biopsy. Fortunately, the operative approaches suitable for one lesion are, in general, suitable for the other.

The central variant of neurofibromatosis (von Recklinghausen's disease) may present with bilateral acoustic tumors in relatively young patients. In patients with neurofibromatosis, acoustic tumors may grow to a large size before producing significant deterioration of hearing. Unfortunately, they are much more likely to invade cranial nerve VIII, and thus hearing conservation is much more difficult to achieve in patients with neurofibromatosis. Patients with this disorder are likely to have neuroma formation involving other peripheral nerves just as they leave the central neuraxis. Many of these formations are intradural. All patients with central neurofibromatosis are also more likely to develop meningiomas that may be multiple (Fig. 16–3).

Treatment. The treatment of choice for most patients with acoustic neuromas is surgical removal. The considerable controversy that has existed since the 1960s regarding the various merits of different approaches is beginning to subside as cooperation between neurosurgeons and otologists becomes the norm.

The translabyrinthine approach is now the technique most frequently used for the removal of acoustic tumors. The advantages of this approach include complete exposure of the internal auditory canal, which permits removal of tumor from the lateral end of the internal auditory canal under direct vision. Good lateral exposure at the same time permits identification of the facial nerve in its labyrinthine portions, where it is least likely to be encased in tumor. Translabyrinthine

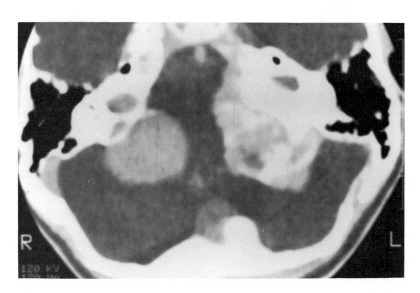

Figure 16–3. Bilateral acoustic neuromas in a 14-year-old child with central neurofibromatosis. The child presented with mild unsteadiness that was most noticeable when he rode his bike. He had almost normal hearing despite these large lesions. A parasagittal meningioma can be seen in the posterior midline. The left cerebellopontine angle mass was surgically removed. Histologic examination showed that this was a mixture of an acoustic neuroma and a meningioma. (CT scan courtesy of Michael Glasscock, Vanderbilt University.)

approaches require no cerebellar retraction and therefore minimize the risk of postoperative cerebellar edema or infarction. Disadvantages include the obligatory sacrifice of hearing, relatively high incidence of postoperative cerebrospinal fluid leakage, and poor exposure of the posterior extension of very large tumors.

Suboccipital approaches offer an excellent view of the cranial nerves and the posterior portions of the tumor. They have a relatively low incidence of cerebrospinal fluid leakage and do not require the obligatory sacrifice of hearing. However, the success rate of conservation of useful hearing when the tumor is larger than 1.5 cm in diameter is less than 5%. The disadvantages of the operation include the necessity for cerebellar retraction or resection, the difficulty of removing tumor in the lateral internal auditory canal, and the late exposure of the facial nerve. The operation was traditionally performed with the patient in a sitting position, which exposes the patient to the risk of an air embolus. Use of the sitting position is becoming less common, and the operation is now most frequently performed with the patient in the supine position. The suboccipital approach is the approach of choice when hearing conservation surgery is to be attempted in a patient whose tumor is larger than 1.5 cm.

The middle fossa approach is used for small tumors when hearing conservation is to be attempted. The approach is difficult, but it offers the following advantages: The entire internal auditory canal can be well visualized from above so that the tumor can be completely removed from the lateral end of the internal auditory canal. Hearing can be conserved because no part of the labyrinth is entered and the cochlear nerve can be preserved. Because the principal portion of the dissection is performed from above, the chances of inadvertently injuring the vasculature of the cochlear nerve is somewhat reduced. The facial nerve is constantly in the field, and the tumor must be removed from underneath it. For this reason, some authors report an increased incidence of facial nerve paralysis when the middle fossa approach is used. Extradural retraction of the temporal lobe can result in subdural or parenchymal hematoma, edema, or a delayed seizure disorder.

Extremely large tumors may be resected by using a combination of the translabyrinthine and suboccipital approaches. This is easy to do because additional bone removal beyond the posterior limits of the sigmoid sinus exposes the suboccipital posterior fossa dura.

Regardless of the approach, the extent of preservation of the facial nerve is a function of tumor size. The facial nerve can be anatomically preserved in 96% of patients with tumors smaller than 1.5 cm in diameter and in 85% of patients with tumors between 1.5 and 2.0 cm in diameter, but in only 60% of patients with tumors larger than 3.0 cm in diameter. In general, anatomic preservation of the facial nerve correlates well with ultimate recovery of facial nerve function, although some patients with anatomic preservation of the nerve never regain function. Paresis of the facial nerve in the immediate postoperative period is the rule. Facial recovery may begin as early as several days after the operation or may be delayed for a year or more. The more rapid the return of facial function is, the better is the ultimate outcome. Some patients have good function in the recovery room but lose it over the ensuing hours or days. Such patients can be expected ultimately to have virtually normal facial function.

In patients who are elderly, who are poor surgical candidates, or who refuse surgery, consideration should be given to either observation of the tumor with serial imaging at 6-month intervals or the use of stereotaxic cobalt 60 radiation therapy. Although stereotaxic radiation therapy (the gamma knife) has been used for almost two decades, its value in the treatment of acoustic tumors remains obscure. Although a significant number of patients experienced tumor regression in an initial group of Swedish patients, notable side effects were relatively common. For this reason, the total dose has been lowered. There is no long-term experience with the new, reduced dosage, and therefore no information on long-term effectiveness of this therapy is available. However, within the first 1 to 2 years after treatment, a significant proportion of patients (about 20%) have experienced tumor regrowth. Many patients lose hearing as a consequence of stereotaxic radio surgery. Facial nerve salvage rates, however, seem to be good. Anecdotal reports by experienced surgeons indicate that surgery after stereotaxic radiation therapy is more difficult to perform, and the chances of salvaging the

the bony ridge separating the jugular fossa from the carotid artery but was not capable of reliably distinguishing chemodectoma from large skull base neuromas. A combination of MRI scanning and enhanced CT now frequently permits not only diagnosis of the lesion but accurate tumor mapping. The presence or absence of intracranial involvement and the involvement of bony structures can be accurately determined. Even so, glomus tumors still usually require arteriographic evaluation, which permits precise identification of feeding vessels. Even if preoperative embolization is not being considered, knowledge of the major sources of arterial inflow permits early isolation and ligation of these vessels during the operative procedure to minimize intraoperative bleeding. The presence and the extent of the tumor within the jugular vein should also be determined arteriographically. The tumor may extend proximally as far as the torcular Herophili and may extend distally below the thoracic inlet. The extent of intraluminal involvement may significantly alter the surgical approach. Intraluminal tumor extension can frequently be determined from the arteriogram. Rapid shunting from the arterial side through the tumor into the vein may opacify the jugular outflow system nicely during the arterial phase of the examination (Fig. 16–7). Careful evaluation of the venous phase of the arteriogram may permit accurate identification not only of intraluminal involvement but also of collateral venous outflow. When this information cannot be determined from the arteriogram, retrograde jugular venography should be performed.

Most large glomus tumors involve the adventitia of the carotid artery. It is useful to determine how far anteriorly and medially a tumor extends along the carotid. In some cases, involvement is limited to the horizontal petrous portion just anterior to the jugular bulb. In others, involvement extends along the carotid arteries through the horizontal petrous portion and up to or into the cavernous sinus. The extent of carotid involvement significantly affects the nature of any surgical procedure.

A variety of classification schemes for glomus tumors have been developed. Currently, the staging system of Fisch and the Glasscock-Jackson staging system are most commonly used. Some controversy exists as to the appropriate management of these slow-growing tumors. Radiation therapy ap-

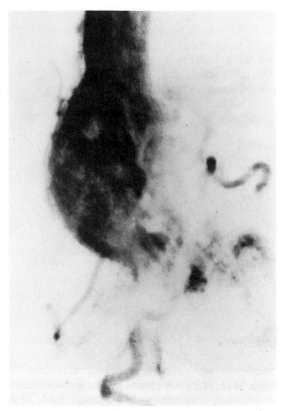

Figure 16–7. Large glomus jugulare. External carotid injection shows early filling of the ipsilateral jugular vein. This is caused by shunting of a large amount of blood through the tumor into the jugular system. The proximal jugular vein, the jugular bulb, and the sigmoid sinus were occluded approximately to the level of the superior petrosal sinus.

pears capable of halting tumor growth for some time in many patients but rarely produces tumor regression. A number of histologic studies have shown that the principal effect of radiation to these lesions is on the supporting vasculature and not directly on the neoplastic tumor cells. Despite the fact that these tumors do not seem to be radiocurable, the radiation therapy literature reports successful control of symptoms in many patients. Some patients have experienced return of cranial nerve function after radiotherapy. Treatment by radiation is not without hazard. The injury to adjacent tissues (cartilage, bone, brain) may progress to actual necrosis. These tumors may start growing again years after apparent radiotherapeutic control. In such cases, surgical resection occurs in a previously irradiated field, and perioperative complications are likely to be higher. Although surgical management provides the best chance of cure, radiotherapy should be considered for patients who refuse surgery, those who have medical conditions that contraindicate surgery, and those who are elderly; it should also be considered as an adjunct in the management of incompletely resected tumors.

Embolization has been advocated in the management of glomus tumors, both as a method of growth control and as an adjunct to surgical removal. These tumors are extraordinarily vascular. Embolization can be extremely difficult because there can be multiple branches of the ipsilateral and contralateral external carotid artery, branches from the vertebral system, and branches off the internal carotid via the meningohypophyseal trunk. Embolization is fraught with the hazard of inadvertent spillage of embolic material into the circulation of the brain and consequent stroke or death. However, successful embolization immediately before the operative procedure can meaningfully reduce intraoperative blood loss. Perhaps most important, it may facilitate precise surgical removal of the tumor, and thus the number of cranial nerves that can be spared is increased. Embolization should be undertaken only by an experienced interventional neuroradiologist. Surgical therapy is the mainstay of treatment for these lesions. These operations are long and complex and frequently involve significant blood loss. Postoperative care is plagued with problems related to lower cranial nerve deficits and cerebrospinal fluid leakage. The approaches to this lesion as they have been worked out principally by Fisch and Glasscock are well described and are reviewed in Chapter 57.

MIDDLE EAR ADENOMA AND ADENOCARCINOMA

The glandular elements in middle ear mucosa may undergo neoplastic change. Such tumors are difficult to sort out pathologically. Benign adenoma must be differentiated not only from adenocarcinomas but also from atypical glomus tumors, carcinoid tumors, choristomas, and mucoepidermoid carcinomas. Primary adenomas and adenocarcinomas of the ear are uncommon, and evaluation of patients with such lesions should include a search for a primary lesion elsewhere. It is difficult for even experienced

pathologists to determine, on the basis of histopathologic criteria, how aggressive the lesions are; therefore, surgical treatment must be based on clinical presentation rather than on histologic findings. The presence of facial nerve paralysis, although unusual, in itself is compatible with the diagnosis of a benign lesion and does not mandate an aggressive resection. Bone erosion is a key variable. In the absence of bone erosion, simple excision with close follow-up is adequate. The presence of bone erosion, however, is evidence of a more invasive neoplasm, and consideration should be given to a more radical surgical extirpation or the use of postoperative radiation therapy, or both.

CARCINOMA

Squamous cell carcinoma of the ear accounts for 5% to 10% of cutaneous malignancies. Many of these lesions are presumed to be a consequence of actinic exposure and thus are more frequent in men and in the later decades of life. Basal cell carcinoma also occurs with some regularity on the auricle. Although basal cell carcinomas do not metastasize, local invasion can be extensive. Basal cell carcinoma may be deeply locally invasive with only minimal surface manifestations. If neglected or inadequately treated, basal cell carcinoma arising in the auricle has considerable lethal potential. Therefore these lesions must receive attention despite the fact that they do not metastasize. Those lesions that involve the lateral portions of the auricle may be treated in the same way as cutaneous carcinomas elsewhere. Wedge resection with an adequate margin is frequently all that is required. Attention should always be given to regional draining lymph nodes. For lesions involving the helix, consideration should be given to the retroauricular nodes or intraparotid nodes. When invasion involves the cartilage or the underlying bone, attention should be directed toward lymph nodes within the neck. Lesions that involve the concha have a distinct propensity for infiltrating the soft tissues of the external auditory canal. Invasion through the fissures of Santorini may result in early bone or parotid gland involvement. Therefore, tumors that arise in the concha must be attended to even when quite small. Involvement of the tissues in the external auditory canal may be occult, and lesions of the concha should be removed only when precise histologic control of margins is possible. This author favors the use of Mohs surgery as the best method of ensuring complete excision with the initial operative procedure. When these lesions recur, they frequently involve the temporal bone, the temporomandibular joint, or the parotid gland, and large, deforming resections may be required.

Squamous cell carcinomas arising within the external auditory canal are relatively uncommon, but when they do occur, early diagnosis is crucial. When pain is associated with chronic otorrhea and granulation tissue is present within the external auditory canal, neoplasm should be considered. Chronic mastoid infective processes and cholesteatoma are rarely painful; the obvious exception is malignant otitis externa. The presence of pain with a chronically draining ear or granulation tissue requires immediate biopsy. Biopsy findings of "granulation tissue" are not a satisfactory explanation of painful otorrhea. The diagnosis should be pursued by repeated biopsy or tympanomastoidectomy. When malignant lesions are limited to the external auditory canal and have not penetrated the tympanic membrane, lateral temporal bone resection ("sleeve" resection of the external auditory canal) may be curative. Once these lesions have spread beyond the external auditory canal, large-scale surgery is required. When the temporomandibular joint is involved, parotidectomy and mandibular condylectomy should be included. Once these tumors have invaded bone in any area, consideration should be given to concomitant neck dissection. If the tumor extends medial to the tympanic membrane or involves the facial nerve, total temporal bone resection is required if a cure is sought. Meticulous radiographic evaluation is essential to planning therapy. Differences in tumor extension of 1 to 2 mm may make great differences in the therapeutic approach required.

MENINGIOMA OF THE TEMPORAL BONE

Meningiomas arise from the endothelial cells within the arachnoid villi. Because arachnoid villi are found in association with the cranial venous sinuses and the cerebral veins, a high percentage of meningiomas arise close to the major dural venous outflow tracts. Only a small proportion of meningiomas involve the temporal bone. They most frequently arise from the middle fossa surface or the posterior fossa surfaces of the petrous portions of the temporal bone. They occasionally arise from the arachnoid villi within the internal acoustic meatus, and they even more rarely occur primarily within the middle ear. Although the vast majority of meningiomas are benign, they can be clinically and histologically malignant.

Approximately 10% to 15% of cerebellopontine angle masses turn out to be meningiomas. It is not yet possible to make this diagnosis preoperatively. Suspicion should be raised when hearing is good, when the mass is placed eccentrically over the internal auditory canal, and when there is no expansion of the internal auditory canal (Figs. 16–8A, 16–8B). Meningiomas are much more likely to invade bone than are neuromas; therefore, they are more likely to invade the cochlea and the middle ear. Meningiomas produce symptoms by involving adjacent nerves. Thus meningiomas of the petrous apex and of the superior surface of the temporal bone are likely to manifest with facial paresthesias or extraocular motor defects. Meningiomas involving the posterior surface of the temporal bone are more likely to manifest with the symptoms of hearing loss and dysfunction of the lower cranial nerves that are indistinguishable from those symptoms produced by neuromas in the same area. Diagnosis of meningioma is frequently made only intraoperatively. Fortunately, meningiomas are generally benign, and local excision, if complete, is curative. Because meningiomas are much more likely to invade surrounding areas of bone and may spread diffusely over the involved meninges (en plaque), excision should include a margin of normal bone and meninges. Margins should be confirmed by intraoperative examination of frozen section. In some cases, histologic differentiation from other lesions, such as schwannoma, is difficult. Diagnosis of malignant meningioma on the basis of histologic criteria may also be problematic.

Petrous Apex Lesions

Infection (petrous apicitis) is less frequent now than it once was, but it still occurs and

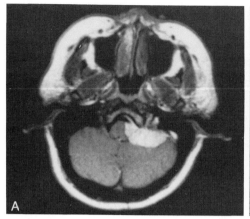
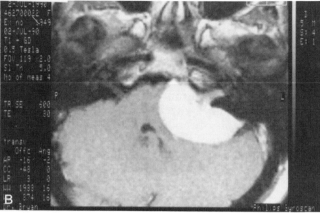

Figure 16–8. *A.* A gadolinium-enhanced MRI scan shows a large cerebellopontine angle tumor. The lesion appears to be broadly based on the dura of the posterior petrosa. *B.* Higher cut from the same MRI scan. The neurovascular bundle passing into the internal auditory canal is well visualized. There is no signal enhancement, which suggests that it is free of tumor. There is no evidence of expansion of the bony internal auditory canal. The fourth ventricle seems to be shifted slightly to the contralateral side. Careful evaluation of the entire scan showed that this tumor was epicentered inferior to the internal auditory canal without evidence of involvement of the canal. The patient had only a 30-db flat neurosensory hearing loss. On the basis of these findings, a preoperative diagnosis of meningioma was made. A suboccipital approach was used to remove this large lesion, and hearing improved after surgery.

should be within the differential diagnosis of abnormalities of this area.

Cholesteatomas arise infrequently, but when they occur they present a difficult surgical problem. They are generally believed to be congenital and arise from embryonic epidermal cell rests. The most common symptom of congenital cholesteatomas of the petrous apex is sensorineural hearing loss, which may be progressive. In this respect, congenital cholesteatomas of the petrous apex are similar to other cerebellopontine angle tumors. Unlike those tumors, however, a relatively high incidence of facial nerve involvement has been reported for congenital cholesteatomas of the petrous apex. Facial nerve paralysis is often preceded by months of facial spasm, which appears to be a consequence of facial nerve irritation produced by cholesteatomas.

The most common primary lesion of the petrous apex is the cholesterol granuloma. This cystic lesion is filled with dark, chocolate-colored fluid containing birefringent cholesterol crystals and hemosiderin. Cholesterol granulomas are thought to be secondary to spontaneous bleeding within the air cells of the petrous apex. Blood breakdown products and cholesterol crystals produce an inflammatory reaction and granuloma formation. Cholesterol granulomas tend to expand and, like other lesions in this area, manifest most frequently with sensorineural hearing

loss. Retro-orbital pain is a relatively common and distinguishing feature of cholesterol granulomas. They are often silent, however, until they have reached an advanced stage of development. They can erode anteriorly around the carotid artery and involve the clivus and the cavernous sinus (Fig. 16–9).

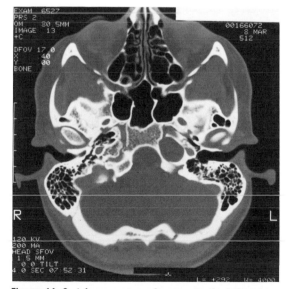

Figure 16–9. A large cyst can be seen in the left petrous apex. Some erosion of the clivus can be detected. The erosive character of this lesion is supported by some mild bowing of the medial wall of the internal carotid canal. This cholesterol granuloma was exteriorized through an infralabyrinthine approach.

Inferior extension may involve the nerves of the jugular foramen and produce symptoms of lower cranial nerve paralysis. Both cholesterol granulomas and cholesteatomas generally remain extradural.

Differentiation between cholesterol granulomas and cholesteatomas can frequently be accomplished radiographically. On MRI scans cholesterol granulomas exhibit a high signal intensity on both T1- and T2-weighted images. Cholesteatomas have high signal intensity on T2-weighted images but only low to moderate signal intensity on T1-weighted images. Because the bone is not visualized, it may be difficult to establish on the basis of MRI whether high-signal areas within the petrous apex are expansive or static erosive. Surgery should be predicated on clear signs of growth seen on the CT scan, on which details of bony anatomy can be conclusive. Evidence of expansion includes involvement of the clivus, posterior expansion with thinning and attenuation of bone, erosion of the jugular tubercle, and displacement of the internal carotid artery.

Cholesterol granulomas are adequately treated by permanent drainage. A variety of operative approaches are available. When hearing is absent, the simplest approach is translabyrinthine exposure of the apical cyst. When hearing is present and to be preserved, a retrolabyrinthine or infralabyrinthine approach is best. A middle fossa approach, with placement of a shunt tube from the petrous apex over the cochlea into the mastoid, provides the least reliable method of drainage and ventilation. Cholesteatomas must be completely removed if a cure is to be achieved, but many cases may be successfully controlled by radical exteriorization. Complete removal of a lesion of the petrous apex is difficult. Extradural operative approaches are best for cholesteatomas because the keratin debris filling these lesions is extremely irritating to the meninges and subarachnoid space. Serious sterile meningitis may occur after gross contamination of the subarachnoid space with keratin debris. Unless the removal of every remnant of the epidermal matrix can be ensured, the petrous apex should be exteriorized through a radical mastoidectomy cavity.

Lifelong, regular cleaning of desquamated epithelium from these permanently exteriorized cysts is essential if complete removal is not achieved.

CHORDOMA

Chordomas are neoplasms that arise from remnants of the notochord. Even though they arise from embryonic tissue and are relatively common in children, the majority are seen in patients of middle age. They may be seen in any portion of the vertebral column. When they are intracranial, they most commonly arise from the midline clival region in the area of the spheno-occipital synchondrosis. Chordomas arising in this area may grow anteriorly and manifest as nasopharyngeal masses, or they may grow posteriorly and produce significant compression and distortion of the brain stem. Histopathologic differentiation from some types of mesenchymal tumors (chondrosarcoma, chondroid chordoma) may be quite difficult.

Chordomas usually manifest with fronto-orbital headache and visual disturbances. Progressive loss of visual acuity, diplopia from extraocular muscle defects, and visual field cuts are common. As this lesion enlarges, it is likely to begin producing progressive impairment of cranial nerves VII and VIII, disorders of pituitary function, and, when growth is anterior and superior, nasal obstruction and anosmia. These tumors may be quite large at the time of diagnosis, and distortion of the brain stem may be dramatic (Fig. 16–10). Although they are not malignant, incomplete surgical resection produces a high rate of local recurrence. Chordomas are relatively radiointensive, and extremely

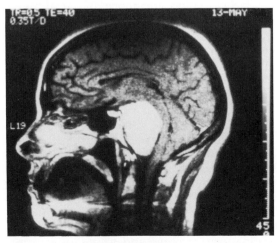

Figure 16–10. Parasagittal MRI scan of a large clival chordoma. There is dramatic distortion and compression of the brain stem. This lesion was successfully extirpated by a transcochlear-translabyrinthine approach.

high doses (7000 cGy) are needed for control. Clival chordomas can be resected transorally or transfacially. Such approaches carry the risk of creating a communication between the subarachnoid space and the nasopharynx. When such communication has developed, organisms that colonize the upper aerodigestive tract can produce intractable and untreatable meningitis and death. To avoid this complication, clival chordomas are often approached transtemporally through a combined translabyrinthine-transcochlear approach.

VASCULAR LESIONS

Anomalies of the posterior venous outflow tract or carotid artery may manifest with temporal bone signs and symptoms. Congenital anomalies of the carotid artery may produce either vascular tinnitus or a visible vascular mass behind the tympanic membrane. Arteriography is diagnostic and should precede surgery for any patient with a suspected vascular lesion. High-riding jugular bulbs are relatively common and are frequently seen as dusky vascular masses behind the inferior-posterior tympanic membrane. In a normal ear, the jugular bulb is usually apparent to an experienced examiner. However, the presence of middle ear effusion may obscure the high jugular bulb, which may then be entered inadvertently during myringotomy. Placement of absorbable packing (Gelfoam) controls bleeding. A high-riding jugular bulb is generally an incidental finding, although occasional patients may complain of vascular tinnitus, and this author has seen two patients in whom the high-riding jugular bulb has obstructed the eustachian tube and caused the formation of posterior-superior retraction cholesteatomas that required tympanomastoidectomy.

Hemangiomas can occur anywhere along the facial nerve, including the internal auditory canal. Hemangiomas of the facial nerve may cause intermittent or permanent facial nerve paralysis when they occur within the fallopian canal. Radiographic evaluation shows dilatation of the fallopian canal in most cases, but exploration of the nerve is occasionally required for establishing the diagnosis. Hemangiomas of the internal auditory canal may produce facial nerve paralysis, hearing loss, or tinnitus. Small lesions are usually not distinguishable from other intra-

canalicular neoplasms before surgical opening of the internal auditory canal.

Arteriovenous malformations of the posterior fossa dura usually manifest as vascular tinnitus. However, when a larger volume of arterialized blood passing into the involved sinus produces retrograde arterial flow in the veins draining the brain, manifestations of increased intracranial pressure such as headache, visual changes, or acute subarachnoid hemorrhage may occur (Fig. 16–11). Physical evaluation usually identifies an objective bruit over the mastoid area. Patients with objective vascular tinnitus should always be studied with arteriography. Although operation is necessary only when the retrograde flow of arterialized blood produces intracranial hypertension or involves draining cortical veins, many patients elect intervention to rid themselves of intolerable vascular tinnitus.

A significant proportion of these arteriovenous lesions can be managed by endovascular neuroradiologic intervention. Arterial or venus embolization can completely eliminate or render asymptomatic many of these

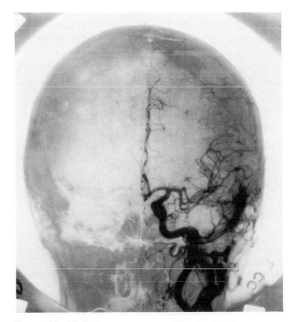

Figure 16–11. Left common carotid injection in a patient with a left-sided dural arteriovenous malformation draining into the midsigmoid sinus. The cortical veins were involved and were exposed to the retrograde flow of arterialized blood under high pressure. High-pressure flow in the thin-walled veins had resulted in two previous episodes of introparenchymal hemorrhage, which left the patient with a significant neurologic deficit. The lesion was removed through a skull base approach.

malformations. Care must be exercised, however, because branches of the internal carotid circulation may be involved in the malformation.

When embolization techniques fail or are contraindicated, surgical therapy may be considered. Ligation of arterial inflow is never adequate, and surgical therapy should be directed toward complete excision of the malformation. This frequently requires removal of a substantial portion of the temporal bone to expose the involved sigmoid sinus, the jugular bulb, and the upper jugular vein, all of which should be removed together.

METASTATIC LESIONS

Metastatic involvement of the temporal bone is uncommon but may arise in three ways. (1) Hematologic dissemination of primary malignancies from other parts of the body is most common with breast, prostate, and kidney malignancies. Hematologic primary malignancies may also involve the temporal bone, as in leukemias, lymphomas, and multiple myelomas. (2) Regional primary tumors may reach the temporal bone by direct extension; examples are squamous and basal cell carcinoma of the overlying skin or upper aerodigestive tract. (3) Primary lesions arising in the parotid gland may reach the temporal bone by direct invasion along preformed neural pathways (Fig. 16–12). The possibilities of metastatic disease must always be considered when the histologic appearance of the temporal bone lesion is unusual.

SUGGESTED READINGS

Bojrab DI, Glasscock ME, Roland PS, Jackson CG: Glomus Tumors of the Temporal Bone: A Self-Instructional Package. Washington, DC: American Academy of Otolaryngology—Head and Neck Surgery Foundation, Inc., 1988.

Fisch U: Infratemporal fossa approach for glomus tumors of the temporal bone. Ann Otol Rhinol Laryngol 91:474–479, 1982.

Gacek RR: Evaluation and management of primary petrous apex cholesteatoma. Otolaryngol Head Neck Surg 88:519–523, 1980.

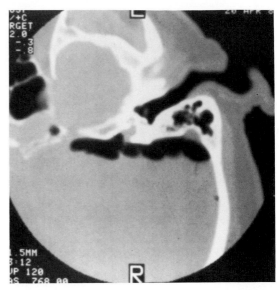

Figure 16–12. Air contrast posterior fossa cisternogram showing tumor in the lateral portions in the internal auditory canal. Operative removal showed this to be squamous cell carcinoma. Repeated MRI scanning revealed a small focus of mucoepidermoid carcinoma in the medial lobe of the parotid gland from which only the squamous portion had metastasized. The patient had a history of facial nerve paralysis that started 2 years before evaluation. One year before evaluation, he sustained complete and total neurosensory hearing loss. Approximately 6 months before evaluation, he developed significant vertigo and ataxia.

Glasscock ME, Hays JW: The translabyrinthine removal of acoustic and other cerebellopontine angle tumors. Ann Otol Rhinol Laryngol 82:415–427, 1973.

Goldenberg RA: Surgeon's view of the skull base from the lateral approach. Laryngoscope 94 (Suppl 36, part 2), 1981.

Jacobson CG: Facial Nerve Paralysis: Diagnosis and Treatment of Lower Motor Neuron Facial Nerve Lesions and Facial Paralysis. Washington, DC: American Academy of Otolaryngology—Head and Neck Surgery Foundation, Inc., 1986.

Kinney SE, Wood BG: Surgical treatment of skull base malignancy. Otolaryngol Head Neck Surg 92:94–99, 1984.

Meyerhoff WL, Roland PS, Mickey B, Schaefer SD: Complications of skull base surgery: Their prevention and management. In Johnson JT, Blitzer A, Ossoff R, Thomas RJ (eds): Instructional Courses (pp. 389–404). Washington, DC: CV Mosby, 1988.

Smith PG, Leonetti JP, Kletzer RG: Differential clinical and radiographic features of cholesterol granulomas and cholesteatomas of the petrous apex. Ann Otol Rhinol Laryngol 97:599–604, 1988.

CHAPTER 17

Facial Nerve Paralysis

Michael J. LaRouere, MD   Jack M. Kartush, MD

ANATOMY

The facial nerve travels a tortuous course from the brain stem through the temporal bone and the parotid gland to reach the facial musculature (Fig. 17–1). After leaving the brain stem ventral to the cranial nerve VIII complex, cranial nerve VII occupies the anterosuperior compartment of the internal auditory canal. Its blood supply in this region arises from a branch of the anteroinferior cerebellar artery. Coursing over the transverse crest anterior to Bill's bar (vertical crest), it then begins its labyrinthine segment. At the entrance to the fallopian canal (the meatal foramen), the diameter of the facial canal is at its narrowest (0.68 mm) (Fisch, 1981). The facial nerve then travels anteriorly, between the labyrinth and the cochlea, to reach the geniculate ganglion. The major source of blood supply to the nerve at this juncture is the labyrinthine artery. A branch of cranial nerve VII that courses anteriorly from the geniculate ganglion and exits the temporal bone through the facial hiatus, is the greater superficial petrosal nerve (Fig. 17–1).

Leaving the geniculate ganglion, the facial nerve turns abruptly posteriorly (its first genu) and enters the tympanic segment of the fallopian canal. This area is marked anteriorly by the attachment of the cochleariform process to the facial nerve sheath. The nerve then travels between the horizontal semicircular canal and the oval window niche to reach its second genu. Approximately 55% of facial nerves are dehiscent within the tympanic segment, and 15% exhibit a bony dehiscence over the geniculate ganglion.

Turning inferiorly, the nerve enters its vertical segment within the mastoid cavity. As the facial nerve descends, it becomes 2 to 3 mm more lateral in position. Near the stylomastoid foramen the nerve begins to curve anteriorly, becoming engulfed by fibers of the digastric tendon. Within the mastoid segment, the facial nerve gives rise to the stapedius and the chorda tympani nerves (Fig. 17–1). These branch points can occur between the second genu and the stylomastoid foramen. The main blood supply within the vertical segment of the nerve arises from the stylomastoid artery.

Exiting at the stylomastoid foramen, between the styloid process and the mastoid tip, the facial nerve emits a branch to the posterior belly of the digastric muscle as it enters the substance of the parotid gland. The nerve then branches at the pes anserinus into temporal and cervical divisions (Fig. 17–1). This branch point occurs at a variable length from the stylomastoid foramen.

Within the bony fallopian canal, the facial nerve is encased in a tough sheath composed of epineurium, through which a capillary network courses, and of periosteum arising from the fallopian canal. This thick sheath serves to protect the facial nerve from trauma and infection, but it may also contribute to ischemic necrosis that results from edematous entrapment. Perineurium and endoneurium also add to the connective tissue barrier.

The function of the facial nerve is to supply motor fibers to the mimetic musculature on the ipsilateral side of the face. It also

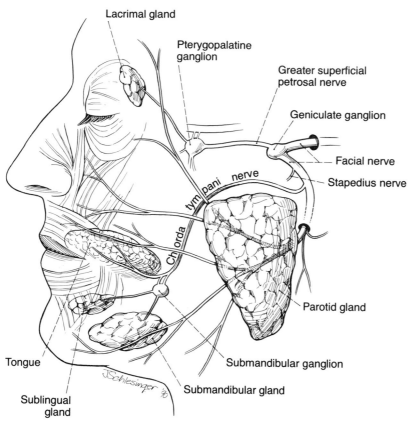

Figure 17–1. Course of the facial nerve demonstrating motor branches to the mimetic musculature; parasympathetic innervation to the submandibular, sublingual, lacrimal, and minor salivary glands; and taste fibers emanating from the anterior two thirds of the tongue.

carries preganglionic parasympathetic fibers, which course through the greater superficial petrosal nerve to synapse in the pterygopalatine ganglion and ultimately innervate the lacrimal gland. Preganglionic parasympathetic fibers also travel through the chorda tympani nerve to synapse in the submandibular ganglion. Postganglionic fibers then supply innervation to the submandibular and sublingual glands (Fig. 17–1). The sensation of taste, from the anterior two thirds of the tongue and palate, is passed through the chorda tympani nerve to its bipolar nuclei in the geniculate ganglion and transmitted to the nucleus solitarius in the brain stem (Fig. 17–1).

NEUROPHYSIOLOGY AND RESPONSE TO INJURY

A nerve action potential can be created by any factor that increases the permeability of the axonal membrane to sodium. These include electrical, mechanical, and thermal stimulation. Once an action potential is initiated, saltatory conduction occurs on either side of the initial area of depolarization, causing current spread in opposite directions: orthodromic (distally) and antidromic (proximally). A compound muscle action potential is typically a broad, multiphasic potential because the nerve is made up of many axons with varying speeds of conduction that depend on their myelin content and diameter. The morphologic characteristics and the amplitude of the compound muscle action potential vary, depending on the type of fibers stimulated as well as on the synchrony of axonal discharge. Large myelinated fibers, which compressive lesions generally affect first, have the lowest thresholds and are responsible for much of the recorded compound muscle action potential.

It is essential to understand the various

classes of nerve injury and their potential outcomes. *Neuropraxia, axonotmesis,* and *neurotmesis* refer to increasing degrees of neural injury as proposed by Seddon (1943). A conduction block, or neuropraxia, implies a mild injury to the nerve without disruption of axonal or connective tissue continuity. Complete or nearly total recovery of function is expected. Axonotmesis implies a more severe injury that may cause wallerian (distal) degeneration of axons. Neurotmesis describes total transection of the nerve.

Sunderland (1978) further classified nerve injury into five groups on the basis of the progressive degree of axonal and connective tissue trauma (Table 17–1). Sunderland class III, IV, and V injuries imply a poorer prognosis for recovery because the axon, which grows at a rate of 1 mm per day, must traverse progressively more scar tissue as the severity of injury increases.

DISORDERS ASSOCIATED WITH FACIAL PARALYSIS

Bell's Palsy

Bell's palsy is an idiopathic peripheral facial nerve paralysis that has a sudden onset. Although the cause of Bell's palsy remains unknown, a viral cause is most likely. Mulkens and colleagues (1980) isolated the herpes simplex virus from a nerve biopsy sample of a patient with Bell's palsy. Several other investigators have demonstrated elevated herpes virus titers in the plasma of patients with Bell's palsy. Other causes that have been championed include vascular compromise and a coldness theory. The latter is supported by the fact that 15% to 20% of patients report that the affected side had been exposed to cold air just before the onset of the paralysis. Despite the cause, the final pathophysiologic characteristic noted in Bell's palsy is edema with entrapment of the nerve in the fallopian canal, most notably at the meatal foramen (Fisch, 1981). Fisch observed increased swelling of the nerve just proximal to the geniculate ganglion in 15 of 16 patients. He also noted an intraoperative electrophysiologic conduction block at this location.

The natural course of Bell's palsy was examined by Peiterson (1982), who studied 1011 patients and found that on presentation, 69% demonstrated complete facial paralysis, whereas 31% had some degree of partial paresis. In 71% of the patients, normal facial function returned spontaneously, whereas 29% experienced some sequelae. No patient remained completely paralyzed. Peiterson found that if recovery began within the first 3 weeks after the onset of paralysis, facial function returned more completely than if recovery began after 3 months of paralysis. Poorer recovery was correlated with advancing age, postauricular pain, an abolished stapedial reflex, or eye dryness. Factors that increase the risk of developing Bell's palsy include diabetes mellitus (four times the normal risk); pregnancy, especially during the third trimester (3.3 times the normal risk); and advanced age. A seasonal increase could not be proved by Adour and Wingerd (1974). In general, bilateral facial paralysis is not Bell's palsy; however, recurrent ipsilateral facial paralysis occurs in approximately 10% of patients with Bell's palsy. May and associates (1984) pointed out that recurrent ipsilateral facial palsy represents a tumor in approximately 30% of such cases. By definition, slowly progressive facial palsy is not Bell's palsy and deserves an extensive diagnostic work-up, as does a palsy without any recovery 6 months after onset. In addition, while studying 500 patients with classic Bell's palsy, May (1986a) found that 20% had an identifiable cause of the paralysis.

Herpes Zoster Oticus

Herpes zoster oticus (Ramsay Hunt syndrome) consists of facial paralysis and auditory and vestibular dysfunction associated with herpetic vesicles of the auricle and the external auditory canal. Several autopsy studies have documented a viral origin for this syndrome, the herpes zoster virus being the primary agent. Esslen (1977) found that more than 40% of patients with herpes zoster oticus have accompanying auditory or vestibular dysfunction; this percentage is much greater than that of similar patients with Bell's palsy.

The facial nerve appears to be more severely damaged in herpes zoster oticus than in idiopathic facial palsy. Histologic studies have demonstrated larger segmental and more intense involvement of cranial nerve

TABLE 17–1. Classifications of Nerve Injuries

Seddon Classification	Sunderland Classification	Pathophysiologic Process
Neuropraxia	I	Physiologic block
Axonotmesis	II	Axons disrupted
	III	Axons and endoneurium disrupted
	IV	Axons, endoneurium, and perineurium disrupted
Neurotmesis	V	Complete transection

VII in herpes zoster oticus. In addition, a greater percentage of patients with herpes zoster oticus showed severe nerve degeneration with electrical testing. In contrast to patients with Bell's palsy, only 30% of patients with herpes zoster oticus recover normal facial function, and thus 70% experience some sequelae.

Melkersson-Rosenthal Syndrome

Melkersson-Rosenthal syndrome consists of intermittent facial nerve paralysis, recurrent swelling of the lips or the face, and a fissured tongue. The syndrome was initially described by Melkersson (1928), and Rosenthal (1931) added a fissured tongue to the description. This complex of symptoms frequently begins in childhood and is more common in females. Swelling (nonpitting edema) generally occurs in the upper lip and most often precedes the facial paralysis. The paralysis usually, but not always, corresponds to the side of the swelling and is recurrent.

The diagnosis of the Melkersson-Rosenthal syndrome is established by history and may be supported by a lip biopsy that reveals granulomatous changes. The origin of this syndrome is unclear, but a motor disturbance of the capillary and arterial network of both the facial nerve and the subcutaneous tissue is assumed. Melkersson-Rosenthal syndrome is differentiated from Heerfordt's disease, which is a rare form of sarcoidosis that causes uveitis, parotitis, fever, preauricular swelling, and facial paralysis.

Traumatic Facial Paralysis

Less than 2% of patients with head injury develop dysfunction of cranial nerve VIII. Trauma, however, is the second leading cause of facial paralysis (after Bell's palsy).

Two pure types of temporal bone fractures are described (longitudinal and transverse), although most clinical fractures are mixed on roentgenographic analysis. Longitudinal fractures are the most common (90%) type of temporal bone fracture but cause facial paralysis in less than 20% of patients who sustain them. In contrast, transverse fractures occur less frequently (10%) but have a 50% incidence of facial nerve involvement.

With both types of fracture, the perigeniculate area is usually the epicenter of injury. Complete nerve transection is more often seen with transverse fractures. An intraneural hematoma is generally associated with a longitudinal fracture. Facial nerve paralysis more often immediately follows a transverse fracture. Adour and colleagues (1977) and other researchers have observed that immediate paralysis after trauma implies a poor functional recovery, whereas delayed onset or incomplete palsy has a better prognosis. Nevertheless, because progressive edema can result in permanent facial paralysis, facial function should be closely monitored electrodiagnostically after injury.

Facial Paralysis Secondary to Infection

Acute otitis media or chronic otitis media without an associated cholesteatoma is a rare cause of facial paralysis, with an incidence of less than 0.1%. The pathophysiologic process proposed by Graham (1977) involves neural edema and vascular insufficiency. Facial paralysis occurs in approximately 1% of patients who present with a cholesteatoma. Pressure and inflammation secondary to the cholesteatoma are thought to cause the facial nerve paralysis. In general, the paralysis is slowly progressive.

Malignant external otitis, described by Chandler (1974), is a chronic pseudomonal infection of the external auditory canal, skin, and temporal bone. It usually occurs in diabetics or immunocompromised persons. Facial paralysis occurs in 40% of patients and is a poor prognostic sign. Until the mid-1980s, the majority of patients who developed facial paralysis died of their infections, and fewer than half of the survivors had normal facial function. The facial nerve is typically involved at the stylomastoid foramen.

Facial Paralysis in Children

As in adults, Bell's palsy is the leading cause of facial paralysis in children, although an identifiable cause is more often found. Traumatic facial nerve injury is most commonly seen in the neonatal period. Smith and colleagues (1981) noted that 80% of neonatal paralysis was secondary to birth trauma. Approximately 90% of affected infants recovered spontaneously.

Congenital facial paralysis can occur in Möbius's syndrome (bilateral facial paralysis and unilateral or bilateral abducens paralysis), in hemifacial microsomia, and in Goldenhar's syndrome. Cardiac defects can occur in association with an isolated ramus mandibularis paralysis.

Tumors and Facial Paralysis

Facial nerve paralysis resulting from neoplasm generally has a gradual onset, but in 10% to 20% of such patients, the onset can be acute. Facial paralysis that does not abate at all after 6 months should be further evaluated in order to rule out neoplastic disease. Benign tumors that cause facial nerve dysfunction are more often intratemporal. These lesions include facial nerve neuromas, acoustic neuromas, petrous apex cholesteatomas and cysts, and glomus tumors. Extratemporal tumors that cause facial paralysis are in general malignant and of parotid origin. The most common parotid tumor that causes facial nerve paralysis is a mucoepidermoid lesion followed by an adenoid cystic carcinoma. Facial paralysis in the presence of a malignant parotid tumor generally carries a poor prognosis.

Iatrogenic Facial Nerve Paralysis

Iatrogenic facial nerve paralysis occurs in approximately 1% to 2% of all otologic sur-

gical procedures. In neuro-otologic procedures, the facial nerve is at increased risk. For small and medium-sized acoustic tumors, the incidence of facial nerve injury is reported to be 13%. Other conditions that result in an increased risk to the facial nerve include congenital atresia, revision surgery, and surgery for recurrent cholesteatoma. Kartush and colleagues (1989) showed that the use of intraoperative facial nerve monitoring can enhance preservation of the anatomic and functional integrity of the facial nerve.

Bilateral Paralysis

Several disorders have been associated with bilateral facial paralysis. These include a variant of sarcoidosis (uveoparotid fever), diabetes mellitus, mononucleosis, and leukemia. Acute idiopathic polyneuritis, or Guillain-Barré syndrome, and various acute toxic polyneuropathies are known to cause facial diplegia.

Lyme's disease is a more recently described cause of bilateral facial paralysis. Approximately 10% of infected patients develop either bilateral or unilateral facial nerve paralysis. The paralysis is often accompanied by other systemic abnormalities. Melkersson-Rosenthal syndrome and, in rare instances, Bell's palsy can be associated with facial diplegia.

DIAGNOSIS

The diagnosis of facial nerve disorders relies on history, physical examination, radiologic examination (computed tomographic scan or magnetic resonance imaging), selected audiometric tests, and special tests related to facial nerve function. The special tests are divided into traditional site-of-lesion testing and electrodiagnostic testing, which are conducted to assess the degree of dysfunction and prognosis for recovery. Controversy exists as to whether every patient presenting with facial paralysis should have a computed tomographic scan or a magnetic resonance imaging scan to rule out neoplasia before a diagnosis of idiopathic facial paralysis is made.

Topognostic Testing

By assessing the function of the accessory branches of the facial nerve, topognostic tests were originally thought to pinpoint the site of lesion in facial paralysis. Clinical experience has demonstrated the limited accuracy of these tests, although they continue to be used by some clinicians and merit discussion.

Of all the topognostic tests, Schirmer's test appears to be the most efficacious. The test is performed by placing filter paper in the fornix of each eye. A reduction in lacrimal secretion by 25% to 30% in one eye or a bilateral reduction (less than 2.5 cm over 5 minutes) is considered abnormal. Fisch (1977) noted that all patients with a 90% reduction on electroneurography (ENoG) had an abnormal result of Schirmer's test; however, not all patients with an abnormal Schirmer's test result had more than 90% reduction on ENoG. ENoG was shown to be a better predictor of ultimate facial function. The authors perform lacrimal testing primarily as a means of assessing the patient's proclivity for exposure keratitis rather than for topognostic or prognostic assessment.

Stimulating the tongue in order to assess the chorda tympani nerve has not proved useful in either predicting the site of lesion or determining the degree of injury to the facial nerve.

Salivary flow testing was introduced by Magielski and Blatt (1958). After the submandibular ducts on each side are cannulated, salivary flow is stimulated, and the outputs of both ducts are compared over a 1-minute period. May and associates (1981) initially found that salivary flow declined earlier in Bell's palsy than did responses on electrical tests. They considered a 25% unilateral reduction predictive of a poor functional recovery. May (1990) more recently retracted this statement because he found that salivary flow testing is no more accurate than guessing.

The stapedius reflex can be measured with standard tympanometric techniques. Koike and colleagues (1977) observed that if the stapedius reflex reappeared within the first 3 weeks after the onset of paralysis, overall prognosis was good. Fisch (1977) found no correlation between ENoG and stapedius reflex results.

Electrical Testing

The aim of electrically testing the facial nerve is to assess the condition of the axons distal to the stylomastoid foramen. Consequently, if the conduction block occurs proximal to the stylomastoid foramen, as it does in more than 90% of facial nerve injuries (Shambaugh and Clemis, 1973), 48 to 72 hours are needed for wallerian degeneration to take place to the extent that the paralysis can be monitored with electrical tests. To circumvent this delay in diagnosis, magnetic stimulation and antidromic stimulation of the facial nerve are being investigated. To date, the mainstays of electrodiagnostic testing include the nerve excitability test (NET), the maximal stimulation test, ENoG, and electromyography.

Nerve Excitability Test

In the NET, or minimal nerve excitation test, percutaneous electrical stimulation is administered to the stylomastoid foramen. As initially described by Laumans and Jongkees (1963), electrical impulses are delivered at increasing levels of current until a facial twitch occurs. A difference of 3.5 mA between the sides of the face is considered a poor prognostic sign. Several problems exist with this testing method, including (1) subjectivity of assessment and (2) the fact that because mainly large myelinated fibers are stimulated as a result of their low threshold, small unmyelinated fibers are not recruited until high current levels are used. Perhaps for these reasons, May and associates (1983) showed that 42% of patients with Bell's palsy had an incomplete recovery despite a normal NET result.

Maximal Stimulation Test

Popularized by May and colleagues (1971), the maximal stimulation test involves a level of electrical stimulation at which point maximal facial movement is observed. Both sides of the face are compared, and movement is judged as equal, slightly decreased, markedly decreased, or absent. May and associates (1983) found that of patients with normal maximal stimulation test results, 92% experienced normal recovery and no patients experienced extremely poor recovery. Of the patients whose responses to maximal stimulation testing were markedly decreased or absent, 86% demonstrated incomplete recovery.

Electroneurography

Whereas the NET and maximal stimulation test entail a subjective appraisal of facial nerve response, ENoG objectively records and quantifies the response. As described by Esslen (1977), ENoG entails supramaximal stimulation at the stylomastoid foramen. A compound muscle action potential is recorded with the use of bipolar surface electrodes placed optimally near the nasolabial groove (Fig. 17–2). Kelleher and coworkers (in press) showed the nasal alae to be the most reliable site for recording consistent waveforms. Kartush and associates (1985) supported Esslen's technique by demonstrating that optimal lead placement, as opposed to standard lead placement, decreased interside variance. Compound muscle action potentials of each side are compared. Fisch (1984) found that the velocity of degeneration, or the number of days that it takes for degeneration to take place, is proportional to the degree of nerve injury. In other words, the more rapidly the nerve degenerates, the worse the underlying nerve injury is. In addition, Fisch noted the endpoint, or percentage of maximal degeneration, to be prognostic of later return of facial function. Fisch (1981) observed that if 95% or more degeneration took place within 3 weeks, 50% of patients with Bell's palsy experienced unsatisfactory return of facial function. Once 90% degeneration was reached, nine of ten patients progressed to more than 95% degeneration within 2 weeks. Fisch (1984) reported that if 90% degeneration of the compound muscle action potential was noted within 6 days after the onset of facial palsy resulting from trauma, a poor return of facial function could be expected.

Early deblocking, or the return of some visible voluntary facial movement, in a previously paralyzed face has been found by Fisch (1984) and others to be a good prognostic sign. Early deblocking, however, may cause a further reduction in the compound muscle action potential, and in this situation, the prognostic value of electrical testing may be clinically misleading. ENoG has been shown to be the most accurate prognostic indicator of all electrical tests, the maximal stimulation test being the next best (May and associates 1983).

Kartush and associates (1987) used ENoG to assess the degree of subclinical facial nerve involvement before cerebellopontine angle and skull base surgery. In addition, ENoG occasionally plays a role in the diagnosis of occult tumors involving the facial nerve (May, 1986b). Initial investigations indicate that ENoG may be beneficial in managing patients with malignant otitis externa (Kartush and Graham, 1990). The progression or the resolution of an underlying neuritis can be monitored by serial ENoG studies to determine the efficacy of treatment. An abnormal ENoG result may prove to be an indication for additional or continued treatment of these patients.

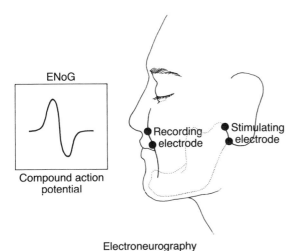

Electroneurography

Figure 17–2. Recording technique for electroneurography. Stimulus intensity is increased at the stylomastoid foramen until maximal amplitude is observed in the recorded compound muscle action potential. (From Kartush JM, Lilly D, Kemink JL: Facial electroneurography: clinical and experimental investigations. Otolaryngol Head Neck Surg 93:516, 1985.)

Electromyography

Electromyography is a recording technique in which the electrical activity in muscles is observed with the use of needle electrodes placed directly into the muscle substance. Electromyography is used to measure the electrical responses (1) during needle insertion, (2) when the patient is at rest, and (3) during voluntary movement. In muscle with

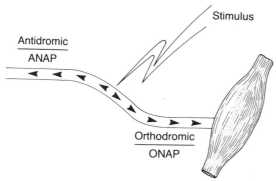

Figure 17–3. Stimulation of a peripheral nerve causes conduction to take place in two directions: (1) orthodromic, or toward the periphery, and (2) antidromic, or in a retrograde manner. (From Kartush J, Prass R: Facial nerve testing: electroneurography and intraoperative monitoring. In Johnson J, Kartush JM, Prass RL [eds]: American Academy of Otolaryngology Head and Neck Surgery Instruction Courses, Vol. I [pp. 231–247]. St. Louis: CV Mosby, 1988.)

normal innervation, voluntary facial motor unit potentials are seen. Esslen (1977) found that the prognosis for a good recovery is increased in idiopathic facial paralysis if voluntary motor unit potentials exist within the first week of paralysis. Fibrillation potentials are indicative of muscle denervation, but because they do not occur until 2 to 3 weeks after the injury, electromyography is of little benefit in determining prognosis within the first weeks of paralysis. Polyphasic reinnervation potentials, or giant waves, indicate nerve regeneration and may occur before the onset of clinically detectable facial movement. Electrical silence indicates complete absence of motor unit end plate activity. Electromyographic recordings are particularly useful for differentiating congenital from traumatic facial paralysis.

Antidromic Potentials

In an effort to diagnose facial nerve degeneration earlier than 48 to 72 hours after nerve injury (during which wallerian degeneration occurs), antidromic, or retrograde, potentials of the facial nerve have been measured (Fig. 17–3). Kartush and associates (1987) found that there is no trans-synaptic conduction of this response, as occurs with evoked auditory brain stem response. Consequently, without a brain stem component, complete transection of the nerve can be associated with little or no change in response amplitude.

Magnetic Stimulation

Magnetic stimulation of the facial nerve is currently being evaluated. A pulsed magnetic field can penetrate skin and bone to induce an in-depth electrical current (Fig. 17–4). Investigations have shown that the facial nerve compound muscle action potential is similar in response amplitude and morphologic characteristics to those obtained with ENoG (Kartush et al., 1989). In addition, latency studies indicate that the magnetically stimulated facial nerve can be depolarized near its root entry zone. This technique may allow for stimulation proximal to the site of most facial nerve injuries and may thus perhaps eliminate the 2- to 3-day delay associated with currently used electrical tests. Further investigations, however, are needed to assess the clinical utility of this technique.

TREATMENT

The treatment of many types of facial nerve paralysis, especially Bell's palsy, remains

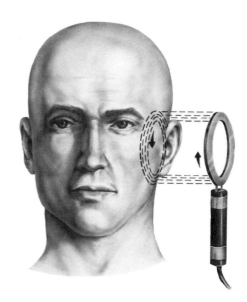

Magnetic transtemporal stimulation

Figure 17–4. Transtemporal magnetic stimulation allows a pulsed magnetic field to induce an in-depth electrical current. (From Kartush JM: Electroneurography and intraoperative facial monitoring in contemporary neurotology. Otolaryngol Head Neck Surg 10:496–503, 1989.)

controversial. Medical, surgical, and expectant treatments have been advocated for idiopathic facial paralysis.

Bell's Palsy

Spontaneous Recovery

As previously outlined, Peiterson (1982) found that 71% of patients with Bell's palsy experienced a complete return of facial function without treatment. Eighty-four percent of patients experienced a satisfactory return of function. In idiopathic facial paralysis, an incomplete palsy typically has an excellent prognosis. In addition, early deblocking, especially within the first 3 weeks of paralysis, is indicative of a good prognosis. The role of electrical testing is to identify the patients with a poor prognosis for whom the following treatment modalities may offer the most benefit.

Medical Treatment

Steroids, including prednisone and adrenocorticotropic hormone (ACTH), have been used in the treatment of idiopathic facial paralysis since 1951. Stankiewicz (1987) reviewed 94 papers associated with steroid use in Bell's palsy and concluded that a statistically definitive study citing a benefit for steroids had not been performed. He found strong trends suggesting that steroids may prevent denervation, lessen synkinesis, hasten recovery, and prevent progression of incomplete paralysis to complete paralysis. He found that steroids do prevent crocodile tearing.

Herpes Zoster Oticus

Medical Treatment

As in Bell's palsy, steroid use in herpes zoster oticus is still disputed. Adour (1977) found that 50% of patients with herpes zoster oticus progressed to total denervation, whereas only 25% did so with steroid treatment.

Acyclovir, a virostatic agent, has been introduced in the treatment of patients with herpes zoster oticus. Dickins and colleagues (1988) found that intravenous acyclovir (10 mg/kg every 8 hours for 7 days) resulted in a marked improvement in facial function over previously tried medications for herpes zoster oticus. Because of a small sample size, his results were not statistically significant. The effects of acyclovir were so rapid and dramatic that Dickins and colleagues strongly believed that acyclovir was responsible for the improvement in the paralysis.

Facial Paralysis in Acute Otitis Media

Medical Treatment

Antibiotics, in conjunction with wide myringotomy, are important in the treatment of facial paralysis associated with acute otitis media. If the paralysis does not abate rapidly, surgical intervention is recommended.

Malignant Otitis Externa

Medical Treatment

Prolonged intravenous antipseudomonal antibiotics are the mainstay of treatment for paralysis associated with malignant external otitis. When facial palsy complicates malignant otitis externa, the authors combine a lateral temporal bone resection and facial nerve decompression with appropriate long-term antibiotics.

SURGICAL THERAPY

Bell's Palsy

The role of surgical therapy in idiopathic facial paralysis remains unsettled. To date, there have been no well-controlled prospective clinical trials to answer the following questions:

1. What are the indications for surgical therapy? (Progression and degree of nerve dysfunction.)
2. What type of decompression is necessary?

Central to these questions is the manner in which recovery of facial function is analyzed. Although no grading system is perfect, adoption of the House Brackman classification (House, 1983) should allow greater uniformity in reporting results.

Since the first attempt at facial nerve decompression, many authors have advocated surgical decompression. Pulec (1966) first described total facial nerve decompression by using the middle cranial fossa approach outlined by House (Fig. 17–5) in conjunction with a transmastoid approach. May (1979) initially found that a transmastoid subtemporal facial nerve decompression favorably influenced the course of idiopathic paralysis and herpes zoster oticus in patients whose testing indicated a poor prognosis. May subsequently retracted this finding after he abandoned his study of facial nerve decompression, citing statistical difficulties in assessing the effects of any treatment of Bell's palsy. His surgical technique, however, did not include decompression of the meatal foramen, which has been shown to be the site of greatest nerve entrapment in Bell's palsy (Fisch, 1981).

Fisch (1981) advocated total facial nerve decompression (middle cranial fossa and transmastoid approaches) if ENoG demonstrated facial nerve degeneration reaching 90% or more within 21 days after the onset of the paralysis. The major limitation of this retrospective study was a small sample size (27 patients). Fisch emphasized that the visible area of greatest edema and the site of an electrophysiologic conduction block appear to be at the meatal foramen. Currently, a multi-institutional study is being conducted to ascertain the role of total facial nerve decompression in idiopathic facial paralysis. In this investigation, ENoG is being used to stratify patients into favorable and poor prognostic groups on the basis of Fisch and Esslen's criteria (B. Gantz, 1990, personal communication).

Traumatic Facial Paralysis

Surgical treatment of traumatic facial paralysis of temporal bone origin is also debated. Several researchers have advocated facial nerve decompression and repair if there are an immediate onset and complete facial nerve paralysis. Currently, Fisch (1984) and others recommend electrical testing with ENoG from the onset of the paralysis, whether the onset is immediate or delayed. Decompression is recommended when denervation reaches more than 90% within 6 days from the onset of the paralysis. Fisch (1984) identified the perigeniculate area as the region of the facial nerve most often injured by temporal bone trauma. Facial nerve paralysis caused by birth trauma may also be followed by serial ENoG as well as electromyography.

Recurrent Facial Palsy

Total facial nerve decompression has been recommended in cases of Melkersson-Rosen-

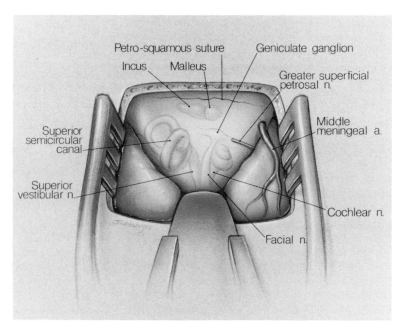

Figure 17–5. Left temporal bone as viewed from the middle cranial fossa with the temporal lobe retracted medially. Note relationship of the facial nerve to the cochlea anteriorly and the superior semicircular canal posteriorly.

Petro-squamous suture

Geniculate ganglion

Incus Malleus

Greater superficial petrosal n.

Middle meningeal a.

Superior semicircular canal

Superior vestibular n.

Cochlear n.

Facial n.

Figure 17–6. Alternatives to direct hypoglossal facial anastomosis. A jump-graft anastomosis spares the majority of the hypoglossal nerve's interlacing fascicles, unlike the split-nerve anastomosis.

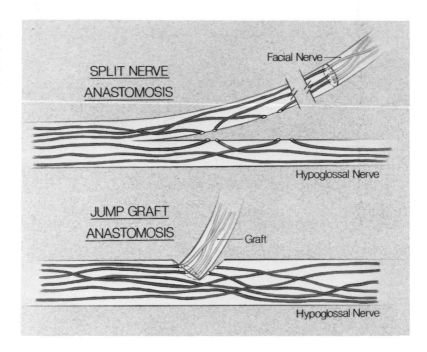

thal syndrome. Nyberg and Fisch (1985) and Graham and Kartush (1988) found that total facial nerve decompression in cases of idiopathic recurrent facial paralysis and Melkersson-Rosenthal syndrome is effective in preventing further episodes of paralysis.

Otitis Media With and Without Cholesteatoma

Complete facial nerve paralysis that results from acute otitis media and does not resolve with antibiotics and wide myringotomy should be treated with mastoidectomy. Neurolysis (opening the nerve sheath) remains controversial. For cases in which facial nerve paralysis results from a cholesteatoma, mastoidectomy with limited decompression has been advocated. The authors' current practice is to open the nerve sheath to identify a plane between the nerve and the cholesteatoma. This permits them to dissect the matrix free. When granulation tissue is present, without a cholesteatoma, a limited decompression without neurolysis is performed.

Neoplasia

Facial nerve paralysis secondary to tumor is usually treated surgically. Parotid cancers af-fecting facial nerve function often require total parotidectomy with partial or total facial nerve sacrifice. Benign tumors causing facial nerve paralysis are usually intratemporal and are removed surgically. These include glomus tumors, acoustic neuromas, and facial neuromas. The role of surgical decompression of facial neuromas without resection is debated.

Facial Rehabilitation

If the facial nerve has been severed, the best return of function is gained with direct repair

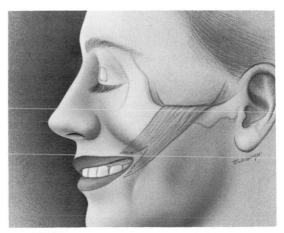

Figure 17–7. Temporalis muscle transposition with overcorrection of the smile. Gold weight implant is shown in the upper eyelid.

Figure 17–8. A mechanically evoked facial nerve response (burst response) is observed during intraoperative manipulation of the facial nerve. (From Kartush JM: Electroneurography and intraoperative facial monitoring in contemporary neurotology. Otolaryngol Head Neck Surg 10:496–503, 1989.)

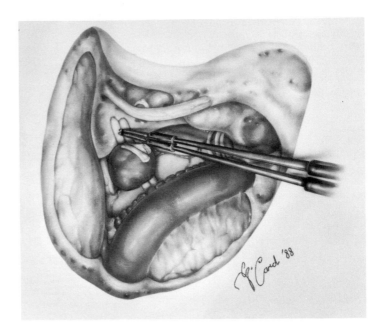

as soon as possible. To avoid undue tension at the anastomotic site, facial nerve transposition or nerve grafting can be used.

Another means of rehabilitating the paralyzed face includes substitution with the hypoglossal nerve. Contraindications to an anastomosis at cranial nerves VII to XII include paralysis of cranial nerve X and neurofibromatosis (May and associates, 1984). Hypoglossal-facial nerve substitution has been a reliable technique for facial reanimation, but 25% of patients complain of spasticity and synkinesis as well as changes in speech and swallowing. M. May (1986, personal communication) introduced a "jump graft" technique (Fig. 17–6) that results in satisfactory facial reinnervation and virtually no gross changes in hypoglossal function. The authors' current practice is to combine half of the hypoglossal nerve with a selective temporalis transposition to the corner of the mouth. This allows immediate reanimation while neural regeneration occurs.

Cross-face nerve grafting, introduced by Scaramella (1971), entails the use of sural nerve jump grafts from the nonparalyzed facial nerve. This technique has met with only marginal success.

Dynamic facial reanimation procedures for patients with facial paralysis and an inadequate peripheral neuromuscular system were popularized by Rubin (1977) and Conley and Gullane (1978). Temporalis muscle transposition is effective in allowing voluntary smiling but does not allow mimetic movements. May (1986b, personal communication) advocated temporalis transposition to the lower face with insertion of gold weights in the upper eyelid to assist with eye closure (Fig.

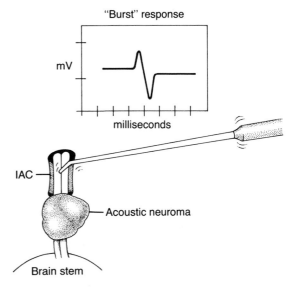

Figure 17–9. Bipolar electrical stimulation of the facial nerve during translabyrinthine removal of a right-sided acoustic neuroma. (From Kartush JM: Electroneurography and intraoperative facial monitoring in contemporary neurotology. Otolaryngol Head Neck Surg 10:496–503, 1989.)

17–7). The ability to rehabilitate the eye independently with a gold weight means that reanimation (using an anastomosis for cranial nerves VII to XII or muscle transposition) can be directed to the lower face, and ocular synkinesis can be avoided. Muscle transposition is generally used in cases of long-standing facial paralysis or lack of a seventh nerve stump for nerve anastomosis. Gold weight insertion can be temporary or permanent, depending on the cause of the paralysis.

Free flaps, involving both vascular or vascular and neural anastomoses, have been employed in the rehabilitation of the paralyzed face. More experience with these techniques is needed.

Intraoperative Facial Nerve Monitoring

Intraoperative monitoring of cranial nerve VII appears to enhance the surgeon's ability to preserve the anatomic and functional integrity of the facial nerve. Monitoring is currently employed during acoustic tumor surgery (Fig. 17–8), vestibular neurectomy, microvascular decompression, and selected otologic surgery.

The goals of facial nerve monitoring during surgery are (1) to permit early nerve identification, (2) to enhance neural preservation by minimizing trauma, and (3) to assess neural integrity after dissection is complete. Both electrically and mechanically (Fig. 17–9) evoked facial nerve electromyographic responses can be visualized as well as acoustically represented. Facial electromyographic signals are amplified and displayed through a loudspeaker in the operating room to provide immediate feedback to the operating surgeon.

SUGGESTED READINGS

Adour KK: Herpes zoster causing facial paralysis: treatment of facial palsy of infectious origin. *In* Fisch U (ed): Facial Nerve Surgery (pp 419–421). Birmingham, AL: Aesculapius, 1977.

Adour KK: Diagnosis and management of facial paralysis. N Engl J Med 307:348–351, 1982.

Adour KK, Bayajian JA, Kahn ZM: Surgical and nonsurgical management of facial paralysis following closed head injury. Laryngoscope 87:380–390, 1977.

Adour KK, Wingerd J: Idiopathic facial paralysis (Bell's palsy): factors affecting severity and outcome in 446 patients. Neurology 24:1112–1116, 1974.

Baker DC, Conley J: Regional muscle transposition for rehabilitation of the paralyzed face. Clin Plast Surg 6:317–331, 1979.

Chandler JR: Malignant external otitis and facial paralysis. Otolaryngol Clin North Am 7:324–383, 1974.

Conley J, Gullane PF: Facial rehabilitation with temporalis muscle. Arch Otolaryngol 104:423–426, 1978.

Dickins JRE, Smith JT, Graham SS: Herpes zoster oticus: treatment with intravenous acyclovir. Laryngoscope 98:776–779, 1988.

Esslen E: The Acute Facial Palsies. Berlin: Springer-Verlag, 1977.

Fisch U: Total facial nerve decompression and electroneurography. *In* Silverstein H, Norrell H (eds): Neurological Surgery of the Ear (pp 21–23). Birmingham, AL: Aesculapius, 1977.

Fisch U: Surgery for Bell's palsy. Arch Otolaryngol 107:1–11, 1981.

Fisch U: Prognostic value of electrical tests in acute facial paralysis. Am J Otol 5(6):494–498, 1984.

Graham MD: Facial paralysis in acute bacterial infections of the ear. *In* Fisch U (ed): Facial Nerve Surgery (pp 204–241). Birmingham, AL: Aesculapius, 1977.

Graham M, House W (eds): Disorders of the Facial Nerve. New York: Raven Press, 1982.

Graham MD, Kartush JM: Total facial nerve decompression for recurring facial paralysis—an update. Otolaryngol Head Neck Surg 101:496–503, 1988.

House JW: Facial nerve grading systems. Laryngoscope 92:1056–1069, 1983.

Kartush JM: Electroneurography and intraoperative facial monitoring in contemporary neurotology. Otolaryngol Head Neck Surg 101:496–503, 1989.

Kartush JM, Bouchard KR, Graham MD, Linstrom CL: Magnetic stimulation of the facial nerve. Am J Otol 10:14–19, 1989.

Kartush J, Graham MD: Rationale and means of preoperative facial assessment. *In* Castro D (ed): Facial Nerve (pp 175–178). Amsterdam: Kugler and Ghedini, 1990.

Kartush J, Lilly P, Kemink J: Facial electroneurography: clinical and experimental investigations. Otolaryngol Head Neck Surg 93:516–523, 1985.

Kartush JM, Niparko JK, Graham MD: Electroneurography: preoperative facial nerve assessment for tumors of the temporal bone. Otolaryngol Head Neck Surg 97:257, 1987.

Kelleher MJ, Gutnich HM, Prass RL: Waveform morphology and amplitude variability in facial nerve electroneurography. In press.

Koike Y, Hojo K, Iwasaki E: Prognosis of facial palsy based on the stapedial reflex test. *In* Fisch U (ed): Facial Nerve Surgery (pp 159–164). Birmingham, AL: Aesculapius, 1977.

Laumans E, Jongkees L: On the prognosis of peripheral facial paralysis of endotemporal origin: II. Electrical tests. Ann Otol Rhinol Laryngol 72:621, 1963.

Magielski JE, Blatt IM: Submaxillary salivary flow: a test of chorda tympani nerve function as an aid in diagnosis and prognosis of facial nerve paralysis. Laryngoscope 68:1770–1789, 1958.

May M: Total facial nerve exploration: transmastoid, extralabyrinthine, and subtemporal indications and results. Laryngoscope 89:906–917, 1979.

May M: Trauma to the facial nerve. Oto Clin North Am 16:661–670, 1983.

May M: Differential diagnosis by history, physical findings, and laboratory results. *In* May M (ed): The Facial Nerve. New York: Thieme Medical Publishers, 1986a.

May M: Tumors involving the facial nerve. *In* May M (ed): The Facial Nerve. New York: Thieme Medical Publishers, 1986b.

May M: Science is for the moment and truth is forever. Otolaryngol Head Neck Surg 102:1–2, 1990.

May M, Blumenthal F, Klein SR: Acute Bell's palsy: prognostic value of evoked electromyography, maximal stimulation and other electrical tests. Am J Otol 5:1–7, 1983.

May M, Blumenthal F, Taylor FH: Bell's palsy: Surgery based upon prognostic indicators and results. Laryngoscope 91:2092–2103, 1981.

May M, Harvey JE, Marovitz WF, Stroud M: The prognostic accuracy of the maximal stimulation test compared with that of the nerve excitability test in Bell's palsy. Laryngoscope 81:931–938, 1971.

May M, Klein SR, Taylor FH: Indications for surgery for Bell's palsy. Am J Otol 5(6):503–512, 1984.

Melkersson E: Ett fallar recidivirande facialispares i samband med angio-neurotiskt odem. Hygeia 90:737, 1928.

Mulkins PS, Blecker JO, Schroder FP: Acute facial paralysis: a virological study. Clin Otolaryngol 5:305–310, 1980.

Nyberg P, Fisch U: Surgical treatment and results of idiopathic recurrent facial palsy. *In* Portman M (ed): Facial Nerve (pp 259–268). New York: Masson, 1985.

Peiterson E: The natural history of Bell's palsy. Am J Otol 4(2):107–111, 1982.

Pulec JL: Total decompression of the facial nerve. Laryngoscope 76:1015–1028, 1966.

Rosenthal C: Klinisch-orbbiologischer boitrag zur konstitutions pathologic gemeninsames auftreten von (rezidivierender familiar er) facialishahmung, aminoneurotischem gesichtsodem and lingua plicata in arthritismusfamiliar. Z Neurol Psychiat 31:475–501, 1931.

Rubin L: Reanimation of the paralyzed face. St. Louis: CV Mosby, 1977.

Scaramella L: L'anastomosi tra i due nervi faccial. Arch Otologie 82:209–215, 1971.

Seddon HJ: Three types of nerve injury. Brain 66:237, 1943.

Shambaugh G, Clemis J: Facial nerve paralysis. *In* Paparella M, Shumrick D (eds): Otolaryngology, vol 2 (p 275). Philadelphia: WB Saunders, 1973.

Smith JD, Crumley R, Harker L: Facial paralysis in the newborn. Otolaryngol Head Neck Surg 89:1021–1024, 1981.

Stankiewicz JA: A review of the published data on steroids and idiopathic facial paralysis. Otolaryngol Head Neck Surg 97:481–486, 1987.

Sunderland S: Nerve and Nerve Injuries, 2nd ed (pp. 133–141). Edinburgh: Churchill Livingstone, 1978.

CHAPTER 18

Vestibular Physiology

Dennis P. O'Leary, PhD

The human vestibular labyrinth, which consists of three semicircular canals, the utricle, and the saccule, provides information for two main functions of the vestibular system: control of posture and coordinated motion. The physiologic mechanisms underlying these functions have been studied as a network of interacting control systems, each of which accomplishes local tasks. For example, the vestibulo-ocular reflex functions mainly to allow clear vision during walking by stabilizing the eyes during faster head movements. Stabilized visual information is useful during locomotion for appropriate body orientation in the environment. In contrast, standing still or walking in the dark does not require vision, but it is accomplished by activation of specific antigravity muscle groups to avoid falling. In this case, proprioceptive information adds an important component to the information from the inner ear. Under normal conditions, the interacting vestibular, visual, and proprioceptive subsystems function in a synergistic manner that is often transparent to the user. For example, it is often said that a normal human is generally unaware of his or her vestibular system until the onset of vestibular disease.

The study of vestibular physiologic mechanisms has advanced through use of control principles derived from engineering, and this usage has also influenced the otolaryngolic approach to diagnostic evaluation. Pathologic vestibular dysfunction can be regarded as a maladjusted control system, and vestibular test results are often expressed in engineering terminology.

Advances in vestibulo-ocular physiology research during the 1970s showed the vestibular system's "plasticity"—that is, the ability to adapt to changing input states by modifying information transmission at the cellular level. In a control framework sense, vestibular plasticity can be compared to a modern rocket control system that can adapt to environmental changes by modifying its control signals to keep the rocket on course. Mechanisms of plasticity are thought to be the basis for clinical compensation for vestibular lesions.

In this chapter, vestibular physiologic processes are examined from a control system perspective, and examples of how this approach has influenced modern diagnostic screening of vestibular disorders are given.

LABYRINTHINE RECEPTORS

Role of the Cupula

The membranous canals enlarge to form an ampulla, which contains hair cells arranged along the surface of a saddle-shaped crista. Extending above the crista is the cupula, a gelatinous membrane whose perimeter is attached to the ampulla (Fig. 18–1). The cupula is labile and subject to shrinkage, which led to earlier misconceptions about its size. Earlier studies based on films of stained cupula implied that the cupula was detached distal to the crista and could be displaced in a way similar to a swinging gate, or "torsion pendulum." This is now considered unlikely, at least during physiologic stimulation, but such large displacements could result from damage through excess pressure. Because of their mathematical simplicity, equations modeling the cupula as a torsion pendulum are still used as physiologic approximations, and they often provide useful parameters for describing physiologic processes.

Cilia extend from the hair cells in the crista into fine channels in the cupula. Because the membranous labyrinth is fixed to the bone, rotational head movements (angular accelerations) result in an inertial lag of endolymph inside the canals in the direction opposite to that of the head. The endolymph exerts pressure on the cupula, distorting it slightly and causing local forces on the cilia within it. The fine movements of the cilia appear to alter ionic conductivities in membrane channels, which results in hair cell stimulation. Figure 18–2 shows a current view of cupular displacement.

Receptor Generator Mechanisms

A static potential gradient occurs in the semicircular canal ampulla, with the endolymph positive in relation to the more negative crista. This potential is thought to act during mechanoelectric transduction as a generator potential, which results in transmission of neurotransmitters at synapses of hair cells to afferent fibers. Postsynaptic potentials in the afferent fibers are thought to modulate the neural impulse activity in the first-order afferent fibers.

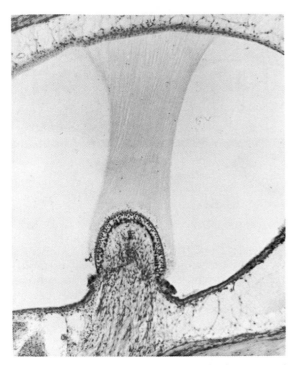

Figure 18–1. A cross-section through the long axis of the ampulla showing the crista-cupula system of the horizontal semicircular canal from a squirrel monkey. Note that the cupula fills the entire lumen of the ampulla. (From Igarashi M: Dimensional study of the vestibular end organ apparatus. *In* The Role of the Vestibular Organs in Space Exploration, NASA Publication No. SP-115 [pp 47–54]. Washington, DC: National Aeronautics and Space Administration, 1966.)

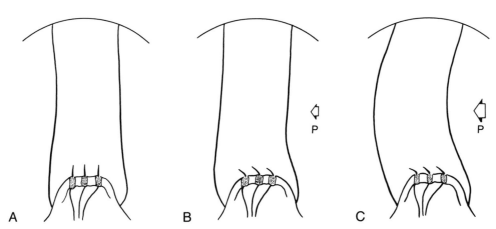

Figure 18–2. A cupula displacement model. *A.* The cupula extends from the elevated crista to the opposite ampullary wall in its resting position so that the cilia tuft essentially projects from the crista to the cupula, where the kinocilium is embedded. *B.* With slight pressures or initial endolymph displacement, the base of the cupula shifts with shearing in the subcupular space. This displacement causes a bowing of only the basal parts of the cupula. *C.* Increased pressure (P) on the endolymph displaces broad areas of the cupula so that the maximal displacement shifts toward the center of the cupula. (From Hillman DE, McLaren JW: Displacement of the semicircular canal cupula during sinusoidal rotation. Neuroscience 4:2001–2008, 1979.)

Neural Response Dynamics

Semicircular Canals

Although the canals themselves are sensitive to angular acceleration, the averaged neural responses were proportional to head velocity. Viscous damping in the receptor was therefore thought to "integrate" head movement accelerations to resemble head velocity. The kinocilia of all hair cells in a crista are morphologically polarized—that is, oriented toward the utricle in lateral canals and away from the utricle in vertical canals (Fig. 18–3). Canal afferent fibers are "functionally polarized" in the sense that cupular motion toward the kinocilia results in increased afferent activity, whereas motion directed away from the kinocilia results in decreased activity. The biophysical basis for this functional bipolarity is currently unknown.

Early studies suggested that the torsion pendulum model was an accurate descriptor of individual afferent response characteristics; all afferent fibers from a canal were thought to carry similar information that was in some sense "averaged" by the brain. But later studies showed that individual afferent fibers differed widely in their response characteristics; an afferent response type topographically correlated with location of innervation in the crista. Studies in lower animals (fish and frogs) showed that afferent fibers that innervated the crest region of the crista responded best to faster head movements, whereas afferent fibers that innervated the crista slopes responded best to slower movements. Similar afferent response differences were found in cats and primates. But such differences cannot be associated directly with the well-known existence of both type I and type II hair cells in mammals. These differences occur also in fish and frogs, which have only type II hair cells. An example of such response diversity is shown in Figure 18–4.

The response differences could reflect mechanoelectrical transduction differences in different receptor regions (e.g., differences that are like the cochlear traveling wave), but this conjecture remains to be clarified. Eighth cranial nerve canal afferent fibers can, however, be considered analogous to cochlear afferent fibers in the following sense. Fast head movements are carried by larger fibers in particular nerve regions, and slow head movements are carried by small fibers localized in other regions; this scenario is analogous to that of fibers with high-tone and low-tone characteristic frequencies in the cochlear nerve.

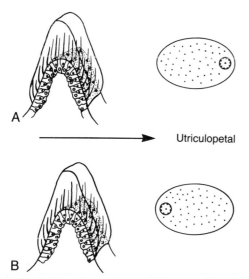

Utriculopetal

Figure 18–3. Schematic representation of orientation of kinocilia in cristae of semicircular canals. In horizontal cristae (A) all kinocilia are oriented toward the utricle, whereas in vertical canals (B) they are oriented away from the utricle. (Adapted from Spoendlin HH: Ultrastructural studies of the labyrinth in squirrel monkeys. In The Role of the Vestibular Organs in the Exploration of Space, NASA Publication No. SP-77 [pp 7–22]. Washington, DC: National Aeronautics and Space Administration, 1965.)

Utricle and Saccule

Each afferent fiber that innervates the macular receptors responds preferentially to a certain direction of net force. This results from innervation of specific regions of hair cells that are morphologically oriented in similar directions. Regional mappings of hair cell orientation within each macula therefore provide an effective guide to net directional sensitivity to regional stimulating forces. Examples are shown in Figure 18–5. A net depolarization occurs in certain regions of the macula during stimulation in a given force direction, and activity in afferent fibers that innervate those regions is increased. Mappings of such so-called functional polarization vectors were determined from single afferent recordings in animal studies, and they provide a rough guide to the expected responses of each afferent fiber under various stimulus conditions (Fig. 18–6). However,

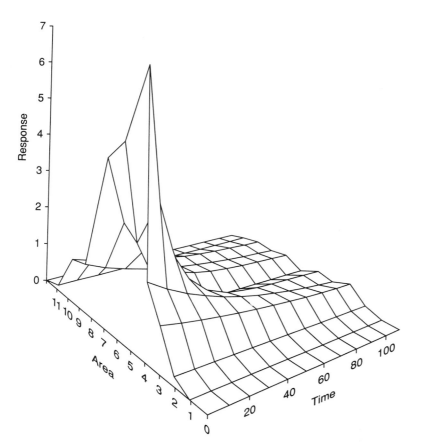

Figure 18–4. A three-dimensional representation of experimental neural impulse activity from the horizontal semicircular canal of the guitarfish after onset of a sudden movement. Response, in units of (impulses/second)/(degrees/second), differs symmetrically in different areas of the nerve near the receptor during a time epoch of 100 milliseconds. A sharp burst of nerve activity occurs from central nerve areas immediately after the movement onset. (From O'Leary DP, Dunn RF: Multiple information channels in guitarfish vestibular receptors. Histologia Medica 1[Suppl]:27, 1985.)

the multiplicity of polarization vectors in these receptors increases their response complexities many times in relation to the bidirectional responses of the canals. The global effect of such complexity on behavioral vestibular responses remains to be explored.

Macular afferent fibers are spontaneously active, with stable activity rates that vary as a function of head position as a static response. Changes in head position by only 1° can result in a detectable static change to a new firing rate; hence their classic designation as gravity receptors. But these afferent fibers also exhibit dynamic characteristics, in the form of patterned variable activity, during head movements. Afferent fibers that innervate regions of greatest hair cell depolarization are therefore the most active, and such regions are thought to vary in dynamic patterns that sweep across the maculae during head movements. Similar response dynamics were found in afferent fibers from both superior and inferior branches of the vestibular nerves, fibers that were thought to derive from the utricular and saccular maculae, respectively. Both utricular and sac-

cular afferent fibers showed similar static and dynamic response characteristics but with orthogonally oriented sensitivity vectors. This suggests that the physiologic mechanisms of both macular receptors are similar and that the receptors carry similar information concerning head position and movement in their respective orientation planes.

Efferent Innervation

Vestibular receptor efferent innervation has been demonstrated anatomically in many studies, but its physiologic significance is currently unclear. Studies in lower vertebrates showed efferent inhibition of afferent responses, whereas similar studies in mammals showed either minimal or even excitatory influences. Moreover, time-related changes in efferent activity were often too slow to significantly affect behavioral head movements. Further studies are required to determine what, if any, effect efferent fibers have on the control of movement or, possibly, even on slower autonomic functions.

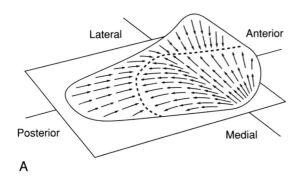

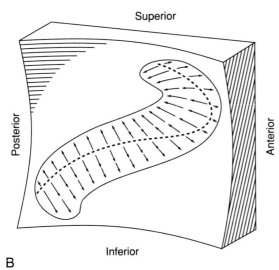

Figure 18–5. Schematic representation of polarization pattern of sensory cells in *(A)* macula utriculi and *(B)* macula sacculi of guinea pig. Arrows indicate the direction of polarization, which spreads up to a certain boundary beyond which the polarization is reversed. In *A*, kinocilia on either side of the dividing line are facing each other, whereas in *B* the kinocilia face away from each other. (Adapted from Spoendlin HH: Ultrastructural studies of the labyrinth in squirrel monkeys. *In* The Role of the Vestibular Organs in the Exploration of Space, NASA Publication No. SP-77 [pp 7–22]. Washington, DC: National Aeronautics and Space Administration, 1965.)

CENTRAL VESTIBULAR NEUROPHYSIOLOGIC PROCESSES

Labyrinthine Input to the Vestibular Nuclei

The four vestibular nuclei are important centers for the coordination of multisensory inputs, particularly somatosensory and visual information, in addition to the roles that they play in various vestibular projection pathways. These nuclei receive projections from all labyrinthine receptors, but the input is organized in specific ways. In some regions, afferent terminations are found from only certain receptors. Other regions share overlapping termination zones of afferent fibers from different canals or share canal and macular afferent fibers. It is useful, however, to summarize the vestibular projection pathways in the schematic manner shown in Figure 18–7.

Lateral (or Deiters') nucleus predominates as a receiving area for the gravity receptors. Utricular and saccular afferent fibers terminate in this nucleus, and studies of both electrical activity and sensitivity to tilt show evidence that this nucleus is an important projection area for the macular receptors. However, this nucleus also receives afferent fibers from all three semicircular canals, which indicates its apparently lesser role as a receiving area for rotational stimuli.

The medial nucleus receives a strong input from all three semicircular canals in its rostral regions. In addition, tilt-sensitive neurons are found throughout the nucleus, but they have much smaller mean response amplitudes than do those of the ventral Deiters' nucleus. Some medial nucleus cells respond to both angular acceleration and tilt. In general, the second-order neurons that receive canal input predominate in the rostral parts of the nucleus, whereas tilt-sensitive neurons are concentrated in the caudal regions.

The descending nucleus receives significant utricular input in addition to saccular input in its rostral regions.

The superior nucleus apparently receives input only from canals, predominantly the vertical canals. Within the subdivisions of the superior nucleus, superior canal responses are found laterally and posterior canal units medially. Studies of natural stimulation indicate relatively few horizontal canal neurons in this nucleus. The major projection of this nucleus is to the extraocular motor nuclei.

Responses to Natural and Electrical Stimulation

The nature of afferent responses differs in different regions of the nuclei. For example, electrical stimulation of afferent fibers from specific receptors has shown detailed patterns of electrical activity, such as field potentials and monosynaptic and polysynaptic convergence, that originate from the various

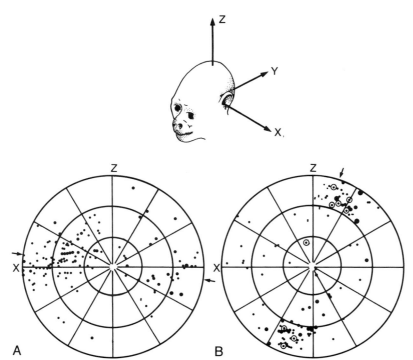

Figure 18–6. Functional polarization vectors from *(A)* 142 units identified as originating from the superior (SN) branch and *(B)* 115 units from the inferior (IN) branch of the squirrel monkey vestibular nerve. X and Z directions correspond with those of the inset monkey's head. Both radial and circular lines demonstrate 30° angular separations, the former in the plane of the page and the latter in directions extending toward (O) and away from (X) the reader. Each point depicts one unit's vector, although vector directions, but not their magnitude, are represented. Small arrows denote median angles of vectors for SN and IN units. Circled points denote units obtained after superior nerve section. (From Fernandez C, Goldberg JM: Physiology of peripheral neurons innervating otolith organs of the squirrel monkey. I. Response to static tilts and to long-duration centrifugal force. J Neurophysiol 39:970–984, 1976.)

receptors and are projected to various nuclear regions. It would be valuable to combine this physiologic information with detailed information from anatomic studies in order to construct a comprehensive control theory model of these nuclei. But the structural and functional complexity of the vestibular projection pathways, combined with their multisensory capabilities, makes comprehensive modeling of these nuclei difficult at present.

Central neurons responding in the same directional sense as first-order afferent neurons are type I; those responding in the opposite sense are type II. Others responding in both directions with increasing activity are type III, and those responding with decreasing activity are type IV. On the basis of vestibular nerve stimulation—that is, differing spontaneous and dynamic response characteristics—type I responses are further cat-

egorized as "tonic" and "kinetic." Central neural responses often occur with a detectable latency (time delay) that reflects the extent of central processing of the information projected from the periphery.

A schematic overview of the reflex connections of each labyrinthine receptor is shown in Figure 18–8. Each receptor has projection pathways extending both rostrally and caudally, although the information from the utricle and the saccule is projected predominantly toward the spinal tracts.

Commissural Activity

The vestibular nuclei communicate through commissural activity, which may influence compensation for unilateral lesions in the following manner. Commissural influence (in the cat) inhibits type I neurons from the

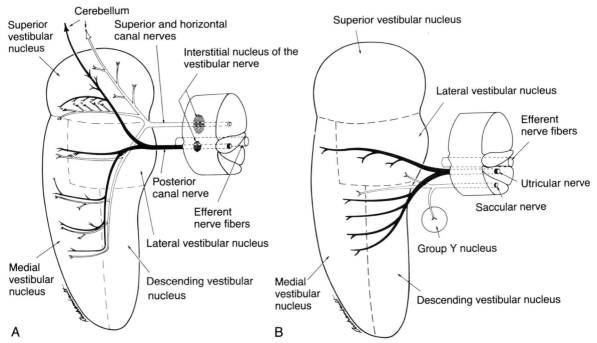

Figure 18–7. Diagram of the central termination of canal afferent fibers *(A)* and macular afferent fibers *(B)* in the vestibular nucleus. (Adapted from Gacek RR: The anatomical-physiological basis for vestibular function. *In* Honrubia V, Brazier MAB [eds]: Nystagmus and Vertigo [pp 3–23]. New York: Academic Press, 1982.)

semicircular canals. This influences the spontaneous activity in vestibular afferent fibers. After unilateral labyrinthectomy, type I responses are observed on the affected side after compensation has taken place, although no input occurs from the ipsilateral labyrinth. The consequent modulation to rotational stimulation is a result of changes in commissural inhibition, which thus demonstrates its potentially powerful influence on compensation.

Stimulation of specific canal nerve branches shows an organization related to natural planes of rotational specificity. Neurons activated from stimulation of the ipsilateral horizontal nerve are selectively inhibited by stimulation of the contralateral horizontal nerve. Neurons innervating the anterior and posterior canals are inhibited by stimulation of the posterior and anterior nerves, respectively.

VESTIBULOSPINAL SYSTEM

Early descriptions of vestibulospinal physiologic mechanisms showed the various postural reflexes that are elicited behaviorally when an animal is placed in various positions in relation to the gravitational vector. More recent descriptions include the interactions of various multisensory and motor subsystems that can act for finer control of posture and movement. A modern description must also include microgravity (i.e., "weightless") environments in the absence of a gravitational reference. Therefore, physiologic control descriptions of vestibulospinal effectors now include a dynamic component that is superimposed on the familiar postural adjustments and can operate even in microgravity conditions.

Mammalian vestibulospinal information is transmitted primarily via three tracts: the *lateral vestibulospinal tract* (LVST), the *medial vestibulospinal tract* (MVST), and the *reticulospinal tract* (RST). Physiologic influences of these tracts have been studied by applying natural or electrical stimulation and recording intracellular synaptic potentials and afferent impulses evoked in motoneurons of the projected pathways.

The Lateral Vestibulospinal Tract. The LVST regulates motor activity in alpha and gamma motoneurons through monosynaptic

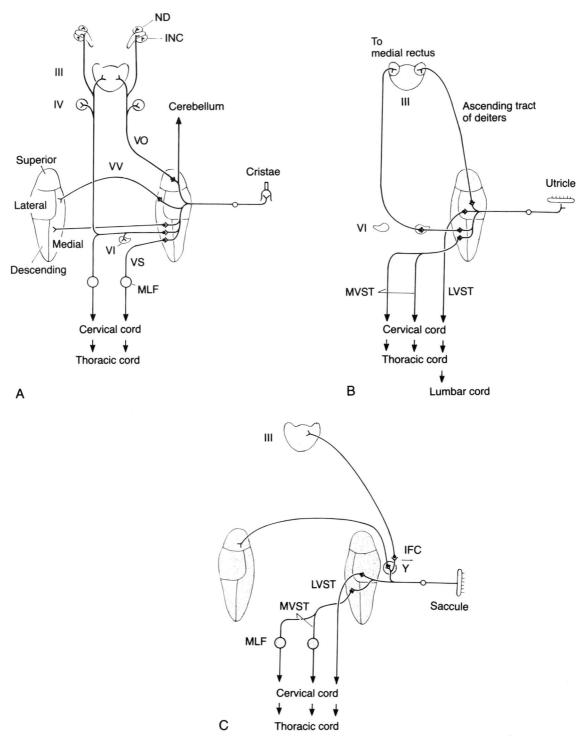

Figure 18–8. Diagram summarizing reflex connections of the cristae *(A)*, the utricle *(B)*, and the saccule *(C)*. ND, nucleus of Darkshevich; INC, interstitial nucleus of Cajal; VO, vestibulo-ocular; VV, commissural; VS, vestibulospinal; MLF, medial longitudinal fasciculus; MVST, medial vestibulospinal tract; LVST, lateral vestibulospinal tract; IFC, infracerebellar nucleus. (Adapted from Gacek RR: The anatomical-physiological basis for vestibular function. *In* Honrubia V, Brazier MAB [eds]: Nystagmus and Vertigo [pp 3–23]. New York: Academic Press, 1982.)

and polysynaptic connections and also through interneurons in segmental reflex pathways. During walking on a treadmill, this regulation can take the form of strong facilitation of gastrocnemius activity during the extension phase, but not during the flexion phase, of the step cycle.

The multisensory processing capability can be illustrated by the following example. The LVST relays information from utricular, saccular, and canal afferent fibers, which can modulate somatosensory excitatory inputs to Deiters' nucleus. But somatosensory information from cerebellar Purkinje cells and fastigial neurons is also relayed by the LVST, with excitatory inputs to Deiters' nucleus.

The Medial Vestibulospinal Tract. The MVST receives monosynaptic and polysynaptic input from labyrinthine receptors projecting to the medial, descending Deiters' nuclei. All three semicircular canals project second-order information to the MVST via the medial nucleus; relatively few cells that are higher than second order are projected. Indirect evidence suggests that at least a small number of MVST neurons receive spinal excitation evoked from proximal limb joints or stimulation of the spinal cord in C-1 to C-3 regions.

In contrast to the LVST, the MVST projects both inhibitory and excitatory information directly to upper cervical and thoracic motoneurons, but apparently not to limb motoneurons. The main control function of the MVST is to relay labyrinthine information, which is then integrated with other inputs in the tract neurons.

Reticulospinal Tracts. Vestibular influences on the RSTs are less understood than those on the other two tracts. However, reticulospinal neurons are excited by stimulation of either the ipsilateral or contralateral vestibular nerves.

VESTIBULO-OCULAR REFLEX

Movements of the eyes result from the actions of six extraocular muscles attached to each eye. The neural signals controlling them derive from four control systems that act together as the *oculomotor system* to command voluntary and involuntary motions of the eyes via a "final common pathway"—the oculomotor nerves: (1) voluntary fast eye movements generated to look at a specific target are under control of the *saccadic* system; (2) slow movements that track a moving target are under control of the *pursuit* system; (3) eye movements that follow moving contrast boundaries in the peripheral visual field are under control of the *optokinetic* system; and (4) eye movements that are compensatory to head movements are *vestibulo-ocular*.

The vestibulo-ocular reflex (VOR) acts to stabilize foveal fixation of the eyes during head movements by causing a counter-rotation of the eyes in order to compensate for rotational movements of the head. This counter-rotation prevents visual images from "moving across the retina" during head movements and thus provides a stable view of the environment during locomotion. Horizontal eye movements, which respond to lateral canal stimulation, occur through projection pathways that are quite different from those carrying information from the vertical canals for vertical and oblique eye movements. These differences are shown schematically in Figure 18–9.

The projection pathways and the physiologic control mechanisms of horizontal VOR eye movements are better known than those of the vertical VOR eye movements. Therefore, VOR modeling, as discussed in the next section, has focused generally on the horizontal VOR.

Central VOR Information Processing

Nerves from the vestibular semicircular canals generally represent head angular velocity information and not position. Therefore, a mathematical integration must occur in the central pathways of the VOR to convert head velocity information to position of the head. A "neural integrator" is assumed to act in parallel with head velocity information relayed through the VOR, to result in precise compensatory movements of the eyes in response to head movements. The neural integrator would prolong the normal response time of the VOR and would result in prolonged neural activity that sustains compensatory eye movements.

Although the location and the structure of a neural integrator in the VOR are at present unknown, the identification of its operational characteristics is useful for testing hypotheses of neural function. For example,

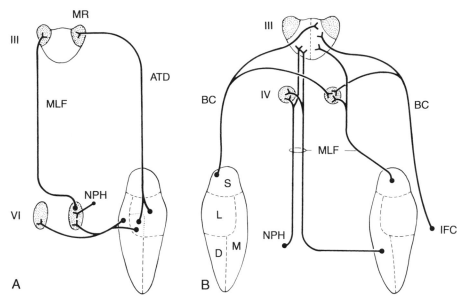

Figure 18–9. Diagram of projection pathways of vestibulo-ocular neurons for horizontal *(A)* and vertical and oblique *(B)* eye movements. MR, medial rectus subnucleus; ATD, ascending tract of Deiters; MLF, medial longitudinal fasciculus; NPH, nucleus praepositus hypoglossi; BC, brachium conjunctivum; IFC, infracerebellar nucleus; S, L, M, D, superior, lateral, medial, and descending vestibular nucleus, respectively. (Adapted from Gacek RR: The anatomical-physiological basis for vestibular function. *In* Honrubia V, Brazier MAB [eds]: Nystagmus and Vertigo [pp 3–23]. New York: Academic Press, 1982.)

such an integration could be performed through actions of a multiple neural circuit, in which a single impulse at the input of a chain of neurons can set up a prolonged train

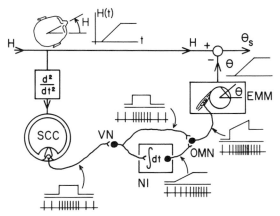

Figure 18–10. The processing of signals in the vestibulo-ocular reflex. Neural signals indicate both actual spike activity and its firing rate. H(t), head position that acts as an input disturbance; SCC, semicircular canals; NI, neural integrator; EMM, eye-movement mechanics; VN, vestibular nucleus; OMN, oculomotor nucleus. (From Robinson DA: Oculomotor control signals. *In* Lennerstrand G, Bach-y-Rita P [eds]: Basic Mechanisms of Ocular Motility and Their Clinical Implications [pp 337–378]. New York: Pergamon, 1975.)

of impulses. This and other hypotheses are the focus of current modeling efforts, which are based both on control theory and, more recently, on neural network computer algorithms. A goal of all such modeling is to incorporate what is known about neural activity at various VOR substages. One such model is shown in Figure 18–10.

Before more complex models can be examined, it is necessary to consider two useful system definitions used to characterize control of the VOR: gain and phase.

Definitions of Gain and Phase. Many vestibular subsystems can be characterized by objective responses (e.g., eye or limb movements) to specific stimuli, such as head or body movements. In contrast, human audiograms are based on subjective responses in the absence of observable effector responses. Vestibular stimulus-response data are used to determine the gain and phase. The system *gain* is defined as the output magnitude divided by the input magnitude. The system *phase* is defined as the time delay of the output in relation to the input; it is expressed quantitatively in degrees, whereby 360° defines one period. Both gain and phase are dependent on the *frequency* of the input, in addition to other possible physiologic factors.

In practice, these quantities are often estimated with computers by using Fourier analysis programs. These system characteristics are illustrated in Figure 18–11, which shows human head and eye velocity trajectories produced during 0.5 seconds of active vertical head shaking. The movements are rapid, with sufficiently small angular displacements to prevent "turning on" the fast eye movement (saccade) generators in the pons; therefore, nystagmus fast components do not occur. The VOR responds to the active head movements by producing compensatory (i.e., opposite polarity) eye movements.

The gain and the phase can be estimated as follows. If A_i is the amplitude of the ith peak and t_i is the time of that peak's occurrence, the period is $t_5 - t_1$ seconds, the frequency is 1/period, the gain is $|A_4/A_3|$, and the phase is $\{[(t_4 - t_1)/(t_5 - t_1)] \times 360°\}$. The average frequency of the head and eye waveforms in Figure 18–11 is slightly greater than 5 Hz (cycles per second) because about 2.5 complete periods occurred within 0.5 seconds. The average gain is less than 1 because peak eye amplitudes are less than the adjacent (reversed polarity) peak head amplitudes within each period. The average phase lag is less than 180° because eye peaks lag behind head peaks of the same polarity by slightly less than half the time between head peaks of the same polarity. Note that the eye peak occurred before the opposite polarity head peak. Does this mean that the "response" occurred before the "stimulus"? No, because the positive eye peak can be viewed as a response to the earlier positive head peak, which for normal subjects is usually a phase delay of 180° to 190°. In contrast, the phase shown in Figure 18–11 is less than 180°, which can occur in certain vestibular disorders. The system characteristics illustrated in Figure 18–11 were recorded from a patient who had been exposed to gentamicin ototoxicity.

Eye Movement Patterns of Response to Rotational Stimuli. Eye movements resulting from low-frequency rotational testing are composed of slow and fast components of nystagmus. (Use of the term nystagmus "fast component" instead of the often-used nystagmus "fast phase" is recommended for avoiding ambiguity with VOR system phase, as discussed earlier.) The slow component is under command of the vestibulo-ocular system, whereas the fast component is commanded by the paramedian pontine reticular formation, a brain stem center that is also responsible for generating saccadic eye movements. The periodic stimulus profile results in frequent changes in the direction of nystagmus, in contrast to the nystagmus "beating" that occurs in caloric testing and can be unidirec-

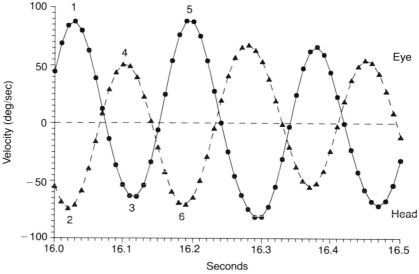

Figure 18–11. Trajectories of head (solid line) and eye (dashed line) velocities sampled at the points shown during 0.5 seconds of active human vertical head and eye movements by a patient exposed to gentamicin ototoxicity. (From O'Leary DP, Davis LL: High-frequency autorotational testing of the vestibulo-ocular reflex. Neurologic Clinics 8[2]:297–312, 1990.)

tional over relatively long time epochs. These directional changes require a specialized form of analysis, in which the fast components are ignored, so that the eye movement responses can be properly related to the input stimuli. In general, it is necessary to identify the beginning and the end of fast components and to eliminate them from further analytic consideration. The slow components are then reconstructed by repositioning the waveform to produce a "cumulative eye position" without fast components. This repositioning usually requires computer analysis of the form shown in Figure 18–12. Gains and phases at various frequencies are then computed and plotted from the cumulative eye position.

Effective modeling of the VOR must include also interactions with the visual system, and, when appropriate, the other oculomotor systems. For example, a current hypothesis is that the brain receives an "efference copy" of eye velocity, which, when added to head velocity information from the VOR, results in the velocity of the environment with respect to the head.

Adaptive Control in the Oculomotor System

The VOR was thought for many years to be a three-neuron reflex arc that operated automatically to stabilize vision through eye movements compensatory for head movements. But this concept was re-examined during the 1970s when it became evident that VOR gain and phase could be modified by changing the apparent size, direction, or both

of objects in the visual field. In human subjects wearing prism goggles that reversed visual field objects right to left (analogous to vision in a mirror), the VOR reacted over time by dramatic changes in how eye movements responded to head motion. Figure 18–13 shows one example in which the eye movement direction reversed after 14 days of continuous reversed vision, with the eyes then moving in the same direction as the head.

The subject's VOR could then compensate correctly for the new visual conditions created by reversing prism glasses. Moreover, this new condition persisted even in darkness, which indicates that major changes had occurred in brain processing in response to the reversed visual field; this phenomenon is known as *neural plasticity*. Time courses of the gain and phase changes are shown in Figure 18–14, in which it is apparent that subsequent removal of the prisms resulted in a return to the normal compensation pattern.

How was this remarkable plasticity accomplished? Extensive research in multiple laboratories demonstrated that additional pathways interact with the classic VOR, in such a way that an error signal, projected from the retina to the brain stem and the cerebellum, carried information that head movement caused blurred vision. This finding suggested an adaptive control model of the VOR, in which adjustment of the conventional VOR control parameters to minimize the error signal was possible. Figure 18–15 shows an expanded view of the rabbit VOR pathways in which the error signal just described

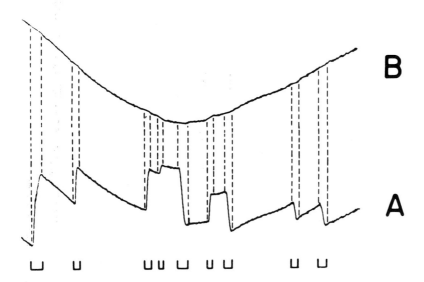

Figure 18–12. Method of reconstructing nystagmus slow phase "cumulative eye position" (CEP) by identifying and removing fast phases. *A.* Eye position responses obtained from an alert rhesus monkey during rotational chair stimulation. *B.* Slow phase CEP after identification and removal of fast phases, and reconstruction of the waveform with a computer algorithm. (From Furman JM, O'Leary DP, Wolfe JW: Application of linear system analysis to the horizontal vestibulo-ocular reflex of the alert rhesus monkey using pseudorandom binary sequence and single frequency sinusoidal stimulation. Biol Cybern 33:159–165, 1979.)

Figure 18–13. Normal *(top)* and fully adapted *(middle)* nystagmoid responses obtained during test stimuli in the dark from one human subject exposed to continuous vision reversal. The adapted response, which was recorded after 14 days of reversed vision, approximates a reversed replica of the normal one. Both records of eye movement are correctly phase-related to the lower record *(bottom)* of stimulus angular velocity. (From Jones GM: Plasticity in the adult vestibulo-ocular reflex arc. Philos Trans R Soc Lond [Biol] 278:319–334, 1977.)

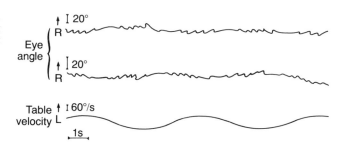

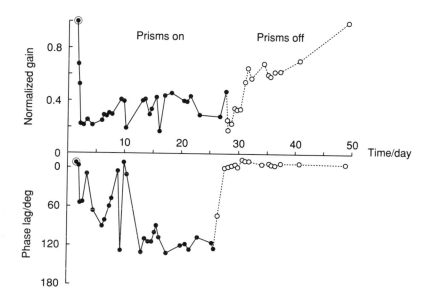

Figure 18–14. VOR phase (lower curve) and normalized gain (upper curve) from one human subject exposed to continuous vision reversal for 27 days (solid circles) and during readaptation after return to normal vision (open circles). Circled points are mean control values obtained just before the patient donned the reversing prisms. Phase is registered in relation to that associated with perfect compensation with normal vision. (From Jones GM: Plasticity in the adult vestibulo-ocular reflex arc. Philos Trans R Soc Lond [Biol] 278:319–334, 1977.)

Figure 18–15. Neuronal diagram of the flocculo-vestibulo-ocular system in the rabbit. It illustrates the possible mechanism of vestibulo-ocular adaptation; the vestibular mossy fiber-granule cell–Purkinje cell pathway through the flocculus acts as a modifiable side path of the VOR arc, and the modification of the side path is effected by retinal error signal conveyed through the pretectal area (inferior olive, IO) climbing fiber pathway. The retinal error signals (RES) monitor mismatching of the VOR to the visual environment. III and VI, oculomotor and adbucens nuclei. (From Ito M: Synaptic plasticity in the cerebellar cortex that may underlie the vestibulo-ocular adaptation. *In* Berthoz A, Melvill Jones G [eds]: Adaptive mechanism in gaze control [pp 213–221]. New York: Elsevier, 1985.)

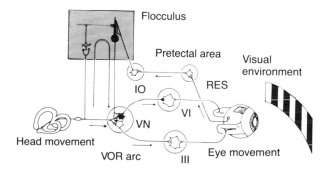

is projected as neural activity through the pretectal area and the inferior olive to the cerebellar flocculus, which then sends a signal to and from the vestibular nuclei.

Adaption of the VOR also occurred when the apparent visual world increased or decreased in size, as a result of the wearing of telescopic lenses. Similar effects were found to occur from combined vestibular-optokinetic stimulation, which resulted in apparent movement of the visual field.

Ablation studies in animals showed that the flocculus of the vestibulocerebellum was necessary for the establishment and maintenance of VOR adaptation. This finding suggested two possibilities: (1) the flocculus may itself be the site of adaptive VOR control, or (2) additional extracerebellar structures with inputs to the flocculus may be the command centers for VOR adaptation.

Investigations of cellular control mechanisms for VOR adaptation have led to suggestions that it is induced by a shift of dominance between two populations of floccular Purkinje's cells, by modulation of information in transmidline coupling pathways through the commissural system, or by both. Experiments are continuing at present to better define the cellular basis of VOR plasticity.

Modeling of adaptive VOR control has expanded to include possible optokinetic influences to better account for slow and fast effects of gain modifications. For example, Figure 18–16 shows a model in which a fast optokinetic system combines with vestibular information to establish appropriate gain and balance adjustments to error signals induced by retinal image slip.

In addition to the VOR, another neural control system helps stabilize object tracking during head movements. The smooth pursuit system operates in a closed loop in which information from the retina is used to control eye movements for tracking moving objects. The relative importance of each system for visual stabilization depends on the frequency range of head motion. The pursuit system is most important for angular head motion frequencies below about 1.0 Hz, whereas stabilization at higher frequencies is determined primarily by the VOR.

Rotational Testing of the VOR

The anatomic and physiologic characteristics of the VOR provide a window into the brain and the inner ear that is invaluable for modern diagnoses of vestibular dysfunction. Clinical caloric and positional testing are widely used, and manuals describing various methods of scoring nystagmus beats are readily available. These methods are largely empirical and are not based in systems and control theory. In contrast, rotational VOR testing methods involve the use of rotational acceleration as a more natural stimulus and of systems engineering concepts such as quantitative data descriptors. The rotational methods and descriptors that are in present clinical use are described as follows.

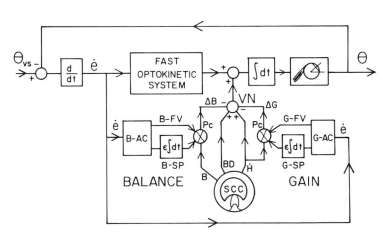

Figure 18–16. Adaptive control of gain and balance in the vestibulo-ocular and optokinetic systems. The semicircular canals (SCC) produce three signals: head velocity (H), a tonic resting-level bias (B), and a possible imbalance or disturbance bias (DB) between the two sides. These signals project directly to the vestibular nuclei (VN) and also through a cerebellar side path that has been artificially divided into a gain and a balance path. Modulation of bias (ΔB) and of gain (ΔG) occurs through Purkinje's cells (Pc), which inhibit the vestibular nuclei. Both systems are activated by retinal image slip ($\dot{e}$), the rate of change of the difference between eye position (θ), and the position of the visual surround (θ_{vs}), through adaptive control pathways for balance (B-AC) and gain (G-AC). Both systems cause fast, visually activated changes in gain (G-FV) and bias (B-FV) and long-term, semipermanent changes (G-SP) and (B-SP) denoted by a small gain (ε) and an integral action. (From Robinson DA: Oculomotor control signals. *In* Lennerstrand G, Bach-y-Rita P [eds]: Basic Mechanisms of Ocular Motility and Their Clinical Implications [pp 337–378]. New York: Pergamon, 1975.)

Sinusoidal Harmonic Acceleration (SHA) Testing. SHA testing was developed in the 1970s by researchers who fastened chairs to platforms designed for industrial use to transform a voltage waveform to rotational velocities. Other stimulus protocols such as velocity ramps, steps, and pseudorandom inputs have been used; however, the SHA protocol, with sequential application of discrete sinusoids at frequencies from 0.01 to about 0.2 Hz, is the main protocol used clinically and available commercially. In practice, these systems have upper frequency limits of about 1.0 Hz.

In SHA testing, the gain is often transformed to decibels by multiplying it by 20 $\log_{10}$ and plotting decibels versus $\log_{10} f$, where f is the stimulus frequency. Phase is usually plotted linearly in degrees versus $\log_{10} f$. These gain and phase plots are defined as Bode plots of a system. It is now common to characterize both normal and pathologic vestibular subsystems by Bode plots, as shown later.

Figure 18–17 shows Bode plots of VOR gain and phase from 50 normal subjects tested on a rotary chair. The mean gains were above 0.4 even at ultralow frequencies of 0.01 Hz (a period of 100 seconds). Why should the vestibular system respond at such low frequencies, which are far below those commonly experienced in daily life? The reason is unclear at present. But low-frequency SHA rotational testing is in current use clinically for diagnostic screening of certain vestibular disorders that can produce abnormal gain and phase patterns at these frequencies.

Active Head Movement VOR Testing. An alternative approach to VOR rotary chair testing is to use voluntary head oscillations with a rotational sensor attached to a head strap as the stimulus monitor. This approach has been used at frequencies from 0.2 to about 6.0 Hz.

It is useful to consider 2 Hz as a functional boundary between lower and higher frequency responses because ocular smooth pursuit is relatively ineffective at stabilizing the eye at frequencies higher than 2 Hz.

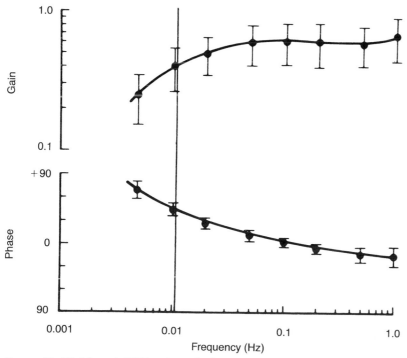

Figure 18–17. Normal VOR gain and phase responses for 50 human subjects tested at six stimulation frequencies in a computerized rotary chair. The vertical line drawn at 45° indicates the corner frequency, derived in systems engineering. Points, means; error bars, plus and minus 1 standard deviation. (From Wall C III: The sinusoidal harmonic acceleration rotary chair test. Neurologic Clinics 8[2]:269–285, 1990.)

Below 2 Hz, the VOR's contribution to visual stabilization can be strongly influenced, or even suppressed, by other competing ocular motor systems or cognitive processes such as imagined targets. Above 2 Hz, the VOR is the system used for visual stabilization, and the VOR is relatively unaffected by the presence or the absence of real or imagined targets at these higher frequencies. In theory, proprioceptors in the neck muscles could influence eye movements during active head movements through the cervico-ocular reflex. However, the gain of the cervico-ocular reflex is so low as to appear insignificant in humans.

The Vestibular Autorotation Test (VAT). The VAT is a relatively new, commercially available computerized system for testing the VOR across a band width from 2.0 to 6.0 Hz. Physiologically, this frequency range is the one most commonly encountered during common behavioral movements such as walking. In the VAT, an auditorily cued sweep frequency of active head oscillations is used as the stimulus. An instrumented head strap worn by the patient is used to record head and eye movements for testing both the horizontal and the vertical VORs. Specialized recording systems inside a portable computer are used for bedside and out-

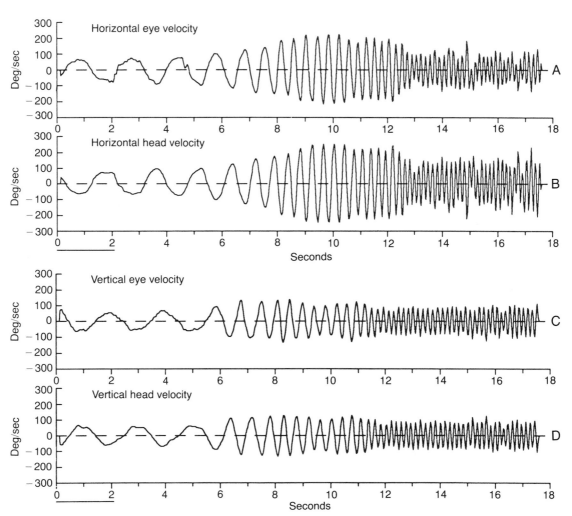

Figure 18–18. Head and eye trajectories during an 18-second vestibular autorotation test (VAT) from a normal subject, showing horizontal eye (*A*), horizontal head (*B*), vertical eye (*C*), and vertical head (*D*) velocity versus time. Bars under the axes indicate the 2-second epochs used for calibrating the electro-oculographic eye movement signals. Note absence of nystagmus at these frequencies and amplitudes. (From O'Leary DP, Davis LL: High-frequency autorotational testing of the vestibulo-ocular reflex. Neurologic Clinics 8[2]:297–327, 1990.)

patient clinical testing. Patients are instructed to fixate on a 1-cm–diameter disk positioned at a known distance from the eyes and to move their heads in synchrony with a computer-generated auditory tone. Each auditory beat cues the subject to perform a smooth head movement over a half-period trajectory. The auditory tone interbeat interval increases in frequency from 0.5 to 0.8 Hz during the initial 6 seconds and then sweeps linearly from 1.0 to 6.0 Hz during the remaining 12 seconds. Data from the first 6 seconds are used only for electro-oculographic calibration, and data from the last 13 seconds are used to compute VOR gains and phases. Each test lasts 18 seconds and is repeated three times in both horizontal (side-to-side) and vertical (up-and-down) head movement planes. Examples of data from one horizontal test and one vertical test are shown in Figure

18–18. Note the absence of nystagmus fast components.

Figure 18–19 shows the range of gain and phase data from horizontal and vertical VATs of 100 normal subjects. The shapes and contours of the horizontal VOR gains and phases differ from those of the vertical VOR gains and phases, which implies that they are commanded by different physiologic control systems. In clinical use, the VAT results from individual patients are compared with the patterns shown in Figure 18–19 as a normal reference.

POSTURAL CONTROL MECHANISMS

Effective stabilization of various parts of the body result from the labyrinthine tonic (or

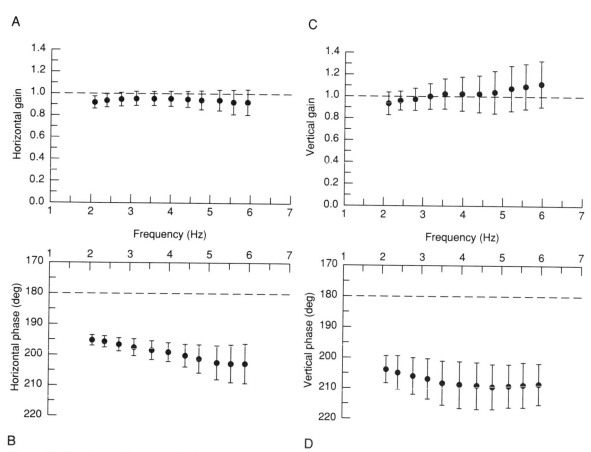

Figure 18–19. Grouped VAT results from 100 normal subjects are shown as horizontal gains *(A)* and phases *(B)* and as vertical gains *(C)* and phases *(D)*. Points, means; error bars, plus and minus 1 standard deviation. (Adapted from O'Leary DP, Davis LL: Vestibular autorotation testing of Meniere's disease. Otolaryngol Head Neck Surg 103:66–71, 1990.)

static) reflexes. A change of head position induces systematic changes in postural reflexes that govern the limbs, the trunk, and the neck. The tonic labyrinthine reflex that controls the position of the neck is considered to be a closed-loop control for holding head position. In contrast, the tonic labyrinthine reflexes operating on the trunk and the limbs are thought to be under open-loop control because the labyrinthine receptors are not necessarily affected by immediate postural changes in the trunk and limbs.

Effects of vestibular lesions on body equilibrium function in animals are minimal after a unilateral saccular macula ablation but marked after utricular ablation. This suggests that the utricle is the more important gravity receptor for the maintenance of body equilibrium.

The variability of postural reflexes in humans was analyzed by recording electromyographic responses of subjects standing on a force-measuring platform, which could be rotated in pitch around an axis aligned with a subject's ankle joints (Fig. 18–20). Tilting the platform toe-up while leaning backward led to an increase of the latency of stabilizing responses from the triceps surae muscle and to a decrease of response latency in the anterior tibial muscle. These latency changes, which functionally destabilize posture, can be suppressed or compensated for by reflexive contractions of antagonists. Rapid postural responses among human leg muscles during standing were activated according to fixed patterns. Extensions to other induced motions reinforced the concept that the resulting patterns of electromyographic activity were highly specific for each kind of displacement and that subjects could reorganize the activity patterns from one form to another even after unexpected stimulus changes.

The specific information used by the brain to determine body position in space depends on environmental conditions. For example, vision provides inaccurate information about a stationary reference when objects in the visual field are moving. This effect is a result of the familiar perceptual illusion of translation while remaining stationary in the presence of a large moving object (e.g., a bus or a railroad car). Similarly, somatosensory information can be inaccurate when the support surface is compliant or moving. The vestibular system therefore serves as an internal reference to resolve multisensory conflicts induced by the environment.

Does VOR plasticity affect postural control? Prolonged optic reversal of vision resulted in marked decrease in the ability of human subjects to maintain balance while standing or walking on flat wooden rails, with eyes open or closed. Results showed systematic pattern of adaptive changes in postural control; the plastic nature of these changes is indicated by their long-term retention and complete reversibility.

Under conditions of a stable visual field and a fixed support surface, the brain uses somatosensory and visual information for spatial reference because these systems are more sensitive than the vestibular system to subtle shifts in body position. During rapid changes in body orientation, the fast-acting muscle proprioceptors provide the greatest sensitivity. Vision is most sensitive to slow changes in orientation. Of course, the vestibular system is also always active, both to resolve any sensory conflicts and to contribute complementary information.

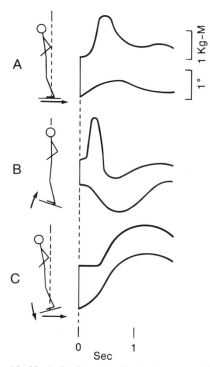

Figure 18–20. Left: three methods for postural stimulation with a moving platform to achieve: anteroposterior (AP) sway (A); ankle rotation (B); and ankle stabilization by platform rotation proportional to the angle of induced AP sway (C). Right: time course of ankle reaction torque on platform base and the AP sway angle are shown for each mode of stimulation. (From Nashner LM: Fixed patterns of rapid postural responses among leg muscles during stance. Exp Brain Res 30:13–24, 1977.)

Postural responses are an ongoing sequence of coordinated muscular contractions. A slight displacement of the body away from vertical results in early, nonvolitional muscle contractions of the legs and trunk within 150 milliseconds of the displacement. These automatic responses are mediated by long-loop pathways involving sensory and motor neural components in spinal pathways, with motor contributions from the brain stem and the cortex.

Two distinct movement patterns (strategies) about the ankles and the hips can occur during automatic postural responses (Fig. 18–21). The ankle strategy is to rotate the body about the ankle joints, whereas the hip strategy is to use corrective movements about the hip and the upper body. The timing and the combination of these patterns are dependent on environmental conditions. For example, the ankle strategy is most effective for small body displacements and a firm support surface.

Dynamic Posturography. The objective testing of sway strategies under various visual and somatosensory conditions is called *dynamic posturography,* and computerized testing systems are now available commercially. They provide two main classes of information: (1) diagnostic information about lesions that involve extravestibular central nervous system pathways or pathways unrelated to the vestibulo-ocular reflex and (2) objective documentation of a functional disability that can assist in the medical manage-

ment, such as tracking changes in response to surgery, pharmaceutic treatment, or physical rehabilitation therapy.

PHYSIOLOGIC CHARACTERISTICS OF CENTRAL VESTIBULAR COMPENSATION

The rehabilitation of patients with vestibular deficits has been re-examined in light of evidence that vestibular compensation could be based on similar mechanisms and time courses, as described earlier, for adaptive plasticity of the VOR. In addition, the compensation process can be affected by conditions immediately after a functional vestibular loss. Compensation can be facilitated by exercise and increased somatosensory and visual exposure. Conversely, it can be reduced by medications, blindfolding, anesthesia, and casts on the hindlimbs of animals. What are the candidate physiologic mechanisms for vestibular compensation?

Compensation for a peripheral vestibular disorder is thought to occur through changes within the central nervous system, as opposed to a correction of the peripheral disorder. The central nervous system regions necessary for compensation are not localized to any specific areas, but they are distributed widely. Experimental studies have shown that lesions in the cerebellum, the brain stem, the spinal cord, and the cerebrum can prevent or impair compensation for peripheral pathologic processes.

Three physiologic mechanisms have been proposed for central nervous system compensation:

1. *Central sensory substitution,* wherein vision and somatosensory information can partially substitute for a lack of dynamic vestibular information following vestibular lesions.

2. *Rebalancing tonic activity in central vestibular centers,* which is based on cerebellar inhibition of the spontaneous activity in the vestibular nuclei of the intact side and is removed gradually as new activity is regenerated in the affected side. The eventual recovery of symmetric activity in the vestibular nuclei is strongly correlated with successful central nervous system compensation.

3. *Physiologic habituation,* a decrease in magnitude of responses to repetitive sensory

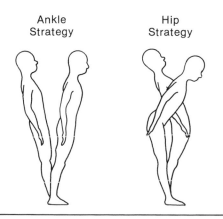

Ankle
Strategy

Hip
Strategy

Figure 18–21. Schematic representations of the ankle and hip strategies of postural movement. (From Nashner LM, Peters JF: Dynamic posturography in the diagnosis and management of dizziness and balance disorders. Neurologic Clinics 8[2]:331–349, 1990.)

stimulation. Two mechanisms are thought to operate: short-term habituation can occur through progressively smaller synaptic potentials in sensory neurons, but long-term habituation is thought to result from effective inactivation of pre-existing synaptic connections between sensory and motor neurons. This could be the basis for the empirical evidence that vestibular patients who are symptomatic during certain head maneuvers can reduce their symptoms by systematically repeating those maneuvers over a sufficiently long time period.

SUGGESTED READINGS

Arenberg IK, Smith DB: Diagnostic Neurotology. Neurologic Clinics 8(2):199–481, 1990.

Berthoz A, Melvill Jones G (eds): Adaptive Mechanisms in Gaze Control. New York: Elsevier, 1985.

Honrubia V, Brazier MAB (eds): Nystagmus and Vertigo. New York: Academic Press, 1982.

CHAPTER 19

Vertigo

Joseph L. Leach, MD   William L. Meyerhoff, MD, PhD

"Deaf, giddy, helpless, left alone, to all my friends a burden grown."—Jonathan Swift, on his own inner ear afflictions

Balance disturbance is one of the most challenging problems faced by the otolaryngologist in everyday practice. The severity of symptoms may range from hardly noticeable alterations in space perception to totally incapacitating vertigo. To further confuse matters, organ systems beyond the confines of the head and neck may be responsible for these symptoms. *Vertigo* is defined as the hallucination or the illusion of motion. This motion may be rotatory or linear. Vertigo is the classic symptom experienced when dysfunction of the peripheral vestibular system occurs and is not synonymous with *dizziness,* the term more commonly used by the patient. Dizziness is less specific and implies any altered sensation of orientation in space. Dizziness may refer to feelings of light-headedness, feeling spacy, faintness, or giddiness. *Light-headedness* is another nonspecific term that can relate to vestibular or nonvestibular dysfunction. All of these symptoms may be aggravated by riding in a car or walking down aisles of a grocery store or in crowds (motion intolerance). *Ataxia* is the failure of muscular coordination and may be present in patients with vestibular disease. *Motion sickness* is the syndrome of sweating, pallor, nausea, and vomiting caused by vestibular overstimulation. *Syncope, fainting,* and *loss of consciousness* are not forms of vertigo and usually indicate disease in the cardiovascular system.

As discussed in Chapter 18, the vestibular system is one of the three systems by which the body orients itself in relation to space. The vestibular system acts in close concert with the proprioceptive and visual systems, and this collaboration is anatomically manifested by the presence of central projections from the vestibular end organ. The cell bodies of the vestibular nerve are located in Scarpa's ganglion and send projections to the brain stem vestibular nuclei (superior, descending, lateral, and medial). The neurons in these nuclei in turn send projections to several central nervous system stations, including connections to the sympathetic nervous system, the dorsal efferent nucleus of the vagus nerve, the salivatory nuclei, the phrenic nuclei, and the nucleus ambiguus. These projections are responsible for pallor and the sensations of sweating, nausea, and excessive salivation that often accompany vertigo. In addition, there are projections to and from the cerebellum that account for ataxia. These projections also serve to suppress vestibular imbalance that occurs when peripheral lesions are present. Projections through the reticular formation to the cerebral cortex account for the perceived sensation of vertigo. Connections with the ocular cranial nerve nuclei (cranial nerves II, III, and VI), via the medial longitudinal fasciculus, are responsible for the production of nystagmus, which is the objective sign of the subjective symptom of vertigo (Fig. 19–1).

DIAGNOSIS OF VERTIGO

When the patient with balance disturbance is evaluated, it is necessary to have an organ-

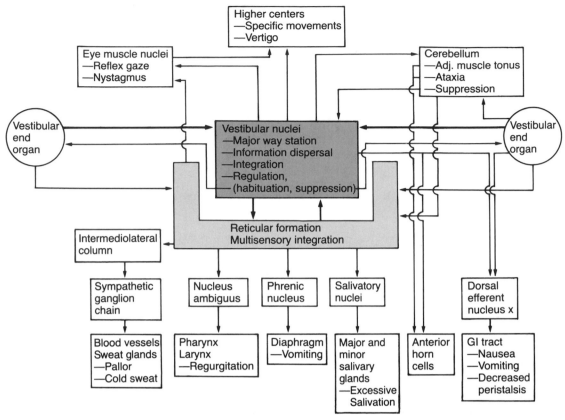

Figure 19–1. Schematic representation of the central projections for vestibular end organ. The arrows represent known tracts. This indicates the high degree to which the vestibular system is integrated into the neuraxis. Under normal circumstances, the vestibular system is principally a proprioceptive one (upper half of schema), but under abnormal circumstances, it initiates considerable motor activity (lower half of schema). (Redrawn from McCabe BF: Vestibular physiology: its clinical application in understanding the dizzy patient. *In* Paparella MM, Shumrick DA [eds]: Otolaryngology. Philadelphia: WB Saunders, 1973.)

ized approach to avoid getting bogged down in a cumbersome history (Table 19–1). It is important to first ascertain the true nature of the complaint and whether it does indeed represent vertigo, light-headedness, ataxia, or syncope. After ascertaining the true nature of the complaint, which may be more difficult than it sounds, the physician should determine the onset, the frequency and the duration of the symptoms, and what factors, if any, precipitate the attacks. It is important to establish the presence of associated symptoms, which may include sweating, pallor, nausea, vomiting, tinnitus, hearing loss, feeling of aural fullness, and otalgia, as well as the impact the disorder is having on the patient's quality of life (Table 19–2). A difference in pitch perception between the two ears or a distortion or a perversion of the appreciation of speech or sound is highly suggestive of cochlear end organ disease.

Tinnitus, when present, also suggests peripheral disease, and it is important to determine whether it is pulsatile, low in pitch, or unilateral or bilateral. True spinning vertigo accompanied by nausea, vomiting, and diaphoresis usually indicates a peripheral vestibular origin, although brain stem and cerebellar ischemia may duplicate these symptoms. Is balance worse when the patient walks to the right or to the left? Does head motion precipitate the attacks? Do friends or family members note any unusual eye movements during these attacks? Are attacks seasonal or related to changes in barometric pressure? The antecedent history can also be of value, and inquiry should be made into the history of ear infection, head trauma, loss of consciousness, whiplash injury, birth defects of the skull, and whether the vertigo was precipitated by exercise, straining, or lifting. Note should be made of underlying medical disorders, including multiple sclerosis, diabetes mellitus, atherosclerotic vascular disease, autoimmune disorders, allergy, endocrine disease, and ocular problems. A drug history is important, and note should be made of the types and amounts of medication taken as well as the amounts of alcohol, caffeine, nicotine, and table salt consumed.

A thorough head and neck examination, including pneumatic otoscopy, tuning fork tests, cranial nerve tests, tests of cerebellar function, and auscultation of the neck is essential to help establish the correct diagnosis. Balance testing may include Romberg's test, past pointing, and gait testing. A complete general physical examination is necessary if one hopes to rule out the presence of associated systemic disease. Laboratory studies rarely pinpoint the source of vertigo but may be of some benefit when suggested by the patient's history and physical examination (Table 19–3). Treponemal testing should be pursued to rule out syphilis as a cause. Antinuclear antibody tests, erythrocyte sedimentation tests, and rheumatoid factor studies help establish the presence of autoimmune diseases. Two studies that are not widely available, the lymphocyte inhibition assay and the migration inhibition test, have been used in certain centers to rule out the presence of autoimmune phenomena directed against the inner ear. Such phenomena should be of concern only in patients with fairly rapidly progressing signs and symptoms. Thyroid function studies and tests for glucose tolerance may uncover an underlying endocrine disorder. Hyperlipidemia and hypercoagulability states may produce vertigo, and appropriate tests may be ordered to rule them out. Spinal fluid protein and cellular analysis may be of some benefit when a central nervous system cause is considered.

Testing of the auditory system encompasses both behavioral and physiologic evaluation. Behavioral studies represent the foundation of an audiologic examination and are supplemented by the physiologic studies. Behavioral studies require a voluntary response from the patient and are therefore subject to the patient's cooperation. They include threshold testing for air and bone as well as testing for speech reception threshold and discrimination. Change in behavioral responses after dehydration can also be measured, and the measurements are helpful when inner ear fluid imbalance is suspected.

Physiologic studies do not require a voluntary response, and therefore the patient's cooperation is not an issue. These studies include tympanometry, which is a measure of tympanic membrane compliance and the characteristics of the stapedial reflex, and the measurement of acoustic emissions and the evoked potentials of electrocochleography (ECochG), auditory brain stem response (ABR), and middle-latency response (MLR), among others.

Essentially, ECochG measures the electric potentials associated with inner ear and auditory nerves. Three parameters are recorded: the cochlear microphonic, the summating potential, and the eighth nerve action potential. The cochlear microphonic is an alternating current response to sound stimuli generated by the hair cells of the organ of Corti. The summating potential, on the other hand, is a direct current response of undetermined origin. The action potential is the cumulative response from thousands of individual nerve fibers in the distal portion of the auditory nerve. The primary component of the action potential is referred to as N1, which is identical to wave I of the ABR and is useful in determining threshold. All these measurements can be obtained either with invasive, transtympanic electrodes or with noninvasive electrodes in the external auditory canal. An increase in the ratio of the summating potential to the action potential has been correlated with labyrinthine causes of vertigo, particularly Meniere's disease and perilymph fistula, and appears to be related to altered basilar membrane biomechanics associated with inner ear fluid imbalance. ECochG can also be used intraoperatively to identify adequate decompression of the endolymphatic space. As with behavioral audiometry, ECochG can be used in conjunction with dehydrating agents. Specific improvement noted in the ratio of summating to action potentials is attributed to lowering of endolymphatic pressure. The degree to which the examining physician uses the supplemental testing is predicated on the index of suspicion.

ABR testing involves monitoring the small electric potentials that arise in the auditory system after acoustic stimulation. A computer uses these potentials to generate a graphic waveform in which wave amplitude varies with time. Various peaks within the waveform correspond to activity at certain locations within the brain stem (e.g., wave I

TABLE 19–1. Vestibular Evaluation

Name _____ Age _____ Date _____

Address _____ City _____ State _____

	Yes	No	
1. Is your dizziness			Give date that your dizziness started:
Lightheadedness	_____	_____	
Swimming sensation	_____	_____	
Wooziness	_____	_____	_____
Faintness	_____	_____	
Blacking out (unconsciousness)	_____	_____	Frequency of attacks:
Turning or spinning	_____	_____	
Side-to-side movement	_____	_____	_____
Up-and-down movement	_____	_____	
Falling sensation	_____	_____	
2. Is your dizziness			
Sudden in onset	_____	_____	
Gradual in onset	_____	_____	
Constant	_____	_____	
In attacks that last			
Seconds	_____	_____	
Minutes	_____	_____	
Hours	_____	_____	
Days	_____	_____	
3. Do you have a warning before an attack?	_____	_____	
4. Is your dizziness accompanied by			
Nausea	_____	_____	
Vomiting	_____	_____	
Rapid heart beat	_____	_____	
Sweating	_____	_____	
5. Is your dizziness related to meals?	_____	_____	

	Yes	No	Yes	No
6. Is it brought on by			Is it made worse by	
Walking	_____	_____	_____	_____
Sitting up	_____	_____	_____	_____
Lying down	_____	_____	_____	_____
Standing	_____	_____	_____	_____
Arising from lying down	_____	_____	_____	_____
Turning	_____	_____	_____	_____
Walking in dark	_____	_____	_____	_____

7. Are you completely free of dizziness between attacks? _____ _____

8. Do you know of anything that will
   Stop your dizziness or make it better _____ _____
   Make your dizziness worse _____ _____

TABLE 19–1. Vestibular Evaluation *Continued*

	Yes	No	
9. Do you suspect a cause for your dizziness?	_____	_____	If yes, what?
			_____
10. Do you have hearing loss in your			
Right ear	_____	_____	
Left ear	_____	_____	
11. Do you have ringing in your ears?			
Right ear	_____	_____	
Left ear	_____	_____	
12. Do you feel pressure in your ears?			
Right ear	_____	_____	
Left ear	_____	_____	
13. Do you have discharge from your ears?			
Right ear	_____	_____	
Left ear	_____	_____	
14. Do you have double or blurry vision?	_____	_____	
15. Were you exposed to any irritating fumes, paints, etc., at the onset of your dizziness?	_____	_____	
16. Do you have any allergies?	_____	_____	
To what? _____			
17. Have you ever injured your head?	_____	_____	
Were you unconscious?	_____	_____	
18. Had you been taking any medications regularly before your dizziness started?	_____	_____	
What? _____			
19. Do you drink alcohol?	_____	_____	
How much? _____			
20. Have you ever smoked or do you now smoke?	_____	_____	
How much? _____			
How long? _____			
21. Have you ever been told you had either high or low blood pressure?	_____	_____	
Which?	High ___	Low ___	

From Vermeersch H, Meyerhoff WL, Boothby R: Vertigo. *In* Meyerhoff WL (ed): Diagnosis and Management of Hearing Loss (pp. 105–125). Philadelphia: WB Saunders, 1987.

TABLE 19–2. Diagnostic Protocol for Vertigo

History

Otolaryngologic History
Establish the nature of dizziness as well as frequency, duration, and precipitating factors
Establish the presence of associated symptoms: hearing loss, otorrhea, head trauma, noise exposure, tinnitus, otalgia, feeling of aural fullness, diplacusis, recruitment, Tullio's phenomenon, nausea, and vomiting

Complete General History
Hypothyroidism, adrenocortical insufficiency, blood dyscrasias, visual disturbance, arteriosclerotic vascular disease, diabetes mellitus, collagenoses, allergy, renal disease, syphilis, and medications

Physical Examination

Otolaryngologic
External ear and tympanic membrane, cranial nerves, spontaneous nystagmus, fistula test, Romberg's test, past pointing, Hennebert's sign, dysdiadochokinesia

General
Vascular and systemic diseases as suggested by history

Neurologic
Cerebellar signs, seizures, multiple sclerosis

Audiologic Test Battery

Tuning fork tests (e.g., Rinne's, Weber's)
Pure tone audiometry
Speech reception threshold
Tone decay tests
Loudness recruitment tests (short increment sensitivity index [SISI] test, alternate binaural loudness balance [ABLB] test)
Von Békésy and comfortable loudness von Békésy tests
Binaural pitch masking
Impedance audiometry and stapedial reflex testing (including stapedial reflex decay)
Auditory brain stem response (ABR)

Electronystagmography

Spontaneous Nystagmus
Provoked Nystagmus
Positional tests
Caloric tests (air caloric and water caloric)
Eye-tracking tests
Optokinetic tests (Bárány)
Calibration
Rotatory testing
Posturography

Radiology

Skull
Mastoid and internal auditory canals
Polytomography of the internal ear
Clivogram (posterior fossa myelogram) and pneumencephalography
Computed tomography
Nuclear magnetic resonance
Angiography
Cervical spine

General Examinations

Cardiovascular (electrocardiogram [EKG])
Hematology (white blood count [WBC], hemoglobin [HGB], sedimentation rate, electrolytes, lipid analysis, coagulation studies)
Endocrine (ACTH, thyroid function tests, diabetes)
Serologic and immunologic evaluation (FTA-ABS, lupus erythematosus cell preparations)
Lumbar puncture (syphilis, multiple sclerosis, culture for meningitis, cell block)
Viral studies (stool, CSF, serum)

From Vermeersch H, Meyerhoff WL, Boothby R: Vertigo. *In* Meyerhoff WL (ed): Diagnosis and Management of Hearing Loss (pp. 105–125). Philadelphia: WB Saunders, 1987.
ACTH, adrenocorticotropic hormone; FTA-ABS, fluorescent treponemal antibody absorption; CSF, cerebrospinal fluid.

TABLE 19–3. Questionnaire for Patients with Balance Disturbance

Name _____ Date _____

The purpose of this questionnaire is to identify difficulties or unsteadiness. Please circle the appropriate answer.

1.	Does looking up increase your problem?	Yes	No	Sometimes
2.	Because of your problem do you feel frustrated?	Yes	No	Sometimes
3.	Because of your problem do you restrict your travel for business or recreation?	Yes	No	Sometimes
4.	Does walking down the aisle of a supermarket increase your problem?	Yes	No	Sometimes
5.	Because of your problem do you have difficulty getting into or out of bed?	Yes	No	Sometimes
6.	Does your problem significantly restrict your participation in social activities such as going out to dinner, to movies, dancing, or to parties?	Yes	No	Sometimes
7.	Because of your problem do you have difficulty reading?	Yes	No	Sometimes
8.	Does performing more ambitious activities like sports, dancing, household chores such as sweeping or putting dishes away increase your problem?	Yes	No	Sometimes
9.	Because of your problem are you afraid to leave your home without having someone accompany you?	Yes	No	Sometimes
10.	Because of your problem have you been embarrassed in front of others?	Yes	No	Sometimes
11.	Do quick movements of your head increase your problem?	Yes	No	Sometimes
12.	Because of your problem do you avoid heights?	Yes	No	Sometimes
13.	Does turning over in bed increase your problem?	Yes	No	Sometimes
14.	Because of your problem is it difficult for you to do strenuous housework or yardwork?	Yes	No	Sometimes
15.	Because of your problem are you afraid people may think you are intoxicated?	Yes	No	Sometimes
16.	Because of your problem is it difficult for you to go for a walk by yourself?	Yes	No	Sometimes
17.	Does walking down a sidewalk increase your problem?	Yes	No	Sometimes
18.	Because of your problem is it difficult for you to concentrate?	Yes	No	Sometimes
19.	Because of your problem it is difficult for you to walk around your house in the dark?	Yes	No	Sometimes
20.	Because of your problem are you afraid to stay home alone?	Yes	No	Sometimes
21.	Because of your problem do you feel handicapped?	Yes	No	Sometimes
22.	Has your problem placed stress on your relationships with members of your family or friends?	Yes	No	Sometimes
23.	Because of your problem are you depressed?	Yes	No	Sometimes
24.	Does your problem interfere with your job or household responsibilities?	Yes	No	Sometimes
25.	Does bending over increase your problem?	Yes	No	Sometimes

corresponds to cranial nerve VIII). The amplitude and latency of these peaks may then be analyzed and compared with normative values and with values obtained from the opposite ear to determine whether any retrocochlear abnormality is present. An increase in the latency between waves I and V, the absence of wave V, and a significant difference in interaural wave V latencies usually indicate retrochlear disease.

Whereas ABR involves the use of the electric readings obtained 2 to 10 milliseconds after the stimulus is presented, the MLR concerns the waveforms produced 12 to 50 milliseconds after the stimulus is presented. The MLR may more accurately reflect the hearing process, but it is prone to interference by muscular stimulation.

Auditory testing is an important aspect in the evaluation of vestibular difficulties because of the anatomic proximity of the two systems and the common fluid that they share. Auditory testing not only is useful in determining the presence or absence of hearing loss but also can help define the site of lesion when hearing loss is present.

Study of the vestibular system is of obvious importance in evaluation of the patient with equilibrium difficulties. Vestibular testing, like auditory testing, includes modalities that require an accurate response and those that do not. Modalities that can provide useful information without a patient's cooperation are electronystagmography (ENG) and sinusoidal harmonic acceleration; platform posturography, in contrast, loses significant value in studies of the patient who is unwilling to cooperate.

Nystagmus is the objective sign of subjective vertigo. Nystagmus is quantified and recorded by ENG. In this method of testing, electrodes are used to detect the electrical potential difference between the retina and the cornea as the eye moves. These movements are then recorded on a polygraph as characteristic sawtooth movements. By convention, the direction of the nystagmus is described as the direction of the fast phase, although it is the slow phase that is generated by the abnormal vestibular imput, and the fast phase merely represents a correction in movement induced by the brain stem.

Before testing, the patient is instructed to avoid drugs or medications that may alter ENG responses. After calibration, the patient's ability to horizontally and vertically track is tested, after which the patient is observed for spontaneous and gaze-induced nystagmus. Positional testing is then performed in an attempt to induce nystagmus. Last, the patient is subjected to caloric stimulation, which involves the use of warm (44°C) and cool (30°C) irrigations of the external auditory canal with either water or air to induce stimulation of the semicircular canals. Comparison of the two ears may reveal either a hypoactive or a hyperactive peripheral vestibular apparatus and can often separate central from peripheral causes.

Simultaneous stimulation of both ears may also be of value in eliciting latent unilateral reduced vestibular response. The nystagmus obtained is then analyzed, and the maximal slow phase velocity is measured for the right side (R) and the left side (L). The difference between sides is then calculated from the formula

$$100 \times (RW + RC) - (LW + LC)/RW + RC + LW + LC,$$

whereas the formula for directional preponderance is

$$100 \times (RW + LC) - (RC + LW)/RW + RC + LW + LC.$$

A difference of 20% to 30% is considered pathologic. Central causes of nystagmus often produce calibration overshoots, opticokinetic abnormalities, poor eye tracking, and failure to suppress the nystagmus with visual fixation. Peripheral lesions manifest as a unilateral reduced vestibular response with caloric stimulation. Positional testing may also delineate peripheral from central causes. A peripheral lesion usually manifests as direction-fixed nystagmus that is preceded by a 15- to 20-second delay in onset that is associated with vertigo, and this nystagmus fatigues with repetition. Positional nystagmus that does not have these characteristics may be central or peripheral in origin. It must be remembered that direction-changing nystagmus can be the result of ethanol alcohol consumption within 24 hours of testing. Fistula testing is a variant of routine ENG and is performed by applying air pressure to the external auditory canal and the eardrum in an attempt to elicit nystagmus. A positive result indicates a fluid imbalance in the inner ear (Meniere's disease, perilymph fistula). Of importance is that despite its value in helping in the diagnosis of vestibular disease, a normal ENG result does not preclude the presence of such disease.

Sinusoidal harmonic acceleration is a rotational test that has been developed to assess the vestibulo-ocular reflex. In comparison with the ENG, this test is potentially more sensitive and allows more precise control of stimuli. Harmonic acceleration tests are undertaken to evaluate the vestibulo-ocular system by analyzing compensatory eye movements in response to clockwise and counterclockwise rotation. Again, the maximal slow phase of the nystagmus is measured, and the difference between right and left is calculated by the formula $100 \times (R - L/R + L)$. Although sinusoidal harmonic testing cannot identify the side of the lesion in unilateral disease, it is very helpful in identifying the presence of disease and following its recovery.

Platform posturography is a modality for evaluating the vestibulospinal reflex and helps differentiate problems of the vestibular system from those of the central nervous system as well as those of the visual and proprioceptive systems (Fig. 19–2). Posturography records the postural sway of a patient on a moving platform. The platform is equipped with strain gauges that measure the torsional forces exerted by the subject's feet. A strain gauge is attached to the subject's hip to measure ankle sway, and another gauge, attached to the back, detects contributions from ankle and hip sway. With movement, readings are taken and analyzed by computer. The effect of visual imput is negated by moving a canopy in synchrony with the platform, and movement of the force plates themselves can deprive the patient of proprioceptive information usually generated by ankle joint angulation. With vestibular dysfunction, the sway becomes more irregular and intense.

An important measurement is the threshold gain, or the amount of motion that induces sway. Another important parameter is the performance index, which is calculated by taking the anteroposterior sway signal and scaling the result as a percentage of the maximal anteroposterior sway possible during in-place standing. A value of zero indicates good stability, whereas a value of 100 indicates that the subject either fell or stepped off the platform. A disadvantage of platform posturography is that although it is possible to quantify the amount of vestibular dysfunction, peripheral and central disorders cannot always be differentiated, nor is it always possible to determine which side is affected more severely. The dynamic platform can also be used to identify body sway in conjunction with the fistula test in patients with fluid imbalance in the inner ear.

Imaging studies have added tremendous benefit to the physician who is charged with evaluating a patient with balance disturbance. These studies are particularly useful when there is a high index of suspicion of a space-occupying lesion, a temporal bone fracture, or congenital anomalies. Computed to-

James W. Aston Ambulatory Care Center

The University of Texas Southwestern Medical Center at Dallas

Audiovestibular Services

5303 Harry Hines Boulevard
Dallas, Texas 75235
214-688-3071

NAME: ____________ EX: ________ DATE: ____________

SS#: ____________

PLATFORM EVALUATION

Sensory Organization Test

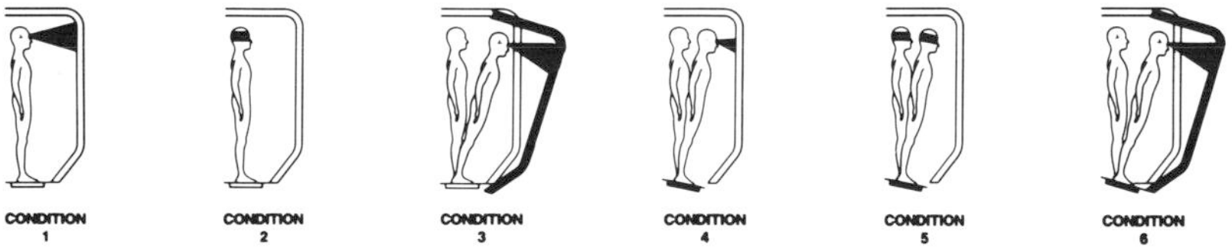

Movement Coordination Test

Symmetry:

Latency:

Amplitude Scaling:

Adaptation:

INTERPRETATION/RECOMMENDATION:

Figure 19–2. Audiovestibular testing.

mography (CT) has largely replaced conventional tomography for evaluating masses or defects in the temporal bone. Magnetic resonance imaging (MRI), particularly when used in conjunction with gadolinium contrast, has become the most sensitive test for diagnosing a tumor of the cerebellopontine angle and, for the most part, has eliminated the need for air and iophendylate (Pantopaque) studies in this region. MRI is also excellent for identifying lacunar infarcts or multiple sclerosis as causes of central vertigo. Radiographs of the cervical spine may be helpful in cases in which there is a history of cervical arthritis or trauma.

Despite extensive study with these techniques, the origin of vertigo may remain in doubt. For certain cases, when the index of suspicion is high, an exploratory tympanotomy may be necessary as a diagnostic modality to rule out a perilymph fistula. Despite technologic advances, exploratory tympanotomy remains the most accurate test for this entity.

SPECIFIC DISORDERS

Infectious Disorders

Bacterial Agents. With the advent of antibiotics, generalized bacterial labyrinthitis has become rare, but its effects can be devastating. Bacterial labyrinthitis most commonly occurs as a sequela of bacterial meningitis; it extends to the inner ear via the internal auditory canal or the cochlear aqueduct. It is common especially in children because of the frequency of meningitis and the patency of the cochlear aqueduct. *Streptococcus pneumoniae* is the most common pathogen. Bacterial meningitis (especially that caused by *Haemophilus influenzae*) can also produce a basal arachnoiditis, which can lead to the formation of adhesions in the region of the cerebellopontine angle. These adhesions may affect both the vestibular and cochlear nerves, causing hearing loss and vertigo. Labyrinthitis may also be otitic in origin, occurring as a sequela of either acute or chronic otitis media. Fistula of the lateral semicircular canal from cholesteatoma is a common cause of focal labyrinthitis, and the inflammatory process is usually sterile, much like the focal labyrinthitis that occurs in the region of the round window membrane in chronic otitis media when bacteria become involved. The responsible agent is most commonly *Streptococcus pneumoniae*. When labyrinthitis is infectious, its process is diffuse, and symptoms, which usually include fever, chills, diaphoresis, nausea, vomiting, vertigo, tinnitus, and profound sensorineural hearing loss, can be severe. Brisk nystagmus is usually present and is typically irritative (toward the affected ear) early in the course of the disease but later becomes paralytic (away from the affected ear). Audiometric studies usually reveal a profound hearing loss, and ENG demonstrates ipsilateral reduced or absent responses in the later stages.

In its focal and less severe forms, serous (sterile) labyrinthitis results from passage of toxic products of otitis media into the inner ear. Passage of infection may occur either through the round window, as mentioned earlier, or through a fistula created by bone erosion. Because the basal turn of the cochlea is usually affected, high-frequency hearing loss is a common symptom, but vertigo may also occur. This vertigo is typically less severe than that produced with bacterial labyrinthitis, and the outlook for recovery is much better. As with early bacterial labyrinthitis, the nystagmus, which is rarely produced, is irritative (toward the affected ear).

Treatment of diffuse bacterial labyrinthitis includes hospitalization, antibiotic therapy, volume repletion, vestibular suppression, and appropriate antiemetics.

Bacterial labyrinthitis secondary to otitis media must be treated surgically. If there is acute otitis media, a wide myringotomy with drainage of pus should be performed. If there is coexistent chronic otitis media, mastoidectomy must be performed once the patient is stable to remove foci of cholesteatoma or granulation tissue. Labyrinthine fistulas caused by cholesteatoma may be present.

Once the source of infection has been removed, the incapacitating vertigo usually subsides within 5 to 7 days. Disequilibrium, especially with position change, persists for several weeks, and recovery from symptoms may never be complete in the older patient. Although there is usually permanent profound sensorineural hearing loss with bacterial labyrinthitis, serous labyrinthitis usually follows a more benign course, in which the vertigo resolves over a shorter time period, and the hearing level (except for the high-frequency loss) usually returns to preinflammation values.

Viral Agents. Viral agents may also cause vertigo by infecting the vestibular nerve and end organ. Viral labyrinthitis may give rise to permanent hearing loss (in about 40% of patients), but the vertigo usually improves over several weeks as the brain stem compensates. Viruses may adversely affect the labyrinth by infecting the endolymphatic space, the perilymphatic space, or the end arterioles of the labyrinth by obstruction with endothelial inflammation. Endolymphatic labyrinthitis is more common than perilymphatic labyrinthitis and typically is caused by mumps, rubella, rubeola, or influenza viruses. Clinical differentiation of these entities is difficult, but treatment of all four is confined to supportive care. Occasionally, delayed hydrops occurs years after viral labyrinthitis. Frequently, there is no hearing in the affected ear, and the patient presents with a feeling of aural fullness and episodic incapacitating vertigo. Patients who fail to improve with nonsurgical care do well with vestibular nerve section.

Vestibular neuronitis or ganglionitis is a less severe form of infection in which hearing is typically spared, although high-frequency audiometry may demonstrate a hearing loss. The disease affects males and females equally, with a predilection for the fourth through sixth decades. Symptoms usually manifest after a viral upper respiratory infection and include vertigo, nystagmus, nausea, vomiting, and diaphoresis. The nystagmus is typically paralytic (away from the affected ear). As with viral labyrinthitis, the vertigo associated with viral vestibular neuronitis typically resolves over a period of weeks, but caloric testing may reveal a unilateral reduced vestibular response that persists indefinitely.

Diagnosis of viral diseases of the vestibular system is difficult and usually not cost effective. Cerebrospinal fluid and stool cultures or serum viral titers may reveal a causative agent, but diagnosis is usually made on the basis of history and physical findings. Treatment for viral vestibular infections is symptomatic (bed rest, volume repletion, vestibular suppressants) because, as a rule, no specific treatment is effective.

One viral infection of the peripheral vestibular system that has shown response to specific therapy is herpes zoster oticus, or Ramsay Hunt syndrome. The infection can cause severe vertigo. It usually begins in the geniculate ganglion and produces the symptoms of facial paralysis, aural pain, sensori-neural hearing loss, vertigo, and vesicular eruptions of the auricle, the external auditory canal, and the tympanic membrane. High doses of corticosteroids and acyclovir (a specific antiviral agent) have been shown to reduce the duration of symptoms, especially the facial paralysis.

Syphilis. Although less common than in previous years, syphilis remains a diagnosis to be considered in any patient with vertigo. Whereas fluctuating progressive hearing loss tends to be the primary symptom of luetic otitis, syphilis may produce vertigo in its secondary, tertiary, or congenital manifestations. Congenital syphilis often manifests with mucopurulent rhinitis (snuffles), saddle nose, frontal bossing, saber shins, and characteristic dental findings. Vertigo and sensorineural hearing loss may be seen. The congenital type of the disease may arise as either a severe early form or a latent, more benign form that commonly affects women in their late 30s.

Secondary syphilis in the form of meningoencephalitis can cause luetic labyrinthitis. More commonly, however, syphilis affects the inner ear in its tertiary forms. The disease causes a neuronitis, degeneration of the end organ, panosteitis, endolymphatic hydrops, and obliterative endarteritis. The osteitis may lead to the presence of tiny perilymphatic fistulas. Application of pressure to the sealed external auditory canal may give rise to nystagmus. This phenomenon, when it occurs in the presence of an intact tympanic membrane, is known as Hennebert's sign. Diagnosis is based on positive results of a flocculation test (Venereal Disease Research Laboratory, rapid plasma reagin), which are not specific but do revert to normal after successful treatment of the disease. Treponemal antibody tests generally are more specific but the results remain positive even in the setting of adequately treated disease. A Western blot assay reportedly detects multiple antibody isotypes to *Treponema pallidum,* which indicate whether the infection is active.

Long-term penicillin administration (lasting 90 days) remains the mainstay of therapy, and high doses of steroids may help improve the aural symptoms. If initial steroid treatment does show some benefit, steroid use may be necessary for a prolonged period. Endolymphatic shunt surgery for patients with luetic vertigo is controversial but might be effective in relieving endolymphatic hydrops produced by the disease.

Fungal Agents. Fungal labyrinthitis is an uncommon cause of vertigo that occurs predominantly in immunosuppressed patients. *Candida, Mucor, Cryptococcus,* and *Blastomyces* species are the most common organisms identified. In spite of aggressive treatment, including amphotericin B and surgical debridement, fungal infection of the labyrinth in a debilitated patient is often a terminal disease.

Allergy and Autoimmune Phenomena

The inner ear may act as a shock organ to both inhalant and food allergens. Food allergies are mediated by a non-IgE pathway in about two thirds of cases. Vertigo, tinnitus, hearing loss, and a feeling of aural fullness may all be relieved by avoidance of the offending allergen. Diagnosis is directed toward allergen identification either by skin testing or by elimination diets. Hyposensitization with allergen extracts may help alleviate vertigo caused by inhalant allergy.

Autoimmune inner ear disease can be either a local manifestation of a systemic disease or a phenomenon confined to the inner ear itself. The typical manifestation is that of rapidly progressive, fluctuating, asymmetric sensorineural hearing loss associated with vertigo. Diagnosis is based on the presence of these symptoms in addition to a beneficial response to steroids and cyclophosphamide, associated autoimmune disorders, and abnormal results of screening blood tests (antinuclear antigen, immunoglobulin level, rheumatoid factor, erythrocyte sedimentation rate). The lymphocyte inhibition assay and the migration inhibition test measure the presence of serum antibodies to inner ear antigens. These tests are believed to have a high predictive value for patients with autoimmune inner ear disease. Treatment consists of steroid therapy, or cytotoxic agents, or both.

Relapsing polychondritis is a systemic disease of probable autoimmune origin that eventually produces cochleovestibular damage in more than 40% of affected patients. Symptoms may include ataxia, vertigo, nausea, and vomiting. Diagnosis is based on the presence of chondritis of one or more organs, polyarthritis, or histologic confirmation. Screening of patients with suspected polychondritis reveals an erythrocyte sedimentation rate often in excess of 100 mm/hour. Treatment is with corticosteroids, nonsteroidal anti-inflammatory agents, sulfones, and cytotoxic agents.

Cogan's syndrome has many characteristics of an autoimmune disease in that it produces a vasculitis. This syndrome may represent a form of periarteritis nodosa. The syndrome includes nonsyphilitic interstitial keratitis, progressive fluctuating hearing loss, tinnitus, and vertigo. Other manifestations may include fever, chills, myalgias, a heart murmur, and leukocytosis. The ENG may show spontaneous nystagmus with the eyes opened or unilateral or bilateral absent responses. Some improvement in symptoms may be noted with steroid or cyclophosphamide administration. The major diagnostic dilemma is in differentiating patients with Cogan's syndrome from patients with otitic syphilis.

Vascular and Hematologic Disorders

Any condition that results in decreased perfusion of the vestibular end organ may produce vertigo, whereas any condition resulting in decreased circulation to the central nervous system may cause vertigo but more commonly results in lightheadedness or a feeling of faintness. Postural change in the elderly patient can lead to the latter and is a frequent cause of lightheadedness and dizziness.

Vertigo is among the more common manifestations of transient ischemic attacks. These attacks may also manifest as dysarthria, dysphagia, circumoral parasthesia, change in vision, or unilateral weakness or numbness. Transient ischemic attacks and their nature resolve within minutes. Diagnosis is confirmed by the presence of associated symptoms. Auscultation may reveal a bruit in the carotid artery, and endarterectomy may improve blood flow to the labyrinth. Vasodilators and prostaglandin inhibitors may also be of some therapeutic value.

Vascular loop has been described as a cause of vertigo and motion intolerance. This condition should be considered in a patient who presents with episodic vertigo and failure to improve with multiple medical and surgical regimens. These patients also frequently complain of motion intolerance as well as grocery store aisle–induced vertigo. The ENG is consistent with a peripheral cause of vertigo. Air cisternogram–computed tomography or magnetic resonance imaging may reveal a vascular structure in contact with the eighth nerve from the root entry zone to the middle of the internal auditory canal. Unfortunately, however, such a finding is present in many normal people and therefore does not imply a causal relationship. The ABR may show increased intervals between waves I and III, giving some additional information on which to base a cause-and-effect relationship. Demyelinization of the nerve secondary to vascular compression has been postulated to be the underlying cause of the vertigo. Relief of symptoms has been obtained with mobilization of the vessel away from the nerve and placement of polytef (Teflon) felt between the nerve and vessels. Selective sectioning of the vestibular nerve may likewise result in the allaying of vestibular symptoms.

Vertigo is a very common, and often early, manifestation of vertebrobasilar artery insufficiency (VBI). VBI is a symptom complex that ranges from lightheadedness to severe vertigo, vomiting, diplopia, dysarthria, vision changes, and, occasionally, drop attacks. VBI is produced by conditions that diminish the blood flow in the vertebrobasilar system, such as strenuous movement of the upper extremities. Atherosclerotic vascular disease is the most common underlying cause. Prostaglandin inhibitors or vasodilators may be of some benefit.

Stroke is another vascular entity that may produce vertigo as one of its manifestations. Occlusion of the posterior inferior cerebellar artery may result in Wallenberg's syndrome (which includes vertigo), nausea, vomiting, dysarthria, dysphagia, ipsilateral Horner's syndrome, and loss of sensation to the ipsilateral face and contralateral body. These associated symptoms may be of secondary importance to the patient and obscured by the vertigo and its attendant vegetative symptoms. Such a situation gives credence to the necessity of obtaining a thorough history before vestibular studies are performed and treatment is prescribed.

Nystagmus directed toward the side of the lesion with the eyes open and away from the lesion with the eyes closed may be present. ENG, if obtained, may produce central findings such as direction-changing positional nystagmus and difficulty tracking. Arteriography confirms the diagnosis of this potentially fatal disease, and neurosurgical intervention may save the patient's life. Small cerebellar infarcts may also produce balance disturbance, and the symptoms may be similar to those of vestibular neuronitis. Cerebellar hemorrhage or infarct may produce vertigo in association with headaches, Cheyne-Stokes respiration, gait abnormalities, and nystagmus. Diagnosis is confirmed by CT or MRI. Treatment for severe lesions includes supportive care, medications to reduce brain edema, and decompressive surgery in selected cases; less severe lesions may be stabilized by vasodilators and prostaglandin inhibitors. Aneurysms of the basilar artery have been reported to cause vertigo, dysphagia, and multiple cranial nerve palsies. Such aneurysms may be identified with CT, MRI or arteriography. Surgical intervention may be necessary.

Vertigo may also be a manifestation of migraine headache. The diagnosis of migraine headache is established by the presence of episodic headaches and any three of the following:

1. Abdominal pain, nausea, and vomiting during the headache.
2. Hemicephalalgia.
3. Pain of a pulsatile quality.
4. Complete relief after a period of rest.
5. Associated aura.
6. Family history of migraine headaches.

When the vertigo is synchronous with the headache and these characteristics coexist, migraine headache as the cause of vertigo can be confirmed. Tinnitus and vertigo are thought to be the effect of constriction of the basilar artery. Vestibular deficits associated with migraine are usually temporary but may be permanent. Symptomatic relief may be obtained with alpha-adrenergic blocking agents, beta blockers, or calcium channel blockers.

The hyperviscosity syndrome refers to symptoms related to elevated blood viscosity. It may be associated with polycythemia, macroglobulinemia, sickle cell anemia, or hypergammaglobulinemia. Symptoms may include vertigo, nystagmus, hearing loss, headache, and vision changes. The pathophysiologic process probably involves sludging of blood in the capillaries and venules in the labyrinth, the vestibular nerve, the vestibular nuclei, or the cerebellum. Diagnosis is made by a high index of suspicion and the appropriate laboratory tests. Symptoms resolve with reduction of blood hyperviscosity.

Leukemia may reduce the oxygen-carrying capacity of the blood to cause hypoxia of the vestibular end organ. There may also be a leukemic infiltrate of the petrous apex of the temporal bone. Hemorrhage into the labyrinth may occur and may result in severe vertigo, nystagmus, tinnitus, and sensorineural hearing loss. Therapy is confined to treatment of the underlying cause, supportive measures, and vestibular suppressants.

Neoplasms

Neoplastic involvement of the central or peripheral vestibular system may give rise to vertigo or, more commonly, ataxia and generalized disequilibrium. Acoustic neuromas account for the majority of masses presenting in the cerebellopontine angle, although meningiomas, neuromas of other cranial nerves, cholesteatomas, glomus tumors, cholesterin granulomas, vascular malformations, and metastatic malignancies may also occur in the same region. The first signs of acoustic neuroma typically include slowly progressive asymmetric sensorineural hearing loss and tinnitus, but vertigo and especially gait disturbance may occur later. Meningioma, the second most commonly occurring mass in the cerebellopontine angle, usually manifests with similar characteristics, although gait disturbance in the absence of hearing loss may be a more prominent early sign.

Neurofibromas of the internal auditory canal are generally bilateral but otherwise manifest in a way similar to that of acoustic neuromas. Cholesteatoma of the petrous apex can manifest with similar characteristics, but facial paralysis may be more common. Screening for all cerebellopontine angle lesions may be performed with ABR and ENG, and diagnosis may be confirmed with contrast medium–enhanced CT or, preferably, gadolinium-enhanced MRI.

Treatment of most tumors of the cerebellopontine angle involves surgical resection through the middle cranial fossa, the suboccipital, or the translabyrinthine approach. The middle cranial fossa approach is an intracranial procedure that enables the removal of small tumors in the internal auditory canal, but the facial nerve may be at some risk. The suboccipital technique is also an intracranial approach that enables removal of tumors near the cerebellopontine angle and entails less risk to the facial nerve. The translabyrinthine approach requires only modest retraction on the dura and the cerebellum and entails the least risk to facial function, but the procedure ablates any residual hearing and is associated with a somewhat higher risk of postoperative cerebrospinal fluid leakage. Radiation and chemotherapy may play a role in the treatment of selected cases. Vertigo is rarely a symptom of central nervous system tumors, although cerebellar and temporal lobe neoplasms frequently produce ataxia.

Trauma

Trauma to the balance system spans the spectrum from a seemingly inconsequential bump on the head to a potentially catastrophic injury. Temporal bone fractures are the result of severe blows to the head and are typically classified as longitudinal or transverse, depending on the axis of the fracture line. Although this classification is important from an academic standpoint, it is also important to recognize that many severe injuries result in a combination of fractures that do not fit in either the pure longitudinal or the pure transverse classification.

Longitudinal fractures are more common than transverse fractures and are produced from blows to the squamous temporal or parietal portion of the skull. The fracture line starts at the mastoid tegmen and runs along the roof of the eustachian tube. A conductive type of hearing loss secondary to ossicular damage or a tympanic membrane tear is usually produced, but the facial nerve, the internal auditory canal, and the labyrinth are typically spared. Blood, cerebrospinal fluid, or both may be noted in the external auditory canal.

Transverse temporal bone fractures result from blows to the frontal or occipital areas of the skull and are more life threatening; consequently, fewer victims of this type of injury live to be evaluated. The fracture line starts at the jugular foramen and extends to the foramen spinosum or lacerum. Facial paralysis and injury to the labyrinth and the internal auditory canal are much more common with this type of fracture, and hematotympanum rather than otorrhea is typical because the tympanic membrane remains intact. Diagnosis of temporal bone fractures may be confirmed with fine-cut CT of the temporal bone. The nystagmus produced is usually paralytic as a result of immediate and irreversible damage to the vestibular end organ. The resultant vertigo is treated with vestibular suppressants and exercises until central compensation occurs. Occasionally, vestibular injury may be incomplete and the vertigo recurrent. Patients in this condition respond well to vestibular nerve section. Excessive use of vestibular suppressants, however, retards vestibular compensation.

Concussion of the brain and the labyrinth may also produce injury to the vestibular system and result in vertigo. Trauma to the cranial contents causes transudate of serum into the perivascular spaces, slowing of circulation, and hemorrhage. This process may involve the labyrinth, the vestibular nerve, and the nuclei or the cerebellum. Findings may range from an isolated nystagmus toward the involved ear to headache, irritability, and poor concentration. Hearing loss may be present in the case of labyrinthine concussion. Diagnosis is based on the history (usually associated with a loss of consciousness), audiologic testing, ENG, and the absence of other pertinent findings on CT or MRI scans. If the associated head injury is not severe, central compensation eventually allows resolution of the vertigo. The prognosis, as is true with other labyrinthine disturbances, is better in the younger patient. Vestibular suppressants may provide symptomatic relief. In some patients, delayed endolymphatic hydrops may develop years after injury. The exact mechanism for this condition is not known, and the treatment is similar to that of Meniere's disease.

Cupulolithiasis, or benign paroxysmal positional vertigo, is the condition proposed to result from displacement of otoconia from the utricular macula into the ampulla of the posterior semicircular canal, which makes that canal a gravity-sensitive organ. Trauma has been proposed as a major cause of otoconial displacement; however, aging, toxins, infections, surgery on the stapes, or vascular insults may also be responsible. Prolonged bed rest may also facilitate deposition of otoconia from the macula to the more dependent posterior semicircular canal. When the affected ear is placed in a dependent position, the otoconia deflect the cupula in an utriculofugal direction, producing nystag-

mus, nausea, and vomiting. Classic benign paroxysmal positional vertigo produces nystagmus that is delayed 15 to 20 seconds after placement of the affected ear in the down position. The nystagmus is also fatigable, short in duration, horizontorotatory in nature, associated with vegetative symptoms, and directed toward the involved ear.

Diagnosis of cupulolithiasis is confirmed by history and the presence of the type of nystagmus just described. ENG may reveal reduced vestibular response on the affected side. Treatment involves elicitation of the vertigo by vestibular exercises; the goal is to hasten the process of central compensation. Cases resistant to nonsurgical treatment after 1 year may be treated by section of the nerve of the singular canal (the nerve that provides innervation from the ampulla of the posterior semicircular canal); results in most instances are good.

Perilymph fistula, although occasionally spontaneous, is usually thought to occur as the result of trauma. When leakage occurs, it is usually through the oval window annulus, the round window membrane, the fissula ante fenestrum, or microfissures in the floor of the round window niche. In rare instances, Hyrtl's fissure may be present. The pressure responsible for the leak may be implosive (such as that produced by a sudden increase in middle ear pressure) or explosive (such as that produced by a sudden increase in the pressure of the cerebrospinal fluid and transmitted through the internal auditory canal or the cochlear aqueduct). Common inciting events include head trauma, strenuous physical exertion, coughing, acoustic trauma, sneezing, straining, scuba diving, and descent in airplanes.

The classic presentation of perilymph fistula is one of fluctuating hearing loss, broadband tinnitus, vertigo or ataxia, and a feeling of aural fullness. Some patients with perilymph fistula may experience Tullio's phenomenon (vertigo induced by loud noise). Most patients suffering from perilymph fistula, however, do not present in the classic manner but rather manifest vaguer symptoms. In children, the condition is especially hard to diagnose. Children who have sudden hearing loss or progressive sensorineural hearing loss with or without disequilibrium must be considered to have perilymph fistula. The diagnosis is especially suggested in children with otorrhea or otorhinorrhea, otologic symptoms, and temporal bone abnormalities that appear on radiographic studies.

Although tinnitus, a feeling of aural fullness, hearing loss, and vertigo are present alone or in combination in most patients with perilymph fistula, the confirmation of fistula on the basis of history alone is very difficult. Physical examination may be equally unrevealing. Findings of audiologic tests and ENG may be inconclusive. Results of the fistula test may be positive but are negative in most cases. Fistula testing in combination with platform posturography is now being used and may prove to be a more accurate method of diagnosis. Radiologic studies are usually normal in the absence of a skull fracture, although in children, Mondini's deformity or a widely patent modiolus or cochlear aqueduct may be present. ECochG, by its ability to detect relative imbalances in inner ear fluids, is currently being investigated as a potential aid in the diagnosis of perilymph fistula. Preliminary studies indicate that ECochG is fairly specific but not sensitive for perilymph fistula and that abnormal ECochG findings revert to normal after oval and round window grafting. Platform posturography and sinusoidal harmonic acceleration tests usually provide nonspecific results. The most accurate test currently available for diagnosing perilymph fistula is exploratory tympanotomy, and even this does not approach perfect diagnostic accuracy.

Treatment of perilymph fistula consists of bed rest with head elevation, sedation, and avoidance of exertion, except in unusual instances in which subluxation, fracture, or dislocation of the stapes footplate is suspected after trauma. Early surgery is indicated for these patients. Grafting of the oval and round window surfaces with an autogenous tissue seal may be indicated for patients who are unresponsive to nonsurgical measures. Surgical repair of a perilymph fistula is associated with a reasonably good prognosis for the resolution of the vestibular symptoms, but the outlook for improvement in hearing is more guarded. Some clinicians perform endolymphatic sac decompression procedures in concert with round and oval window grafting for cases of perilymph fistula that coexist with Meniere's disease. As with adults, diagnosis of perilymph fistula is based primarily on a high index of suspicion. Grafting may halt the progression of sensorineural hearing loss but is generally more effective in ameliorating vestibular symptoms.

Related to the syndrome of perilymph fistula in children may be the large vestibular aqueduct syndrome. Implosive forces may cause stepwise fluctuating sensorineural hearing loss and vertigo. Symptoms are often instigated by relatively minor head trauma. Diagnosis is made with CT scans. Optimal treatment of this entity has not been established, although suboccipital plugging of the vestibular aqueduct has been successfully tried in at least one severe case.

Iatrogenic injury to the inner ear may result in vertigo. During the course of ear surgery, the labyrinth may be inadvertently entered; this leads to sensorineural hearing loss and vertigo. Such injuries should be grafted with a tissue seal within 24 hours.

Injuries to the neck may also be associated with vertigo by mechanisms that remain unclear, although faulty spinocerebellar communication has been considered. The vertigo is usually self-limited but may reappear with neck rotation. Treatment consists of vestibular suppressants, muscle relaxants, physical therapy, and a soft cervical collar.

Toxic Agents

Balance disturbance may result from any drug that damages the vestibular end organ. Pharmacologic agents that adversely affect the inner ear include aminoglycoside antibiotics, quinine, salicylates, alkylating agents (such as cisplatin), loop diuretics, and occasionally oral contraceptives. The adverse effect of these agents is usually dose-related and enhanced by underlying renal compromise, advanced age, noise exposure, and concomitant administration of other vestibulotoxic drugs. Balance disturbance may be accompanied by high-pitched tinnitus and hearing loss. Streptomycin, gentamicin, and tobramycin are among the aminoglycoside antibiotics that cause vestibular injury before cochlear injury. The mechanism of injury of aminoglycoside antibiotics is by destruction of vestibular hair cells. The loop diuretics, such as ethacrynic acid and furosemide, create toxic effects on the stria vascularis and dark cells of the utricle, which cause defects in fluid regulation; the primary effect of quinine is thought to be on the vestibular nerve and vestibular nuclei. The site of action for salicylate-induced balance disturbance has not yet been defined. Most vestibulotoxic drugs (except quinine, salicylates, and oral contraceptives) have an irreversible effect on the vestibular end organ. Treatment consists of discontinuing the offending agent and supportive care. In the case of effects from aminoglycoside antibiotics, adequate hydration and drug level monitoring are recommended as prophylactic measures.

Balance disturbance has also been reported to occur after exposure to toxins such as carbon monoxide, heavy metals (lead, mercury), alcohol, and tobacco. The effect of these agents is believed to be on the vestibular nerve or the membranous labyrinth, although it is not well understood.

Metabolic Abnormalities

Hypothyroid patients have been observed to manifest vertigo and hearing loss. The mechanism of action for this phenomenon is unknown, but symptoms do improve with thyroid replacement in a certain percentage of these patients. Not only may symptoms include vertigo and hearing loss, but some patients complain of tinnitus and a feeling of aural fullness as well. The diagnosis is usually suspected as a result of the presence of other symptoms of hypothyroidism, such as weight gain, skin dryness, and constipation. The diagnosis is confirmed with laboratory tests of thyroid hormone levels.

Diabetes mellitus may cause unsteadiness through a variety of mechanisms. Problems with insulin regulation may lead to hypoglycemia, which can cause lightheadedness and faintness. In addition, small vessel disease associated with diabetes may result in ischemia to involved neurons and neuroepithelium, and the primary neuropathy associated with diabetes may affect the vestibular nerves. High glucose concentrations within the inner ear may also alter vestibular function. When associated with retinopathy and peripheral proprioceptive defects, vestibular deficits in the diabetic patient become even more devastating. Diagnosis is generally made from results of serum glucose tolerance tests, and treatment involves dietary control, oral hypoglycemic agents, or insulin therapy.

Adrenocortical insufficiency (Addison's disease), a cause of postural hypotension, can result in vertigo. Theories about the pathophysiologic processes include abnormal glucose metabolism, lowered serum sodium levels, end organ hypoxia secondary to vasospasm, and altered function at the neural junction. Diagnosis is based on findings of systemic manifestations of the disease and confirmed by abnormal cortisol levels stimulated by adrenocorticotropic hormone (ACTH). Treatment consists of steroid replacement.

Epilepsy

Epileptic seizures often are preceded by transient vertigo, and vertigo may be the only symptom of seizure disorder. The latter condition is most commonly a result of seizures within the cortical representation of vertigo in the temporal lobe. Temporal lobe epilepsy may manifest with episodic vertigo and the absence of sensorineural hearing loss. Only a few patients' histories reveal an association with nausea or vomiting, but auditory and visual hallucinations and loss of consciousness are often present. ENG may demonstrate nystagmus that worsens with attempts at visual fixation. Diagnosis is based on electroencephalogram and ENG findings. Treatment is with anticonvulsant agents.

Congenital and Neonatal Disorders

Several neonatal and congenital abnormalities of the inner ear may manifest as vertigo or nonspecific balance disturbance. The patent cochlear aqueduct and the Mondini deformity have already been discussed. The Michel type of deformity is a complete lack of development of the inner ear and is extremely rare. The Mondini-Alexander type is a maldevelopment of the cochlear and vestibular end organs. The Bing-Siebenmann type is a malformation of the membranous labyrinth with preservation of the bony labyrinth. These morphologic abnormalities may occur alone or as part of a syndrome.

Of the hereditary syndromes, Usher's syndrome is the one most commonly associated with ataxia and vestibular dysfunction. The mode of inheritance is usually autosomal recessive, and associated findings include retinitis pigmentosa and sensorineural hearing loss. Waardenburg's syndrome is an autosomal dominant disorder characterized by hypertelorism, a confluent eyebrow, and a white forelock. Vestibular dysfunction is present in the majority of afflicted patients.

The Arnold-Chiari malformation is a herniation of the cerebellum through the foramen magnum and may produce oscillopsia (visual jumbling of objects) and gait unsteadiness. Findings may include spontaneous downbeat nystagmus, lower cranial nerve palsies, and ataxia. CT scans or, preferably, MRI may demonstrate herniation of the cerebellar tonsils through the foramen magnum. Treatment involves decompression of the foramen magnum region.

Miscellaneous Disorders

Multiple sclerosis is a chronic disease associated with numerous areas of demyelinization within the central nervous system. Vertigo is the presenting symptom of multiple sclerosis in 5% to 10% of these patients and eventually manifests in 30% to 50% of patients. Nystagmus is present in up to 70% of those afflicted. Internuclear ophthalmoplegia, the pathognomonic eye movement disorder of multiple sclerosis, develops as a result of involvement of the median longitudinal fasciculus. The internal rectus on one side is weak, and the external rectus on the other side is paralyzed. ENG may reveal dissociated nystagmus on lateral gaze and pendular nystagmus. Magnetic resonance imaging is now the study of choice for diagnosis of multiple sclerosis, although ABR and visual evoked response can be helpful. Immunosuppressive agents may improve the vertigo.

Dandy's syndrome refers to the symptom complex resulting from bilateral absence of labyrinthine function. This most commonly results from tumor- or drug-induced destruction of the vestibular system, although idiopathic peripheral vestibular degeneration may produce the same symptoms. Symptoms include oscillopsia and disequilibrium when the patient is walking in the dark. Treatment includes reassurance that the natural compensatory processes will gradually reduce the problem. Labyrinthine exercises may enhance the development of neck reflex control of eye movement. The prognosis is improved if the patient is young, if the onset is insidious, and if tumor involvement is the cause of the disease.

Persistent mal de debarquement syndrome is a disorder consisting of sensations of imbalance lasting months to years after a period of motion exposure. Classically, after a pleasure cruise, patients complain that they still sense the ship moving. Some patients may demonstrate direction-changing positional nystagmus on ENG, but other studies are generally unrewarding. Treatment for this disorder has not been standardized, but vestibular exercises may be of benefit. Some patients with this symptom complex have been found to have perilymph fistula.

The degenerative processes associated with aging have been associated with balance disturbance. Because of the symmetric nature of the disease process, ataxia is more common, but vertigo may occur as well. Aging may produce cell loss at the end organ, neuronal loss, demyelination, and synaptic changes. Despite the association with aging, a specific cause of vertigo can be found in the majority of elderly patients, and the physician should search diligently for an underlying etiologic process. Treatment of the underlying cause may alleviate symptoms. When coupled with other neurosensory deficits, balance disturbance can be disabling in the elderly, and recovery is hindered by poorer vestibular suppression in this age group.

Childhood is also associated with specific vestibular disorders. Benign paroxysmal vertigo of childhood is characterized by multiple brief episodes of vertigo with nystagmus in patients under the age of 4 years. A related phenomenon is paroxysmal torticollis of infancy, in which children experience attacks of head tilting at varying intervals during the day. Results of the physical examination, the ENG, the audiogram, and the encephalogram are usually normal for both disorders. The etiologic process of each entity is unknown but may be related to migraine. Treatment is supportive because the diseases are self-limited.

Vertigo occasionally is a manifestation of labyrinthine otosclerosis (otosclerotic inner ear syndrome). The otospongiotic process may alter the circulatory or metabolic functions of the bony labyrinth and create sensorineural hearing loss, vertigo, or unsteadiness. Diagnosis is made from history, audiometric findings, radiographic studies, and occasionally exploratory tympanotomy. Sodium fluoride, calcium gluconate, and vitamin D may help prevent progression of the otospongiotic foci and alleviate the vertigo. Stapedectomy may relieve vertigo caused by otosclerosis in a certain number of patients. Preoperatively, however, the surgeon must be sure that endolymphatic hydrops is not present because of the increased risk to the inner ear when stapedectomy is performed in the presence of this condition. ECochG and dehydration tests may help in this regard.

Vertigo that is psychogenic may be difficult to distinguish from psychologic disorders secondary to vertigo. Most patients with Meniere's syndrome manifest symptoms of depression or neurosis. It is therefore critical to label vertigo as psychogenic only after an aggressive search for other causes has been conducted. True functional vertigo is often bizarre in nature; rarely is it of the true spinning type. Often the attacks are described as being continuous and associated with out-of-body experiences. Hyperventilation is a common finding in this group of patients. After a thorough work-up for an underlying organic cause has proved negative, these patients are best managed by a psychiatrist. Biofeedback may play a role in therapy.

Meniere's Syndrome

Meniere's syndrome is a symptom complex arising from endolymphatic hydrops, which produces distention of the membranous labyrinth. The classic symptoms of Meniere's syndrome are fluctuating sensorineural hearing loss initially in the low frequencies, a feeling of aural fullness, tinnitus, and episodic vertigo. The distinction of Meniere's disease (idiopathic endolymphatic hydrops) and Meniere's syndrome is made only after other causes of endolymphatic hydrops (such as infection, allergy, trauma, and hormonal dysfunction) have been ruled out. The vertigo associated with endolymphatic hydrops usually lasts several hours and may be associated with nausea and vomiting. After the attacks, the patient is left with tinnitus and unsteadiness for several days. The hearing loss often resolves slowly after each episode, but over time, the hearing gradually deteriorates. The contralateral ear may become involved in up to 40% of cases. Occasionally, tinnitus, hearing loss, and a feeling of aural fullness may occur by themselves (cochlear Meniere's syndrome), or the vertigo may be present alone (vestibular Meniere's syndrome). Another variant is known as Lermoyez's syndrome, wherein the hearing and the tinnitus actually improve after the attack of vertigo. The crisis of Tumarkin is yet another variant that includes falling that is caused by loss of extensor tone in association with the vertiginous episodes. If cases of incomplete symptoms are followed long enough, most develop the complete quadrad.

The diagnosis of Meniere's syndrome is based on history, with some help from audiometric and ENG findings. Audiometry usually demonstrates a "Pike's Peak" pattern or sensorineural loss in the low frequencies that may involve all frequencies as the disease progresses. The audiogram may demonstrate improvement in pure-tone hearing and in speech discrimination after administration of dehydrational agents (such as glycerol or urea), which theoretically reduce the amount of endolymphatic hydrops. Recruitment is usually present, and diplacusis (the perception of different pitches in each ear) may also be found. The ENG may be normal or may show reduced vestibular response or directional preponderance to caloric stimulus. The ABR is usually normal. ECochG may show an elevation of the ratio of summating potential to action potential. There is, however, no absolute diagnostic test for Meniere's syndrome.

On histopathologic examination, the early stages of Meniere's syndrome demonstrate bulging of Reissner's membrane, but as the disease progresses, this bulging is accompanied by degeneration of the hair cell population in the organ of Corti. The saccule and the cochlea are usually more involved than the utricle and the semicircular canals. Temporal bones may reveal sclerosis and obliteration of the endolymphatic duct and sac.

Treatment of Meniere's syndrome initially includes avoidance of caffeine, nicotine, and salt. Diuretics may also be prescribed in hopes of lowering the endolymphatic pressure. Vestibular suppressants, such as meclizine, scopolamine, and diazepam may relieve the symptoms of vertigo. For patients who experience acute incapacitating episodes, tranquilizers may be administered intravenously in a hospital setting. Histamine, administered subcutaneously, intravenously, or sublingually, has been advocated as a treatment for the vertigo associated with Meniere's syndrome. The mode of action of histamine is unclear. Aminoglycoside antibiotics (streptomycin, gentamicin) may be administered intramuscularly or intravenously in a monitored setting in order to ablate the vestibular function of the end organ in patients with bilateral disease. This ablative form of therapy must be followed by careful audiometric testing to prevent cochleotoxicity. Oscillopsia and ataxia may be side effects of aminoglycoside vestibular ablation. In a large percentage of patients, Meniere's syndrome is self-limited, and no further treatment is indicated.

The surgical therapy of Meniere's syndrome remains controversial, but most otologists agree that surgery remains a valuable alternative if medical therapy fails. Decompression of the endolymphatic sac has been shown to be successful in ameliorating the vertiginous episodes in approximately 60% to 80% of patients, and improvement in hearing occurs in about 25%. Advantages of the endolymphatic sac procedure include its low morbidity and nondestructive nature. The incidence of total sensorineural hearing loss with the procedure is less than 5%. Decompression of the endolymphatic system may also be achieved by placement of a stainless steel tack through the oval window into the saccule or through the basilar membrane via the round window. Chances of relieving the vertigo are very good, but it is almost certain that hearing loss will result from these latter procedures. Cryosurgery has been used to create small fistulas between the endolymphatic and perilymphatic systems. Facial nerve paralysis is a definite possibility with this procedure, and cryosurgery for endolymphatic hydrops is not widely used.

Many practitioners feel that endolymphatic decompression surgery is not efficacious in patients with poor hearing, longstanding Meniere's syndrome, or a history of unsuccessful decompression surgery. For these patients, section of the vestibular nerve is another surgical option. There are several ways in which this may be performed, including the translabyrinthine, middle cranial fossa, retrolabyrinthine, and retrosigmoid (suboccipital) approaches. Patients with no serviceable hearing usually get relief from total ablation of inner ear function by labyrinthectomy via the external auditory canal or the transmastoid route. A small percentage of these patients experience no relief of vertigo with labyrinthectomy alone, and many clinicians prefer to resect the vestibular nerve during the same procedure. Both approaches offer a better than 90% chance of relieving vertigo, little risk to the facial nerve, and relief of tinnitus in some cases. The transmeatal route is more direct and faster and is associated with a lower likelihood of cerebrospinal fluid leakage. A disadvantage of this approach is that the cochlear nerve is cut, and future efforts at cochlear implantation are prevented. Another drawback is that the vestibular nerve must be sectioned lateral to Scarpa's ganglion, which may possibly lead to neural regrowth. Disadvantages of using the transmastoid route include the need for packing the mastoid cavity with abdominal fat.

Middle fossa vestibular nerve section is an intracranial approach whereby a window of bone from the squamous temporal area is temporarily removed and the internal auditory canal is unroofed. The vestibular nerves are then cut; this procedure yields a better than 90% chance of relief of vertigo. There is a small chance of hearing loss, temporal lobe injury, and cerebrospinal fluid leakage and a very real possibility of transient facial nerve paralysis. The middle fossa approach may be used in a patient with a radical mastoid cavity or chronic otitis media.

The retrolabyrinthine approach involves removal of bone between the posterior semicircular canal and the sigmoid sinus, dissection along the posterior petrous bone, and section of the vestibular nerves at the cerebellopontine angle. An abdominal fat graft is used to fill the mastoid cavity. This technique is faster and easier than the middle fossa approach and associated with less hearing loss and less facial paralysis. There is a lower (70% to 90%) chance of relief of vertigo with this procedure, perhaps because it is more difficult to visualize a distinct cleavage plane between the vestibular and cochlear nerves near the medial internal auditory canal. The possibility of cerebrospinal fluid leakage is somewhat higher with this technique.

The retrosigmoid internal auditory canal approach was devised to allow better visualization of the cleavage plane between the cochlear and vestibular nerves. Bone is temporarily removed from behind the sigmoid sinus and the cerebellum is decompressed and retracted medially. The posterior wall of the internal auditory canal is removed, and the vestibular nerves are sectioned. This method affords a higher cure rate and a smaller chance of cerebrospinal fluid leakage than does the retrolabyrinthine approach, but it takes more time and involves more risk to the labyrinth. The chances of postoperative facial weakness are greater because the facial nerve must be dissected off the vestibular nerve. This operation should not be performed on elderly patients, on patients with neck stiffness or headaches, or on patients who have radiographic demonstration of a high-riding jugular bulb. Many patients complain of severe, long-standing headaches after this procedure.

TREATMENT OF VERTIGO IN GENERAL

As outlined earlier, the treatment of vertigo should be directed toward the specific cause. At times, however, a definitive diagnosis cannot be made, and nonspecific therapy must be instituted. In general, it is wise to discuss with the patient general lifestyle measures that may help alleviate the symptoms of vertigo. Included among these are judicious diet, sufficient rest, and exercise. Avoidance of undue stress, alcohol, tobacco, excessive salt, and caffeine is also indicated. Changes at the workplace may be necessary to prevent accidents by employees with vertigo who are required to operate heavy machinery. Some benefit may be attained in some cases of position-oriented vertigo by having the patient purposefully reproduce the activity that precipitates the vertigo.

Several medications are available to help relieve vertigo. Included among these are the tranquilizers diazepam and droperidol, which are especially valuable in relieving acute attacks. Little is known about the mode of action by these drugs in relieving vertigo, but it is believed that the effect probably occurs in the central nervous system. Diazepam in addition appears to have a direct depressant effect on the vestibular nuclei. Vasodilators (smooth muscle relaxers) are especially beneficial in cases of atherosclerotic vascular disease and cases of central vertigo.

Anticholinergic agents are effective in controlling vertigo and motion sickness. Again, the specific site of activity is unknown, but these drugs probably affect the central nervous system. Scopolamine may be delivered transcutaneously or sublingually to alleviate symptoms. Patients should be warned of the possibility of blurred vision, dry mouth, and palpitations in association with these medications.

Antihistamines (meclizine, diphenhydramine) also appear to have anticholinergic properties whose site of action is probably the central nervous system. This class of drugs is very effective in reducing vertigo, nausea, and vomiting. Drowsiness is a frequent side effect of the antihistamines that makes this class of drug unpopular with many patients.

Vestibulotoxic drugs, such as the aminoglycoside antibiotics, can be given to patients with bilateral disease or disease in only the hearing ear to ablate the vestibular end organ. Streptomycin and gentamicin are ototoxic agents that usually affect vestibular function before hearing. Both drugs may be given systemically or by infusion into the middle ear. Drug levels and renal function should be carefully monitored with this type of therapy. These drugs have also been administered intratympanically with some success.

Surgical therapy may be indicated by a specific type of underlying disease, or it may be indicated when the cause of vertigo is nonspecific. As mentioned earlier, stapedectomy occasionally relieves vertigo associated with a vestibular focus of otospongiosis, and singular nerve section has been effective in alleviating benign paroxysmal positional vertigo. Endolymphatic sac decompression procedures are thought to help resolve vertigo by equalizing pressure within the endolymphatic space. Vestibular neurectomy reduces end organ imput and allows relief of vertigo in a large percentage of cases. Labyrinthectomy may be carried out when preservation of hearing is not a consideration.

SUGGESTED READINGS

Baloh WB, Sloane PD, Honrubia V: Quantitative vestibular function testing in elderly patients with dizziness. Ear Nose Throat J 68:935–939, 1989.

Belal A: Dandy's syndrome. Am J Otol 1:151–156, 1980.

Black FO, Peterka RJ, Elardo SM: Vestibular reflex changes following aminoglycoside induced ototoxicity. Laryngoscope 97:582–586, 1987.

Brown JJ, Baloh RW: Persistent mal de debarquement syndrome. Am J Otolaryngol 8:219–222, 1987.

Busis SN: Diagnostic evaluation of the patient presenting with vertigo. Otolaryngol Clin North Am 6:3–23, 1973.

Clemis JD: Cochleovestibular disorders and allergy. Otolaryngol Clin North Am 7:757–780, 1974.

Filipo R, Lazzari R, Barbara M, Franzese A, Petruzzellis MC: Psychologic evaluation of patients with Ménière's disease in relation to therapy. Am J Otol 9:306–309, 1988.

Harker LA, Rassekh CH: Episodic vertigo in basilar artery migraine. Otolaryngol Head Neck Surgery 96:239–250, 1987.

Harrison MS, Dix MR: Vestibular neuronitis. In Dix MR, Hood JD (eds): Vertigo (pp. 167–176). New York: John Wiley, 1984.

Healy GF, Friedman JM, Strong MS: Vestibular and auditory findings of perilymph fistula: a review of 40 cases. Trans Am Acad Ophthalmol Otol 82:44–49, 1976.

Hughes GB: Current controversies in autoimmune inner ear disease. Insights Otolaryngol 2(6), 1987.

Jackler RK, De La Cruz A: The large vestibular aqueduct syndrome. Laryngoscope 99:1238–1243, 1989.

McCabe BF, Gantz BJ: Vascular loop as a cause of incapacitating dizziness. Am J Otology 10:117–120, 1989.

Schuknecht HF: Cupulolithiasis. Arch Otolaryngol 90:113–126, 1969.

Silverstein H, Norell H, Haberkamp T: A comparison of retrosigmoid IAC, retrolabyrinthine, and middle fossa vestibular neurectomy for treatment of vertigo. Laryngoscope 97:165–173, 1987.

Sloane PD, Balch RW, Honrubia V: The vestibular system in the elderly. Am J Otolaryngol 10:422–429, 1989.

Vermeersch H, Meyerhoff WL, Boothby R: Vertigo. In Meyerhoff WL (ed): Diagnosis and Management of Hearing Loss (pp 105–125). Philadelphia: WB Saunders, 1987.

CHAPTER 20

Tinnitus

William L. Meyerhoff, MD, PhD   Brock D. Ridenour, MD

The word *tinnitus* (tĭ-nī′təs) is derived from the Latin verb *tinnire*, "to jingle." In the past, tinnitus aurium has been used to designate sounds perceived to originate from one or both ears, whereas *tinnitus cranii* (cerebri) has been used to describe sound that is nonlocalized or sensed within the head. The present usage of the word tinnitus is more inclusive, however, and refers to an auditory perception of internal origin that is undesirable and annoying to the patient but rarely heard by others.

Random sampling of the population reveals that almost 40 million Americans suffer from sustained periods of tinnitus and that approximately 20% of these people sense a serious decrease in the quality of their life as a result of this affliction. Significant sleep disturbance is reported by 16 million tinnitus sufferers in the United States alone, and approximately 1 million Americans with tinnitus are virtually incapacitated by their symptoms. The almost ubiquitous nature of tinnitus is well recognized, and the complete absence of tinnitus is considered quite rare. Approximately 95% of individuals experience some form of auditory perception when they are placed in an anechoic chamber. Speculation regarding the source of this phenomenon includes the resting discharge of cochlear hair cells, the molecular motion of air within the middle ear or anechoic chamber, and the presence of circulating blood in or near the organ of Corti. Fortunately, most people are not conscious of their tinnitus because of the masking effect of ambient noise. Although tinnitus is known to occur in all age groups, the majority of sufferers are between the ages of 40 and 80 years. In one study, tinnitus

was found to be present in approximately 25% of healthy elderly patients with no history of noise exposure, ototoxic medications, or systemic disease. As a rule, males and females are equally affected. Although the prevalence of tinnitus in the pediatric population is difficult to assess, previous estimates have most likely understated the problem. Of all the aural symptoms, tinnitus has the capacity to be the most devastating. This distressing situation may affect concentration, productivity, and interpersonal relationships. Patients experience anxiety, frustration, insecurity, and despair. Of patients complaining of severe tinnitus, approximately one third have been shown to demonstrate criteria for the diagnosis of major depression. The occasional patient considers suicide.

Approximately 50% of patients with tinnitus localize the noise to a specific ear, whereas the remaining 50% identify the sound as coming from both ears or the head in general. Approximately 25% of patients describe tinnitus in a simple form such as a pure tone. The majority (70%) of all sufferers describe their tinnitus as steam escaping, ringing, or buzzing. Still others describe their tinnitus in terms of more complex or diversified sounds such as the ocean rumble or the chirping of a cricket. In a study of noise-induced tinnitus with human volunteers, George and Kemp (1989) essentially confirmed these statistics. Approximately 22% of the study patients noted a tonal quality to their tinnitus, whereas 78% described their perceived sound as noisy or complex. Most patients experience tinnitus of a constant duration; however, tinnitus may be intermittent or pulsatile with fluctuations in intensity and quality, depending on the etiologic factor. Tinnitus must be differentiated from auditory hallucinations, which are more complex sounds, such as voices and music, and which suggest drug intoxication or psychiatric disturbance. It must also be distinguished from autophony, the hearing of one's own voice and respiratory sounds as a result of a conductive hearing loss or a patulous eustachian tube.

In an attempt to better classify tinnitus, matching techniques have been employed to gain useful objective information not available in the patient's history. The major problem in successfully matching tinnitus is having available a sufficient variety of sound stimuli so that a match can be found. Basic audiometers provide tones of an octave or a half-octave and are capable of generating at least one form of noise. More complex models may have, in addition, several noises (white, complex or sawtooth, speech spectrum, or narrow band), warble tones, and continuously variable tones and noises. Many matching techniques involve the use of a predetermined set of frequencies that are presented to the patient at approximately 10 db above measured threshold. The subject is required to choose the frequency most similar to the perceived tinnitus. The next presentation includes the patient's frequency choice from the previous trial along with a different (modified) choice at the opposite end of the frequency spectrum. This bracketing sequence continues until the pitch of the patient's tinnitus is approximated. A specific tinnitus match may then be made by use of a pulsed monaural tone; the final frequency adjustments are controlled by the patient. A series of consecutive frequency matches is then completed.

Previous reports by Burns (1984) and Penner (1987) have shown that considerable variation may occur in a series of pitch matches made by a patient with subjective tinnitus. The average standard deviation measured by these investigators varied from 15% to 20%. Penner (1983) stressed the importance of checking each pitch match for the possibility of octave confusion. After the spectrum of external sound best matching the pitch of the tinnitus has been determined, a determination of loudness level is made. Loudness matching in decibels above threshold (sensation level) is performed at a frequency corresponding to the pitch of the tinnitus.

Matching tinnitus to an external sound results in a frequency range from near 0 Hz to over 10,000 Hz with a fairly even distribution and a peak incidence between 3000 and 5000 Hz. More than 80% of patients with tinnitus demonstrate an identifiable band width of 2400 Hz or less. In his audiometric study of 200 patients, Reed (1960) found that tinnitus associated with conductive hearing loss tended to be of lower frequency than was that associated with sensorineural hearing loss. He also noted that patients with low-frequency or narrow-band tinnitus generally experienced a greater loudness of tinnitus than did their respective counterparts. The determination of band width and objective loudness, however, was not found to correlate with diagnosis, type of deafness, or site of origin.

Other investigators have begun quantifying tinnitus by use of the loudness balance procedure as previously outlined. In a large study by Meikle and colleagues (1984), 79% of patients had loudness matches concentrated in a narrow range between 0 and 6 db. The low magnitude of the tinnitus is especially surprising because these patients were symptomatic and attended a large tinnitus clinic. Comparing the objective magnitude of their tinnitus with a subjective severity scale showed no correlation; more than 50% of the patients rated their tinnitus as severe. Previous studies have confirmed this lack of agreement between perceived severity and loudness. Pitch was also found to have no influence on perceived severity, and surprisingly, patients with constant tinnitus did not judge their tinnitus to be more severe than did patients with intermittent symptoms. However, some correlation with perceived severity was noted in patients with duration of tinnitus greater than 5 years and in patients demonstrating complex tinnitus consisting of four to five distinct entities.

Several investigators have noted that conventional methods for loudness matching may be flawed by the measurement of loudness at a frequency corresponding to the patient's tinnitus. Because patients frequently have a significant hearing loss in this region, loudness matching is likely to be influenced by the presence of recruitment. In the presence of an abnormal growth of loudness, small changes in sensation level may represent an inordinately rapid growth in perceived loudness. A proposed alternative method is to perform loudness matching at a frequency in which the patient's hearing is normal. Proponents of this method feel that loudness measured in this fashion is more likely to be consistent with severity as perceived by the patient. Against this recruitment theory, however, is a study by George and Kemp (1989) in which noise-induced tinnitus was measured in normal-hearing patients. The phenomenon of recruitment was eliminated in this study because no subjects displayed elevated tone thresholds. Again, no correlation was found between the matched loudness of tinnitus and severity as perceived by the patient.

Although many tinnitus sufferers do not complain of hearing loss, the majority have an identifiable impairment in hearing. The basis for this paradox comes from the preservation of hearing in the speech frequencies. In other situations, such as listening to music, the listener may have control of the spectral composition of the signal or may be uninterested or inattentive to imbalances. The perceived pitch of tinnitus associated with sensorineural hearing loss often lies within a region approximately one third down the sloping audiometric curve. There is lack of agreement as to whether the frequency of tinnitus corresponds to the frequency of maximal hearing loss. There does appear to be some relationship in certain cases of identifiable cause, such as noise-induced hearing loss in which increased auditory thresholds and tinnitus both occur in the high frequencies. Similarly, early in the course of Meniere's disease, both hearing loss and tinnitus tend to be in the low frequencies.

ETIOLOGY

There are nearly as many proposed classification systems for tinnitus as there are suggested forms of treatment. A site-of-lesion classification system may be helpful in guiding a systematic evaluation of a patient. Another useful classification proposed by Fowler (1944) divides tinnitus into vibratory and nonvibratory forms (Table 20–1). Vibratory tinnitus is that caused by real sound, mechanical in origin, arising within or in proximity to the ear. Vibratory tinnitus is frequently objective, which signifies that it may be heard by an observer, with or without the aid of amplification. Nonvibratory tinnitus

TABLE 20–1. Tinnitus

Vibratory
  Vascular disorders
    Arteriovenous malformation
    Carotid occlusive disease
    Aneurysm
    Venous hum
    Glomus tumor
    Dehiscent jugular bulb
    Persistent stapedial artery
    Abnormal mastoid emissary vein
    Arteriovenous fistula
    Benign intracranial hypertension
    Paget's disease
  Neuromuscular
    Palatal myoclonus
    Stapedial muscle spasm
    Tensor tympani muscle spasm
    Temporomandibular joint dysfunction
  Miscellaneous
    Patulous eustachian tube
    Middle ear inflammation or cholesteatoma
    Spontaneous otoacoustic emissions (SOAEs)
Nonvibratory
  Peripheral
    External auditory canal
    Middle ear
    Cochlea
  Central
    Auditory nerve
    Brain stem
    Central auditory pathways

does not result from real sound generation but is the manifestation of neural excitation from within the auditory system. Nonvibratory tinnitus can be divided into peripheral and central types, depending on the site of origin. Nonvibratory tinnitus is always subjective, which means that it can be heard only by the patient.

Vibratory tinnitus generally has a more easily identifiable cause than does nonvibratory tinnitus and therefore has a more rational basis for treatment. Pathologic states responsible for vibratory tinnitus are usually vascular or neuromuscular in nature or result from an abnormally patent eustachian tube. Work by Penner (1988) provided good evidence that spontaneous otoacoustic emissions may, in some instances, be responsible for the presence of annoying vibratory tinnitus. When the source of vibratory tinnitus produces sufficient mechanical energy to be heard by others, tinnitus becomes objective. If energy is insufficient, however, tinnitus remains subjective. Nonvibratory tinnitus, although more common than vibratory tinnitus, is not as well understood and has a more obscure origin. Nonvibratory tinnitus may be simply classified, however, according to the anatomic site of origin. Peripheral mechanisms relate to the cochlea and auditory nerve; central processes involve the brain stem and higher auditory pathways.

Vibratory Tinnitus

Regional vascular disorders with associated increased turbulent blood flow often result in tinnitus as the first or most prominent symptom. Transmission of turbulent sound energy through the skull is believed to occur in some patients with critical stenotic lesions of the common or internal carotid vessels. Occasionally, tinnitus may occur contralateral to these lesions as a result of an intracranial steal phenomenon or through compensatory blood flow in the opposite system. Arteriovenous malformations involving the supratentorial and infratentorial meningeal vessels frequently demonstrate outflow through the lateral sinus and are another source of vascular tinnitus (Figs. 20–1, 20–2). These lesions must be distinguished from vascular neoplasms (Fig. 20–3) (paraganglio-

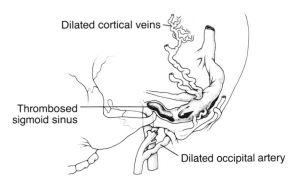

Figure 20–2. Schematic representation of the arteriovenous malformation shown in Figure 20–1. Note the dilation and immediate filling of the lateral sinus. (Courtesy of Peter Roland, MD.)

mas), aneurysmal dilations, severe high-output anemias, thyrotoxicosis, abnormal mastoid emissary veins, aberrant vessels (internal carotid, persistent stapedial artery, dehiscent jugular bulb), middle ear inflammation, Paget's disease, or arteriovenous fistula following trauma. All can create enough mechanical energy to result in the auditory perception of sound. Tinnitus in such cases is frequently

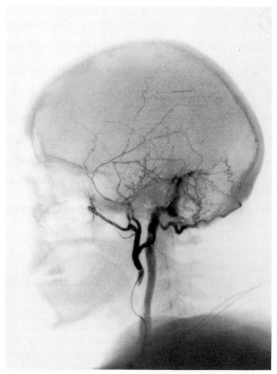

Figure 20–1. Arteriovenous malformation demonstrating supratentorial and infratentorial feeding vessels from the external carotid artery. (Courtesy of Peter Roland, MD.)

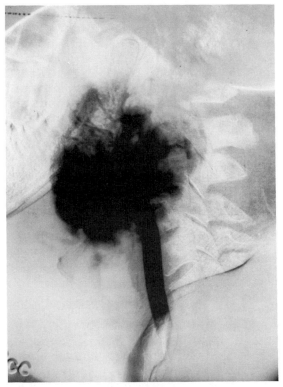

Figure 20–3. Arteriogram demonstrating a large glomus tumor of the lateral neck and skull base. (Courtesy of Peter Roland, MD.)

pulsatile and synchronous with the heart beat. Another not too infrequent cause of pulsatile tinnitus is benign intracranial hypertension. This is often a diagnosis of exclusion and typically occurs in obese women presenting with headache, nausea, vomiting, diplopia, and transient visual obscurations. Diagnosis is confirmed on the basis of increased intracranial pressure and normal cerebrospinal fluid constituents with no evidence for ventricular enlargement or an intracranial mass. Tinnitus is attributed to turbulent blood flow in the jugular bulb in the presence of elevated interstitial fluid pressures, and therefore ipsilateral jugular vein compression diminishes tinnitus. Vibratory tinnitus may also arise as a result of the interference of laminar flow in the jugular vein as it curves around the lateral process of the atlas. Turning the head toward the affected side or applying pressure over the carotid sheath frequently decreases or eliminates tinnitus originating in this fashion and aids in the diagnosis. Ipsilateral internal jugular vein ligation can be performed in severe cases; however, the efficacy of this procedure has not been determined. Hentzer (1968) followed 13 patients with venous hum tinnitus over a 15-year period. In five patients, tinnitus resolved spontaneously, whereas only one of four surgical patients demonstrated long-term benefit.

Clonic muscular contractions of the tensor tympani, stapedius, tensor veli palatini, or levator veli palatini muscles may result in a clicking sound that can be heard by the patient and the examiner alike. This sound usually has a rate faster than the corresponding pulse and may demonstrate a wide range of activity, averaging between 40 and 200 contractions per minute. Occasionally, this form of tinnitus may be altered by a conscious effort on the patient's behalf. Movement of the tympanic membrane or palate may be observed and recorded by tympanometry or electromyography, respectively. These recordings are found to be synchronous with the tinnitus. Intracranial neoplasms, cerebrovascular disorders, multiple sclerosis, and psychogenic disorders have all been implicated as underlying causes for these neuromuscular problems. In the absence of an identifiable etiologic factor, this form of tinnitus may be eliminated by surgical lysis of the stapedial tendon and tensor tympani muscle. Finally, tinnitus may occur as a result of stapedius contraction that is simultaneous with movement of mimetic musculature. This has been observed as a sequela of Bell's palsy in which misdirection occurs between nerve fibers innervating stapedial and mimetic muscles. Yamamoto (1985) measured auditory threshold shifts and middle ear compliance changes during voluntary facial movement by these patients.

The eustachian tube, which is normally closed, may become abnormally patent or patulous. The nasopharyngeal air turbulence of respiration may then be transmitted through the patent eustachian tube, which results in another form of vibratory tinnitus. Otoscopy and tympanometry reveal respiratory-associated tympanic membrane movements. This condition may result in autophony and is generally seen after a large and rapid weight loss, in patients using birth control pills or other forms of estrogens, or during the postpartum period. Placing the head in a dependent position may cause local venous engorgement and closure of the eustachian tube, with resultant temporary cessation of symptoms. Autophony may be relieved by placement of tragal cartilage in the tympanic orifice of the eustachian tube. However, middle ear effusion may be a complication of this procedure. Finally, developments in otoacoustic emissions have led to the discovery of another potential source of vibratory tinnitus. Otoacoustic emissions are believed to represent an aspect of cochlear biomechanical processing that is responsible for the high sensitivity, sharp tuning, and wide dynamic range of the human ear.

Spontaneous otoacoustic emissions (SOAEs) represent one recognized form of these unusual acoustic energies and can be detected by inserting a miniature microphone in the external auditory meatus. Studies have shown that anywhere from 28% to 50% of men and 56% to 70% of women have measurable SOAEs, the great majority of which are not implied in the pathogenesis of tinnitus. Penner (1988) showed by deductive reasoning that SOAEs may be linked to the presence of annoying tinnitus in rare patients, if strict criteria are applied. Patients should demonstrate tinnitus matching that correlates closely with the recorded frequency of the SOAEs (2% to 3% variability). Suppression of all tinnitus should be anticipated when a 20-db frequency-specific (same-frequency SOAE) masking tone is used but not when a 90-db pure tone of unrelated frequency is applied. Finally, the subjective loudness of tinnitus in either ear should correspond to measured values of the SOAEs. Identifying patients with tinnitus related to SOAEs may have important therapeutic applications, because SOAEs are abolished by the simple administration of salicylates. More recently, Penner (1990) estimated the prevalence of SOAE-related tinnitus to be approximately 4% among a group of 96 volunteer tinnitus sufferers.

Nonvibratory Tinnitus

Many disorders have been associated with nonvibratory tinnitus, and most entail associated hearing loss at the cochlear level (Table 20–2). Among the most common causes of tinnitus and associated sensorineural hearing loss are those produced by aging, vascular changes, and past noise exposure. However, the understanding of this symptom is far from complete and has led to considerable speculation into the possible sites of origin and pathophysiologic mechanisms of this phenomenon. It appears that nonvibratory tinnitus may arise spontaneously from aberrant neural activity within the auditory pathways and may occur independently of auditory stimulation. This abnormal neuronal

TABLE 20–2. Nonvibratory Tinnitus

Bell's palsy
Benzodiazepine withdrawal
Conductive hearing loss
Labyrinthitis
  Allergic
  Viral
  Bacterial
  Spirochetal
Medications
Meniere's disease
Metabolic disorders
  Diabetes mellitus
  Hypothyroidism
Middle ear inflammation
Otosclerosis
Perilymph fistula
Presbycusis
Trauma
  Head
  Acoustic
Tumor
  Facial nerve neuroma
  Eighth nerve tumor
  Temporal lobe neoplasm
Vascular insufficiency
Vitamin or trace metal deficiency
Vascular compression of the cochleovestibular nerve

activity may be interpreted by higher cortical centers as sound.

A neurogenic cause for tinnitus of middle ear origin was first hypothesized by Lempert (1946), and this formed the basis for a procedure aimed at removing the tympanic plexus (tympanosympathectomy). Lempert postulated that certain patients with chronic ear infection could experience tinnitus as a result of a ganglionitis of the tympanic plexus. Inflammatory, electrical, or chemical stimulation of the plexus was believed to result in tonic impulse transmissions to the inner ear through the round and oval window. Of 15 patients treated by tympanosympathectomy, 10 were reported to experience complete relief of their tinnitus. Tsyganov (1968), in an attempt to reproduce Lempert's results, was able to achieve reduction of tinnitus in 50% of his patients by chemically lysing the tympanic plexus. Trowbridge (1949) also believed in an intimate connection among the glossopharyngeal, trigeminal, and sympathetic fibers of the tympanic plexus and the inner ear. He believed that pathologic changes of the middle ear or neighboring structures could result in impulse formation in the tympanic plexus and lead to tinnitus or, in cases of more intense stimulation, pain. This proposed pathophysiologic process could explain tinnitus associated with Costen's syndrome. This syndrome is poorly understood and includes temporomandibular joint dysfunction with associated pain, limitation of motion, headache, tenderness over the muscles of mastication, joint crepitus, and, in about 25% of the cases, the aural symptoms of tinnitus, hearing loss, otalgia, and disequilibrium. Treatment directed toward the joint dysfunction itself usually relieves or reduces the aural symptoms.

According to another hypothesis, nonvibratory tinnitus may result from increased spontaneous activity of auditory neurons as a result of hyperactivity of cochlear hair cells. Such hyperactivity was the basis for the leaky hair cell theory of Davis (1954): that injured hair cells have an increased spontaneous firing rate. Similarly, Bredberg and colleagues (1972) demonstrated noise-induced morphologic changes in the stereocilia of experimental cats that were postulated to result in decoupling between hair cells and the tectorial membrane. Partial decoupling of only a small segment of the basilar membrane could theoretically result in a tonal or narrow-band tinnitus, whereas broad-band tinnitus may result from longer regions of partial decoupling. Tonndorf (1976) expanded this theory to explain the generation of tinnitus in patients with Meniere's disease. He reasoned that during an acute episode of endolymphatic hydrops, the static displacement of the basilar membrane produces a shearing displacement between hair cells (stereocilia) and the overlying tectorial membrane. Because displacement is greatest in the apical region, decoupling in this segment should result in low-frequency noise production (roaring), which is typical among patients with Meniere's disease.

If increased spontaneous cochlear (hair cell) activity is to be implied in the etiology of tinnitus, then peripheral destructive procedures such as labyrinthectomy and cochleovestibular nerve section should ameliorate tinnitus. Several authors including House and Brackmann (1981) observed that tinnitus may persist in certain patients despite these ablative procedures. This has led to support for the concept of central tinnitus. According to this theory, the site of tinnitus may begin peripherally and later induce long-term changes in central activity that cannot be corrected with cochlear nerve sectioning. This mechanism for tinnitus generation has been compared with the development of "phantom limb" pain that develops after the removal of the limb.

Another proposed theory for explaining nonvibratory tinnitus has been developed in an animal model by Sasaki and associates (1981). They hypothesized that functional cochlear integrity is necessary for maintaining appropriate central inhibitory influences with the auditory system. When afferent auditory signals are altered by pathologic changes at the cochlear level, inhibitory influences are diminished and secondary auditory neurons are released into tonic hyperactivity (deafferentation). The authors used C-2-deoxyglucose as a method of mapping cellular metabolism in the brain. After cochlear nerve sectioning in the guinea pig, Kauer and coworkers (1982) found an early reduction in neural activity in auditory nuclei connected to the lesioned ear. A paradoxical increase in activity of these auditory nuclei was later noted after a latency of 3 to 14 days. They suggest that this may be analogous to the pathogenesis of tinnitus in the human being. If such is the case, patients with tinnitus are not very dissimilar from patients who have suffered injury to other sensory nerves and, after healing, experienced pain. This pain (tinnitus) is thought to result from spontaneous discharge from deafferented secondary neurons.

Finally, a small number of patients may experience nonvibratory tinnitus as the result of vascular compression of the cochlear division of cranial nerve VIII. Jannetta (1967) introduced the concept of vascular decompression for cranial nerve maladies. He theorized that mechanical compression of a cranial nerve at the nerve entry zone by elongated arteries may occur after sagging of the brain with aging, with resultant hyperactivity dysfunction of that nerve (ephaptic conduction or short-circuiting). It is known from previous studies that compression of cranial nerves is more likely to be symptomatic when it occurs proximal to the Obersteiner-Redlich zone, where axons are insulated by central myelin produced by oligodendroglia. Because the transition zone for cranial nerve VIII is in the auditory meatus, the entire intracranial portion of cranial nerve VIII is sensitive to compression.

The lack of total understanding of nonvibratory tinnitus is evidenced by its multiple and varied explanations. The literature is concerned primarily with clinical and theoretical impressions and has little factual basis. This may be partially explained by the fact that tinnitus is primarily a subjective complaint for which objective indicators are usually sparse and also the fact that a proven animal model has been difficult to develop.

PATIENT EVALUATION

The evaluation of a patient with tinnitus begins with a thorough history. Attempts should be made to ascertain the age of onset, mode of progression, family history, and association with hearing loss, vertigo, and aural fullness. Subjective information should be collected regarding the location of the tinnitus, its pitch, the relative complexity (pure tone, complex), the pattern (continuous, intermittent, pulsatile, clicking, blowing), the intensity, and the duration. The effect of ambient noise on intensity should be noted, and a subjective severity scale should be administered. This information is important for epidemiologic considerations and for providing an accurate description of the patient's symptoms and response to therapy. To date, no correlation has been made between the patient's subjective description of the tinnitus and the underlying etiologic factor or site of lesion.

Additional history should include information regarding any aural discharge, head injury, noise exposure, previous ear surgery, or exposure to ototoxic drugs. The patient should be asked about possible precipitating events (e.g., Valsalva's maneuver) and signs and symptoms of any disorder with which tinnitus is known to be an associated symptom. A thorough drug history with specific reference to the ingestion of new medications, quinine, and nonsteroidal anti-inflammatory drugs or to the recent cessation of benzodiazepine usage is essential. A complete neuro-otologic and head and neck examination should be performed, with special emphasis on auscultation of the mastoid tip, ear, skull, and neck. Sismanis (1989) encouraged the use of a modified electronic stethoscope (auscultoscope) as a routine procedure on patients with pulsatile tinnitus. Inspection of the auricle, external auditory canal, and tympanic membrane should be completed along with tuning fork examination and pneumatic otoscopy. Patients should be screened for hypertension and evidence of cardiovascular disease.

A wide range of diagnostic modalities is available for the study of patients with tinnitus. In patients demonstrating audible tinnitus (objective) or in patients whose history and physical examination suggest an underlying mechanical basis, specific testing should be undertaken to identify the responsible process. Angiography confirms the presence of vascular anomalies, stenotic segments, or tumors. Tympanometry helps to identify subtle changes in tympanic membrane compliance or myoclonus of the stapedial muscle, the tensor tympani muscle, or the muscles of the palate. Once myoclonus has been identified, the etiologic factor should be searched for (intracranial neoplasm, multiple sclerosis, cerebrovascular disorders, psychogenic causes). Audiometric assessment is essential for the patient suffering nonvibratory tinnitus. Pure-tone audiometry should be performed; however, atypical patients with normal octave and semioctave audiometry may have a localized hearing loss detected only with the use of sweep frequency von Békésy audiometry. The discovery of a hearing loss warrants evaluation and management as though hearing loss were a coexistent complaint. More serious disease is suggested by the presence of unilateral, asymmetric, fluctuating, or progressive hearing loss. Tympanometry should be performed, and speech discrimination should be tested in and out of noise. The short increment sensitivity index and alternate binaural loudness balance may be used to demonstrate recruitment, which suggests a cochlear site of lesion. Retrocochlear disease may be implied in the patient who experiences rapid tone decay, absent stapedial reflexes, and an abnormal auditory brain stem response.

Further investigations into known causes of tinnitus should be dictated by the index of suspicion aroused by the history, the physical examination, and the audiometric profile. Electronystagmography and platform posturography may demonstrate simultaneous pathologic processes of the vestibular system. Electrocochleography has been useful in the diagnosis of Meniere's disease and may have some application in patients suspected of having perilymph fistula. Measurement of SOAEs may prove helpful in patients with normal hearing and complaints of low-frequency tinnitus; however, this procedure is not yet widely accepted.

Metabolic disorders should be considered, and laboratory data should include a complete blood count, thyroid function tests, and a measure of fasting blood glucose levels. All patients should have a serologic test for syphilis. Pfister (1989) concluded that late neurologic manifestations resembling neurosyphilis, including the development of tinnitus, may develop in Lyme's borreliosis. Testing for antibodies against *Borrelia burgdorferi* should be considered in patients with suggestive histories. Computed axial tomography demonstrates many intracranial neoplasms and offers detail of the tympanic cavity, petrous bone, and skull base. Magnetic resonance imaging offers superior visualization of tumors involving the facial nerve and the cerebellopontine angle. Use of the contrast agent gadolinium enhances the sensitivity of this modality. Tinnitus matching (pitch and loudness) is important in patients thought to have tinnitus from SOAEs and in those patients considered candidates for therapeutic masking. Psychoacoustic testing (frequency and loudness matching) may also be used to assess the effect of various treatment modalities such as biofeedback. A Minnesota Multiphasic Personality Inventory and a psychologic evaluation as proposed by

House (1978) may have prognostic as well as diagnostic value for some patients.

TREATMENT

When discussing tinnitus, it is important to realize that tinnitus is a symptom and not a disease. Therefore, no single modality of treatment is expected to be successful in all patients. Many patients have already compensated for their tinnitus in a healthy and socially acceptable fashion and require little or no additional treatment. In most cases, all that is needed is a thorough explanation and reassurance against a more serious illness. However, other patients require treatment in order to be brought to a functional level. No patient should ever be told that the situation is hopeless or that no helpful treatment is readily available.

Several therapeutic modalities are available to the patient, not all of which are mutually exclusive and none of which offers a panacea. They include various medications, surgery, hearing aids, masking devices, biofeedback, hypnosis, acupuncture, psychotherapy, and electric stimulation. It must be remembered that patients with tinnitus do have a perplexing problem, and even if a treatable cause is not uncovered, these patients should not be abandoned.

Surgical Therapy

Surgical therapy plays a role in the treatment of most forms of vibratory tinnitus as well as in space-occupying lesions of the cerebellopontine angle, temporal lobe neoplasms, perilymph fistula, vascular compression of the cochlear nerve, and conductive hearing loss. The results of many neuro-otologic procedures on tinnitus have been discovered serendipitously while the procedures were being directed primarily at control of vertigo and tumor removal. At present, there is little evidence in the otologic or neuro-otologic literature to suggest the efficacy of surgical treatment aimed primarily at the treatment of tinnitus. An exception to this rule, however, may exist in the patient with suspected vascular compression of the cochleovestibular nerve bundle.

Vibratory tinnitus resulting from arteriovenous malformation, carotid occlusive disease, vascular tumor, and traumatic arterio-venous fistula usually resolves after successful management of the underlying pathologic process. Accordingly, Gardner (1984) reported a 61% improvement in tinnitus after the resection of large glomus tumors with skull base involvement; an 83% improvement was achieved for tumors confined to the middle ear space. Somewhat less predictable results can be anticipated in tinnitus that is frequently associated with otosclerosis. A successful stapedectomy can now be performed in over 90% of cases; however, an improvement in tinnitus has been reported in only 35% to 75% of oval window surgery.

In Meniere's disease, surgical treatment results are difficult to assess in light of the fluctuating natural history of the disease process. Operations on the endolymphatic sac, stellate ganglion sympathectomy, and intermittent repetitive sacculotomy have all provided relief of tinnitus in 30% to 50% of patients with Meniere's disease. Labyrinthectomy alone sacrifices hearing and has demonstrated very poor results with regard to tinnitus control (8% to 16%). Selective vestibular nerve section in a patient with useful hearing can be performed through either a middle fossa or a retrolabyrinthine approach with a 50% chance of improving tinnitus. Why this procedure is effective for tinnitus in some patients remains uncertain; however, success may be explained by the presence of cochleovestibular anastomotic fibers and cochlear efferent fibers in the vestibular nerve. Translabyrinthine vestibular neurectomy also sacrifices hearing and is effective in approximately 50% of patients with Meniere's disease with tinnitus. Several authors have shown figures supporting the view that translabyrinthine section of both the cochlear and vestibular nerves results in an improved chance of controlling tinnitus while decreasing the risk of worsening tinnitus (Fisch, 1976; Glasscock et al., 1980; House and Brackmann, 1981; Silverstein et al., 1986). This suggests that patients with incapacitating vertigo, profound sensorineural hearing loss, and complaints of tinnitus should be considered for cochleovestibular nerve section. Some caution should be exercised, however, because sectioning of the cochlear nerve prohibits future use of other modes of therapy such as a cochlear implant.

Although translabyrinthine acoustic neuroma surgery is essentially equivalent to a cochleovestibular neurectomy, the results for tinnitus are less reliable, and in a large percentage of patients, the procedure may result in a worsening of symptoms. House and Brackmann (1981) reviewed 500 patients who underwent translabyrinthine tumor removal and found that whereas 40% of patients improved after surgery, 50% complained of worsening tinnitus. Gardner (1984) reported that 62% of patients improved after tumor removal; Silverstein and colleagues (1986) noted only a 25% improvement rate. Results for tinnitus appear to be similar regardless of whether the cochlear nerve is left intact during surgery.

In 1981, Jannetta reported 11 patients who underwent vascular decompression of cranial nerve VIII solely for the management of tinnitus. Five of 11 patients were cured or improved by the procedure, whereas six experienced no relief. It is not clear whether these failures resulted from poor selection of patients, central patterning of tinnitus, or failure to allow adequate time for improvement. Meyerhoff and Mickey (1988) reported suggested guidelines for the selection of patients most likely to benefit from this procedure. They suggested that patients must have incapacitating tinnitus associated with unilateral high-frequency sensorineural hearing loss and retrocochlear audiometric findings. Furthermore, patients must have normal psychiatric and neuro-otologic examinations, and magnetic resonance imaging must show no evidence of other disease. With use of these criteria, Meyerhoff and Mickey were successful in the treatment of two patients who were incapacitated by tinnitus.

Tinnitus may also be a prominent symptom in patients with idiopathic perilymph fistula and has been reported by some authors to be present in up to 95% of patients. Data specifically relating the effect of surgical management on tinnitus are not widely available because most patients undergo surgery for hearing loss or balance disorder. These figures will most likely become more available in the near future.

Medical Therapy

A large variety of medications have been advocated for the treatment of tinnitus. Some medications are directed toward the proposed pathophysiologic mechanisms for the production of tinnitus, whereas others are provided to help the patient better tolerate the situation. Agents aimed at increasing blood flow have been advocated on the basis of the theory that end organ or central auditory ischemia may be responsible for some forms of tinnitus. These medications have included adrenergics, adrenergic-blocking agents, antiadrenergics, cholinomimetics, anticholinesterase agents, cholinolytics, smooth muscle relaxants, plasma polypeptides, and vitamins. In a review of the relative efficacy of these medications and their potential benefits and potential side effects, Snow and Suga (1975) concluded that papaverine hydrochloride was the most efficacious in increasing blood flow to the cochlea.

Vitamins, including vitamin A, vitamin C, vitamin B_{12}, and nicotinic acid, and trace metals such as zinc and copper have been suggested for their beneficial effect on vascular integrity. Magnesium sulfate, barbiturates, meprobamate, and reserpine have all been used at some time for their depressant effect on the central nervous system.

Local anesthetics, especially the derivatives of para-aminobenzoic acid (procaine), and the aminoacyl amide group (lidocaine, lignocaine) have been advocated for the treatment of tinnitus on the basis of their ability to decrease sensory activity at a central level. Intravenous administration of these agents has provided reliable temporary improvement in a large majority of patients, although they have no proven therapeutic efficacy in long-term therapy. Their short duration of effect and poor biologic availability with oral administration make these agents impractical. Success with intravenous lidocaine has led to interest in other orally available local anesthetics as well as several anticonvulsive medications and membrane stabilizers. Tocainide, carbamazepine, primidone, aminooxyacetic acid, and taurine have all been used with sporadic success. However, the high incidence of side effects and the inconsistency of results have limited their usage. In one study, the efficacy of transtympanic lignocaine administered by iontophoresis was studied. No benefit from this therapy could be assessed, and there was no evidence for penetration of the middle ear space or circulation by the medication.

Masking

According to Vernon and Schleuning (1978), masking for the relief of tinnitus was mentioned as early as 400 B.C. Masking tinnitus is performed by amplifying environmental noise or by the introduction of artificial noise by a masking device. Hearing aids are a simple form of masking whereby ambient noise is amplified in the frequencies pertaining to hearing loss. Hearing aids have been shown to be of benefit in patients with mild hearing loss, with unilateral hearing loss, and with tinnitus accompanying "burnt-out" cases of Meniere's disease in which a severe to profound sensorineural hearing loss exists.

A tinnitus masker may be tried in patients who do not receive benefit from a standard hearing aid or in patients with annoying tinnitus and normal hearing. Patients with mild tinnitus who are troubled only in quiet environments are often satisfied by the addition of a comforting background noise. Others require the use of a tinnitus masker designed to produce a masking tone or noise corresponding to the measured pitch of the patient's tinnitus. For tinnitus in the range of spectral capability, the masking generator is modified to produce as little noise as necessary for overcoming the tinnitus. Some patients may experience the added benefit of postmasking suppression of their tinnitus, referred to by Feldman (1971) as residual inhibition. This does not occur in all patients and may persist for extremely variable lengths of time. Some patients have found that inexpensive portable radios such as the Sony Walkman may effectively act as maskers, whether recorded noise, tones, or music is used. Masking is not without limitation, however. If tinnitus occurs in the frequency range necessary for speech discrimination, masking may further decrease understanding in an otherwise functional ear. The tinnitus of certain patients is particularly difficult to mask, and the patients are believed to be suffering from tinnitus of a central origin. Experience to date suggests that masking devices benefit approximately 10% to 15% of carefully selected tinnitus sufferers.

Electric Stimulation

Many studies have been performed to assess the effects of electric stimulation on tinnitus. Stimuli consisting of both direct and alternating current have been applied to various sites within the middle ear and the inner ear with varying results. House (1976) gave the first reports of tinnitus being suppressed by a cochlear implant. More recent data have

shown that up to 75% of patients receiving cochlear implantation for profound sensorineural hearing loss may experience incidental relief of tinnitus. Thedinger and associates (1985) reported several patients who underwent placement of cochlear implants specifically for tinnitus. Results in these patients were less promising, however, and caution against the routine use of cochlear implantation for the management of tinnitus.

Biofeedback

In many cases, the disability attributed to tinnitus is related more closely to the patient's psychologic reaction to tinnitus than to the tinnitus itself. The fact that many people with tinnitus function very well suggests that an individual's reaction to a life situation plays an important role.

The purpose of biofeedback is to learn voluntary control of an unconscious or an involuntary process such as stress. The primary focus of biofeedback is on relaxation achieved through teaching the patient to control certain parameters such as skin temperature and muscle tension. By combining relaxation techniques with self-control strategies, patients are better able to develop coping techniques for dealing with this inescapable, adverse condition.

Studies have shown that biofeedback does not result in physiologic alteration of tinnitus, according to psychoacoustic measurements of tinnitus pitch and loudness. Instead, patients are generally more relaxed and confident in their ability to cope with tinnitus. Most patients realize their increased capacity to control problems of sleep, headache, tension, and dizziness.

The results of biofeedback on the treatment of tinnitus are encouraging because they demonstrate that significant relief can be achieved by some patients. Studies have shown that up to 80% of patients treated by biofeedback report improvement; 15% of patients report total relief.

Miscellaneous Therapies

Other therapies for tinnitus have included acupuncture, hypnotherapy, diet, and holistic medicine. Because there exist few therapeutic approaches to tinnitus that can reliably result in alleviation, careful explanation of the symptom with reassurance adds immeasurably to the art of caring for patients. If the physician or the audiologist cannot fulfill these needs, support groups and psychotherapy may be beneficial.

SUGGESTED READINGS

Bredberg G, Ades HW, Engstrom H: Scanning electron microscopy of the normal and pathologically altered organ of Corti. Acta Otolaryngol 301(Suppl):3–48, 1972.

Burns EM: A comparison of variability among measurements of subjective tinnitus and objective stimuli. Audiology 23:426–440, 1984.

Davis H: Tinnitus—new aspects on etiology and management: physiological aspects. Trans Am Acad Ophthalmol Otolaryngol 58:527–528, 1954.

Feldman H: Homolateral and contralateral masking of tinnitus by noise bands and by pure tones. Audiology 10:138–144, 1971.

Fisch U: Surgical treatment of vertigo. J Laryngol Otol 90:75–86, 1976.

Fowler EP: Head noises in normal and in disordered ears. Arch Otolaryngol 39:498–503, 1944.

Gardner G: Neurotologic surgery and tinnitus. J Otolaryngol 9(Suppl):311–318, 1984.

George RN, Kemp S: Investigation of tinnitus induced by sound and its relationship to ongoing tinnitus. J Speech Hear Res 32:366–372, 1989.

Glasscock ME, Davis WE, Hughes GB, Jackson CG: Labyrinthectomy versus middle fossa vestibular nerve section in Meniere's disease. A critical evaluation of relief of vertigo. Ann Otol Rhinol Laryngol 89:318–324, 1980.

Hentzer E: Objective tinnitus of the vascular type. Acta Otolaryngol 66:273–281, 1968.

House JW: Treatment of severe tinnitus with biofeedback training. Laryngoscope 88:406–412, 1978.

House JW, Brackmann DE: Tinnitus: surgical treatment. Ciba Found Symp 85:204–216, 1981.

House WF: Cochlear implants. Ann Otol Rhinol Laryngol 85(Suppl 27):3–93, 1976.

Jannetta PJ: Arterial compression of the trigeminal nerve at the pons in patients with trigeminal neuralgia. J Neurosurg 26:1159–1162, 1967.

Jannetta PJ: Neurovascular compression in cranial nerve and systemic disease. Ann Surg 192:518–525, 1981.

Kauer JS, Nemitz JW, Sasaki CT: Tinnitus aurium: fact . . . or fancy. Laryngoscope 92:1401–1407, 1982.

Lempert J: Tympanosympathectomy. Arch Otolaryngol 43:199–212, 1946.

Meikle MB, Vernon J, Johnson RM: The perceived severity of tinnitus. Otolaryngol Head Neck Surg 92:689–696, 1984.

Meyerhoff WL, Mickey BE: Vascular decompression of the cochlear nerve in tinnitus sufferers. Laryngoscope 98:602–604, 1988.

Meyers D: Tinnitus. Hosp Med 11:55–56; 62–64, May 1975.

Penner MJ: Variability in matches to subjective tinnitus. J Speech Hear Res 26:263–267, 1983.

Penner MJ, Burns EM: The dissociation of SOAEs and tinnitus. J Speech Hear Res 30:396–403, 1987.

Penner MJ: Audible and annoying spontaneous otoacoustic emissions. Arch Otolaryngol Head Neck Surg 114:150–153, 1988.

Penner MJ: An estimate of tinnitus caused by spontaneous otoacoustic emission. Arch Otolaryngol Head Neck Surg 116:418–423, 1990.

Pfister HW, et al: Latent Lyme neuroborreliosis: presence of Borrelia burgdorferi in the cerebrospinal fluid without concurrent inflammatory signs. Neurology 39:1118–1120, 1989.

Reed GF: An audiometric study of two hundred cases of subjective tinnitus. Arch Otolaryngol 71:95–104, 1960.

Sasaki CT, Babitz L, Kauer JS: Tinnitus: development of a neurophysiologic correlate. Laryngoscope 91:2018–2024, 1981.

Silverstein H, Haberkamp T, Smouha E: The state of tinnitus after inner ear surgery. Otolaryngol Head Neck Surg 95:438–441, 1986.

Sismanis A, Williams GH, King MD: A new electronic device for evaluation of objective tinnitus. Otolaryngol Head Neck Surg 100:644–645, 1989.

Snow JB, Suga F: Control of the microcirculation of the inner ear. Otolaryngol Clin North Am 8:455–466, 1975.

Thedinger B, House WF, Edgerton B: Cochlear implant for tinnitus: case reports. Ann Otol Rhinol Laryngol 94:10–13, 1985.

Tonndorf J: Endolymphatic hydrops: mechanical causes of hearing loss. Arch Otorhinolaryngol 212:293–299, 1976.

Tonndorf J: Acute cochlea disorders: the combination of hearing loss, recruitment, poor speech discrimination, and tinnitus. Ann Otol 89:353–358, 1980.

Trowbridge BC: Tympanosympathetic anesthesia for tinnitus aurium and secondary otalgia. Arch Otolaryngol 50:200–215, 1949.

Tsyganov AI: Anesthesia of the tympanic plexus in the treatment of subjective tinnitus. Arch Otolaryngol 87:127–131, 1968.

Vernon J, Schleuning A: Tinnitus: a new management. Laryngoscope 88:413–419, 1978.

Yamamoto E, Nishimura H, Hirono Y: Occurrence of sequelae in Bell's palsy. Acta Otolaryngol (Stockh) 446(Suppl):93–96, 1988.

Yamamoto E, Nishimura H, Iwanaga M: Tinnitus and/or hearing loss elicited by facial mimetic movement. Laryngoscope 95:966–970, 1985.

PART THREE

Nose, Paranasal Sinuses, and Nasopharynx

CHAPTER 21

Congenital Lesions

Dennis M. Crockett, MD   Steven P. Peskind, MD

Congenital lesions of the nose, the naso-pharynx, and the paranasal sinuses are relatively uncommon, and their diagnosis, work-up, and eventual surgical management are often challenging to the head and neck surgeon. The newborn infant is an obligate nasal breather because of the proximity of the soft palate to the tongue base and the supraglottic larynx. Therefore, many infants with these lesions present with nasal airway obstruction and respiratory distress, and this is why the head and neck surgeon is called for an evaluation. The purpose of this chapter is to discuss differential diagnosis, radiographic assessment, and surgical management of lesions that manifest in the nose, the naso-pharynx, and the paranasal sinuses of the newborn infant and the young child. Paranasal embryologic development is an important consideration because many of these lesions result from aberrations of facial development.

EMBRYOLOGIC CONSIDERATIONS

Accurate evaluation and management of congenital lesions of the nose, the nasopharynx, and the paranasal sinuses by the head and neck surgeon depend on a thorough knowledge of the embryologic processes of the paranasal region. The embryologic development of the nose cannot be understood without regional considerations of simultaneous cranial-oral-facial induction and development. These primary events occur between the fourth and eighth weeks of fetal development. Within the early developing brain,

so-called organization centers induce the cartilaginous and bony structures of the midface and the developing sensory organs. As the forebrain develops, the olfactory bulbs begin to protrude and take their superior position in relation to the developing nasal structure.

Simultaneous midfacial development contributes to the evolving nasal structures. Three developing facial projections define nasal structure: the frontonasal process, the maxillary process, and the mandibular process; the last two are derived from the first branchial arch. The frontonasal process develops over the forebrain and contributes to the development of the forehead. This ecto-dermally derived structure also contributes to the development of the nasal olfactory placodes, which are induced by their proximity to the developing olfactory nerves. Proliferation of these placodes gives rise to the medial and lateral nasal prominences. These prominences then surround the nasal pit, which ultimately becomes the nares.

The frontonasal, maxillary, and mandibular prominences merge and eventually complete the formation of the central facial structure. Fusion of the medial nasal prominence with the maxillary prominence contributes to development of the upper maxilla and the philtrum of the upper lip. Intraorally, the primary palate is derived from proliferation of the medial nasal process and contributes to the intermaxillary segment and the four incisor teeth.

Concomitantly with facial events, processes within the primitive oral cavity contribute to nasal and nasopharyngeal development. The precursor of the oral cavity begins as the stomodeum. With further fetal growth, a secondary membrane of ectodermal origin, known as the oropharyngeal membrane, develops. Simultaneously, by the fourth week of development, the endodermally derived foregut, or primitive pharynx, is in opposition with the oropharyngeal membrane, which disintegrates and forms a cavity between the mouth and the pharynx. The nasopharynx and the oropharynx are then divided into separate anatomic compartments, with the development of the primary and secondary palates. The secondary palate is derived from the palatine shelves, which develop from the maxillary prominences and proliferate from a vertical/lateral position to a medial/horizontal position. Completion of the palate thus concludes development of the nasal floor.

During the ongoing fusion of the midfacial structures, further nasal differentiation may be examined in terms of extranasal and intranasal events. Externally, the frontal prominence contributes to the forehead and nasal bridge. The two medial nasal prominences then fuse to form the nasal tip and the columella. The lateral prominences develop into the alar cartilages. Intranasally, the frontonasal process contributes to the development of the nasal capsule, the precartilaginous anlage for the forming nasal cartilaginous structures. This capsule develops a medial portion and a lateral portion that consist of the mesethmoid, which is the nasal septal precursor, and the lateral ectethmoid, which contributes to the conchae of the lateral nasal wall. Early in nasal development, the primitive nares are separated from the oral region by the oronasal membrane. The simultaneous development of the palatal shelves with disintegration of the membrane then forms the choanae. Failure of this membrane to disintegrate is postulated as a cause of choanal atresia.

The septal cartilage initially develops from the mesethmoid in a superior to inferior direction. When the palatal shelves close, the oral cavity and nasopharynx are defined. Ossification of the mesethmoid cartilage then results in the perpendicular plate of the ethmoid, a septal component, and the crista galli. Posteriorly, the vomer is produced by membranous ossification of connective tissue instead of cartilage. The vomer begins as two vomerine bones that fuse before birth and thus contribute to the bony septum.

Understanding the embryogenesis of the cranium, as well as of the bony and cartilaginous nasal structures, provides insight into the formation of the most common midline nasal masses: the dermoid sinus cyst, the glioma, and the encephalocele. One theory of congenital nasal masses is that in the course of development, two potential spaces exist: the fonticulus frontalis, between the frontal and nasal bones, and the prenasal space, between the nasal cartilages. Dural projections are postulated to have been in contact with each of these spaces, which in normal development are obliterated. The dural connection related to the cribriform plate area projects through the prenasal space via the foramen cecum. Lack of obliteration of these spaces would then allow dural and neural elements to protrude, as in the case of encephaloceles and gliomas. Connection of these projections with nasal dermal elements would explain dermoid cysts.

Another congenital nasal mass that may be explained on the basis of its embryologic development is congenital obstruction of the nasolacrimal drainage system. The nasolacrimal duct begins in the nasolacrimal groove between the maxillary and lateral nasal prominences. It begins as a solid tube of tissue that, with time, canalizes to form a duct connecting the conjunctivae to the internal nose. This duct usually becomes fully patent within the first month of the postpartum period, but the process may take several months. Obstruction may occur proximally in the region of the lacrimal sac to distally at the level of the nasal mucosa, which results in fluid accumulation and cyst formation that may extend intranasally.

When the intranasal structures are established, development of the paranasal sinus begins. In the third to fourth month of fetal development, mucous membranes infiltrate the cartilaginous structures of the lateral nasal wall by the process of primary pneumatization. During further growth, secondary pneumatization occurs with sinus infiltration of bony structures. The maxillary sinus initially pneumatizes in the ectethmoid cartilage at about 10 weeks of gestation. Secondary pneumatization begins around the fifth month. After birth, the sinuses begin to grow by resorption of the maxillary walls. The floor of the maxillary sinus moves inferiorly with further bony resorption and tooth eruption. The ethmoid sinuses begin with primary pneumatization of the ectethmoid at 4 months of gestation. Secondary pneumatization then proceeds from birth to age 2 years. The cells of the anterior ethmoid are postulated to invade the frontal bone, thus creating the frontal sinus. The sphenoid sinus begins to develop from the sphenoethmoidal recess at about the fourth month of gestation. Secondary pneumatization is then completed by age 6 to 7 years.

NASAL EXAMINATION IN THE NEONATE AND THE YOUNG CHILD

If a perinasal congenital lesion is suspected, intranasal examination is necessary for two reasons: (1) to assess the degree of nasal obstruction present and (2) to help assess the anatomic extent of the lesion. Intranasal examination in a newborn infant or a young child should be performed in a setting in which oxygen, suction, and proper resuscitation equipment are readily available. Proper sized laryngoscopes and endotracheal tubes and rigid bronchoscopes are set up before the examination to be available in cases in which acute airway obstruction is a possibility. It is entirely appropriate to perform the examination for certain worrisome cases in the operating room with the help of an anesthesiologist.

Neonates and young children are kept on NPO (nothing by mouth) status for 3 hours before the procedure. No oral or intravenous sedation is used. For topical intranasal anesthesia and vasoconstriction, a neurosurgical pledget is soaked in a half-and-half mixture of 4% lidocaine hydrochloride solution and 0.25% phenylephrine hydrochloride and then inserted into one nasal fossa. Five minutes is allowed to elapse, the pledget is removed, and the same procedure is accomplished for the other nasal fossa.

Assistants are needed for stabilizing the child's head and body, and the nasal fossas and the nasopharynx are examined with either a flexible nasopharyngolaryngoscope or a rigid fiberoptic telescope. After examination of the nose and the nasopharynx, the oropharynx, the hypopharynx, and the larynx may be visualized and examined.

EVALUATION AND MANAGEMENT OF SPECIFIC CLINICAL ENTITIES

Nasal Dermoid Sinus Cyst

The nasal dermoid sinus cyst is a cyst or a sinus tract, or both, that is lined by epithelium, and it may contain any number of skin adnexal structures (hair and hair follicles, eccrine glands, sebaceous glands). This lesion is distinguished from the epidermoid cyst, which is lined by a simple squamous epithelium that contains no skin appendages. The nasal dermoid sinus cyst may be seen clinically as a cyst and a sinus tract, with or without an external opening; as an isolated subcutaneous cyst; or as a sinus tract and a fistula alone. According to embryologic considerations, nasal dermoid sinus cysts may develop anywhere from the base of the columella to the anterior cranial fossa. Typically, if a cyst and a sinus tract are both present, the cyst occurs in either the medial canthal area or the supratip region, and the external opening is found in the supratip region. One or two hairs commonly protrude from the external cutaneous opening of the sinus tract. With large cysts, a widened nasal dorsum may be noted. Nasal dermoid sinus cysts may extend deeply to involve soft tissue and cartilaginous and bony components of the paranasal region, and they may extend intracranially. The cyst component may expand with time, may cause local erosion of bone, and is subject to recurrent infection.

Before any planned biopsy or surgical excision, accurate radiographic evaluation is an essential part of the work-up of a paranasal mass in a newborn or a young child. If an intracranial connection exists, blind operative intervention may result in an inadvertent and unrecognized cerebrospinal fluid leakage. Direct coronal computed tomography is probably the initial study of choice. Sequential scans may delineate the path of the nasal dermoid sinus cyst by demonstrating erosion of the nasal and lacrimal bones, as well as a bone defect in the base of the skull if an intracranial connection exists. Other computed tomography findings may include widening of the nasal septum and the bony septum, as well as a bifid crista galli. Unfortunately, unossified areas in the cribriform plate and in the fovea ethmoidalis are common in the newborn infant and may confound the computed tomographic evaluation. Magnetic resonance imaging has been used to supplement the computed tomographic findings if an intracranial connection is suspected. Magnetic resonance imaging delineates both the intracranial and the extracranial components of the soft tissue mass and is capable of showing the dermoid sinus cyst in the sagittal, coronal, and axial planes.

Complete surgical excision is the treatment of choice for the nasal dermoid sinus-cyst. After radiographic evaluation, the surgical approach is planned. If an intracranial connection is known or strongly suspected, neurosurgical consultation is obtained. The neurosurgeon completes an intradural or an extradural approach and identifies the cyst in the anterior cranial vault. This is followed by delivery of the cyst into the intranasal field. The head and neck surgeon completes excision from below. If the dermoid sinus cyst is in the midline and lower two thirds of the nose, and if there is no or minimal involvement of overlying skin, a single midline vertical incision incorporating the fistula opening is the approach of choice and yields the best cosmetic result in the authors' experience (Fig. 21–1). For cysts overlying the nasion, a horizontal incision probably yields the best cosmetic result. When the sinus cyst is off the midline, or when there is overlying cutaneous involvement, the head and neck surgeon must be creative and use the principles and dynamics of local skin flaps for the best possible cosmetic result (Fig. 21–2).

Congenital Nasolacrimal Duct Drainage System Cyst

Failure of canalization of the nasolacrimal duct drainage system may occur proximally (lacrimal canaliculi and sac) or distally (at the nasal mucosanasolacrimal duct epithelium interface) and result in fluid accumulation and cyst formation. As noted by Berkowitz and colleagues (1990), several terms have been used to describe this clinical entity and include dacryocystocele, mucocele, and amniotocele; however, the term congenital nasolacrimal duct drainage system cyst is preferred. Depending on the site of obstruction, infants with these lesions may present with dacryocystitis, epiphora, or an intranasal mass (unilateral or bilateral) that causes nasal obstruction and respiratory distress. Treat-

ment of epiphora and dacryocystitis is conservative, with massage and antibiotics if indicated. However, infants who present with respiratory distress as a result of obligate nasal breathing must first be evaluated with nasal endoscopy. This procedure may reveal a cystic mass projecting beneath the inferior turbinate. Because this lesion may be confused with gliomas and encephaloceles, a computed tomography or a magnetic resonance imaging scan may then be performed to assess for intracranial and bony abnormalities. In children in whom respiratory distress is life threatening and unresponsive to conservative management, recommended surgical therapy includes intranasal marsupialization, which decompresses the cyst and relieves nasal obstruction. After surgery, the child should be monitored closely for further symptoms of respiratory distress. The nasal cavity should be reinspected endoscopically and irrigated with saline until crusting is controlled and the operative site is healed.

Gliomas and Encephaloceles

Gliomas and encephaloceles are usually considered together, and they present a continuum, according to their embryogenesis. Although they are histologically identical, gliomas lack an intracranial connection, whereas encephaloceles represent a protrusion of brain through a bone defect and maintenance of a cerebrospinal fluid connection to the subarachnoid space. The term *glioma* is considered a misnomer because these lesions are not true neoplasms. Histologically, gliomas represent heterotopic neurotissue that is predominantly glial.

Slightly fewer than two thirds of gliomas manifest extranasally, one third manifest intranasally, and the remainder manifest both externally and intranasally. Approximately 15% to 20% of gliomas maintain a fibrous stalk connection with the dura, and there may be an associated bone defect in the base of the skull. Extranasal gliomas usually manifest in the region of the glabella, are firm and reddish, are lobular to palpation, and are noncompressible (Fig. 21–3). The overlying skin may contain telangiectases, and they do not pulsate or transilluminate. Intranasal gliomas have a similar appearance but are smoother and may be difficult to differentiate from encephaloceles.

Nasal encephaloceles may manifest exter-

Text continued on page 456

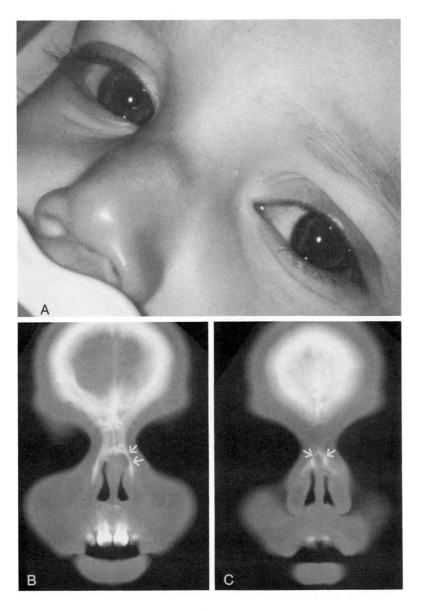

A

B

C

Figure 21–1. *A.* Nasal dermoid sinus cyst involving the middle third of the nose. *B to E.* Sequential direct coronal computed tomography scans and magnetic resonance imaging scans of the lesion demonstrate erosion of the nasal bones, but no intracranial extension. *F.* Design of incision and after cyst excision. Note erosion of nasal bones. *G.* Postoperative result 8 weeks later.

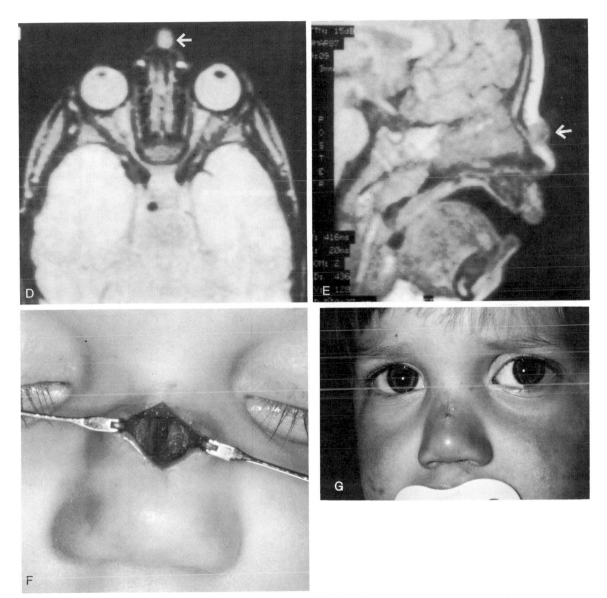

Figure 21–1. *Continued*

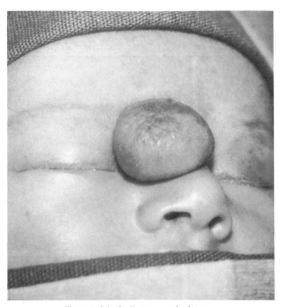

Figure 21–3. Extranasal glioma.

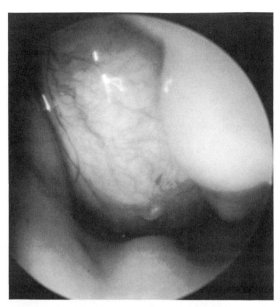

Figure 21–4. Fiberoptic transnasal telescopic view of basal encephalocele.

nally, intranasally, or in both locations. Anatomically, nasal encephaloceles have been classified as (1) sincipital (frontoethmoid), which usually manifest externally with an associated bone defect that corresponds to the foramen caecum between the frontal and ethmoid bones, and (2) basal, which usually manifest intranasally and are associated with defects in the cribriform plate, the superior orbital fissure, or the posterior clinoid fissure.

Frontoethmoid encephaloceles typically appear in the region of the glabella, are bluish, are soft and compressible to palpation, and transilluminate. Unlike gliomas, they may elicit a positive result on Furstenberg's test (expansion of the mass with compression of the jugular veins). Basal encephaloceles have characteristics that are similar to those of intranasal masses (Fig. 21–4). Both types may be associated with expansion of the bony nasal vault and hypertelorism.

Radiographic evaluation of encephaloceles should include computed tomography to delineate the bony craniofacial configuration, as well as magnetic resonance imaging to demonstrate the anatomic extent of the encephalocele (Fig. 21–5). Suspected gliomas should be evaluated first with computed tomography. Magnetic resonance imaging may be used to prove or disprove suspected intracranial connection.

Extranasal gliomas are treated by an extra-

cranial approach, which includes excision of the lesion and use of appropriate local skin flaps for the best cosmetic result. The surgical approach for intranasal gliomas depends on their size and anatomic extent. Endoscopic sinus surgery instruments and technique may be used for small intranasal gliomas that

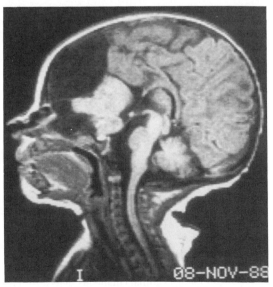

Figure 21–5. MRI scan of frontoethmoidal encephalocele. (Courtesy of Marvin Nelson, Department of Radiology, Children's Hospital of Los Angeles.)

have been shown by radiographic studies to be completely extracranial. A lateral rhinotomy approach, limited to the alar crease if possible, or a facial degloving approach may be used for large intranasal gliomas (Fig. 21–6).

All encephaloceles require neurosurgical consultation, and the intracranial removal always precedes the extracranial repair. Depending on the size and extent of the encephalocele, extracranial repair may be performed concomitantly with the intracranial removal or deferred to a later date.

Teratomas

Unlike the nasal dermoid sinus cyst, which contains ectodermal and mesodermal embryologic components, true teratomas are composed of all three germ layers. The neck and the nasopharynx are the most common sites of presentation for teratomas of the head and the neck. If confined to the nasopharynx, teratomas may be confused with gliomas and encephaloceles. Larger teratomas may be associated with variable craniofacial deformity. Histologically, they are composed of well-differentiated tissues, with a predominance of neuroectodermal and neural tissues.

Clinically, teratomas usually manifest at birth and cause significant airway obstruction in the newborn. They are discovered during nasal examination. Radiographic evaluation should include computed tomography to delineate the anatomic and bony extents of the lesion. If an intracranial connection is sus-

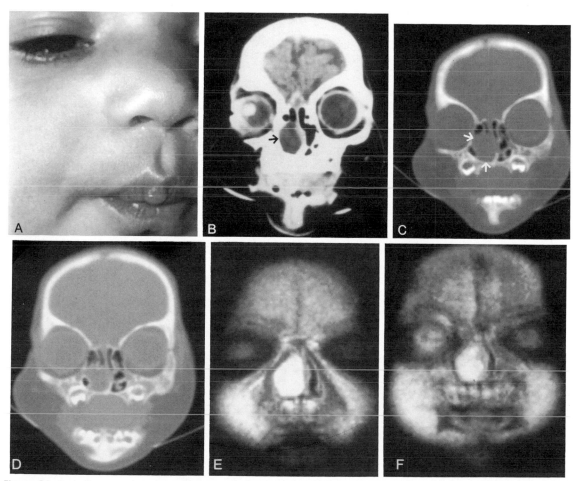

Figure 21–6. *A.* Preoperative view of intranasal glioma with widening of the nasal dorsum. *B* to *D.* Sequential direct coronal CT scans show doubtful intracranial connection. *E* to *G.* MRI scans confirm the intranasal anatomic extent and the absence of an intracranial connection. *H, I.* Design of incision to follow the alar crease for adequate exposure and intranasal excision of the glioma.

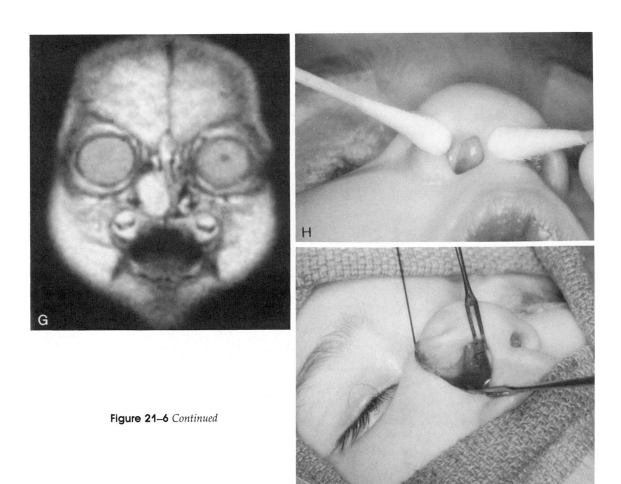

Figure 21–6 *Continued*

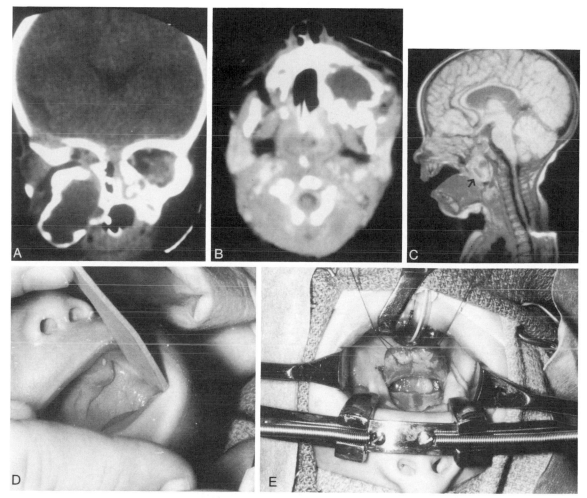

Figure 21–7. *A, B.* CT scans show anatomic extent of a large teratoma involving the nose, the nasopharynx, and the maxilla. *C.* Sagittal MRI scan demonstrates nasopharyngeal component of the teratoma. *D.* Intraoperative photograph shows extension of the teratoma into the gingival buccal sulcus. *E.* Transpalatal exposure of the nasopharyngeal component of the teratoma.

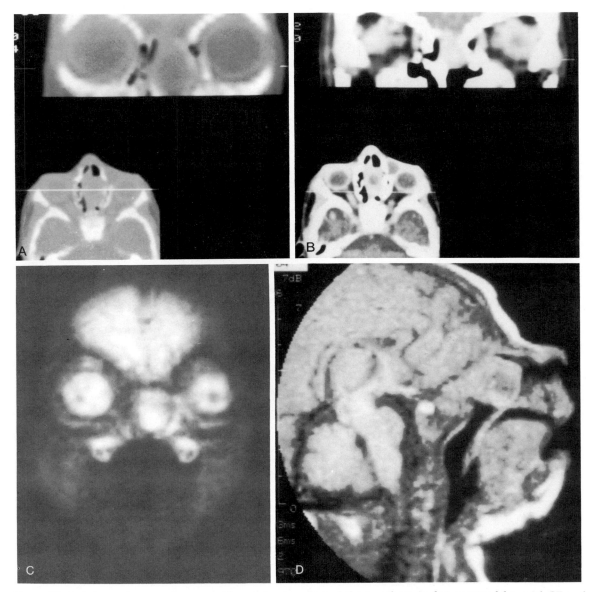

Figure 21–8. Intranasal mesenchymoma. The anatomic extent of the neoplasm is demonstrated by axial CT and coronal re-formations (*A, B*) and by coronal sagittal MRI (*C, D*).

TABLE 21–1. Other Congenital Benign and Malignant Neoplasms of the Nose, Nasopharynx, and Paranasal Sinuses

Benign
Hamartoma
Hemangioma/vascular malformation
Nasopharyngeal dermoid ("hairy polyp")
Fibrous tumors
Mesenchymoma
Melanotic neuroectodermal tumor of infancy
Lateral/median fissural cysts of maxilla
Nasopharyngeal (Tornwaldt's) cyst

Malignant
Teratocarcinoma
Fibrosarcoma
Rhabdomyosarcoma

pected, magnetic resonance imaging is useful.

As with the nasal dermoid sinus-cyst, as well as gliomas and encephaloceles, the choice of surgical approach depends on the anatomic extent of the teratoma. At the authors' institution, a facial degloving approach, in combination with transpalatal exposure, has been used to adequately remove teratomas involving the nose, the nasopharynx, and the adjacent paranasal sinuses and maxilla in two patients (Fig. 21–7).

Other Benign and Malignant Neoplasms

Various other benign and malignant neoplasms may manifest in the nose, the nasopharynx, or the paranasal sinuses (Fig. 21–8). Although rare, these neoplasms should be included in the differential diagnosis of an obstructing paranasal mass in the newborn. They may be difficult to distinguish from gliomas, encephaloceles, and teratomas on the basis of their external appearance. As with the lesions already discussed, adequate radiographic evaluation (computed tomography and magnetic resonance imaging) is necessary before surgical intervention. Table 21–1 is a list of other benign and malignant neoplasms of the nose, the nasopharynx, and the paranasal sinuses that have been reported on a congenital basis.

SUGGESTED READINGS

Batsakis J: Teratomas of the Head and Neck. *In* Batsakis J: Tumors of the Head and Neck (pp. 155–162). Baltimore: Williams & Wilkins, 1979.

Berkowitz RG, Grundfast KM, Fitz C: Nasal obstruction of the newborn revisited: clinical and subclinical manifestations of congenital nasolacrimal duct obstruction presenting as a nasal mass. Otolaryngol Head Neck Surg 103:468–471, 1990.

Hengerer AS, Oas R: Congenital Anomalies of the Nose: Their Embryology, Diagnosis and Management. Washington, DC: American Academy of Otolaryngology–Head and Neck Surgery Foundation, 1987.

Hughes GB, Shapiro G, Hunt W, et al: Management of the congenital midline nasal mass: a review. Head Neck Surg 1:222–233, 1980.

Lusk RP, Lee PL: Magnetic resonance imaging of congenital midline nasal masses. Otolaryngol Head Neck Surg 95:303–306, 1986.

Lusk RP, Muntz HR: Nasal obstruction in the neonate secondary to nasolacrimal duct cysts. Inter J Pediatr Otorhinolaryngol 13:315–322, 1987.

Sessions RB: Nasal dermal sinuses—new concepts and explanations. Laryngoscope 92(Suppl):1–28, 1982.

Sperber GH: Craniofacial Embryology. Boston: Wright, 1989.

CHAPTER 22

Anatomy and Physiology of the Nose and Paranasal Sinuses

Steven D. Schaefer, MD   Maher Sesi, MD

The anatomy and physiology of the nose and paranasal sinuses has gained a great deal of interest and importance over the last several decades. Cosmetic surgery of the nose has increased dramatically. This has caused the rhinoplastic surgeon to study more carefully and precisely the anatomy of the nose and its supporting structures. The intranasal surgeon has developed a more acute awareness of the physiologic characteristics of the nose. The otolaryngologist, the neurologist, and the neurosurgeon have become interested and more concerned with problems of the olfactory system. An acute interest in sinus surgery has developed with the blossoming of endoscopic sinus surgery in the United States. Thus from many aspects, study of the anatomic and physiologic characteristics of the nose and paranasal sinuses has taken on more importance.

THE NOSE

Anatomy of the Nose

The nose is a pyramidal structure; its pointed tip or apex projects anteriorly, and its base is attached to the facial skeleton. Superior to the apex is the dorsum of the nose, which leads to the root of the nose, where the dorsum merges with the forehead (Fig. 22–1). The *columella* extends from the apex of the nose posteriorly and strikes the center of the lip at the base of the nose. On either side of the columella are the right and left anterior nares. The nares are bounded laterally and laterosuperiorly by the alae of the nose and inferiorly by the floor of the nose. The base of the nose is actually pear-shaped and is called the *piriform aperture*. The superior and lateral margins are formed by the frontal processes of the maxilla and the nasal bones, which also create the bony vault of the nose. The base is formed by the alveolar process of the maxilla. In the midline is the anterior nasal spine. The superior border of the nasal bones forms a suture with the frontal bone and is an important point of support for the bony nasal vault because of the buttress formed by the underlying nasal spine of the frontal bone. Also acting as a buttress for the nasal bones is the perpendicular plate of the ethmoid bone. The midline point at which the nasal bones meet the frontal bone is termed the *nasion*. The *rhinion* is the inferior point of the midline suture between the nasal bones where they meet the upper lateral cartilages.

The cartilaginous vault consists of the upper lateral cartilages and adjacent portion of the cartilaginous septum. The *lobule* is the portion of the nose that includes the tip, the lower lateral cartilages, the alae, the vestibular regions, and the columella. The upper

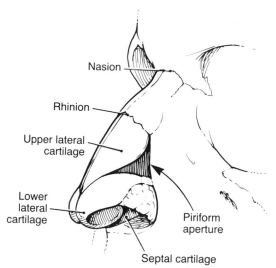

Figure 22–1. Anatomy of the external nose.

lateral cartilages attach to the undersurface of the nasal bones and form the cartilaginous portion of the dorsum of the nose. Inferiorly or caudally they lie under the craniad portion of the *lower lateral cartilages*. In some individuals this relationship does not exist, and thus the support of the external nose is potentially less secure at this point. Between the upper and lower lateral cartilages laterally are found one or more sesamoid cartilages. The lower lateral cartilages are also paired and consist of a medial and lateral crus with a dome between them. The lower lateral cartilages are horseshoe-shaped. The medial crus enters the skin of the columella, where it articulates loosely with its sister crus of the opposite side. Posterior to the columella is the nasal septum. Within the nares, the skin of the vestibule changes abruptly at the limen vestibuli from a stratified nonkeratinizing epithelium to the typical ciliated columnar respiratory epithelium.

The *alar muscles* consist of two sets: the dilators and the constrictors. The dilators are made up of the dilator naris (anterior and posterior), the procerus, and the quadratus labii superioris alaeque nasi. The constrictors or compressors of the nose are composed of the nasalis and the depressor septi.

The *septum* divides the nose into right and left nasal cavities. The septum is formed superiorly by the perpendicular plate of the ethmoid bone and inferiorly and posteriorly by the vomer, the maxillary crest, the palatine crest, and the sphenoidal crest. Ante-

riorly the septum is formed by the quadrilateral cartilage, the columella, and the premaxilla.

The nasal cavities begin at the piriform aperture anteriorly and end posteriorly at the choanae. The roof of the nasal cavity is formed anteriorly by the nasal bones, the nasal spine of the frontal bone, the body of the ethmoid, and the body of the sphenoid bone. The cribriform plate forms the major portion of the roof of the nose. Posteriorly the roof slopes down to the choanae. The floor of the nose is formed by the palatal process of the maxilla and the horizontal process of the palatal bone posteriorly. The lateral wall of the nasal cavity is formed from several bones: the nasal surface of the maxilla, the lacrimal bone, the superior and middle turbinates of the ethmoid bone, the inferior turbinate, the perpendicular plate of the palatine bone, and the medial pterygoid.

The *turbinates* (or conchae) each form a passage (or meatus) between the lateral nasal wall and the concha (Fig. 22–2). The space between the inferior turbinate and the floor of the nose is called the inferior meatus. The space between the middle turbinate and the inferior turbinate is the middle meatus, and the space between the middle and superior turbinates is the superior meatus. Occasionally, a fourth turbinate called a supreme turbinate is observed.

The *inferior turbinate* is the largest of the three. It accepts the drainage of the nasolacrimal duct, which is located on the lateral wall 3 to 3.5 cm behind the posterior margin of the nostril. The middle meatus accepts the drainages from the frontal and maxillary sinuses and from the anterior ethmoid cells. It is also the most complex of the three meatuses and is described later. The superior meatus accepts drainage from the posterior ethmoid cells by one or more orifices of variable size into the central portion of the meatus. Above and behind the superior turbinate but in front of the body of the sphenoid is the *sphenoethmoid recess*, into which opens the sphenoid sinus.

Both the middle and inferior turbinates are covered with pseudostratified ciliated columnar epithelium. The stroma of the middle turbinate is characterized by the presence of glands, whereas that of the inferior turbinate is characterized by many blood lakes. These blood lakes, or venous plexuses, constitute the erectile tissue of the nose. They are distributed chiefly along the inferior border of

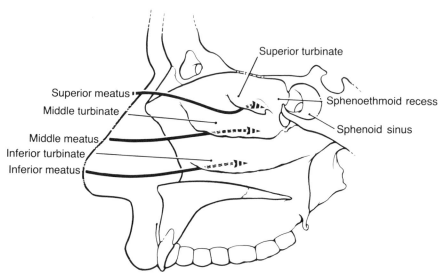

Figure 22–2. Arrows are directed at the appropriate meatus lateral to the turbinate.

the inferior turbinates and the posterior portions of the inferior and middle turbinates. The nares are composed of anterior and posterior nares. The anterior nares provide communication of the nasal cavity with the outside. They are considerably smaller than the posterior nares. The posterior nares (or choanae) through which the nasal fossae and the nasopharynx communicate are apertures located on either side of the nasal septum. Each opening is formed inferiorly by the horizontal plate of the palatine bone, medially by the vomer, superiorly by the sphenoid and the ala of the vomer, and laterally by the medial pterygoid plate of the sphenoid. They are 2.5 cm in height and 1.25 cm in width.

Blood Supply to the Nose

The blood supply to the external nose is derived from branches indirectly derived from the external carotid artery as well as from branches of the *ophthalmic artery*, which is a branch of the internal carotid artery. The *facial artery* branches that supply the external nose include the superior labial artery, which supplies the ala of the nose, and the lateral nasal artery, which supplies the ala of the nose and the bridge of the nose (Fig. 22–3). The dorsal nasal artery, which is a terminal branch of the ophthalmic artery, supplies the dorsum of the nose. Venous drainage of the external nose is by way of veins that accompany these arteries. Blood supply to the in-

ternal nasal cavity is also derived indirectly from the internal carotid artery via the ophthalmic artery and from the external carotid system via the *maxillary artery* (Fig. 22–4). In the orbit, the ophthalmic artery gives off the anterior and posterior ethmoid arteries. Each of these arteries pierces the frontoethmoid suture, the anterior ethmoid foramen being 14 to 22 mm posterior to the maxillolacrimal suture, and the posterior ethmoid foramen being 3 to 13 mm (average 10 mm) posterior to the anterior ethmoid foramen and only 3 to 8 mm (average 5 mm) in front of the optic nerve. The *anterior ethmoid artery* supplies the anterosuperior portion of the septum and the lateral walls of the nose. The smaller *posterior ethmoid artery* supplies a smaller region in the posterosuperior region of the nose in the region of the superior concha.

The maxillary artery enters the pterygopalatine fossa and divides into branches, of which the terminal artery is the sphenopalatine artery, which passes through the sphenopalatine foramen into the nasal cavity behind the posterior end of the middle turbinate. The sphenopalatine artery divides into the posterolateral nasal arteries, which supply the lateral nasal wall, and into the posterior septal arteries, which supply the septum. Branches of the septal sphenopalatine artery traverse the septum to enter the incisive foramen and emerge onto the palate in the oral cavity. The anterosuperior part of the septum is also supplied by the anterior

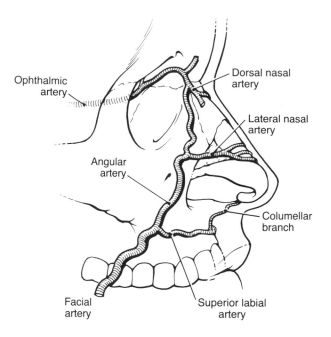

Figure 22–3. Blood supply to the lateral nasal wall. Note septal branches of the ethmoid and sphenopalatine arteries.

ethmoid artery. The vestibule of the nose is supplied by terminal branches of the arteries mentioned as well as by the nasal branches of the superior labial artery. The anterior septum is thus an important site of anastomosis between the branches of the ophthalmic artery of the internal carotid system and the maxillary and facial arteries of the external carotid system. The site of anastomosis of these vessels on the anterior septum has been called *Kiesselbach's plexus* or *Little's area*. This is the most common site for nosebleeds.

Venous drainage of the nasal cavity follows the arteries just named. Veins in the roof of the nasal cavity follow the ethmoid veins into the orbital cavity, where they become tributaries of the ophthalmic veins. These usually course into the *cavernous sinuses* and become part of the drainage pattern of the dural venous sinuses. The posterior portion of the nasal cavity drains via the sphenopalatine vessels into the pterygopalatine fossa and subsequently into the pterygoid plexus. The anterior portion of the nasal cavity drains into the anterior facial veins

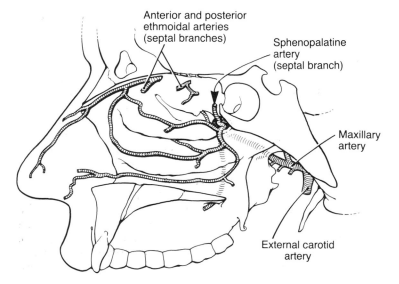

Figure 22–4. Blood supply to the external nose.

and then into either the external or internal jugular vein. Because both the pterygoid venous plexus and the ethmoid veins have communications with the dural venous sinuses and because the veins of the nose are lacking in valves, infections in the nose or sinuses may spread into the adjacent orbital tissues or intracranially with disastrous clinical consequences.

Nerve Supply to the Nose

The motor supply to the muscles of the nose is from the *buccal branches* of the facial nerve. In addition to the olfactory nerve, the sensory nerves to the nose consist of branches of the maxillary and ophthalmic divisions of the *trigeminal nerve* (Fig. 22–5). The first branch of the trigeminal nerve, the *ophthalmic*, gives rise to the nasociliary nerve, of which the chief branches are the anterior ethmoid nerve, the posterior ethmoid nerve, and the infratrochlear nerve. The infratrochlear nerve supplies part of the skin of the side of the nose. The external nasal nerve, which is a branch of the anterior ethmoid nerve, supplies the skin of the lower part of the dorsum of the nose. The anterior ethmoid nerve divides into medial and lateral nasal branches. The medial branch supplies the anterior part of the septum; the lateral branch supplies a similar part of the lateral wall and is also the source of the external nasal nerve. A large medial branch of the *maxillary nerve* (or sec-

ond division of the trigeminal nerve) arises in the pterygopalatine fossa and enters the nasal cavity in the sphenopalatine foramen, where it divides and contributes branches to the mucosa on both the lateral and septal walls of the nasal cavity. The branch on the lateral wall forms the posterolateral nasal nerves. These nerves course anteriorly in the mucosa over the inferior and middle turbinates. The branch to the nasal septum is called the *nasopalatine nerve*. It continues anteriorly as a major nerve in the mucosa, supplying branches to the septal area. It exits the nose via the incisive foramen, where it communicates with the anterior palatine nerves.

The *maxillary division* of the trigeminal nerve also gives rise to the posteroinferior nasal nerves, which after entering the nose via the sphenopalatine foramen provide sensation to the inferior turbinates. The *infraorbital nerve* emerges from the infraorbital foramen from the maxillary nerve. It terminates in the skin with an external nasal branch that supplies the lateral aspect of the bridge of the nose and both the external and internal surfaces of the ala of the nose.

In the pterygopalatine fossa, a number of dental branches arise from the maxillary division of the trigeminal nerve. The posterosuperior alveolar nerve arises from the maxillary nerve in the pterygopalatine fossa and exits via the pterygomaxillary fissure. It supplies the roots of the posterior teeth as well

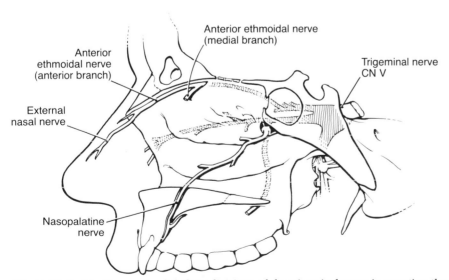

Figure 22–5. Maxillary and ophthalmic divisions of the trigeminal nerve innervating the nose.

as the buccal gingiva associated with these teeth. After the maxillary nerve enters the infraorbital canal, a middle superior alveolar nerve is given off to the bicuspids. Distal to this is an anterosuperior alveolar nerve, which supplies the incisors and the canines. In the pterygopalatine fossa, a palatine branch descends from the maxillary nerve to form the greater and lesser *palatine nerves* at the greater and lesser palatine canals. These supply the palatal mucosa and gingiva from the molar teeth to the first bicuspid.

The *sphenopalatine ganglion* (pterygopalatine ganglion) appears to be functionally associated with the maxillary division of the trigeminal nerve, suspended by the pterygopalatine nerves in the fossa. It is, however, a parasympathetic ganglion of the facial nerve. It lies deeply within the pterygopalatine fossa just lateral to the sphenopalatine foramen. The preganglionic parasympathetic innervation of the nasal mucosa begins in the superior salivatory nucleus, and the fibers are carried via the greater superficial petrosal nerve through the pterygoid canal until it synapses in the sphenopalatine ganglion. The postganglionic parasympathetic fibers leave the sphenopalatine foramen and follow the various branches of the maxillary division of the trigeminal nerve to provide parasympathetic flow to the lacrimal gland and to mucosal glands of the nasal fossa, palate, and pharynx. General sensory fibers to the nasal mucosa as well as parasympathetic secretomotor fibers to the mucous glands of the nasal mucosa are also carried with these nerves.

Sympathetic innervation starts as the preganglionic sympathetics from the thoracic spinal cord to the superior cervical sympathetic ganglion. The postganglionic fibers form the internal carotid nerve, which accompanies the internal carotid artery into the skull. After traversing the carotid canal, some of the fibers form the *deep petrosal nerve,* which joins the greater superficial petrosal nerve in the pterygoid canal to form the nerve of the *pterygoid canal.* These postganglionic fibers distribute via branches of the maxillary nerve to blood vessels of the oral and nasal mucosa as vasomotor fibers.

Parasympathetic fibers to the lacrimal gland are also contained in the nerve of the pterygoid canal. After synapsing in the sphenopalatine ganglion, the postganglionic fibers join the zygomatic branch of the maxillary nerve to the zygomaticotemporal nerve.

Just before the point at which the zygomaticotemporal nerve leaves the orbit, the postganglionic secretomotor fibers leave the nerve to enter the lacrimal gland.

The *olfactory nerve* descends through the cribriform plate (lamina cribrosa) from the undersurface of the olfactory bulb and is distributed to the mucous membrane covering the upper portion of the superior turbinate and corresponding portion of the septum. The terminal nerve, originating from the terminal ganglion medial to the olfactory bulb, sends three or four rami through the anterior portion of the cribriform plate to the anterosuperior portion of the cartilaginous septum. The nerve anastomoses with the nasopalatine and ethmoid nerves.

Histologic Characteristics

The nasal fossa, nasopharynx, and paranasal sinuses are lined with continuous mucous membrane of varying thickness and character. Anteriorly in the nasal vestibule, cuboid squamous epithelium is found. Above the level of the superior turbinate, olfactory epithelium is found; below this level, respiratory epithelium is found. The respiratory epithelium consists of tall, columnar, pseudostratified ciliated cells with goblet cells and brush cells bearing microvilli. The mucosa of the sinuses is the same as but thinner than that of the nasal fossa and contains fewer glands. The olfactory epithelium is brownish in color and consists of supporting cells, basal cells, and olfactory cells. In the tunica propria, numerous branched glands of Bowman are found.

Physiologic Characteristics of the Nose

Olfaction

The olfactory epithelium consists of three types of cells: supporting cells, basal cells, and olfactory cells. The olfactory nerve cells are bipolar cells. The dendrite extends to the olfactory epithelium, where an olfactory rod or vesicle is formed. Attached to this vesicle are six to eight nonmotile cilia. Somehow the olfactory nerve is stimulated, and an impulse travels to the olfactory bulb and then to the axon of the olfactory cell. The axons join to form about 20 filaments, the fila olfactoria, that pass through the cribriform plate to enter the olfactory bulb in the brain. The next order neurons form the olfactory tract to pass to the piriform cortex and the brain. Also, the trigeminal nerve sends fibers to the olfactory epithelium, but they respond to sensory and not odorous stimuli.

Unfortunately, it is not known how the olfactory sense functions in humans. Evidence to date has not shown a specific receptor for each type of odor or chemical stimulus. One theory is that the molecular quality perceived as odor lies in certain vibrational movements of the odorous molecules. However, the nature of this sense is not known. The just-noticeable difference in odor *is* known to require approximately a 30% change in intensity. It is also known that there are extensive connections between the olfactory centers and other portions of the brain (hypothalamus, brain stem, caudate nucleus, internal capsule, limbic system, uncus and hippocampus of the temporal lobe, thalamus, and frontal lobe); the effect of odors on taste and appetite, the role of olfaction in the reproductive process, and the systemic effect of olfaction have been well documented.

The role of the rhinologist in studying olfaction has been growing. Knowledge of anosmia, dysosmia, cacosmia, and hyposmia disorders and etiologic factors is growing. To be smelled, a substance must be not only volatile but also soluble in water and lipids. Anosmia can be caused by anything that causes trauma to the olfactory epithelium and disrupts this simple principle. Etiologic agents include viral infection; trauma to frontal lobe, cribriform plate, or the nose itself; tumors of the frontal lobe; nasal polyps or sinusitis; or industrial fumes, such fumes being of growing concern in the realm of workers' compensation.

Airway

The nose is essentially a respiratory organ that provides a passageway for the incoming and outgoing air. The air pathway is determined largely by the upward direction of the anterior nares and the shape of the nasal vault. The air stream enters vertically and then turns about 90° posteriorly to travel through the nose. Then it turns another 90°

when it reaches the nasopharynx. The expiratory route is essentially the opposite but has some eddying that is caused by the nasal valve; eddying also results from septal deviations.

The air stream is narrow, being less than 1 to 2 mm. At the anterior nasal valve, the cross section of the airway is 10 to 40 mm and is the narrowest portion of the respiratory tract. The nose provides about 50% of the total respiratory tract resistance. The linear air speed is greatest at the anterior nasal valve, reaching 3.3 m/second at an inspiratory flow rate of 200 mL/second.

Another factor affecting the diameter of the nasal vault is the nasal cycle. This is defined as the congestion and decongestion of the cavernous tissues of the nasal conchae. This cycle is present in 80% of people with normal nasal function. Every 30 minutes to 3 hours, the turbinates on one side decrease in size while those on the other side increase. The total nasal cross-sectional area remains the same.

Particle Removal

The nose cleanses inspired air before it reaches the lungs. The nasal mucosa is effective in filtering out particles in the air of 4.5 μm and above; over 95% of these particles are filtered out and carried away by the mucous blanket. The cilia move the mucus at about 6.7 mm/minute and beat at a rate of 160 to 1500 beats/minute. About 1 quart of mucus is produced per day. The mucin is composed of mucopolysaccharides and mucoproteins. Mucus is predominantly water and about 3% mucin and 1% salts; when the mucus reaches the nasopharynx, it passes downward undetected.

Humidification

Air entering the nose is warmed and humidified before reaching the lungs; the nose is very efficient at both these tasks. Air entering the nose at temperatures of −5°C to 55°C is brought to 31°C to 37°C on entering the pharynx. The nose is able to saturate inspired air with water so that the air arrives to the lungs at 100% humidity; on expiration, some of this water is returned to the nose. Humidification occurs by evaporation from the mucous blanket.

Defense Against Infection

The nasal mucosa accomplishes this function by two major mechanisms: (1) the mucous blanket moves infective particles such as viruses and bacteria out of the nose and into the stomach before they can penetrate, and (2) nasal mucus contains antibodies against viruses and bacteria.

Mucous Blanket. The mucous blanket is a thin, sticky, tenacious adhesive sheet; its pH is about 7 in a healthy person. It contains water, salts, mucin, and IgA. It is found throughout the nose (except the vestibule), the sinuses, the middle ear, the eustachian tube, and the bronchial tree. The beating of cilia propels the blanket of mucus and trapped foreign bodies to the esophagus, where it is swallowed or expectorated. Thus the mucus flows backward and downward; the flow from the sinuses is toward the ostia and then backward and downward. Mucus is produced by both mucous and serous glands and principally by goblet cells of the mucosa.

Two layers of the mucous blanket have been identified. There is a deeper, less viscid layer and a superficial, more viscid layer into which the tips of the cilia penetrate. Insoluble particles are caught on the superficial layer and propelled by the cilia. Soluble particles reach the deeper layer and are evacuated along with it.

The mucociliary transport is really two systems working together. It is dependent on the actively beating cilia that propel the mucus. The deeper layer also moves posteriorly but is less well understood. The speed of the mucociliary transport varies from 1 to 20 mm/minute for healthy persons. The flow of blood supply is from posterior to anterior, whereas that of mucus is from anterior to posterior; thus this is an efficient way for humidifying the inspired air.

Pterygopalatine Fossa

Description of the anatomy of the nose and nasal cavity cannot be complete without discussion of the pterygopalatine fossa. This fossa is an elongated triangular area that lies between the posterior border of the maxillary sinus and the pterygoid process. Its boundary is formed medially by the perpendicular plate of the palatine bone and superiorly by the inferior portion of the sphenoid bone. The sphenopalatine foramen is situated at the junction of the roof and medial walls, close to the posterior tip of the middle turbinate. Through this foramen pass most of the vessels and nerves to the nasal cavity. The sphenopalatine ganglion is just lateral to the foramen. Also communicating with the sphenopalatine space is the foramen rotundum, through which pass the maxillary nerve, the pharyngomaxillary fissure, and the infraorbital fissure. Inferiorly, the greater and lesser palatine canals communicate with the fossa. Within the fossa are the second and third divisions of the *trigeminal nerve* as well as the *vidian nerve*.

THE PARANASAL SINUSES

The paranasal sinuses are among the most poorly described anatomic sites within the human body because of the great variations between individuals and the inconsistency of terminology in describing these structures. The problems in terminology arose from initial confusion about the origin of individual sinuses and the debate among surgeons in the preantibiotic era about the treatment for acute and chronic sinusitis. From the preantibiotic era came a consensus that the sinuses could best be understood by study of their embryology, and from that came the foundations of modern sinus surgery. In the context of modern endoscopic sinus surgery, the importance of treating ethmoid disease as the source of maxillary or frontal sinusitis came as early as 1916 when J. Parsons Schaeffer stated that "the maxillary sinus is often a cesspool for infectious material from the sinus frontalis and certain of the anterior group of the cellulae ethmoidales." Such is an example of knowledge lost and rediscovered when new interest in the sinuses arose after advances in instrument technology and the work of modern sinus surgeons (Wigand et al., 1978; Messerklinger, 1985).

Embryology and Development of the Sinuses

The primordia (anlagen) of the sinuses originate rather late during the prenatal period.

During the first and second months of embryonic life, the main features of the nasal cavity are differentiated. The sinuses arise as local epithelial sprouts or recesses of the nasal mucosa after the second month. The recesses later become the ostia of the various sinuses. In the third fetal month, an evagination, or bud, in the infundibulum gives rise to the maxillary sinus. At birth, the sinus has a volume of 6 to 8 mL but is fluid filled, which makes interpretation of plain film radiography difficult. The sinus then undergoes two periods of rapid growth, one between birth and 3 years and the other between 7 and 12 years. After the second period of growth, subsequent expansion involves pneumatization of the alveolar process of the maxilla. All growth is completed by adulthood and results in descent of the maxillary sinus floor from 4 mm above the floor of the nose between birth and 8 to 9 years of age to 4 to 5 mm below this site in the adult (Van Alyea, 1951).

The *sphenoid sinuses* originate in the third fetal month as paired evaginations of the mucosa of the sphenoethmoid recess and undergo essentially no growth until the age of 3 years. After this period, the sinus begins to pneumatize the sphenoid bone, and by age 7 years, the sinus begins to extend posteriorly toward the sella turcica. It may reach its final form and extent between ages 12 and 15 years or may continue to develop into adulthood to involve the basisphenoid; any possible arrest in development accounts for the tremendous variation in the size of the sinus.

Of all the paranasal sinuses, the *ethmoid sinus* has the greatest variation. The anterior cells of this sinus first appear in the third fetal month as evaginations (also termed pits or furrows) of the lateral nasal wall adjacent to the middle meatus. The origin of these pits is the *frontal recess*, which in turn originates from the middle meatus. The posterior group of cells arises from the superior meatus. At birth, the anterior (or anteromedial cells, depending on the division of the sinus into two or three parts) ethmoid sinus measures 2 mm × 2 mm × 5 mm, and the posterior group of cells measures 2 mm × 4 mm × 5 mm. At this time, the ethmoids are fluid filled and are difficult to recognize on routine radiographic examination. They may be visualized on routine films at age 1 year and then only if they are well developed. Growth of the cells is relatively rapid, espe-cially in the second year of life. By the 12th year, the ethmoids have reached nearly adult size; expansion during puberty involves primarily bone outside the ethmoid capsule.

The *frontal sinus* has several possible origins, each of which influences the relationship of the sinus to the lateral nasal wall, particularly in the embryologic anterosuperior extension of the middle meatus, the frontal recess. The development of the frontal sinus is initiated in the fourth fetal month when the entire nasofrontal area is represented by the frontal recess. Each frontal sinus may have a different origin and a unique communication within the middle meatus. Kasper (1936) found the most common origin of the frontal sinus to be pits or furrows in the frontal recess that were rudimentary anterior ethmoid cells (described previously as frontal recess cells). The more remote or lateral these pits are from the ethmoid infundibulum, the more lateral are the frontal sinuses and their communications with the nose. When the sinus arises from the ethmoid infundibular cells, the connection with the nose tends to be more in line with the ethmoid infundibulum. Far less common is the frontal sinus that is derived from direct extension of the entire frontal recess. At birth, the sinus has little clinical relevance, often being indistinguishable from the anterior ethmoid cells. By age 12 years, the frontal sinus is still somewhat smaller than adult size, and growth is completed before 20 years of age.

Anatomy of the Paranasal Sinuses

In the adult, the ethmoid sinuses form a pyramid, the wider base being located posteriorly and the entire sinus measuring 4 to 5 cm anteroposteriorly, 2.5 cm in height, and 0.5 cm anteriorly and 1.5 cm posteriorly in width. The roof of the sinus, the fovea ethmoidalis, extends 2 to 3 mm above the more medial cribriform plate. The lateral wall of the sinus, the *lamina papyracea*, forms the most constant part of the sinus. The actual reported size of the sinus and the number of cells vary with each series, with a range of 4 to 17 cells per person. The fact that the sinus is known as the ethmoid labyrinth attests to the intricacy of the structure and challenges the understanding of the anatomy.

The classification proposed by Ritter in

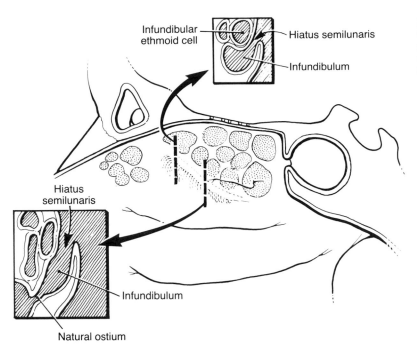

Infundibular ethmoid cell

Hiatus semilunaris

Infundibulum

Hiatus semilunaris

Infundibulum

Natural ostium

Figure 22–6. Anatomy of ostiomeatal complex. Cross sections are illustrated at the site of the ethmoid and maxillary infundibulum.

1978 most clearly conveys the origin and drainage of the ethmoid cells. The most anterior cells are the *frontal recess cells*, whose numbers range from zero to four. These cells arise from the anterosuperior growth of the ethmoid into the frontal bone. They may come to rest within the frontal bone, forming the frontal sinus; give rise to a *bulla,* or bulge, into the frontal sinus floor; or form supraorbital ethmoid cells as they pneumatize the orbit. The number of *infundibular cells* ranges from one to seven, and they are the next most anterior cells. The most constant of these cells are those that form the extramural cells, the *agger nasi,* through the pneumatization of the lacrimal bone. These cells are located on the lateral nasal wall immediately anterior to the middle turbinate. They drain into the ethmoid infundibulum, which is a pouch or a trough that ends superiorly in the frontal recess, and in some people these cells may be the origin of the frontal sinus. The *bullar cells,* ranging in number from one to six, are the most constant of the anterior ethmoid cells and form a partial sphere lateral to or beneath the middle turbinate, the bulla ethmoidalis. These cells drain into the middle meatus via ostia that lie superiorly, posteriorly, and parallel to the hiatus semilunaris.

The *hiatus semilunaris* is the entrance of a curved groove between the bulla ethmoidalis, which borders it posteriorly, and its anterior border, which is a ridge of bone formed by the ascending process of the maxilla, the *uncinate process* (Fig. 22–6). The groove is known as the *infundibulum.* Superiorly, the hiatus communicates with the ethmoid infundibulum. The uncinate process is also either a semilunar structure that ranges from nearly flat to 4 mm in height or a projection into the nasal cavity that is 14 to 22 mm in length. The uncinate process is immediately posterior to the agger nasi cells and therefore may not be visualized easily in the lateral nasal wall.

On the medial, superior surface of the bulla is a furrow, the suprabullar furrow, that can evaginate to form suprabullar ethmoid cells within the ethmoid and adjacent bones. The conchal cells invade the middle turbinate, and when these cells are located in the anterior aspect of the turbinate, they are referred to as *conchae bullosa.* The middle turbinate is the medial appendage of the nasal wall and overhangs the bulla ethmoidalis, the hiatus semilunaris, and the uncinate process. Anteriorly, the middle turbinate is attached superiorly to the cribriform plate. The major attachment of the middle turbinate to the ethmoid capsule and the *lamina papyracea* is formed by the ground plates or lamella. The most important of these, the ground or *basal lamella,* separates the anterior ethmoids from the posterior ethmoids. The number of posterior ethmoid cells ranges from one to seven, and they not only invade the posterior ethmoid capsule but may also invade the middle turbinate, sphenoid, maxillary, and palatine bones. At the junction of the lamina papyracea and the frontal bone, the posterior ethmoid artery enters the posterior ethmoids approximately 3 to 8 mm anterior to the optic nerve. In rare cases, the optic nerve may be surrounded by posterior extramural ethmoid cells. Both the anterior and posterior ethmoid arteries lie at the articulation of the lamella of the middle and superior turbinates with the lamina papyracea.

The adult *frontal sinus* is described as measuring 28 mm high, 24 mm wide, and 20 mm deep. The sinus is compartmentalized further by intrasinus septi and marginated by irregular bone. The communication of this sinus with the nose is usually described as a distinct *nasofrontal duct*. More often, this is not the case; the sinus instead drains by an ostium that can vary from 2 to 10 mm in size (and on average is less than 5 mm). The connection with the nose may be directly through the frontal recess or through the anterior ethmoid cells. There is significant variability in the accessibility of this passage via the nose, depending on the origin of this sinus.

In the adult, the *maxillary sinus* can be described as being triangular, measuring 25 mm along the anterior limits of its base, 34 mm deep, and 33 mm high. The sinus can be partially compartmentalized by septa, and in rare cases, separate cavities can exist in the posterior part of the sinus. A primary or natural ostium is located in the superior aspect of the medial wall of the sinus and drains into the ethmoid infundibulum or the hiatus semilunaris. Although actual numbers differ, most ostia are in the region of the posterior half of the infundibulum, posterior to the midpoint of the bulla ethmoidalis. The ostium tends to be elliptical, measuring 1 to 20 mm in length. In 15% to 40% of individuals, accessory ostia are found. These ostia may be located in the infundibulum of the membranous region of the medial sinus wall, which is only a reduplication of the mucosa of the sinus and the lateral nasal wall. This region is inferior to the uncinate process and superior to the insertion of the inferior turbinate.

The average *sphenoid sinus* in the adult measures 20 mm high, 23 mm deep, and 17 mm wide. The volume varies from 0.1 mL to 30 mL, the average ranging from 5 to 7.5 mL. As the sinus expands, vessels and nerves in the lateral aspect of the body of the sphenoid bone come to lie as indentations in the wall of the sinus. Thus anatomic dissections performed by various authors have revealed a projection of the internal carotid artery, the optic nerve indentation, and the vidian nerve indentation. Researchers have also found thinning of the superior wall, which may separate the sinus from the dura by only 1 mm. Approximately 22% of skulls have an intrasinus septum. The sphenoid ostium drains by a single ostium into the sphenoethmoid recess. The ostium is 2 to 3 mm in diameter and may be either round or elliptical. The sinus depends on mucociliary flow for drainage, inasmuch as the ostium is typically 10 to 15 mm from the floor of the sinus or 8 mm from the cribriform plate (range 1 to 15 mm) and 5 mm lateral to the nasal septum. The middle turbinate may make visualization of this ostium difficult. The ostium actually tends to be more often inferior than superior to the average location, lying at an angle of 30° to the floor of the nose. Various measurements have been reported because of this difficulty in visualization. Dixon (1937) noted that the sphenoid ostium was 7 cm from the anterior nasal spine. He also found that the pituitary fossa is 8.5 cm from the anterior nasal spine.

Physiology of the Paranasal Sinuses

The sinuses are lined with respiratory epithelium. Under this is a tunica propria formed with fibroelastic tissue containing mucous and serous glands. The secretions of these glands combine and form a mucous blanket that covers the epithelium. This blanket and the ciliated epithelium form the mucociliary system. The mucosa is supplied by both parasympathetic and sympathetic innervation. With stimulation, parasympathetic innervation causes an abundant watery flow, whereas sympathetic innervation causes a mucinous secretion. The epithelial lining of the sinuses helps supply the nose with a steady covering of mucus to help it warm and humidify the inspired air.

Mucous Blanket

The sinuses are capable of secreting antibacterial and antiviral substances to be carried into the nose. The majority of inspired particulate matter is deposited on the anterior end of the middle and inferior turbinates and in the middle meatus; the chemicals in the sinus tend to flow toward these areas, thus helping the nose to cleanse the inspired air. Seventy percent to 80% of all particles 3 to 5 μ in diameter are deposited in the nose. Only particles less than 1 μ can pass through the nose. The mucous blanket contains mast cells, polymorphonuclear leukocytes, eosinophils, lysozyme, IgA, IgG, and interferon. The mucous blanket has an upper layer that is highly viscous, elastic, and tenacious; the lower layer is of lower viscosity, which enables the cilia to move the blanket forward. The speed of flow differs in different areas. In the maxillary and frontal sinuses, the direction of flow of the mucus is circular or spiral, centering at the natural ostium. In the ethmoid and sphenoid sinuses, the flow is directed toward the natural ostium. The mucous blanket is renewed every 10 to 15 minutes.

The cilia function best in a humid environment. When the relative humidity drops below 50%, ciliary activity is impaired, as it is when the temperature drops below 18°C. Decreased ciliary activity may allow easier penetration and proliferation of bacteria and viruses. Viral disease causes cellular necrosis, which acts as an excellent culture medium for bacteria. Thus 24 to 48 hours after the onset of acute viral infections, there is evidence of a bacterial component. The mucociliary system attempts to prevent bacterial superinfection and is usually successful. Chronic infection results when the system fails. Failure results from a severe infection, from anything occluding sinus drainage so that the mucous blanket cannot cleanse the sinus, or from ciliary stasis.

Sinus Obstruction

The maxillary sinus empties into the middle meatus in the area of the hiatus semilunaris. Partial or complete block of the natural ostium is usual in either acute or chronic disease. The anterior ethmoid cells empty into the infundibulum along with the frontal sinus. Secretions from here drain across the maxillary ostium. Thus anything causing obstruction in the area of the hiatus semilunaris may obstruct these three sinuses.

Chronic or chronic-recurrent sinusitis therefore implies a breakdown in the mucociliary system. This breakdown usually involves the anterior ethmoids because of location and anatomic structure. Chronic infection here produces edema of the surrounding mucosa, with subsequent block of frontal, maxillary, and anterior ethmoids. The posterior ethmoids may drain through the anterior ethmoids or posteriorly. The sphenoid sinus drains independently, but its ostium may be obstructed by edema involving the posterior ethmoids or the posterior middle turbinate.

Sinus Function

The function of the sinuses is unknown. Studies have shown that they probably do not impart a resonance to the voice as was once thought. Another function that has been stated is to warm and humidify inspired air, but the air exchange between the nose and sinuses makes this function insignificant in comparison with the function of the nose. Because the sinuses have such a small volume (45 mL), it appears that they do not regulate intranasal pressure. Sinuses do form some sort of shock absorber, but the effectiveness depends on the degree of pneumatization.

The sinuses secrete some mucus to help the nasal cavity, but this is a small amount of the total secreted. However, the location of the ostia is such that the nose is supplied with the mucus it needs where it is needed most. This is the area of the middle meatus.

CONCLUSION

Although a great deal is known about the anatomic and physiologic characteristics of the nose, there is much to be learned. The sense of smell and the exact neural understanding for olfaction must be discovered. The realm of endoscopic sinus surgery has greatly increased the understanding of the mechanics and anatomy of the paranasal sinuses. The realm of rhinology and allergy has just been opened, and further research is being conducted throughout the world. The study of rhinology and sinus disease has an exciting future in the field of otolaryngology.

SUGGESTED READINGS

Dixon FW: A comparative study of the sphenoid. Ann Otol Rhinol Laryngol 46:687–698, 1937.

Hollingshead WH: Anatomy for Surgeons: The Head and Neck. Hagerstown, MD: Harper & Row, 1968.

Kasper KA: Nasofrontal connections. A study based on one hundred consecutive dissections. Arch Otolaryngol 23:322–343, 1936.

Messerklinger W: Endoskopische Diagnose und Chirurgie der rezidivierenden Sinusitis. *In* Krajina Z (ed): Advances in Nose and Sinus Surgery. Zagreb, Yugoslavia, Zagreb University, 1985.

Meyerhoff WL: Physiology of the nose and paranasal sinuses. *In* Paparella M, Shumrick D (eds): Otolaryngology (pp 297–318). Philadelphia: WB Saunders, 1980.

Rice D, Schaefer SD: Endoscopic Sinus Surgery. New York, Raven Press, 1988.

Ritter FN: The Paranasal Sinuses: Anatomy and Surgical Technique, 2nd ed. St. Louis, CV Mosby, 1978.

Schaeffer JP: The genesis, development, and adult anatomy of the nasofrontal region in man. Am J Anat 20:125–143, 1916.

Van Alyea OE: Nasal Sinuses: An Anatomic and Clinical Consideration, 2nd ed. Baltimore: Williams & Wilkins, 1951.

Wigand ME, Steiner W, Jaumann MP: Endonasal sinus surgery with endoscopical control: from radical operation to rehabilitation of the mucosa. Endoscopy 10:255–260, 1978.

CHAPTER 23

Nasal Obstruction

Eugene B. Kern, MD

Can you remember when you had your last upper respiratory tract infection? Did you experience difficulty breathing? Were you breathing through your mouth? Was this difficulty breathing through the nose associated with dry mouth, dry lips, or disturbed sleep? Persons who come to a physician with the chief complaint of a stuffy nose, nasal obstruction, or difficulty breathing through the nose may also experience shortness of breath.

Nasal airway obstruction is a common and usually a disturbing symptom. The external nose may provide a clue as to whether a previous nasal trauma has produced a nasal deformity. The patient's history is extremely important because the diagnosis of allergic, vasomotor, or drug-induced nasal obstruction can be suggested by or made from the history. A history of previous nasal surgery or nasal trauma may mean that the nasal airway obstruction is a result of a nasal septal perforation or still uncorrected abnormality or sequelae, such as scar tissue from surgical or nonsurgical trauma. It is important to have a conceptual etiologic framework and to use a systematic approach in dealing with patients who complain of nasal airway obstruction so that an accurate diagnosis can be made and proper treatment can be rendered.

Nasal obstructions may be divided into those that are caused by mucosal changes, structural changes, or both (Table 23–1). The mucosal changes may be physiologic (nasal cycle and positional) or pathologic (viral, bacterial, fungal, allergic, vasomotor, rhinitis medicamentosa, hypertrophied mucosa, and atrophic mucosa). The structural changes capable of producing nasal airway obstruction may involve the septum (nasal septal deformities, nasal septal trauma, septal hematoma, septal abscess, and septal perforation) or new growths (nasal polyps, papillomas, inverting papillomas, and other benign or malignant tumors). In addition, other miscellaneous causes may produce nasal airway obstruction (hypertrophied adenoids, foreign body, choanal atresia, intranasal scars, alar collapse, and some other rare causes).

Pathologic nasal airway obstruction can be simplified into abnormalities that can be seen (anterior abnormalities) and those that cannot be seen (posterior abnormalities).

Anterior causes of nasal airway obstruction that can be seen on anterior rhinoscopy with or without telescopes may include both mucosal and structural disturbances. The visible mucosal disturbances are changes that occur at the time of involvement and include viral rhinitis, bacterial rhinitis, and fungal rhinitis. In these cases, clear or mucopurulent discharge with red, swollen, edematous (boggy) turbinates is visible. During the active period (exacerbation) of allergic or vasomotor nasal reactions, clear secretions with pale violescent, swollen, edematous (boggy) turbinates can be seen. If the nose is quiescent (remission), a person with allergic or vasomotor nasal reactions may have a normal-appearing mucosa. Persons with rhinitis medicamentosa, hypertrophied mucosa, or atrophic mucosa are found on examination to have apparent mucosal changes. In rhinitis medicamentosa, the mucosa is usually red and may be granular in appearance, whereas in hyperplastic mucosa, the mucosa appears pale, with or without some polypoid changes, and also may be granular. In

TABLE 23–1. Causes of Nasal Obstruction

General Causes
 Mucosal
 Structural
 Mixed
Specific Causes
 Mucosal
  Infectious diseases
   Viral infections
   Bacterial infections
   Fungal infections
  Allergic nose
  Vasomotor nose (vasomotor rhinopathy,
   vasomotor rhinitis, or nonallergic rhinitis)
  Rhinitis medicamentosa
  Hypertrophied mucosa–hypertrophied turbinates
  Atrophic mucosa, nasal atrophy, atrophic rhinitis,
   and ozena
 Structural
  Nasal septal abnormalities
   Deviation or bend
   Obstruction
   Impaction
   Nasal valve
   Compression of the middle turbinate
  Nasal trauma
  Septal hematomas
  Septal abscess
  Septal perforations
  Nasal polyps
  Papillomas
  Inverting papillomas
  Other benign tumors: (1) nasal gliomas and
    (2) juvenile angiofibromas
  Malignant tumors
 Mixed
  Hypertrophied adenoids
  Choanal atresia
  Intranasal synechia, scars, and stenosis
  Narrow nose syndrome
  Alar collapse
  Others (rare)
  Foreign bodies

atrophic mucosa the mucosa can be pink, but it is usually thin, and, depending on the degree of atrophy, it may have associated fetid crusts.

The structural disturbances that can be seen (and sometimes are seen only after topical decongestion of the nose) include anterior septal abnormalities (areas 1, 2, and 3), midseptal and posterior septal abnormalities (areas 4 and 5), septal hematoma, septal abscess, septal perforation, nasal polyps, nasal tumors, and intranasal scars (Fig. 23–1).

Posterior causes of nasal airway obstruction that are visible on posterior rhinoscopy in the nasopharynx may include hypertrophied adenoids, posterior septal abnormali-ties (area 5), choanal atresia, choanal polyps, and tumors.

Pathologic features that cannot be seen and that can produce nasal airway obstruction include allergic and vasomotor nasal reactions during remission. These reactions also include chronic sinusitis, because the results of an intranasal examination may be normal ("cannot be seen" disease), and yet a person with chronic sinusitis can complain of nasal airway obstruction. Roentgenograms (plain and computed tomographic scans) are helpful in making the diagnosis. Facial paralysis, scleroderma, interruption of sympathetic nerves (Horner's syndrome), and, more commonly, use of systemic medications such as antihypertensive agents (rauwolfia derivatives) are causes of nasal obstruction resulting from something that cannot be seen on nasal examination.

The most frequent error is to miss structural pathologic features on nasal examination because the nose has not been topically decongested and re-examined. Another common problem is to miss pathologic features of the valve because a nasal speculum or telescope has been introduced too far into the vestibule and has occluded and bypassed the valve region. Therefore, if the patient's symptom of nasal obstruction cannot be explained, the nose and the nasopharynx should be decongested and re-examined, and the valve region should be checked. If the examination is still noncontributive to explaining the symptoms, pathologic conditions that cannot be seen (allergic or vasomotor reactions in remission, systemic medications like antihypertensives) should be suspected, and sinus radiographs should be obtained to rule out chronic sinusitis.

In summary, nasal obstruction may result from mucosal changes, or structural changes, or both. Usually the pathologic process can be seen on anterior nasal examination or posterior nasopharyngeal examination. If a cause for the nasal obstruction cannot be seen, re-examination should be conducted after topical decongestion and sinus roentgenograms (direct coronal computed tomographic scans are preferable) should be ordered and obtained to rule out chronic sinusitis; other causes of pathologic conditions that cannot be seen should be considered.

MUCOSAL CAUSES OF NASAL OBSTRUCTION

Physiologic Considerations

Nasal Cycle

The physiologic alteration of congestion and decongestion of the nasal turbinates is termed the nasal cycle. Approximately 80% of the population have an active nasal cycle. If you test your own nose, you will find that breathing may be more difficult on one side, and the sides will switch after approximately 2 to 4 hours. The importance of the nasal cycle is that the total nasal resistance remains somewhat constant in the normal healthy person. The total nasal resistance, or breathing through both nares, is lower than the resistance of either one of the sides. This situation allows for the changing volumes of erectile tissue (turbinates) of the two sides of the nose to continue to function in a rhythmic cycle of congestion and decongestion without producing the symptoms of total nasal airway obstruction. Thus a patient who informs the physician that first one nostril and then the other stops up is usually describing a normal physiologic phenomenon.

Positional

Positional nasal airway obstruction is another normal physiologic phenomenon. When a person lies on one side, that side (the dependent side) tends to become obstructed. This seems to be more prevalent in persons who have a nasal airway abnormality: an upper respiratory tract infection, a septal deformity, or some other nasal airway obstruction. A person who has, for example, a left-sided nasal airway obstruction resulting from a septal problem or polyps sleeps mainly on the left side, because when sleeping on the right (or open) side, the right side becomes obstructed as a result of the dependent positional phenomenon. Thus there is a tendency to rotate onto the left side so that unobstructed breathing can occur. Persons with nasal airway obstruction tend to favor or sleep on the side of the obstruction, especially if the obstruction is unilateral.

Persons who sleep supine or horizontal on the bed or with less than a 30° elevation off the bed may complain of nasal airway obstruction. This is caused by an increase in venous pressure of the turbinates and is one of the reasons why persons with nasal airway obstruction may sleep on one or two pillows. This orthopnea (dyspnea when in the supine position) can usually be relieved when the patient sits up above 30° from the horizontal position or stands up.

Infectious Diseases

Viral Infections

There are many causes of the common cold, also termed viral rhinitis, upper respiratory tract infection, acute rhinitis, or acute coryza. Hundreds of rhinoviruses have been proved to be causal factors in the production of this viral upper respiratory tract disorder, including adenoviruses, influenza and parainfluenza viruses, rhinoviruses, respiratory syncytial viruses, and certain types of coxsackieviruses and echoviruses. To determine the exact etiologic agent, isolation of the virus and serologic testing are necessary. These procedures are usually not practical in the everyday practice of medicine and are used mainly in epidemiologic studies. Each episode of a common cold seems to be virus type specific, which is why persons can have multiple upper respiratory tract infections caused by various etiologic agents and substrains within a specific group.

There is no conclusive evidence that lowering the body resistance, lowering the body temperature, or exposure to cold water or chilling air induces an upper respiratory tract infection. Some evidence suggests that these exposures decrease the defensive mechanisms in the nose that preclude the local invasion of the nasal mucosa by the viruses in question. Other evidence suggests that certain states of health can predispose people to upper respiratory tract infections. For example, irritating fumes, pollutants, and even cigarette smoke have been implicated as possible factors in the production of upper respiratory tract infections. Once an upper respiratory tract infection caused by one or more of the various viral groups occurs, bacterial complications involving the sinuses, nasal pharynx, adenoids, eustachian tube, oropharynx, tonsils, trachea, or even the bronchi and lungs can appear. This is especially true in the pediatric population and particularly in the age group of neonates to 2-year-olds. Predisposing factors in young children include crowded living conditions (including day care centers) and the possibility that early discontinuation of breast feeding leaves the infant with less antiviral and antibacterial protection. Bacterial complications of viral rhinitis occur more frequently in older, debilitated patients with chronic pulmonary disorders or those with immunodeficiency syndromes (e.g., AIDS).

Symptom Complex. Usually patients with upper respiratory tract infections have a symptom complex that includes rhinorrhea, sneezing, nasal airway obstruction, sore throat, and systemic findings of lethargy, fatigue, myalgia, and headache. Temperature is usually normal in the adult, whereas in the child it ranges from above 37.7°C to 38.8°C or 39.4°C in most instances. Adults usually complain of loss of the sense of smell or taste and may also complain of disturbed sleep. Constant sneezing, nose blowing, sniffling, irritation and redness of the nose and upper lip that result from constant wiping, and dryness of the lips that is caused by mouth breathing all can be found as the disorder progresses. Discharge from the nose becomes thicker and, if bacterial contamination supervenes, becomes mucopurulent. Barring any serious complications, the course usually terminates after 4 to 14 days. A summary of symptoms is listed in Table 23–2.

Differential Diagnosis. Allergic rhinitis

TABLE 23–2. Frequency of Common Cold Symptoms

Symptoms	Frequency (%)
Severe	
Nasal discharge	100
Nasal obstruction	99
Moderate	
Sore or dry throat	96
Malaise	81
Postnasal discharge	79
Headache	78
Cough	76
Mild	
Sneezing	97
Feverishness	49
Chilliness	43
Burning eyes and mucous membranes	28
Aching muscles	22

From Kleinfeld C: Handbook of Nonprescription Drugs, 5th ed. Washington, DC: American Pharmaceutical Association, 1977.

(seasonal or perennial) has no systemic involvement. The same is true of vasomotor nose and cerebrospinal fluid rhinorrhea. Examination that shows the mucosa to be hyperemic and reveals the symptom complex is usually enough to make the diagnosis of the common cold. A specific etiologic diagnosis is rarely practical and is impossible unless the virus is isolated from acute and convalescent serum samples. The diagnosis therefore rests on the basis of history, physical findings, and the absence of the persistence of symptoms that might occur in other disorders. For example, upper respiratory tract infection symptoms and rhinorrhea may occur in persons who have bacterial streptococcal pharyngitis, diphtheria, measles, or pertussis (whooping cough), and thus confusion may occur in these conditions with the rhinorrhea of the common cold. Lymphocytosis may be present in the other disorders but is not common in the uncomplicated upper respiratory tract infection. The so-called flu is usually caused by an influenza virus, and the symptoms may be more dramatic and fulminating and can possibly be fatal. Worldwide epidemics occur, but mortality is an unlikely outcome.

Prophylaxis. Various measures have been undertaken to prevent the common cold, including vaccines and high doses of specific vitamins. None have been proved in a double-blind study to be efficacious in preventing the common cold. Production of vaccines to the large variety of strains of viruses that produce the common cold is impractical.

Treatment. Treatment of the febrile patient centers on the high intake of fluid. The diet should be light, especially when anorexia occurs. Bed rest is advisable, along with symptomatic medication for pain, headache, and fever (Table 23–3). Should cough ensue, codeine or some other cough suppressant can be useful (Table 23–4). The antihistamine decongestants are sometimes effective in drying the nasal mucosa. Topical nasal sprays are not recommended for adults. Decongestants can be used in infants, especially for feeding; 0.025% or 0.125% phenylephrine sprayed into the nose just before feeding can help. Inhalations provided by a vaporizer with cold water can be useful, especially in the person who has lower airway involvement. Antibiotic drugs are not recommended

TABLE 23–3. Common Nonprescription Drugs Used for the Common Cold

Product (Manufacturer)	Dosage Form	Ingredients			
		Sympathomimetic	*Antihistamine*	*Analgesic*	*Other*
Alka-Seltzer Plus (Miles)	Effervescent tablet	Phenylpropanolamine bitartrate, 26.5 mg	Chlorpheniramine maleate, 2.1 mg	Aspirin, 324 mg	—
Allerest (Pharmacraft)	Time capsule	Phenylpropanolamine hydrochloride, 50 mg	Pyrilamine maleate, 15 mg; Methapyrilene fumarate, 10 mg	—	—
Bayer Children's Cold Tablets (Glenbrook)	Tablet	Phenylpropanolamine hydrochloride, 3.125 mg	—	Aspirin, 81 mg	—
Chlor-Trimeton Decongestant (Schering)	Tablet	Ephedrine, 60 mg	Chlorpheniramine maleate, 4 mg	—	—
Colrex (Rowell)	Capsule	Phenylephrine hydrochloride, 5 mg	Chlorpheniramine maleate, 2 mg	Acetaminophen, 300 mg	Ascorbic acid, 200 mg
Contac (Menley & James)	Time capsule	Phenylpropanolamine hydrochloride, 50 mg	Chlorpheniramine maleate, 4 mg	—	Belladonna alkaloids, 0.2 mg
Coricidin (Schering)	Tablet	—	Chlorpheniramine maleate, 2 mg	Aspirin, 325 mg	Caffeine, 30 mg
Coricidin "D" (Schering)	Tablet	Phenylpropanolamine hydrochloride, 1.25 mg	Chlorpheniramine maleate, 2 mg	Aspirin, 325 mg	—
Coricidin Demilets (Schering)	Children's chewable tablet	Phenylephrine hydrochloride, 2.5 mg	Chlorpheniramine maleate, 0.5 mg	Aspirin, 80 mg	—
Coricidin Medilets (Schering)	Children's chewable tablet	—	Chlorpheniramine maleate, 0.5 mg	Aspirin, 80 mg	—
CoTylenol (McNeil)	Tablet	Phenylephrine hydrochloride, 5 mg	Chlorpheniramine maleate, 1 mg	Acetaminophen, 325 mg	—
Demazin (Schering)	Syrup repetabs	Phenylephrine hydrochloride, 2.5 mg/5 mL, 20 mg/tablet	Chlorpheniramine maleate, 1.0 mg/5 mL, 4 mg/tablet	—	Alcohol, 7.5% (syrup)
Dristan (Whitehall)	Tablet	Phenylephrine hydrochloride, 5 mg	Phenindamine tartrate, 10 mg	Aspirin	Caffeine; aluminum hydroxide; magnesium carbonate
Fedrazil (Burroughs Wellcome)	Tablet	Pseudoephedrine hydrochloride, 30 mg	Chlorcyclizine hydrochloride, 25 mg	—	—
Neo-Synephrine Elixir (Winthrop)	Liquid	Phenylephrine hydrochloride, 5 mg/5 mL	—	—	Alcohol, 8%
Novafed (Dow)	Syrup	Pseudoephedrine hydrochloride, 30 mg/5 mL	—	—	Alcohol, 7.5%
Novafed A (Dow)	Syrup	Pseudoephedrine hydrochloride, 30 mg/5 mL	Chlorpheniramine maleate, 2 mg/5 mL	—	Alcohol, 5%
Novahistine Elixir (Dow)	Syrup	Phenylpropanolamine hydrochloride, 18.75 mg/5 mL	Chlorpheniramine maleate, 2 mg/5 mL	—	Alcohol, 5%
Ornex (SmithKline Consumer)	Capsule	Phenylpropanolamine hydrochloride, 18 mg	—	Acetaminophen, 325 mg	—
Sine-Off (SmithKline)	Tablet	Phenylpropanolamine hydrochloride, 18.75 mg	Chlorpheniramine maleate, 2 mg	Aspirin, 325 mg	—
St. Joseph Cold Tablets for Children (Plough)	Tablet	Phenylpropanolamine hydrochloride, 3.125 mg	—	Aspirin, 81 mg	—
Sudafed (Burroughs Wellcome)	Tablet; syrup	Pseudoephedrine hydrochloride, 30 mg/tablet or 5 mL	—	—	—
Triaminic (Dorsey)	Syrup	Phenylpropanolamine hydrochloride, 12.5 mg/5 mL	Pheniramine maleate, 6.25 mg/5 mL; Pyrilamine maleate, 6.25 mg/5 mL	—	—
Triaminicin (Dorsey)	Tablet	Phenylpropanolamine hydrochloride, 25 mg	Chlorpheniramine maleate, 2 mg	Aspirin, 450 mg	Caffeine, 30 mg
Triaminicin Chewables (Dorsey)	Chewable tablet	Phenylpropanolamine hydrochloride, 6.25 mg	Chlorpheniramine maleate, 0.5 mg	—	—
4-Way Cold Tablets (Bristol-Myers)	Tablet	Phenylephrine hydrochloride, 5 mg	—	Aspirin, 324 mg	Magnesium hydroxide, 125 mg; White phenolphthalein, 15 mg

TABLE 23–4. Cough Suppressant Dosages

| | Dosage | | |
| | Adults | *Children* | |
Drug and Category	*Adults*	*6 to 12 years*	*2 to 6 years*
Codeine (I)	10 to 20 mg every 4 to 6 hours (not to exceed 120 mg/24 hours)	5 to 10 mg every 4 to 6 hours (not to exceed 60 mg/24 hours)	2.5 to 5 mg every 4 to 6 hours (not to exceed 30 mg/24 hours)
Dextromethorphan (I)	10 to 20 mg every 4 hours or 30 mg every 6 to 8 hours (not to exceed 120 mg/24 hours)	5 to 10 mg every 4 hours or 15 mg every 6 to 8 hours (not to exceed 60 mg/24 hours)	2.5 every 4 hours or 7.5 mg every 6 to 8 hours (not to exceed 30 mg/24 hours)
Diphenhydramine hydrochloride (I)	25 mg every 4 hours (not to exceed 150 mg/24 hours)	12.5 mg every 4 hours (not to exceed 75 mg/24 hours)	6.25 mg every 4 hours (not to exceed 37.5 mg/24 hours)
Noscapine hydrochloride (III)	15 to 30 mg every 4 to 6 hours (not to exceed 180 mg/24 hours)	7.5 to 15 mg every 4 to 6 hours (not to exceed 90 mg/24 hours)	3.75 to 7.5 mg every 4 to 6 hours (not to exceed 45 mg/24 hours)

As proposed by the Food and Drug Administration Over-The-Counter Panel on Cold, Cough, Allergy, Bronchodilator, and Anti-Asthmatic Drugs.

From Kleinfeld C: Handbook of Nonprescription Drugs, 9th ed. Washington, DC: American Pharmaceutical Association, 1977.

unless there is fever associated with a bacterial complication.

Bacterial Infections

In a primary or a secondary bacterial infection in the nose, discharge is usually mucopurulent. Its color is predicated on the type of organism that is invading the nasal tissues. Bacterial rhinitis frequently leads to sinusitis. In the broad spectrum of bacterial disorders involving the nose, most are caused by gram-positive organisms.

The most common of the gram-positive organisms that produce infectious diseases in the nose are coagulase-positive staphylococci. These organisms may appear in and about the anterior nares and may also be present in the nasopharynx, especially in physicians, nurses, and other medical personnel. Some strains of staphylococci are penicillin-resistant.

Streptococcal organisms come in three strains. Further classification is based on carbohydrate in a particular bacterial cell wall that allowed grouping into A through O (Lancefield's typing). Streptococci can produce rhinitis, with rhinorrhea and febrile illness including nausea, vomiting, headache, and malaise. However, the usual findings include a sore throat and signs of pharyngeal involvement. The stuffy nose alone or rhinitis alone is not characteristic of this type of infection. Pneumococcal organisms may also involve the nose, but this is un-

likely. *Staphylococcus epidermidis* (*albus*) may also involve the nose, but this too is an extremely uncommon occurrence.

Gram-negative organisms may also produce bacterial rhinitis. The most common organism of this group in the upper midwestern United States is *Haemophilus influenzae*. The other organism that is gram negative and capable of producing nasal infection is *Escherichia coli*. Tuberculosis, tularemia, and plague are unlikely causes of clinical rhinitis. When they do occur, they are usually part of a generalized systemic disorder. Treatment is based on control of systemic symptoms and specific antibiotics against the cultured organisms.

When a mucopurulent discharge is present in a patient who is ill or who is not responding to conventional treatment, culture of the nasal discharge is in order. Material for culture can be obtained from the patient's nose conveniently in a routine clinical setting. It is possible with adequate lighting to visualize the region of the middle meatus and to obtain a culture from that region when a patient has signs or symptoms of acute or recurrent suppurative rhinosinusitis. When necessary, cultures should be grown for general bacteria, acid-fast bacilli, and fungi. Another culture should be performed specifically for anaerobic organisms, especially when a patient has a severely toxic condition or is threatened with regional, intracranial, or ophthalmologic complications. Smears might also be helpful in these instances to identify the organism so that adequate antibiotic therapy can be instituted immediately, while the cultures are maturing.

An underlying disorder should be sought in persons with recurrent rhinosinusitis. Diabetic patients, patients who have been on a long-term regimen of steroid therapy, and patients with a generalized debilitating systemic disorder are only some of those more likely to be susceptible to recurrent infections. Remember to question the patient about previous immunizations.

Further mention must be made of pertussis produced by *Haemophilus pertussis* (*Bordetella pertussis*). This organism usually involves the region of the nasopharynx. The patient may have symptoms that are similar to those of upper respiratory viral inflammations, such as sneezing, lacrimation, anorexia, and rhinorrhea. The paroxysmal night-time cough, however, becomes prominent, and the diagnosis should be made on the basis of the leukocytosis and a lymphocytosis with positive sputum cultures. Thus when patients fail to respond to conservative measures, cultures, complete blood cell count, and other studies should be considered.

Primary tuberculosis occasionally occurs in young children and is seen initially as an upper respiratory tract infection. This is important to remember when persons who are exposed to tuberculosis are treated. Appropriate studies, including chest roentgenograms, smears, cultures, and tuberculin skin testing, are necessary for arriving at the correct diagnosis. Both leprosy and tuberculosis may involve the nose and cause chronic destruction of nasal tissues, but their occurrence is unusual in North America.

Fungal Infections

Fungal diseases rarely involve the nose, except when they are secondary invaders in debilitated patients. Fungi are opportunistic pathogens and are most likely to be found in persons who have underlying systemic disorders, such as uncontrolled diabetes and leukemia, or in patients treated with immunosuppressive agents, antimetabolites, corticosteroids, or ionizing irradiation. These opportunistic infections can occur in the nose and the sinuses together; phycomycosis, cryptococcosis, nocardiosis, aspergillosis, and candidiasis are the most common. Blastomycosis and histoplasmosis also may be

seen. Of these, phycomycosis (mucormycosis) or rhinocerebral phycomycosis can occur in the nose and the sinuses. It may produce a purulent drainage from the nose and also necrotic destruction of the septum, the palate, and the orbital contents, including the sinuses. Rhinocerebral phycomycosis is usually fatal and occurs most often in diabetics with ketoacidosis. These people should receive treatment for the diabetes along with administration of amphotericin B for the fungal infection. It should be remembered that these are opportunistic fungi, and so samples obtained from a draining nose or sinus should be sent for general culture and culture for acid-fast bacilli, fungi, and anaerobes, especially in extremely ill patients or patients with underlying diabetic ketoacidosis.

Pseudomonas, Klebsiella, Proteus, Enterobacter, Serratia, Paracolobactrum, and *Escherichia* are all organisms that can produce hospital-acquired infections. In general, this is a rare development in the nose or the paranasal sinuses; however, these possibilities should be suspected in a person who is ill and has a secondary infection in the region of the nose and paranasal sinuses. Appropriate cultures should be done. Protozoal infections or diseases produced by worms rarely involve the nose or the paranasal sinuses.

In summary, when a patient with pain, fever, weight loss, constitutional disturbances, and nasal and paranasal sinus inflammation fails to improve, cultures should be performed for all possible causes while an underlying systemic disorder is searched for. When a patient fails to improve, consultation with other specialists should be considered.

Allergies as a Cause of Nasal Infection

Basic to the understanding of the clinical features of the allergic nose is knowledge of the allergic mechanism. The inflammatory response induced by the antibody-antigen reaction is caused by the release of chemical mediators. Histamine, serotonin, acetylcholine, bradykinin, slow-reacting substance of anaphylaxis, prostaglandins, rabbit aorta–contracting substance, and eosinophil chemotactic factor are just a few of these vasoactive chemical mediators of the allergic reaction. In the mast cells in the connective tissue (also called tissue basophils), there are granules that contain the vasoactive amines such as histamine. The antibody reacts with a specific antigen in the region of the mast cell surface. This interaction between antibody and antigen causes release of these vasoactive substances, such as histamine, which are the chemical prototype for this discussion.

Histamine release from the mast cells produces smooth muscle contraction, increased glandular secretion, and vasodilation. It is not important for the clinician to be aware of the nuances of the immune response because much of the information is still unknown or poorly understood. The basic principle is that the antibody-antigen interaction produces a release of histamine and other mediators of vasodilation.

It is important to realize that the histamine and the other vasoactive substances produce (1) the vasodilation that causes the nasal airway obstruction and (2) the increased glandular secretion that produces the runny nose (rhinorrhea); the transudation of fluid produces the interstitial edema. This edema and rhinorrhea are probably responsible for sneezing and itching of the nose. These symptoms are usually exacerbated at night or in the recumbent position, and the patient may also experience irritability, fatigue, anorexia, depression, loss of the sense of well-being, and a host of other secondary or tertiary symptoms related to oral respiration (mouth breathing).

In summary, in allergic rhinitis, the antigen stimulates a sensitive nasal respiratory epithelium that induces antibody production, namely of IgE. The IgE synthesis occurs in the lymphoid tissues—in the plasma cell. The IgE antibody has an affinity for the receptor sites on mast cells and basophilic leukocytes. The IgE antibody and antigen interaction occurs on the mast cells and promotes the release of pharmacologic mediators that produce vascular dilation, glandular secretion, and smooth muscle contraction. These mediators include histamine and histaminelike substances.

History (Seasonal Allergic Rhinitis and Perennial Allergic Rhinitis)

Seasonal allergic rhinitis usually involves a specific time of year when symptoms are more severe and this is usually related to pollination of trees, grasses, or weeds. The severity of the symptoms may vary from year to year, depending on the intensity of the allergen concentrations in the environment.

Perennial allergic rhinitis is usually caused by house dust, molds, or animal danders. It is important to search for an etiologic factor in the patient's environment. Various clues may be evident from the history as to when the symptoms occur, where they occur, and what makes them worse.

Evaluation of patients with allergic rhinitis depends in large measure on obtaining an accurate history. Try to determine whether the person has seasonal or perennial allergic rhinitis. It is important to recognize that rhinorrhea, sneezing with nasal obstruction, and intense pruritus of the palate, the pharynx, and the eyes are all characteristics of allergy. Many patients have a history of infantile eczema, asthma, bronchospasm, urticaria, and hives, along with a family history of allergic rhinitis. The physician should look for the seasonal variations in symptoms that will help determine the correct diagnosis. For example, are the symptoms worse at a particular time of year? This may help determine whether the cause is allergic in nature. Are the symptoms made worse during the season of pollination of trees, grasses, or weeds, or are the symptoms present year round but also associated with seasonal flares? In this situation, the patient may have perennial allergic rhinitis with coexisting seasonal allergic rhinitis.

Symptoms

In allergic rhinitis, the symptoms are produced by antigens that are inhalants (such as tree, grass, and weed pollen; dust; molds; and animal hair), ingestants, injectants, or infectants. The effect of the inhalants (also called aeroallergens) is usually worse on a day that is dry and windy or during the morning hours in a specific pollinating season. Patients with allergic rhinitis usually have associated ophthalmologic problems. Increase in lacrimation and itchiness of the eyes are frequent. The hallmark of allergic rhinitis is recurrent sneezing, which usually is staccato and rapid in succession. Thus sneezing, nasal obstruction (stuffy nose), nasal discharge, and an itchy nose and itchy eyes are part of the allergic rhinitis syndrome.

Examination

Symptoms are mainly confined to the patient's eyes, ears, nose, roof of mouth, and throat and occasionally involve the lower airway. During the acute stage of allergic rhinitis, the patient usually has rhinorrhea, recurrent sneezing, and pale, boggy nasal mucosa. The person often complains of itchiness of the palate and irritation of the eyes. The patient may experience a flare of urticaria or atopic dermatitis. It is important to recognize that patients with allergic rhinitis do not usually have manifestations of a bacterial inflammatory response unless they have complications such as nasopharyngitis, otitis media, rhinosinusitis, or bronchitis. Most children with rhinorrhea frequently rub their noses upward, performing the so-called allergic salute.

The physical findings observed in the patient include mouth breathing caused by edema of the turbinates. Usually the deep vessels of the turbinates are congested because of vascular dilation, but constriction of the superficial vessels of the turbinates causes the pallor. Secretions are thin and watery as a result of histamine-stimulated glandular secretion. A mucopurulent discharge usually suggests a secondary infection. Lacrimation is frequent, and conjunctivitis or chemosis may also occur.

Diagnosis

Diagnosis of allergic rhinitis is facilitated by the history of seasonal flares. An estimate should be made of whether the symptoms are worse when the patient is indoors or outdoors. History is the cornerstone of diagnosis. A suggestive history in association with positive skin testing that substantiates the existence of IgE antibodies fixed to the skin in sensitive persons establishes the diagnosis. The diagnosis may be a seasonal allergic rhinitis or perennial allergic rhinitis, or both. The stimulus is related to tree, grass, and weed pollen in seasonal allergic rhinitis, whereas in perennial allergic rhinitis the stimulus is usually related to house dust, molds, and animal danders. It should be remembered that the patient may have both seasonal and perennial allergic rhinitis! The radioallergosorbent test is a useful in vitro test that measures the quantity of IgE antibodies. The test is based on the fact that IgE antibodies from a patient's serum bind to the test antigen and this then reacts with a radiolabeled antibody to IgE.

Skin tests to determine the degree and the extent of the patient's sensitivity should be ordered when the patient is extremely symptomatic or when the condition cannot be controlled by antihistamine decongestants given orally. Tests should be ordered to substantiate the diagnosis of allergic rhinitis because some patients with vasomotor nose (to be described) have seasonal variations caused by temperature changes. If the patient is very sensitive, the antigens should be given by scratch and not intradermal testing.

Course

Allergic rhinitis usually occurs in patients under the age of 20 years. Remissions can occur and are more likely to do so in seasonal allergic rhinitis than they are in perennial allergic rhinitis. Asthma develops in fewer than 10% of patients with allergic rhinitis. Sinusitis is a rare complication of seasonal allergic rhinitis, although in patients with perennial allergic rhinitis, a postnasal discharge and mucosal changes in the sinuses commonly develop, and acute and chronic suppurative sinusitis can also develop. In patients who have nasal allergies, nasal polyps develop infrequently. Some asymptomatic patients have positive skin tests for allergens. Some of the patients may go on to develop allergic rhinitis, although no reason for this occurrence is known. Symptoms of allergic rhinitis (seasonal or perennial) may be mild and can range from minor irritation to marked irritability, fatigue, lethargy, and disturbance in the person's entire sense of well-being and functioning. There is great individual variability.

Management

The mainstay of medical management is avoiding the allergen! Avoidance is the preferred method of treatment for seasonal and perennial allergic rhinitis. If this is either impractical or impossible because of work-related situations or physical presence in an endemic area, then medication is used for prophylactic and symptomatic relief. Medical treatments are grouped into the following categories:

1. Sympathomimetics
2. Antihistamines
3. Cromolyn sodium (Intal, Aarane)
4. Steroids
    Topical sprays

Dexamethasone (Decadron, Turbinaire)
Beclomethasone dipropionate (Vanceril)
Flunisolide (Nasalide)
Systemic steroids
  Oral
  Intramuscular
  Intranasal
5. Immunotherapy (hyposensitization, desensitization "shots")

The basic principle underlying the medical management (aside from avoidance) is to counteract the physiologic effects of the vasoactive mediator release that is initiated by the interaction between the antigen and IgE. Sympathomimetics and anti-inflammatory agents (steroids) are used to counteract the effects of the active mediators after they are released. Antihistamine drugs should be used prophylactically to inhibit the effects of histamine. Cromolyn is used to block mediator release from the mast cells. Thus medical treatment is directed toward counteracting, inhibiting, or blocking the active mediators by using sympathomimetics and anti-inflammatory drugs (steroids), antihistamines, and cromolyn, respectively. All have a role in the amelioration of the patient's symptoms.

Sympathomimetics. Sympathomimetic agents have both alpha-adrenergic and beta-adrenergic activity. The classic prototype is epinephrine (Table 23–5). Its primary action is to produce contraction of smooth muscle of the blood vessels in the nasal mucous membrane. This produces nasal vasoconstriction that helps to decrease the airway obstruction and allows the patient to breathe more freely. Occasionally, these sympathomimetic medications produce side effects, such as tachycardia, increase in blood pressure, and stimulation of the nervous system with irritability and nervousness. In general, the sympathomimetic agents may be administered either orally or topically, but oral medications are preferred because they may counteract the drowsiness and lethargy induced by the various antihistamines. The use of topical sympathomimetics is to be avoided because rhinitis medicamentosa can occur. A pernicious cycle follows repeated topical use of sympathomimetics: the topical sympathomimetic agents produce vasoconstriction; after this pleasing decongestion, severe vasodilation or rebound vasodilation can occur and thereby exacerbate the symptoms of nasal obstruction. The patient then uses the

medication once again and enters the cycle of decongestion followed by rebound vasodilation and requires more decongestion and recurrent use of topical medicine. Patients can become habituated to the sympathomimetic nose drops or sprays. They find it difficult to refrain from using these drops or sprays, which provide temporary respite from oppressive nasal obstruction.

Antihistamines. There are approximately six major pharmacologic families of antihistamines. The antihistamines are competitive inhibitors and therefore must be given prophylactically to be most effective. Of the major classes of antihistamines, there is a wide variation in individual response to drug efficacy and undesirable side effects. An antihistamine preparation that is effective for one person may cause the annoying side effects of drowsiness, dryness of mouth, dysuria, palpitations, hypertension, headaches,

TABLE 23–5. Sympathomimetics: Dosages

Pseudoephedrine Hydrochloride
Indications
For symptomatic relief of nasal congestion

Administration and Dosage
Adults, 60 mg every 4 hours
Children 6 to 12 years, 30 mg every 4 hours
Children 2 to 6 years, 15 mg every 4 hours

Trade name

Sudafed:	Tablets, 30 mg, 60 mg
Novafed:	Timed-release capsules, 120 mg
Pseudo-Bid:	Timed-release capsules, 120 mg
Pseudoephedrine HCl:	Liquid, 30 mg/5 mL
Novafed:	Liquid, 30 mg/5 mL
Sudafed Syrup:	Liquid, 30 mg/5 mL

Phenylpropanolamine Hydrochloride
Indications
Nasal congestion associated with the common cold, vasomotor rhinitis, sinusitis, nasopharyngitis, or allergic conditions

Administration and Dosage
Adults, 25 mg every 4 hours, or 50 mg every 8 hours
Children 6 to 12 years, 12.5 mg every 4 hours or 25 mg every 8 hours
Children 2 to 6 years, 6.25 mg every 4 hours or 12.5 mg every 8 hours

Trade Name

Phenylpropanolamine hydrochloride	Tablets, 25 mg, 50 mg
Propadrine	Capsules, 25 mg, 50 mg; elixir, 20 mg/5 mL and 16% alcohol in 473 mL

insomnia, nervousness, blurred vision, or diplopia in another.

The major groups of antihistamines are essentially made up of a large heterocyclic benzene structure. The major groups include the alkylamines, the ethanolamines, the ethylenediamines, the phenothiazines, the piperazines, and a miscellaneous group of drugs (Table 23–6). Because individual response varies so widely, three different antihistamine medications from these groups should be tested as an initial trial. The author prefers to prescribe the combination drugs (antihistamines and sympathomimetics together) because the antihistamines may produce sedation, whereas the sympathomimetics may produce stimulation (Table 23–7). The sympathomimetic combination can alleviate some of the sedative problems of the antihistamines. When three different antihistamine groups are tried simultaneously, the patient should be informed that no one specific medication works in all patients. After a 4-day trial with each different type of medication, the most satisfactory medication for the patient (relief of symptoms and minimal side effects) is the medication of choice. The patient should then be instructed to continue to use this medication for the symptomatic period.

An initial trial in adults would include the following medications:

TABLE 23–6. Antihistamine Drugs

Drug (by Chemical Class and Category)	Trade Name
Alkylamines	
Chlorpheniramine	Chlor-trimeton, Teldrin
Brompheniramine	Dimetane
Dexbrompheniramine	Disomer
Dexchlorpheniramine	Polaramine
Dimethindene	Forhistal
Triprolidine	Actidil
Triprolidine and pseudoephedrine	Deconamine
Brompheniramine, phenylephrine, and phenylpropanolamine	Dimetapp
Dexbrompheniramine and pseudoephedrine	Disophrol, Drixoral
Chlorpheniramine, phenindamine, and phenylpropanolamine	Nolamine
Chlorpheniramine and pseudoephedrine	Novafed A Capsules
Ethanolamines	
Diphenhydramine	Benadryl
Carbinoxamine	Clistin
Doxylamine	Decapryn
Carbinoxamine and pseudoephedrine	Rondec T
Ethylenediamines	
Tripelennamine	Pyribenzamine
Methapyrilene	Histadyl
Tripelennamine and ephedrine	Pyribenzamine with ephedrine
Pyrrobutamine and cyclopentamine	Co-Pyronil
Histamine H$_1$-Receptor Antagonists	
Astemizole	Hismanal
Terfenadine	Seldane
Phenothiazines	
Methdilazine	Tacaryl
Promethazine	Phenergan
Chlorpromazine	Thorazine
Trimeprazine	Temaril
Piperazines	
Hydroxyzine	Atarax
Cyclizine	Marezine
Meclizine	Bonine
Miscellaneous	
Cyproheptadine	Periactin
Clemastine fumarate	Tavist

Modified from Kleinfeld C: Handbook of Nonprescription Drugs, 5th ed. Washington, DC: American Pharmaceutical Association, 1977.

TABLE 23–7. Commonly Used Preparation: Antihistamine Decongestants

Drug Name	Antihistamine	Sympathomimetic	Dosage Forms	Adult Dose
Actifed	Triprolidine, 2.5 mg	Pseudoephedrine, 60 mg	Tablets Syrup (child)	1 tablet tid 1 tsp tid
Benadryl	Diphenhydramine, 25 mg or 50 mg	—	Capsules 50 mg Elixir 12.5–25 mg (child)	1 capsule tid or qid 1 tsp tid
Chlor-trimeton	Chlorpheniramine, 4 mg, 8 mg, 12 mg	—	8 mg, 12 mg Repetabs 2 mg, Syrup (child)	1 tablet bid or tid 1 tsp qid
Co-Pyronil	Pyrrobutamine, 15 mg Methapyrilene, 25 mg	Cyclopentamine, 12.5 mg	Capsules Syrup	1 or 2 capsules bid or tid 0.5 or 1 tsp bid or tid
Deconamine	Chlorpheniramine, 4 mg	D-Pseudoephedrine, 60 mg	Tablet Capsules Elixir (child)	1 tablet tid or qid 1 capsule bid or tid 0.5 or 1 tsp tid or qid
Demazin	Chlorpheniramine, 2 mg	Phenylephrine, 10 mg	Repetabs Syrup (child)	1 or 2 tablets tid or tid 1 or 2 tsp every 3 to 4 hours
Dimetane	Brompheniramine, 8 and 12 mg	—	Extentabs 2 mg Elixir (child)	1 tablet bid or tid 1 to 2 tsp tid or qid
Dimetapp Extentabs	Brompheniramine, 12 mg	Phenylephrine, 15 mg Phenylpropanolamine, 15 mg	Extentabs Elixir (child)	1 tablet bid or tid 1 tsp tid
Disophrol Chrontabs	Dexbrompheniramine, 6 mg	D-Isoephedrine, 120 mg	Tablets	1 tablet bid or tid
Drixoral	Dexbrompheniramine, 6 mg	D-Isoephedrine, 120 mg	Tablets	1 tablet bid or tid
Isoclor	Chlorpheniramine, 10 mg	Pseudoephedrine, 65 mg	Time capsules Liquid (child)	1 capsule bid 1 tsp qid
Neotep	Chlorpheniramine, 9 mg	Phenylephrine, 21 mg	Granucap	1 capsule bid
Nolamine	Chlorpheniramine, 4 mg Phenindamine, 24 mg	Phenylpropanolamine, 50 mg	Tablet	1 tablet bid or tid
Novafed A	Chlorpheniramine, 8 mg	Pseudoephedrine, 120 mg	Capsules Liquid (child)	1 capsule bid 1 tsp qid
Ornade	Chlorpheniramine, 8 mg	Phenylpropanolamine, 50 mg	Spansule	1 spansule bid
Polaramine	Dexchlorpheniramine, 6 mg	—	Repetabs 4 mg, tablets Syrup (child)	1 repetab bid or tid 1 tablet tid or qid 0.5 tsp tid or qid
Propadrine	—	Phenylpropanolamine	Capsules 25 mg Capsules 50 mg Elixir 20 mg (child)	1 capsule qid 1 capsule tid 1 tsp tid
Pyribenzamine	Tripelennamine, 25 mg, 50 mg	—	Tablets Elixir (child)	1 tablet tid or qid 0.5 tsp tid or qid
Pyribenzamine with ephedrine	Tripelennamine, 25 mg	Ephedrine, 12 mg	Tablets	1 tablet qid
Rondec T	Carbinoxamine, 4 mg	Pseudoephedrine, 60 mg	Tablet Syrup (child)	1 tablet qid 0.5 tsp qid
Singlet	Chlorpheniramine, 8 mg (plus acetaminophen 500 mg)	Phenylephrine, 40 mg	Tablet	1 tablet tid or qid
Sinubid	Phenyltoloxamine, 66 mg (plus acetaminophen, 300 mg; phenacetin, 300 mg)	Phenylpropanolamine, 100 mg	Tablets	1 tablet bid
Sudafed	—	Pseudoephedrine, 30 mg, 60 mg	Tablets Syrup (child)	1 tablet qid 1 tsp qid
Teldrin	Chlorpheniramine, 8 mg, 12 mg	—	Capsules	1 capsule bid

Bid, twice a day; tid, three times a day; qid, four times a day.

1. Dexbrompheniramine (Disophrol Chrontab Tablets), one every 8 to 12 hours for 4 days;
2. Brompheniramine (Dimetapp Extentabs), one every 8 to 12 hours for 4 days;
3. Chlorpheniramine (Deconamine SR Capsules), one every 12 hours for 4 days.

If these are unsuccessful, another trial could include the following medications:

1. Phenindamine (Nolamine Tablets), one every 8 to 12 hours;
2. Chlorpheniramine (Novafed A Capsules), one every 12 hours;
3. Carbinoxamine (Rondec Tablets), one every 6 hours;
4. Dexchlorpheniramine maleate (Polaramine Repetabs Tablets), one every 12 hours, and with Polaramine (antihistamine) add

propanolamine (Propadrine), 50 mg every 12 hours;

5. Terfenadine (Seldane), 60 mg, one every 12 hours;

6. Astemizole (Hismanal), 10 mg, one daily taken on an empty stomach.

The medication that was once successful may become ineffective because tolerance develops or the patient becomes "resistant." A different antihistamine compound may be used again on a trial basis until a satisfactory medication is found. This new antihistamine is used until the patient again becomes tolerant. It is possible to return to the original antihistamine-sympathomimetic combination that was successful at first.

It is also important to recognize that antihistamines may produce other disturbing side effects, such as impotence, difficulty in urination, and incoordination. The symptom that is most relieved by the antihistamine-decongestant combination is the nasal discharge rather than the nasal congestion. The antihistamines usually alleviate neither the tearing of the eyes (epiphora) nor the itching of the eyes. Should these conditions occur, a topical adrenergic antagonist for the eye symptoms is useful. An epinephrine solution sold over the counter, such as naphazoline hydrochloride (Vasocon), is useful and beneficial for relief from itchy eyes.

Cromolyn Sodium. The exact mechanism of action of cromolyn sodium is not known, although it is thought that this medication can be successful in the treatment of perennial and seasonal allergic rhinitis by preventing the release of histamine and other amines from the mast cells. The drug prevents the degranulation of mast cells, which in turn prevents the subsequent release of the toxic amine mediators. Disodium cromoglycate is a powder and comes in 2% or 4% solutions. It may be sprayed with an insufflator that dispenses 20-mg doses and can be used four to six times daily. No systemic toxic effects have been reported, although occasionally headache, nasal dryness, and irritation may occur. The overall efficacy of this drug is good.

Topical Steroids. Another nasal steroid for topical application is dexamethasone. Each puff administers approximately 0.08 mg of dexamethasone. The patient uses two puffs three times a day in each nostril; thus in one day a total of 12 puffs are used (about 1.0 mg of dexamethasone). Some of the steroid is absorbed systemically, in a range of 0.3 to 0.5 mg, or approximately half of the intranasal dose, which is equivalent to approximately 2 to 4 mg of prednisone. This drug may cause partial adrenal suppression, which returns to normal after the drug has been discontinued.

Beclomethasone dipropionate has the reported advantage of being effective without producing adrenal suppression. Some work has suggested that the inhaled beclomethasone in the treatment of chronic asthma is similar in effect to alternate-day prednisone treatment on hypothalamic-pituitary-adrenal function. Two puffs of beclomethasone nasal spray in each nostril four times a day, used during the ragweed season, have been helpful in controlling symptoms. Each puff administers 50 μg. The maximal daily dose should not exceed 20 puffs, or 1000 μg (1 mg), in adults, and the drug also may be used to treat other types of seasonal allergic rhinitis.

The topical steroids are useful against nasal congestion but less so against nasal discharge. Consequently, a combination of antihistamines that are useful against the discharge and of topical steroids that are useful against the nasal congestion may be useful and effective for both symptoms. The topical steroids may be effective in the treatment of rhinitis medicamentosa and may be used until the patients are no longer suffering the effects of the topical sympathomimetic spray-rebound phenomenon.

Systemic Steroids. At least for seasonal allergic rhinitis, systemic steroids given orally can be extremely effective in severe cases for a short time. Prednisone, in an initial dose of 60 mg and then the same maintenance dosage for 5 days, can be extremely helpful.

An intramuscular injection of 12 mg of betamethasone (Celestone), either alone or in combination with other medications (antihistamine sympathomimetics), also can be extremely effective in the control of seasonal allergic rhinitis.

Intranasal injections of steroids in the form of triamcinolone acetonide may give excellent results in allergic rhinitis, although visual disturbance can occur after corticosteroid injections of the turbinate, including transient blurring or, rarely, permanent blindness. After a vasoconstrictor has been applied topically to diminish vascular absorption by closure of the submucosal vessels, injections should be administered slowly, with minimal pressure, along several points in the turbinates. A 25-gauge, 2.75-cm needle should be used.

Subsequently, the effects of steroids may diminish. Thus an initial effective steroid treatment may be followed by less effective or less dramatic results, despite repeated steroid therapy. Why this occurs is unknown. It is also important to realize that the complications of long-term steroid therapy may include cataracts, osteoporosis, ulcer disease, and diabetes, which are serious problems, especially as a result of treatment of allergic rhinitis.

Immunotherapy. Immunotherapy (hyposensitization, desensitization "shots") is not the most ideal type of treatment because of the cost, discomfort, time, and variable degree of efficacy. When should immunotherapy be considered? Patients who are suffering and who are incapacitated either because they cannot avoid the antigen or because their condition cannot be controlled by medication alone require both medication and immunotherapy. Medication alone essentially has diminished the extensive need for the expensive immunotherapy, but until more effective medications with fewer undesirable side effects are obtained, immunotherapy probably still will be used.

Although there has been controversy concerning the documented efficacy of this type of treatment, it is likely to remain popular. It is thought that blocking antibodies are formed by the desensitization treatment. There is no adequate information to determine whether immunotherapy reduces the risk of the development of asthma in patients with allergic rhinitis, although some observers think that immunotherapy for allergic rhinitis does reduce the risk of asthma in patients under the age of 25 years. It is known, however, that immunotherapy can diminish the intensity of hay fever (pollen reaction), and the clinical application must be tempered by convenience for the patient and expense of the required multiple injections.

. The general principle, for drugs or immunization, is to use the minimal effective dose for the shortest effective period so as to keep the patient symptom-free for the longest time. Animal danders can be avoided in the home environment. The inhalant allergens—namely, the weeds, grasses, trees, molds, and house dust—are the allergens most successfully treated by immunotherapy. If the patient has seasonal allergic rhinitis for 2 weeks per year, then immunotherapy is probably not justified, because other medical measures are usually successful.

Vasomotor Rhinopathy, Vasomotor Rhinitis, or Nonallergic Rhinitis as a Cause of Nasal Obstruction

So-called vasomotor nose is a multifaceted response to various nonallergic stimuli. It can be experienced as a nasal airway obstruction produced by the patient's awareness of the normal nasal cycle. Actually, vasomotor nose is a diagnosis made by exclusion. First, nasal obstruction resulting from the normal nasal cycle or from dependent positions that may also be a normal physiologic phenomenon is ruled out. Second, allergic nose (seasonal or perennial) is ruled out.

It is well known from animal studies that the vasculature of the nose receives both adrenergic and cholinergic innervation. This autonomic nervous system control of the vasculature in general and of the venous sinusoids in particular allows the engorgement mechanisms of the turbinates to be understood. Cholinergic stimulation produces vasodilation and thus engorged or swollen turbinates. The result is a nasal passage that is obstructed. Stimulation of the cervical sympathetic nerves produces nasal vasoconstriction and associated nasal patency.

It is thought that the autonomic nervous system, because of its influence and control of the nasal vascular mechanisms, can produce symptoms similar to those of allergic rhinitis. Vasomotor rhinopathy is caused by a disturbance in the autonomic nervous system and is termed vasomotor dysfunction. These vasomotor reactions are primarily the result of parasympathetic stimulation (or sympathetic inhibition) that causes the vasodilation, increased vascular permeability with edema, and increased glandular secretion.

When the mechanisms of action in allergic rhinitis are compared with those in vasomotor nose, the allergic reaction is found to be the result of the antibody-antigen interaction, with release of mediators produce dilation of arterioles and capillaries with increased permeability and transudation of fluid and edema. This results in the symptoms of nasal airway obstruction, sneezing, and itching. The release of mediators also increases the glandular activity and increases secretions that result in the symptom of rhinorrhea. In a typical vasomotor reaction, autonomic nervous system dysfunction produces increased parasympathetic action (decreased sympathetic action), which in turn produces dilation of arterioles and capillaries with increased permeability; this in turn leads to transudation of fluid and edema, which cause nasal airway obstruction, sneezing, and itching. The increased parasympathetic activity increases glandular activity and produces increased nasal secretions, with the resulting symptom of rhinorrhea. In essence, the allergic reaction and the vasomotor dysfunction produce similar symptoms by different mechanisms. In the allergic reaction, the mechanism is antibody-antigen interaction, whereas in the vasomotor reaction, it is autonomic nervous system dysfunction.

Symptoms

Patients with allergic rhinitis or vasomotor rhinitis are sometimes difficult to distinguish because their symptoms are quite similar: namely, nasal obstruction, rhinorrhea, and sneezing. Patients with allergic rhinitis usually have more itching and recurrent staccato-like sneezing. This is generally not present or as prominent in vasomotor nose. In Table 23–8, allergic rhinitis is compared with vasomotor rhinopathy.

Because the mechanism of action for vasomotor nose is through the autonomic nervous system with hypothalamic participation, it is understandable that an emotional disturbance may become associated with the symptom of nasal airway obstruction through the autonomic nervous system.

Vasomotor reactions may be caused by autonomic nervous system dysfunction; in addition, nasal obstruction, rhinorrhea, and sneezing may be caused by irritative, physical, endocrine, and other factors. The nose may be sensitive to hormonal influences because nasal vasomotor reactions may be related to pregnancy or to oral contraceptives. Fortunately, the "rhinitis" of pregnancy is

TABLE 23–8. Comparisons of Allergic Rhinitis and Vasomotor Nose

Allergic Rhinitis	Vasomotor Nose
Nasal Symptoms	
Nasal obstruction, rhinorrhea, sneezing	Nasal obstruction, rhinorrhea, sneezing
Associated Symptoms	
Lacrimation, itching	Usually none, but can be same as allergic rhinitis
Mechanism	
Antibody-antigen reaction	Autonomic nervous system dysfunction
Etiologic or Precipitating Factors	
Allergens (antigens)	Nonallergic causes
Inhalants: pollens from trees, grasses, weeds; molds, house dust; animal danders	Mechanical irritation, smoke, dust, smog, humidity (lack), climate
Ingestants: wheat, eggs, fish, medications	Physical factors: temperature (cold), air conditioning, cold floors, hot foods
Injections: medications	Emotion: anxiety, guilt, rage, sexual excitement ("honeymoon nose")
	Endocrine: pregnancy, menstruation, diabetes, hypothyroidism
	Other: beer drinking (allergy uncertain), anemia, nephritis, medications
Occurrence	
Intermittent (seasonal)	Intermittent (seasonal)
Constant (nonseasonal; perennial)	Constant (nonseasonal; perennial)

relieved soon after delivery and is probably related to a hormonal imbalance. Patients with hypothyroidism are known to have "rhinitis," although the exact mechanism of the production of the "rhinitis" in hypothyroidism is unknown. Reserpine (a rauwolfia agent) and propranolol, which are used to treat cardiovascular disease, can produce chronic nasal obstruction.

After perennial and seasonal allergic rhinitis, infectious disorders, foreign bodies, nasal polyps, intranasal anatomic (septal) deformities, atrophy, tumors, and rhinitis medicamentosa have been ruled out, approximately 60% of cases of nasal airway obstruction are undiagnosed rhinitis. These undiagnosed cases usually come under the heading of vasomotor nose.

Patients with a history of vasomotor nose

may describe an unusual sensitivity to environmental irritants, to cold floors, to air conditioning, or to changes in humidity. This nonallergic rhinitis is usually associated with symptoms of nasal airway obstruction and profuse rhinorrhea. There are usually no seasonal variations, but the symptoms may mimic perennial allergic rhinitis; however, because there may be exacerbations and remissions, they may also mimic seasonal allergic rhinitis. This mimicking occurs when patients are sensitive to temperature changes associated with seasonal variations. Some workers think that ingested foods rarely cause allergic rhinitis, although this is an area of controversy. The patients with vasomotor nose do not usually have a positive family history for allergy. They describe the onset of their irritative phenomenon as having occurred in adulthood. Sneezing is rare, and itching is uncommon. Nonallergic rhinitis with eosinophilia has been introduced into the literature (Mullarkey, 1988). This condition frequently is associated with nasal polyps and usually can be treated successfully with both topical and systemic steroids. For a summary of the characteristics of the various types of common so-called rhinitis, see Table 23–9.

Physical Examination

On physical examination, the nasal turbinates may be pale, swollen, and polypoid.

Eosinophils may be present in nasal secretions, as they may also be present in allergic rhinitis (perennial or seasonal). The eosinophils originate in the bone marrow and contain histaminase and a granule known as major basic protein. Eosinophils are attracted by various antigen-antibody complexes and also by complement. Their exact role in the allergic reaction is obscure, although there is indirect evidence that they may tend to modulate the immediate type of hypersensitivity reaction. It is thought that the eosinophil may inactivate certain of the vasoactive amines, although why the eosinophil is also present in vasomotor nose is unknown.

Diagnosis

The diagnosis of vasomotor nose is one of exclusion. After the historical facts are obtained, the physical examination can be similar or exactly identical to that of patients with allergic rhinitis (seasonal and perennial). The roentgenographic changes of thickened sinus mucosal membrane are nonspecific and nondiagnostic. Many patients with vasomotor nose have polyps, and they have a higher incidence of associated asthma than do patients with allergic rhinitis. These patients do not have any immunologic evidence of antibodies to allergens. It should be remembered that allergic rhinitis and vasomotor nose can occur together. After every other cause of nasal obstruction and nasal dis-

TABLE 23–9. Characteristics of Various types of Rhinitis

| Characteristic | Infectious | Allergic | | Nonallergic (Vasomotor) |
		Seasonal	Perennial	
Etiology	Respiratory infection	IgE-mediated immunologic reaction	IgE-mediated immunologic reaction	Autonomic nervous system disorder
Seasonal pattern	Often worse in winter	Yes	Present year round	Worse in changing seasons
Recurrences	Clears completely	Mild symptoms between attacks	Mild symptoms between attacks	Frequently continues
Family history of allergy	Occasional	Common	Common	Occasional
Systemic symptoms	Common	Rare	Rare	Rare
Other allergic symptoms (asthma, eczema)	Occasional	Common	Common	Occasional
Pruritus	No	Yes	Yes	Mild or absent
Fever	Occasional	No	No	No
Conjunctivitis	No	Yes	Yes	No
Discharge	Mucopurulent	Waterlike	Waterlike	Waterlike
Paroxysmal sneezing	No	Yes	Yes	Yes

From Kleinfeld C: Handbook of Nonprescription Drugs, 9th ed. Washington, DC: American Pharmaceutical Association, 1977.

charge has been ruled out, vasomotor nose can be diagnosed by exclusion.

Management

Medical. Management is predicated on whether the individual has significant symptoms. It is extremely important to ask the patient, "How much is this condition bothering you?" If the patient is markedly disturbed by the nasal airway obstruction (and many are), then a sequence of treatment is indicated.

Medical management can be effective. Avoidance of the precipitating factor is of primary importance. Certainly if the etiologic factor is a medication, such as a reserpinelike drug or oral contraceptives, then avoidance is suggested. If the patient is pregnant, she can be reassured that the problem is short term and that topical medication can be used prudently. The response to the antihistamines is usually fair to poor, whereas the response to the sympathomimetics may be of limited value. However, a trial period is recommended (see Table 23–7 for selection of medication). There is no response to immunotherapy because the mechanism of symptom production is not based on an antibody-antigen reaction. Cromolyn also has no use in vasomotor nose because the condition is not a result of the antibody-antigen interaction.

Topically applied corticosteroids, such as beclomethasone, may yield excellent results because of their anti-inflammatory properties. Steroids applied orally, intramuscularly, or intranasally may also produce an excellent response for the same reasons. Only in severe cases, however, should steroids be used.

Communication and discussion with the patient are an extremely important part of medical management, especially if no underlying abnormality can be determined. The concept of an exaggerated normal nasal reaction should be discussed. For example, it should be explained to the patient that some persons have noses that are sensitive to environmental stimuli, just as some patients have skin that is sensitive to sunlight. Persons with nasal sensitivity may be irritated by air conditioning or air pollution (smog or smoke). If the concept of biologic variability and nasal sensitivity is explained, the patients can better understand their disturbance. Insight can be helpful to accepting and living with the disorder.

In summary, medical management is based on communication with the patient (enlightenment), avoidance of the precipitating factor, a trial of orally administered medications (antihistamine decongestants), and, for severe disturbances, a trial of steroids. If this procedure is not successful and long-term hypertrophic changes have occurred, then surgical management is indicated, especially if there are concomitant polyps and chronic suppurative rhinosinusitis.

Surgical. As far as surgical management is concerned, when turbinate hypertrophy occurs, conservative management is recommended. Only limited partial resections of the posterior tips of the inferior turbinates or conservative partial resection of the turbinate tissue yields good results. Freezing and electrocautery of the turbinates have been advocated, and results have been favorable in some reports. Because the physiologic concept of autonomic nervous system dysfunction is involved in vasomotor nose, some workers have used vidian neurectomy with limited success. This cutting of the vidian nerve controls the watery discharge but not the nasal obstruction. If nasal polyps are present, the nasal airway obstruction should be removed.

Complications

The complications of vasomotor nose usually include nasal polyps and asthma. Aspirin sensitivity, nasal polyps, and asthma frequently coexist. Why this occurs is still an enigma. Patients with vasomotor nose are more likely to have asthma and nasal polyps than are patients with allergic rhinitis. With the development of polyps comes the associated recurrent chronic sinusitis, which needs treatment as indicated by the extent and nature of the disease.

Finally, if a patient does not respond to medical management and conservative surgical management, and if allergy evaluation is not definitive, the physician should consider sending the patient to a food allergist, even though such a course is controversial, especially if the symptoms are severe and cannot be relieved.

Rhinitis Medicamentosa

In patients who use phenylephrine or other types of topical decongestants in spray or nose drop form, there is a possibility, with prolonged use, that a rebound phenomenon will develop. After the short period of vasoconstriction that occurs with the topical decongestants, this rebound phenomenon, or vasodilation, leads to a series of events in which the medication is overused. The short period of vasoconstriction after the application of the decongestant is again followed by vasodilation, which causes nasal airway obstruction and motivates the patient again to use the topical decongestant. This dependence on topical vasoconstrictors is termed rhinitis medicamentosa.

In general, nasal sprays or nose drops should be used only rarely (perhaps no more than 3 consecutive days several [three or four] times a year). This is true for infants with upper respiratory tract infections who need to breathe while they are being fed. Occasional use of nasal sprays is indicated for relief of severe nasal obstruction in persons with allergic rhinitis or to facilitate nasal decongestion in persons with acute rhinosinusitis (Table 23–10).

Etiology and Symptoms

Rhinitis medicamentosa usually occurs in a patient who has allergic rhinitis, vasomotor nose, or an upper respiratory tract infection and who uses the decongestant to ameliorate the symptom of nasal obstruction. The obstruction is caused either by the underlying pathologic condition or by the rebound phenomenon secondary to prolonged abuse of nose drops.

Diagnosis

Diagnosis is usually made on intranasal inspection (hypertrophied mucosa) and on the basis of the history of the abuse of the topically applied decongestant to the nasal mucosa.

Management

The pillar of management is discontinuation of the topical decongestant and treatment of any underlying pathologic condition. One method of helping the patient is an intramuscular injection of 12 mg of betamethasone. Another method is the topical use of beclomethasone. The patient can be instructed to use the nose drops in only one nostril to prove that the rebound effect does occur. The hope is that the untreated nostril (the one not being decongested) will return to normal in 7 to 21 days. Of course, it is important to examine the patient and to manage the underlying nasal pathologic condition, whether it is an allergic or a vasomotor nose or concomitant nasal airway obstruction that results from a structural abnormality, such as nasal septal deformity.

Hypertrophied Mucosa: Hypertrophied Turbinates

Hypertrophy of the turbinates can cause upper airway obstruction and all of the related symptoms, ranging from those that are annoying to those that severely disturb the patient's sense of well-being. Hypertrophied turbinates may be related to abuse of nose drops (rhinitis medicamentosa). There also may be enlargement or hypertrophy of the turbinates as a result of mucosal swelling or edema secondary to polypoid changes related to allergic or vasomotor nose.

Symptoms

Symptoms generally relate to nasal airway obstruction or to the underlying disorder, or both. If it is an allergic or a vasomotor nose, the concomitant sneezing, itching, and nasal discharge, along with the problem of nasal airway obstruction, are usually apparent. On occasion, if the middle turbinate is enlarged, middle turbinate compression syndrome can occur. This diagnosis is established by the clinical evidence that the middle turbinate can press against the septum and produce some symptoms that usually are related to neuronal or reflex responses. The symptoms of this syndrome range from pain and headache to systemic disturbances. Anesthetization of the middle turbinate with 5% (50 mg/mL) cocaine often relieves the pain, the headache, or other local symptoms.

Diagnosis

The diagnosis of hypertrophied turbinates or compression of the middle turbinate is made on the basis of inspection and shrinkage.

TABLE 23–10. Common Topical Nasal Decongestants

Product (Manufacturer)	Application Form	Sympathomimetic	Preservative/ Antiseptic	Other
Afrin (Schering)	Nasal spray, nose drops	Oxymetazoline hydrochloride, 0.5 mg/mL	Benzalkonium chloride, 0.2 mg/mL; phenylmercuric acetate, 0.02 mg/mL	Sorbitol, 40 mg/mL; glycine, 3.8 mg/mL; sodium hydroxide
Benzedrex (Smith Kline & French)	Inhaler	Propylhexedrine, 250 mg	—	Aromatics
Coricidin (Schering)	Nasal spray	Phenylephrine hydrochloride, 5 mg/mL	—	—
Dristan (Whitehall)	Inhaler, nasal spray	Propylhexedrine (inhaler), phenylephrine hydrochloride (spray)	Benzalkonium chloride (spray)	Pheniramine maleate (spray), menthol, eucalyptol, methyl salicylate
Forthane (Lilly)	Inhaler	Methylhexaneamine, 250 mg	—	Menthol, 32 mg; aromatics
Neo-Synephrine Hydrochloride (Winthrop)	Nasal spray, nose drops, nasal jelly	Phenylephrine hydrochloride, 0.25 and 0.5% (spray); 0.125, 0.25, 0.5, and 1% (drops); 0.5% (jelly)	Benzalkonium chloride, 0.2% (spray)	Methyl salicylate, menthol, camphor, eucalyptol, (spray)
Privine (Ciba)	Nose drops, nasal spray	Naphazoline hydrochloride, 0.05%	Benzalkonium chloride, 1:5,000	—
Sine-Off Once-A-Day (Menley & James)	Nasal spray	Xylometazoline hydrochloride, 0.1%	—	Menthol, eucalyptol, camphor, methyl salicylate
Tuamine (Lilly)	Inhaler	Tuaminoheptane (equivalent to Tuamine), 325 mg	—	Menthol, 32 mg; aromatics
Vicks Sinex (Vick)	Nasal spray	Phenylephrine hydrochloride, 0.50%	Cetylpyridinium chloride, 0.04%; thimerosal, 0.001%	Methapyrilene hydrochloride, 0.12%; menthol; eucalyptol; camphor; methyl salicylate
4-Way (Bristol-Myers)	Nasal spray	Phenylephrine hydrochloride, 0.05%; naphazoline hydrochloride, 0.05%; phenylpropanolamine hydrochloride, 0.2%	—	Pyrilamine maleate, 0.2%

Usually after shrinkage the middle turbinate is still pressed against the septum, and the polypoid or hypertrophic changes of the mucosa of the turbinates persist.

Management

Medical. Nonsurgical management revolves around the treatment of the underlying condition. If hypertrophic changes are present, they are usually irreversible and require some type of surgical management to decrease the size of the turbinates, especially if there is significant nasal airway obstruction. At times, cautious and judicious injection of 20 mg of triamcinolone acetonide into each turbinate may be helpful. On rare occasions the mucosa of the septum may be cobblestoned or exhibit marked hypertrophic changes, and 20-mg injections of triamcinolone acetonide are unrewarding; thus limited surgical resection is warranted to improve the nasal airway to relieve obstructive symptoms.

Surgical. Surgical management is based

on debulking the polypoid hypertrophic mucosa, especially if there are posterior or mulberry tips of the inferior turbinates. These posterior portions of the inferior turbinates can be resected with a snare without producing severe atrophic changes. Removal of an entire inferior turbinate for benign disease is strongly discouraged because removal of an inferior turbinate can produce nasal atrophy and a miserable person. Such people unfortunately are still seen in the author's offices; these people are nasal cripples.

Other surgical management includes freezing, electrocoagulation, or careful, limited, and judicious submucosal resection of the hyperplastic turbinate tissue. These procedures should be performed by experienced surgeons.

Atrophic Mucosa, Nasal Atrophy, Atrophic Rhinitis, and Ozena

Early nasal atrophy can occur either as part of the aging process or as the result of nasal trauma. It is important to recognize that even a minor injury sustained many years before the onset of nasal atrophy may be responsible for this clinical syndrome. Atrophic rhinitis actually is a final stage of nasal atrophy, and the most extreme form is ozena.

In cases of ozena, a host of bacterial organisms frequently are found, and the nose is filled with hard, mucopurulent, fetid crusts. The exact causes, aside from the trauma or inflammatory response, may be metabolic or endocrine disturbances with superimposed chronic bacterial infection.

Nasal obstruction to breathing occurs along with the foul, odoriferous crusts and associated epistaxis. The patient also suffers from psychic disturbances. Various speculations have been offered, although there is no specific known cause for ozena, except for the atrophy that can occur after extensive nasal surgery with indiscriminate removal of normally functioning nasal tissue. This may be necessary for management of malignant nasal tumors but is rarely justified for benign nasal disease. The diagnosis is usually made on examination of the nose. An underlying disorder, such as Wegener's granulomatosis or another chronic inflammatory reaction, must be excluded. The patient may also have an external nasal deformity that results from atrophy of intranasal structures, especially the septal cartilage, with loss of support. The external nasal deformity is usually a saddle nose.

A biopsy specimen usually shows squamous metaplasia of the nasal tissues, atrophy of the submucosa, and perivascular infiltration with fibrosis. The mucosa is frequently thin and ulcerated, and atrophy with destruction of all of the intranasal tissues can also occur.

Management

Medical. Medical management is usually centered on cleansing and nasal douching. In more extreme forms, the recommended medications and cleansing for persons who have marked atrophic rhinitis or ozena are listed as follows.

Medications:

1. Premarin spray, 25 mg; streptomycin, 10 g; and saline, 100 mL (a No. 127 DeVilbiss atomizer is needed); solution needs to be refrigerated.
2. 25% Glucose and 75% glycerin, 120 mL (to be placed on a cotton-tipped swab).
3. Oil of sesame, 120 mL, and four drops oil of rose geranium (administered by an eyedropper).

Treatment:

1. The patient fills a 90-mL ear syringe with one part 3% hydrogen peroxide and two parts water. Each nostril is irrigated once, followed by irrigation by one syringe full of clear water in each nostril.
2. Two sprays of the conjugated estrogens (Premarin) and streptomycin are applied in each nostril.
3. The nose is swabbed with a cotton-tipped swab soaked with glucose and glycerin.
4. The eyedropper is filled with oil of sesame and rose geranium, and the contents of one full dropper are introduced into each nostril.

(Salt water occasionally may be used instead of peroxide. It should be prepared as about 0.25 tsp of salt to 1 cup of water. If this amount of salt is irritating, less should be used.)

Surgical. Surgical management is based on the principle of introducing autogenous or allograft material into the nose to narrow the nasal cavity. The patient will have a sense of improved respiration because a resistance has been created. Multiple operations are usually required over several years to produce enough submucosal scar tissue to narrow the nose sufficiently. Other surgical management is usually cosmetic, especially if there has been collapse of the nose with a saddle nose deformity. An iliac bone graft can be useful. These procedures should be undertaken by surgeons who are familiar with difficult nasal reconstructive procedures. The results can be quite rewarding, especially if a bone graft is needed and is introduced successfully.

STRUCTURAL CAUSES OF NASAL OBSTRUCTION

In addition to mucosal causes, nasal airway obstruction can be caused by nasal structural changes. The intranasal or the external bony and cartilaginous changes are usually apparent to the naked eye and frequently produce symptoms that are surgically reversible. The most common cause of a nasal septal deformity is trauma, which may be intrauterine or may occur during parturition or, more likely, during early childhood or later in life. Many nasal septal deformities are associated with external nasal deformities, and often the patient has no recollection of when the traumatic event occurred. There is no question that a nasal septal deformity can be an important contributor to nasal airway obstruction.

Nasal Septal Abnormalities

Deviation or Bend

Some mild deviation of the nasal septum is an expected finding on a normal examination. One to 2 mm from the midline is within normal limits and cannot be considered abnormal, unless the nasal valve area is obstructed.

Obstruction and Impaction

A nasal septum that touches the lateral wall of the nose is considered a nasal obstruction. The nose must be sprayed with a topical decongestant, such as 1% phenylephrine, and then should be re-examined. If the septum no longer touches the lateral nasal wall,

the septal deformity is termed a *nasal septal obstruction*. However, if the nasal septal deformity is still in contact with the lateral wall of the nose after the nose has been sprayed with a topical decongestant, the condition is referred to as a *nasal septal impaction*.

The Nasal Valve

The normal nasal valve subtends an angle of approximately 10° to 15° between the caudal end of the upper lateral cartilage and the nasal septum. The nasal valve area extends from the region of the caudal end of the upper lateral cartilage in its relationship to the nasal septum medially and laterally to the bony point of the piriform aperture and the soft fibrofatty tissue in this region; it is bounded below by the floor of the nose and posteriorly by the head of the inferior turbinate (Kasperbauer and Kern, 1987). When the nasal valve is abnormal, symptoms can be produced by an already collapsed valve or because of increased collapsibility of the valve. The major symptom of narrowing of the valve is nasal airway obstruction. Many patients with a narrowed nasal valve report that pulling on the face laterally improves the nasal air flow. This is a positive Cottle's sign and usually indicates that the nasal valve is at fault (Heinberg and Kern, 1973).

Diagnosis. The diagnosis of nasal septal abnormalities is made from a history of nasal obstruction and from physical examination. The caudal end of the septum, or area 1, can be seen and palpated without the use of expensive equipment. Area 2 or the valve area can often be observed just by peering into the nose with a penlight directed at the region of the valve (Fig. 23–1) or by using the tip of a nasal speculum.

Symptoms. Symptoms of nasal septal deformities may be nonexistent or may range from mild to a marked bilateral nasal airway obstruction with subsequent mouth breathing and findings distant from the nose, including restless sleep, irritability, aprosexia nasalis, and even a disturbance in a person's sense of well-being. Nasal airway obstruction alone can have a profound and deleterious effect on an otherwise normal person.

Management. The management ranges from doing nothing if the patient essentially

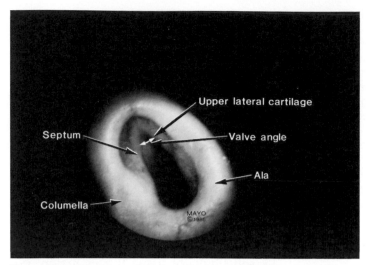

Figure 23–1. Overview of the nasal valve. When a nasal speculum is used, care must be taken not to obscure the nasal valve. Sometimes vibrissae may need to be trimmed to visualize the nasal valve angle. The nasal valve is best examined without the introduction of any instrument into the nose. The nasal valve area is bounded by the nasal septum, the caudal end of the upper lateral cartilage, the soft fibrofatty tissue overlying the piriform aperture, the floor of the nose, and posteriorly by the head of the inferior turbinate. This area is shaped like an inverted cone or teardrop with a slitlike apex, which is called the nasal valve angle and normally subtends an angle of 10° to 15°. Example of a left nostril demonstrating the septum, the upper lateral cartilage, the valve angle, the ala, and the columella. (From Kasperbauer JL, Kern EB: Nasal valve physiology: implications in nasal surgery. Otolaryngol Clin North Am 20:699–719, 1987. Reprinted by permission of the Mayo Foundation.)

is asymptomatic to extensive nasal septal and pyramid surgery (Kern, 1977; Lipton and Kern, 1990). An important aspect is the extent to which the symptoms bother the patient. These operations should be performed by a surgeon who is knowledgeable about nasal respiratory (breathing) surgery.

The primary indication for surgical treatment of the deviated septum is nasal airway obstruction. Other indications occur in persons who have epistaxis; in these cases, surgery on the septum is needed for removing a deformity to gain access to a bleeding site. An operation may be necessary because the deformity predisposes to recurrent rhinosinusitis or because of significant abnormalities that not only interfere with nasal airway function by producing nasal obstruction but also produce such symptoms as headache and facial pain. Another indication for a nasal septal operation is to gain access to the sphenoid for sphenoid sinus lesions or access to the sella turcica and pituitary gland. By far the most important indication for nasal septal surgery is nasal airway obstruction to breathing!

The Submucous Resection. The submucous resection is an operation that reached its culmination in the pioneering days early in the 20th century. In general, this operation has been supplanted by nasal septal reconstruction. The resected septum is now reconstructed so that the normal rigid midline structure is reconstituted.

Complications. Complications usually include bleeding, collapse of the nose, infection, or persistent obstruction by incomplete removal of the nasal septal airway obstruction. Development of a nasal airway obstruction during the healing phase can be caused by development of intranasal scar tissue that produces subsequent nasal airway obstruction.

Usual Results of Nasal Septal Reconstruction. Depending on the degree of disease, most patients can expect an improvement in the nasal airway after reconstruction (Mertz et al., 1984; Gordon et al., 1989; Slavit et al., 1991). Exact numbers are not available, but a likely range is approximately 80% to 90% improvement of the nasal airway, a 1% to 2% chance of immediate complications, and probably a 5% to 15% chance that a secondary procedure may be required for cosmetic or functional airway dysfunction, or both.

Aftercare. Packing or intranasal stents or supports are usually maintained in place for 5 to 7 days, depending on the extent of the procedure, and the patient usually wears an external nasal dressing. Ecchymosis or edema of the face rarely occurs unless the external pyramid is mobilized. Some type of protection should be worn at night for approximately 6 weeks. The patient should be advised not to lift any weight over 9 kg (20 pounds) for several weeks because the strain of lifting may induce bleeding. In addition, the patient should not engage in any activity (including strenuous sexual activity) that increases the heart rate for approximately 10 to 14 days after the operation until all the packings and dressings are removed and the wounds have healed. Normal activities may be resumed within 10 to 20 days.

Compression of the Middle Turbinate

Frequently, a middle turbinate may be bullous (concha bullosa) or enlarged and may compress the nasal septum, producing symptoms such as pain, headache, recurrent sinusitis, or possibly even distant reflex responses. Anesthetization of the turbinate usually relieves most of these local symptoms, and surgical decompression is warranted when the patient experiences such relief on several occasions.

Nasal Trauma

Nasal trauma usually refers to acute nasal injury. Trauma that has occurred previously usually represents either a cosmetic or a nasal respiratory (breathing) problem. An acute nasal injury can produce an upper airway obstruction as a result of a septal, upper lateral cartilage, or bony dislocation or hematoma, or combinations of each. Important parts of the history are the time of the insult, the instrument, and the intensity of the blow. In most cases of nasal injury, it is advisable to obtain exact details, and photographic recordings of the patient's face are mandated, especially when legal actions may be insti-

tuted. Frequently, patients and their families do not notice their abnormalities or facial asymmetry unless the difference is pointed out on a photograph or with the aid of a mirror.

Nasal injuries are probably the most frequent of all facial injuries. Often the injury may be considered too trivial to warrant treatment; at other times the injury may be so extensive that multiple surgical procedures are required. Head and facial injuries may be so severe that nasal injuries are neglected because neurologic deficits have required neurosurgical intervention or other surgical procedures to maintain life.

Age Ranges. Nasal trauma to infants during delivery is usually easy to reduce, especially during the immediate postpartum period, although some dislocations reduce spontaneously. Digital manipulation frequently reduces the septal dislocation because the major portion of the infant's nose is cartilaginous.

In children, the injuries are sometimes overlooked because they are considered minimal; however, growth and developmental potential allow these so-called minor injuries to become significant respiratory or cosmetic deformities later in life. Thus in childhood, dislocations that produce nasal airway obstruction should be reduced immediately after the injury. Acute nasal trauma in adults also should be reduced promptly to obviate functional nasal respiratory and cosmetic abnormalities. The diagnosis of nasal trauma is usually made by history and physical examination. A history of epistaxis after the injury usually connotes an injury to the nasal mucosa. Edema, ecchymosis, crepitus, obvious external deformity, and a history of epistaxis are important clues, and intranasal examination is mandatory to rule out septal trauma and septal hematomas.

Roentgenograms. Roentgenograms of the facial bones and nasal bones can be obtained mainly for legal purposes, although the information that they provide is usually only incidental to the clinical evaluation. Roentgenograms should not influence the final course of management because they never supplant the history or the extranasal and intranasal examination. The determination of whether an operation should be performed is based not on the roentgenographic findings but on the clinical findings. In particular, a patient can have a septal or upper lateral cartilage fracture, dislocation, or hematoma in the presence of a negative roentgenogram.

Lacerations. External lacerations are usually a good indication that the underlying tissues have been injured. These should be cleansed and closed primarily if surgery on the nose is not planned. Closure of an external laceration may be delayed if immediate surgery is planned. At the time of surgery realignment or removal of these fragments may be performed through these wounds. All possible soft tissues should be saved, and repairs should be made by meticulous approximation. A tetanus booster should be given as indicated.

Intranasal lacerations should be approximated and sewn to prevent postoperative scarring and resultant nasal airway obstruction.

Management. If after external and intranasal examination a fracture dislocation of the septum or external nose is found, with or without a septal hematoma, surgical management of the acute injury is required in order to avoid or reduce functional (breathing) or cosmetic disturbances. In the author's opinion, manipulation of the nose on unfamiliar patients is probably best carried out in an operating room after adequate decongestion and anesthetizing of the patient. Administration of cocaine and injection of anesthesia are usually adequate to allow elevation of a displaced nasal bone fragment. For extensive exploration, general anesthesia is best, especially in children and in agitated people with extensive injuries. Patients with injuries that include loss of tissue, mucosal tears, or septal dislocation require the care of specialists who are interested in and competent in treating nasal facial trauma.

Several hours after the nasal trauma, edema and ecchymosis usually develop and make the diagnosis a bit more difficult. If the patient is seen before extensive edema and ecchymosis occur, it is possible to make a diagnosis and perform a definitive procedure; however, if edema and ecchymosis prevent an adequate evaluation, intranasal examination should still be undertaken, the nose should be lightly packed (put to rest), and tape dressings and stents should be placed on the nose to reduce discomfort. The patient should be given medication for pain and can be re-examined 1 week later. These procedures are of course acceptable after an intranasal examination demonstrates no evidence of a septal dislocation, a septal mucosal laceration, or a septal hematoma. The physician should also be aware of the possibility of leakage of cerebrospinal fluid with nasofacial injuries.

It is much easier to obtain adequate local and topical anesthesia in an operating room. If the patient is unknown to the attending physician and has a severe nasal trauma with epistaxis and fracture dislocation of the septum and external nose, with laceration of the external skin and the nasal mucosa, repair in an emergency room or in an office setting is extremely difficult. Operating room intervention by an experienced intranasal surgeon is preferable in this situation. The office or emergency room is suitable for a closed reduction of an external nasal bone depressed fracture, if adequate anesthesia and sedation can be safely administered. If after adequate decongestion and proper examination a septal dislocation or laceration of nasal mucosa is observed, the operating room allows the option of making incisions or other manipulations without compromise.

Immobilizing the fragments and open reduction may be necessary for the best results. A nasal fracture that is not immediately corrected but is held in an abnormal position by subsequent scar tissue makes "simple" reduction much more difficult at a later date; therefore, nasal injuries generally should be evaluated thoroughly and treated as soon as possible to avoid future cosmetic and breathing abnormalities.

Pediatric Nasal Injuries. Nasal injuries in the pediatric age group are common. A minimal injury in a child can produce a delayed functional or cosmetic abnormality. It may be extremely difficult, if not impossible, to examine the young child without general anesthesia. It is wise and prudent, especially if the nasal injury has produced a gross external abnormality, to take the patient to the operating room and examine the nose while the child is under general anesthesia. If there is any question about the extent of the injury, a colleague who is familiar with intranasal surgery should be consulted. Injury to a growing nose may produce either cartilaginous overgrowth or retardation of growth.

Even a minimal injury in a child can produce a septal hematoma; therefore, the intranasal structures must be thoroughly evaluated before definitive treatment can be intelligently undertaken. (The possibility that the child has been abused should be considered, especially in cases of facial injuries.)

Careful and timely intervention in children with severe nasal injuries should be no more deleterious to the growth, development, and function of the nose than the original injury itself. When the intervention is handled by a competent nasal surgeon who uses the concepts of reconstruction, adequate nasal growth and development and improved respiratory function can be anticipated, although the family should be advised of the possibility of the necessity of a subsequent operation. Treatment of complications of nasal septal injury and external nasal injury is much more difficult than providing adequate initial management.

Septal Hematomas

The most common cause of septal hematoma is septal trauma, either surgical or nonsurgical, usually caused by the nonsurgical blow to the nose, either accidental or as part of an altercation.

Diagnosis. The diagnosis of a septal hematoma is made on inspection; a wide midline septal area results from the accumulation of blood beneath the septal mucosa in the septal space. On palpation of the septal mucosa with a cotton carrier or cotton swab, the septum is soft and compressible.

Management. After nasal anesthesia is administered, the hematoma is aspirated, and a small anterior nasal packing is introduced. If injury is extensive, with septal dislocation and bleeding, then exploration is warranted. A small incision can also be made to evacuate the hematoma, and packs can then be introduced to prevent reaccumulation of blood in the septal space. It is important to recognize the presence of an underlying fracture dislocation of the septum or external nose, for this too may require formal surgical management. A septal hematoma that is not evacuated may lead to pressure necrosis of the septal cartilage, loss of nasal support, and collapse of the nose. Septal abscess can also occur as a result of an undrained septal hematoma.

Septal Abscess

When the septal space becomes infected after a surgical or nonsurgical trauma, a septal abscess can develop. The destruction of the septum secondary to septal abscess can be rapid and devastating. Not only can loss of the septal structures, subsequent collapse of the nose, and a septal perforation occur, but the infection can also spread beyond the confines of the nose and even produce (rarely) a serious intracranial complication.

Diagnosis. The diagnosis is usually made in a patient who has suffered a previous trauma to the nose, either surgical or nonsurgical, and who then experiences a septic course with pain, fever, heat, redness, tenderness, and nasal airway obstruction, with or without purulent discharge.

Management. Management involves diagnostic incision and drainage, cultures, and specific antimicrobial agents; because most of the organisms are gram-positive, an antibiotic against the gram-positive organisms is mandatory (after the cultures have been taken). Intravenously administered crystalline penicillin G, 1 to 5 million units every 4 to 6 hours, is a good initial treatment while culture and sensitivity reports are awaited. If the abscess is extensive and the patient does not respond well to incision and drainage, the care of a physician who is specialized in the field of nasal surgery may be required.

Septal Perforations

The most common etiologic factor in septal perforations is trauma, either surgical or nonsurgical, including submucous resection or other types of nasal surgery. Nonsurgical trauma may include digital trauma, electrocautery, cocaine abuse, chemical inhalants (sulfuric acid, mercurials, arsenicals, cyanamides, chemical fumes, and acids), and inflammatory conditions. These inflammatory conditions include bacterial infections, such as gram-positive or gram-negative organisms secondary to septal abcess, and rare problems such as tuberculosis and syphilis. Fungal infections certainly may also produce nasal septal perforations, along with granulomatous disorders such as Wegener's granulomatosis and sarcoidosis. In about 25% of patients, the cause is unknown.

Diagnosis. Diagnosis is usually easily made on inspection of the nasal septum. Perforations may be extremely small or extremely large, ranging from 1 mm (pinpoint) up to and including loss of almost the entire nasal septum. If the nose is not sprayed with a topical vasoconstrictor, a smaller and more posterior perforation may be overlooked. Biopsy may be required to rule out sarcoidosis, Wegener's granulomatosis, and polymorphic reticulosis.

Symptoms. The symptoms vary, but the most common are recurrent intermittent epistaxis, crusting, and nasal airway obstruction. Some persons with septal perforations are asymptomatic and require merely the establishment of an etiologic diagnosis (if possible) and reassurance.

Management. Medical management is directed toward treatment of the underlying cause and also toward management of crusting and bleeding. Bland ointments (such as petroleum jelly), good humidification, and possible irrigation with glucose and glycerin solution or nasal washes can be useful as temporary measures in the management of symptomatic patients. Nonsurgical closure with the introduction of Silastic buttons has been useful in reducing the amount of epistaxis and crusting and is successful in about 70% of the cases (Kern et al., 1977; Hanson et al., 1986; Kern, 1988). This procedure should be introduced by a person who is able to use a headlight, a nasal speculum, and bayonet forceps simultaneously. Surgical closure can be successful when the perforations are less than 2 cm. The chances for success decrease with the increasing size of the perforation. Many patients prefer medical management or the use of a Silastic button for the control of crusting and bleeding. The septal button can be considered a first alternative to surgery. For perforations larger than 3 cm, a custom-made septal Silastic button has been helpful.

New Growths

Any space-occupying new growth in the nose, whether benign or malignant, may obstruct the nasal airway. The benign tumors are much more common than malignant lesions of the internal nose.

Nasal Polyps. The exact origin and mechanism of the development of nasal polyps are still unknown, but their formation is probably a nonspecific response to nasal mucosal inflammation.

Nasal polyps occur in persons who have a history of allergic or vasomotor rhinitis and are probably more prevalent in persons who have vasomotor nose than in those who have allergic rhinitis. The main symptoms are related to nasal airway obstruction. On occasion they produce or are associated with chronic rhinosinusitis, and on even rarer occasions, they may produce destruction of bone and widening of the midfacial area.

The asthma triad—intrinsic asthma (nonallergic asthma), aspirin sensitivity, and nasal polyps—has been known for many years. Persons with these conditions usually have vasomotor nose, nonallergic asthma, and aspirin sensitivity. The aspirin sensitivity can usually produce a bronchospastic attack.

Cystic fibrosis can occur concomitantly in patients with nasal polyps, especially in the younger age group; therefore, a teenager or a preteenager with nasal polyps is considered to have cystic fibrosis until it is proved otherwise.

Antral choanal polyps are another entity. They are usually large polypoid masses that originate in the maxillary sinus, grow through the ostium of the maxillary sinus, and may appear as a pedunculated or single polypoid lesion obstructing the nose and hanging down into the choana posteriorly.

Diagnosis. Diagnosis is usually made by history and physical examination. As in any other physical examination of the nose, it is important to decongest the nose and also to look into the nasopharynx to observe the area of the choana and the posterior tips of the inferior turbinates. Benign nasal polyps are yellow to gray, translucent, grapelike masses in the nose and should not be mistaken for the inferior turbinate, which is usually pink and on the lateral nasal wall opposite the midline nasal septum.

Management. Various nonsurgical treatments have been tried for nasal polyps, including intrapolyp injection of steroids, topical steroid sprays, and systemic steroid injections. The degree of success with topical and systemic steroids is variable. Once the polyps are well established, medical treatment is usually unsuccessful. It is currently thought that there is decreased recurrence once the nasal polyps have been removed, if topical beclomethasone is sprayed into the nose.

In general, the treatment of choice is surgical. Removal of a single polyp with a snare can be done in the physician's office while the patient is under local and topical anesthesia. If the polypoid disease is extensive and is seen to involve maxillary, ethmoid, and sphenoid sinuses on direct coronal sinus computed tomographic scans, then intranasal ethmoidectomy and intranasal maxillary antral windows (middle meatal antrostomy) with polypoid tissue resection are the surgical treatment that is indicated. The sphenoid sinuses should be opened if they are involved with polypoid disease. A recurrence rate of 30% warrants further operation. The patient must be informed that the disorder can recur and that subsequent procedures may be required over an extended time. All nasal polyps must be sent for microscopic pathologic investigation because on occasion the "garden variety," or "allergic polyp," is not benign.

Papillomas

Papillomas are benign, wartlike tumors that occur either on the nasal septum or on the lateral wall of the nose and produce nasal airway obstruction and intermittent bleeding. A simple excision with electrocautery of the base of the lesion is usually the only procedure that is required. Histologic evaluation is important to be sure that the lesions are not the inverting type of papilloma.

Inverting Papillomas. Inverting papillomas can occur concomitantly with nasal polyps and have a propensity for recurrence. They occur predominantly in males, but they have a marked tendency to recur in females. They also have a propensity to occur with malignant squamous cell nasal tumors. They occur most frequently on the lateral wall of the nose and may also produce nasal airway obstruction, intermittent bleeding, or both. Many of these patients have had a previous nasal operation. Treatment is usually by a

major wide nasal surgical excision through an external nasal lateral rhinotomy approach. All polyps removed in the physician's office should be sent for histologic evaluation to be certain that the patient does not have inverting papilloma or an associated malignancy. The overall recurrence rate for inverting papillomas is approximately 30%, and it is greater in women than in men by 2:1. The associated malignancy rate ranges from 5% to 15%. Lifelong follow-up examinations are mandatory.

Other Benign Tumors

Nasal Gliomas. Nasal gliomas are developmental abnormalities of neurogenic origin with no malignant potential. Biopsy is necessary for establishing the diagnosis. Excisional biopsy usually offers complete cure, although a frontal craniotomy is necessary for those persons who have nasal gliomas with intracranial connection or an associated cerebrospinal fluid rhinorrhea or recurrent episodes of meningitis. Symptoms are usually those of an intranasal mass, an external nasal mass, or respiratory distress, especially if a nasal glioma occurs in infants who have a large intranasal mass and associated nasal airway obstruction. Children with intranasal masses should be referred to a competent nasal surgeon for evaluation and treatment.

Juvenile Angiofibroma. Juvenile angiofibromas are histologically benign tumors and may produce a triad of nasal airway obstruction, epistaxis, and nasal drainage. They occur exclusively in teenage boys and primarily in the nasopharynx and extend out of the sphenopalatine foramen into the lateral or infratemporal fossa. It is extremely rare for the tumor to occur after the age of 25 years. Diagnosis is usually made by inspection of the intranasal space and the nasopharynx. Conventional roentgenograms of the sinus, submental vertex views, and tomograms, with the knowledge of the history of nasal obstruction and epistaxis in a teenage boy with a nasal mass, help establish the diagnosis. Angiography is not essential for the diagnosis. Biopsy should not be performed in the office because torrential lethal hemorrhage may occur. A suspicious intranasal mass in a teenage boy should be evaluated by a competent specialist. Treatment is surgical and should be performed by an experienced nasal surgeon. Radiation is not considered a primary treatment modality, especially with the risks to the preadult patient. Most (90%) boys with this tumor survive and are free of disease after operation; however, intracranial extension of the tumor can lead to hemorrhage, and these patients may exsanguinate during the operation.

Other rare tumors do occur but are not important in this discussion.

Malignant Tumors

Malignant tumors of the nose and paranasal sinuses usually grow insidiously. The symptoms are usually related to the mass effect and their location. If they extend into the intranasal space, they produce nasal airway obstruction, epistaxis, or both. They may produce other symptoms related to their location, including facial paresthesia, proptosis, pain, and other findings related to the spread to contiguous structures. These tumors may be classified as squamous cell epitheliomas, glandular tumors that include the cylindromas (adenocystic adenocarcinomas), melanomas, and other rare tumors.

Squamous cell carcinoma of the septum is usually either an exophytic or ulcerative type of lesion. These lesions bleed easily and may be associated with pain. Diagnosis is based on histologic examination after biopsy. Five-year survival rates for malignant tumors in these regions are variable, but they are under 50%.

Squamous cell cancers of the sinuses are insidious and may grow in the sinal recesses to a large size before their presence is detected. Their undetected growth is an important factor in reducing the survival rates.

Patients with nasal obstruction, facial pain, epistaxis, and paresthesias of the face need a full evaluation, including sinus films and intranasal and nasopharyngeal examination, to find an early cancer of the nose and sinuses.

At times it is difficult to classify these tumors into clear-cut histologic entities. Metastasis may occur. Combined wide surgical resection and preoperative radiation provide the only chance to improve the dismal survival rate. Preoperative radiation is excellent, because this saves eyes and palates that might otherwise be compromised as a result of surgery. The surgery (lateral rhinotomy) is then performed to determine the extent of

the disease and to see whether the tumor is still present. The same is true with cancer of the nasal septum. High-voltage radiation should be considered in nonresectable lesions or in lesions that are surgically inaccessible. A large number (approximately 20% to 30%) of patients have metastatic disease. Patients with large, fungating tumors usually have a shorter survival time than patients with small, sessile lesions that are diagnosed early and are widely excised.

Malignant melanomas, although uncommon in the nose and paranasal sinuses, can occur as darkly pigmented, fleshy nasal masses. They, like most tumors, have a better prognosis when they arise in the nose than when they arise in the sinuses because the early appearance of symptoms leads to early diagnosis. Surgical therapy, combined with planned preoperative irradiation, offers the best survival prognosis. Local recurrence is a problem, and repeated surgical procedures, irradiation, and chemotherapy may be necessary. Uncontrolled local disease or distant metastases, as in most other malignant tumors, usually result in death. Metastatic tumors can also occur in the nose and paranasal sinuses. Suspicion should be raised if a patient has had a primary cancer diagnosed at another site, such as the breast, the gastrointestinal tract, or the genitourinary tract, and now has new nasal or sinus tumors.

Cancer in the nose and paranasal sinuses should be suspected in patients who have nasal obstruction (of recent onset), epistaxis, pain, or associated strange new symptoms in and about the face and eyes. The nose should be examined, and roentgenograms (computed tomographic scans) of the sinuses should be performed. Biopsy of a suspicious intranasal lesion should be carried out in the operating room by an experienced surgeon.

Miscellaneous Causes of Nasal Airway Obstruction

Hypertrophied Adenoids. Hypertrophied adenoids, especially in the younger patient, may be another common structural cause of nasal airway obstruction. The patient may have a host of symptoms, ranging from snoring and sleep disturbance to increased irritability. It is usually the patient's parents who are aware of the symptoms while the patient is sleeping. A diagnosis may be established by rhinomanometry (nasal breathing tests), or by study of the nasopharynx by indirect mirror examination, or both. Frequently, visualization of an enlarged adenoidal mass on nasopharyngeal examination is extremely difficult in the gagging, squirming child; however, diagnosis may be possible through shrinkage of the nasal mucosa and direct observation of the nasopharynx through the nose. Lateral roentgenograms of the neck frequently demonstrate the enlarged adenoidal tissue. Treatment is adenoidectomy.

Choanal Atresia. Choanal atresia is thought to be the result of a developmental arrest during gestation. Bilateral choanal atresia usually is manifest at birth. The patient may have cyanosis and failure to breathe, because the infant must breathe through the nose in order to suckle effectively. Bilateral choanal atresia is an emergency and treatment should be instituted immediately. Unilateral choanal atresia may be missed for many years, because the patient usually does not have notable nasal respiratory problems at birth, as occur in the case of the bilateral choanal atresia. The patient with unilateral atresia may have unilateral mucopurulent nasal discharge with persistent rhinorrhea and intermittent obstructive symptoms.

The diagnosis of bilateral choanal atresia is usually made in the neonate when the physician is unable to pass a nasal catheter (No. 6 French) through the nasal chambers. Decongestion can be effected with 0.125% phenylephrine, and the nose can be directly examined either with an otoscope or with a nasal speculum and headlight. Another diagnostic modality may include contrast radiography or methylene blue instilled into the nose to prove the presence of the choanal atresia.

Once the diagnosis has been made, surgical management is the treatment of choice, although conservative measures may be used, such as an oral airway and feeding by lavage. Concomitant or associated anomalies should be looked for in infants with choanal atresia. Before operation is undertaken, a thorough medical examination must be carried out to determine whether other life-threatening anomalies are present. A transnasal microsurgical approach is probably better than transpalatal surgery, but once the diagnosis is made, the patient should be referred to a surgeon who has experience in this type of reconstructive rhinologic surgery.

Intranasal Synechia, Scars, and Stenosis. Intranasal synechia, scars, and stenosis may also cause nasal airway obstruction and all of the disturbing symptoms secondary to upper airway obstruction.

Etiology. The most common cause is traumatic injury followed by an inflammatory response, including scarring. The traumatic injury may be surgical, occurring during an operative intervention on the nose when two raw surfaces from the septum or the lateral wall of the nose form fibrous adhesions during healing and produce synechia or scars. Nonsurgical trauma from automobile injuries or other blunt trauma to the nasal structures may produce mucosal tears or injury of the lateral wall of the nose, with subsequent development of synechia, scars, and stenosis.

Other nonsurgical injury may occur during nasotracheal intubation or the passing of nasogastric tubes. Attempts at passing transnasal tubes may produce injury to the nasal mucosa, especially if there is a marked deviation of the nasal septum. Bleeding may occur, and the two raw traumatized surfaces on the septum and lateral wall of the nose may heal together. If extreme difficulty in passing a nasal tube occurs, a colleague who is familiar with the variations in intranasal anatomy should be consulted.

Diagnosis. The diagnosis is usually made on direct inspection of the intranasal space before and especially after decongestion. It is important to examine the region of the valve, especially in persons who have had previous rhinoplasty or other intranasal surgery because scars may occur anteriorly. A nasal speculum should not be introduced into a person's nose before an examination of the valve region; otherwise, the anterior scars, synechia, or stenosis may be missed.

Symptoms. Symptoms usually depend on the degree and the site of obstruction. If the obstruction is significant and is anteriorly placed, nasal respiratory insufficiency or nasal airway obstruction, mouth breathing, dyspnea, and disturbed sleep may be the symptoms that the patient complains of most bitterly. This is especially true if the patient has experienced a recent surgical or nonsurgical injury. Patients frequently complain when they have a sudden onset of difficulty breathing through the nose, because it is distressing to most people.

Management. Management is surgical and depends on correcting the underlying cause.

Synechia, scars, and stenosis may be surgically repaired, although the results are best when injured nasal mucosa is repaired primarily.

The Narrow Nose Syndrome. The narrow nose syndrome is a constellation of symptoms that revolves around nasal airway obstruction. The patient usually has varying degrees of nasal respiratory difficulty. The cause may be congenital, hereditary, traumatic, or surgical (commonly after rhinoplasty). The nasal pyramid may have been fractured inward to narrow the nose intentionally. If this narrowing has been overdone, the patient suffers from nasal airway obstruction. Nonsurgical nasal trauma is also a common cause, although these same symptoms of nasal airway obstruction can be seen in certain persons with a highly arched narrow nose.

Alar Collapse. Collapse of the alar cartilages may produce nasal airway obstruction. The cause is usually previous injury, resorption of most of the cartilage, loss of cartilaginous resilience, or a family predisposition to a thin lower lobular cartilage with a narrowed vestibule. Diagnosis is made on observation of the person during quiet respiration. As the negative pressure is increased, the lobule, or ala, draws closer to the septum and effectively shuts off the inflow of air. Management is usually surgical, although other methods have been used by patients, such as stents, straws, dilators, and even toothpicks, to hold the ala open to avert the uncomfortable symptoms of nasal airway obstruction.

Others (Rare). Nasal obstruction can occur without an obvious intranasal cause. In cases of facial nerve paralysis, the dilator naris muscle may also be paralyzed. The patient may therefore complain of nasal airway obstruction. In addition, if the greater superficial petrosal nerve is involved with the facial nerve paralysis, the glandular secretion is reduced, and the patient may have a dry nose and complain of a sense of nasal airway obstruction.

Scleroderma involves the facial structures. The tissues of the face are taut, and the patient may also describe symptoms related to nasal airway obstruction.

When there is superior cervical ganglion involvement, regardless of the cause, or after section of the superior cervical ganglion, the patient may have parasympathetic stimulation that is unopposed, and he or she complains of symptoms related to nasal airway obstruction.

Foreign Body. Although a foreign body is not strictly a structural case of nasal obstruction, its presence, especially in children, can produce nasal obstruction. Such a factor should be suspected, especially if there is a unilateral mucopurulent nasal discharge. Diagnosis may require decongestion of the nose, and removal of the object (in patients under the age of 5 years) may require general anesthesia.

SUGGESTED READINGS

Gordon ASD, McCaffrey TV, Kern EB: Rhinomanometry for preoperative and postoperative assessment of nasal obstruction. Otolaryngol Head Neck Surg 101:20–26, 1989.

Hanson RD, Facer GW, Kern EB: Prosthetic closure of septal perforations. OTO '87 1:2–5, 1986.

Heinberg CE, Kern EB: The Cottle sign: an aid in the physical diagnoses of nasal airflow disturbances. Rhinology 11(3):89–94, 1973.

Kasperbauer JL, Kern EB: Nasal valve physiology: implications in nasal surgery. Otolaryngol Clin North Am 20:699–719, 1987.

Kern EB: Surgery of the nasal valve. In Sisson GA, Tardy ME Jr (eds): Plastic and Reconstructive Surgery of the Face and Neck: Proceedings of the Second International Symposium, Vol 2 (pp 43–59). New York: Grune & Stratton, 1977.

Kern EB: Nonsurgical closure of nasal septal perforations. In Rees TD, Baker DC, Tabbal N (eds): Rhinoplasty: Problems and Controversies: A Discussion With the Experts (pp 262–268). St. Louis: CV Mosby, Company, 1988.

Kern EB, Facer GW, McDonald TJ, Westwood WB: Closure of nasal septal perforations with a silastic button: results in 45 patients. Oto Rhinol Laryngol Dig 39:9–17, 1977.

Lipton RJ, Kern EB: Nasal septal reconstruction. In Pillsbury H (ed): Operative Challenge in Otolaryngology/Head and Neck Surgery (pp 219–233). Chicago: Year Book Medical Publishers, 1990.

Mertz JS, McCaffrey TV, Kern EB: Objective evaluation of anterior septal surgical reconstruction. Otolaryngol Head Neck Surg 92:308–311, 1984.

Mullarkey MF: Eosinophilic nonallergic rhinitis. J Allergy Clin Immunol 82:941–949, 1988.

Slavit DH, Facer GW, Kern EB: Total nasal septal reconstruction with caudal end transplant. Paper presented at the American Rhinologic Society Spring Meeting, Waikoloa, HI, May 9, 1991.

CHAPTER 24

Epistaxis

Richard L. Mabry, MD, FACS

INCIDENCE AND SEVERITY

The entity of nasal bleeding encompasses the entire spectrum of severity from minor to catastrophic. It can represent a nuisance or a nightmare for both patient and physician. The great majority of episodes of epistaxis are never treated by a physician; they cease spontaneously or are controlled with self-help measures. Almost without exception, these situations represent bleeding from sites in the anterior nose that lend themselves to easy access for self-treatment. Should treatment by a physician be required, anterior epistaxis is by far the easiest type to manage.

Less frequently, epistaxis is of the posterior variety. In virtually every instance, it requires the intervention of a physician. The location of the bleeding source hinders both accurate diagnosis and appropriate treatment. In addition, this category of nosebleed is most often seen in elderly patients with concomitant medical problems such as hypertension and arteriosclerosis, which further impede control of the bleeding. The degree of bleeding in posterior epistaxis is often underestimated because much of the blood is swallowed. This may allow the problem to go unchecked longer than would the more obvious anterior bleeding.

ANATOMY

The anatomic structure of the nasal cavity makes epistaxis likely and yet renders it difficult to treat. The nasal septum is almost never without spurs and deflections, which

contribute to crust formation and make surface vessels more vulnerable to rupture but less accessible for proper visualization and treatment. The areas beneath the turbinates may be the site of bleeding, but they cannot be readily visualized without significant intranasal manipulation (which is doubly difficult when it is attempted during active bleeding). Although the entire nasal cavity is not a small space, access is via relatively small anterior nares, which hinder both visualization and manipulation. Only since the 1980s, with the common usage of fiberoptic nasal endoscopes, has this problem been overcome to some degree.

Not only is the nose extremely vascular, but the lack of muscles surrounding intranasal blood vessels eliminates the potential for spontaneous cessation of bleeding by local muscular contraction. Most anterior epistaxis originates from Little's area, which is on the anterior nasal septum. A venous plexus (Kiesselbach's plexus) in this location is particularly vulnerable to trauma and is responsible for most anterior nosebleeds. In addition, however, anterior epistaxis may originate from other areas of the cartilaginous septum, from the inferior turbinates, from the anterior portion of the middle meatus, or from branches of the anterior ethmoid artery that supply the anterior roof of the nasal vault (Fig. 24–1).

The exact localization of the site of posterior epistaxis is often difficult. The more common sites are from high and posterior septal spurs, from Woodruff's plexus (located under the posterior half of the inferior turbinate), and from the posterior portion of the middle meatus and the sphenopalatine re-

Figure 24–1. Blood supply of the nasal septum and lateral nasal wall.

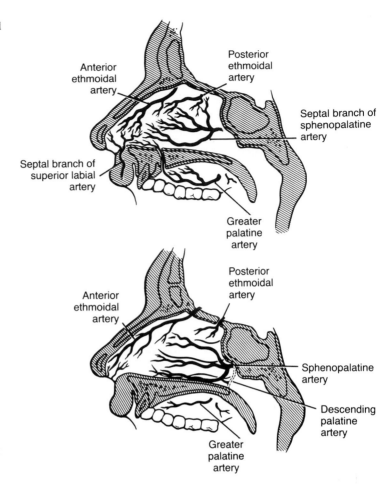

cess. The vessels usually responsible for posterior epistaxis are the sphenopalatine, greater palatine, and pharyngeal arteries.

More details on the anatomy and vasculature of the nose are given in Chapter 22.

CAUSES OF EPISTAXIS

The causes of epistaxis may conveniently be divided into *direct* and *indirect*. Indirect causes are those circumstances and conditions that contribute to the development or persistence of nosebleeds. An understanding of these factors is important in the prevention of epistaxis as well as its treatment.

The direct or proximate cause of most epistaxis is some type of trauma. This may be self-inflicted (nose picking), iatrogenic (surgery, intranasal manipulation), or a result of external forces (fractures involving the nose or paranasal sinuses, rapid pressure changes such as barotrauma). Other in-

stances of epistaxis are due to spontaneous rupture of intranasal vessels. In this circumstance, additional predisposing and contributory factors are almost always present.

A number of factors may contribute indirectly to the presence and persistence of epistaxis. The first such group may be classified as *vascular*. Arteriosclerosis and hypertension, the two prime examples in this category, prevent vessel contraction that would normally slow bleeding and furnish an abnormally high pressure head for sustaining bleeding once it has begun. Similar circumstances are seen as a result of diabetic vasculopathy and coarctation of the aorta.

Hematologic disorders that aggravate or prolong nasal bleeding include the entire spectrum of coagulopathies and clotting disorders (e.g., hemophilia). Primary blood disorders such as leukemia may be marked by frequent episodes of nasal bleeding. In addition, many medications exert a significant effect on blood clotting and may act as anticoagulant agents although they are administered for some other purpose entirely. For instance, one should not forget that aspirin, even in small but regular doses, can significantly prolong prothrombin time and contribute to frequent nosebleeds.

An associated inflammatory condition may contribute to epistaxis, either through the increased blood flow noted locally with an infectious process such as sinusitis or a generalized febrile illness or through the nasal trauma associated with frequent or forceful nose blowing (which often marks the course of such illnesses). Chronic inflammatory conditions of the nose and sinus may result in the formation of nasal polyps, and these frequently bleed because of local mechanical trauma.

In addition to polyps, other neoplasms, either benign or malignant, are potential sources of bleeding from the nose and sinuses. Repeated epistaxis without an obvious source or cause should suggest the need for a thorough evaluation of the paranasal sinuses and "hidden" regions of the nose through computed tomography scans and fiberoptic endoscopy for ruling out an otherwise inapparent neoplastic process.

Two instances of *hormonal* factors that may cause or aggravate epistaxis are worthy of mention. In pregnancy, because of increased cardiac output and marked engorgement of the nasal mucosa, epistaxis is a frequent occurrence. This is often aggravated by rhinitis of pregnancy, addiction to nose drops with rebound rhinitis, and other nasal problems common in pregnancy. Instances of vicarious menstruation from aberrant tissue in the nasal turbinates have been described. Such occurrences are exceedingly rare, but the periodicity of bleeding suggests the diagnosis, and confirmation is made through turbinate biopsy.

The final group of factors contributing indirectly to epistaxis is the large group of *local* causes. One of the most important such factors is crusting, which can be caused by inadequate ambient humidity (desert climate, heated air), by the drying effect of certain drugs (antihistamines, antidepressants, anticholinergics), by exposure to chemicals or irritating fumes (such as smoke and dust), or by impairment of local intranasal humidification caused by a septal deviation or perforation. Rhinitis medicamentosa (which results either from rebound from topical nasal decongestants or from such systemic medications as beta blockers and some antihypertensive agents) causes turbinate engorgement and may aggravate nasal bleeding.

NONSURGICAL MANAGEMENT OF EPISTAXIS

Prevention

Folk medicine advocates prevention of epistaxis by wearing or carrying a piece of carnelian (red quartz), which is said to be effective by "stopping the blood from rising." Failing the efficacy of such a maneuver, a number of other preventive measures may be recommended to patients who are subject to or at risk for epistaxis.

One of the major causes of epistaxis is parching of the nasal membranes during winter or in dry climates. Therefore, patients should be advised to use humidifiers as necessary to combat dryness in the home (especially in the bedroom) and to use intranasal saline sprays frequently for the same purpose. Petrolatum or a similar bland ointment applied gently within the anterior nares once or twice a day is also helpful. (The oft-mentioned risk of lipid pneumonia from aspiration of large amounts of intranasal petroleum products used at bedtime is probably overrated, especially if prudence is exercised in the amount of ointment applied.) Irritants, such as smoke and chemical fumes, should be avoided as much as possible. In addition, the frequency and duration of use of decongestant nasal sprays should be limited because the rebound phenomenon may promote epistaxis.

For minimizing traumatic epistaxis, physicians should give their patients instructions in the proper technique of nose blowing. Specific warnings about vigorous efforts, especially during times of nasal irritation, should be delivered. Patients taking salicylates or anticoagulants should be warned that they are more vulnerable to epistaxis than are persons with normal coagulation mechanisms and that they should take precautions accordingly. Because hypertension accentuates the degree of epistaxis, appropriate medical management of elevated blood pressure is essential.

Attempts at prevention notwithstanding, the practicing otolaryngologist will continue to encounter patients with epistaxis. The balance of this section deals with the systematic management of this problem.

Initial Treatment

The aim of therapy is to localize the bleeding site and to achieve hemostasis in some manner. However, the very first maneuver must be the application of an apron or a gown to the patient and the provision of a towel and an emesis basin. This is accompanied by the donning of protective gear by the physician. Whereas formerly only esthetic considerations made a gown and gloves desirable, universal precautions for minimizing potential exposure to acquired immunodeficiency syndrome (AIDS) when dealing with blood mandate goggles or glasses and suggest the advisability of a mask.

Although it is not always necessary, instances of epistaxis marked by profuse bleeding (especially posterior epistaxis) and involving apprehensive or hypertensive patients often call for the administration of a systemic analgesic or anxiolytic agent. A time-tested preparation, morphine sulfate, 10 mg intramuscularly, is often helpful in these situations and provides both analgesia and sedation. For sedation alone, diazepam is an excellent choice. However, the physician must be aware of the potential for oversedation to produce respiratory depression.

A *topical anesthetic* is usually helpful. A 4% solution of cocaine hydrochloride (keeping the amount applied less than 5 mL) serves not only as an anesthetic agent but also as an excellent vasoconstrictor (see following section on local measures).

The final initial preparations include provision of good *illumination* and adequate *suction*. A headlight is much more effective in dealing with instances of epistaxis than is the more traditional head mirror, which requires frequent readjustment of the light source or mirror angulation as the patient's position changes. The suction should be strong enough to keep a dry field even in the presence of brisk bleeding and should be connected to a large Frazier (or similar) suction tip.

Localization of Bleeding Site

Once initial preparations are complete, the first task is localization of the bleeding site,

if possible. The site and pressure head of the bleeding source dictate all further therapy.

Ideally, the patient should be placed in an upright position. If it is necessary to deal with epistaxis when the patient is supine, head elevation of 60° or more makes examination and manipulation easier, but more important, it minimizes posterior "rundown" and the attendant choking and gagging that often make treatment of epistaxis so trying.

The cooperative patient should be asked to clear all clots from the nose and nasopharynx by vigorous blowing into a towel. If this is not possible, suction should be used to accomplish this. In a few gratifying instances, this simple measure is rewarded by cessation of active bleeding! However, even in these situations, the bleeding source should be located and appropriate measures taken to prevent recurrence of bleeding.

At this point, topical cocaine (or a similar anesthetic solution) is applied. Suction is then advanced posteriorly and superiorly within the bleeding nostril until the area of bleeding is identified. If it is impossible to localize a site, it is usually necessary to progress directly to nasal packing. However, if one can identify the bleeding source, specific local measures are worthwhile.

Topical Vasoconstrictors. Topical cocaine not only acts as an anesthetic but also supplies local vasoconstriction. However, it may be necessary to apply a more powerful vasoconstrictor. Historically, epinephrine, 1:1000, has been applied on cotton pledgets for this purpose. In more recent years, oxymetazoline (either on pledgets or sprayed throughout the nasal cavity) has become popular, serving as an effective vasoconstrictor but with the added advantages over epinephrine of lessened hypertension and tachycardia and a prolonged period of action.

If vasoconstrictor-soaked pledgets are applied over the bleeding site and local pressure is maintained (with an instrument or by external nasal pinching), some episodes of anterior epistaxis can be controlled. Nevertheless, additional definitive measures are suggested, even if such initial success occurs.

Topical Hemostatic Agents. If clot removal and application of topical vasoconstrictors either diminish the amount of bleeding or cause cessation, it may be helpful to apply agents that hasten clotting and form a protective barrier. These include cellulose preparations (Surgicel, Oxycel), topical thrombin, microfibrillar collagen (Avitene), and epsilon-aminocaproic acid (EACA). A remedy not much used at present but often effective is the topical application of porcine strips (small strips of salt pork). This material does hasten clotting, and for years most emergency room refrigerators contained a small piece of frozen salt pork from which strips were shaved when the need arose.

Cauterization. The next method ordinarily employed is some means of cauterizing the bleeding point. In the past, this involved a chromic acid bead, which was fashioned by heating chromic acid powder within a loop on the end of a metal applicator. This method has now been largely replaced by the silver nitrate applicator. Success in using chemical cautery is often dependent on maintaining a dry field with good suction in order to adequately cauterize the bleeding point. For more diffuse areas, application of Monsel's solution (saturated solution of ferric subsulfate) may be effective in achieving local cautery.

Thermal cautery from a heated metal probe has given way to electrodesiccation by use of an electrocautery unit. The most efficient way of employing this method is by the use of a combined suction-cautery tip, which can clear blood from the field and allow accurate cauterization of the bleeding site. This maneuver requires the use of a local anesthetic because it is often quite painful. In addition, great care must be taken to avoid injudicious or prolonged cauterization, lest septal perforations or nasal synechiae result.

Extreme and unusual cases of epistaxis may yield to cauterization with use of the laser. The argon, neodymium-YAG and KTP lasers seem best suited for this application. The most common indication for laser therapy in epistaxis is bleeding that results from hereditary hemorrhagic telangiectasia involving the nasal cavity. More comments on the use of lasers in epistaxis are found in the section on surgical management.

Nasal Packing

Anterior epistaxis from a venous source can usually be controlled by the measures already described. However, instances of bleeding from an arterial source or that stems from an area within the nasal cavity not readily accessible for visualization and manipulation usually require some form of tamponade. Nasal packing may take many forms and can be classified according to the site of application: anterior or combined anterior-posterior.

Anterior nasal packing is most commonly carried out by use of half-inch–wide ribbon gauze. This may be plain selvage or a nonsticking synthetic. Insertion and removal of the packing are facilitated by lubrication, either petrolatum or in the form of an antibiotic ointment (such as neomycin-polymyxin [Neosporin] ointment). Antibiotic ointments prevent the foul odor usually associated with nasal packing left in situ for several days. Too copious an application of a petroleum-based ointment to packing is said to carry the risk of myospherulosis (a localized foreign body reaction).

The method of inserting an anterior pack varies with the preference of the physician and is affected by the haste with which it is necessary to control bleeding. In general, the gauze is grasped approximately midway between the two free ends with a bayonet forceps, and the first loop of gauze is wedged into the posterosuperior portion of the nasal cavity, after which subsequent loops are layered from superior to inferior (Fig. 24–2). Doubling the gauze allows it to be placed and removed more quickly. After the packing has reached the area of the vestibule, it

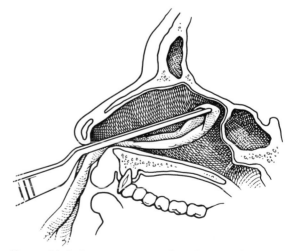

Figure 24–2. First step in nasal packing with ribbon gauze; the doubled gauze strip is wedged firmly into the posterior-superior portion of the nasal cavity. Subsequent loops are layered from superior to inferior.

should be snugly tamped down (packing tends to loosen spontaneously within a few hours), with a cotton plug placed in the external naris for further pressure. A gauze drip pad can then be placed beneath the nose and held in place by tape, which comes from below the nose up along either side to the radix, forming a sling. This is not easily dislodged, it exerts continued gentle pressure on the packing, and it does not move with facial motions as does tape placed from cheek to cheek.

A relatively new innovation in anterior packing is a highly compressed polymer (Merocel) prepared as a nasal tampon that is inserted into the nasal cavity and then hydrated (by added saline or by blood), with expansion and the application of local pressure. A number of different shapes and sizes of nasal tampons are available, many of which have incorporated a silicone nasal tube for allowing some nasal breathing while the nose is packed. (This feature may not be desirable in the treatment of epistaxis because there is a tendency for blood to leak from the posterior nares into the tube and be expelled anteriorly, which distresses the patient and the family.) One design, the Doyle tampon, is said to exert pressure sufficient for control of even some posterior bleeding points (Fig. 24–3). Although they are much easier and less traumatic to insert and remove than is conventional gauze anterior packing, these nasal tampons may not exert sufficient pressure for adequate tamponade of brisk bleeding sites.

Posterior nasal bleeding sites require a buttress in the nasopharynx, not so much for exerting pressure against the sphenopalatine artery branches in this region as for allowing firm anterior packing to be placed without the risk of prolapse into the nasopharynx. The classical *posterior pack* is a rolled mass of lamb's wool, folded gauze, or a doubled portion of tampon held by umbilical tape or strong suture, which is tied in place over an anterior bolster. Some buttresses modify the shape of the pack to a conical plug, which snugly fills the choana without undue nasopharyngeal pressure.

For placing a posterior pack, a rubber catheter is inserted into one nostril (if the pack is for one side only) or in each nostril (if the pack is to block both choanae). The catheter is then grasped with a hemostat as it appears below the edge of the soft palate and is pulled out the mouth. Two of the three strings that have been attached to the posterior pack are tied to the catheter (one to each catheter if two are used). The catheters are then withdrawn, and the guide strings are grasped firmly in one hand. With the index finger of the other hand, the physician maneuvers the pack behind the soft palate and seats it firmly in the nasopharynx. With continued traction exerted on the guide strings (by an assistant or the physician), tight gauze anterior packing is placed. If a unilateral pack is placed, the guide strings are tied firmly over a rolled gauze pad placed over the external naris as a bolster. If bilateral packs are used, the gauze pad is placed over the columella and the strings are tied. For prevention of columellar damage, some authors advocate placing a fragment of tongue depressor within the pad to keep the strings from cutting into soft tissue. The third string on the posterior pack, which had been left hanging into the pharynx, can be brought out the mouth and taped to the cheek, or cut and allowed to hang into the pharynx. This string is later used to remove the posterior pack (after the anterior strings are cut and the anterior packing is removed).

Considering the trauma involved for both patient and physician in placing a conventional posterior pack, it is not surprising that alternative means of packing continue to be sought. Indeed, the number of new types of posterior pack being developed reflects the shortcomings of those already in existence. A Foley catheter (inserted via the nose into the nasopharynx and inflated with water or saline solution) has been advocated as an easy and effective substitute for conventional posterior packs. It has been said that air, rather than saline or water, should be used

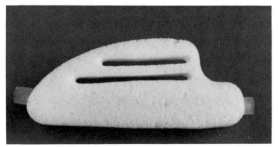

Figure 24–3. Doyle design Merocel nasal tampon, after expansion by hydration. The unhydrated, compressed tampon is easily inserted and usually expands as a result of hydration by blood, although saline may be applied to hasten the process.

for inflation of the catheter because the weight of the liquid can pull the balloon inferiorly, away from the desired area of tamponade. Although it is easier to insert and remove, the Foley balloon does not always exert the firm, even pressure needed in this area. Also, the length of catheter left sticking out the anterior naris presents a cumbersome appearance.

Less cumbersome and more effective than a Foley catheter is the Gottschalk Nasostat, which features an inflatable balloon designed to exert pressure on the sphenopalatine artery as it enters the nasal cavity posteriorly (Fig. 24–4A). Although requiring additional, separate anterior packing if other vessels are involved, the Nasostat features a noncollapsible bulge in the catheter that abuts the anterior naris to hold the device firmly in place.

Other inflatable nasal catheters for control of anterior and posterior epistaxis are available (Fig. 24–4B). These may be made of rubber or silicone and often include a central lumen for nasal respiration. Such devices are quickly inserted and removed, and the posterior and anterior balloons may be inflated separately to the precise amount of pressure desired. They furnish good postnasal pressure, but overinflation must be avoided to prevent pressure necrosis if they remain in place for any length of time. In general, bulging of the soft palate is a sign of overinflation of any of these devices.

Possible Complications. Patients requiring posterior packing are obvious candidates for hospitalization because of the severity of their bleeding and the potential for complications. If packing (either anterior alone or in combination with a posterior pack) is nec-

essary for the control of epistaxis, several associated measures are necessary. Because of the complications of infection, antibiotics are usually administered. In addition to the expected problems of otitis media and sinusitis, intranasal packing may be followed by toxic shock syndrome because of absorption by the body of an endotoxin produced by certain strains of *Staphylococcus aureus*. Although up to 40% of healthy persons are nasal carriers of *Staphylococcus*, not all *S. aureus* species produce the endotoxin. The theoretic risk of toxic shock syndrome from nasal packing is on the order of 2%. However, because of the severity of the illness, coverage with antistaphylococcal antibiotics (such as a cephalosporin or an antistaphylococcal penicillin) is advised while packs are in place.

For combating the potential complications of hypoventilation and hypoxia, close monitoring of the airway and arterial blood gases is necessary, especially in patients requiring combined anterior-posterior packing. If supplemental oxygen by mask is given (usually in a 40% concentration), close observation for further respiratory depression resulting from removal of the respiratory drive (by lowering the pCO$_2$) is necessary. For the same reason, sedatives should be administered with caution; remember that agitation may be due to hypoxia rather than pain.

Other Measures. Other, more general measures are employed as appropriate. These include restriction of activity, elevation of the head, and the local application of ice to the face. If posterior packing is in place, observation for palatal bulging (indicating excessive pressure) and for laceration or excessive pressure on the columella from the

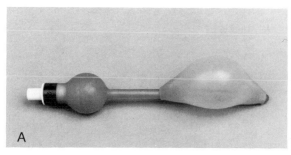
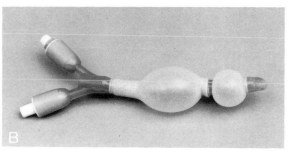

Figure 24–4. *A*, The Gottschalk Nasostat has an inflatable posterior bulb, but it requires anterior ribbon gauze packing if anterior bleeding is present. The anterior noncollapsible bulb forms a buttress between pack material and the anterior nares. *B*, The inflatable pack has separate inflation ports for the anterior and posterior balloons.

guide strings is necessary. In addition to oxygen supplementation, humidification of inspired air is necessary for combating the dryness that results from obligatory mouth-breathing. Obviously an intravenous line should be started early in the treatment of severe epistaxis for the replacement of fluids and the administration of blood should it be necessary.

Consultation with an internist and other appropriate specialists is advisable at this point. In addition to the continued medical management of any existing medical problems, fluid and electrolyte balance and hematologic parameters must be carefully evaluated and monitored.

A hematologic evaluation is important in any patient with unexplained, recurrent, or prolonged nasal bleeding. This may be begun by the otolaryngologist, but assistance should be sought from a hematologist as necessary. To evaluate each phase of hemostasis would require a test to measure the formation of hemostatic plugs (platelet count and appearance, bleeding time), the generation of thrombin (partial thromboplastin time to measure the intrinsic pathway and prothrombin time for the extrinsic pathway), and the thrombin-fibrinogen reaction and the stability of the resultant fibrin clot (thrombin time and plasma clot stability). Other more specific tests may be ordered on the basis of clinical knowledge of the patient and the results of these initial tests.

Pack Removal. The length of time nasal packing is left in place varies with individual circumstances and the physician's personal preference. In general, packs should be left in place at least 24 to 48 hours after the cessation of active bleeding. A good general rule is that no patient ever bled because packs were left in too long! Pack removal should be performed in a setting in which pack reinsertion can be quickly carried out should rebleeding occur, and patients should be observed closely (either at home or in the hospital setting) for at least 24 hours after pack removal before being allowed to gradually resume activity.

Alternative Measures

Because of the discomfort and potential complications associated with nasal packing, or because packing is not always effective in controlling severe instances of epistaxis, alternative measures may be considered.

Some physicians believe that if simple anterior packing is ineffective, packing under anesthesia is worthwhile. They believe that this allows tighter and more effective tamponade. However, if it is elected to take the patient to surgery and use a general anesthetic, surgical measures (see the next section) are more appropriate.

For posterior bleeding, pterygopalatine fossa injection has been advocated. This is performed with a 22-gauge spinal needle via the greater palatine foramen with injection of approximately 3 mL of 2% lidocaine with 1:100,000 epinephrine. The pressure from the injected material, in addition to the vasoconstrictor effect of the epinephrine, affects the sphenopalatine artery in this area. This may afford temporary or (in a few instances) lasting relief from bleeding. It can be helpful by slowing down bleeding until posterior packing can be placed or definitive surgery performed. Great care must be exercised to avoid the orbit with this maneuver, and visual loss is a potential complication of pterygopalatine fossa injection.

Treatment of severe posterior epistaxis by cryotherapy has been described as free of many of the complications associated with packing or surgery. Hicks reported his experience of more than 20 years and described this alternative method of treatment as quite effective (Hicks and Norris, 1983). Although not universally successful, it is worthy of consideration as an alternative to surgical intervention.

Yet another alternative means of treating severe posterior epistaxis is localization of the bleeding site by arteriography, followed by selective embolization. Because of the potential complications of amaurosis, hemiplegia, failure to control bleeding, and even death, this procedure is most often used only when more conventional measures have failed.

SURGERY FOR EPISTAXIS

The most common indication for surgery in the patient with epistaxis is failure of medical management to control the problem. However, some physicians believe that severe bleeding episodes should be managed with surgical intervention as soon as possible, in light of the discomfort, possible prolonged hospital stay, and potential complications associated with packing. In general, surgery is considered after failure of conservative measures, in the presence of pulmonary or cardiovascular problems that make complications of prolonged posterior packing likely, and when circumstances make transfusion difficult (e.g., rare blood type). The timing of surgery and the choice of procedure remain controversial. This section addresses the various modalities currently employed and their proper application.

Vessel Ligation

The easiest vessel to ligate for control of nasal bleeding is the external carotid artery. Exposure of this vessel is not difficult, especially for the surgeon familiar with its anatomy from head and neck surgery, and the technical aspects of the procedure are relatively simple. The surgeon should always identify several branches of the external carotid before ligating it for avoidance of the catastrophic mistake of ligating the internal carotid (which does not branch within the neck). However, because of anastomotic vessels plus blood supply via the ethmoid system, this ligation alone is often unsuccessful in controlling nasal bleeding.

In order to ligate the feeder vessels to the nose as close to their terminus as possible, ligation of the internal maxillary artery has been advocated as the preferred procedure for vascular interruption in epistaxis. This is typically done through a transantral approach with use of the operating microscope. After the medial half of the posterior antral wall has been removed and the pterygopalatine periostium opened, the maxillary artery is identified in the pterygopalatine fat. After identification of the main artery, microclips are applied to the main trunk proximal to the descending palatine and again as far medially as possible, on the descending palatine branch distally, and on all identifiable remaining branches (Fig. 24–5). Creation of a large nasoantral window prevents postoperative hematoma formation.

In an attempt to make transantral vessel ligation even simpler, Simpson and associates (1982) described a technique of sphenopalatine artery ligation through the posteromedial antral wall, with bypassing of the pterygomaxillary space for ligation of the

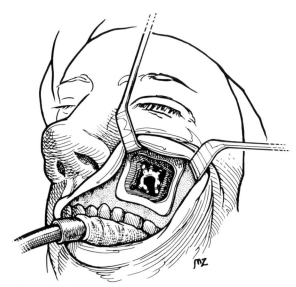

Figure 24–5. Schematic depiction of the anatomy of internal maxillary artery ligation.

sphenopalatine at its most distal point. Intraoral ligation of the maxillary artery has been suggested by Maceri (Maceri and Makielski, 1984). This interrupts the vessel between the first and second parts and seems an appropriate alternative when the transantral approach cannot be employed (because of massive fracture, tumor, aplasia).

The complications reported in association with transantral vessel ligation include paresthesia or anesthesia of the cheek, periorbital hematoma, ophthalmoplegia, temporary or permanent diplopia, and blindness. In addition, ligation of the internal maxillary or sphenopalatine artery alone may not control bleeding.

In instances of bleeding from high in the nose, and when there is any reason to suspect that internal maxillary artery ligation alone will be ineffective, ligation of the anterior ethmoid artery is advised. Some physicians recommend that this procedure be performed routinely with all maxillary or sphenopalatine artery ligations, whereas others judge every case individually. After an incision has been made along the side of the nose near the inner canthus of the eye, careful dissection of the periostium reveals the anterior ethmoid artery as it crosses from the orbit to the interior of the nose (Fig. 24–6). It can be doubly ligated or doubly clipped and need not be transected. Although some authors suggest otherwise, the posterior eth-

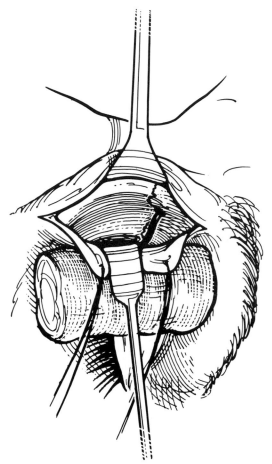

Figure 24–6. Schematic depiction of the anatomy of anterior ethmoid artery ligation.

moid artery need not always be ligated and should be avoided when possible because of its proximity to the optic nerve. After ethmoidal artery ligation, careful reapproximation of the periostium is necessary for avoidance of postoperative diplopia.

There exist differences of opinion about leaving nasal packing in place after vessel ligation for epistaxis. The surgeon is guided ultimately by individual experience but should consider that if packs are left in place after surgery, removal should be possible if there is no bleeding for 24 to 48 hours after the procedure.

The existence of significant collateral circulation to the nasal cavity can be deduced by the absence of tissue necrosis after unilateral ligation of both the internal maxillary artery (and its branches) and the anterior ethmoid artery. Vessel ligation does not completely deprive the nasal cavity of its blood

supply, but it simply decreases the pressure head involved. There may be instances when vessel ligation is ineffective. In addition, consideration is now more often being given to procedures that identify the bleeding site and deal with it specifically by means of cautery.

Selective Cauterization of Bleeding Site

Anderson and associates (1984) have presented a method of systematically searching under anesthesia for bleeding sites in instances of posterior epistaxis. In their series, bleeding had not been controlled by nasal packing, or it recurred when it was removed; nasal anatomy prevented proper pack placement; or significant cardiovascular or pulmonary insufficiency made use of posterior packs undesirable. The nasopharynx and posterior choanae are examined in the fashion of an adenoidectomy, and bleeding sites are cauterized with a disposable, malleable suction electrocautery. If bleeding continues from within the nose, the nasal cavity is examined, and septoplasty is performed if necessary to allow adequate visualization. Bleeding sites are cauterized in a similar manner. If bleeding appears to be coming from beneath a turbinate, medial infracture of that structure allows access. Anderson and associates reported good results with this technique, and the author's experience parallels theirs.

More recent literature reports detail the use of rigid fiberoptic endoscopes combined with a malleable electrocautery tip for endoscopic identification and selective cauterization of intranasal bleeding points.

The most common use of the laser for control of intranasal bleeding is in instances of diffuse bleeding that results from hereditary hemorrhagic telangiectasia. The technology of the laser (especially the argon or KTP laser) is advocated as equally effective or more effective than electrocautery in controlling intranasal bleeding from more mundane causes. At present, work is under way by some investigators to link rigid intranasal endoscopes with lasers for use in the management of epistaxis.

Combination of Methods

Epistaxis often requires not just one method for control but a combination of many approaches. Such a special case is hereditary hemorrhagic telangiectasia. Nasal bleeding that results from this disorder may resist the physician's best efforts, and repeated bleeding marks the course of the disease. In addition to the classical chemical and electric cautery techniques and nasal packing, embolization and vessel ligation may eventually be required. Hormonal therapy with estrogen has been used in some instances. Smaller areas of telangiectasia may respond to laser photocoagulation; septal dermoplasty has been advised for larger bleeding areas.

SUGGESTED READINGS

Anderson RG, Shannon DN, Schaefer SD, Raney LA: A surgical alternative to internal maxillary artery ligation for posterior epistaxis. Otolaryngol Head Neck Surg 92:427–433, 1984.

Chandler JR, Serrins AJ: Transantral ligation of the internal maxillary artery for epistaxis. Laryngoscope 75:1151–1159, 1965.

Fairbanks DN: Complications of nasal packing. Otolaryngol Head Neck Surg 94:412–415, 1986.

Hicks JN, Norris JW: Office treatment by cryotherapy for severe posterior nasal epistaxis—update. Laryngoscope 93:876–879, 1983.

Jacobson JA, Kasworm EM: Toxic shock syndrome after nasal surgery. Arch Otolaryngol Head Neck Surg 112:329–332, 1986.

Mabry RL: Management of epistaxis by packing. Otolaryngol Head Neck Surg 94:401–403, 1986.

Maceri DR, Makielski KH: Intraoral ligation of the maxillary artery for posterior epistaxis. Laryngoscope 94:737–741, 1984.

Marcus MJ: Nasal endoscopic control of epistaxis—a preliminary report. Otolaryngol Head Neck Surg 102:273–275, 1990.

McDonald TJ, Pearson BW: Follow-up on maxillary artery ligation for epistaxis. Arch Otolaryngol 106:635–638, 1980.

Parkin JL, Dixon JA: Argon laser treatment of head and neck vascular lesions. Otolaryngol Head Neck Surg 93:211–216, 1985.

Simpson GT, Janfaza P, Becker GD: Transantral sphenopalatine artery ligation. Laryngoscope 92:1001–1005, 1982.

Strutz J, Schumacher M: Uncontrollable epistaxis: angiographic localization and embolization. Arch Otolaryngol Head Neck Surg 116:697–699, 1990.

Wurman LH, Sack JG, Flannery JV Jr, Paulson TO: Selective endoscopic electrocautery for posterior epistaxis. Laryngoscope 98:1348–1349, 1988.

apy is unsuccessful or if the complications of the disease require it.

Chronic sinusitis should be treated after the overlying acute disease has been successfully treated. The underlying chronic process should be thoroughly evaluated by complete nasal examination or endoscopic examination or both. A CT scan in the coronal plain is necessary for complete evaluation of the sinuses. The diagnosis of chronic sinusitis is made on the basis of the history, physical examination, and CT findings.

Once the diagnosis of chronic sinusitis is made, the patient may be treated according to the diagnosed underlying etiologic agent. Treatment of this disease may include a combination of antibiotics, steroids (both intranasal and systemic), antihistamines and decongestants (topical and systemic), allergy desensitization, and control of the environment.

Surgery may be indicated and consists of various "traditional procedures," or "functional endoscopic sinus surgery." Treatment is decided on the basis of the extent of the disease and the diagnosed etiologic agent. Surgical therapy should also be based on the extent of the patient's disease; however, it is recommended that the surgeon use the procedure with which he or she is most familiar.

NASAL POLYPOSIS

Nasal polyposis remains a challenge to the treating physician. Infection, allergy, trauma, chemicals, metabolic disease, and psychogenic factors have all been implicated as etiologic agents among many. However, the pathophysiologic mechanism and pathogenesis are still unclear. Diagnosis is made on the basis of a thorough history, a comprehensive physical examination, and a CT scan.

On pathologic examination, the nasal polyp represents a focal reactive prominence of the lamina propria mucosae. A variable pronounced edema with an inflammatory infiltrate and proliferation of connective tissue fibroblasts can be visualized. Mucous glands can be found in all nasal polyps.

Treatment of nasal polyposis is directed toward the underlying etiologic agent. A well-organized medical plan is still the treatment of choice and includes all of the same modalities as used for the treatment of chronic sinusitis. Should medical therapy

fail, surgical management is recommended. It is important, however, to treat the underlying cause of the polyps, for if the polyps are removed and the underlying cause is untreated, there is a greater chance that the polyps will return.

WEGENER'S GRANULOMATOSIS

Wegener's granulomatosis is an unusual disease; however, it is not rare. The etiologic agent is unknown, but the disorder may represent an unusual form of an autoimmune disease. The disease is certainly a multisystem disorder and may be fatal. It is characterized by a focal necrotizing vasculitis that may affect the upper and lower respiratory tracts, the skin, the joints, and the kidneys. Wegener's granulomatosis is now best regarded as a clinical continuum or spectrum.

Adults are usually affected; however, the disease may be diagnosed in children. The onset is usually gradual, with multiple organ systems involved; however, on occasion it may be fulminant. The usual presentation starts with the development of a granulomatous condition in the upper respiratory tract followed by bronchitis, pneumonia, and glomerulonephritis. Each of these conditions may be found alone or in any combination except glomerulonephritis; the kidney cannot be involved alone because focal necrotizing glomerulitis is nonspecific. Death may occur from uremia if treatment fails.

Initially, the patient may present to the otolaryngologist with a painful ulcer of the nose or a granular draining otitis media and hearing loss that is unrelentingly progressive and unresponsive to treatment. These lesions may be infected secondarily by *Staphylococcus aureus* or *Pseudomonas aeruginosa*. Pansinusitis is quite common. In order of frequency, the maxillary sinuses are most often involved, followed by the ethmoid, frontal, and sphenoid sinuses. The eyes may be involved in up to 40% of the cases; this involvement may be primarily vascular or by contiguousness to adjacent upper airway lesions. Ocular lesions include corneoscleral ulceration, necrogranulomatous keratitis, granulomatous sclerouveitis, and conjunctivitis with occasional proptosis and pseudotumor of the orbit. Cutaneous involvement is said to occur in up to 50% of patients, but muscle involvement is uncommon. Cardiac manifestations include vasculitis of the coronary vasculature, valvulitis, and pericarditis. Nervous involvement occurs in 25% to 50% of patients; a mononeuritis complex is not an infrequent finding. Pulmonary lesions are almost invariably involved, and changes range from small subclinical lesions to multiple nodular lesions.

Diagnosis is made on the basis of a nasal or lung biopsy that reveals necrotizing granulomas with giant cells and widespread areas of vasculitis. A renal biopsy may demonstrate a glomerulitis and vasculitis with immune complex deposits in the vascular walls. Laboratory tests are not specifically diagnostic, although an elevated erythrocyte sedimentation rate, hypergammaglobulinemia, and anergy are usually present.

True Wegener's granulomatosis is sensitive to cyclophosphamide therapy. Reports indicate that in most cases, long-term remissions and even cures can be achieved with the use of this drug. In patients with fulminating disease, especially with renal failure, treatment is started with large doses of prednisone. This therapy is continued until the disease is under control. The erythrocyte sedimentation rate and the creatinine level are monitored for evaluating response to treatment. When these are controlled, cyclophosphamide therapy is instituted. Radiation has failed to alter the course of this disease. There are other alternative drugs for patients who cannot tolerate cyclophosphamide. In these patients, azathioprine, chlorambucil, methotrexate, and cyclosporine have been used. Plasmapheresis has also been tried. However, use of these drugs and procedures is still experimental.

MIDLINE (LETHAL, NONHEALING) GRANULOMA

Midline (lethal, nonhealing) granuloma is characterized by ulceration and induration in the tissues of the nose or nasopharynx; it extends into the adjacent structures and results in the gradual destruction of the tissues of the midface. Despite the name *midline lethal granuloma*, not all cases are lethal, and not all are granulomatous.

Clinically, the most common symptom is nasal obstruction. The patient may present with an ulceration, associated discharge or epistaxis, or pain. The lesions may be preceded by a long nasal prodrome, and the nasal lesions can be locally ulcerative and destructive or may be diffuse. In the upper aerodigestive tract, polymorphic reticulosis involves the nasal cavity and paranasal sinuses, larynx, tracheobronchial tree, palate, pharynx, and nasopharynx. The nasal lesions are often bilateral. Like Wegener's granulomatosis, but unlike idiopathic midline granuloma, the systemic complaints of polymorphic reticulosis are out of proportion to the nasal complaints. The symptoms include malaise, fatigue, night sweats, and fever.

As the disorder progresses, lesions are observed in the skin, lungs, and lymph nodes. Death may occur in a matter of months or after many years and is usually secondary to meningitis, pneumonia, debilitation, or uncontrolled hemorrhage. The patients affected by midline lethal granuloma are usually younger than are those with Wegener's granulomatosis. Men are more commonly affected than are women by a 3:1 ratio.

According to Batsakis (1979), midline (nonhealing) lethal granuloma appears histologically as three definable lesions. The first definable lesion appears as a localized destructive lesion characterized by nonspecific acute and chronic inflammation and necrosis. Granulomas and giant cells are infrequent. There is no atypical cellular infiltrate unless the lesion is in transition to the second type of lesion.

The second definable lesion is a pseudolymphomatous tissue reaction called polymorphic reticulosis by some authors and lymphomatoid granulomatosis by others. There is abundant clinical and histologic evidence that polymorphic reticulosis is linked closely to lymphoma. On histologic examination, a characteristic atypical and polymorphic lymphoreticular infiltrate is seen. An angiocentric growth pattern may simulate a vasculitis; however, there is absence of fibrinoid necrosis in the vessel walls.

The third lesion of this continuum appears as an extranodal lymphoma. Transitional forms of this disease clearly exist, and this fact along with difficulties in histopathologic interpretation makes this group of lesions some of the most difficult to diagnose.

Midline lethal granuloma responds to large doses of irradiation (4000 to 6000 cGy). It has a good prognosis should the disease be localized. Dramatic long-term remissions can be achieved with large doses of local irradiation. The prognosis is not quite as good in patients with systemic disease. Chemotherapeutic agents have not been useful in treating this disease.

TUBERCULOSIS

In the absence of pulmonary tuberculosis, nasal involvement is extremely rare. The other part of the upper airway that is involved is the larynx. Nasopharyngeal or nasal involvement is usually characterized by nasal discharge, pain, or partial obstruction. The lesion may present as a beefy red, edematous nodular area with associated exudate, crusting, or bleeding. Progression to ulceration of the cartilaginous septum may occur rapidly. The nasal floor and bony septum are rarely involved. A granulomatous growth or polyp most commonly originating on the nasal septum or inferior turbinate may be the presenting lesion, but in most cases a positive chest film accompanies this disease.

If tuberculosis is suspected either from history or from an accompanying positive chest film, further evaluation should include smears and cultures of sputum and nasal drainage, followed by biopsy for evidence of tuberculous granulomatous reaction and acid-fast bacilli.

The histopathologic features include a typical granuloma, the center of which usually liquefies and is thus termed caseous necrosis. Pale epithelial cells with giant cells surround the center. The outer layer has lymphocytes, histiocytes, and fibrosis. Current therapy consists of isoniazid and rifampin.

SARCOIDOSIS

Sarcoid is a granulomatous disease of unknown origin with significant upper airway involvement. It seems to affect mostly American Blacks and Scandinavians. When it involves the nose and paranasal sinuses, the typical symptom is that of nasal obstruction. Epistaxis, nasal pain, and anosmia are also found. The nasal mucosa is usually dry and crusting. Yellow subcutaneous nodules are characteristic and probably represent submucosal granulomas. Intranasal sarcoid has a predilection for the septum and inferior turbinates. Bone involvement is rarely seen.

Nasal synechiae may form between the inferior turbinate and the nasal septum. The disease may cause a nasal septal perforation as well.

Very often the nodular corrugated appearance may be confused with changes seen with vasomotor rhinitis. The differential diagnosis may be narrowed by the history and the lack of vasoconstriction with topical agents. Other findings usually include a positive chest film and cervical adenopathy.

Patients often complain of malaise, low-grade fever, and weight loss. The disease is often characterized by disseminated granulomatous lesions that can involve any tissue in the body. The symptoms in the more progressive stages involve the pulmonary, hepatic, renal, splenic, visceral, and optic systems.

The nasal biopsy typically reveals submucosal noncaseating granuloma composed of epithelioid cells and multinucleated giant cells. A positive elevated angiotensin-converting enzyme is indicative. Other laboratory abnormalities, such as elevated liver function tests and elevated serum and urinary calcium levels, may be found. Serum immunoglobulin levels, particularly that of IgG, may be elevated. The Kveim test is positive in 80% of patients, but it should not be performed except in research centers.

Systemic steroids may be used to treat sarcoid when systemic organs are involved. When the disease is confined to the nose, topical steroids have been effective.

SYPHILIS

Syphilis can occur in any age group. Primary syphilis may appear as a lesion (chancre) on the external nose or inside the vestibule. However, it most commonly manifests on the skin. The intranasal chancre appears as a hard, nonpainful, ulcerated papule usually associated with an enlarged rubbery nontender node, which usually occurs approximately 3 weeks after exposure. Secondary lesions, on the other hand, are not seen intranasally. However, nasal involvement is usually seen in tertiary or latent syphilis. The lesions seen in these later stages, which usually occur years after the disease has been contracted, involve both the bony and cartilaginous nasal septum. The lesion may even erode through the hard palate. This may lead to a saddle nose deformity. Congenital syphilis, nicknamed the "snuffles," appears between birth and 2 years of age. It is characterized by a marked rhinitis, with nasal obstruction secondary to the mucosal inflammation and a mucopurulent discharge that is often bloody. If this goes unrecognized, it can cause a chondritis and an osteitis that can also lead to a saddle nose deformity. The secondary lesions and congenital lesions are both highly contagious. Other stigmata of the disease include interstitial keratitis, sensorineural deafness, and Hutchinson's incisors (Hutchinson's triad), rhagades, mulberry molars, and saber skin.

A nonspecific lymphoplasmacytic perivascular inflammatory cell infiltrate is histologically visualized. Proliferation of the small vessel endothelium is noted. Special stains reveal the *Treponema pallidum* organisms. The serum obtained from the primary lesion may be dark stain–positive for *T. pallidum*. The antibody tests, however, are usually negative for 8 to 12 weeks. During the secondary stage, the VDRL (Veneral Disease Research Laboratory) test is uniformly positive, and the FTA-ABS (fluorescent treponemal antibody absorption test) is likely to be reactive.

The recommended treatment is with penicillin. Erythromycin may be substituted in patients with a penicillin allergy. With successful treatment, reagin test titers decrease only slowly, but the FTA-ABS levels are unaffected.

NASAL DISEASES UNCOMMON IN THE UNITED STATES

Atrophic Rhinitis

Atrophic rhinitis is characterized by progressive chronic inflammation, atrophy, and fibrosis affecting the respiratory mucosa, submucosa, seromucinous glands, nasal vasculature, and underlying periosteum and bone. An excessively patent nasal passage with crusting and squamous metaplasia results in a fetid odor from the foul mucus and a loss of the sense of smell. The mucosa is pale, shiny pink, and covered with foul-smelling crusts. Bleeding may occur on its removal.

There is no pathognomonic histopathologic change, nor has any specific bacteria been cultured. This disease probably represents an end stage of prolonged infection.

Many treatments have been recommended; however, none has proved to be completely effective. Frequent nasal irrigations and good nasal hygiene are only partially helpful. Implant operations work initially, but extrusion rates have been high. Closure of the nostrils in stages either totally or to a diameter of 3 mm has been successful; however, closure is recommended for a period of 3 years for the results to be worthwhile. Long-term follow-up is still needed to evaluate this modality.

Rhinoscleroma

Rhinoscleroma is endemic to subtropical countries in Africa, Asia, South and Central America, and Eastern Europe. In the United States, it is seen more frequently in the southwest and western regions where the hygiene is poor. *Klebsiella rhinoscleromatis* is the etiologic organism and almost always affects the nose. The infection usually begins anteriorly as a firm submucosal plaque and expands into hard nodules that obstruct the nostrils. The final stages may cause disfigurement of the nose and consist of fibrosis and stenosis.

On histologic examination, the lesion usually shows a chronic granulomatous mass consisting of lymphocytes, plasma cells, and fibrosis with prominent histiocytic cells and Mikulicz cells. Culture yields positive results in more than 95% of patients and is diagnostic.

The recommended treatment consists of streptomycin and tetracycline for 4 weeks, followed by a repeat course 1 month later. Surgical correction of the scarring with the use of buccal mucosa grafts and polymeric silicone has been successful for reconstructing the lining of the nose.

Leprosy

Leprosy is endemic to warm, medically deprived areas. *Mycobacterium leprae* is the etiologic agent, and this organism is attracted to subcutaneous nerves and secondarily to the skin and mucosa of the upper respiratory tract. Occasional cases occur in Texas, Louisiana, California, and Hawaii. There are two principal forms of this disease. Tuberculoid leprosy is a relatively benign and self-limiting form affecting people who are relatively resistant to the offending organism. The nose is less commonly involved in this form, and patients usually present with an anesthetic macular plaque. Biopsy of the cutaneous involved nerve, which is often enlarged and palpable, demonstrates a noncaseating granuloma. These patients have a positive lepromin skin test.

Lepromatous leprosy is a disseminated form occurring in patients with a low resistance to *M. leprae* as demonstrated by a negative lepromin test. In this form, the bacteria can be found in all of the tissues of the body. Physical examination reveals nodules that have a tendency to form in the skin of the cooler regions of the body. These nodules appear as small, multiple macules or papules that can coalesce to form thickened plaques or nodules. They are commonly found on the alae of the nose, lips, ears, and forehead and thus cause the characteristic leonine facies. Intranasal, oropharyngeal, and laryngeal mucosal lesions can occur. The lesions of the nose appear as red granular ulcers and may result in a septal perforation. The diagnosis may be made by Ziehl-Neelsen stains of the scrapings or by identification of the bacteria on biopsy.

Treatment includes good nasal hygiene and the long-term administration of dapsone.

Fungal Infections

Fungal infections have become more common in the United States with the ever-increasing population of immunocompromised patients. Among the more commonly seen fungal infections of the nose and paranasal sinuses are rhinosporidiosis, blastomycosis, mucormycosis, and aspergillosis. Diagnosis is made by history, physical examination, cultures, histologic examination, and radiologic evaluation that includes CT studies.

There are four forms of fungal sinusitis: mycetoma, invasive, indolent, and allergic. Sinus mycetoma or "fungal ball" is unilateral, and there is usually no bone destruction. On pathologic examination, there is a closely packed, tangled mass of fungal hyphae without allergic mucin. This mass is resistant to conservative management and requires surgical removal.

The invasive form of fungal sinusitis can be either slowly or rapidly progressive. In immunocompromised patients, it tends to be quite aggressive. Initially one sinus may be involved with soft tissue necrosis, granulomatous reaction, and fibrosis that may progress to bone and soft tissue invasion with extensive bone destruction. Aggressive debridement with systemic antifungal therapy is indicated in these patients.

The indolent form of fungal sinusitis usually appears first as a chronic unilateral sinusitis in an immunocompromised host. A chronic fibrosing granulomatous inflammatory process with multinucleated giant cells is seen in histologic examination. Surgical debridement is necessary to treat this form of fungal infection.

Allergic Fungal Sinusitis. The fourth form of sinusitis is allergic fungal sinusitis. This form occurs in atopic patients and affects multiple sinuses. The patients present with a history of asthma and regularly have nasal polyposis. The inflammatory process affects multiple paranasal sinuses. The sinusitis is recalcitrant and recurrent despite treatment with multiple antibiotics and surgical procedures. There may be laboratory evidence of an allergic state.

On radiographic examination, opacification without bone destruction is evident. The CT scan appearance of decreased density or low attenuation found with chronic sinusitis is distinctly different from the increased density or high attenuation seen with fungal disease.

There is no tissue invasion on histologic examination. The inspissated mucoid material, termed allergic mucin, is histologically similar to the material observed in the bronchi of allergic bronchopulmonary aspergillosis. The mucin contains aggregates of inflammatory cells, most of which are eosinophils. A laminated arrangement to mucin is visualized. Charcot-Leyden crystals are numerous, and special staining often discloses fungal hyphae.

Among the diverse agents responsible are *Bipolaris spicifera*, *Alternaria tenuis*, *Curvularia lunata*, and *Aspergillus flavus*. Interestingly, specific IgG antibody appears to be the most markedly elevated. Specific IgE is elevated but not usually to the same degree.

This type of sinusitis is best treated by eliminating the offending mold from the environment if possible. Where elimination or avoidance is not possible, immunotherapy and steroids may be effective.

Rhinosporidiosis

Rhinosporidiosis is a granulomatous disease caused by the fungus *Rhinosporidium seeberi*.

It is endemic to poor areas in Sri Lanka, Africa, and India. It commonly presents in young adult males from India who are found to have an irregular dull pink to red polyp or mass that bleeds and is friable. Nasal obstruction, epistaxis, and purulence are common symptoms. Spores are present on pathologic examination and are diagnostic. Pseudoepitheliomatous squamous cell metaplasia overlies numerous globular cysts termed sporangia. A granulomatous reaction is also usually evident.

No medical therapy is available, and complete surgical excision of the lesion is the treatment of choice.

Blastomycosis

This disease is rare and is caused by the fungus *Blastomyces dermatitidis*. It was originally referred to as Gilchrist's disease or North American blastomycosis, but it can be found in South America and Africa as well. Missouri, Mississippi, and the Ohio River valley are areas where this disease is most commonly found. The portal of entry is the pulmonary system, and hematogenous spread typically leads to dissemination. The patient usually presents with a cough and a low-grade fever. A cutaneous verrucous ulcer with a serpiginous border is usually seen. These ulcers may involve the nose with extension into the nasal mucous membranes. Isolated intranasal involvement is rare. A mucosal verrucous growth with scarring may be present.

On histopathologic examination, this lesion resembles well-differentiated carcinoma. The diagnosis can be made on the basis of sputum cultures or biopsy, which typically reveal the doubly refractile broad-based buds with giant cells. Culture on Sabouraud's medium as well as fungal stains should be performed. Amphotericin B is the drug of choice for treatment.

Mucormycosis

Mucormycosis is seen mostly in patients with underlying debilitating illnesses or those taking immunosuppressive agents. It is also seen in the diabetic population. The infecting organisms are species of *Absidia*, *Mucor*, or *Rhizopus*. These species are saprophytes of soil, manure, and fruits and may inoculate the nasal cavity by inhalation. Hyperglycemia, ketosis, and acidic blood pH may enhance invasion by these organisms.

The disease may be characterized by acute rhinosinusitis, facial cellulitis, and gangrenous mucosal changes. The nasal mucosa becomes characteristically brick-red or black, which may be followed by a dense, mycelial matrix varying from white to gray. The organism invades along vascular channels, and it has a predilection for the internal elastic lamina of arterial structures. This is the reason for orbital and intracranial spread resulting in blindness, ophthalmoplegia, and hemiplegia. Ischemic infarction is a result of arterial occlusion. Venous drainage may produce thrombosis and hemorrhagic necrosis.

The organisms appear histologically as variably sized and shaped, irregularly branching nonseptate hyphae. The organisms may also be cultured.

The treatment consists of surgical debridement and drainage. The organisms thrive in necrotic tissue, and vascular thrombosis may interfere with the transport of medicine. Thus all of the necrotic material must be debrided. Amphotericin B is the drug of choice, and heparinization may be helpful. Diabetes or any underlying debilitating disease must be controlled for an improved prognosis.

Aspergillosis

This is the most common fungus infecting the nose and paranasal sinuses. It is caused by one of six *Aspergillus* species, all of which are saprophytes of the soil. These spores are then inhaled. Nasal obstruction from mucosal edema and mucopurulent nasal discharge are usually the presenting symptoms. Occasionally, a false membrane from matted fungal filaments forms. Gray and black membranes are associated with *A. fumigatus* and *A. niger*, respectively.

A characteristic wide-branching septate hypha is seen on histologic examination. A chronic inflammatory reaction with interspersed spores that range in size and appearance occurs. These range from small round cells with clear cytoplasm to large cysts filled with thousands of small, newly developed spores. Cultures can be obtained from tissue specimens.

Although this fungus usually appears in the chronic form, it may infect the debilitated or immunosuppressed patient. If this occurs, the disease may become aggressive, causing an infection resembling mucormycosis. In this case, a relentlessly progressive vasculitis and thrombosis with necrosis is the result.

In the chronic form, aspergillosis is not life-threatening and should be treated by debridement and local therapy. In the acute life-threatening disease, prompt debridement with systemic amphotericin B administration is necessary.

SUGGESTED READINGS

Batsakis JG: Tumors of the Head and Neck, Clinical and Pathological Considerations (pp 492–500). Baltimore: Williams & Wilkins, 1979.

Fauci AS, Wolff SM: Wegener's granulomatosis and related diseases. DM 23:1–36, 1977.

Fauci AS, Johnson RE, Wolff SM: Radiation therapy of midline granuloma. Ann Intern Med 84:140–147, 1976.

Friedmann I, Osborn DA: Pathology of Granulomas and Neoplasms of the Nose and Paranasal Sinuses. Edinburgh: Churchill Livingstone, 1982.

Hoekstra JA, Fauci AS: The granulomatous vasculitides. Clin Rheum Dis 6:373–388, 1980.

Josephson JS: The role of endoscopic sinus surgery for the treatment of nasal polyposis. Otolaryngol Clin North Am 22:831–840, 1989.

Kennedy DW, Zinnreich ST: The functional endoscopic approach to inflammatory sinus disease: current perspectives and technique modifications. Am J Rhinol 2:89–96, 1988.

McDonald TJ: Manifestations of systemic disease. In Cummings CW, Fredrickson JM, Harker LA, et al (eds): Otolaryngology—Head and Neck Surgery (pp 597–609). St. Louis: CV Mosby, 1986.

Ritter FN: Surgical management of paranasal sinusitis. In Cummings CW, Fredrickson JM, Harker LA, et al (eds): Otolaryngology—Head and Neck Surgery (pp 937–944). St. Louis: CV Mosby, 1986.

CHAPTER 26

Neoplastic Diseases

Dale H. Rice, MD

Understanding the natural history of tumors of the paranasal sinuses, nasal cavity, and nasopharynx requires a thorough knowledge of the anatomy, which will not be covered extensively in this chapter. This knowledge is also essential for proper treatment. These neoplasms account for less than 1% of all malignancies and approximately 3% of all carcinomas of the upper aerodigestive tract. Eighty percent of carcinomas in the nose and paranasal sinuses involve the maxillary sinuses; most of the remainder occur in the ethmoid sinuses. Carcinoma of the frontal sinus or the sphenoid sinus in isolation is rare. The disease is usually discovered when it is still regional, but bone destruction is present in 70% to 80% of cases.

These tumors are usually at a locally advanced stage when first diagnosed, partly because of the patient's delay in seeking evaluation. This delay averages 3 to 6 months and may occur in part because initial symptoms seem trivial. Because of this advanced stage of diagnosis, 60% to 75% of patients die within 5 years, usually of local spread.

It is well established that exposure to the sintering and roasting of nickel increases the risk of squamous cell carcinoma of the nasal cavity and maxillary sinus, whereas exposure to wood dust and the chemicals used in furniture making increases the risk of adenocarcinoma of the ethmoid sinus one-thousandfold. Additional occupations at risk include boot makers, shoemakers, mustard gas and isopropanol workers, and "luminizers" exposed to ionizing radiation from radium.

SIGNS AND SYMPTOMS

Cancer of the nasal cavity is predominantly a disease of males, probably because of occupational exposure. Most victims are over the age of 50 years. The initial symptoms depend on the site of origin and direction of extension of the tumor. The most common presenting symptom is unilateral nasal airway obstruction often associated with purulent or hemorrhagic discharge. Other common symptoms result from extension of the carcinoma into the cheek, through the palate, or into the orbit (Fig. 26–1). Oral symptoms occur in 25% to 35% of patients and include dental pain, loosening of teeth, malocclusion, mass in the palate, or change in the fit of dentures. Nasal symptoms occur with extension into the nose and usually include nasal obstruction with watery to purulent rhinorrhea and intermittent epistaxis. These symptoms occur in 50% of patients. Ocular symptoms occur in approximately 25% and include exophthalmos, diplopia, and visual impairment as well as epiphora. Facial symptoms result from extension of the neoplasm into the cheek and include the presence of a mass and anesthesia or paresthesia of the infraorbital nerve. Posterior extension leads to trismus through involvement of pterygoid muscles.

TREATMENT

The proper treatment for a given sinus tumor depends on a full knowledge of the histologic type and its natural history as well as exact

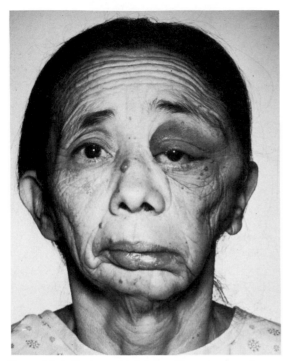

Figure 26–1. Patient with left maxillary sinus carcinoma invading cheek and orbit.

knowledge of the full extent of the tumor. In general, planned combined therapy is the treatment of choice, under the presumption that the tumor is in fact resectable. There is some debate as to whether preoperative or postoperative radiation therapy is best; both have some advantages. The general tendency has been to use postoperative radiation therapy. Whereas this makes the dosimetry more difficult, it does presumably eliminate the potential for geographic miss because the full extent of the tumor should be known postoperatively. Erosion of the base of the skull, extension of the neoplasm into the nasopharynx, fixed cervical metastases, and systemic metastases signal almost certain incurability. Cervical metastases, even if not fixed, indicate a poor prognosis. Increasingly, skull base invasion is being treated with planned craniofacial resection, which produces an improved survival rate.

CARCINOMA OF THE NASAL CAVITY

Carcinomas of the nasal cavity, like other carcinomas, occur more commonly in men and in middle age or later; 85% are squamous cell carcinomas, and 5% are bilateral. A history of smoking is common, as is a history of chronic sinusitis, although the incidence of chronic sinusitis seems to be similar to that in the general population. Fifty percent of these lesions arise on the turbinate, followed in order of frequency by the septum, the vestibule, the posterior choanae, and the nasal cavity floor. These lesions are often diagnosed relatively early and can be managed equally well by resection or radiation. Larger lesions are more successfully treated with planned combined therapy.

Esthesioneuroblastoma is an uncommon tumor first described by Burger and associates in 1924 (Batsakis, 1979). This tumor arises from the olfactory epithelium and thus may arise from the upper third of the nasal septum, the superior or supreme turbinate, or the cribriform plate. It occurs over a wide range of ages; two thirds of the patients are between the ages of 10 and 30 years. Because of its rarity, good treatment data are difficult to obtain, but most authors favor a craniofacial excision with or without postoperative irradiation.

CARCINOMA OF THE MAXILLARY SINUS

Maxillary sinus carcinomas account for 80% of all sinus cancers; of these, 80% are squamous cell carcinomas. Ninety-five percent of the patients are over the age of 40 years, and as previously mentioned, there is an increased incidence in those with heavy metal exposure, especially to nickel. The initial symptom generally depends on which wall of the maxillary sinus is breached by the tumor first; this breaching leads to some dysfunction of structures on the other side of the wall. Approximately 40% to 60% of the patients present with facial asymmetry, tumor extension into the oral cavity, and a tumor visible in the nasal cavity. At least one of these signs is present in 90% of patients. Likewise, bone destruction is visible on the computed tomographic scan in 90%. Nodal metastases markedly lower the cure rate, and there is a twofold increase in nodal metastases with oral cavity invasion. Planned combined therapy is preferred; there is an overall 5-year survival in unselected cases of 25% and 45% in patients who have resectable lesions and are treated with planned combined therapy.

CARCINOMA OF THE ETHMOID SINUSES

Ethmoid sinus carcinoma is the second most common of the paranasal sinus carcinomas (Fig. 26–2). The most common initial complaint is nasal obstruction with or without rhinorrhea. Other common symptoms include displacement of the globe with proptosis and diplopia, broadening of the nasal dorsum and anosmia, and extension into the anterior cranial fossa. Principles of treatment are the same as those of the maxillary sinus; the overall 5-year survival rate is 20% to 25%.

CARCINOMA OF THE FRONTAL AND SPHENOID SINUSES

Primary cancers of the frontal and sphenoid sinuses are rare. These areas are usually involved secondarily by tumors in the ethmoid sinus or the nasopharynx. To date, somewhat more than 100 cases of frontal sinus carcinoma have been reported, but most of them also involved the ethmoid sinuses and are thus suspect. The initial signs and symptoms are those of acute frontal sinusitis with erosion of bone that occurs rapidly; few patients survive more than 2

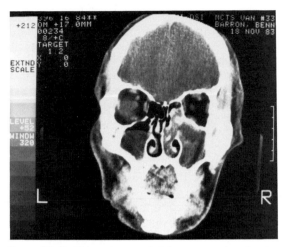

Figure 26–3. Coronal computed tomogram showing inverted papilloma of the right nasal cavity with secondary obstructive maxillary sinusitis.

years. Primary carcinoma of the sphenoid sinus is much more difficult to diagnose, and these patients usually have involvement of the nasopharynx or sphenoethmoidal recess. The most common clinical signs and symptoms involve the eye and the cranial nerves of the cavernous sinus. Occasionally, chronic headache is the first symptom. Survival is unusual.

OTHER TUMORS OF THE NASAL CAVITY

The majority of tumors of the nasal cavity and paranasal sinuses are squamous cell carcinomas and adenocarcinomas. A wide variety of benign and malignant tumors may also occur but are much less common.

Probably the most common miscellaneous tumor is the inverted papilloma (Fig. 26–3). This tumor is benign and has an initial symptom of nasal obstruction in 65% of cases; 63% of patients have had previous nasal operations, including polypectomy, septoplasty, or a sinus procedure. The majority of these lesions arise on the lateral nasal wall. A variable percentage of these lesions are associated with squamous cell carcinoma (8% to 50%). The preferred treatment is medial maxillectomy and en bloc ethmoidectomy through a lateral rhinotomy approach. When this is done, the recurrence rate is approximately 13%.

Chondrosarcomas may occur in the nasal

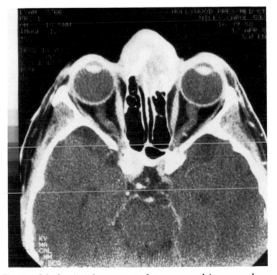

Figure 26–2. Axial computed tomographic scan showing adenoid cystic carcinoma of the left ethmoid sinus.

cavity and sinuses. These tumors tend to be advanced at the time of the diagnosis, and posterior spread adversely affects prognosis. The proper treatment is complete resection; no cures have been reported with positive margins. The overall 5-year survival rate is 50% to 60% but many of these patients eventually die of the disease after longer follow-up.

Primary lymphomas of the sinus are rare (Fig. 26–4). The majority are histiocytic lymphomas, and the preferred treatment is radiation therapy; the 5-year survival rate is 26%. The most common cause of death is the development of disseminated disease.

The first case of leiomyosarcoma involving the nasal cavity and paranasal sinuses was reported in 1958, and there currently have been fewer than 20 reported cases; the average age of the patients is 50 years, and the sex distribution is equal (Fig. 26–5). These tumors are radioresistant, and the best treatment is wide excision. The prognosis is poor.

Approximately 20 cases of hemangiopericytoma and an additional 23 cases of "hemangiopericytoma-like" neoplasms have been reported. There are clearly benign and malignant varieties, but they cannot be distinguished histologically. These tumors tend to occur in the sixth to seventh decades with an equal sex distribution. The most common initial symptoms are nasal obstruction and epistaxis. The preferred treatment is wide excision.

With the exclusion of adenocarcinomas, mucous gland neoplasms of the nasal cavity and paranasal sinuses are uncommon. The most common of these is the adenoid cystic

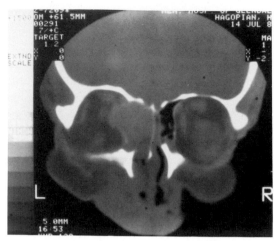

Figure 26–5. Coronal computed tomogram of patient with leiomyosarcoma of the left ethmoid sinus.

carcinoma, followed by the pleomorphic adenoma, the mucoepidermoid carcinoma, and the undifferentiated carcinoma. These tumors tend to be more aggressive than are their counterparts in the major salivary glands, but this may in part reflect delayed diagnosis. The 10-year survival rate for patients with adenoid cystic carcinoma is 7%.

Malignant melanomas of the mucosa of the nasal cavity and paranasal sinuses are uncommon. Before 1969, only 97 cases had been reported. The average age at onset is older than that of patients with cutaneous melanoma; only 20% of these melanomas occur in patients under 50 years of age. The prognosis is poor, with a mean survival of 2.3 years. Wide excision is the only effective treatment.

Fibro-osseous lesions form a large number of sometimes confusing disease processes. Osteoma is the most common lesion involving the sinuses. It has a predilection for the frontoethmoid suture (Fig. 26–6), and there are two types: the cortical osteoma, which appears round or lobulated with ivorylike density; and the cancellous osteoma, which is much less dense and is sometimes mistaken for a soft tissue mass. These are usually incidental findings on radiography. If treatment is indicated, local excision is curative.

Although fibrous dysplasia is not a tumor, it behaves in a tumorlike fashion. It tends to occur in children and young adults with a female preponderance (Fig. 26–7). The initial symptom is usually facial asymmetry, which is painless. The radiologic appearance is char-

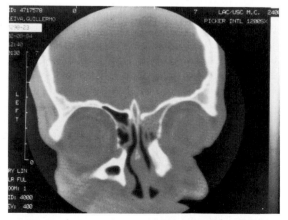

Figure 26–4. Coronal computed tomogram of patient with Burkitt's lymphoma of the left ethmoid sinus.

acteristic, with a homogeneous radiopaque lesion shown with poorly defined margins. Growth of the lesion often stops in the postadolescent period, and treatment should be conservative excision in order to maintain facial symmetry. Irradiation should not be used because of the risk of later development of osteosarcoma. The ossifying fibroma tends to occur in the same age group as does fibrous dysplasia, with the same female preponderance. Swelling, which is painless, produces facial asymmetry. This lesion tends to be more locally aggressive and should be treated with complete excision. True giant cell tumors are rare neoplasms of cryptogenic histogenesis. These lesions are locally invasive, and treatment is wide excision. Osteosarcomas of the facial bones tend to occur in an older age group than do osteosarcomas of the long bones, with an average age of 31 years. Most patients present with a swelling or a mass that is often painful. The prognosis is poor; the 5-year survival rate is 19% to 30%. The only chance for cure is complete excision.

NEOPLASMS OF THE NASOPHARYNX

Ninety-five percent of all tumors of the nasopharynx are squamous cell carcinomas. The only other tumors to occur with any regularity are the juvenile nasopharyngeal angiofibroma and the chordoma.

The juvenile nasopharyngeal angiofibroma is an uncommon tumor that occurs

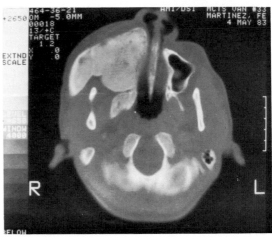

Figure 26–7. Axial computed tomographic scan of patient with fibrous dysplasia of the right maxilla.

almost exclusively in adolescent males. The most common initial symptom is epistaxis unrelated to trauma. Although the tumor is benign, it is locally aggressive and invades the nasal cavity, the orbit, and the cranial cavity if left untreated. For the less extensive lesions, complete resection can generally be done with little or no morbidity. There is considerable disagreement over proper treatment once intracranial spread has occurred. Many physicians favor a craniofacial resection, whereas others favor radiation. Despite the fact that the tumor is benign and radiation therapy should be ineffective, good results have been reported with use of this modality. Because these patients are young, the risk of the later development of malignant neoplasms is considerable and should be considered in the treatment decision.

The chordoma is a rare tumor arising from remnants of the primitive notochord; 45% occur in the nasopharyngeal area, whereas 55% occur in the sacrococcygeal region. This tumor is histologically benign but locally aggressive and often far advanced at the time of presentation. Because of this, complete excision is usually impossible. The tumor is also radioresistant, and because of that and its local aggressiveness, treatment usually eventually fails. There are two histologic types of chordoma: the chordoma and the chondroid chordoma. The mean survival for the chordoma is slightly more than 5 years; the mean survival for the chondroid chordoma is slightly more than 15 years.

It is now well known that squamous cell

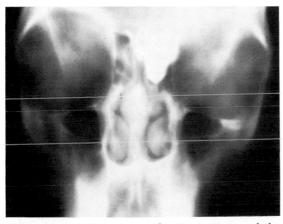

Figure 26–6. Polytomogram showing osteoma of the frontoethmoid area.

carcinoma of the nasopharynx has an increased incidence in the non-Japanese Asian races with a very high incidence in the southern Chinese, particularly in and around Hong Kong. This tumor is associated with the Epstein-Barr virus; all patients have elevated titers to this virus. The incidence of this tumor in the United States is less than 1% of all tumors, whereas it accounts for 18% of all tumors in Hong Kong; 50% of the oncology beds in Hong Kong are occupied by patients with this disease. It is now known that one of the etiologic factors is salted fish in the diet of southern coastal China.

The nasopharynx is a relatively silent anatomic site; the presenting symptom in 75% of patients is a neck mass in the jugulodigastric region. Approximately 25% of patients have metastases to the posterior triangle of the neck initially, but the majority metastasize to the jugulodigastric region initially. Local symptoms include serous otitis, unilateral nasal airway obstruction, bilateral nasal airway obstruction, hyponasal speech (rhinolalia clausa), and cranial neuropathies. Approximately 16% of the patients present with a sixth nerve palsy, and 14% present with a fifth nerve palsy. Involvement of each of the 12 cranial nerves has been reported as the initial symptom for this disease, however. A more ominous finding is destruction of the base of the skull on radiologic evaluation.

The initial treatment for patients with this disease is radiation therapy, with bilateral ports from the skull base to the clavicles. Most patients have clinically apparent neck disease; of those who do not, the majority have microscopic disease. A common problem is persistent neck disease after a full course of radiation therapy. In that setting, it is best to perform a biopsy of the nasopharynx first. If the nasopharynx biopsy is positive, nothing should be done, because the primary lesion will be fatal before the neck disease is. If the nasopharyngeal biopsy is negative, a neck dissection should be performed, with recognition that despite the negative biopsy, some of these patients have recurrence in the nasopharynx at a later date.

Resection has been proposed for selected patients who fail to improve with radiation therapy. Initial results have been encouraging, but the proper place of surgery in this disease has yet to be fully determined.

SUGGESTED READINGS

Adams GL: Malignant tumors of the nose and paranasal sinuses. *In* Kagan AR, Miles J (ed): Head and Neck Oncology. New York: Pergamon Press, 1989.

Batsakis JG: Tumors of the Head and Neck. Baltimore: Williams & Wilkins, 1979.

Shah JP, Galich JH: Craniofacial resection for malignant tumors of ethmoid and anterior skull base. Arch Otolaryngol 103:514, 1977.

Vaughan TL: Occupation and squamous cell cancers of the pharynx and sinonasal cavity. Am J Ind Med 16:493, 1989.

Yu-Hua H, Giu-Yi T, Yu-Qin Q, et al: Comparison of pre- and postoperative radiation in the combined treatment of carcinoma of the maxillary sinus. Rad Oncol Biol Phys 8:1045, 1982.

PART FOUR

Oral Cavity, Oropharynx, Hypopharynx, and Salivary Glands

CHAPTER 27

Anatomy and Physiology of the Oral Cavity

William C. Ardary, MD, DDS

The oral cavity, the initial portion of the digestive system, plays a functional role in the ingestion and digestion of food. Through the act of mastication, food is mixed with saliva and broken down into smaller particles that are subsequently transported to the stomach by peristaltic muscle contractions of the esophagus. The oral cavity, an integral portion of the stomatognathic system, also functions in deglutition, speech articulation, and respiration.

The oral cavity proper and the vestibule form the mouth (Fig. 27–1). The vestibule is bounded externally by the lips and cheeks and internally by the alveolar process, gingiva, and teeth. Frenula join the upper and lower lips and the cheeks to the gingiva. The oral cavity proper is the more central region of the mouth and is bounded by the hard and soft palate superiorly; by the tongue, the lower jaw, and the mucosa of the floor of the mouth inferiorly; and by the oral pharynx posteriorly.

LIPS AND CHEEKS

The lips and cheeks (Fig. 27–2) form the orifice of the mouth and are composed of four distinct tissue layers: an outer cutaneous, a deeper muscular, a submucosal glandular, and an inner mucosal layer. Functionally, the lips and cheeks play an important role in mastication, assisting the tongue in the transfer of food between the vestibule and oral cavity. They also have a role in speech articulation.

Lip Anatomy

The most prominent external feature of the lips is the vermilion mucosa, which merges with the outer skin to form a transitional region termed the vermilion border. Anatomic landmarks of the upper lip (Fig. 27–3) include a central philtrum depression, which is bordered by a left and right philtrum eminence, and a curving region of the vermilion border called the Cupid's bow. The Cupid's bow unites with its opposite counterpart in the midline to form the vermilion

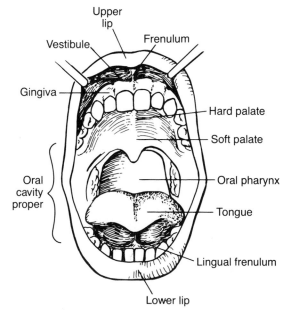

Figure 27–1. The mouth from an anterior view.

Figure 27–2. Median section of the lower lip illustrating the four distinct tissue layers: cutaneous, muscular, glandular, and mucosal.

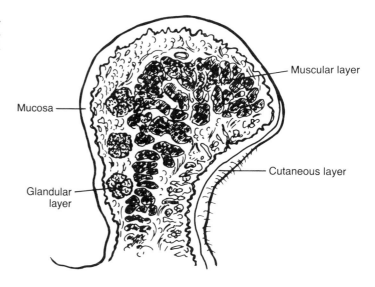

tubercle. Internally, the vermilion mucosa merges with the oral mucosa, forming the so-called wet-dry line. The submucosa of the lips contains the labial salivary glands.

Cheek Anatomy

The cheeks are structurally similar to the lips. They form the lateral borders of the mouth. The external skin and internal mucosal linings enclose the buccal fat pad and the principal muscle of the cheek, the buccinator. The parotid duct (Stensen's duct) pierces the buccal mucosa and enters the mouth at the level of the upper second molar tooth. Buccal salivary glands are contained within the submucosal tissues.

Muscles of Lips, Cheeks, and Perioral Region

The oral musculature (Fig. 27–4) includes muscles of the aperture and muscles of the lips and cheeks. The predominant muscle within the lips is the orbicularis oris, which encircles the oral aperture. The function of this muscle is to close and protrude the lips. Supplementary muscles of the face work in concert with the orbicularis oris to move the lips and mouth.

Five facial muscles converge at the angle region of the oral aperture. They are the levator anguli oris, zygomaticus major, risorius, platysma, and depressor anguli oris. Their fibers merge and interlace with fibers of the orbicularis oris.

The levator anguli oris arises from the canine fossa of the maxilla and inserts into the superior aspect of the angle of the mouth. Its function is to elevate the angle of the mouth. The zygomaticus major, which joins the orbicularis oris on its lateral aspect, originates from the zygoma. It is the predominant muscle functioning during the act of smiling. Originating from the lateral facial fascia and joining together with the posterior fibers of the platysma is the risorius muscle. This muscle functions predominantly during laughter. The depressor anguli oris originates from the anterior mandible and attaches to the inferior aspect of the angle region of the mouth. The function of the depressor anguli oris is to depress the corner of the mouth.

Additional muscles of the upper lip include the levator labii superioris alaeque nasi, the levator labii superioris, and the zygoma-

Figure 27–3. Anatomic landmarks of the upper lip.

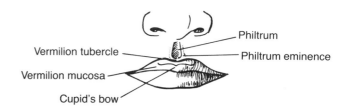

Right lateral   Left lateral

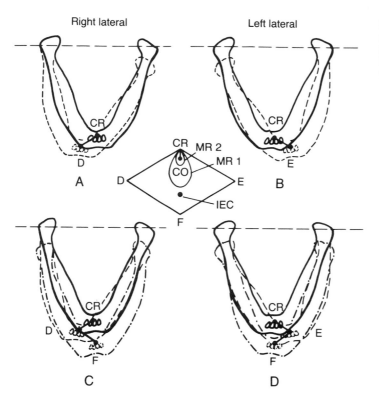

Figure 27–11. Border movement of the mandible in the horizontal plane. *A.* Right laterotrusion. *B.* Left laterotrusion. *C.* Left laterotrusion with protrusion. *D.* Right laterotrusion with protrusion.

fossa, and the ligamentous attachments of the temporomandibular joint. These anatomic characteristics influence the position of ridges and grooves on the teeth. Anatomic factors influencing mandibular movement in the sagittal and frontal planes include the angle and degree of slope of the articular eminence and the degree of overbite and overjet of the anterior teeth. The slope characteristics of the articular eminence and the amount of anterior overbite and overjet determine cusp height and fossa depth. The amount of anterior overbite and overjet controls the magnitude of disocclusion between the posterior teeth, which ultimately determines the height of the cusps and the depth of the fossas on the posterior teeth. The degree and the angle of the posterior slope of the articular eminence also influence cusp height and fossa depth. The steeper the slope is, the greater are cusp height and fossa depth.

The process of mastication is thought to be dependent on the occlusion. However, this concept is somewhat controversial; various studies have shown that the actual contact of the teeth is minimal while food is being chewed and occurs to a greater degree during deglutition. The amount of occlusal

contact that occurs during mastication is influenced to a great degree by the nature and consistency of the food being chewed. During the chewing cycle, the teeth are brought together more frequently in lateral and centric occlusal positions, especially as the food is broken down into smaller pieces.

Interdigitation of the teeth can occur on both the working and nonworking sides of the occlusion. The working or functioning side of occlusion is the side of mandibular movement in which the buccal cusps of the lower molars oppose the buccal cusps of the upper molars. On the balancing or nonfunctioning side of occlusion, the lower buccal cusps are positioned against the inclines of the maxillary lingual cusps. Bilateral mastication in which the working and nonworking sides of occlusion are alternated has been determined to be the most efficient form of chewing.

Mastication can be divided into various stages. The first stage is called the preparatory phase. Food is taken into the oral cavity and positioned by the cheeks and tongue on the working side of occlusion. The preparatory stage is followed by food contact and the beginning of the crushing phase. In this phase, food is broken down into smaller particles by either unilateral or bilateral mastication. When the food particles become small enough, the teeth begin to contact and the grinding phase begins. The grinding phase is characterized by frequent interdigitation of the mandibular and maxillary molars, which results in the milling of food to a size suitable for swallowing. Mastication is terminated by centric occlusal contact of the dentition and swallowing of the food bolus.

Masticatory function is variable between individuals, and at times there is no clear distinction between the various phases. Masticatory effectiveness is influenced by the area of occlusal contact, which is dependent on the number of teeth, the position of the teeth, and the presence of occlusal interferences.

Nerve Supply to the Gingiva, Alveolar Processes, and Teeth

The trigeminal nerve (cranial nerve V), via its maxillary and mandibular branches, provides sensory innervation to the teeth, gingiva, and alveolar processes of the maxilla and mandible (Fig. 27–12). The maxillary division of the trigeminal nerve enters the pterygopalatine fossa after exiting from the foramen rotundum. Within this fossa, several

branches are given off. The zygomatic nerve is the first branch; it enters into the orbit through the inferior orbital fissure. Ganglionic branches to the sphenopalatine ganglion are given off next. Distal to the ganglionic branches, one or two posterior superior alveolar nerves are usually present; they are the last of the nerve branches within the pterygopalatine fossa and enter the maxilla via the posterior alveolar foramina. The maxillary division continues anteriorly to enter the inferior orbital fissure and from this point on is referred to as the infraorbital nerve. Within the inferior orbital fissure, the middle and anterior superior alveolar nerves originate.

The mandibular division of the trigeminal nerve emerges at the base of the skull from the foramen ovale. It splits into an anterior and posterior division. The posterior division divides to form the lingual and inferior alveolar nerves. The inferior alveolar nerve enters the mandible via the mandibular foramen. Its terminal branch, the mental nerve, emerges from the mental foramen.

In the maxilla, the molars, their supporting alveolar bone, and the labial gingiva opposite the molars are innervated by the posterior superior alveolar nerve. The premolars and adjacent labial gingiva and alveo-

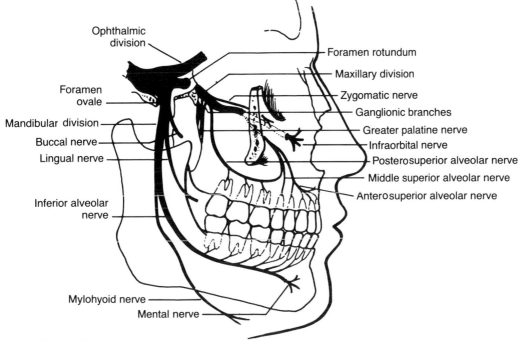

Figure 27–12. The trigeminal nerve.

lar process are supplied by the middle superior alveolar nerve. In the anterior maxilla, general sensation to the canine and incisor teeth as well as to the labial gingiva and to the alveolar process opposite these teeth is provided by the anterior superior alveolar nerve. The palatal gingiva and the alveolar process opposite the maxillary molars and premolars are innervated by the greater palatine nerve. The anterior palatal mucosa and the alveolus from the canines to the central incisors are supplied by the nasopalatine nerve.

In the mandible, the inferior alveolar nerve innervates all of the teeth. The buccal gingiva, the mucosa of the vestibule, and the lateral aspect of the alveolar process in the posterior region of the mandible opposite the molars and premolars are supplied by the buccal nerve. Anteriorly, the labial gingiva, the mucosa of the anterior vestibule, and the alveolus adjacent to the canine and central incisors are innervated by the mental nerve. The lingual nerve supplies the alveolar process, gingiva, and mucosa on the lingual aspect of the mandible as well as the mucosa of the floor of the mouth.

Arterial Supply to the Gingiva, Alveolar Processes, and Teeth

The vascular supply to the mandible and maxilla, including the gingiva, alveolar processes, and teeth, is provided by the maxillary artery (Fig. 27–13). Originating from the external carotid artery within the parotid gland, the maxillary artery passes deep and medial to the subcondylar region of the mandible and then enters into the infratemporal fossa. Within this fossa, the external pterygoid muscle serves as an anatomic landmark that can be used to divide the maxillary artery into three specific regions. The first part of the artery lies anterior to the muscle; the second part traverses across its surface; and the third part, the terminal portion of the vessel, enters the pterygopalatine fossa. Branches of the first part of the maxillary artery include the deep auricular, tympanic, middle meningeal, accessory meningeal, and inferior alveolar arteries. The second part of the maxillary artery supplies the muscles of mastication as well as the buccinator. Vessels within this division are the masseteric, deep temporal, pterygoid, and buccal arteries. The terminal branches of the maxillary artery

arise within the pterygopalatine fossa and include the posterior and middle superior alveolar, pterygoid, infraorbital, descending palatine, and sphenopalatine arteries. These vessels are accompanied by branches of the maxillary nerve and exit the fossa through foramina in the posterior maxilla.

The greater palatine artery supplies the mucosa, glands, and gingiva of the posterior two thirds of the hard palate. The nasopalatine artery, a branch of the sphenopalatine artery, nourishes the mucosa and gingiva of the anterior palate. The superior alveolar arteries provide vascularity to the gingiva, alveolar processes, and teeth of the maxilla. The maxillary molars, supporting alveolar bone, and gingiva are supplied by the posterior superior alveolar artery. The posterior maxillary labial gingiva and mucosa receive additional blood flow from the buccal artery. The blood supply to the premolars and anterior teeth, as well as their supporting alveolar bone and gingiva, is derived from the middle and anterior superior alveolar arteries. The anterior labial gingiva and mucosa also obtain a portion of their blood supply from the superior labial artery, a branch of the facial artery.

The predominant blood supply to the mandible, including the teeth, gingiva, and alveolar processes, is derived from the inferior alveolar artery. Additional vascularity to the mandible is provided by perforating blood vessels arising from the muscles that attach to its cortical surface. The inferior alveolar artery enters the mandible through the mandibular foramen. It continues anteriorly within the mandibular canal, giving off dental and septal branches that supply the molar and premolar teeth as well as the supporting alveolar bone and gingiva. Terminal branches of the inferior alveolar artery include the mental and incisive arteries. The incisive artery, through its dental and septal branches, supplies the anterior mandibular teeth, supporting alveolar bone, and gingiva.

THE PALATE

The palate forms the superior boundary of the oral cavity (Fig. 27–14). It is divided into two distinct regions: the hard palate and the soft palate. The hard palate forms the anterior two thirds of the palate and is bony in character. The posterior third of the palate is

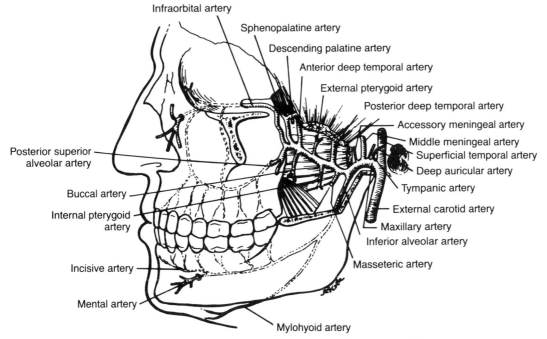

Figure 27–13. The maxillary artery and vascular supply to the maxilla and mandible.

the soft palate and is composed of muscles and the palatine aponeurosis.

The hard palate is lined by a keratinized stratified squamous epithelium. On the basis of the nature of the submucosal tissues, the hard palate can be divided into an anterior fatty region and a posterior glandular region. Surface anatomic landmarks of the hard palate include the incisive papilla, anterior folds of mucosa called rugae, a midline palatal raphe, and the gingiva. The osseous portion of the hard palate is composed of the palatine processes of the maxilla anteriorly and the horizontal plates of the palatine bones posteriorly. Palatal to the third molar, two osseous foramina can be identified. The larger anterior opening is called the greater palatine foramen. The greater palatine vessels and nerve exit at this point. The smaller posterior opening is referred to as the lesser palatine foramen, in which the lesser palatine vessels and nerve emerge. The anterior palate also has an osseous opening that is known as the incisive foramen. It is located in the midline

Figure 27–14. The palate, which forms the superior border of the oral cavity, is divided into the hard and soft palates.

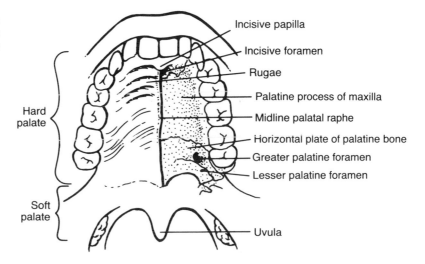

just posterior to the maxillary incisors. The nasopalatine nerve and vessels traverse through this orifice.

The soft palate, a pliable posterior extension of the hard palate, is confluent with the pharynx laterally. Posteriorly, it terminates as a free margin. The central pendulant portion of the posterior margin of the soft palate is called the uvula. Overlying the muscular layer of the soft palate is a surface layer of mucosa composed of a nonkeratinized epithelium. Deep to the mucosa, a glandular submucosal tissue layer is present.

Muscles of the Soft Palate

The soft palate is composed of the confluence of five pairs of muscles: the tensor veli palatini, levator veli palatini, palatoglossus, palatopharyngeus, and musculus uvulae (Fig. 27–15).

The tensor veli palatini originates from the scaphoid fossa, the spine of the sphenoid bone, and the lateral sides of the auditory tube. Its tendon wraps around the hamulus of the pterygoid, joining in the midline with its counterpart from the opposite side to form the palatal aponeurosis. Its function is to tense the soft palate and open the auditory tube during deglutition.

The levator veli palatini originates from the petrous portion of the temporal bone and the medial side of the auditory tube. Its fibers join in the midline with those of the opposite side. Contraction results in elevation of the soft palate.

The tonsillar pillars are formed by the palatoglossus and the palatopharyngeus muscles. The palatoglossus (anterior tonsillar pillar) arises from the anterior surface of the soft palate and inserts into the dorsum and lateral aspect of the tongue. Contraction of this muscle produces a decrease in the anterior opening of the fauces as well as an elevation of the tongue posteriorly. The palatopharyngeus (posterior tonsillar pillar) originates from the soft palate. It inserts on the posterior border of the thyroid cartilage and aponeurosis of the pharynx. Its function is to narrow the oropharyngeal isthmus and elevate the larynx during swallowing.

The final pair of muscles forming the soft palate are the uvular muscles. Their origin is from the posterior nasal spine and palatine aponeurosis. They insert into the mucosa of the uvula. The function of these muscles is to elevate the uvula.

Nerve Supply to the Palate

The sensory nerve supply to the hard palate is derived from the nasopalatine nerve (anterior third) and the greater palatine nerve (posterior two thirds). The greater palatine nerve arises from the pterygopalatine (sphenopalatine) ganglion within the ptery-

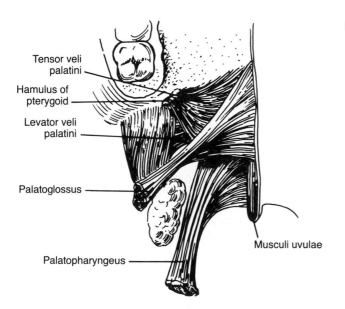

Figure 27–15. The musculature of the soft palate.

Tensor veli palatini

Hamulus of pterygoid

Levator veli palatini

Palatoglossus

Musculi uvulae

Palatopharyngeus

gopalatine fossa. It descends within the greater palatine canal to reach the hard palate through the greater palatine foramen. The nasopalatine nerve, a branch of the maxillary nerve, departs through the sphenopalatine foramen, traverses across the roof of the nasal septum, and travels along the vomer within the mucoperiosteum. It exits through the incisive foramen to supply the anterior portion of the hard palate.

The soft palate receives its sensory nerve innervation from two sources: the lesser palatine nerve and the glossopharyngeal nerve (cranial nerve IX). The lesser palatine nerve, a branch of the maxillary nerve, arises within the pterygopalatine fossa from the pterygopalatine (sphenopalatine) ganglion and exits through the lesser palatine foramen. It supplies general sensation to the soft palate. The glossopharyngeal nerve, via its tonsillar branch, provides additional sensory innervation to the soft palate.

The motor innervation to all of the muscles of the soft palate, except the tensor veli palatini, is from the pharyngeal plexus. The pharyngeal plexus is composed of contributions from the sympathetic, glossopharyngeal, vagus, and spinal accessory nerves. The tensor veli palatini is supplied by motor fibers of the mandibular division of the trigeminal nerve (V_3).

Arterial Supply to the Palate

The blood supply to the palate (Fig. 27–16) is derived from the greater palatine artery, the lesser palatine artery, the nasopalatine artery, and the ascending palatine branch of the facial artery. The greater and lesser palatine arteries originate from the maxillary artery within the pterygoid fossa. They descend within their own canals, emerging from the greater and lesser palatine foramina, respectively. The greater palatine artery vascularizes the bone, mucosa, glands, and gingiva of the posterior two thirds of the hard palate. The anterior third of the hard palate is supplied by the nasopalatine artery, a branch of the sphenopalatine artery. The soft palate receives its blood supply from two sources, the lesser palatine artery and the ascending branch of the facial artery. After emerging from the lesser palatine foramen, the lesser palatine artery courses posteriorly to nourish the soft palate. The lesser palatine artery supplements the ascending branch of the facial artery, which provides the predominant blood supply to the soft palate.

Figure 27–16. Palatal blood supply.

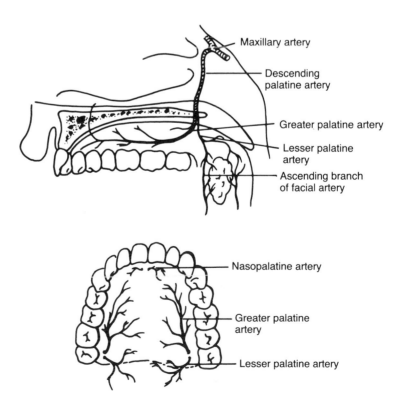

Maxillary artery

Descending palatine artery

Greater palatine artery

Lesser palatine artery

Ascending branch of facial artery

Nasopalatine artery

Greater palatine artery

Lesser palatine artery

FLOOR OF THE MOUTH

The floor of the mouth (Fig. 27–17) and the tongue form the inferior boundary of the oral cavity proper. Inferior to the mucosa of the floor of the mouth is the sublingual space. This U-shaped region is bounded laterally by the body of the mandible; inferiorly by the mylohyoid muscle; medially by the genio-hyoid, genioglossus, and hyoglossus muscles; and superiorly by the mucosa of the floor of the mouth. The primary contents of the sublingual space include the sublingual gland, the sublingual artery and vein, the lingual nerve, the hypoglossal nerve, the deep portion of the submandibular gland, and the duct of the submandibular gland (Wharton's duct). The sublingual space, which is in reality a potential space, is filled with a loose connective tissue matrix. It becomes a true space only when the loose connective tissue is broken down by an invading infectious process, such as occurs in Ludwig's angina, a cellulitis of the floor of the mouth usually arising from a carious lower molar.

Anatomic landmarks of the mucosa of the floor of the mouth include the lingual frenum, a fold of mucosa extending from the tongue to the floor of the mouth; two sublingual papillae, which are just anterior to and on each side of the lingual frenum; the ducts of the submandibular glands, which open on each papilla; and the plica sublingualis, which is formed by the superior aspect of the sublingual gland. The plica sublingualis is actually a ridge of tissue extending posteriorly from the sublingual papilla. It contains between six and eight sublingual gland ducts that open along its crest.

The sublingual space is bounded laterally by the lingual aspect of the body of the mandible. To understand the anatomic relationships of the sublingual space, it is important to review the medial surface anatomy of the mandible (Fig. 27–18). Medial surface landmarks include the inferior and superior genial tubercles, digastric fossa, mylohyoid line, sublingual gland fossa, submandibular gland fossa, lingula and mandibular foramen, mylohyoid groove, coronoid process, mandibular notch, mandibular condyle, and areas of attachment for the pterygomandibular raphe and the medial pterygoid muscle.

Muscles of the Floor of the Mouth

The medial and inferior borders of the sublingual space are formed by the muscles of the floor of the mouth (Fig. 27–19). The paired mylohyoid muscles limit the inferior extension of the sublingual space and form the actual floor of the mouth. Originating from the mylohyoid line on each side of the mandible, they insert into the body of the hyoid bone as well as into the midline raphe. The raphe extends from the hyoid bone to its attachment in the midline on the medial side of the anterior mandible. The function of the mylohyoids is to elevate the hyoid bone, base of the tongue, and floor of the mouth.

The geniohyoid, genioglossus, and hyoglossus muscles contribute to the medial border of the sublingual space. The geniohyoid muscle, a paired muscle, originates from the

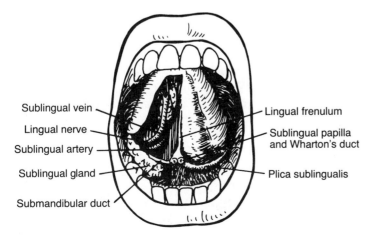

Figure 27–17. The floor of the mouth.

Sublingual vein

Lingual nerve

Sublingual artery

Sublingual gland

Submandibular duct

Lingual frenulum

Sublingual papilla and Wharton's duct

Plica sublingualis

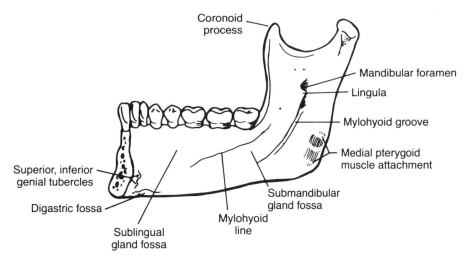

Figure 27–18. Anatomic landmarks of the medial surface of the mandible.

inferior genial tubercle and inserts into the anterior surface of the body of the hyoid bone. Contraction of this muscle elevates the tongue and hyoid bone. Originating from the superior genial tubercle is the paired genioglossus muscle, one of the extrinsic tongue muscles. It has a dual insertion into the body of the hyoid bone and into the base of the tongue. The function of its posterior fibers is to protrude the tongue, whereas the anterior fibers produce tongue retraction and depression. The hyoglossus, also a paired extrinsic muscle of the tongue, originates from the body of the greater cornu of the hyoid bone and inserts into the side of the tongue. Contraction of this muscle produces tongue depression.

Nerve Supply to the Floor of the Mouth

The lingual nerve, a branch of the mandibular division of the trigeminal nerve, provides general sensory innervation to the floor of the mouth, the anterior two thirds of the tongue, and the lingual gingiva of the mandible. After emerging from the anterior fibers of the medial pterygoid muscle in the poste-

Figure 27–19. Musculature of the floor of the mouth.

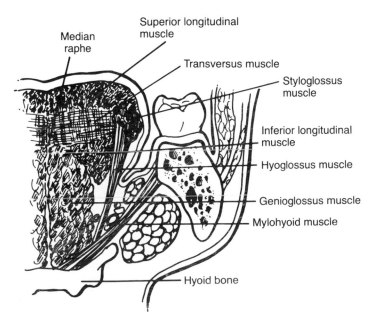

rior region of the mandible, it enters the floor of the mouth inferior to the superior constrictor and superior to the mylohyoid. In its course anteriorly, it crosses over the submandibular duct, traveling with the duct for a short distance on its lateral side. It then passes underneath and crosses the duct medially to enter the anterior portion of the tongue and sublingual region.

The motor supply to the muscles of the floor of the mouth is derived from three nerves. The mylohyoid muscle is supplied by the mylohyoid nerve, a branch of the mandibular division of the trigeminal nerve. The genioglossus and hyoglossus muscles are innervated by cranial nerve XII, the hypoglossal nerve. Cervical fibers from C_1, which join with the hypoglossal nerve, supply the geniohyoid.

Arterial Supply to the Floor of the Mouth

The arterial supply to the floor of the mouth, sublingual region, and sublingual gland is derived from the sublingual artery. The sublingual artery is one of the terminal branches of the lingual artery.

THE TONGUE

The tongue (Fig. 27–20), which is predominantly a muscular structure, functions in mastication, taste, speech articulation, and deglutition. The tongue is composed of an anterior portion called the body, or anterior two thirds, of the tongue. It is separated from the posterior third or root of the tongue by a V-shaped line termed the terminal sulcus. The foramen cecum, which is a remnant of the thyroglossal duct, is located at the angle of the terminal sulcus.

Developmentally, the anterior and posterior portions of tongue are derived from different embryologic structures. The body of the tongue is formed from the floor of the developing pharynx and originates predominantly from the first branchial arch. The posterior third of the tongue originates from the third branchial arch and is formed from the anterior wall of the developing pharynx. This dissimilarity in developmental origin explains the structural, topographic, and functional differences between the anterior two thirds and the posterior third of the tongue.

The mucosa of the anterior two thirds of the tongue differs widely in structure and is made up of four types of papilla. The filiform papillae, which are epithelial-lined connective tissue projections, give the tongue its characteristic appearance. Located on the dorsal surface of the oral portion of the tongue, they are slender, thread-shaped structures devoid of any taste buds. Interspersed between the filiform papillae are red, mushroom-shaped structures called fungiform papillae. They are red because their core is composed predominantly of vascular

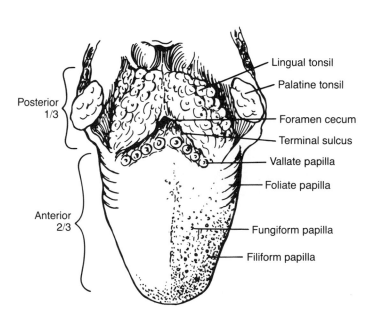

Figure 27–20. The tongue.

Posterior 1/3

Anterior 2/3

Lingual tonsil

Palatine tonsil

Foramen cecum

Terminal sulcus

Vallate papilla

Foliate papilla

Fungiform papilla

Filiform papilla

elements. They are found only on the dorsal surface of the tongue and usually contain one to three taste buds. The vallate papillae are found in a V-shaped configuration in front of the terminal sulcus. They are circular structures that contain many taste buds within the epithelium of their lateral surface. Located along the lateral border of the tongue are the foliate papillae. They are narrow vertical folds of mucous membrane and are not well developed in humans. Taste buds, however, are contained within the epithelium of the foliate papillae.

The mucosa of the posterior third of the tongue is devoid of papillae. The surface of the tongue in this area is composed of oval, irregularly shaped structures called the lingual follicles. These follicles contain lymphoid tissue and are surrounded by a crypt. Mucous glands deposit their secretions into these crypts. Collectively, the lingual follicles form the lingual tonsil.

The ventral tongue mucosa is smooth, and papillae are absent. The lingual vein can be identified on each side of the undersurface of the tongue.

Muscles of the Tongue

The musculature of the tongue is composed of three paired extrinsic muscles and three paired intrinsic muscles (Fig. 27–21). Separating these paired muscles and located in the midline is the septum of the tongue. The extrinsic muscles originate outside the body of the tongue. Therefore, contraction of these muscles can change the shape of the tongue as well as move it bodily. Conversely, the intrinsic muscles originate and insert entirely within the confines of the tongue. The resultant contraction of these muscles can therefore only produce a change in tongue shape.

The extrinsic tongue muscles are the genioglossus, hyoglossus, palatoglossus, and styloglossus. The genioglossus muscle has a dual insertion into the body of the hyoid bone and the base of the tongue. The function of its posterior fibers is to protrude the tongue; the anterior fibers produce tongue retraction and depression. The hyoglossus originates from the body of the greater cornu of the hyoid bone and inserts into the side of the tongue. Contraction of this muscle results in tongue depression. The palatoglossus, the muscular component of the anterior tonsillar pillar, arises from the anterior surface of the soft palate and inserts into the dorsum and lateral aspect of the tongue. The function of this muscle is to decrease the anterior opening of the fauces and elevate the tongue posteriorly. The styloglossus originates from the anterior border of the styloid process and inserts into the side of the tongue. Its function is to retract and elevate the tongue.

The intrinsic tongue muscles are the longitudinal, transverse, and vertical. The longitudinal muscle is divided into a superior and an inferior division. The superior division arises from the submucous region of the posterior portion of the tongue. The inferior division originates from the inferior aspect of the tongue between the genioglossus and hyoglossus muscles. Both divisions insert

Figure 27–21. Musculature of the tongue.

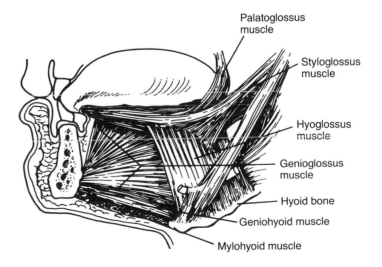

Palatoglossus muscle

Styloglossus muscle

Hyoglossus muscle

Genioglossus muscle

Hyoid bone

Geniohyoid muscle

Mylohyoid muscle

into the tip of the tongue. Contraction of this muscle produces tongue shortening and turning up of the tip. The transversus has its origin from the median fibrous septum. It inserts into the dorsal and lateral portions of the tongue. The function of this muscle is to narrow and elongate the tongue. The verticalis originates from the mucous membrane on the dorsum of the anterior tongue and inserts into the undersurface of the tongue. Contraction of this muscle flattens and broadens the tongue.

Nerve Supply to the Tongue

The sensory nerve supply to the tongue can be explained on the basis of the developmental differences that exist between the anterior two thirds and the posterior one third of the tongue. Recall that the anterior two thirds of the tongue is derived from structures of the first and second branchial arches (mandibular division of the trigeminal and facial nerves, respectively). The posterior third is formed from structures derived from the third and fourth branchial arches (glossopharyngeal and vagus nerves, respectively). Therefore, general sensation to the anterior two thirds of the tongue is supplied by the third division of the trigeminal nerve, specifically the lingual nerve. In addition, taste to the anterior two thirds of the tongue is supplied from the chorda tympani (cranial nerve VII) via the lingual nerve. Both general sensation and taste to the posterior third of the tongue are derived from the glossopharyngeal nerve. The mucosa of the valleculae is innervated by the internal laryngeal nerve, a branch of cranial nerve X.

The motor innervation to the musculature of the tongue, both intrinsic and extrinsic, except the palatoglossus, is provided by the hypoglossal nerve. The palatoglossus is innervated by the pharyngeal plexus.

Arterial Supply to the Tongue

The arterial supply to the tongue is obtained chiefly from the lingual artery. Arising from the external carotid artery at the level of the greater horn of the hyoid bone, the lingual artery passes deep to the hyoglossus to enter into the tongue. Two dorsal lingual arteries originate posteriorly to supply the root of the tongue as well as the palatine tonsil. The lingual artery continues anteriorly, bisecting into two terminal branches: the deep lingual artery and the sublingual artery. The deep lingual artery vascularizes the anterior two thirds of the tongue. The sublingual artery supplies the floor of the mouth.

SUGGESTED READINGS

Angle EH: Classification of malocclusion. Dent Cosmos 41:248–264, 1899.

Angle JL: Factors in temporomandibular joint form. Am J Anat 83:223–246, 1948.

Castelli W: Vascular architecture of the human adult mandible. J Dent Res 42:786–792, 1963.

DuBrul EL: Sicher's Oral Anatomy, 7th ed. St. Louis: CV Mosby, 1980.

Gysi A: The problem of articulation. Dent Cosmos 52:1, 1910.

Posselt U: Studies in the mobility of the human mandible. Acta Odont Scand 10(Suppl 10):3–160, 1952.

Posselt U: Physiology of Occlusion and Rehabilitation, 2nd ed. Philadelphia: FA Davis, 1968.

Ramford SP, Ash MM: Occlusion, 3rd ed. Philadelphia: WB Saunders, 1983.

Stalland H, Steward CE: Concepts of occlusion. Dent Clin North Am 591–606, November 1963.

Starkie C, Stewart D: The intramandibular course of the inferior dental nerve. J Anat 65:319–323, 1931.

Strong LM: Muscle fibers of the tongue functional in consonant production. Anat Rec 126:61–71, 1956.

CHAPTER 28

Salivary Glands: Anatomy and Physiology

Theda C. Kontis, MD   Michael E. Johns, MD

A comprehensive knowledge of salivary gland anatomy and physiology is essential for the head and neck surgeon. The salivary glands have important anatomic relationships with significant structures in the head and neck and provide the environmental milieu for the oral cavity; therefore, an understanding of glandular development is important in the study of tumor histogenesis. In humans, the major salivary glands consist of the paired parotid, submandibular, and sublingual glands. The minor salivary glands are composed of hundreds of glandular rests that line the entire oral cavity.

DEVELOPMENTAL ANATOMY

The major salivary glands develop early in embryonic life as outpouchings of stomodeal ectoderm (oral epithelium) into the surrounding mesenchyme (Fig. 28–1). The primordial tissues originate at the sites of the eventual duct orifices within the oral cavity. The primordium grows and branches; lumina eventually form by central cell death and degeneration. The cells further develop into elaborate tubuloacinar systems, and the most distal acinar cells differentiate into secretory cells. The surrounding mesenchymal tissue completely envelops the lobulated gland to form a connective tissue capsule.

The minor salivary glands arise from both the oral ectoderm and the nasopharyngeal endoderm, although no histologic differences are seen in the adult glands. Their development is similar to that of the major salivary glands; however, the ductal system is less developed. The acinar elements differentiate into both serous and mucus-secreting cells, forming simple tubuloacinar systems.

Parotid Gland

The parotid anlage is the first of the major salivary glands to appear in embryonic life, at 4 to 6 weeks of development. The paired primordial tissues originate on the buccal mucosa and grow posteriorly along the lateral aspect of the masseter muscle toward the mandibular ramus. As the gland grows posteriorly, the facial nerve is simultaneously developing and advancing anteriorly, eventually becoming surrounded by glandular tissue. The mesenchymal capsule is formed later in development and entraps lymph nodes as it condenses around the gland. In addition, it sends projections into the gland to form the connective tissue that creates the interlobular septa. As the ductal structures differentiate, the terminal ducts dilate to form serous secreting cells, whereas the proximal duct becomes the main glandular duct.

Submandibular Glands

The paired submandibular gland anlages are seen late in the sixth week of development. These primordia arise in the floor of mouth and grow inferoposteriorly, deep to the my-

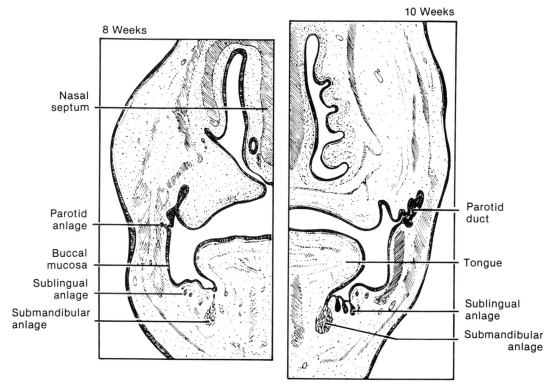

Figure 28–1. Growth of the major salivary glands at 8 and 10 weeks of embryonic life.

lohyoid muscle. The proximal tissue becomes the main duct, and terminal ducts differentiate into serous and mucus-secreting cells.

Sublingual Glands

The final salivary glands to develop are the sublingual glands, which appear in the eighth week of development. The glands arise from 10 to 20 primordia, each with separate ducts, and lie on the floor of the mouth along the course of the submandibular anlage. The glands are surrounded by a common mesenchymal capsule. The secretory elements consist mostly of mucus-secreting cells, but they also contain serous secreting cells.

ANATOMY OF SALIVARY GLANDS

Parotid Gland

The parotid gland is the largest of the salivary glands, weighing 14 to 28 g and measuring roughly 6.0 cm (height) × 3.5 cm (width). The gland is irregularly triangular or wedge-shaped and lies deep to the preauricular skin and fatty subcutaneous tissue. The parotid gland is unilobular; however, the facial nerve subdivides the gland, by definition, into a large supraneural component and a smaller infraneural component (Fig. 28–2). The supraneural gland lies adjacent to the masseter muscle and extends superiorly to the zygoma. The infraneural gland lies medial to the angle of the mandible and extends medially toward the styloid process and the pharyngeal wall. The isthmus of the gland is described as the constriction of the gland between the mandibular ramus, the masseter muscle, and the posterior belly of the digastric muscle.

Stensen's duct (the parotid duct) arises from the anterior border of the gland, approximately 1.5 cm below the zygoma. Accompanied by the buccal branch of the facial nerve, the duct traverses the masseter muscle and the buccal fat pad, coursing a distance of approximately 1.0 cm. Next, the duct turns medially and pierces the buccinator muscle to open intraorally in the buccal mucosa. The duct orifice can be located intraorally at the tip of a small papilla of mucosa opposite the

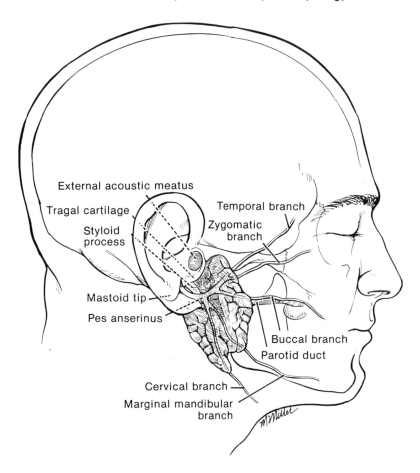

second upper molar. Topographically, the course of the duct lies along a line drawn from the floor of the external auditory canal anteriorly toward the oral commissure. The duct is approximately 4 to 6 cm long and 0.5 mm in diameter. Occasionally, an accessory parotid duct accompanies the main duct and drains into it directly.

Parotid Compartment: Anatomic Relationships

The parotid compartment is described as the triangular space that contains the parotid gland, with its associated nerves, blood vessels, and lymphatic vessels. The musculoskeletal boundaries of the parotid compartment are, in essence, the anatomic relationships of the gland itself.

The superior boundary of the parotid compartment is the zygomatic arch. The posterior border is formed by the cartilaginous and bony portions of the external auditory canal; however, a tail of parotid tissue extends inferiorly toward the mastoid process and overlaps the sternocleidomastoid muscle. The floor of the compartment is bounded by the styloid process, the styloid muscles, the internal carotid artery, the internal jugular vein, and the transverse process of the atlas (which can occasionally be mistaken for a parotid tail tumor when palpated). The anterior margin of the gland forms a diagonal from the posterior to superior boundaries and lies superficial to the masseter muscle.

The parotid compartment is subdivided into a nerve compartment (superficial portion), a venous compartment (middle portion), and an arterial compartment (deep portion). The nerve compartment contains the facial, greater auricular, and auriculotemporal nerves. The venous compartment contains the superficial temporal vein; this vein joins the internal maxillary vein to form the posterior facial vein (retromandibular vein), which lies deep to the facial nerve in the substance of the gland. The posterior facial vein then divides into an anterior branch and a posterior branch, and the latter joins the posterior auricular vein (at the lower pole of the gland) to form the external jugular vein. The deep arterial compartment is composed of the external carotid artery, which divides into the internal maxillary and superficial temporal arteries.

The parotid gland, although unilobular, may contain extensions or processes of glandular tissue. The superficial gland may possess a condylar process (extending toward the temporomandibular joint), a meatal process (lying in the incisure of the cartilaginous portion of the external auditory canal), and a posterior portion (positioned between the mastoid process and the sternocleidomastoid muscle). The infraneural gland may contain two processes: the glenoid process and the stylomandibular process. The former projects toward the glenoid fossa, and the latter extends toward the stylomandibular ligament. The clinical relevance of the deep process relates to parapharyngeal extensions of tumors and abscesses.

Fascial Relationships

The parotid fascia is a continuation of the superficial layer of the deep cervical fascia and is divided into superficial and deep fascial layers. The superficial fascia is an extension of the fascia surrounding the sternocleidomastoid muscle posteriorly and the masseter muscle anteriorly. The fascia extends superiorly to the zygoma and lies just deep to the preauricular skin and the subcutaneous fat. The dense fibrous superficial fascia lies on the lateral aspect of the parotid gland and sends fascial extensions deep into the gland. These septa join the stroma of the gland at the level of the facial nerve and prevent development of a plane between the gland and the fascia. In addition, the compartmentalization of the gland by this inelastic fascia prevents stretch of the glandular capsule in response to a suppurative or similar rapidly expanding process. For this reason, prompt surgical drainage of suppurative parotid disease is mandatory.

The deep layer of parotid fascia extends from the fascia of the posterior belly of the digastric muscle. This looser layer forms the stylomandibular membrane, which attaches to the angle of the mandible anteriorly, the stylomandibular ligament inferiorly, and the styloid process posteriorly (Fig. 28–3). The stylomandibular membrane separates the parotid gland from the submandibular gland.

Occasionally, the stylomandibular process of the parotid gland can herniate through a weakness in the stylomandibular membrane and lie in the parapharyngeal space, adjacent to the lateral pharyngeal wall. Tumors in this region can be seen intraorally and are described as dumbbell-shaped or round, depending on the tumor's relationship to the stylomandibular membrane.

Facial Nerve

Before surgical manipulation of the parotid gland, the surgeon must be well acquainted with the course of cranial nerve VII, the great motor nerve of the face. The facial nerve exits the skull base via the stylomastoid foramen just posterolateral to the styloid process and anterior to the insertion of the posterior belly of the digastric muscle into the mastoid tip. As the nerve exits the stylomastoid foramen, it gives off three motor branches: to the posterior auricular muscle, to the posterior belly of the digastric muscle, and to the stylohyoid muscle. The main nerve trunk, approximately 2 to 3 mm in diameter, courses anteroinferiorly and laterally to enter the posterior border of the parotid gland, superficial to the external carotid artery and the posterior facial vein.

Once the nerve has entered the parotid gland, it branches at the pes anserinus ("goose's foot") into two major divisions: an upper division (temporofacial) and a lower division (cervicofacial). The pes usually is located approximately 1.3 cm away from the nerve's exit from the stylomastoid foramen. The two divisions again subdivide, but in a more variable pattern. Five classic major subdivisions are identified: temporal, zygomatic, buccal, marginal mandibular, and cervical. The branches then course through the substance of the gland to exit anteriorly and innervate the muscles of facial expression. The temporal branch crosses the zygomatic arch to innervate the temporal region, the zygomatic branch supplies the region lateral to the orbit, the buccal branch supplies the nose and mouth, the mandibular branch innervates the muscles of the lower lip and the chin, and the cervical branch innervates the platysma muscle. There is, however, substantial cross-innervation to the same muscles and communications between branches. The internerve communications are most often seen between buccal and temporozy-

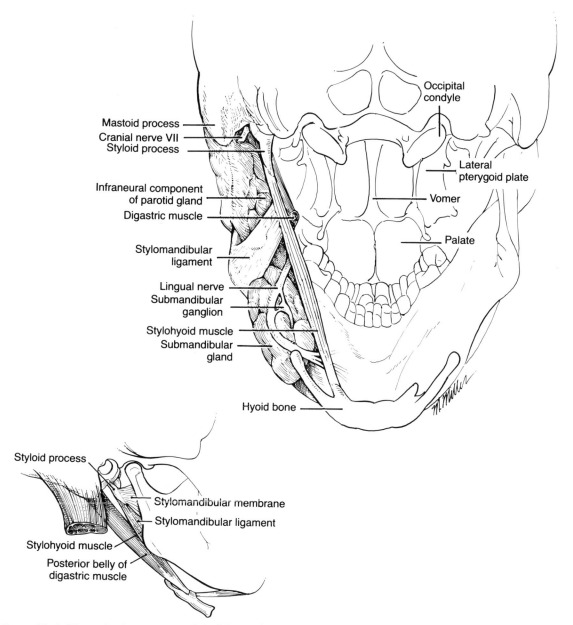

Figure 28–3. View of inferior aspect of skull base, showing parotid and submandibular glands. Note the course of the lingual nerve (inset). The stylomandibular membrane attaches to the mandible, the stylomandibular ligament, and the styloid process and separates the parotid and submandibular glands.

gomatic branches and rarely between marginal mandibular and cervical branches (Fig. 28–4).

Although great anatomic variation exists, there are some constant relationships that are of benefit to the surgeon, especially when tumor distorts the normal anatomy. The buccal branch runs parallel and just superior to the parotid duct. The duct can be located 1.5 cm inferior to the zygomatic arch. The buccal branch can be identified anteriorly and then followed posteriorly to the main trunk of the facial nerve. Similarly, the temporal branch can be found at the superior aspect of the gland, running parallel to the superficial temporal artery and vein. The marginal mandibular branch can be found at the inferior border of the parotid gland, running superficial to the posterior facial vein.

The main trunk of the facial nerve can be

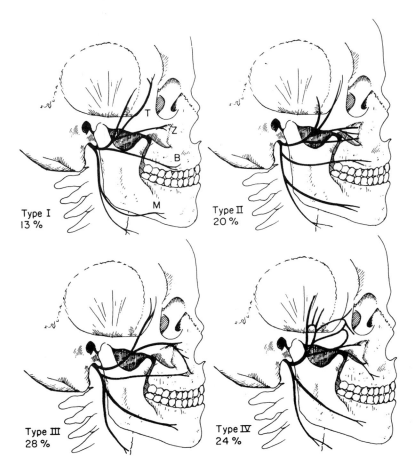

Figure 28–4. Common variations in branching of the facial nerve. (From Johns ME: The salivary glands: anatomy and embryology. Otolaryngol Clin North Am 10:261–271, 1977.)

identified by its constant relationship to the styloid process and by the insertion of the digastric muscle into the mastoid process. By careful dissection at the posterior border of the parotid gland, the wall of the external auditory meatus can be followed to the tragal "pointer." This pointer is a projection of conchal cartilage that points medially in the direction of the nerve as it exits the stylomastoid foramen. In addition, the nerve's main trunk lies 6 to 8 mm anteroinferior to the tympanomastoid suture line. Certain situations, such as bulky tumors, make identification of the main trunk of the nerve impossible. On occasion, such situations require that mastoidectomy be performed in order to identify the vertical portion of the facial nerve and its exit from the stylomastoid foramen.

Greater Auricular Nerve

The greater auricular nerve, the largest branch of the cervical plexus, is generally identified and sacrificed during parotid surgery. It provides sensation to the posterior

surface of the auricle and the ear lobule. It travels between the sternocleidomastoid muscle and the platysma, passes around the posterior border of the sternocleidomastoid muscle, and then is directed cephalad toward the auricle, where it branches just inferior to the external auditory canal. This nerve is often harvested and used for facial nerve grafting.

Auriculotemporal Nerve

The auriculotemporal nerve is a branch of the third or mandibular division of the trigeminal nerve, which exits the skull base at the foramen ovale. The auriculotemporal nerve courses posterolaterally and splits to surround the middle meningeal artery. Anterior to the external auditory canal, the nerve turns superiorly and follows the superficial temporal vessels to innervate the scalp. During its course, the nerve passes through the deep portion of the superior aspect of the parotid gland and is prone to injury during parotidectomy.

The auriculotemporal nerve carries postganglionic parasympathetic fibers from the otic ganglion to the parotid gland. These secretomotor fibers stimulate gland secretion. When the nerve is injured at operation, aberrant innervation to the skin can occur and result in gustatory sweating, or Frey's syndrome.

Arterial Supply

The major arterial supply to the parotid gland is from the external carotid artery, which runs in the deep portion of the gland parallel to the mandibular ramus. At the level of the condyle, it divides into its two terminal branches: the maxillary and superficial temporal arteries. Before bifurcating, the artery gives off a small postauricular artery, which then gives off (1) a stylomastoid branch that enters the stylomastoid foramen deep to the facial nerve and (2) an auricular branch that supplies the anterior mastoid tip. A branch of the superficial temporal artery, the transverse facial artery, runs with the transverse facial vein and supplies the parotid gland, the parotid duct, and the masseter muscle. It runs anteriorly parallel to and between the zygomatic arch and the parotid duct.

Venous Drainage

The venous drainage of the parotid gland is via the retromandibular (posterior facial) vein, which empties into both the internal and external jugular systems. The retromandibular vein is formed from the union of the superficial temporal and internal maxillary veins. It travels in the parotid tissue posterior to the mandibular ramus and lateral to the external carotid artery but medial to the facial nerve, and it emerges at the lower border of the gland. The vein joins the postauricular vein to form the external jugular vein. In addition, the retromandibular vein joins the anterior facial vein to form the common facial vein, which empties into the internal jugular system.

Lymphatics

Two layers of lymph nodes are present in the parotid gland. The superficial nodes lie under the superficial parotid fascia and number from 3 to 20. These nodes receive lymphatic drainage from the external auditory canal, the auricle, the temporal region of the scalp, the eyelids, the lacrimal glands, and the parotid gland itself. The second layer of nodes consists of several nodes buried deep in parotid tissue. These nodes receive drainage from the parotid gland, the external auditory canal, the middle ear, the nasopharynx, and the soft palate. Both systems drain into the superficial and deep cervical nodes.

Submandibular Gland

The submandibular (submaxillary) gland is the second largest of the major salivary glands and usually weighs 10 to 15 g. It contains both serous and mucus-secreting acini. The gland lies medial and inferior to the ramus of the mandible and wraps around the posterior aspect of the mylohyoid muscle, creating a superficial and a deep lobe (Figure 28–5). The gland lies mainly in the submandibular triangle whose boundaries are formed by the body of the mandible and anterior and posterior bellies of the digastric muscle (Figure 28–6). Often the gland extends below the lower boundaries of the triangle and always extends upward along the medial aspect of the mandible. The posterior aspect of the gland lies adjacent to the posterior digastric and stylohyoid muscles.

The superficial portion of the gland extends medially toward the genioglossus muscle to lie in the lateral sublingual space. The deep portion of the gland lies inferior to the mylohyoid muscle and constitutes the bulk of the gland. The deep portion is covered by the superficial layer of the deep cervical fascia, the platysma muscle, the superficial fascia, the subcutaneous tissue, and the skin. The superficial layer of the deep cervical fascia, which extends from the hyoid bone to the mandible, splits to surround the gland.

Wharton's duct (the submandibular duct) runs from the deep hilum of the gland anteriorly along the medial surface of the gland between the mylohyoid and hyoglossus muscles and then onto the genioglossus muscle. It is approximately 5 cm long and opens lateral to the lingual frenulum at the floor of the mouth. Important anatomic relationships exist along the course of the duct: the hypoglossal nerve lies inferiorly and the lingual nerve lies superiorly.

The submandibular gland receives both sympathetic and parasympathetic innervation. Much of the parasympathetic nerve supply is from the facial nerve via the chorda

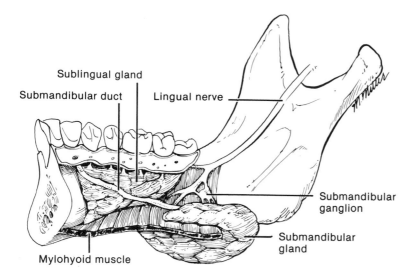

Sublingual gland

Submandibular duct

Lingual nerve

Submandibular ganglion

Submandibular gland

Mylohyoid muscle

Figure 28–5. View of the medial aspect of the mandible showing the superficial and deep lobes of the submandibular gland. Note the courses of the submandibular duct and the lingual nerve. The sublingual gland is also seen with multiple ducts opening along the floor of the mouth.

tympani. This nerve carries preganglionic parasympathetic fibers to the submandibular ganglion via the lingual nerve. The postganglionic parasympathetic fibers originate in the submandibular ganglion and pass to the gland to stimulate the secretion of watery saliva. The submandibular ganglion lies on the hyoglossus muscle at the posterior aspect

of the mylohyoid muscle and is attached to the gland and to the lingual nerve by short rootlets. The postganglionic sympathetic fibers originate in the superior cervical ganglion and travel to the gland with the lingual artery to stimulate the secretion of thick mucoid saliva.

The major arterial supply to the subman-

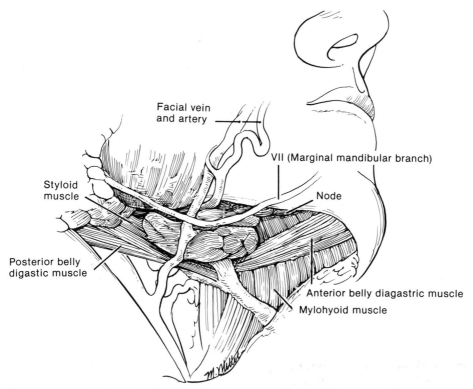

Facial vein and artery

VII (Marginal mandibular branch)

Styloid muscle

Node

Posterior belly digastic muscle

Anterior belly diagastric muscle

Mylohyoid muscle

Figure 28–6. The submandibular triangle lies between the mandible and the digastric muscle. Note the relationship of the marginal mandibular nerve to the facial vein.

dibular gland is via the facial artery, which grooves the deep portion of the gland as it courses anterosuperiorly. At the superior aspect of the gland, the artery turns outward and passes around a notch in the body of the mandible anterior to the masseter muscle, thereby supplying the face. A small branch of the facial artery, the submental artery, runs with the nerve to the mylohyoid muscle along the mylohyoid muscle and also supplies the submandibular gland. The venous drainage is via the anterior facial vein, which lies on the superficial layer of cervical fascia.

Unlike the parotid gland, the submandibular gland does not have lymph nodes within the glandular tissue; rather, nodes lie on the gland just deep to the cervical fascia. The nodes drain into the deep cervical lymphatic system and the jugular chain.

Sublingual Gland

The sublingual gland is the smallest of the major salivary glands, weighing approximately 2 g. The gland is primarily mucus secreting and lies deep to the mucous membrane of the floor of the mouth. The gland is bordered laterally by the mandible and the genioglossus muscle and inferiorly by the mylohyoid muscle (Fig. 28–5). The submandibular duct and the lingual nerve run between the gland and the genioglossus muscle. Unlike the other major salivary glands, no true fascial capsule surrounds the sublingual gland.

The ductal system of the gland is composed of 10 to 12 ducts (ducts of Rivinus) that exit the superior surface of the gland and open along the sublingual fold, or plica, of the floor of the mouth. Occasionally, one or more of these ducts may join to form the major sublingual (Bartholin's) duct, which empties directly into the submandibular duct.

The innervation to the sublingual gland is identical to that of the submandibular gland. The gland receives its postganglionic parasympathetic secretory innervation from the submandibular ganglion via the lingual nerve. The sympathetic fibers reach the gland via the facial artery.

The major blood supply to the sublingual gland is from the sublingual branch of the lingual artery and the submental branch of the facial artery. The venous drainage is via the corresponding veins. Lymphatic drainage is to the submandibular nodes.

Minor Salivary Glands

The minor salivary glands are small glands located throughout the oral cavity and number 600 to 1000. They are individual mucous, serous, and mixed glands that are concentrated in the buccal, labial, palatal, and lingual regions. In addition, they are located in the superior pole of the tonsils (Weber's glands), in the tonsillar pillars, in the base of the tongue, and along the inferolateral aspect of the tongue. Tumors of the minor salivary glands are most often seen in the glands located in the palate, the upper lip, and the cheeks.

Each minor salivary gland has its own duct that opens directly into the oral cavity. The vascular supply and lymphatic drainage correspond to those that supply the region of the oral cavity where the glands are situated. The lingual nerve supplies the parasympathetic innervation to all the glands except the glands of the palate, which receive their innervation from the sphenopalatine ganglion via the palatine nerves.

PHYSIOLOGY

The function of the major and minor salivary glands is to produce saliva. Saliva is secreted during the oral phase of deglutition, at which time it acts to lubricate food; it has multiple protective functions as well. The 24-hour volume of salivary secretion has been estimated at 1000 to 1500 mL. Without stimulation, the submandibular glands produce 69% of the total flow; the parotid glands, 26%; and the sublingual glands, 5%. Both the parasympathetic and the sympathetic divisions of the autonomic nervous system stimulate active glandular secretion. The glands can secrete saliva at a maximal rate of approximately 1 mL/minute/g of gland. In addition, they have a high rate of metabolism; blood supply to the glands has been shown to increase tenfold when the glands are fully stimulated.

Functions of Saliva

Digestive

The primary function of saliva is to aid in the mastication of foods. Both the high water content of saliva and the salivary mucins (glycoproteins produced by the submandibular, sublingual, and minor salivary glands) moisten and lubricate foods to facilitate their ingestion.

Carbohydrate digestion is initiated in the oral cavity by the action of salivary amylase. Like pancreatic amylase, salivary amylase is an alpha-1,4-glucan 4-glucanohydrolase (molecular weight, 45,000), which hydrolyzes the alpha-1,4 linkages and the alpha-1,6 linkages at branch points to produce maltose and a variety of oligosaccharides. It functions optimally at a pH of 6.9; however, activity has been demonstrated between pHs of 4 and 11. Salivary amylase is inactivated by the acidic pH of the stomach, and carbohydrate digestion is therefore somewhat limited. Activity has been demonstrated to continue for several hours in the inner aspects of the gastric bolus, which is somewhat protected from the gastric acidity.

Amylase constitutes the major protein fraction of parotid saliva and is also seen, to a lesser extent, in submandibular saliva. Its concentration is independent of salivary flow rates. The importance of salivary amylase in carbohydrate digestion has been debated. In view of the continued action on the gastric bolus, carbohydrate breakdown can be as much as 75% complete. In addition, salivary glands hypertrophy in patients with excessive starch intake. However, patients who do not produce saliva do not show signs of carbohydrate deficiency; pancreatic amylase alone is sufficient for starch breakdown.

Saliva also assists in the perception of taste by dissolving food and allowing chemical stimulation of taste receptors. Saliva from the minor salivary glands continuously irrigates the taste papillae so that subsequent taste stimuli can be detected. In addition, the concentrations of glucose and sodium in the saliva are below taste thresholds and actually enhance taste perception by eliminating the possibility of competition at the receptor sites.

Mechanical Protection

The mucins in saliva become concentrated on the oral mucosa and protect the surfaces from desiccation and chemical irritation. Saliva also cools hot foods, buffers chemicals, and provides constant lavage in the oral cavity. When the glands are unstimulated, they produce saliva at a low-flow steady rate that serves to debride foods, epithelial debris, and bacteria from the oral cavity.

Anticariogenic Protection

Most clinicians are well aware of the prevalence of dental caries in patients with xerostomia. Saliva not only is important in the prevention of caries but also has been shown to play an active role in the enamel formation of maturing teeth. Immature teeth incorporate inorganic ions from saliva (calcium, fluoride, phosphate, magnesium) that contribute to the maturation of enamel. Research has also shown that early dental lesions become remineralized by the incorporation of salivary calcium.

Antibacterial Protection

The major antibacterial compounds of saliva (lysozyme, secretory IgA, thiocyanate-dependent factor, and histidine-rich peptide) function by preventing bacterial adhesion, agglutinating microorganisms, and inhibiting cell multiplication. Lysozyme causes lysis of bacteria presumably by activating autolysins. Bacteria are aggregated by the actions of mucin and lysozyme. Secretory IgA is the major immunoglobulin found in exocrine secretions (tears, respiratory mucosa, colostrum, and saliva). Secretory IgA is synthesized by plasma cells in the parotid and submandibular glands and interferes with bacterial adherence. In addition, thiocyanate dependent factor (salivary peroxidase) interferes with cell metabolism by attacking a currently unknown target in the bacterial cytoplasm. The histidine-rich peptide of parotid saliva also has been shown to have bactericidal and antifungal effects. None of these compounds, however, has been shown to affect oral hygiene to a significant degree.

Antineoplastic Protection

Experiments have shown that animals with chemically induced xerostomia have more malignancies than do control animals when chemical carcinogens are introduced. This finding suggests that the buccal mucin layer may serve as an important antineoplastic barrier.

Homeostasis

With loss of body fluids, the salivary glands become dehydrated and decrease their resting rate of flow, which causes the sensation of dryness of mouth (thirst). In addition, salivary glands are signaled by osmotic changes detected by the hypothalamus and by volemic changes detected by the renin-angiotensin system. Mercury, lead, sulfa, iodine, morphine, and antibiotics are actively excreted into the saliva; however, their excretion does not appear to play an important role in homeostasis. Manifestations of these excretions are seen as lead deposition in the gingiva and as mercury poisoning stomatitis.

Viruses can also be excreted into the saliva. The rabies and poliomyelitis viruses have been isolated from saliva and can be transmitted in this manner. Research on the human immunodefiency virus (HIV) suggests that it, too, is excreted into the saliva of infected individuals. All patients seropositive for HIV have been shown to possess secretory IgA antibodies to viral proteins in their whole saliva. However, data on whether the virus can be transmitted by this route are lacking.

Hormonal Function

The major hormones of the salivary glands are nerve growth factor and epidermal growth factor. Nerve growth factor promotes the growth of sensory and sympathetic nerve cells; its removal (by the use of antisera) causes sympathetic nervous cell atrophy. Interestingly, removal of the salivary glands does not significantly affect the development of the sympathetic nervous system. These data suggest that the nerve growth factor is

made elsewhere and probably is merely released from the salivary glands.

Epidermal growth factor has been identified as human urogastrone, a polypeptide found in high concentration in the urine. It has been isolated from submandibular and parotid saliva and appears to play a role in gastric and duodenal cytoprotection by inhibiting gastric acid secretion.

Production of Saliva

The Secretory Unit

The secretory unit of the salivary gland is defined as the acinus, the secretory tubule, and the collecting duct. Saliva secretion is an active process that begins in the acinus (proximal) and is modified by the ducts (distal).

The tubuloacinar systems of the parotid and submandibular glands are complex. The abundant acini secrete saliva, which travels via the intercalated ducts to the many intralobular ducts. These ducts then empty into a smaller number of interlobular ducts, which in turn empty into a single, large-caliber collecting duct (Fig. 28–7). The intralobular and interlobular ducts are considered the secretory tubules because they play an important role in salt and water transport. The sublingual tubuloacinar system differs in that the interlobular ducts empty into 10 to 12 separate collecting ducts.

The acinar cells and proximal ducts are surrounded by myoepithelial cells that contract to expel preformed secretions. The pa-

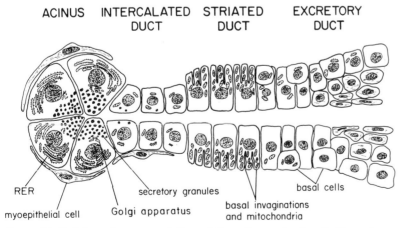

Figure 28–7. Schematic representation of the salivary gland unit. The primary secretion is formed by the acinar cells and modified to a hypotonic fluid as it passes through the ducts. (From Regizi JA, Batsakis JG: Histogenesis of salivary gland neoplasms. Otolaryngol Clin North Am 10:297–307, 1977.)

rotid acinar cells are entirely serous cells and secrete saliva that is devoid of mucins. The submandibular and sublingual glands produce mixed and mucous saliva, respectively, and therefore a more viscous saliva.

The minor salivary glands contain acinar cells that are serous, mucous, or mixed. Their collecting ducts are rudimentary at best. Little is known about their secretory capabilities.

The Secretory Process

In early theories of salivary secretion, it was presumed that saliva production was a passive process that involved the ultrafiltration of plasma. It is now clear that cell synthesis and active transport are the mechanisms for saliva production. The acinar cells produce the primary secretion, whose osmolality and major electrolyte composition are similar to those of plasma. The tubular cells then make considerable modifications in the salivary electrolytes as the saliva flows by, producing a hypotonic fluid.

At low salivary flow rates, acinar cell metabolism is aerobic. However, at higher flow rates, anaerobic metabolism predominates, which results in increased levels of lactate and decreased levels of glucose in the saliva.

Primary Secretion

The term *primary secretion* refers to the fluid produced by the acinar cells into the ductal lumen. The acinar cells of the salivary gland histologically resemble other protein-secreting cells. Study of the acinar cell ultrastructure demonstrates abundant endoplasmic reticulum, Golgi bodies, and secretory (zymogen) granules. The secretory granules provide most of the organic components of the primary secretion. Serous acinar cells produce secretory granules with amylase, whereas mucous cells produce the glycoprotein mucin.

Studies of the electrical properties of the acinar cells have demonstrated that active ion transport is also involved in the secretory process. The resting membrane potential of acinar cells is between -20 and -35 mV. Upon stimulation by the autonomic nervous system, the acinar cells hyperpolarize; that is, the resting potential becomes even more negative as a result of the efflux of K^+ and the influx of Cl^-. This occurrence is contrary

to the action of other excitable cells in the body, which depolarize when stimulated. The hyperpolarization of acinar cells is known as the secretory potential.

Multiple ion channels have been identified at the basolateral plasma membrane of the acinar cell (Fig. 28–8). The major channels are a Ca^{2+}-activated and a voltage-activated K^+ channel (blocked by tetraethylammonium), an $Na^+/K^+/2Cl^-$ cotransporter (blocked by loop diuretics), and an Na^+/K^+ adenosinetriphosphatase (ATPase) (energy requiring, and blocked by ouabain). Neurotransmitters produced by cholinergic stimulation bind cell receptors at the basal membrane of the acinar cell. This stimulation then causes two transduction mechanisms to occur: generation of adenosine 3',5'-cyclic monophosphate (cAMP) and breakdown of plasma membrane polyphosphoinositides. The cAMP signals the initiation of intracellular secretory events. The polyphosphoinositides cause a release of intracellular Ca^{2+}. This intracellular calcium is required for the transport of Cl^- from the apical membrane into the ductal lumen and for the release of potassium at the basal membrane. In addition, the $2Cl^-/Na^+/K^+$ cotransport channel replenishes the Cl^- supply. The Na^+/K^+ ATPase breaks down adenose triphosphate and transports $3Na^+$ out of the cell and $2K^+$ into the cell. Two other channels in the membrane consist of an Na^+/H^+ antiport and a Cl^-/HCO_3^- antiport, which serve to replenish intracellular Na^+ and Cl^-.

The result of these ion movements is a net increase in Cl^- entering the cell and a recirculation of K^+. Because of the lumen negativity, Na^+ diffuses between the acinar cells into the ductal lumen to maintain electrical equilibrium. Water, too, diffuses transcellularly into the lumen to maintain osmotic equilibrium. The primary secretion produced by the acinar cells has the following ion concentrations: 150 mmol/L of Na^+, 136 mmol/L of Cl^-, and 14 mmol/L of HCO_3^-. The fluid produced by the acinus is isotonic to plasma.

Ductal Secretion

The ducts that transport the primary secretion alter its composition by secretion of electrolytes, water, and organic solutes and by the resorption of electrolytes and water. The events that occur at the ductal level are not well understood. What is clear, however,

Figure 28–8. Summary of cellular events in the salivary gland acinar cell. Neurotransmitter (NT) stimulates the production of cAMP, which signals the initiation of intracellular secretory events. NT also stimulates the breakdown of polyphosphoinosidides (PI), which release intracellular Ca^{++}. Calcium is required for the secretion of K^+ and Cl^-. The lumen negatively allows for the passive diffusion of Na^+.

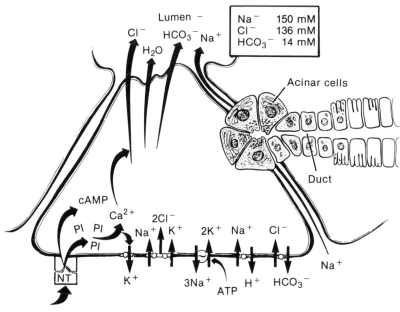

Na⁻	150 mM	
Cl⁻	136 mM	
HCO₃⁻	14 mM	

is that the net change in electrolyte composition is closely related to the rate of salivary flow. When this rate is low, there is ample time for ion exchange. When flow is rapid, however, there is less time for ion transfer, and so the final saliva is more like the primary secretion. At any flow rate, the saliva produced is always hypotonic to plasma.

However, at higher flow rates, the tonicity is also higher. At maximal salivary flow rates, the salivary tonicity is approximately 70% of that of plasma.

The net effects of ductal transport are a decrease in sodium concentration and an increase in potassium levels. Studies of rat submandibular gland saliva (Fig. 28–9) have

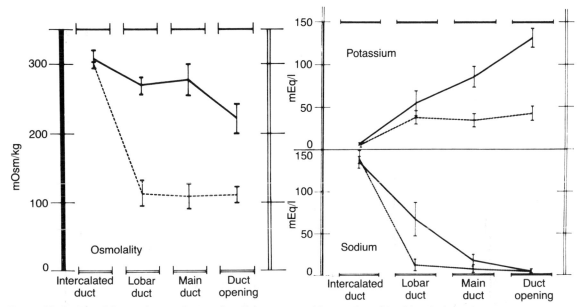

Figure 28–9. Osmolality and potassium and sodium concentrations at four ductal levels from the rat submandibular gland, with (dotted line) and without (solid line) stimulation. (From Young JA, Schögel E: Micropuncture investigation of sodium and potassium excretion in rat submaxillary saliva. Pflueger Arch Ges Physiol 1966, 291:85–98.)

shown initial concentrations of sodium and potassium to be 150 mEq/L and 10 mEq/L, respectively, and final concentrations to be 5 mEq/L and 40 mEq/L, respectively. Osmolality was measured to decrease from 300 mOsm/µg to 100 mOsm/µg. At high flow rates, the sodium concentration is higher because there is less time for absorption. At low flow rates, potassium reaches a steady state and can attain concentrations as high as 130 mEq/L.

Localization studies to identify the sites of electrolyte and organic solute secretion in the dog parotid gland are shown in Figure 28–10. In these experiments, the appearance times of radioisotopes in the saliva after arterial injection were analyzed. Central to the studies was the fact that blood flow in the periductal capillaries is countercurrent to the direction of salivary flow. The isotope therefore reaches the distal segments before the proximal ducts and the acini. The results showed that water enters the duct most distally, followed by the anions, the cations, iodide, and finally urea. The long potassium curve suggests that acinar secretion is also involved. The rapid decline in the T_2O curve

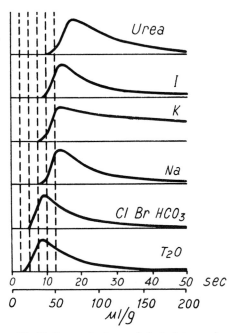

Figure 28–10. Concentrations of electrolytes and organic solutes in dog parotid saliva after interarterial injection of those substances. Note the progressive latency in appearance from T_2O to urea. (From Burgen ASV, Emmelin N: Physiology of the Salivary Glands. London: Edward Arnold, 1961.)

suggests that either rapid dilution or exchange with nonlabeled H_2O from the blood has occurred.

Autonomic Innervation

Parasympathetic Nervous System

The preganglionic parasympathetic neurons originate in the salivary nuclei of the brain stem and enter the salivary glands in their sensory nerves. The auriculotemporal nerve (branch of cranial nerve V_3) carries postganglionic fibers from the otic ganglion to the parotid gland. The chorda tympani (branch of cranial nerve VII) carries postganglionic fibers from the submandibular ganglion along the lingual nerve to the sublingual and submandibular glands. In addition, some preganglionic fibers to the submandibular gland synapse in ganglion cells in the hilum of the gland, known as Langley's ganglion.

The major neurotransmitter of the parasympathetic nervous system is acetylcholine. Receptors for acetylcholine are either muscarinic or nicotinic; however, in salivary gland stimulation, the muscarinic receptors seem to play a dominant role at the ganglion synapses. Although acetylcholine is secreted at the terminal end of the postganglionic axon, no true synapse exists. The neurotransmitter is released proximal to the secretory cells, and stimulation is via neurotransmitter diffusion.

Stimulation of salivary gland secretion by the parasympathetic nervous system produces an abundant, watery saliva, which persists for as long as the stimulation is present. Anticholinesterases prolong the effects of acetylcholine at the receptor sites. Atropine, on the other hand, competes with acetylcholine for the receptor at the ganglionic level and thus blocks gland stimulation. Atropine has been used as an antisialogogue, but scopolamine and methscopolamine, which function similarly, are more effective and produce fewer anticholinergic side effects. The effects of atropine can be reversed by citric acid administration, which causes copious secretion; this has been called the atropine paradox.

Sympathetic Nervous System

The sympathetic nerves arise in the superior cervical ganglion and enter the salivary glands with their arterial supplies: along the lingual artery to the submandibular gland, along the facial artery to the sublingual gland, and along the external carotid branches to the parotid gland. Stimulation of this branch of the autonomic nervous system is supplemental to parasympathetic gland stimulation rather than antagonistic, as once was believed. The sympathetic stimulation of the glands produces a scant, viscous saliva rich in organic and inorganic solutes. Secretion ceases entirely, however, with prolonged stimulation.

The major neurotransmitter for this system is norepinephrine. It has classically been held that only the sympathetic nervous system causes contraction of the myoepithelial cells of the acinar units; however, parasympathetic fibers have also been shown to innervate the cells and cause contraction.

The synapses of the sympathetic nervous system are adrenergic, and receptors are either alpha or beta, types 1 and 2. Alpha-1 receptors are responsible for vasoconstriction and the contraction of smooth muscles. The alpha-2 receptors are presynaptic and serve a regulatory function. The beta-1 and beta-2 receptors are involved in cell secretion, which they accomplish by creation of the intracellular chemical messenger cAMP.

Regulation of Secretion

The interplay between the sympathetic and parasympathetic nervous systems in the regulation of salivary secretion is not well understood. It is currently believed that during the ingestion of food, the salivary reflex elicited is actually the result of complex coordination between the two systems at the level of the secretory cells and the myoepithelial cells. Their contribution to ductal secretion, however, is currently unknown.

Historically, salivary secretion was believed to result from parasympathetic stimulation. Sympathetic stimulation was thought to have an inhibitory effect on secretion because of vasoconstriction. According to current theories of salivary secretion, the parasympathetic nervous system is primarily responsible for physiologically stimulated salivary secretion. The sympathetic system actually augments this secretion by stimulation of myoepithelial cell contraction and by the increased secretion of amylase. It also provides a resting vasomotor tone.

Studies of dog submandibular glands have shown that stimulation of the beta-adrenergic sympathetic nervous system causes glandular secretion. Stimulation of the alpha receptors causes vasoconstriction and myoepithelial contraction. However, stimulation of the dog parotid gland by the sympathetic nervous system alone did not result in stimulation; only after a brief stimulation of the parasympathetic nervous system did sympathetic nervous system stimulation effect secretion. Therefore, it is believed that the sympathetic system actually augments the parasympathetic stimulation; this cooperation is known as augmented secretion. This augmented saliva has been shown to have an increased concentration of amylase in comparison with saliva elicited by simple parasympathetic stimulation alone. The sympathetic nervous system is responsible for contraction of the myoepithelial cells and exocytosis of preformed secretions and thus serves not only to increase the volume of flow but also to alter the fluid composition.

Although myoepithelial cell contraction is part of the salivary reflex, vasoconstriction is not. In the mid-1800s it was shown that strong stimulation of the sympathetic nervous system caused decreased salivary flow as a result of vasoconstriction. However, this effect was subsequently found to be caused by direct stimulation of the alpha-1 receptors, rather than being a direct result of the physiologic salivary reflex. The sympathetic system provides a resting vasomotor tone to the blood vessels of the salivary glands. Section of the sympathetic nerves results in an increased blood flow by removal of the vascular tone. On the other hand, parasympathetic denervation does not cause a decrease in glandular blood flow; this indicates that no vasodilatory tone is provided by this system. There is thus no antagonism between the two systems even at this level.

Denervation studies have shown that the cells actually become more sensitive to sympathetic and parasympathetic neurotransmitters after interruption of either system. When parasympathetic axons are sectioned, there is an increase in secretion. In the late 1800s this was believed to be secondary to the removal of inhibitory neurons. Today this so-called paralytic salivary secretion is explained initially by a leakage of neurotransmitter from the degenerating nerves (2 days) and then by an increase in circulating catecholamines released by the adrenal glands. An increase in secretory cell sensitivity to these circulating neurotransmitters has been shown and can persist for years. This mechanism potentially explains the rebound increase in secretion seen after atropine inhibition (atropine paradox).

The glands respond to sympathectomy similarly by increasing their sensitivity to both acetylcholine and epinephrine. After long-term sympathectomy, the concentration of amylase has been shown to increase in parotid saliva. The glands thus have complex systems that can re-equilibrate after neuronal injury.

Secretion from the minor salivary glands is not affected by atropine administration or by denervation. The minor glands secrete spontaneously even after excision.

The salivary glands, in time, atrophy after denervation. Studies have shown that after sympathectomy of the parotid gland, there is a 10% decrease in glandular weight, as opposed to a 30% decrease after parasympathectomy. Interestingly, when both sympathetic and parasympathetic stimuli were removed, only a 4% decrease in gland weight was observed.

Salivary Flow Rates

Salivary flow rates in the unstimulated gland are estimated at approximately 0.001 to 0.2 mL/minute/gland. Flow rates in the stimulated gland rise to 0.18 to 1.7 mL/minute/gland. The daily volume of saliva produced is estimated at 1.0 to 1.5 L, or an average flow of 1 mL/minute. When unstimulated, the submandibular gland provides 69% of flow; the parotid gland, 26%; and the sublingual gland, 5%. However, under stimulation the parotid gland supplies the bulk of the flow. With or without stimulation, the minor salivary glands produce 7% to 8% of total flow.

The mechanism responsible for the sensation of a dry mouth is not clearly defined. It is possible that it is related to the amount of hydration of the oral mucosa, but the degree of mucosa dehydration that causes the sensation of a dry mouth is unknown. It may be that xerostomia is the result of salivary flow rates below the rate of water absorption and evaporation.

Conversely, hypersecretion of saliva is viewed either in terms of excessive flow rates of up to two times normal or as being secondary to flow rates exceeding the capacity for swallowing. In humans with ptyalism (drooling), parasympathetic denervation by section of the tympanic plexus has been used therapeutically. Although tympanic neurectomy is successful for short-term management, long-term results have not been consistent. Some surgeons opt to perform rerouting of the bilateral parotid duct or ligation procedures with or without bilateral removal of the submandibular gland.

Alterations in Flow and Composition

Although control of salivary gland secretion and rate of flow are controlled by the autonomic nervous system, multiple factors have been shown to influence this control.

Psychic

Pavlov was perhaps the first to show a correlation between salivation and the psyche. In his famous experiments, dogs salivated profusely at the sound of a bell, which was paired with the delivery of food. In humans, the thought of food similarly stimulates salivary secretion; however, the sight of food generally does not.

Fear has been shown to cause sympathetic vasoconstriction of the glandular vessels and produces the well-known sensation of a dry mouth. This physiologic phenomenon was recognized in ancient times and was used as a primitive lie detector test. The accused person was to hold a cup of dry rice in the mouth. If he or she was guilty, the low salivary flow rate caused by fear would enable him or her to expel all the rice from the mouth. If he or she was innocent, the increased salivary flow rate would transform the rice into a gummy mass that could not be completely expelled.

Decreased flow rates are also seen in manic-depressive patients. In the depressed phase, flow rates are very low. In the manic phase, flow rates are higher than in the depressed phase but still well below normal.

Patients with anorexia nervosa or bulimia also complain of xerostomia. This may, in part, be caused by dehydration secondary to laxative and diuretic abuse as well as by decreased fluid intake. Interestingly, these patients occasionally develop hypertrophy of the salivary gland (parotid and submandibular), which persists even after they are cured of the disease. This has potentially devastating effects on persons whose primary disease was centered on their body image.

Circadian Rhythm

A diurnal variation in salivary secretion has been reported with decreased production in the morning and increased production in the afternoons. During sleep, parotid secretion ceases, and submandibular and sublingual flow rates approach zero. The minor salivary glands produce spontaneous secretions that are not subject to diurnal variation. Patients with Addison's disease do not show diurnal salivary flow rates; this suggests that variations in aldosterone levels may play a role in these circadian rhythms.

Aging

Salivary flow is age-dependent. From ages 5 to 29, flow rates increase; after age 29, rates fall. The decline in secretion may be a result of atrophy of acinar cells and their replacement by fat cells. In addition, calcium concentration increases from ages 5 to 49.

Radiation

When salivary glands are included in the ports for radiation therapy, there is an almost logarithmic decrease in salivary secretion. Flow rates have been estimated to be as low as 0.1 mL/minute. Alterations in taste discrimination occur by the second week of radiation therapy. The amount of recovery and the potential for recovery have been debated. In general, these patients do not regain normal secretory function. In addition, radiation alters the composition of saliva; the saliva tends to be more viscous and can interfere with talking or swallowing.

Diet

Different foods have also been implicated in affecting salivary composition. The ingestion of meats causes the secretion of a thick, mucin-rich saliva, which facilitates swallowing. In experiments in which sand was placed in subjects' mouths, the saliva produced was thin and protein-poor and thus assisted in lavage of the oral cavity.

The type of carbohydrate does not appear to influence the concentration of amylase in the saliva. Long-term studies in populations with high carbohydrate intake, however, have shown higher concentrations of salivary amylase in comparison with populations with low carbohydrate intake.

Drugs

Drugs that affect salivary flow rates can occur either centrally or peripherally. Stimulatory drugs may act centrally, may mimic the autonomic neurotransmitters, or may prolong the action of the neurotransmitters. Inhibitory drugs act as central nervous system depressants, block the ganglionic receptors, or block the peripheral receptors.

SUGGESTED READINGS

Anatomy

Grant JCB: An Atlas of Anatomy, 6th ed. Baltimore: Williams & Wilkins, 1972.

Pansky B, House EL: Review of Gross Anatomy, 3rd ed. New York: Macmillan, 1975.

Physiology

Proceedings from the 10th International Conference on Oral Biology-Saliva and Salivary Glands [special issue]. J Dent Res 66(2), 1986.

the thyroarytenoid, cricothyroid, lateral cricoarytenoid, and interarytenoid muscles. Additional protection of the laryngeal inlet is provided by the false vocal cords, which approximate, and by the epiglottis, which retroflexes. These actions result in "gutter" formation on both sides of the larynx, which allows food to enter the piriform sinuses and bypass the airway. Simultaneously, inhibitory impulses come from the central respiratory center, causing cessation of breathing and thereby preventing inhalation. Other muscles, such as the palatopharyngeus and salpingopharyngeus, elevate the pharynx while the mylohyoid muscle pulls the hyoid bone and larynx superiorly and anteriorly into a position beneath the tongue base. This action and glottic closure are very important factors that prevent aspiration.

As the pharyngeal phase progresses, peristaltic actions of the superior, middle, and inferior constrictor muscles move the bolus into the hypopharynx, where contact with the pharyngeal wall elicits relaxation of the upper esophageal sphincter. This sphincter is made up by muscle fibers of the cricopharyngeus and inferior constrictor muscles, is 3 to 4 cm in length, and normally maintains a muscular tone of about 30 to 40 cm water pressure.

The last phase of swallowing is the esophageal phase in which peristaltic waves and gravity move the bolus from the hypopharynx to the stomach. Several clinically important areas of esophageal constriction include the upper esophageal sphincter, the thoracic inlet, the aortic arch, the tracheal bifurcation, and the lower esophageal sphincter. Normally, the primary wave of peristalsis generates 100 cm of water pressure and moves the bolus of food the length of the esophagus within 6 to 9 seconds. A second wave that is triggered by increased midesophageal pressure can occur when food is still in the esophagus after the primary wave. There exists a protective mechanism in which the upper esophageal sphincter opens when 25 cm of water pressure exists in the pharynx, whereas it takes 100 cm of water pressure from below to open this sphincter. Likewise, much less pressure in the esophagus is required to open the lower esophageal sphincter than is required in the stomach to open it and cause reflux.

HISTORY

The symptom of dysphagia is not pathognomonic for any specific disease. Fortunately, most patients can impart more detail than the simple statement that they have difficulty swallowing. The physician thus begins with a thorough history, which allows him or her to develop differential diagnoses. Specific questions are appropriate and can lead to clues that implicate some diagnoses and eliminate others. For example, time of onset and progression of a symptom might infer a foreign body in a patient who suddenly develops dysphagia during a meal, whereas slow, progressively worse dysphagia over several months might portend a malignancy or a neuromuscular disorder. In either case, specific questioning is useful. The questionnaire shown in Table 29–1 is a good starting point for most patients. Either early in the history or sometime later during the physical examination, patients often voluntarily point to a level in their upper aerodigestive tract where they perceive the obstruction or dysfunction to be. It is important to realize that this information can be misleading because the level at which the patient has symptoms may not be the same level at which disease exists.

Because the list of diseases that can cause dysphagia is so extensive, it may be useful to organize the etiologic factors into categories. Even after a thorough history, pinpointing the diagnosis is often very difficult. The possibilities, however, can usually be narrowed to one or more of the categories in Table 29–2.

A patient's age is usually a key point in determining whether dysphagia is acquired or congenital. There are exceptions, but most congenital problems of the upper aerodigestive tract are discovered at an early age. For an infant, the history may be limited to difficulty feeding, regurgitation, recurrent pneumonia, or failure to thrive. Physical examination is much more informative, and radiography can identify the problem in most cases. Congenital defects of the esophagus that can manifest these symptoms include esophageal cysts and duplication, atresia and tracheoesophageal fistulas, stenosis and webs of the esophagus, and vascular rings. In the oral cavity and pharynx, defects such as cleft palate may be obvious at birth, but

TABLE 29-1. Dysphagia Questionnaire

History
1. Do you have difficulty swallowing? _____ yes _____ no
2. Is your difficulty in swallowing constant? _____ Or is it present only when eating or drinking? _____
3. Is the difficulty worse for solids? _____ liquids? _____ The same for both solids and liquids? _____
4. When did it start? _____
5. How long have you had difficulty swallowing? _____
6. Does anything improve your swallowing? _____ If so, what? _____
7. Does anything make it more difficult to swallow? _____
8. Is your swallowing problem intermittent or constant? _____
9. Do you have any vomiting? _____
10. Does food or drink sometimes go down your windpipe or cause you to choke? _____
11. Is it painful to swallow? _____ If so, where is the pain, and does it radiate anywhere? _____
12. Do you have hoarseness? _____
13. Have you had shortness of breath, noisy breathing, or cough? _____
14. Have you coughed up any blood? _____
15. Have you noticed any knots or nodules in your neck? _____
16. Do you wear dentures? _____
17. Have you had any recent dental work? _____
18. Have you had any chest pain? _____
19. Have you had any night sweats, chills, or fever? _____ If known, how high did your temperature go? _____
20. Have you had any unplanned or unexpected weight gain or loss? _____
21. Have you been intolerant of temperature changes? _____
22. Has your appetite increased? _____ decreased? _____
23. Have you been tired and lethargic? _____ or have you felt energetic? _____

Past Medical History
1. Have you had any prior surgery; especially chest, neck, throat, or thyroid surgery? _____ Please describe any surgery: _____
2. Have you ever had a malignancy? _____ If so, where? _____
3. Have you ever had radiation therapy? _____ If so, to what part of your body? _____
4. Are you currently on any medications? _____ If so, what are they? _____
5. Do you have or have you ever had any chronic illness, such as diabetes, strokes, heart disease? _____ If so, what was it? _____

laryngeal clefts can go undiagnosed for years. Definitive diagnosis of laryngeal clefts requires direct laryngoscopy.

Acquired causes of dysphagia, which are far more common than are congenital causes, are more often diagnosed in older children and adults. They can also be further subclassified into one or more subcategories (Table 29–2). One of these subcategories, trauma, can lead to scarring that results in strictures. Examples include esophageal burns from caustic ingestion, perforations from instrumentation, radiation therapy, and pharyngeal surgery. Strictures from these etiologic factors may also be classified as mechanical obstruction. Recurrent laryngeal nerve paralysis as a complication of thyroidectomy or chest surgery could be considered a traumatic cause, but in these cases, aspiration rather than obstruction is more likely the chief complaint.

Infectious or inflammatory causes of dysphagia are very common and often associated with pain, fever, chills, malaise, or lethargy. Acute tonsillitis of either the palatine or the lingual tonsils can cause difficulty in swallowing and may be the most common cause of odynophagia and referred otalgia. A patient who has a peritonsillar abscess classically presents with severe dysphagia and dysarthria ("hot potato" voice). Another lesion that typically causes pain during swallowing and sometimes referred ear pain is laryngeal contact ulcer. The classical case is a young, aggressive, male professional who complains of unilateral throat pain that is aggravated by swallowing and radiates to the ipsilateral ear. The patient often points directly at the larynx on the affected side.

TABLE 29-2. Dysphagia Categories

Acquired causes
  Trauma
    Internal
    External
  Infection/inflammation
  Obstruction
  Neoplasms
    Benign
    Malignant
  Neurologic/neuromuscular
Congenital causes

and the examiner's fingers can be placed over the suprahyoid muscles to determine tone and strength as well as laryngeal elevation during the swallow. Another maneuver that may cue the examiner to a postcricoid mass is absence of a laryngeal click. Normally, this click is elicited by grasping the thyroid cartilage and rocking the larynx from side to side over the vertebral column. Also, patients who have Zenker's diverticulum occasionally complain of a foul taste developing in their mouth during the neck examination. This is thought to be caused by expelling of undigested food out of the diverticulum during palpation of the neck.

RADIOGRAPHIC STUDIES

Radiographic studies are an essential part of the work-up for nearly all patients with dysphagia and in many cases yield the definitive diagnosis without the need for formal endoscopy. In selected cases, plain radiographs can be as enlightening as contrast radiography. A chest radiograph with posteroanterior and lateral views is imperative in looking for tracheal deviation, lung masses, and mediastinal abnormalities. Likewise, a soft tissue lateral radiograph of the neck is the procedure of choice for diagnosis of supraglottitis. It is also very useful in diagnosis of retropharyngeal abscesses and foreign bodies. An additional advantage that radiography has over endoscopy is the capability to demonstrate the dynamics of swallowing. Of the various radiographic procedures for studying the swallowing mechanism, the mainstay is fluoroscopic pharyngoesophagography, which permits scrutiny of deglutition from the mouth to the stomach. Providing a permanent record and being able to review an examination have made motion-recording pharyngoesophagography extremely important. Video is the most popular recording method today because it provides instant replays while the patient is still in the examining suite. It is especially good for looking at the pharynx and the cervical esophagus, where the bolus passes very rapidly.

Several radiographic methods exist for examining the esophagus under fluoroscopic control. Obstructive lesions of the esophagus, such as cancers, strictures, and webs, are well delineated by full-column esophagography. This method, however, is not ad-

equate for small lesions. Air-contrast esophagography is much better for small mucosal abnormalities but has the disadvantage of a low sensitivity for picking up distal esophageal abnormalities such as hiatal hernias and varices. The mucosal-relief radiographic examination is a third method for viewing the esophagus and is very good for seeing varices in the distal esophagus but is poor for strictures, diverticula, or any lesion that requires esophageal distention for visualization.

As with esophagography, air-contrast pharyngography provides the best mucosal detail of the hypopharynx. The procedure is performed by having the patient swallow barium and then blow through closed lips (a modified Valsalva maneuver). This causes distention of the hypopharynx and piriform sinuses with air that gives a good contrast with the barium. A second helpful maneuver that results in widening of the vallecula and epiglottis is to have the patient phonate the vowel *e*. Figure 29–1 shows an air-contrast pharyngoesophagogram of a patient with Zenker's diverticulum.

Although the cricopharyngeal sphincter is

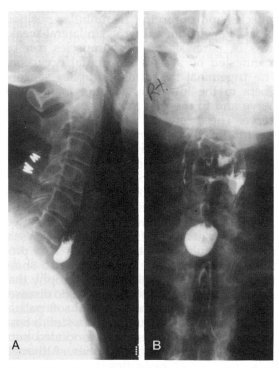

Figure 29–1. Pharyngoesophagography of a patient who complained of dysphagia and postprandial regurgitation of undigested food. *A.* Lateral view *B.* Anteroposterior view.

closed during a modified Valsalva maneuver, it should open completely during full-column contrast pharyngography. If the pharyngoesophageal sphincter does not completely relax, a typical finding is that of a smooth posterior indention in the barium column at about the level of the sixth cervical spine. In some conditions, spasm of the cricopharyngeus muscle actually causes spillage of the contrast material into the larynx. Figure 29–2 shows a pharyngoesophagogram from a patient who had chronic dysphagia and aspiration after undergoing resection of a posterior pharyngeal wall cancer. Pooling of the barium in the vallecula and piriform sinuses and spillage into the layrnx are easily seen. The asymmetry of the piriform sinuses is due to postoperative scarring.

Computed tomography scanning and magnetic resonance imaging are two other modalities that can be useful in the work-up of a patient with dysphagia. They are most helpful for delineating the extent of mass lesions, either external to the digestive tract or within it. The great vessels, thyroid gland, lymph nodes, and other anatomic structures juxtaposed to the aerodigestive tract are well delineated. When these studies are used in conjunction with physical examination and endoscopy, the accuracy of cancer staging is markedly improved.

ENDOSCOPY

Endoscopy of the upper aerodigestive tract is not necessary in all dysphagia cases. When it is indicated, however, it should be preceded by appropriate radiographic studies. For patients who require formal laryngoscopy and pharyngoscopy for oropharyngeal dysphagia, it is equally important to perform a complete esophagoscopy because esophageal lesions and diseases can affect the pharyngeal phase of swallowing. Likewise, when rigid or flexible esophagoscopy is planned for a suspected esophageal lesion, thorough inspections of the pharynx and larynx are imperative. These can be performed with a laryngoscope before rigid esophagoscopy or with a fiberoptic nasopharyngoscope before fiberoptic esophagoscopy. Other types of endoscopy, such as bronchoscopy in a case of tracheoesophageal fistula or nasopharyngoscopy for a suspicious nasopharyngeal mass, are done on an individual

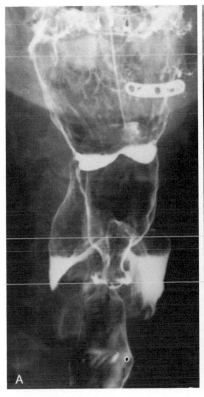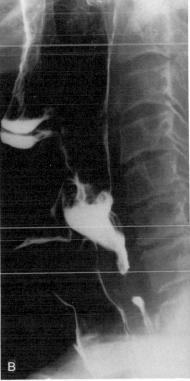

Figure 29–2. Pharyngoesophagography *A.* Anteroposterior view: pooling in the piriform sinuses and vallecula. *B.* Lateral view: review of the videofluoroscopy revealed that the pharyngoesophageal segment never relaxed. A cricopharyngeal myotomy improved swallowing.

case basis, depending on symptoms and other findings.

Endoscopy is most informative in cases of obstructing lesions of the pharynx or the esophagus and in assessing mucosal surfaces. For example, esophagoscopy with biopsy is the most sensitive test for diagnosis of esophagitis and its complications. In addition, therapeutic endoscopic procedures are often performed immediately after diagnostic endoscopy. Foreign bodies are usually removed as soon as they are identified, and after biopsy of a malignancy, endoscopic laser treatment can be performed for palliation or to improve the airway. Esophagoscopy is also sometimes indicated for motor disorders as well as for obstructing lesions. It may be necessary, for example, to rule out an underlying gastroesophageal cancer in a case in which radiography demonstrates achalasia.

MANOMETRY

Esophageal manometry is the most definitive procedure for diagnosis of esophageal motility disorders. When history, physical examination, or radiography implicates a motility disorder, manometry is indicated to assess peristaltic activity and record amplitude and duration of contractions. Classical manometric findings in patients who have achalasia are complete lack of esophageal peristalsis, an elevated lower esophageal sphincter pressure, and impaired relaxation of the lower esophageal sphincter during swallowing. Some patients have weak, low-amplitude contractions that are uncoordinated and ineffective. Any patient with classical achalasia symptoms of dysphagia, postprandial regurgitation of undigested food, and noncardiac chest pain should undergo manometry in addition to esophagography.

Esophageal manometry in patients who have gastroesophageal reflux is a less informative diagnostic tool. Although lower esophageal sphincter hypotension can sometimes be demonstrated in these patients, the test does not provide a definitive diagnosis. It can be of help, however, in identifying patients who might benefit from fundoplication surgery. In one study of reflux patients undergoing fundoplication, preoperative manometry showed that patients with hypotensive lower esophageal sphincter pressures respond favorably to the surgery.

Although manometry is rarely used clinically to evaluate the pharyngeal phase of swallowing, the introduction of manofluorography simultaneously combines measurements of pharyngeal pressures with videofluorography of bolus transit. Because pressures at different levels of the pharynx can be correlated with the anatomic structures producing them, the pharyngeal bolus transit can be analyzed by studying pressure gradients. Manofluorography identifies two functional regions, the oropharynx and pharyngoesophageal segment, that are primarily responsible for generating these pressures. From preliminary investigations, it appears that the major force in the oropharynx is generated by the tongue's acting as a piston and pushing the bolus down through the cylinder-like pharynx. Simultaneously, elevation of the larynx enhances the opening of the pharyngoesophageal segment, with creation of a relative negative pressure. Although the pharyngeal constrictors have been thought to be responsible for stripping the bolus down the pharynx by peristaltic actions, it is now thought by some investigators that these muscles serve more as a clearing-out force than as a major driving force. Because manofluorography combines pressure recordings with a visual radiographic view, it has the potential for better identifying patients who will benefit from a cricopharyngeal myotomy.

GLOBUS HYSTERICUS

Although a discussion of every cause of dysphagia is beyond the scope of this chapter, globus hystericus is an exception because it is one of the most common diagnoses in outpatient clinics and is in a category by itself. Dysphagia patients who undergo a work-up that is found to be completely normal are often diagnosed as having globus hystericus or psychogenic dysphagia. The typical chief complaint is a persistent pharyngeal foreign body sensation, sometimes described as a fullness or tightness in the throat. This sensation is often relieved by swallowing, which is why many clinicians do not consider this symptom to be true dysphagia. Esophagography can be normal or can reveal a smooth cricopharyngeal bar, which implicates cricopharyngeal muscle spasm. In either case, as long as the patient is not experiencing dysphagia while eating, a conservative approach to management is indicated. Counseling is often worthwhile because patients frequently are afraid they have cancer, or they can relate the onset of symptoms to psychologic stress. Occasional histories reveal depression, for which psychiatric consultation is offered. Follow-up examination is usually scheduled in 2 to 4 weeks. If the patient is not improved, radiographic studies are ordered, and the workup proceeds according to what is found.

SUGGESTED READINGS

Backer CL, Ilbawi MN, Idriss FS, DeLeon SY: Vascular anomalies causing tracheoesophageal compression. Review of experience in children. J Thorac Cardiovasc Surg 97:725–731, 1989.

Bass NH: Neurogenic dysphagia: diagnostic assessment and rehabilitation of feeding disorders in the neurologically impaired. Adv Clin Rehabil 2:186–228, 1988.

Kristensen S, Sander KM, Pedersen PR: Cervical involvement of diffuse idiopathic skeletal hyperostosis with dysphagia and rhinolalia. Arch Otorhinolaryngol 245:330–334, 1988.

Marshall JB: Dysphagia. Diagnostic pitfalls and how to avoid them. Postgrad Med 85:243–245; 250; 260, 1989.

Marshall JB: Gastroesophageal reflux disease. Medical aspects. Postgrad Med 85:92–100, 1989.

Marshall JB: Diagnosis of esophageal motility disorders. Postgrad Med 87:81–84; 89–90; 92–94, 1990.

McConnel FM, Cerenko D, Jackson RT, Hersh T: Clinical application of the manofluorogram. Laryngoscope 98:705–711, 1988.

McConnel FMS, Cerenko D, Jackson RT, Guffin TN: Timing of major events of pharyngeal swallowing. Arch Otolaryngol Head Neck Surg 114:1413–1418, 1988.

Ogorek CP, Fisher RS: Detection and treatment of gastroesophageal reflux disease. Gastroenterol Clin North Am 18:293–313, 1989.

Okamura H, Tsutsumi S, Inaki S, Mori T: Esophageal web in Plummer-Vinson syndrome. Laryngoscope 98:994–998, 1988.

Ott DJ: Radiologic evaluation of esophageal dysphagia. Curr Probl Diagn Radiol 17:1–33, 1988.

Raufman JP: Odynophagia/dysphagia in AIDS. Gastroenterol Clin North Am 17:599–614, 1988.

Reynolds JC, Parkman HP: Achalasia. Gastroenterol Clin North Am 18:223–255, 1989.

Sonies BC, Baum BJ: Evaluation of swallowing pathophysiology. Otolaryngol Clin North Am 21:637–648, 1988.

Triadafilopoulos G: Nonobstructive dysphagia in reflux esophagitis. Am J Gastroenterol 84:614–618, 1989.

CHAPTER 30

Congenital Lesions of Oral Cavity, Oropharynx, Hypopharynx, and Salivary Glands

Michael D. Maves, MD, FACS   John A. Stith, MD

An orderly work-up and an evaluation of congenital disorders of the oral cavity, the oropharynx, the hypopharynx, and the salivary glands begin with an understanding of the embryology and anatomy of the region, followed by a knowledge of the syndromes and conditions that can be encountered. Treatment is planned to correct or minimize the effects of such disorders on the life of the affected person.

EMBRYOLOGY

In the 14-somite human embryo, the primitive pharyngeal entoderm contacts the ectoderm to form the buccopharyngeal membrane. This membrane ruptures at the end of the third week of embryologic development to establish an opening between the stomodeum and the foregut.

By the fifth week, a series of pharyngeal arches and clefts are evident. The first pharyngeal arch is composed of (1) a small dorsal portion, the maxillary process, and (2) the much larger ventral portion, the mandibular process. With further development, the cartilage of this first arch, Meckel's cartilage, gives rise to the malleus and the incus. The remainder of the cartilage largely disappears, but part of it undergoes fibrous transformation and forms the sphenomandibular ligament. The mesodermal tissue surrounding the cartilage gives rise to the mandible through intramembranous ossification. The muscles of the first arch, the muscles of mastication, and the anterior belly of the digastric muscle are innervated by the nerve of the first arch, the mandibular branch of the trigeminal nerve (cranial nerve V3).

The anterior two thirds of the tongue forms from two lateral lingual swellings and one medial swelling, the tuberculum impar, after the fourth week of embryologic development. The mesoderm responsible for this structure is derived from the first arch. The mucosa covering the tongue also arises in the first arch and is innervated by the mandibular branch of the trigeminal nerve.

The first pharyngeal pouch contributes mainly to the development of the middle ear cavity at the distal portion of the tubotympanic recess, but the proximal portion communicates with the pharynx to form the pharyngotympanic (eustachian) tube.

The remaining four pharyngeal arches contribute important structures mainly to the ear and the larynx. The second arch contributes to the upper body and lesser horn of

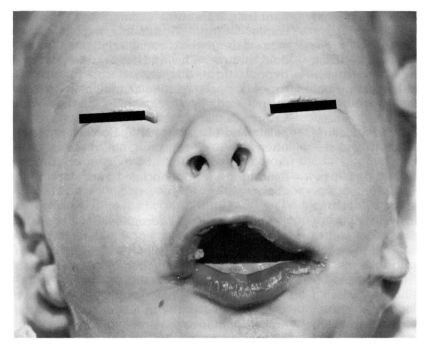

Figure 30–1. Macrostomia in a child with Goldenhar's syndrome.

tion and cardiac deformities, are associated with Down's syndrome. The nasopharynx is narrow, and many patients may not respond to adenoidectomy even though they have pronounced nasal airway obstruction. A fissured tongue is frequently observed. The middle third of the face is often hypoplastic, and the ear canals are small. Affected children tend to have more middle ear disease than do normal children. Even though the nasopharynx is constricted, patients may respond to tonsillectomy and adenoidectomy if they have adenotonsillar hypertrophy and an airway problem. Results of palatopharyngoplasty for correction of snoring or pharyngeal respiration are unpredictable, and in some refractory cases, the surgeon may have to resort to tracheotomy.

Other Syndromes

Hurler's Syndrome (Mucopolysaccharidosis I-H). This disorder is characterized by thickened facial features, mental retardation, and macroglossia.

Peutz-Jeghers Syndrome. Facial features include pigmented lesions that appear on the inside of the cheek but are rarely present on the tongue or the floor of the mouth. The lesions are usually brown to bluish, especially in patients who have intestinal polyps. About 50% of these patients have cutaneous manifestations.

Marfan's Syndrome. This disorder is inherited as an autosomal dominant trait; its features include a high palatal arch; long, narrow teeth; and occasionally malocclusion. Affected persons also have mandibular prognathism.

Osteogenesis Imperfecta. The tarda form is inherited as an autosomal dominant with condylar deformity, prognathic mandible, depressed zygoma, and dentinogenesis imperfecta. More than half of these patients have otosclerosis with stapedial fixation.

Facial Hemiatrophy. This term refers to atrophy of half of the facial structures. Expression and severity are variable. The condition is usually not present at birth, but it becomes apparent in childhood and adolescence. The retardation of growth of the hemiface results in distortion and malocclusion of the dental arches.

Turner's Syndrome. Mandibular hypoplasia and high or cleft palate are features seen in this sex-linked disorder.

Cleidocranial Dysplasia. Clavicular aplasia with delayed ossification of the fontanelles and an exaggerated development of the cranium are the features of this disorder. The patients also have high arched palates with submucous or frank clefts of the palate.

Congenital Anomalies of the Oral Cavity

A variety of common and unusual disorders may be noted in the oral cavity. Hemangiomas may occur on any of the cutaneous and mucous membrane surfaces of the lips, the cheeks, or the oral cavity and are an example of so-called congenital tumors. Treatment is usually conservative inasmuch as many of these hemangiomas spontaneously involute with time. Unfortunately, there is typically a period of growth before regression takes place; this growth may force the treating physician to intervene. Large lesions that show a more aggressive growth pattern may require treatment with steroids, laser, or, occasionally, excision.

The term *macrostomia* refers to exaggerated size of the oral aperture. Although macrostomia may be a component of many congenital syndromes that affect the head and neck (Goldenhar's syndrome, Treacher Collins syndrome), this disorder may also occur in isolation. Treatment may be supportive in terms of altering the feeding regimen of the child, or the condition may require formal operative repair.

Lip pits and sinuses also represent abnormalities that are frequently seen in congenital syndromes of the head and neck. They are usually seen on the lower lips of affected persons and may communicate with minor salivary glands. Excision is the treatment of choice, if warranted.

Dental abnormalities may accompany many congenital syndromes of the head and neck, or they too may occur in isolation. Supernumerary teeth are frequently seen in such abnormalities and are treated with extraction, prosthodontia, or orthodontia. Less commonly seen are teeth deformed by congenital syphilis.

Macroglossia is also a common entity encountered in congenital disorders of the oral cavity, such as those of trisomy 21. However, individual variations in the size of the tongue are noted and may be ascribed to differences in inherited patterns of tongue size. Lymphangiomas of the tongue may mimic simple macroglossia in their early stages, but later the typical features of such an abnormality become obvious. Lymphangiomas of the tongue have a strawberry appearance with irregularities of the papilla over the area of involvement. Imaging studies such as computed tomography or magnetic resonance imaging (MRI) almost always demonstrate more involvement of the tissues in the head and neck than is clinically apparent.

Massive enlargement of the tongue from lymphangioma may necessitate airway intervention such as tracheotomy or resection of the excessive tongue tissue. Use of laser or constricting sutures to prevent hemorrhage is essential. The massive tongue may give rise to dental abnormalities as a result of the pressure of the tongue on the anterior dental arches. The plastic deformation of these structures may require formal treatment at a later time (Fig. 30–2).

A short lingual frenulum or a bifid tongue may be the cause of articulation difficulties in the child and may require surgical repair. Consultation with a speech pathologist is essential for determining the degree of impairment and for continuing treatment afterward.

Median rhomboid glossitis represents a failure of posterior lingual development; a denuded area appears in the posterior aspect of the dorsum of the tongue. No treatment of median rhomboid glossitis is required.

A lingual thyroid gland is a thyroid gland that did not descend from its embryonic origin at the foramen caecum. As the child becomes older, the ectopic thyroid gland tissue at the base of the tongue enlarges, causing dysphagia and dysarthria. Treatment consists of surgical resection, surgical translocation of the thyroid gland to the submandibular area, or suppression of swelling with thyroid hormone.

Congenital Anomalies of the Mandible and Maxilla

Abnormalities of the mandible and the maxilla are usually associated with other congenital syndromes, such as the malar hypoplasia in Treacher Collins syndrome and the mandibular hypoplasia in the Pierre Robin anomalad. Fortunately, isolated abnormalities of the upper and lower dental arches are few and may almost always be related to facial

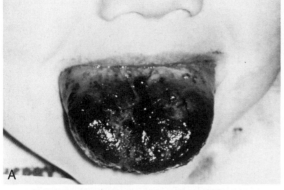

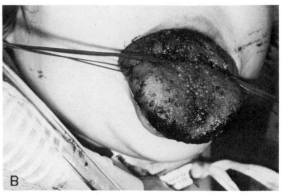

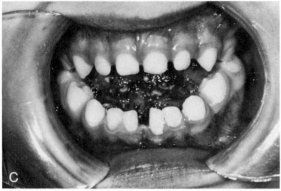

Figure 30–2. *A.* Child with hemangioma of the tongue. The tongue cannot retrude into the mouth. *B.* Excision of anterior tongue with circumferential sutures used for hemostasis. *C.* Postoperatively, the tongue can be positioned in the mouth, but there has been deformation of the dental arches with an open bite deformity caused by the pressure from the tongue. Note the wide interdental spaces.

clefts. A high arched palate is a common problem noted in children and may be regarded as one extreme on a continuum of cleft disorders. Similarly, a short palate (or megapharynx) may represent a failure of complete embryologic development (Fig. 30–3).

Congenital syngnathia, or fusion of the mandible and the maxilla, is an extremely rare congenital abnormality of the mouth. The degree of fusion between the mandible and the maxilla may be slight or may involve nearly the entire dental arch (Fig. 30–4). Considerations of feeding, airway maintenance, and facial growth all play a role in the decision to treat such patients.

Congenital Anomalies of the Pharynx

Teratomas, chordomas, cystic hygromas, and craniopharyngiomas are all congenital tumors that may be noted at birth and require treatment, depending on the degree of functional impairment (Fig. 30–5).

Vallecular cysts are common in children but only infrequently cause any functional problem and almost never require treatment. In contrast, pharyngeal atresia with a failure

of communication between the oral cavity and the pharynx must be recognized immediately and treated early to ensure the newborn's survival.

Choanal atresia is a failure of the buccopharyngeal membrane to disappear; this failure results in lack of communication between the nasal and pharyngeal cavities. Unilateral cases may go unrecognized at first and, when discovered, treated electively, whereas bilateral choanal atresia is an emergency that must be addressed at birth. Because the neo-

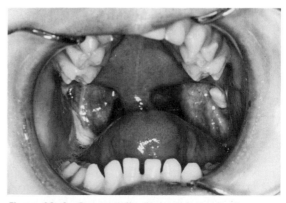

Figure 30–3. Congenitally short, deformed palate.

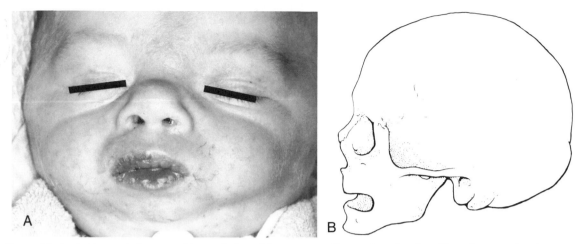

Figure 30–4. *A.* Congenital syngnathia, or fusion of the upper and lower dental arches. Note the poor development of the lower face. *B.* Schematic illustration of the fusion of the mandible and maxilla in the patient.

nate is an obligate nasal breather, a means of establishing the nasal airway must be sought. Perforation of the atresia plate with stenting offers an immediate airway and a possible long-term solution to the abnormality. The nasal stent is removed in 3 months, when the child is able to breathe through the mouth and the emergency of neonatal nasal respiration is no longer a threat. If the nasal airway remains patent after stent removal, then no further treatment is required. If the atresia recurs, however, a formal transpalatal repair is conducted when the patient is 4 or 5 years old.

Congenital Anomalies of the Salivary Glands

The parotid glands are affected more frequently by cysts and congenital lesions than

are any of the other salivary glands (Fig. 30–6). Cysts of the parotid gland are important because they account for 2% to 5% of all parotid gland lesions. Congenital cysts of the parotid gland are of ectodermal origin and may be divided into dermoid cysts, branchial cleft cysts, brachial pouch cysts, and congenital duct cysts.

Dermoid cysts commonly occur as isolated

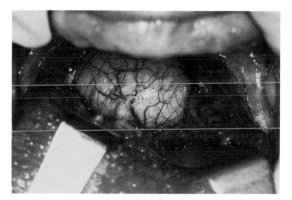

Figure 30–5. Pharyngeal teratoma in an infant who presented with feeding difficulties and respiratory embarrassment.

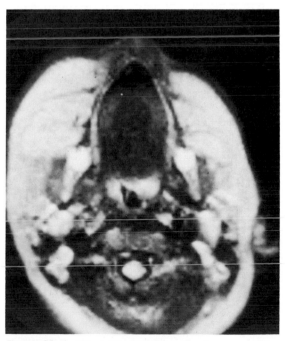

Figure 30–6. Magnetic resonance imaging scan demonstrating asymmetry of the parotid glands as a result of fatty infiltration.

masses within the substance of the parotid gland. Complete removal with protection of the facial nerve is required. These cysts typically contain keratinized squamous epithelium with skin appendages.

Lesions of the first branchial cleft may be classified as either type I or type II, according to Work (1977). Type I cleft cysts appear as sinus tracts or swellings in the region of the posterior conchae or anterior to the tragus. They are duplication anomalies of the membranous external auditory canal and occur deep within the tissues adjacent to the external canal and parotid. Their location can be variable with respect to the facial nerve. Microscopic evaluation reveals that the type I cyst contains only squamous epithelium, without appendages.

Type II cysts are also duplication cysts of the external auditory canal, but they are differentiated from type I cysts by the presence of skin appendages, revealed in histologic examination. Two germinal layers, the ectoderm and the mesoderm, contribute to form these cysts. A sinus stoma and tract are not uncommon findings in the upper portion of the neck at the level of the hyoid bone. The facial nerve is in intimate contact with type II cysts also. Type II cysts occur much less frequently than type I cysts.

A cyst of the first branchial pouch may occur in the region of the parotid gland. Such cysts are rare and usually located deep in the retromandibular area near the middle ear and the eustachian tube.

Congenital ductal cysts cause enlargement of the parotid gland. The diagnosis can be confirmed by MRI and fine-needle aspiration if necessary. These retention cysts may require either no treatment or parotidectomy with preservation of the facial nerve if infection or recurrence becomes a problem.

SUGGESTED READINGS

Cotton RT, Zalsal GH: Non-cleft disorders of the oral cavity and oropharynx. *In* Cummings CW, Fredrickson JM, Harker LA, et al (eds): Otolaryngology—Head and Neck Surgery (pp 1169–1184). St. Louis: CV Mosby, 1986.

Morgan DW, Pearman K, Raafat F, et al: Salivary disease in childhood. Ear Nose Throat J 68:155–159, 1989.

Myer C, Cotton RT: Salivary gland disease in children: a review. Clin Pediatr 25:353–357, 1986.

Parkin JL: Congenital malformations of the mouth and pharynx. *In* Bluestone CD, Stool S (eds): Pediatric Otolaryngology (pp 912–923). Philadelphia: WB Saunders, 1983.

Ward RF, April M: Teratomas of the head and neck. Otolaryngol Clin North Am 22:621–629, 1989.

Wilson DB: Embryonic development of the head and neck: part 3, the face. Head Neck Surg 2:145–153, 1979.

Work WP: Cysts and congenital lesions of the parotid gland. Otolaryngol Clin North Am 10:339–343, 1977.

CHAPTER 31

Diseases of the Oral Mucous Membranes

Terry D. Rees, DDS, MSD

The mucous membranes of the oral cavity are susceptible to numerous disease processes, many of which the otolaryngologist may be called upon to diagnose and manage or to refer to other medical or dental specialists. This review of oral mucosal diseases is limited to mucocutaneous disorders, infectious diseases, and keratinization disorders.

MUCOCUTANEOUS DISORDERS

Lichen Planus

Lichen planus (LP) is a chronic, inflammatory mucocutaneous disease of unknown etiology. It is estimated to affect approximately 1% of the population, but racial differences may occur. The disease may affect skin or oral mucosa alone or concomitantly, and genital lesions occur in a small percentage of patients.

Cutaneous lesions are generally transient or recurrent. They manifest as keratotic, violaceous, pruritic plaques occurring most commonly on flexor surfaces. Conversely, oral lesions assume a variety of clinical appearances, and lesions may persist for years. Oral lesions most commonly affect persons between the ages of 40 and 70 years; there is a slight predilection for females.

Oral lesions often manifest as papular, reticular, or plaquelike white lesions that are usually asymptomatic, although patients may complain of a rough texture to the involved oral tissues (Figs. 31–1, 31–2). In contrast, LP also may occur in atrophic, ulcerative, or bullous forms, which are often quite painful (Figs. 31–3, 31–4). Atrophic LP appears as diffuse, erythematous lesions that frequently occur in apposition to reticular lesions. The reticular form of LP occurs most commonly, whereas bullous LP is rarely encountered. One longitudinal study confirmed that LP may manifest in variable combinations of the clinical forms over time. For purposes of this discussion, atrophic, ulcerative, or bullous LP is described under the broad term erosive lichen planus.

LP can occur on any intraoral surface, but the buccal mucosa and mandibular vestibule are, by far, the most frequent sites. Erosive lichen planus may occur, however, with nearly equal frequency on gingiva or buccal mucosa. In general, lesions on the gingiva tend to be erosive in nature, perhaps because

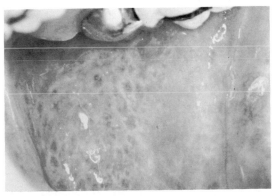

Figure 31–1. Reticular lichen planus of buccal mucosa.

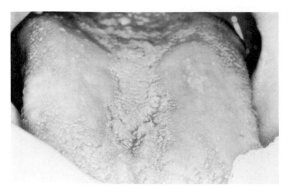

Figure 31–2. Plaquelike lichen planus on dorsum of tongue.

of the traumatic stresses imposed on these tissues during mastication and oral hygiene procedures (Fig. 31–5).

On histologic examination, papular, reticular, and plaque LP lesions exhibit epithelial acanthosis and hyperorthokeratosis or hyperparakeratosis. Epithelial rete ridges assume a saw-toothed configuration, and liquefaction degeneration occurs in the basal cell layer. A dense band of lymphocytic (T-cell) infiltration is found in the connective tissue immediately subjacent to the basement membrane. In atrophic LP, the histologic appearance is somewhat modified by a generalized attenuation of the epithelial stratum spinosum and by the absence of hyperkeratinization (Fig. 31–6). The clinical occurrence of ulcerations or bullae in erosive lichen planus is associated with more pronounced liquefaction degeneration of the basal cell layer, which causes the epithelium to become detached from the underlying connective tissue.

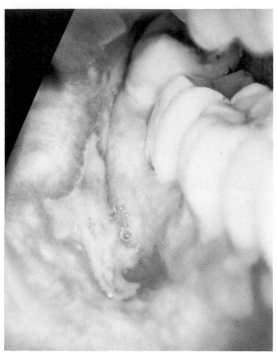

Figure 31–4. Severe atrophic lichen planus with ulceration.

The lymphocytic infiltrate found in LP is suggestive of a localized cell-mediated immune response, and it occurs in other mucocutaneous diseases such as lupus erythematosus and erythema multiforme. A lichenoid form of epithelial dysplasia or malignancy may be encountered, and so a precise diagnosis is essential. A similar lichenoid reaction may also occur in graft-versus-host disease after bone marrow transplantation.

Direct immunofluorescence is of value in confirming the diagnosis of LP. The presence of a linear pattern of antifibrin or antifibrinogen in the basement membrane zone and the occasional presence of immune reactive cytoid bodies in lesional tissue are highly suggestive of, but not diagnostic for, LP (Fig. 31–7). These immunofluorescence findings may also be evident in other mucocutaneous diseases, most notably lupus erythematosus.

Lichenoid drug-induced tissue reactions may produce clinical, histologic, and immunofluorescence features identical to those of idiopathic LP. Most commonly, these reactions have occurred in response to antimalarial drugs, antihypertensive medications, or nonsteroidal anti-inflammatory agents. Dental restorative materials have occasionally

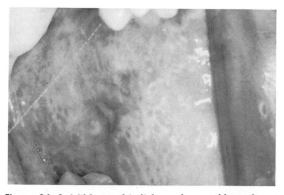

Figure 31–3. Mild atrophic lichen planus of buccal mucosa.

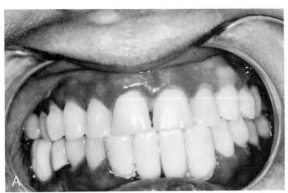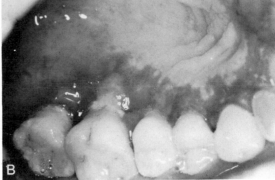

Figure 31–5. Desquamative gingivitis in erosive lichen planus. *A.* Facial view. *B.* Palatal view.

been implicated as causative allergens, although this concept remains controversial.

A number of case reports and small studies have suggested an association between LP and a variety of systemic diseases. Concomitant presence of LP with diabetes mellitus or chronic inflammatory liver disease has been described, but one comparison of LP patients with age- and sex-matched non-LP controls failed to reveal a significant difference. The existence of an overlap of lichen planus with lupus erythematosus, however, has been suggested.

The relationship between oral LP and squamous cell carcinoma has been controversial. LP has been implicated as a precancerous condition in many case reports and some prospective studies. Other authors, however, have challenged these reports and suggested

that many of these lesions have actually represented lichenoid epithelial dysplasia on initial biopsy instead of LP.

Dysplastic changes, however, have been documented on occasion in LP, especially erosive lichen planus. Holmstrup and associates (1988) followed 611 LP patients for 1 to 26 years (a mean of 7.5 years) and found that 1.5% of patients developed squamous cell carcinoma (Fig. 31–8). This represents a

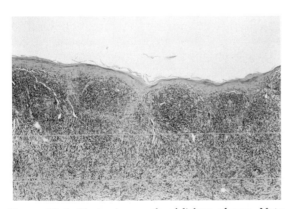

Figure 31–6. Photomicrograph of lichen planus. Note saw-toothed epithelial rete ridges and liquefaction degeneration of basal cells. A dense zone of inflammation is evident in the lamina propria immediately subjacent to the basement membrane. (Photomicrograph courtesy of John Wright, Baylor College of Dentistry, Dallas, Texas.)

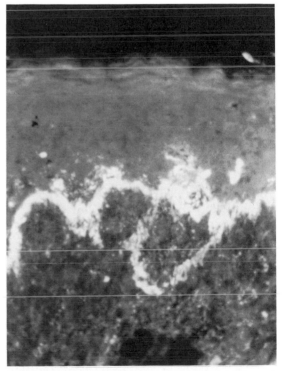

Figure 31–7. Immunofluorescence of lichen planus. A linear pattern of antifibrinogen is evident in the basement membrane zone.

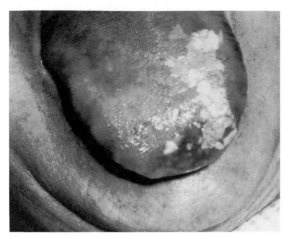

Figure 31–8. Squamous cell carcinoma arising in a lichen planus lesion of 10 years' duration.

fifty-fold increase in malignant changes among LP patients over those in the same age groups in the general population and fulfills the World Health Organization criteria for a premalignant condition.

Because oral LP has a variety of clinical appearances, its accurate diagnosis is dependent on careful evaluation of clinical, histologic, and immunofluorescence findings. White lesions of LP must be differentiated from genokeratotic conditions, such as white sponge nevus, hereditary benign intraepithelial dyskeratosis, dyskeratosis congenita, and lichen sclerosus et atrophicus, and from leukoplakia, hyperkeratosis, scars from cheek biting, or leukoedema. Erosive lesions must be distinguished from lupus erythematosus, erythema multiforme, secondary syphilis, candidiasis, migratory glossitis, or erythema migrans. Gingival LP may manifest as desquamative gingivitis and must be differentiated from bullous or cicatricial pemphigoid, pemphigus vulgaris, psoriasis, or contact allergy.

Proper management of oral LP requires the elimination of factors potentially causing lichenoid reactions, the elimination of local irritants, and the effective use of therapeutic agents. Complete remission may occur in some patients, but none of the treatment methods currently in use is predictably curative. Although the plaque form of LP is generally asymptomatic, it may harbor undetected dysplastic changes; therefore, treatment may be indicated. Surgical excision of small plaquelike lesions is often feasible, and

some success has been achieved with the use of systemic or topical retinoic acids. Lesions tend to return, however, when treatment is terminated. The association of systemic retinoids with fetal deformities must always be considered when women of child-bearing age are treated.

Other therapies have produced mixed results. These include dapsone or the antifungal drug griseofulvin. Good success has been reported in a small group of patients who used an oral rinse of cyclosporine. This treatment method is worthy of further study.

The most successful treatment results have been achieved with use of topical, intralesional, or systemic corticosteroids. High-potency topical agents such as fluocinonide, betamethasone dipropionate, or clobetasol have been demonstrated to be effective; intralesional corticosteroid injections are often beneficial for refractory lesions. Diffuse or inaccessible lesions are usually responsive to short tapering regimens of systemic corticosteroids, but long-term systemic therapy is occasionally necessary. In some instances, immunosuppressive drugs such as azathioprine or cyclophosphamide have been successfully used alone or in combination with corticosteroids. Once severe lesions have been controlled, recurrence can usually be prevented by the use of high-potency topical corticosteroids as needed.

Cicatricial Pemphigoid

Cicatricial pemphigoid (CP), or benign mucous membrane pemphigoid, is a chronic vesiculobullous disorder of the elderly that usually affects mucous membranes. Oral lesions are almost invariably present, sometimes accompanied by involvement of the conjunctiva, skin, genitalia, rectum, nares, larynx, or esophagus. Oral lesions rarely scar on healing, but eye involvement can lead to symblepharon formation (Fig. 31–9) and blindness; laryngeal or esophageal lesions may result in stricture formation. CP-like lesions may occur in childhood, but most affected persons are 50 years of age or older; the disease has a predilection for females over males of approximately 2:1.

Oral lesions are very common, and any mouth tissue may be involved (Fig. 31–10). The gingiva, however, is the most frequent oral site, with involvement in 95% or more of reported cases (Fig. 31–11). Gingival le-

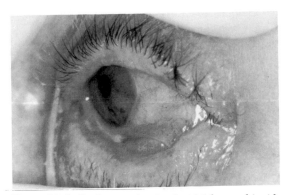

Figure 31–9. Ocular scarring in cicatricial pemphigoid.

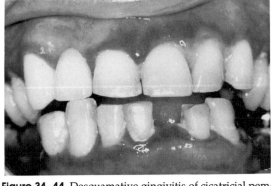

Figure 31–11. Desquamative gingivitis of cicatricial pemphigoid.

sions usually feature loss of the epithelial surface in response to trauma (Nikolsky's sign), leaving raw, painful erythematous surfaces (Fig. 31–12). Blistering and ulceration may occur in other oral sites. Untreated lesions may undergo remission and exacerbation, or they may remain constant for many years. Although CP lesions may occur first or exclusively on extraoral mucosa, the oral cavity is often the first or the only site.

CP is an autoimmune disorder, although CP-like lesions have been induced by a few drugs such as practolol, clonidine, and penicillamine. On histologic examination, CP features a subbasilar split that leads to separation of epithelium from underlying connective tissue (Fig. 31–13). If a bulla is present in the biopsy specimen, the intact basal cell layer may be evident above the separation. On ultrastructural examination, the separation is found within the basal lamina.

Direct immunofluorescence is very helpful in diagnosis of CP. Typically, an intact lesion

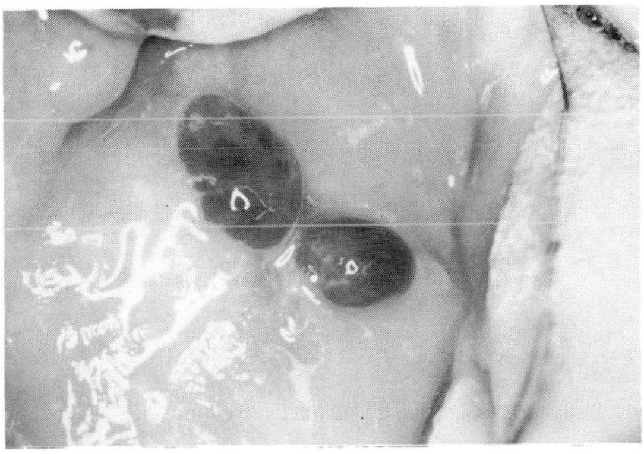

or uninvolved tissue reveals the presence of immunoglobulins (especially IgG), complement (usually C3), and fibrin deposits arranged in a linear pattern at the basement membrane zone (Fig. 31–14). If epithelial separation has occurred in the lesion, however, direct immunofluorescence findings are negative. Consequently, perilesional tissue should be included in the biopsy. Serum indirect immunofluorescence reveals circulating immunoglobulins only 20% to 30% of the time.

Differential diagnosis of CP includes bullous pemphigoid (BP), pemphigus vulgaris, erosive lichen planus, linear IgA disease, and epidermolysis bullosa acquisita. Direct immunofluorescence is often required to establish the diagnosis, although epidermolysis bullosa acquisita can be distinguished from pemphigoid only by use of immunoelectron microscopy. BP and CP have identical histologic and immunologic features. Clinically, CP involves skin less extensively and tends to heal with scarring. BP can affect the oral mucosa, however, and eye lesions are common to both disorders. BP and CP may represent different manifestations of the same disease.

Treatment of CP is dependent on the severity and responsiveness of the lesions. Topical or intralesional corticosteroids are beneficial for localized lesions, but systemic intervention is usually required. Dapsone has proved quite successful, but corticosteroids or combination therapy with prednisone plus immunosuppressive agents may be necessary. When possible, drugs suspected as etiologic factors should be discontinued. Early ophthalmologic evaluation is essential for ensuring detection and treatment of any ocular involvement.

Figure 31–10. Localized blood-filled bulla of cicatricial pemphigoid of buccal mucosa.

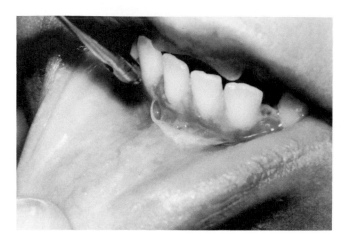

Figure 31–12. Positive Nikolsky's sign to blast of air in gingival cicatricial pemphigoid.

Bullous Pemphigoid

BP is a chronic subepidermal blistering disease that usually affects the elderly. It is an autoimmune disorder characterized by formation of tense bullae, which usually heal without scarring. It may involve a variety of sites on skin; mucous membrane lesions, including ocular ones, are common. Pemphigoid-like lesions have been reported in patients treated with phenacetin, penicillin, practolol, fluorouracil, ultraviolet light, and furosemide.

Mucosal lesions may occur in 10% to 40% of patients; the oral cavity is the usual site of involvement. On occasion, oral lesions precede cutaneous and other manifestations. More commonly, however, the skin is the site of the initial lesion. Oral lesions are usually small or large bullae that may remain intact for long periods and then rupture, leaving a raw, painful, denuded surface. Le-

sions usually occur on the palate, floor of the mouth, tongue, or buccal mucosa. Gingival lesions may manifest as desquamative gingivitis.

Diagnosis of BP is based on the identification of the histologic and immunofluorescence features previously described for CP, plus distinct clinical features. Immunoelec-

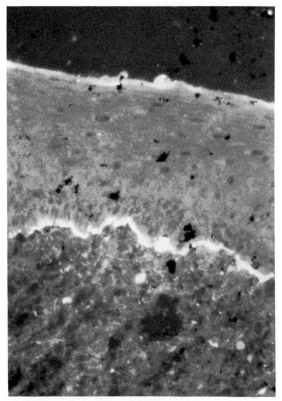

Figure 31–14. Direct immunofluorescence of cicatricial pemphigoid. Note linear pattern of immunoglobulin and complement in basal membrane zone.

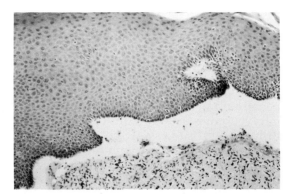

Figure 31–13. Photomicrograph of cicatricial pemphigoid. Note subbasilar separation of epithelium from connective tissue.

tron microscopic studies have identified a bullous pemphigoid antigen located in the lamina lucida of the basal zone. The antigen is apparently produced by basal keratinocytes.

Circulating immunoglobulins reactive to basement membrane zone antigen are present in approximately 70% of BP patients on indirect immunofluorescence examination. The serum titer of immunoglobulins does not necessarily correlate with the degree of disease activity, but the titer may decrease or disappear during remission.

BP must be differentiated from CP, dermatitis herpetiformis, linear IgA disease, epidermolysis bullosa acquisita, and herpes gestationis. In children, skin manifestations must be distinguished from chronic bullous disease of childhood. All of these diseases are similar on histologic and direct immunofluorescence examination, so diagnosis must be based on careful evaluation of the clinical, microscopic, and immunofluorescence features.

Once diagnosed, BP is usually treated by systemic corticosteroids alone or in combination with immunosuppressive agents. Cyclosporine may be effective, and some patients respond to sulfapyridine or dapsone. Plasma exchange may occasionally be necessary, and successful management has been reported with use of tetracycline hydrochloride and niacinamide alone or in combination. The rationale for such therapy is based on evidence that niacinamide blocks mast cell degranulation and protease release from leukocytes, whereas tetracyclines cause suppression of leukocytic chemotaxis.

IgA Diseases

Several distinct clinical syndromes feature linear deposits of IgA in the basement membrane zone. Three of these conditions, linear IgA disease, dermatitis herpetiformis, and childhood cicatricial pemphigoid, may display oral lesions. Dermatitis herpetiformis is a papulovesicular skin disorder characterized immunologically by C3 and granular deposits of IgA in the basement membrane zone. Skin lesions are often seen on the extensor surfaces and sometimes the face. Oral lesions are relatively rare, but they may manifest as erosions, bullae, vesicles, or fissured lesions, and they may occur on any oral mucosal surface. Frequently, oral lesions are localized

at sites of trauma, and they may occasionally precede skin manifestations.

The association of dermatitis herpetiformis with celiac disease is well established, and identification of circulating antigliadin antibodies is of diagnostic value. The mainstay of treatment is dapsone or other sulfones in combination with a gluten-free diet.

Childhood cicatricial pemphigoid is an IgA-associated subepidermal blistering disease of young children, which may feature extensive mucous membrane involvement. Oral vesiculoulcerative lesions are relatively common. There is no evidence of gluten-sensitive enteropathy. The condition differs from classical CP in its onset before the age of 18 years, in the presence of prominent cutaneous eruptions, and in its immunopathologic manifestations.

Linear IgA disease has clinical features very similar to those of BP or CP. Patients with linear IgA disease develop small tense skin bullae, which histologically demonstrate infiltration of polymorphonuclear leukocytes and large mononuclear cells into the blister cavity. Suprabasal lamina blisters are evident on electron microscopy; immunoelectron microscopy reveals IgA deposits at the basal surface of the basal keratinocytes and hemidesmosomes. The condition may occur in children, but it is more common among adults. Mucosal lesions may occur, and oral and ocular involvement is relatively common. Some patients present with oral lesions alone characterized by desquamative gingivitis. Linear IgA disease does not respond to a gluten-free diet, and dapsone is the treatment of choice.

Epidermolysis Bullosa Acquisita

Epidermolysis bullosa acquisita is a rare, acquired mechanobullous disease resembling dystrophic epidermolysis bullosa. It can affect children as well as adults; in most instances, concomitant systemic diseases are present. These may include amyloidosis, cystitis, inflammatory bowel disease, multiple myeloma, systemic lupus erythematosus, rheumatoid arthritis, and psoriasis. Diagnostic criteria include deposition of IgG in a linear pattern in the basement membrane zone as identified by direct immunofluorescence; subepithelial blister cleavage beneath the lamina densa on electron microscopy; and deposition of IgG beneath the lamina densa as demonstrated by immunoelectron microscopy.

Epidermolysis bullosa acquisita may result in oral lesions, including gingival erosions or vesicles with additional erosions or ulcerations of the tongue, soft palate, buccal mucosa, and lips. Nikolsky's sign may be present.

Ocular lesions may occur, sometimes leading to blindness. The presence of eye, skin, and oral bullous lesions suggests that epidermolysis bullosa acquisita may mimic CP or BP. The importance of epidermolysis bullosa acquisita as a marker for significant systemic disease suggests that, on occasion, differentiation should be attempted by use of immunoelectron microscopy. Treatment includes corticosteroid therapy, combination therapy, dapsone, vitamin E, gold sodium thiomalate, or plasma exchange therapy.

Pemphigus Vulgaris

The term *pemphigus* refers to a group of autoimmune bullous diseases that affect skin and mucosa. The group includes pemphigus vulgaris, pemphigus foliaceus, pemphigus vegetans, and pemphigus erythematosus. Pemphigus vulgaris is by far the most common form. It is characterized histologically by acantholysis that leads to intraepithelial blistering. Untreated pemphigus vulgaris has a very high mortality rate (70% to 100%). Since the advent of corticosteroid therapy, however, mortality has decreased markedly.

Pemphigus vulgaris can occur at any age, but lesions most frequently develop between the fourth and sixth decades. Clinically, it presents as bullae, which cover large areas of skin, especially on the trunk. Ruptured bullae leave eroded, painful, weeping surfaces, which lose fluids and electrolytes and may easily become secondarily infected. Nikolsky's sign is usually present. Oral lesions are very common, and the oral cavity is the initial site of involvement in more than half of reported cases. Involvement of other mucous membranes, including the esophagus, the larynx, the pharynx, the vagina, and the rectum, is also common. Oral lesions are similar to those on skin; bullae develop quickly and rupture, leaving eroded painful surfaces with ragged borders (Fig. 31–15). Gingival involvement may manifest as desquamative gingivitis, and on occasion this is the only oral manifestation (Fig. 31–16).

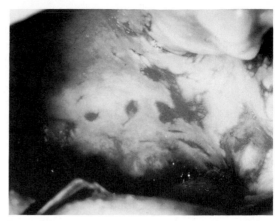

Figure 31–15. Pemphigus vulgaris lesion of soft palate.

Pemphigus vegetans is an uncommon variant of pemphigus vulgaris in which rupture of the initial bullae is followed by the development of fungating masses or vegetations. In the oral cavity, elevated white plaques develop; they sometimes can be scraped away (Fig. 31–17). Tongue, gingival, buccal, labial, and palatal lesions have been described.

Pemphigus foliaceus is a relatively mild form of the disease that features the development of scales rather than blisters. Pemphigus erythematosus manifests with mild bullae and erythematous or crusted skin lesions. It may be a localized variant of pemphigus foliaceus. The oral cavity is rarely or never involved in either pemphigus foliaceus or pemphigus erythematosus.

On histologic examination, pemphigus vulgaris and pemphigus vegetans manifest

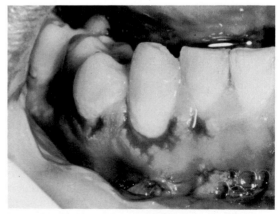

Figure 31–16. Pemphigus vulgaris lesion of mandibular gingiva.

Figure 31–17. Pemphigus vegetans lesion on ventral surface of tongue.

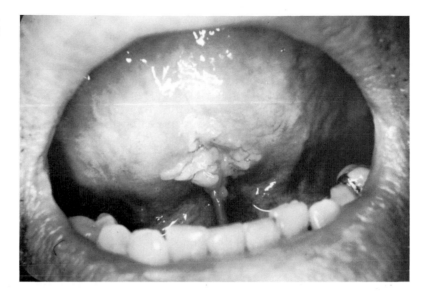

as suprabasilar bullae resulting from acantholysis (Fig. 31–18). The epithelial intercellular bridges are lost, and the bullous cavity contains free-floating Tzanck cells. The inflammatory infiltrate is primarily mononuclear; occasionally, eosinophils and neutrophils are present. In pemphigus vegetans, eosinophil-rich abscesses are sometimes noted intraepithelially.

Direct immunofluorescence reveals a distinct pattern of immunoglobulins and C3 in the intercellular spaces of the epithelium (Fig. 31–19). Positive direct immunofluorescence results can usually be obtained in both lesional or normal skin and mucosa. Circulating IgG autoantibodies are detected by indirect immunofluorescence in most instances of cutaneous pemphigus vulgaris. Early oral lesions, or lesions confined to the oral cavity,

however, may not elicit an elevation in serum antiepithelial antibodies. A variety of drugs, including captopril and penicillamine, may produce pemphigus vulgaris–like lesions.

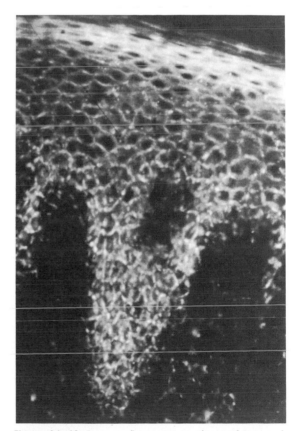

Figure 31–19. Immunofluorescence of pemphigus vulgaris reveals IgG and complement in the intercellular substance of the epithelium.

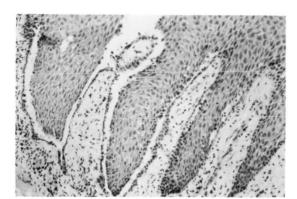

Figure 31–18. Photomicrograph of pemphigus vulgaris. Note intraepithelial separation.

Rifampin may exacerbate skin lesions in pemphigus vulgaris, possibly by increasing the metabolism of corticosteroid.

Diagnosis of pemphigus is dependent on identification of the histologic and direct immunofluorescence features described and is supported by elevated serum antiepithelial titers. Systemic corticosteroid therapy has been the cornerstone of treatment for many years. Others have described successful treatment with gold, immunosuppressive agents, and combination therapy with both corticosteroids and immunosuppressant agents. Oral lesions can often be managed with low to intermediate systemic corticosteroid therapy coupled with a high-potency topical agent such as fluocinonide.

Lupus Erythematosus

Lupus erythematosus is an autoimmune disease that may involve multiple body systems. It affects skin, mucous membranes, and internal organs and is more common in women, especially Black women, than in men. It commonly affects people between the ages of 20 and 65 years. Discoid lupus erythematosus exclusively involves mucocutaneous tissues. The oral cavity may be affected exclusively or may be the site of initial lesions. Oral discoid lupus erythematosus is sometimes difficult to differentiate from lichen planus or leukoplakia, and the presence of skin lesions may simplify the clinical diagnosis. Skin and oral discoid lesions may be present, however, in the systemic form of the disease.

Systemic lupus erythematosus may involve any or most organ systems. Oral lesions are present in 25% to 40% of patients with systemic lupus erythematosus. Distinguishing clinical features include a malar rash, discoid plaques on the face and scalp, and alopecia. Renal involvement is common, and a variety of hematologic and neurologic disorders may occur.

Typical oral lesions of lupus erythematosus feature a central erythematous erosion or ulceration surrounded by radiating keratotic striae on the perimeter of the lesions (Fig. 31–20). Generalized erythematous oral lesions may also occur with or without ulcerations, and leukoplakic plaques may be present. The gingiva may appear erythematous and desquamative (Fig. 31–21), but more commonly, lesions are located on the hard and soft palate, buccal mucosa, and vermilion border of the lips.

Definitive diagnosis of oral discoid lupus erythematosus is based on clinical, histologic, and immunologic data. Microscopic examination features hyperkeratosis with keratin plugging accompanied by atrophy of rete ridges, liquefaction degeneration of the basal layer of epithelium, and thickening of the basement membrane. A bandlike inflammatory infiltrate is evident in the lamina propria. Many of these features, of course, are very similar to oral lichen planus. The histologic presence of patchy PAS (periodic acid Schiff)

Figure 31–20. Oral lesion of discoid lupus erythematosus. Note erythematous center with radiating peripheral white striae.

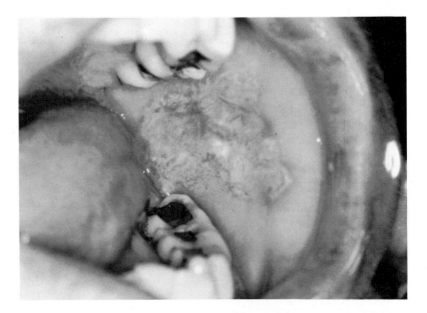

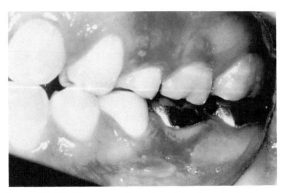

Figure 31–21. Desquamative gingivitis of systemic lupus erythematosus.

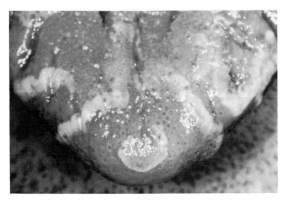

Figure 31–22. Benign migratory glossitis of dorsum of tongue.

positive deposits in the lamina propria immediately subjacent to the epithelium is a helpful diagnostic feature.

Direct immunofluorescence discloses granular deposits of immunoglobulin, C3, and fibrinogen in the basement membrane zone and superior lamina propria. This so-called lupus band may be present in uninvolved skin or mucosa in systemic lupus erythematosus.

Systemic lupus erythematosus is the prototypical autoimmune disease. Circulating antibodies have been identified against a variety of autoantigens. Tissue injury may be mediated by circulating immune complexes and by local formation of immune complexes. Drug-induced lupus erythematosus–like lesions have been described; reactions to procainamide and hydralazine are quite common.

On some occasions, atypical oral lupus erythematosus is indistinguishable from oral lichen planus, and treatment must often be empiric. Oral and skin lesions may respond to topical or intralesional corticosteroids, but results are unpredictable. Antimalarial drugs sometimes produce satisfactory results, as do systemic corticosteroids and immunosuppressive or cytotoxic drugs.

Psoriasis

Psoriasis is an idiopathic disease that has been estimated to affect between 1% and 2% of the world population. It occurs less frequently on dark-complexioned people and is more common in colder climates. Skin lesions manifest as well-circumscribed localized or generalized erythematous papules and plaques covered with white scales and

often affect the scalp, elbows, knees, and sacrum. Lesions appear to occur as a result of accelerated epithelial mitosis, probably induced by immunologic mechanisms. Arthritis may be a feature of the disease, and the temporomandibular joint may be involved.

Psoriasiform lesions of oral mucosa manifest as irregular erythematous areas with raised white to yellow irregular or serpiginous borders (Figs. 31–22 to 31–24). They have been described as representative of four disease entities: psoriasis, Reiter's syndrome, benign migratory glossitis (geographic tongue), and stomatitis areata migrans (ectopic geographic tongue). These conditions have virtually identical microscopic features of epithelial parakeratosis, acanthosis, and spongiosis; elongated and thickened rete ridges; and lymphocytic infiltration of the submucosa. Polymorphonuclear leukocytes are found migrating through the epithelium and occasionally forming intrapapillary microabscesses.

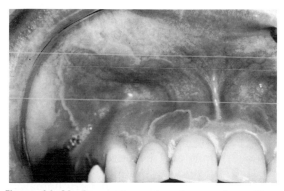

Figure 31–23. Stomatitis areata migrans of maxillary gingiva and alveolar mucosa.

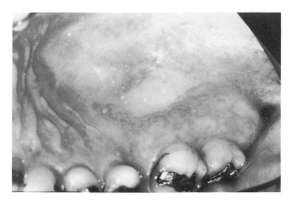

Figure 31–24. Psoriasiform lesions of palate.

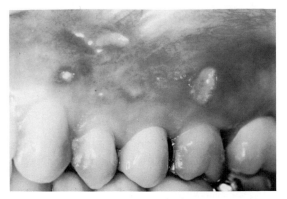

Figure 31–25. Minor recurrent aphthous stomatitis.

Differentiation between Reiter's syndrome and psoriasis is based on the presence or absence of other signs and symptoms associated with Reiter's disease. Benign migratory glossitis manifests as psoriasiform lesions confined to the dorsal surface of the tongue, whereas stomatitis areata migrans can affect any other oral tissue. Benign migratory glossitis and stomatitis areata migrans have been reported with significantly increased incidence in psoriatics, although geographic tongue most commonly occurs in nonpsoriatic patients. Incidence of fissuring of the tongue may also be increased in psoriatics. Gingival psoriasiform lesions may give the appearance of desquamative gingivitis, although lesions are usually painless. In most instances, direct immunofluorescence is negative for oral lesions, but occasionally, immunofluorescent confirmation is possible on the basis of the presence of immunoreactants in the stratum corneum.

Treatment for oral psoriasiform lesions is usually unnecessary, but lesions may respond to topical or systemic retinoids or, occasionally, corticosteroids.

Recurrent Aphthous Stomatitis

Recurrent aphthous stomatitis is an oral ulcerative condition affecting up to 20% of a given population. Lesions usually first appear within the first three decades of life. Episodes are sporadic, and the frequency of lesions diminishes with age. Recurrent aphthous stomatitis occurs in three forms: minor, major, and herpetiform (Figs. 31–25 to 31–27). Minor aphthae are small, shallow ulcerations with slightly raised erythematous borders. The central ulcer is usually covered by a yellow-white pseudomembrane. Lesions are generally no larger than 5 mm in size, and they heal without scarring in 10 to 14 days. This is the most frequently encountered form of aphthae.

Major aphthous stomatitis was previously known as periadenitis mucosa necrotica recurrens or Sutton's disease. Ulcerations are usually larger than 0.5 cm in diameter and indurated with irregular borders. Lesions may persist for a month or more and frequently heal with scarring. They tend to be few in number, but the patient is rarely in remission because new ulcers form before the older lesions have healed.

Herpetiform aphthae are small, multiple ulcerations that occur in crops throughout the oral cavity. Ulcers are painful, and they tend to heal in 7 to 10 days without scarring. One hundred or more ulcers may be present simultaneously, and they tend to enlarge by coalescence. Lesions similar to those of herpetic stomatitis may appear, but no vesicles

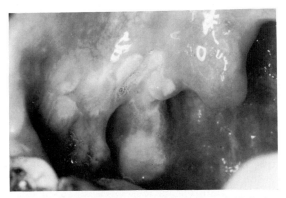

Figure 31–26. Major recurrent aphthous stomatitis lesion of soft palate and pharynx.

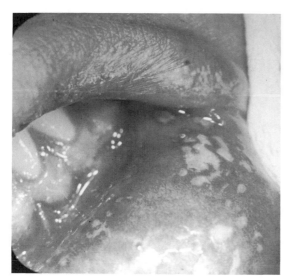

Figure 31-27. Herpetiform recurrent aphthous stomatitis.

are found in herpetiform aphthous stomatitis.

Characteristically, recurrent aphthous stomatitis affects mucosa that is not firmly bound to bone. Occasionally, however, gingival or palatal sites are involved. On microscopic examination, the epithelium is ulcerated and covered by a fibrinous exudate. The underlying connective tissue is infiltrated by polymorphonuclear leukocytes and plasma cells.

The condition is idiopathic, although some evidence links recurrent aphthous stomatitis with antigen-dependent cellularly mediated cytotoxicity. Psychologic stress or minor traumatic injury is often a precipitating factor, and hypersensitivity to various foodstuffs has been implicated. Nutritional deficiencies of iron, folic acid, or B_{12} are found singularly or in combination in a significant percentage of patients, and replacement therapy may result in remission or marked improvement. Gluten-sensitive enteropathy may also be associated with the occurrence of oral ulcerations.

Differential diagnosis includes Behçet's syndrome, erythema multiforme, ulcerative colitis, Crohn's disease, celiac disease, malabsorption syndrome, blood dyscrasias, or the mucocutaneous disorders previously discussed.

Treatment for recurrent aphthous stomatitis should include a detailed search for contributing etiologic factors. An antimicrobial topical rinse (chlorhexidine gluconate) is often beneficial in shortening the duration of ulcers and altering their clinical manifestations. Topical corticosteroids have proved successful, but systemic corticosteroids may be necessary in management of major aphthae or other refractory lesions. Topical tetracycline may be particularly effective in management of herpetiform lesions.

Behçet's Syndrome

Behçet's syndrome is a muco-oculocutaneous syndrome that may include arthralgia/arthritis, central nervous system involvement, intestinal ulcers, and orchitis/epididymitis. Oral aphthous ulcerations and ocular lesions often appear first; genital ulcerations, skin lesions, and arthritis follow. The mean age of onset is 30 years. In western countries, it is more prevalent among women than among men.

Behçet's syndrome is idiopathic, but a genetic predisposition has been suggested, and hypersensitivity reactions appear to play a role in pathogenesis.

Oral lesions of Behçet's syndrome may be managed as described for recurrent aphthous stomatitis. Disseminated or more resistant lesions are best treated with systemically administered corticosteroids either alone or in combination with other immunosuppressive agents. Cyclosporine, chlorambucil, thalidomide, and colchicine have also been used with success.

Erythema Multiforme

Erythema multiforme is an acute inflammatory dermatologic disorder that manifests with distinctive cutaneous lesions with or without mucosal involvement. It primarily affects children, adolescents, and young adults. The milder form manifests as symmetric erythematous wheals on the skin that are surrounded by a circumferential halo (target lesions). The oral cavity is often affected and, on occasion, may be the only site of involvement. Lesions appear as bullae that burst rapidly and leave erythematous erosions and ulcerations, which develop a grayish pseudomembrane and a hemorrhagic crust. The lips are often involved (Fig. 31-28).

Major erythema multiforme (Stevens-Johnson syndrome) may extensively involve

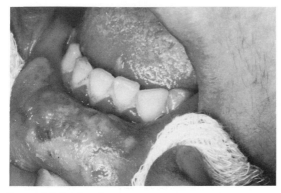

Figure 31–28. Erythematous, crusting erythema multiforme lesions of lip and oral mucosa.

the skin and mucous membranes. Lesions affect the genitalia and conjunctiva as well as the oral cavity, and multisystem involvement may be found. Both forms tend to recur, but recurrences are more common in erythema multiforme minor. Toxic epidermal necrolysis (Lyell's disease) may represent an even more severe form of erythema multiforme.

The condition may be precipitated by iatrogenic (drug-induced) or infectious agents, but on most occasions, no etiologic factor can be identified. Drug-induced erythema multiforme was first associated with the sulfonamides, but many additional drugs have since been implicated, including antibiotics, anticoagulants, and several miscellaneous agents.

Erythema multiforme is often preceded by bacterial or viral infections, most commonly *Mycoplasma* pneumonia or herpes simplex virus infection. Typically, herpes labialis or genitalis may occur 2 to 3 weeks before the outbreak of the disease, which suggests a postinfectious hypersensitivity reaction.

Clinically, prodromal symptoms sometimes occur 1 to 14 days before the onset of erythema multiforme. These may include fever, headache, and general malaise with or without nausea, vomiting, and diarrhea. Prodrome is followed by onset of lesions, which, if untreated, may continue to develop for 10 days to several months. Healing may occur 2 to 3 weeks after onset, but the duration of untreated lesions may be quite prolonged.

The histopathologic features of erythema multiforme are not specific. Either intraepithelial or subbasilar bulla formation may occur, and a perivascular monocytic inflammatory infiltrate is evident. Ultrastructural examination may reveal both the basal lamina and keratinocytes to be undergoing degeneration and necrosis. Direct immunofluorescence reveals perivascular and basement membrane zone deposits of immunoglobulins and complement, accompanied by occasional cytoid bodies. Indirect immunofluorescence is negative.

Erythema multiforme can be differentiated from most other bullous diseases by its acute onset, by the presence of target lesions, and, occasionally, by the presence of slight fever. Therapy often includes administration of systemic corticosteroids, but such treatment is controversial in major erythema multiforme because of the possibility of opportunistic infections, which may be life-threatening. Oral erythema multiforme must be differentiated from primary herpetic gingivostomatitis before the administration of corticosteroids, and so early treatment is often palliative until the diagnosis is clear. Acyclovir may be useful in management of recurrent or chronic oral erythema multiforme that occurs in association with previous herpes simplex outbreak. Drug-associated erythema multiforme is managed by withdrawal of the implicated agent.

INFECTIOUS DISEASES

Candidiasis

Candida albicans is found as an oral commensal in 30% to 60% of healthy mouths. Exposure to the organism often occurs at an early age, and many neonates develop oral thrush in the first few days of life. Several other species of *Candida* are capable of causing disease, but most oral lesions are manifestations of *Candida albicans*. Candidal species become oral pathogens in the presence of altered local or systemic host factors. Local factors may include xerostomia, smoking, or wearing of dentures. Iron deficiency may adversely affect host resistance, and endocrine disorders often predispose a person to candidal infections. The prolonged use of antibiotics, corticosteroids, or antineoplastic drugs may also serve as a predisposing factor. Whereas candidal infections are common in patients with weakened immune defenses, they are especially prevalent in those with altered cellularly mediated immunity, such as acquired immunodeficiency syndrome

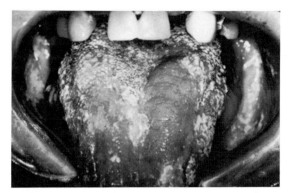

Figure 31–29. Acute pseudomembranous candidiasis (thrush).

(AIDS) patients. Under such circumstances, the oral candidiasis may predispose to fungemia or local spread to the esophagus, epiglottis, larynx, or lymph nodes.

Acute pseudomembranous candidiasis (thrush) is the most common form, manifesting as superficial, confluent, white, elevated plaques that can be wiped away, leaving an erythematous bleeding surface (Fig. 31–29).

Acute atrophic candidiasis (antibiotic sore mouth) manifests as painful, sometimes bleeding erosions of the mucosa (Fig. 31–30). This form of candidiasis is often associated with the use of broad-spectrum antibiotics, but similar lesions may be precipitated by corticosteroid administration.

Chronic atrophic candidiasis (denture sore mouth) may affect the majority of denture wearers, especially those with full dentures. It often occurs in the elderly, but it can affect patients of any age; the upper dentures are most commonly involved. The condition often presents as asymptomatic erythema

and edema of the palatal mucosa. Deep tissue invasion of the causative organism does not seem to occur, although *Candida* can be cultured from the tissue side of the denture and from the superficial surfaces of the involved tissues. The infection responds to antifungal therapy, but treatment must be directed toward both the involved mucosa and the denture itself.

Angular cheilitis features erythematous soreness and fissuring at the external corners of the mouth. Lesions usually occur bilaterally, and they are often induced by loss of vertical dimension of dentures or natural dentition or by habitual licking of the corners of the mouth. Patients may suffer from underlying predisposing systemic disorders such as anemia, neutropenia, diabetes mellitus, or human immunodeficiency virus (HIV) infection.

Medium rhomboid glossitis is an erythematous, raised or flat, sometimes painful lesion in the middorsum of the tongue. It was once believed to represent a developmental defect of the tuberculum impar, but more recent evidence indicates that candidal infection is implicated in some, but not all, such lesions (Fig. 31–31).

Chronic oral multifocal candidiasis features multiple, localized, red, nodular or plaquelike lesions within which candidal species can be isolated. The condition appears to be related to smoking. *Candida* may be the causative agent or coagent, but it is possible that the fungi secondarily invade established lesions, as has been demonstrated with some mucocutaneous disorders.

Chronic hyperplastic candidiasis (candidal

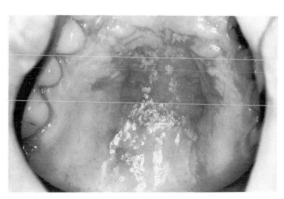

Figure 31–30. Acute atrophic candidiasis of palate (antibiotic sore mouth).

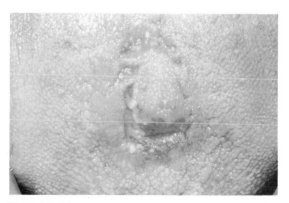

Figure 31–31. Medium rhomboid glossitis-like lesion of dorsum of tongue associated with localized candidal infection.

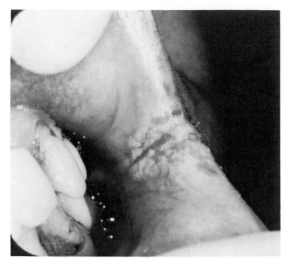

Figure 31–32. Chronic hyperplastic candidiasis (candidal leukoplakia) of corner of mouth.

leukoplakia) manifests as raised, white mucosal patches that may be clinically indistinguishable from other leukoplakia. Lesions may appear as homogeneous white plaques or as mixed erythroplakic-leukoplakic, speckled lesions (Fig. 31–32). The lesions may display epithelial dysplasia and should be considered premalignant. Reports have suggested that candidal leukoplakia is responsive to fluconazole therapy.

Chronic mucocutaneous candidiasis is a persistent form of candidal infection that features lesions of the oral cavity, the skin, the vagina, and the nails in patients suffering from a variety of irreversible, immunologic abnormalities primarily involving T lymphocytes. Lesions may initiate in the oral cavity as pseudomembranous candidiasis and gradually involve extraoral sites (Fig. 31–33). The condition may be familial (autosomal recessive), but it is often associated with an endocrinopathy such as hypoparathyroidism, Addison's disease, hypothyroidism, or diabetes mellitus.

The severity, type, and chronicity of candidal infections may determine the choice of therapy. Common forms of oral candidiasis are generally responsive to topical antifungal agents such as nystatin or clotrimazole. Recurrence is common, however, if the underlying predisposing factors have not been eliminated. Ketoconazole and fluconazole are effective systemic agents that are usually well tolerated. Chronic mucocutaneous candidiasis is sometimes successfully managed with systemic amphotericin B or ketoconazole. The condition often relapses, however, when therapy is discontinued. Treatment of chronic mucocutaneous candidiasis with fluconazole has not yet been reported.

Herpesviruses

The herpesviridae include the herpes simplex viruses (HSV), types 1 and 2; herpes varicella-zoster virus; cytomegalovirus; and Epstein-Barr virus. All are capable of causing oral disease.

The highest rate of infection for HSV is in the first 5 years of life, but a second high rate is associated with the onset of sexual maturity. Most oral infections are caused by HSV-1, even among populations with frequent oral-genital contact. HSV-2 can also cause oral lesions, and, conversely, up to one third of genital HSV infections are caused by HSV-1.

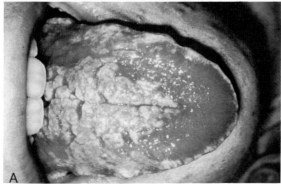
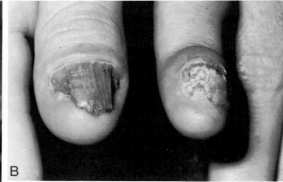

Figure 31–33. Chronic mucocutaneous candidiasis. (Photograph courtesy of William H. Binnie, Baylor College of Dentistry, Dallas, Texas.) *A.* Tongue lesions. *B.* Involvement of fingernails.

Primary herpetic gingivostomatitis features multiple oral vesicles and ulcers, severely inflamed gingiva, cervical and submandibular lymphadenopathy, and elevated temperature; it is usually readily diagnosed on the basis of the clinical features. In some instances, however, acute necrotizing ulcerative gingivitis may be superimposed and thereby make diagnosis difficult. Primary HSV infection may be more severe when it affects adults.

Recurrent HSV infections tend to occur at or near the site of initial infection, and chronic or progressive HSV infections are seen in immunocompromised patients. The acute vesicular eruptions of recurrent herpes resemble the primary lesions, except that they tend to be more localized and heal more rapidly. One third to one half of the general population experiences recurrent herpes labialis (Fig. 31–34).

After initial infection, latency is established when the virus follows neurons to an immunoprivileged site such as the trigeminal ganglion. HSV may be reactivated by a variety of stimuli: trauma, emotional stress, anesthetic injections, exposure to ultraviolet light, immunosuppression, and trigeminal nerve decompensation. Reactivation most commonly results in development of herpes labialis, but intraoral occurrences have been described, especially in leukemic or immunocompromised patients.

Management of oral HSV infection is predicated on an accurate diagnosis. The differential diagnosis includes severe gingivitis, aphthous stomatitis, bacterial stomatitis or pharyngitis, acute necrotizing ulcerative gingivitis, herpangina, erythema multiforme, varicella zoster infection, and vesiculobullous diseases.

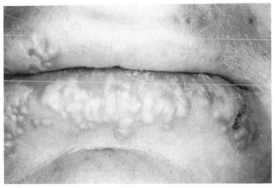

Figure 31–34. Recurrent herpes labialis of lower lip.

Diagnosis is based on the characteristic clinical presentation. In an immunocompromised host, however, unusual clinical features may include development of chronic ulcers and nodular tongue lesions. Viral culturing and viral typing are reliable diagnostic techniques; cytologic examination of Tzanck's smear, Papanicolaou's smear, and biopsies for the presence of inclusions and multinucleated cells can be of some value. Serologic testing for antibody titers at onset and after convalescence is moderately accurate but primarily of epidemiologic value. Assay techniques involving enzyme-linked immunosorbent assay or immunofluorescence assay are rapid and nearly as sensitive as is viral isolation.

Palliative and supportive care remains essential in management of primary or recurrent oral HSV infections. A soft diet and a soothing mouth rinse are helpful. One such mouth rinse consists of one part antihistamine elixir mixed with two parts kaolin and pectin (Kaopectate) and three parts distilled water. The need for analgesics and antipyretics varies from patient to patient.

A wide variety of agents have been proposed for management of herpes labialis, but most have not been demonstrated to be reliably effective. Topical idoxuridine or topical acyclovir is occasionally of benefit in herpes labialis, but not predictably so. Systemic administration of acyclovir may reduce the duration of viral shedding in primary herpetic gingivostomatitis, but the clinical course is not significantly altered. Acyclovir is, however, beneficial for immunocompromised patients in prevention or treatment of herpetic infections, although resistant viral strains have been reported.

Herpes Varicella-Zoster

Primary infection with herpes varicella-zoster virus may occur asymptomatically or result in varicella (chickenpox), which often includes manifestations of oral vesicles or ulcerations. More commonly, however, herpes zoster is the varicella-zoster virus infection encountered in the oral cavity. The maxillary and mandibular divisions of the trigeminal nerve may be involved, leading to ipsilateral oral lesions with or without facial involvement. Prodromal pain and paresthesia occur in affected sites and are followed a few days later by a vesicular eruption, which crusts and heals in 3 to 4 weeks. Treatment for oral varicella-zoster virus infection has often proved difficult. Advances in therapy, however, offer promise. Vidarabine, acyclovir, and alpha-interferon have all proved reasonably successful in treating immunocompromised patients with varicella infection, but acyclovir is probably the drug of choice in localized oral herpes zoster lesions.

Human Cytomegalovirus

Primary infection with cytomegalovirus may occur asymptomatically or with influenza-like symptoms. When disseminated cutaneous manifestations are present, however, mucosal ulcerations may occur. Cytomegalovirus mononucleosis may present with oral features that include petechiae of the soft palate and discrete vesiculoulcerative lesions of the soft palate, the buccal mucosa, and, occasionally, the gingiva. Cytomegalovirus becomes latent after the primary infection, and the latent virus may be harbored in the oropharyngeal epithelial cells or tonsillar lymphocytes. Reinfection with a different cytomegalovirus strain may occur, and reactivation is common in conjunction with immunosuppression or malignancy. Cytomegalovirus infection is highly prevalent among AIDS patients, and the occurrence of persistent, large, indurated oral, esophageal, or oropharyngeal ulcerations in an HIV-positive person should be viewed with suspicion. Treatment is difficult, although new experimental antiviral agents show promise.

Epstein-Barr Virus

The Epstein-Barr virus is believed to be the causative agent in mononucleosis and Burkitt's lymphoma. After acute infection, it becomes latent and may reside in the epithelial cells of the oropharynx and salivary glands. The virus may be shed in saliva and possibly in other body fluids. Primary Epstein-Barr virus infection may occur symptomatically in infants and small children, but in adolescents or adults, it typically manifests as infectious mononucleosis. The characteristic features of that disease include malaise, cervical lymphadenopathy, pharyngitis, palatal petechiae, and oral ulcerations.

Epstein-Barr virus appears to be the causative agent in oral hairy leukoplakia among HIV-positive persons. This condition features the formation of elevated white or yellow plaques primarily on the lateral border of the tongue. It is believed to be a predictor of pending transformation to outright AIDS. Hairy leukoplakia has been reported to have been successfully treated with acyclovir, but treatment is primarily supportive in nature.

Acquired Immunodeficiency Syndrome

AIDS results in profound impairment of cellular immunity that often predisposes the patient to oral malignancy or potentially life-threatening opportunistic infections. Two strains of the human immunodeficiency retrovirus (HIV) are capable of causing immune system impairment. The disruption of T lymphocytes and the resultant secondary disruption of B lymphocytes serve to place the infected person at increased risk for disseminated opportunistic infections. Secondary viral infections in patients with AIDS may significantly influence the clinical features of the disease because viruses stimulate HIV replication and death of infected cells. Secondary viruses may also contribute to the development of malignant disorders in the immunocompromised host. For example, Epstein-Barr virus infection of B cells in HIV-infected hosts may stimulate the development of Burkitt's lymphoma or other lymphoproliferative disease.

Oral manifestations often appear early in HIV infection, and nearly all AIDS patients have oral disease during their illness. Cervical or submandibular lymphadenopathy may occur during the initial acute HIV-related illness or at any stage of the disease. Oral candidiasis may be the first sign of HIV infection; it occurs more frequently with increasing severity of immune system suppression. Acute pseudomembranous candidiasis (thrush) is the most common presentation, and persistent or recurrent infection may indicate the presence of esophageal candidiasis.

Early HIV-related oral candidiasis is usually responsive to antifungal drugs, but lesions tend to recur after treatment is discontinued. Ketoconazole is effective, but resistant candidal strains may develop. In addition, HIV-positive patients may be especially susceptible to liver damage with prolonged use of ketoconazole. Fluconazole offers great promise in management of HIV-related oral candidiasis.

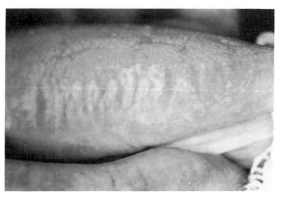

Figure 31–35. Hairy leukoplakia of lateral border of tongue.

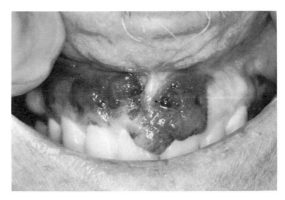

Figure 31–36. Kaposi's sarcoma of maxillary anterior gingiva.

Hairy leukoplakia is an oral condition unique to HIV-infected or otherwise immunocompromised patients. It features nonremovable white patches usually on the lateral border of the tongue (Fig. 31–35). Lesions are often bilateral and painless and vary in severity. The presence of the condition may portend future transition to full-blown AIDS. Lesions are occasionally found on other oral sites, including the buccal mucosa and palate. Hairy leukoplakia is often secondarily infected with *Candida;* lesions may improve but not resolve with antifungal therapy. On histologic examination, vacuolization of oral epithelial cells is associated with human papilloma virus infection; however, human papilloma virus has been excluded in the etiology of hairy leukoplakia because substantial evidence implicates the Epstein-Barr virus as causative. Resolution of lesions has been achieved with acyclovir therapy and with the use of topical retinoids. Treatment may not be necessary, however, unless lesions are symptomatic.

AIDS-associated Kaposi's sarcoma is an angiosarcoma that affects a significant percentage of AIDS patients, often causing lesions in the oral cavity. Oral lesions usually manifest as blue, purple, or red macules, papules, or nodules. They must be differentiated from localized pigmentations, hemangiomas, or pyogenic granulomas, and they are most commonly found on the palate or gingiva. Kaposi's sarcoma occasionally occurs in renal transplant patients and other patients receiving immunosuppressive therapy, which suggests a relationship between the malignancy and an altered immune system. Oral lesions of Kaposi's sarcoma may

interfere with function or create an unesthetic appearance (Fig. 31–36). In these circumstances, lesions can be debulked by means of radiation therapy or laser surgery. Reduction in lesion size can also be achieved by use of vinblastine injections. Other oral malignancies believed to be more common among AIDS patients include squamous cell carcinoma and malignant lymphoma.

Periodontal disease may be more prevalent among HIV-positive persons. Immunocompromised patients may experience an increased incidence of acute necrotizing ulcerative gingivitis (Fig. 31–37). Others develop a chronic persistent erythematous gingivitis, which may be associated with increased gingival recession. A unique HIV-related periodontitis features extensive alveolar bone destruction with a necrotic gingivitis superimposed (Fig. 31–38). Lesions may be confined to localized areas of the periodontium, or they may be more generalized in

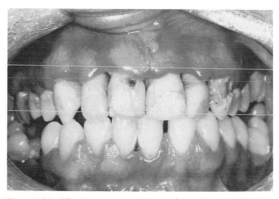

Figure 31–37. Acute necrotizing ulcerative gingivitis in an HIV-positive patient.

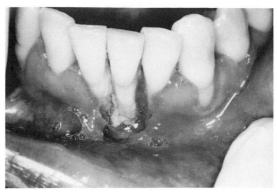

Figure 31–38. HIV-related periodontitis. Note severe localized destructive periodontitis.

severely immunocompromised persons. The periodontal lesions are often quickly and progressively destructive, but they may undergo periods of remission and exacerbation. Therapy includes local debridement of lesions with periodontal scalers and irrigation with antimicrobial solutions such as povidone-iodine (Betadine) or chlorhexidine. Meticulous oral hygiene must be achieved. Systemic antibiotics are not recommended because of the risk of opportunistic infections. One-time use of topical antibiotics, however, may be beneficial. The microbial flora of HIV-related periodontitis appears to involve microorganisms commonly found in rapidly destructive periodontal disease or in acute necrotizing ulcerative gingivitis.

At least 30 oral lesions have been identified in association with HIV infection, including viral infections such as herpes simplex and cytomegalovirus; bacterial infections such as actinomycosis and mycobacteriosis; fungal infections such as cryptococcosis and histoplasmosis; neurologic disturbances such as trigeminal neuropathy and facial paralysis; and miscellaneous conditions such as recurrent aphthous stomatitis, xerostomia, and salivary gland enlargement.

KERATINIZATION DISORDERS

A variety of disorders affect the keratinization process of oral epithelium. Most commonly these disorders are associated with development of white lesions. Heritable genokeratoses may cause diffuse benign white lesions affecting most oral tissue surfaces as well as extraoral mucous membranes and skin or nails. These conditions include white sponge nevus, hereditary benign intraepithelial dyskeratosis, pachyonychia congenita, dyskeratosis congenita, and keratosis follicularis. Histologic features are hyperortho- or hyperparakeratosis and variable degrees of benign dyskeratosis. In general, no treatment is required for these diseases, but in some instances, concomitant systemic disorders may be present and require management.

The term "leukoplakia" signifies a white patch of oral mucosa that cannot be rubbed away and that does not represent a recognized disease such as lichen planus or candidiasis. Such lesions feature hyperkeratosis on microscopic examination, and they may be associated with chronic mechanical irritation, smoking, and use of smokeless tobacco or with development of epithelial dysplasia or squamous cell carcinoma. Erythroplakia is a red lesion of oral mucosa of no apparent cause and not representative of an identified disease entity. On histologic examination, it often demonstrates variable degrees of epithelial dysplasia. Erythroplakic lesions may occur alone or in association with leukoplakia. Unidentified red or white lesions should be viewed with suspicion as potential premalignant or malignant conditions. Biopsy should be considered, with treatment predicated on histologic findings.

SUGGESTED READINGS

Axell T, Henricsson V: The occurrence of recurrent aphthous ulcers in an adult Swedish population. Acta Odontol Scand 43:121–125, 1985.

Bhogal B, Wojnarowska F, Marsden RA, et al: Linear IgA bullous dermatosis of adults and children: an immunoelectron microscopic study. Br J Dermatol 117:289–296, 1987.

Dreizen S: Oral candidiasis. J Am Med 77:28–33, 1984.

Economopoulou P, Laskaris G: Dermatitis herpetiformis: oral lesions as an early manifestation. Oral Surg Oral Med Oral Pathol 62:77–80, 1986.

Holmstrup P, Thorn JJ, Rindum J, Pindborg JJ: Malignant development of lichen planus–affected oral mucosa. J Oral Pathol 17:1–7, 1988.

Huff JC: Antiviral treatment in chicken pox and herpes zoster. J Am Acad Dermatol 18:204–206, 1988.

Laskaris G, Triantafyllou S, Economopoulou P: Gingival manifestations of childhood cicatricial pemphigoid. Oral Surg Oral Med Oral Pathol 66:349–352, 1988.

Lesher JL Jr: Cytomegalovirus infections and the skin. J Am Acad Dermatol 18:1333–1338, 1988.

Lozada F, Silverman S: Erythema multiforme. Clinical characteristics and natural history in fifty patients. Oral Surg 46:628–636, 1978.

Mashkilleyson N, Mashkilleyson AL: Mucous membrane manifestations of pemphigus vulgaris. A 25-year survey of 185 patients treated with corticosteroids or with combination of corticosteroids with methotrexate or heparin. Acta Derm Venereol (Stockh) 68:413–421, 1988.

Medenica-Majsilovic L, Fenske NA, Espinoza CG: Epidermolysis bullosa acquisita. Direct immunofluorescence and ultrastructural studies. Am J Dermatol 9:324–333, 1987.

Pindborg JJ: Classification of oral lesions associated with HIV infection. Oral Surg Oral Med Oral Pathol 67:292–295, 1989.

Pogrel MA, Cram D: Intraoral findings in patients with psoriasis with a special reference to ectopic geographic tongue (erythema circinata). Oral Surg Oral Med Oral Pathol 66:184–189, 1988.

Rawls WE, Hammerberg O: Epidemiology of the herpes simplex viruses. Clin Dermatol 2:29–45, 1984.

Schiffman L, Giansiracusa D, Calabro JJ, et al: Behçet's syndrome. Compr Ther, 12:62–66, 1988.

Schiodt M: Oral manifestations of lupus erythematosus. Int J Oral Surg 13:101–147, 1984.

Silverman S Jr, Gorsky M, Lozada-Nur F, Liu A: Oral mucous membrane pemphigoid. A study of sixty-five patients. Oral Surg Oral Med Oral Pathol 61:233–237, 1986.

Syrjanen S, Laine P, Valle S-L: Demonstration of Epstein-Barr virus (EBV) DNA in oral hairy leukoplakia using in situ hybridization with a biotinylated probe. Proc Finn Dent Soc 84:127–132, 1988.

Thorn JJ, Holstrup P, Rindum H, Pindborg JJ: Course of various clinical forms of oral lichen planus. A prospective follow-up study of 611 patients. J Oral Pathol 17:213–218, 1988.

Ullman S: Immunofluorescence and diseases of the skin. Acta Derm Venereol 140(Suppl):1–31, 1988.

Venning VA, Frith PA, Bron AJ, et al: Ocular and oral involvement in bullous and cicatricial pemphigoid: a clinical and immunopathological study. Br J Dermatol 115(Suppl 30):19–20, 1986.

CHAPTER 32

Cancer of Oral Cavity and Oropharynx

Lanny Garth Close, MD   Norris K. Lee, MD

ANATOMY

Malignant neoplasms arising in the oral cavity and the oropharynx are unique in terms of clinical presentation, patterns of spread, and response to treatment according to the location of the primary tumor. Therefore, a discussion of cancer of this area requires that the oral cavity and the oropharynx be divided into specific sites.

The oral cavity extends from the lips anteriorly to the faucial arch posteriorly. It has been divided into the following sites: lip, floor of mouth, oral tongue, gingiva, retromolar trigone, buccal mucosa, and hard palate. Likewise, the oropharynx includes the soft palate, the tonsillar pillars, the palatine tonsils, the base of tongue, and the posterior oropharyngeal wall. Cancer of the lip is specifically excluded from further discussion in this chapter.

LYMPHATIC DRAINAGE

The lymphatic drainage system of the oral cavity and the oropharynx is rich and extensive. Structures of the oral vestibule and the upper and lower alveolar ridges are drained by a submucosal capillary lymphatic plexus into the submental and submandibular lymph nodes. The hard palate is drained by lymphatics to the upper jugular, submandibular, and retropharyngeal lymph nodes. Lymphatics are especially abundant in the submucosa of the oral tongue and drain to the submandibular and internal jugular nodes. Contralateral spread of disease can occur from primary sites on the tongue, especially after infection, surgery, or irradiation has disturbed normal lymphatic flow. The floor of the mouth is drained by lymphatic channels posteriorly into the deep cervical nodes or laterally into the submandibular and internal jugular lymph nodes. Buccal mucosal lymphatic drainage is primarily to the submandibular nodes.

The primary lymphatic drainage flow of the oropharynx is into the jugulodigastric nodes in the upper jugular chain. In addition, the soft palate, the lateral and posterior oropharyngeal walls, and the base of the tongue drain into the retropharyngeal and parapharyngeal lymph nodes that lie adjacent to the internal carotid artery and internal jugular vein. The most superior and lateral node has been named the node of Rouviere. The lymphatic flow from these nodes drains into the jugulodigastric and posterior cervical group of nodes. Bilateral or contralateral spread of disease is common in cancers that arise near the midline of the base of the tongue and the soft palate.

A knowledge of the patterns of lymphatic drainage is important in the assessment of patients with cancer of the oral cavity and the oropharynx. The location of a clinically positive cervical lymph node in the patient may provide a clue to the location of the primary lesion.

ETIOLOGY

Whereas the etiology of cancer of the oral cavity and oropharynx is uncertain, there is clear evidence linking certain cultural and environmental factors to the incidence of these neoplasms. The use of tobacco in any form is directly related to the incidence of intraoral squamous cancer. For example, cigarette smokers are six times more likely to develop oral cancer than are nonsmokers. According to one study, patients who have been successfully treated for an oral cancer and who continue to smoke have a 40% chance of developing a second primary cancer in comparison with only 6% for those who stop smoking.

Raw tobacco, in the form of either chewing tobacco or snuff, has been closely linked to squamous cell carcinoma of the oral cavity. Tumors usually involve the buccal and alveolar mucosa, corresponding to the placement of the quid. Although cigarette consumption per capita is decreasing in the United States, the use of smokeless tobacco has actually risen, especially in school-age children. The association of tobacco with oral cancer is no surprise to a head and neck surgeon, as evidenced by one report that only 3.4% of more than 900 patients with squamous cell carcinoma of the upper aerodigestive tract had never used tobacco.

The use of alcohol, particularly in large quantities, has been linked to cancer of the upper aerodigestive tract. The addition of alcohol to tobacco is especially devastating; the incidence of oral cancer is reported to be 15 times greater in people who use both substances excessively than in people who neither smoke nor drink. It is postulated that alcohol acts primarily as a cocarcinogen or a promoter in these patients.

Exposure to ultraviolet radiation has been implicated in cancer of the lip, particularly the lower one. Other factors that are suspected of causing but have not yet been proved to cause oral squamous cell carcinoma are metabolic and dietary deficiencies. One study suggests that increased consumption of fruit and vegetables decreases the likelihood of oral cancer. Retinoic acid, a vitamin A analog, has been shown to have some protective effect against cancer of the oral cavity. Conversely, poor oral hygiene and persistent mechanical irritation from sharp teeth or ill-fitting dentures have been impli-cated as causal factors. In addition, occupational exposure to certain chemicals such as isopropyl oils, sulfuric acid, and nickel are thought to be risk factors for cancer in this area.

PATHOLOGY

Nonmalignant Lesions

Papillomas. Papillomas are usually asymptomatic, small (<8 mm in diameter), pedunculated, and located on the faucial arches, the soft palate, or the tonsillar fossas. They can be single or multiple and are usually adequately treated by simple excision. On histologic examination, they are similar to papillomas of the larynx or cervicovaginal tract: hypertrophic epithelium overlying a fibrovascular core. The human papilloma virus is the causative agent, although the exact type is variable. This is the same viral family associated with plantar warts, verruca vulgaris, condylomata acuminata, inverting papillomas of the sinonasal area, verrucous carcinoma, and some squamous cell carcinomas of the upper aerodigestive tract. Therefore, papillomas are theoretically contagious, but the host tissue must be permissive. Most papillomas remain benign and do not recur; however, malignant transformation can occur, usually associated with human papilloma virus 16, and sometimes associated with a history of irradiation exposure.

Tori. Tori of the mandible and hard palate are common and easily recognized as bony-hard excrescences along the inner plate of the lower alveolus or the midline of the hard palate. Usually they are asymptomatic and need no treatment, although many patients are referred to otolaryngologists for evaluation of a possible submucosal tumor. The overlying mucosa occasionally can become atrophic and is more susceptible to mechanical trauma from hard foods such as pizza crusts, bones, and the like. When tori fall within radiotherapy fields, they should be burred down because breakdown of the overlying mucosa predisposes the underlying bone to osteoradionecrosis.

Necrotizing Sialometaplasia. This entity is a benign lesion of the minor salivary glands that can be easily confused with a malignancy. The cause of this lesion is unknown.

Although it is most commonly reported as a reaction to injury to the mucosa (usually iatrogenic), it can occur spontaneously. Its rapid course is suggestive of an inflammatory, rather than neoplastic, process. It presents clinically as an ulcerated lesion. On histologic examination, it can be confused with squamous cell or mucoepidermoid carcinoma by a pathologist who is unfamiliar with the condition. Its clinical significance lies in the fact that the otolaryngologist must be aware of its benign nature and self-limited course, in order that deforming surgery be avoided.

Miscellaneous. Lipomas and fibromas are not uncommon and can be managed expectantly. Hemangiomas, likewise, can be diagnosed clinically and observed. Symptomatic hemangiomas are usually large, may be associated with bleeding and cosmetic deformity, and occur almost exclusively in the pediatric age group. Surgery is reserved for symptomatic lesions, because the majority regress by age 6 years. Lymphangiomas can also manifest as a submucosal mass. Surgical excision is recommended when lesions are small because they tend to grow larger as the child ages. Pyogenic granulomas appear as tender, exophytic, bleeding masses, which are not always associated with trauma that the patient can remember. Excisional biopsy is curative and diagnostic. Multiple neuromas should alert the surgeon to the possibility of multiple endocrine neoplasias; an evaluation for concomitant pheochromocytoma and medullary thyroid carcinoma is required.

Malignant Lesions

Nonsquamous Cancers. Carcinoma of a minor salivary gland can be present anywhere in the oral cavity or the oropharynx. The large majority of these lesions are malignant, usually adenoid cystic or mucoepidermoid. Wide excision and a selective, regional nodal dissection are indicated. Often, this requires partial maxillectomy or mandibulectomy. Adenoid cystic carcinoma requires sampling of any potentially involved nerves and aggressive surgical management, including an attempt to obtain a clear margin up to the skull base, if possible. Chasing the tumor intracranially, however, is futile. Although photons and electrons are not too effective, adjuvant irradiation (XRT) is recommended for any cancers involving nerves, bone, surgical margins, or nodes and any tumor greater than 2 cm in diameter. Neutron beam therapy has been suggested as a more effective modality, but it is cumbersome and not widely available.

Melanoma of the oral mucosa is much less common than its cutaneous counterpart. It should not be confused with melanosis of the oral mucosa, which is found almost universally in Black people. Other entities to be considered in the differential diagnosis include dental amalgam tattoo and vascular lesions. Any dark pigmented lesion in a White person, regardless of age, should be biopsied. For the diagnosis of melanoma, wide local excision is recommended, and palpable neck adenopathy should be resected with an appropriate neck dissection. If clinical findings are negative, the neck may be managed expectantly, although this point is controversial.

Granular cell tumors occur most commonly in the tongue. They may be exophytic or submucosal and seldom are associated with any significant symptoms. They are not cancerous and have no metastatic potential. Simple wide local excision is the proper treatment.

Lymphoma occasionally presents as enlargement of lymphoid tissue in some or all components of Waldeyer's ring, in the appropriate age group. Unilateral enlargement of a tonsil should always suggest this diagnosis. The tumor may be surprisingly large with few associated symptoms, most commonly dysphagia, dysarthria, or hyponasality. Other nodal groups should be evaluated for determination of which would be the easiest to biopsy. A posterior triangle node can be easily biopsied under local anesthesia, if the spinal accessory nerve is carefully avoided. On occasion, an axillary or epitrochlear node biopsy carries less morbidity than does general anesthesia and a tonsillectomy. Care should be taken to excise an entire node in order that the pathologist can study the nodal architecture and perform special stains or other examinations.

Premalignant Squamous Lesions. The spectrum of disease associated with squamous cell carcinoma ranges from premalignant, reversible lesions to locally aggressive carcinoma to frankly malignant carcinoma capable of metastasis. Premalignant lesions are classified by clinical appearance. *Leukoplakia* is strictly a clinical term referring to a white patch of mucosa that cannot be rubbed off without bleeding and does not include candidiasis, lichen planus, or white sponge nevus. Mechanical trauma from dentures or teeth at the occlusal plane may cause leukoplakic lesions. On histologic examination, leukoplakic lesions may display hyperkeratosis, parakeratosis, acanthosis, dysplasia, or any combination of these abnormalities. Dysplasia is classified by degree (mild, moderate, or severe) and should be considered premalignant although reversible. Malignant transformation occurs in 17% to 36% of dysplastic lesions, depending on the length of follow-up and other factors yet to be identified. Multiple factors at the molecular, cellular, extracellular, and immunologic levels are probably responsible for transformation. Biopsy of suspicious lesions is recommended, and dysplasia should be followed closely. Some patients may present with very large areas of involvement with leukoplakia; biopsy of all involved areas is impossible, impractical, and inefficient in such patients. Close follow-up and biopsy of the thicker, elevated, or erythroplastic areas are recommended.

Erythroplasia, or *erythroplakia,* refers to a mucosal patch that is redder than normal. It may occur in combination with leukoplakia or alone. Often there is epithelial atrophy, and carcinoma in situ may already be present. This lesion is a more significant premalignant lesion than is leukoplakia because it is more commonly associated with progression to invasive squamous cell carcinoma.

Squamous Cell Carcinoma. More than 95% of malignant tumors of the oral cavity and oropharynx are squamous cell carcinoma arising from oral mucosa. Typically, oral squamous carcinoma manifests as an obvious ulcerative lesion with a heaped-up border. It is friable and usually infiltrative by palpation. On occasion, tumors can protrude above the surface of adjacent mucosa as an exophytic lesion, but more commonly lesions infiltrate deeply with minimal projection above the surface and are termed endophytic. Endophytic lesions generally carry a more grave prognosis. Whereas squamous cancer of the oropharynx is frequently thought to be more aggressive than is oral cavity cancer, this aggressive character is more likely the result of the advanced stage of most cancers arising in the oropharynx at the time of diagnosis.

Verrucous carcinoma is a variant of squamous carcinoma that can occur in the oral cavity. On histopathologic examination, this lesion consists of well-differentiated squamous epithelium with a sharply circumscribed, pushing rather than infiltrating deep margin. Verrucous carcinomas do not metastasize to regional nodes or distant sites unless invasive squamous carcinoma is present in the lesion. It has been associated with human papilloma virus 16, which may be a causative agent. Biopsy of the lesion may confuse the surgeon because of the pathologist's insistence that the specimen is benign. These lesions frequently grow to large dimensions because of repeated biopsies that are reported as benign. In such cases, the diagnosis is made clinically by the surgeon, who notes aggressive local growth. Wide local excision is adequate therapy. Prophylactic neck dissection is not necessary.

Squamous carcinoma is subclassified according to the degree of differentiation. Low-grade squamous carcinoma is characterized by minimal dysplasia, keratinization, and few mitoses. High-grade tumors have cellular and nuclear pleomorphism with negligible keratinization. Frequency of mitoses, depth of infiltration, and microvascular invasion have been associated with regional node metastases and prognosis. It is generally observed, however, that the prognosis of an individual patient is dependent more on the extent of disease at the time of diagnosis than on the microscopic appearance of the primary tumor.

Lymphoepithelioma is a variant of squamous cell carcinoma that usually occurs in the palatine or lingual tonsils. It represents a poorly differentiated carcinoma with attendant lymphocytes scattered throughout the lesion. The clinical behavior of this cancer differs from that of most squamous cell carcinomas in that this cancer is more often associated with early nodal and distant metastases. It is particularly responsive to radiation therapy.

Squamous cell carcinoma of the oral cavity and the oropharynx tends to remain localized to the primary and regional node sites. Distant metastases occur relatively late in the course of the disease and are associated with recurrent disease above the clavicle in the vast majority of patients. The incidence of distant metastasis ranges from 10% to 45%, depending on whether clinical disease or incidental autopsy findings are considered. The pharynx, the base of tongue, and the anterior tongue, in decreasing order, have the highest likelihood of distant metastasis. Because local and regional therapy has proved effective in controlling disease, it is anticipated that a larger population of patients will fail to benefit from treatment at distant sites. Most distant metastases occur in the lung, the liver, and the bone.

Multiple primary cancers may occur synchronously or metachronously. The diagnosis of a second primary depends on specific criteria: both tumors must be clearly malignant on histologic examination, each must be separated anatomically from the other without any submucosal connection or intraepithelial neoplastic changes, and the possibility that one might represent a metastasis from the other must be excluded. The incidence of a second primary lesion is reported as 5% to 30% and is higher for lesions of the oropharynx than for those arising in the oral cavity.

PREOPERATIVE EVALUATION

When the patient with cancer of the oral cavity or the oropharynx presents at the surgeon's office, a full history should be obtained from the patient and should include the duration of the presenting complaint and related symptoms of dysphagia, dysarthria, otalgia, cranial nerve hypoesthesias, headaches (skull base involvement), and hearing loss (eustachian tube obstruction). The patient may have noted advanced physical signs, including loose teeth, trismus, voice change, neck mass, cranial nerve palsies, or skin involvement. A history of tobacco use in any form predisposes the patient to squamous cell cancer, especially in conjunction with alcohol consumption. A history of premalignant oral lesions or cancer is important. In women, a history of cervicovaginal papillomas or cancer may be suggestive of related lesions in the upper aerodigestive tract.

In obtaining the usual medical history, the surgeon should pay special attention to diseases related to tobacco and alcohol abuse because so many lesions are related to the use of these substances. A history of hypertension, stroke, myocardial infarction, arrhythmias, renal disease, peripheral vascular disease, emphysema, lung cancer, or other pulmonary disease should be explicitly determined. A general, qualitative assessment of exercise tolerance should be obtained. Although all patients are treated with prophylactic antibiotics, it is good practice to know whether a patient has any prosthetic valves or implants. Because of the length of some of these operative procedures, a history of pulmonary emboli is important to know. Clotting disorders or ingestion of aspirin or other nonsteroidal anti-inflammatory medication should be discovered and, if possible, discontinued no later than 2 weeks before surgery. Systemic use of steroids increases the chances of fistula formation; because this usually cannot be discontinued, arrangements must be made to provide a large dose of steroids ("stress dose") intravenously, intraoperatively, and postoperatively until the patient resumes enteral alimentation. If the patient is malnourished, consideration should be given to placing a nasogastric tube during the first office visit. Many patients will not have stopped their alcohol consumption by the time of the operation. These patients may be managed with either intravenous diazepam, lorazepam, or chlordiazepoxide. Often, a smoother course without fear of respiratory depression or hypersomnolence is achieved with intraoperative 5% ethanol drip intravenously. The usual postoperative dose is 30 mL/hour, which can be titrated up or down until the patient feels normal and then can be decreased 5 mL daily until it is tapered off. Finally, the patient often needs adequate pain relief for the interim between diagnosis and treatment.

Preoperative blood values that should be routinely obtained include complete blood count, platelet count, prothrombin and partial thromboplastin times, and template bleeding time for patients taking aspirin or related medications; electrolyte, glucose, urea nitrogen, and creatinine level determinations; liver function tests; and, often, arterial blood gas analyses on room air. Pulmonary function should be assessed clinically; if it is thought to be borderline, spirometry tests with and without bronchodilators should be obtained. An electrocardiogram is essential for any patient who is over 40 years of age or who has any history of or is suspected of having cardiac disease. In such cases, formal cardiologic consultation is mandatory preoperatively. A chest film is also essential, both for the anesthesiologist and to rule out any synchronous lung primary or metastatic lesion.

TREATMENT OF THE NECK

The single most important predictor of prognosis in squamous cell cancer of the oral cavity and the oropharynx is the status of the cervical lymph nodes. Proper treatment of the neck with clinical and subclinical disease is essential because recurrence in the neck usually portends death from the disease. The appropriate treatment of neck disease is controversial because of the variable presentation of these cancers, the variable incidence of occult neck disease, the different biologic behavior of cancers from different sites, the variable status and the current indeterminability of patient immune parameters, and the various kinds of neck dissection procedures available.

Certainly, all clinically palpable neck disease should be surgically extirpated. Whether such an operation entails a classical, radical neck dissection or a selective, function-sparing, modified neck dissection depends on the surgeon's training and experience. The classical radical neck dissection should include all nodal tissue from the submental, submandibular, upper, middle, and lower jugular chains and from the entire posterior triangle as well as the sternocleidomastoideus, the internal jugular vein, and the spinal accessory nerve from the jugular foramen to its insertions in the trapezius. Nodal groups not removed by a classical radical neck dissection include those of the retropharyngeal, paratracheal, superior mediastinal, buccal, facial, periparotid, postauricular, and suboccipital regions. Modified neck dissections were envisioned and designed to decrease the morbidity associated with sacrifice of the soft tissue components of the radical neck dissection. There is good evidence that preservation of the sternocleidomastoideus, spinal accessory nerve, and internal jugular vein does not compromise the oncologic purity of the operation as long as the original tenets of Bocca are strictly followed; that is, the nodal tissue must be removed by not violating the fascial planes that envelop them. Any intraoperative evidence of extranodal disease, however, should mandate local resection of whichever soft tissue structure is involved: nerve, muscle, or vessel. In other words, resection of disease takes precedence over preservation of function.

Because the morbidity associated with a modified neck dissection is relatively low, the efficacy of surgical treatment of the N0 neck is a pertinent question. In terms of disease control, waiting for nodal metastases to develop has been shown to be inferior to prophylactically removing the nodal groups most at risk. Predicting which primary sites and which nodal groups are most likely to be involved with metastases has been based on large retrospective studies. In addition to the radial tumor dimension, certain histopathologic parameters have been positively associated with an increased incidence of regional nodal metastases. These parameters include depth of invasion and microvascular involvement. Most squamous cell cancers of the inferior part of the oral cavity that are deeper than 3 mm thick should have neck dissections, if they can be performed with minimal morbidity. The nodal groups that should be addressed for the anterior oral tongue, the anterior floor of the mouth, and the anterior gingiva are the submental region, the submandibular region, and the upper and middle jugular chains. For lesions at these sites approaching the posterior oral cavity and the retromolar trigone, the upper posterior triangle should also be dissected; such a dissection is termed the *supraomohyoid* neck dissection in the literature. Lesions of the posterior oral tongue may sometimes involve the nodes of the low jugular chain, if there are suspicious nodes found higher in the jugular chain during the dissection. If the low jugular chain or the upper posterior region is involved, the entire posterior triangle should be dissected; this procedure completes a formal "functional" neck dissection. Lesions of the hard palate rarely metastasize; operations for lesions of size T2 and greater should include a supraomohyoid neck dissection.

Lesions of the oropharynx are more likely to metastasize than are oral cavity primary lesions. However, because of the different biologic behavior of these lesions, surgical treatment is not always the first modality. Tonsillar cancer commonly produces cystic metastases, which should not be confused with branchial apparatus cysts. Cancers of the tonsil and oropharyngeal wall, especially exophytic forms, seem to respond well to external beam radiotherapy if they are size

T1 or T2. The neck is given a curative dose of radiotherapy during treatment of the primary lesion. If the neck is clinically N0, then the neck is definitively treated. If the neck is clinically N1, the adenopathy will likely respond well. For more extensive neck disease, further surgical treatment will likely be necessary. This should not be undertaken until 6 weeks after the end of radiotherapy, because the effects of XRT on the primary lesion are not fully known until that time. For tonsillar or oropharyngeal wall cancer larger than T2, the surgical approach to the primary lesion necessitates a neck dissection; the nodal groups to be addressed are the submandibular region, the upper and middle jugular chains, and the upper and middle posterior triangle. In addition, detectable retropharyngeal nodes should be removed.

Cancers of the soft palate are surgically treated but have a low metastatic potential; lesions T2 and larger should include removal of the upper and middle jugular, the upper and middle posterior triangle, and the retropharyngeal chain of nodes, if possible. Lesions of the base of tongue have a high incidence of cervical node metastases that are often bilateral. Small lesions sometimes are treated by XRT definitively; the necks are treated surgically only in case of XRT failure. Larger lesions are treated surgically, and the nodal groups to be included in the neck dissections include the submandibular region, the upper and middle jugular chains, and the upper and middle posterior triangles, bilaterally. If there is obvious nodal involvement of the middle jugular nodes, the lower jugular chain should also be dissected.

For lesions approaching the midline, treatment for bilateral metastases must be considered, and different modalities may be used for each side of the neck. In cases in which combined therapy (surgery plus postoperative XRT) is mandatory and assumed preoperatively, and the clinical findings for the contralateral neck are negative, control of disease in the contralateral neck with XRT alone is probably adequate. If the preoperative hope is that surgical therapy alone will be adequate, then contralateral neck dissection is indicated with the definitive operation. If the primary resection will cause edema or obstruction of the contralateral Wharton's duct, removal of the contralateral submandibular triangle is advised in order to circumvent future confusion between the obstructed gland and metastases.

Because important therapeutic decisions are based on the pathologic findings, communication with the pathologist is essential. The surgical specimen from the neck should be brought to the pathology laboratory and oriented for the pathologist. The nodal groups should be delineated so that useful pathologic information about the patient's stage of disease can be elicited. By convention, cervical lymph nodes are divided into levels. Level I includes the contents of the submandibular and submental triangles. Levels II, III, and IV represent, respectively, the upper, middle, and lower jugular chains, and level V represents the posterior triangle.

In general, survival of patients with regional node metastases is approximately half that expected if the cancer were confined to the primary site. When nodal metastases are multiple, low in the neck, or contralateral, or when disease extends beyond the lymph node capsule (extracapsular spread), survival is further compromised, and the patient's disease is rarely controlled by surgery alone.

RADIOTHERAPY AND CHEMOTHERAPY

Definitive radiotherapy (XRT) is usually accomplished by external beam application of photons, from either a cobalt (^{60}Co) source or a linear accelerator. XRT should be used either as definitive therapy or as an adjunctive modality postoperatively. There is no longer any indication for a preoperative, noncurative dose of XRT or for split-course radiotherapy in the treatment of cancer in the oral cavity or in the oropharynx. Most small primary lesions of these sites respond to definitive XRT, but surgery is recommended in most cases as a first line of treatment because it represents a simple, expeditious treatment that provides valuable pathologic information and does not require special care or management of the teeth. Although the visible and symptomatic sequelae of XRT are its most obvious morbid consequences, the most important disadvantage of XRT is the fact that it can be used only once. In a population of patients with a 20% incidence of second primary lesions and a higher incidence of recurrence with many lesions, XRT must not be used casually too early in the treatment course.

Lesions that are recommended to be

treated by XRT as a primary modality with curative intent include exophytic T1 and T2 tonsil cancer and T1, T2, and sometimes T3 oropharyngeal cancer. Exophytic lesions seem to respond to XRT more favorably than do endophytic ones. Lesions of the tonsil that invade the tongue base respond more poorly and often recur in the tongue. Occasionally, a small (T1) cancer of the base of the tongue can be treated by XRT.

Adjunctive XRT is recommended for any lesion, size T3 or larger, of the oral cavity or the oropharynx. For lesions of size T1 or T2, the decision to prescribe adjunctive XRT is based on histopathologic criteria. Indications for XRT, based on findings at the primary site, include close or involved surgical margins, perineural or microvascular invasion, or bone invasion. Indications based on findings in the neck specimen include involvement of more than one node, involvement of a node at the lowest point of dissection (e.g., the middle jugular chain), involvement of a node that is not in the primary echelon of drainage, extranodal extension, or soft tissue involvement. The XRT fields should cover the entirety of the operative field and the neck. The XRT should always begin within 6 weeks of the operative date, if at all possible. The prompt administration of postoperative XRT may occasionally necessitate its administration in the face of incompletely healed incisions or persistent fistulas.

Pre-XRT evaluation must include dental consultation. Osteoradionecrosis is a fearsome complication and must be avoided. When combined therapy is planned, teeth suspected of being susceptible to osteoradionecrosis should be extracted either before or during the definitive surgery. Fluoride carriers help prevent caries postoperatively. The patient must be informed that lifelong good dental care is essential, and dentists providing future dental treatment should be warned not to perform extractions or significant dental manipulations at any time after XRT.

While the patient is undergoing XRT, follow-up visits should be performed every 1 to 2 weeks. Caloric intake should be monitored. Poor nutrition may predispose the patient to intolerance of XRT, leading the radiotherapist to break regimen and compromise treatment. If weight loss is significant (>10 lb, or >4.5 kg), consideration should be given to placement of a small-bore nasogastric tube until the radiation effects subside. If a long period of inability to feed by mouth is anticipated,

placement of a feeding gastrostomy is helpful and easily tolerated; this can be placed as an open procedure or percutaneously with the help of an endoscope or a fluoroscopically competent radiologist.

Post-XRT follow-up should include timely evaluation of thyroid function, beginning 3 months after the end of XRT and every 4 to 6 months thereafter. If the XRT fields extended up to the skull base, pituitary function needs to be routinely monitored.

The role of chemotherapy in the treatment of cancer of the oral cavity and the oropharynx has not yet been determined. Although patients whose tumors respond to chemotherapy (especially complete responders) have an improved survival and disease-free interval, no prospective randomized study to date has demonstrated evidence that survival of patients treated with chemotherapy is better than that of those who receive conventional treatment. At this time, neoadjuvant chemotherapy should probably not be used outside of prospective, randomized clinical trials. More specific information regarding chemotherapy of head and neck cancers is contained in Chapter 56.

SQUAMOUS CELL CARCINOMA

Floor of Mouth

The floor of the mouth is the region bounded by the lingual plates of the mandible laterally and the tongue medially; it extends from the anterior tonsillar pillars on both sides to the anterior midline. The anterior part of this area is easily inspected, but more persistence is needed to examine the posteriormost extent. Although anterior lesions are first seen by the patient, by an internist, or by a dentist, the otolaryngologist is often the only physician to visualize the posterior floor of mouth. This is best done with two tongue depressors, one retracting the tongue medially and one pulling the oral commissure laterally. Bimanual palpation should be a part of the examination of all patients with oral cavity cancer.

Squamous cell carcinoma of this region manifests most commonly in the sixth and seventh decades, at a median age of 60 years. Men are affected more than twice as frequently as are women. Lesions are clinically graded by the American Joint Committee on

Cancer Staging criteria of 1988 (Table 32–1). The visible part of cancer of the floor of the mouth often does not represent the entirety of the tumor. Lesions T2 and larger often have submucosal components that are best

TABLE 32–1. Staging of Oral Cavity/ Oropharyngeal Cancer

Primary Tumor (T)

TX	Primary tumor cannot be assessed
T0	No evidence of primary tumor
Tis	Carcinoma in situ
T1	Tumor 2 cm or less in greatest dimension
T2	Tumor more than 2 cm but not more than 4 cm in greatest dimension
T3	Tumor more than 4 cm in greatest dimension
T4	(Oral cavity) Tumor invades adjacent structure, e.g., through cortical bone, into deep (extrinsic) muscle of tongue, maxillary sinus, skin
T4	(Oropharynx) Tumor invades adjacent structures, e.g., through cortical bone, soft tissue of neck, deep (extrinsic) muscle of tongue

Regional Lymph Nodes (N)

NX	Regional lymph nodes cannot be assessed
N0	No regional lymph node metastasis
N1	Metastasis in a single ipsilateral lymph node, 3 cm or less in greatest dimension
N2	Metastasis in a single ipsilateral lymph node, more than 3 cm but not more than 6 cm in greatest dimension; or in multiple ipsilateral lymph nodes, none more than 6 cm in greatest dimension; or in bilateral or contralateral lymph nodes, none more than 6 cm in greatest dimension
N2a	Metastasis in single ipsilateral lymph node more than 3 cm but no more than 6 cm in greatest dimension
N2b	Metastasis in multiple ipsilateral lymph nodes, none more than 6 cm in greatest dimension
N2c	Metastasis in bilateral or contralateral lymph nodes, none more than 6 cm in greatest dimension
N3	Metastasis in a lymph node more than 6 cm in greatest dimension

Distant Metastasis (MO)

MX	Presence of distant metastasis cannot be assessed
M0	No distant metastasis
M1	Distant metastasis

Stage Grouping

Stage 0	Tis	N0	M0
Stage I	T1	N0	M0
Stage II	T2	N0	M0
Stage III	T3	N0	M0
	T1	N1	M0
	T2	N1	M0
	T3	N1	M0
Stage IV	T4	N0, N1	M0
	Any T	N2, N3	M0
	Any T	Any N	M1

evaluated by bimanual palpation; the extent of invasion of the tongue root or base can be palpated by placing the external fingers above the hyoid bone. The lingual plate of the mandible is relatively resistant to early cancer invasion, but the periosteum is not. Involvement of the periosteum should be suspected if the lesion is not easily mobile, even if the mucosal abnormality does not reach the alveolar mucosa.

Radiologic evaluation of the extent of early bone invasion is critical for lesions that approach the mandible. Dental occlusal view films have the advantage of demonstrating the inner cortex with a single view. Panorex evaluation delineates the location of the inferior alveolar canal; this information is valuable in the edentulous patient in whom partial mandibulectomy is being considered. In addition, unilateral widening of the canal may indicate perineural invasion. Computed tomography (CT) scans of the area can accurately depict depth of tumor invasion and can depict even minimal cortical bone erosion, provided that thin bone-window slices are obtained in the proper plane. CT scans also show how much tongue involvement exists. It is important to know the extent of marrow involvement in cancers that have progressed through the lingual plate; these margins can best be evaluated by magnetic resonance imaging (MRI) findings, especially with T1-weighted imaging. The role of nuclear bone scans is minimal.

The treatment of choice for all squamous cell cancers of the floor of the mouth is surgical, with adjunctive, postoperative XRT as indicated. All surgical manipulations of the aerodigestive tract are covered prophylactically with antibiotics, usually metronidazole and a second-generation cephalosporin or clindamycin alone. Superficial lesions can be resected transorally and reconstructed by primary closure, split-thickness skin graft, or dermal graft or left to granulate by secondary intention.

Invasion of any significant portion of tongue warrants cautious surgical extirpation. The degree of invasion of the tongue musculature by any cancer is notoriously difficult to determine. A principal reason for recurrence at the primary site is an inadequate deep margin of resection. It is rarely possible for the surgeon to identify the exact site of an initially positive frozen section deep margin. Thus resection of additional tissue, resulting in a subsequently negative margin, cannot be done with assurance, and adjunctive XRT is indicated. It is important to perform this part of the operation by palpation of normal tongue and use of electrocautery for a clean surgical field. Posteriorly, sacrifice of the lingual nerve is not uncommon. Anteriorly, sacrifice of the hypoglossal nerve is acceptable on one side, but care should be used in order to attempt preservation of the contralateral cranial nerve XII if possible.

Lesions with periosteal invasion should be carefully evaluated as the periosteum is being stripped off the bone; if there appears to be any involvement of the inner aspect of the periosteum, then consideration should be given to bone resection. If such is the case anteriorly, resection of just the lingual plate or just the alveolus can be attempted in order to preserve the integrity of the anterior mandibular arch, which is very difficult to reconstruct well. Posterior lesions involving the periosteum can be resected with a segment of the upper aspect of the posterior mandibular body and the anterior aspect of the ascending ramus. Such mandible-saving procedures are more tenuous and ill-advised in long-edentulous patients who have had resorption of the vertical dimension of their mandibular bodies and therefore have little reserve of bone strength. Preoperative Panorex evaluation helps determine whether a marginal mandibulectomy is feasible. A segmental resection of mandible and reconstruction (discussed in the following section) is preferred to a postoperative mandibular fracture. If all the bone is resected down to the inferior alveolar nerve canal, it is advisable to reconstruct with a flap with some thickness because a simple skin graft will leave a bare sensory nerve, which will cause postoperative pain. Some of these mandibular procedures can be performed through the transoral approach, but visualization may be compromised. In such a case, the surgeon should use a lip-splitting or pull-through approach rather than risk a recurrence at the primary site, which would necessitate an extensive mandibulectomy.

Any involvement of bone requires resection of a full-height portion of bone (segmental mandibulectomy). For such exposure, a lip-splitting approach is unexcelled, although healing of the lip and the flap is suboptimal because of less venous and lymphatic drainage. An apron flap can be lifted, in the subperiosteal plane, up as high as the condyle, but exposure is difficult to accomplish without the aid of two experienced assistants. A margin of 2 cm of healthy bone is usually adequate. Any resection posterior to the premolar area should usually encompass the entirety of the posterior mandible, including the condyle and the coronoid, especially in elderly, edentulous patients. Such a defect rarely causes any significant masticatory dysfunction. The mentum will swing to the side of the defect, causing a slight cosmetic deformity, but the total shift is rarely more than 2 cm. Occasionally, patients complain of temporomandibular joint pain in the contralateral joint, which is usually managed conservatively. In younger, dentate patients, there may be a greater effort at reconstruction of proper occlusion. In such cases, preservation of the condyle and upper ascending ramus is advisable, with reconstruction either immediate or delayed. If delayed reconstruction is to be performed, proper occlusion can be ensured by fashioning mandibular reconstruction plates before the resection. These plates are likely to make adjunctive XRT difficult, but there is no good alternative. In addition, with a plate in place, a soft tissue flap is necessary for coverage and closure.

Segmental mandibulectomy of the anterior mandibular arch continues to be a difficult reconstructive problem, which will be discussed later in this chapter. Inadequate reconstruction can lead to oral commissure incompetence, drooling and subsequent skin excoriation, speech and swallowing dysfunction, and depression resulting from disfigurement and societal estrangement. Use of a mandibular plate, even if it is wrapped in a large muscle flap, is complicated by plate exposure and fistulization in a high (>60%) percentage of cases.

Palpable neck metastases should be resected along with the primary lesion. The issue of prophylactic neck dissections is addressed in the section Treatment of the Neck. Adjunctive XRT should be initiated by the sixth or, at the very latest, eighth postoperative week, even in the presence of complications, if there is to be any hope of cure.

Eradication of this disease should approximate 80% to 90% for stage I and stage II disease at 5 years. Stage III disease is associated with a 65% survival rate and stage IV with a 33% survival rate, even with combined therapy.

Oral Tongue

The peak incidence of tongue cancer is in the sixth and seventh decades of life, but studies have shown an increased incidence in people 40 years of age or younger. Tongue cancer in this younger age group is frequently advanced by the time of presentation, is difficult to control, and tends to occur without an associated history of tobacco or alcohol use. Aggressive surgical treatment appears to meet with greater success than does irradiation in this select group of patients. Reviews of patients with tongue cancer have also demonstrated a steadily increasing proportion of females (now approximately 30%) with this disease, presumably a reflection of an increased use of tobacco and alcohol by women.

Most cancers of the oral tongue involve the lateral or ventral surfaces; involvement of the dorsum or midline is unusual. Early lesions are frequently asymptomatic, and pain is commonly associated with larger tumors. Local anesthesia, paresthesia, and bleeding are infrequent; patients often do not present for treatment until one or more regional lymph nodes are clinically involved. Late symptoms include pain perceived as otalgia, difficulty with articulation and swallowing, and weight loss.

Examination of the patient with cancer of the oral tongue most commonly shows an ulcerative lesion of the lateral or ventral tongue, usually without evidence of surrounding leukoplakia or erythroplakia. Pain associated with the lesion often limits tongue mobility. Bimanual palpation of the tongue and the floor of the mouth delineates the infiltrative, deep margin of the cancer and confirms involvement of contiguous structures such as the adjacent floor of the mouth, the inner table of the mandible, or the tonsillar pillar. In patients with no apparent ulcer or mucosal abnormality, a minor neoplasm of the salivary gland must be considered. Massive tumors can extend into surrounding soft tissues such as the deep intrinsic tongue muscles, the base of the tongue, and the mandible to the degree that the exact primary site of the neoplasm cannot be ascertained and differentiation between direct extension of disease and regional node involvement can be difficult. Radiologic evaluation of the primary and regional nodes by contrast medium–enhanced CT or MRI can delineate the extent of disease, the involvement of surrounding structures, and the spread to regional nodes. Such studies should be performed before biopsy in order to avoid hemorrhage-related artifact.

At the time of presentation, most cancers of the oral tongue tend to be early-stage disease, and only one third of patients have clinically apparent regional node involvement. Evidence of distant metastasis is exceptionally rare at the time of initial evaluation.

Either partial glossectomy or irradiation represents satisfactory management of a T1 cancer of the tongue, although surgery alone represents a simple, expeditious treatment that does not require special care or management of the teeth. Small, anterior tumors (T1 and some T2) can be resected and the defect closed primarily with little attendant morbidity. More extensive cancers (T3 and T4) require sacrifice of greater portions of the tongue, which leads to more significant postoperative functional disability. Reconstruction of the defect by use of skin grafts or flaps is often required. Direct invasion of the mandible requires a segmental mandibulectomy, whereas resection of the inner table or the rim alone (marginal mandibulectomy) is probably sufficient for tumor resection when the cancer approaches but does not invade bone.

Neck dissection is indicated for any patient with clinical evidence of cervical node involvement. Treatment of the neck with clinically negative findings is addressed in the section Treatment of the Neck. Postoperative XRT should be administered according to guidelines given in the section Radiotherapy and Chemotherapy and should be initiated no later than 6 to 8 weeks after surgery.

The 5-year disease-free survival rate of patients with oral tongue cancer is roughly 40%. The cause of death in most patients treated for tongue cancers is locoregional failure, and only 15% of patients die of clinically apparent distant metastasis. Up to 30% of patients develop a second primary cancer, usually in the upper aerodigestive tract. Survival is affected by stage of disease, the presence of histologically positive cervical nodes, and the presence of extracapsular spread of nodal disease. The combination of surgery plus radiation therapy may favorably influence survival of patients with more advanced disease.

Gingival Retromolar Trigone

Lesions of this area include those originating on the alveolus or posterior to the last molar. Men and women are affected in approximately equal ratios; the mean age is in the sixth decade. Patients commonly present with bleeding lesions or loose teeth. Involvement of the inferior alveolar nerve can be suspected in a patient with anesthetic teeth or mentum. Preoperative evaluation of the extent of proximal trigeminal involvement can be assisted by MRI scan.

The primary modality of therapy is surgical if there is no intracranial involvement. Retrograde clearance of the nerve should be attempted, up to the foramen ovale; chasing the tumor into the gasserian ganglion is not fruitful. Anterograde spread of the cancer out of the mental foramen also must be considered and removed. On occasion, very large tumors invade the soft tissues of the chin, and reconstruction may involve skin coverage. Lateral spread into the buccal area must be carefully resected. Lesions with posterior invasion manifest with symptoms that suggest a tonsillar primary, which is discussed later in this chapter.

Bone invasion is associated even with small lesions because of the proximity of the mandible. Evaluation of the mandible and marrow is performed as described in the section on lesions of the floor of the mouth. The extent of mandibulectomy is likewise guided by the same principles as those used with floor of mouth lesions. Resection of retromolar trigone lesions almost always requires a posterior mandibulectomy.

Indications for surgical treatment of the neck are the same as those outlined for floor of mouth lesions. Histopathologic findings at the primary site and in the neck dictate the need for adjunctive, postoperative radiotherapy.

Reconstruction can often be simple primary closure if the primary lesion is not too wide. If a marginal mandibulectomy is performed, a split-thickness skin graft can suffice. For a larger defect, the radial forearm free flap is the preferred flap because of its reliability, thinness, and pliability. Unfortunately, this technique is not widely available yet. Various pedicled muscle–soft-tissue flaps are also reliable although accompanied by some oral dysfunction. Large through-and-through defects can usually be reconstructed with a pectoralis major myocutaneous flap with a split-thickness skin graft on the outside.

The survival rate at 2 years is good in comparison with other oral cavity sites. Stage I disease can be associated with a 2-year survival rate of nearly 100%, stage II with 75%, stage III with 60%, and stage IV with 50%.

Buccal Mucosa

The median age of onset for cancer of the cheek or the buccal mucosa is in the seventh decade, and its occurrence in a patient under 40 years of age is rare. This site is an uncommon one for patients in the United States: this cancer represents approximately 5% of cancers of the oral cavity. The great majority of patients with cancer of the buccal mucosa are male.

Alcohol and tobacco consumption are closely linked to cancer of the buccal mucosa. In India, where tobacco chewing is common, the incidence of buccal mucosal cancer is second only to that of cancer of the tongue among oral cavity sites. Many buccal cancers occur along the occlusal line of the cheek, the area of buccal mucosa opposite the point at which the upper and lower teeth articulate. This fact suggests that trauma from sharp or broken teeth or from ill-fitting dentures may be a causative factor.

Early cancer of the buccal mucosa is seldom symptomatic, and delay in diagnosis of 6 to 12 months is common, as evidenced by the fact that approximately half of patients present with disease at stage III or greater. Anterior lesions usually manifest early and are less commonly associated with regional node disease, which, when present, is often confined to the submandibular triangle. More posterior cancers are more often advanced and can involve the adjacent buccinator, the masseter, and the pterygoid muscles, causing pain and trismus. Cancers located posteriorly are more commonly associated with regional node involvement, usually the upper jugular nodes. Overall, approximately one third of patients with cancer of the buccal mucosa present with cervical node metastasis.

Cancers of the buccal mucosa are more often associated with leukoplakia than are other oral cancers. They usually begin as small, ulcerated lesions with surrounding induration, although superficial papillary or verrucous cancers can occur, usually in association with the use of smokeless tobacco. In rare instances, patients may present with far-advanced cancer with severe trismus and through-and-through involvement of the cheek. Visual and bimanual examination of the patient with buccal mucosal cancer helps to delineate the extent of tumor involvement, but CT or MRI evaluation is indicated to determine involvement of the maxilla or mandible as well as regional node spread.

T1 cancer of the buccal mucosa may be satisfactorily treated with either primary irradiation or transoral excision. Surgery offers the advantage of simplicity and does not require special treatment of the teeth. Small defects can be closed primarily and larger ones resurfaced with a skin graft, preferably dermal or full-thickness, for avoiding contracture and subsequent trismus. More extensive lesions, especially those that invade the bone of the maxilla or the mandible, cannot be treated effectively with irradiation and require primary surgery and immediate, one-stage reconstruction. Neck dissection is indicated in any patient with clinically positive nodes or when there is a high likelihood for nodal involvement in the clinically negative neck. Postoperative irradiation is probably indicated for advanced disease (stage III or stage IV) or for the specific indications listed in the section Radiotherapy and Chemotherapy.

The 5-year disease-free survival rate for patients with cancer of the buccal mucosa is 35% to 40%. Survival varies according to the stage of disease, the thickness of the primary, the presence of histologically positive nodes, and the presence of extracapsular spread of nodal disease.

Hard and Soft Palate

Squamous cell carcinoma represents a smaller percentage of all palate tumors because of the correspondingly larger number of other histopathologic types, mostly minor salivary gland cancers. Squamous cell cancer of the hard palate is primarily a disease of the elderly, usually men in their seventh decade of life. The same lesion located on the soft palate, however, usually manifests in a younger age group, averaging in the fifth and sixth decades. The manifestation is usually an ulcerated lesion that does not heal over a course of several months. Necrotizing sialometaplasia must be ruled out by history and biopsy. Advanced lesions may manifest with oronasal or oroantral fistulas. Neural extension along the palatine nerves causes pain. A mucosal abnormality of the hard palate may represent a "tip of the iceberg" phenomenon, the bulk of the tumor being an antral cancer.

Radiologic examination with CT is best for evaluating the amount of superior invasion into the sinus and nasal cavity and the amount of bone invasion. Skull base invasion at the eustachian tube contraindicates surgical therapy.

The primary modality of therapy for both hard and soft palate squamous cell cancers is surgery. Transoral resection of small lesions is possible. If the soft palate can be left intact during resection of hard palate lesions, speech and deglutition rehabilitation is much simplified. For lesions of the soft palate, usually the majority of the soft palate should be resected, even if the uvula is not involved. Although several pedicled flaps have been described for palatal reconstruction, the easiest and fastest reconstructive method is the palatal obturator. For this reason, it is preferable to attempt to save at least two maxillary teeth for anchoring the prosthesis; permanent screwing of the prosthesis into the palate has also been described.

Larger lesions require an infrastructure maxillectomy that can sometimes be performed transorally but usually require more exposure, such as through a Weber-Ferguson or a facial degloving approach. If there is posterior extension into the pterygoid region, a formal maxillectomy is necessary.

Preoperative evaluation by a dental colleague is essential. Many of the patients need combined therapy. Indications for postoperative XRT are the same as those for both primary and regional disease. The incidence of regional metastases to the neck is low enough that prophylactic neck dissection is not recommended. Clinically palpable neck disease should, of course, be resected, with the fact borne in mind that the primary echelon of drainage is the retropharyngeal nodal chain, which is not usually surgically addressed.

Cure rates for 5 years can be expected to be 75% for stage I, 50% for stage II, 35% for stage III, and less than 15% for stage IV disease. Lack of local control at the skull base is the reason for low survival rates of patients with advanced disease.

Tonsillar Fossa/Faucial Pillars

Squamous cell cancer of the tonsillar fossa or faucial pillar affects men more than twice as often as women. The mean age at diagnosis is 58 years. A lesion of this area manifests as a sore throat, dysphagia, odynophagia, or otalgia. More advanced lesions cause trismus as the pterygoid musculature becomes involved. In turn, the presence of trismus makes examination more difficult. Hence these lesions are often underestimated clinically. Bimanual examination is mandatory although uncomfortable for the patient. Involvement of the trigeminal nerve branches causes anesthesia along the alveolus, the teeth, or the chin; anesthesia of the ipsilateral tongue signifies lingual nerve involvement in the parapharyngeal space. Larger, deeper lesions may involve the major vessels.

Adequate evaluation of a lesion in this area requires a CT scan with intravenous contrast material. Special attention should be paid to the amount of skull base involvement, to whether the internal carotid artery is clear, and to the amount of tongue invasion. Intracranial, eustachian tube, or significant nasopharyngeal involvement is a contraindication to surgical therapy.

Early lesions (T1 or T2) can be treated with definitive, high-dosage radiotherapy in an attempt to save the patient a major operative procedure. Lesions that are exophytic on gross examination seem to respond well to XRT. Lesions that creep down onto the glossopalatine fold, or with frank tongue involvement, are more likely to fail to respond to XRT; the site of failure is in the tongue musculature.

Larger or infiltrating lesions require combined therapy (surgery plus postoperative XRT). Surgical approach to the tonsillar area requires partial mandibulectomy, and a lip-splitting incision may be required for adequate exposure. Resection of the maxillary tuberosity (partial maxillectomy) is required for lesions that extend onto the upper gingiva. If there is tongue involvement, the tongue margin must have more than adequate clearance for disease-free survival. If there is carotid involvement, preoperative occlusion studies can be helpful in determining whether sacrifice of the internal carotid will be tolerable, but the chance of cure is low.

If surgery is planned as the primary modality of treatment, regional metastases are addressed as outlined in the section Treatment of the Neck. If the primary lesion is amenable to XRT as a definitive measure, disease in the neck is treated concomitantly with XRT. However, small primary lesions can be associated with large nodal disease, and metastatic deposits greater than 3 cm are not likely to be controlled with XRT alone. Postirradiation surgical resection of such neck disease is often necessary, in which case either a radical or a full, functional dissection of all nodal groups in the neck is recommended. Surgical salvage should not be attempted until 6 weeks have elapsed after XRT is completed, in order to determine whether any surgical treatment of the primary site is also necessary. From a histopathologic perspective, the full effects of radiation cannot be determined until this time period has passed. Some surgeons advocate performing the neck dissection first, with XRT planned as the definitive modality for the primary site. The only advantage of such a schedule is the ease of dissection of an untreated neck in comparison with dissection of an irradiated neck. The disadvantages include the theoretically decreased efficacy of XRT in a neck rendered surgically hypoxic and the distinct possibility of XRT failure at the primary site, which would necessitate another operation for treatment of the persistent primary lesion.

Prognosis for cancers originating at this site is not good. Stage I disease can be expected to entail a survival rate of 65% to 75%, regardless of modality, and that of stage II is approximately 50%. The higher stages are associated with skull base invasion and recurrence, and 5-year survival is less than 20% for stage IV disease.

Base of Tongue

Cancer of the base of tongue tends to occur in older patients; the peak incidence is in the sixth and seventh decades. Men are more commonly affected than are women in a ratio of 2:1. Early cancers are asymptomatic; tumors often reach a considerable size before becoming clinically apparent. A vague discomfort or irritation is frequently the earliest complaint, usually followed by pain when the cancer becomes deeply infiltrative. Referred otalgia is common and indicates advanced disease. Infiltration of the pterygoid muscles can lead to trismus, and extensive invasion of the base of the tongue can restrict tongue mobility, with production of dysarthria and dysphagia. Large tumors are usually associated with decreased oral intake, weight loss, and malnutrition.

Patients with cancer of the base of tongue usually present late; advanced tumors outnumber early lesions in the ratio of 4:1. Approximately 80% of patients with cancer of the base of the tongue present with clinical evidence of regional node disease, and 20% have bilateral neck metastasis.

A patient suspected of having cancer of the base of the tongue should undergo a complete head and neck examination. The base of the tongue is difficult to evaluate by visual examination, and palpation provides better assessment. Unfortunately, patients with trismus are difficult to examine visually or by palpation. Often, patients have difficulty protruding the tongue and have impaired sensation of the ipsilateral tongue, the teeth, and the mental nerve distribution. An indirect mirror or fiberoptic examination is essential for determining the inferior extent of disease as well as the competency of the larynx. Patients with cancer of the oral cavity or the oropharynx usually have a history of tobacco and alcohol use, and a thorough history and a physical examination along with appropriate evaluation of the teeth, the lungs (chest film and pulmonary functions), the cardiovascular system, the liver, and the kidneys is recommended. Although less than 5% of patients have evidence of distant metastasis, an appropriate laboratory screen for such should be included in the patient's evaluation.

Often, a tongue base neoplasm cannot be adequately assessed by office examination, and an examination under anesthesia is required. A direct laryngoscopy and esophagoscopy can be performed at that time to look for a second or a third primary lesion, which has been reported in approximately 10% of these patients. A contrast medium–enhanced CT scan or MRI delineates the three-dimensional extent of disease, depicts involvement of surrounding soft tissue and bony structures, and confirms spread to regional nodes.

Small, superficial cancers of the tongue base are rare and can be cured by either irradiation or surgery. As noted earlier, the vast majority of cancers of the tongue base are advanced; approximately 80% have spread to regional nodes by the time of presentation. Single-modality treatment for this advanced disease is not recommended. Surgical resection of advanced cancer of the tongue base requires a total or supraglottic laryngectomy in combination with the glossectomy. A supraglottic laryngectomy can be considered in the relatively young, healthy patient with good pulmonary function as long as residual tongue base with an intact hypoglossal nerve can be preserved on at least one side. It is preferable to perform a total laryngectomy for prevention of severe aspiration if pulmonary function is compromised, a large portion of the base of tongue must be sacrificed, and both hypoglossal nerves must be removed, or else laryngeal competency is compromised. In questionable cases, a feeding gastrostomy can be added to the treatment regimen in order to provide nutrition either temporarily (e.g., during postoperative irradiation) or on a permanent basis. If cancer has spread to involve the mandibular body or the pterygoid muscles, a segmental resection of the involved portion of the mandible should also be performed. Usually a myocutaneous flap is required to reconstruct the base of tongue defect after tumor resection.

Neck dissection is indicated for any patient with clinical evidence of cervical node involvement or for large or deeply infiltrative primary lesions. Bilateral neck dissection (sparing the internal jugular vein on one side) should be considered for tongue base cancers that approach or cross the midline.

Postoperative irradiation is indicated in the management of advanced tongue base cancer. Margins are almost impossible to assess in every dimension after resection of infiltrative cancer of the tongue. Indications for postoperative XRT are otherwise as listed in the section Radiotherapy and Chemotherapy. Primary reconstruction at the time of surgical resection is essential in order to begin postoperative irradiation within 6 weeks of tumor resection.

The 5-year disease-free survival rate for patients with tongue base cancer is approximately 20%. Interestingly, survival for any stage of tongue base cancer is comparable with that for the corresponding stage of oral tongue cancer. The decreased overall survival rate for tongue base cancer is therefore a reflection of the advanced stage of disease at presentation.

Oropharyngeal Wall

Cancer arising from the lateral or posterior pharyngeal wall is rare, accounting for approximately 10% of cancers of the oropharynx. Early lesions are asymptomatic and may reach a considerable size before manifesting any symptoms. Approximately 60% of such patients present with clinical evidence of cervical node disease at the time of presentation. Most patients have advanced cancer when first seen; 80% present with tumors greater than 4 cm in diameter.

Direct examination of the oropharynx allows visualization of most cancers of the oropharyngeal wall, especially when the tongue is depressed. Indirect mirror examination or fiberoptic nasopharyngoscopy permits a more thorough examination of the lateral and posterior pharyngeal walls. Palpation of the pharyngeal wall, especially under general anesthesia, allows the examiner to determine mobility of the tumor over the prevertebral musculature. Tumors of the pharyngeal wall frequently have submucosal spread or even skip areas, and an examination under anesthesia is valuable in determining extension of disease. Likewise, CT or MRI is extremely useful in determining the extent of disease, third dimension involvement (including prevertebral fascia, vertebral bodies, and the skull base), and regional node disease. Because oropharyngeal wall cancers tend to metastasize to retropharyngeal, parapharyngeal, and even deep parotid lymph nodes, these radiologic studies are essential in determining the presence of otherwise unassessable nodal disease. As with other oropharyngeal primary cancers, the examiner must evaluate the patient for multicentric cancers.

Small, exophytic lesions of the oropharyngeal wall can be treated equally effectively with irradiation or surgery. High lesions can be resected transorally and the defect allowed to heal by secondary intention. More low-lying lesions are more amenable to resection by means of a lateral pharyngotomy or transhyoid pharyngotomy. If surgery is to be considered for larger lesions or patients with clinical or radiologic evidence of regional node metastasis, a neck dissection should include removal of parapharyngeal and retropharyngeal nodes in the vicinity of the cancer. Larger lesions, especially those approaching or involving the skull base, should be considered for a curative dose of irradia-

tion because attempts at surgical resection in this area are frequently met with incomplete tumor removal and increased morbidity. In most cases, provisions for alternative means of nutrition such as a feeding gastrostomy should be considered in order to decrease the morbidity of treatment for advanced lesions, whether the treatment is irradiation, surgery, or a combination of the two.

Although the 5-year disease-free survival rate for small, exophytic lesions of the oropharyngeal wall is as high as 75%, the great majority of lesions are advanced, and the overall survival rate for 5 years is approximately 20%. Local and regional node recurrent disease is the most common cause of death. The reader is directed to the treatment algorithm (Fig. 32–1) on the following page for a summary of treatment recommendations for cancers according to site.

SURGICAL RECONSTRUCTION

The surgical resection of cancer of the oral cavity and the oropharynx can result in significant functional and cosmetic deficits. The degree of difficulty with articulation and swallowing after partial glossectomy depends on the amount of tongue removed as well as the mobility of the remaining tongue. A loss of the gingivolabial or gingivobuccal sulcus can result in drooling and the improper fitting of dentures. Whereas resection of a small segment of mandible at the body/angle area does not alter facial contour to a great degree, drifting of the mandible or trismus can significantly affect mastication. Resection of greater segments of the mandible, especially the anterior arch, can be devastating in terms of both appearance and function. Removal of tongue base or tonsil cancers can significantly affect deglutition, cause life-threatening aspiration, and result in trismus. The devastating effects of a total glossectomy on swallowing and communication are well known.

Under ordinary circumstances, surgical resection of cancer of the oral cavity or the oropharynx represents the initial or primary form of treatment. It is necessary under this circumstance to perform a definitive, one-stage reconstruction during the primary surgery to allow postoperative irradiation in a timely fashion. The need for success of such reconstruction is obvious, because flap necro-

Primary Site	Stage (TNM)	Surgery								XRT***	
		Primary	Neck node levels**						Retropharyngeal	Adjunct	Definitive
			I	II	III	IV	V-A	V-B			
Oral cavity FOM	I-II	✓	✓	✓	✓					✓	
Tongue alveolus buccal mucosa RMT	III IV	✓	✓	✓	✓	✓				✓	
Hard palate	I-II	✓									
	III-IV	✓		✓	✓	✓			✓	✓	
Tonsil	I										
	II*(exoph)										✓
	II*(endo)	✓	✓	✓	✓		✓			✓	✓
	III-IV	✓	✓	✓	✓	✓	✓	✓		✓	
BOT	I										✓
	II-IV	✓		✓	✓	✓	✓	✓		✓	
Oropharyngeal wall	I-II										✓
	III-IV	✓		✓	✓	✓	✓	✓		✓	

KEY: FOM, floor of mouth; RMT, retromolar trigone; BOT, base of tongue.

*Stage II tonsil cancers can be considered exophytic (exoph) or endophytic (endo). Exophytic cancers tend to respond more favorably to XRT.

**Regional nodal levels at greatest risk are marked. Neck dissection and XRT should remove at least these levels, and more, if clinically indicated. Level V is subdivided into nodes above nerve XI (A) and nodes inferior to nerve XI (B).

***Adjunctive XRT is usually given postoperatively. It is always indicated for T_3- and T_4-sized primary lesions. Additional indications are based on the following adverse histopathologic findings:
(1) At the primary site: + or close margin, angioinvasion, neuroinvasion, bone invasion, or submucosal lymphatic spread.
(2) In the neck specimen: extracapsular spread, more than one node involved, + node beyond the primary echelon of drainage, + node at the lowest level of dissection.

Figure 32–1. Treatment algorithm.

sis, sepsis, and fistula may result in an unwanted delay in the initiation of XRT. Thus a thorough preoperative evaluation of the patient must include consideration of all factors related to the success of treatment including the patient's health, ability to withstand prolonged anesthesia and blood loss, emotional and intellectual abilities, motivation and expectations, and the need to return to active employment. In addition, the status of the patient's dentition, airway, and nutritional needs must be considered. Alternative methods of reconstruction can then be determined, with avoidance of any compromise of surgical resection to fit some preconceived reconstructive plan. Experience suggests that the simplest methods of reconstruction usually result in the best functional results.

Small to moderate-sized defects of the oral cavity and the oropharynx are best closed by primary closure as long as maintenance of tongue mobility or an adequate gingivobuccal or gingivolingual sulcus is not compromised. Defects of the hard palate, the soft palate, and the posterior pharyngeal walls after intraoral resection can be allowed to heal by secondary intention unless significant contracture is likely. Skin grafts, either split-thickness, full-thickness, or dermal, can provide satisfactory coverage of defects. Stenting or quilt techniques for maintaining grafts in proper position are necessary depending on location. Once again, the surgeon must consider the potential ill effects of scar contracture on subsequent function.

Larger defects usually require placement

of vascularized skin, soft tissue, and muscle, depending on the size and location of the defect. Myocutaneous flaps have largely supplanted other flaps such as the deltopectoral, forehead, and tongue flaps in the reconstruction of defects of the oral cavity and the oropharynx. These reconstructive options, which include the pectoralis major, trapezius, latissimus dorsi, and scapular myocutaneous flaps, bring an abundant blood supply and are more reliable, effective, and predictable than is the deltopectoral flap. One disadvantage in the oral cavity and the oropharynx is the fact that these flaps replace resected tissue with large, inanimate, insensate blocks of tissue that compromise rehabilitation of swallowing and speech.

Free microvascular flaps represent an additional reconstructive method for defects in this area. They have the advantage of providing vascularized skin and bone in an almost limitless variety of thickness, size, and pliability for allowing reconstruction of defects heretofore considered unreconstructable. The radial forearm flap, for example, represents the ideal flap for reconstruction of small defects of the floor of mouth, which can include small segmental defects of the mandible. The free jejunal graft is ideal for reconstruction after a total laryngopharyngectomy, provided that postoperative irradiation is carefully administered.

Reconstruction of the mandible represents a complex problem. Although the new techniques of myocutaneous and microvascular free flaps as well as osteointegrated implants provide some solutions, satisfactory reconstruction of a tooth-bearing mandible with adequate strength, with satisfactory sulci, and without excessive soft tissue bulk remains a challenge. Many patients, for example, cannot withstand the increased operating time and greater blood loss associated with complex reconstruction. The resurgence of interest in the use of mandibular replacement plates demonstrates the need for simple, expeditious reconstruction of the mandible in some patients.

REHABILITATION AND FOLLOW-UP

Reconstruction of large defects in the oral cavity or the oropharynx with myocutaneous or free microvascular flaps cannot fully restore the patient's ability to masticate, swallow, and speak. Many patients need a palatal drop prosthesis that can provide the palatoglossal contact necessary for initiating deglutition. As the edema and flap bulk resolve in the postoperative period, the prosthesis needs to be modified several times. It is extremely difficult for the patient to keep a palatal prosthesis in place if there are no upper teeth for anchoring. Use of a permanent screw into the palate has been reported.

Physical rehabilitation by a therapist trained in speech and swallowing is important. If possible, the first contact with the patient should be made preoperatively. Physical examination and fluoroscopic evaluation of deglutition determine the regimen of rehabilitation on an individual basis.

All neck dissections are attended by some morbidity. A modified neck dissection in which the spinal accessory nerve has been skeletonized in order to clean out the accessory chain of nodes results in temporary shoulder pain and trapezius weakness. Passive and active range-of-motion exercises for the shoulder, with a trained physical therapist if necessary, should prevent a frozen shoulder and worsening pain. If a radical neck dissection has been performed, formal physical therapy consultation should be obtained in order to train the patient in the use of accessory muscles and prevention of a frozen shoulder.

All patients with squamous cell cancer should be followed indefinitely. In the first 2 years, adequate follow-up can be every 1 to 2 months after therapy. After 2 years, visits can be decreased to every 6 months until the 5-year milestone. After 5 years, the patient can be considered cured and should be followed once a year. The purpose of follow-up is to evaluate functional recovery and to rule out locoregional recurrence. Second primary cancers of the upper aerodigestive tract can be expected to be found in 15% to 20% of cases; it is hoped that they are found early enough to be treatable. A chest film is obtained yearly to rule out a second primary or metastasis. Postradiotherapy patients must have thyroid function studies, and if they were radiated at the skull base, pituitary functions should be checked on a routine basis. Every opportunity should be used to help the patient abstain from tobacco abuse, because the majority of patients with second primary cancers are those who continue smoking.

SUGGESTED READINGS

Byers RM: Modified neck dissection: a study of 967 cases from 1970 to 1980. Am J Surg 150:414–421, 1985.

Byers RM, Newman R, Russell N, Yue A: Results of treatment for squamous carcinoma of the lower gum. Cancer 47:2236–2238, 1981.

Byers RM, Wolf PF, Ballantyne AJ: Rationale for elective modified neck dissection. Head Neck Surg 10:160–167, 1988.

Callery CD, Spiro RH, Strong EW: Changing trends in the management of squamous carcinoma of the tongue. Am J Surg 148:449–454, 1984.

Close LG, Burns DK, Reisch J, Schaefer SD: Microvascular invasion in cancer of the oral cavity and oropharynx. Arch Otolaryngol 113:1191–1195, 1987.

Close LG, Merkel M, Burns DK, Schaefer SD: Computed tomography in the assessment of mandibular invasion by intraoral carcinoma. Ann Otol Rhinol Laryngol 95:383–388, 1986.

Connolly GN, Winn DM, Hecht SS, et al: The reemergence of smokeless tobacco. N Engl J Med 314:1020–1027, 1986.

Crile G: Excision of cancer of the head and neck. JAMA 47:1780–1788, 1906; JAMA 258:3286–3293, 1987.

Hodge KM, Flynn MB, Drury T: Squamous cell carcinoma of the upper aerodigestive tract in nonusers of tobacco. Cancer 55:1232–1235, 1985.

Kaplan R, Million RR, Cassissi NJ: Carcinoma of the tonsil: results of radical irradiation with surgery reserved for radiation failure. Laryngoscope 86:600–607, 1976.

Lindberg R: Distribution of cervical lymph node metastases from squamous cell carcinoma of the upper respiratory and digestive tracts. Cancer 29:1446–1449, 1972.

Medina JE, Dichtel W, Luna MA: Verrucous-squamous carcinomas of the oral cavity. Arch Otolaryngol 110:437–440, 1984.

Shah JP, Candela FC, Poddar AK: The patterns of cervical lymph node metastases from squamous carcinoma of the oral cavity. Cancer 66:109–113, 1990.

Shaha AR, Spiro RH, Shah JP, Strong EW: Squamous carcinoma of the floor of the mouth. Am J Surg 148:455–459, 1984.

Silverman S, Gorsky M, Lozada F: Oral leukoplakia and malignant transformation. Cancer 53:563–568, 1984.

Slaughter DP, Southwick HW, Smejkal W: "Field cancerization" in oral stratified squamous epithelium. Cancer 6:963–968, 1953.

Spiro RH, Huvos AG, Wong GY, et al: Predictive value of tumor thickness in squamous carcinoma confined to the tongue and floor of the mouth. Am J Surg 152:345–350, 1986.

Vikram B, Strong EW, Shah JP, Spiro RH: Failure in the neck following multimodality treatment for advanced head and neck cancer. Head Neck Surg 6:724–729, 1984.

Vikram B, Strong EW, Shah JP, Spiro RH: Failure at distant sites following multimodality treatment for advanced head and neck cancer. Head Neck Surg 6:730–733, 1984.

Vikram B, Strong EW, Shah JP, Spiro RH: Second malignant neoplasms in patients successfully treated with multimodality treatment for advanced head and neck cancer. Head Neck Surg 6:734–737, 1984.

CHAPTER 33

Nonneoplastic Salivary Gland Diseases

Stanley W. Coulthard, MD

Nonneoplastic salivary gland disease confronts the head and neck physician with a difficult diagnostic differential. Multiple disease processes of the salivary glands manifest in a similar manner. The most common presentation of a salivary gland problem, whether neoplastic or nonneoplastic, is swelling of the salivary gland involved. The swelling may be associated with pain, fever, or systemic signs and symptoms. The physician must decide on the basis of these fairly general findings in the history and physical examination which is most likely, a neoplasm or a nonneoplastic process. The outline of possibilities is quite diffuse.

Even though there are thousands of salivary glands in the head and neck, the nonneoplastic diseases generally manifest themselves in the major salivary glands. Usually the parotid or submandibular glands are involved. Most of the nonneoplastic disease processes are results of problems within the complex ductal system in the major glands. Strictures, stones, or parenchymal change may cause ductal compression, obstruction, or infection within the ducts.

The distinction between a neoplasm and a nonneoplastic disease is important because the neoplasms are treated surgically; the nonneoplastic diseases are in general treated medically, at least in the early phases. Because nonneoplastic diseases basically manifest in the major salivary glands, any surgery in these areas deals with major nerves of the head and neck region. In the parotid region, the facial nerve is always at risk with a surgical approach; in the submandibular region, the ramus mandibularis of the facial nerve, the hypoglossal nerve, and the lingual nerve are at risk.

INFECTIOUS DISEASE

Acute Viral Infection

The most commonly recognized infectious disease of the salivary glands is viral. Mumps, an acute nonobstructive inflammatory disease, usually manifests in the parotid gland but may be seen in the submandibular and sublingual glands. History of acute onset of general malaise, salivary gland swelling, and redness of the punctum of the gland is helpful in the diagnosis of the disease. Usually the swelling and discomfort last for 7 to 10 days, and treatment is supportive. During the period of infection, the saliva is clear. Definitive diagnosis requires the examination of acute and convalescent sera. The most difficult long-term problem that follows mumps is the obstructive chronic sialadenitis syndrome. This is caused by the initial infection but manifests many months or years later as a chronic problem.

Acute Bacterial Infection

The anatomy of the major salivary glands is a complex system of small interconnecting

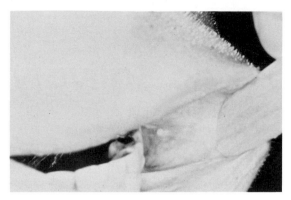

Figure 33–1. The drainage of pus from Stensen's duct in a case of acute suppurative sialadenitis.

ducts that are constantly flushed with saliva. When the salivary flow is slowed or obstructed for various reasons, the patient is prone to the development of a bacterial infection. The classical example of acute suppurative sialadenitis is in the elderly, debilitated person who is dehydrated. This condition is known as surgical parotitis because in the past, postoperative patients were known to develop this problem during a period of dehydration.

The manifestation of acute sialadenitis is swelling of the involved gland with general malaise and fever. Tenderness and erythema may also be present. The pathognomonic feature of this disease is the suppurative drainage that usually can be expressed from the punctum of the gland (Fig. 33–1). The patient is systemically ill and may have high fever, chills, and sepsis. The skin over the gland becomes reddened and hot with an increasing tenseness. The manifestation of an abscessing gland in the major salivary glands is somewhat paradoxical because of the intense investment of the glands with the deep cervical fascia. The multiple investments of fascia with compartments cause the gland to become more tense when a suppurative process is developing, and it is not until very late in the suppurative process that all of the fascial compartments are broken down and the gland becomes fluctuant. The physician must use other signs to determine the advisability of drainage in an acute suppurative process. This decision is usually made on the basis of lack of clinical response to medical management. Medical management consists of a broad-spectrum antibiotic directed at the most commonly identified

pathogens in this process, *Staphylococcus aureus*, *Haemophilus influenzae*, and *Streptococcus pneumoniae*. Usually treatment with cephalosporin or penicillin is started immediately, and a culture is obtained if possible. The patient should be placed on parenteral hydration, heat treatments with massaging of the gland, and sialagogues if they are tolerated.

When vigorous medical management does not cause lysis of fever or improvement in the clinical status of the patient, drainage of the gland should be accomplished, usually within 24 to 48 hours. In the parotid gland, a modified Blair incision is used for wide exposure of the entire gland by elevation of an anterior flap (Fig. 33–2). The fascia of the parotid is then incised, which allows blunt entry into the parenchyma of the gland. Care should be taken to cut only superficially in the fascia and to spread in the direction of the facial nerve fibers. Frequently, only minimal drainage is obtained from the gland when this procedure is followed. The drain-

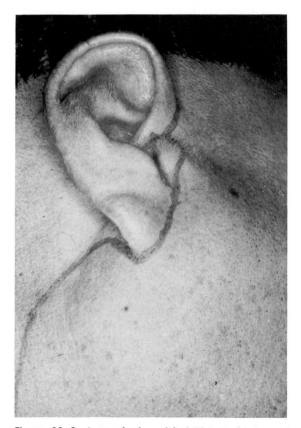

Figure 33–2. A standard modified Blair incision used for exposure of the parotid gland.

age may be not suppurative but of a more serous nature. This is sometimes distressing to the surgeon, who expects to find a well-established suppurative process with pus. Even though the drainage may appear minimal, the procedure usually reverses the signs and symptoms of infection, and the patient improves dramatically. During the process, a drain should be placed at several sites and brought out through the wound.

Drainage of the submandibular gland is based on the same criteria and should be performed through an incision that is approximately two fingers' breadths below the mandible. The gland should be drained in the same way that the parotid is, with a drain left in place and brought out through the wound.

Chronic Sialadenitis

Recurrent infections of either the parotid or the submandibular gland may occur and manifest as a suppurative process. This may become such a difficult problem for the patient that surgical removal of the gland is advisable. Certainly the medical management of the problem should be exhausted before surgery. Thus if surgery is recommended, it is extremely difficult and may require extensive dissection and effort to preserve the facial nerve. Also, removal of as much of the glandular tissue as possible is necessary for preventing recurrence of the chronic sialadenitis.

Chronic recurrent sialadenitis may occur in children or adults and may represent a post-mumps type of process. This is an instance in which observation and good counseling of the patient are necessary. Usually, for both adults and children, a discussion of the problem and a stressing of the importance of medical management, both in the acute infectious phase and in the quiescent phase, achieves improved results. Certainly the patient and the family must realize that stasis in the gland along with poor hygiene and poor hydration predisposes the patient to the problem. The actual acute exacerbation of the sialadenitis in chronic sialadenitis should be treated with a broad-spectrum antibiotic, heat, massaging of the gland, sialagogues, and hydration.

Sialectasis

Sialectasis is a chronic enlargement of segments of the salivary ductal system. As the

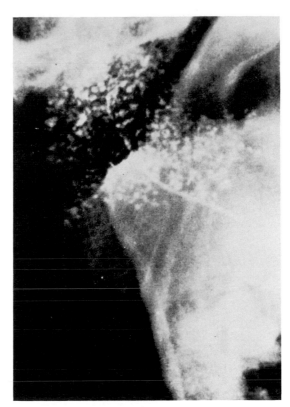

Figure 33–3. A radiograph demonstrating punctate sialectasis.

saccules develop, stasis of the salivary secretions occurs and leads to infection. Patients with sialectasis manifest recurrent sialadenitis as previously described. The difference is the abnormal structural change that causes punctate dilation in the patient with sialectasis.

Development of the sialectasis may be congenital or acquired. In order to make a definitive diagnosis, sialography is necessary. The sialogram demonstrates the classic punctate lesion (Fig. 33–3). A medical evaluation, including testing for autoimmune disorders, should be included in the work-up.

Granulomatous Infections

Tuberculosis may manifest as an acute or a chronic infection of the major salivary glands. Usually the parotid is involved (Fig. 33–4), but the submandibular gland may be infected. The patient may have no other indications of tuberculosis. Skin testing should be used in the evaluation. Surgery may also be necessary for obtaining tissue for microscopic evaluation and culture. If surgery is performed, it is preferable to remove the

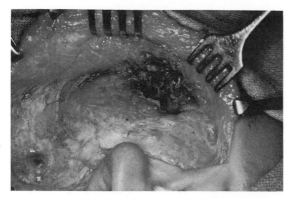

Figure 33–4. An abscess cavity identified in a tuberculous parotitis.

lesion completely, if possible. Chemotherapy should be used regardless of local surgical care.

Chronic infections may develop fistulous tracts to the skin and have drainage.

Atypical mycobacterial infection may manifest in the same way, but often the skin test is negative. Treatment is variable, and conservative excision or curettage is often adequate.

Cat Scratch Fever

Cat scratch disease is a necrotizing granuloma that is directly related to exposure to an animal bite. The causative agent is unknown, but there is a definite history of animal exposure. The manifestation is neck node swelling and major salivary gland involvement. Medical management with local care is recommended.

Actinomycosis

Actinomycosis is caused by an organism that is casually introduced through a dental route. Dental work or chewing on weeds and grasses may be associated with subsequent disease. The disease, once it is in the tissues, causes an extensive invasive sclerotic process. Swelling, with possible pain and typical acute sialadenitis, is the usual presentation. Fistula formation may occur and result in drainage. Drainage from the wound shows a characteristic organism. Once the diagnosis is made, long-term antibiotic therapy, sometimes for many months, is indicated.

Sarcoidosis

Sarcoidosis, uveoparotid fever or Heerfordt's disease, manifests when the uveal tract, the lacrimal gland, and the salivary gland are involved. The parotid gland is usually involved, but all glands may be affected. Once diagnosis is confirmed by biopsy, treatment is supportive.

Sialolithiasis

The pathophysiologic mechanism of stone formation is thought to be stasis with formation of a nidus of mucus, or a bacterial plug, which then acts to precipitate calcium or sodium phosphate salt stones. The growth of the stone and the resulting obstruction lead to sialolithiasis and to a more vicious cycle of obstruction and infection. Symptoms and signs of sialolithiasis are directly related to the degree of obstruction carried by the process. Symptoms include swelling, which is dependent on the degree of systemic infection, and local manifestations of infection. If the stone can be released either spontaneously or by manipulation, improvement should be immediate. Certainly one of the most rewarding procedures is the extraction of a stone from either Stensen's or Wharton's duct with subsequent release of pressure, saliva, and pus. Often it is a solitary calculus located at the ostium (Fig. 33–5). Stones may be identified by radiographic examination (Fig. 33–6). Multiple stones in the duct or gland frequently necessitate surgical removal of the gland (Fig. 33–7). If no further duct manipulation is possible, surgery is necessary. Removal of stones within the gland, or 2 cm or more away from the punctum, is indicated because of the possibility of vessel or nerve injury if intraoral opening of the duct is accomplished. Certainly, if chronic glandular changes have occurred secondary to recurrent infection, the gland should be removed through an external approach.

OBSTRUCTIVE DISEASE

Kussmaul's Disease

Kussmaul's disease, or sialodochitis fibrinosis, develops when mucous plugs form in the collecting system of the major salivary glands. A predisposing factor is dehydration,

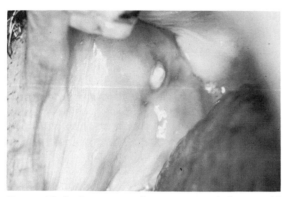

Figure 33–5. A stone at the punctum of the parotid duct.

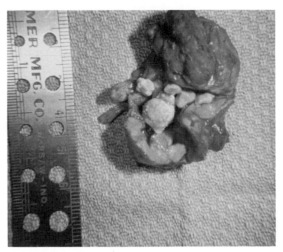

Figure 33–7. The submandibular gland with multiple stones removed surgically.

which may result from fluid restriction or medications. Swelling of the glands may be recurrent and extremely painful when the ductal system is blocked and pressure develops. Diagnosis is confirmed by massaging mucous plugs from the gland. General medical management of the problem with hydration, massaging, and sialagogues is indicated.

Ductal Strictures

Ductal strictures from a variety of etiologic factors, such as trauma, infection, and developmental anomalies, may cause drainage problems and lead to all the signs and symptoms recognized.

The diagnosis of ductal obstruction may require sialography. Sialography may result in an intense inflammatory response in the gland and, ultimately, a suppurative infec-

tion. After a sialogram, vigorous hydration and gland massaging should be accomplished. If the patient has persistent problems with a strictured duct, surgery may be performed. Strictures at the punctum or within 2 cm of the opening may be treated intraorally with a marsupialization of the duct by incising the lumen and allowing drainage. If the stricture is farther within the gland, more extensive surgery with removal of the gland through an external approach is recommended. The reason for external approach with deep strictures is the possibility of vessel and nerve damage with deep gland manipulation. Ductal ligation with low-dosage radiation therapy may be used to cause gland atrophy and decrease in gland activity. This would be more appropriate for the patient who is not able to tolerate surgery.

Strictures may also be secondary to trauma. Trauma to the duct may be initially managed by identifying the duct and stenting the duct with polyethylene catheter (Fig. 33–8). If subsequent stricturing occurs, a gland removal may be necessary.

Cystic Lesions

Abnormal ductal structures with cyst formation may be a result of developmental anomalies or acquired problems. Some cysts may manifest at birth or shortly afterward. These are usually retention cysts with thin walls. In the sublingual area, they are called ranulas. The cyst is filled with mucus and may

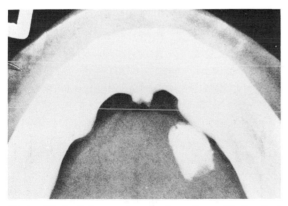

Figure 33–6. A large stone in the submandibular duct demonstrated radiographically.

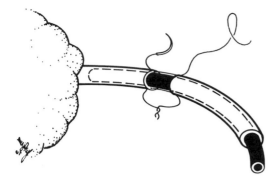

Figure 33–8. Suturing the salivary duct over a polyethylene stent is a method of repair after trauma.

be drained or surgically removed (Fig. 33–9). Many techniques have been described for drainage of cysts or ranulas. The principle of drainage is marsupialization for allowing a chronic opening of the cyst. In general, keeping this type of cyst open is difficult, and surgical removal is more definitive.

Congenital cysts of the parotid have been classified as dermoid, branchial cleft, branchial pouch, and congenital ductal cysts. Walter Work further classified branchial cleft cysts into type I and type II. The branchial cleft lesions are important because of the difficulty in diagnosis and treatment. Swelling is the usual initial manifestation with varying degrees of infectious manifestations.

The Differential Between Type I and Type II

First branchial cleft defects depend on an embryologic germ layer origin. The type I lesions are a duplication of the membranous external auditory canal and may present anywhere around the ear. This anomaly arises from the ectodermal elements only. If infection occurs, broad-spectrum antibiotics and, frequently, drainage are indicated before definitive surgical excision. The best possible surgical field must be obtained to allow complete removal of the congenital cyst and yet protect the facial nerve. The cyst may be in any possible relationship with the facial nerve, which must always be considered at risk during a surgical procedure. This is particularly true when infection has been present.

Type II first branchial cleft cysts are not as common as type I clefts and include ectodermal and mesodermal elements; they are duplication defects of the external canal and auricle. The ectoderm may contain its appendages, such as hair follicles, sebaceous glands, and sweat glands. Infection is frequently associated with swelling and may result in a draining sinus in the area of the ear, the parotid gland, or the upper neck (Figs. 33–10 to 33–12). Ear drainage from a sinus tract draining into the external canal has been the presenting sign of a first branchial cleft defect. Probing of the canal defect may reveal a tract into the parotid or the neck (Fig. 33–12). A radiographic study of the sinus tract may be helpful (Fig. 33–6).

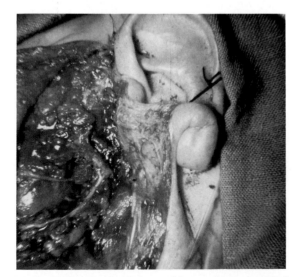

Figure 33–9. An exposed parotid cyst during surgical excision.

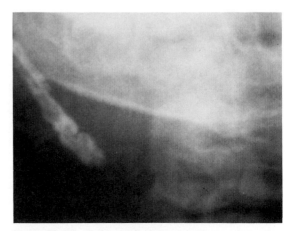

Figure 33–10. Radiograph demonstrating a sinus tract associated with a first branchial sinus.

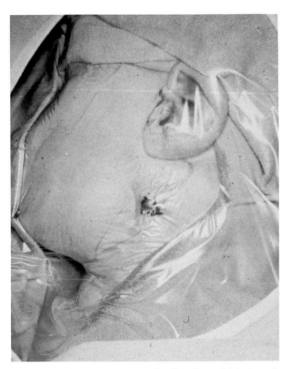

Figure 33–11. Presentation of a first branchial sinus in the neck.

Immunologic Manifestations

The classic immunologic disease causing salivary gland manifestations is Sjögren's syndrome. The term *Sjögren's syndrome* has come to refer to a systemic involvement of autoimmune nature that may have local or systemic manifestations. Presenting symptoms of xerostomia, keratoconjunctivitis, and a systemic autoimmune process confirm the usual disease. A lymphoid component, locally and systemically, may be present and may have a relationship to the increased incidence of lymphoproliferative malignancy in these patients. Manifestations of Sjögren's syndrome are conveniently classed as primary when only local disease is present and as secondary when a systemic autoimmune process is present. Many terms are used to refer to Sjögren's disease, such as sicca complex or sicca syndrome. The addition of the term *primary* or *secondary* clarifies the classification.

The clinical features of the sicca problems from Sjögren's syndrome, whether primary or secondary, are xerostomia and keratoconjunctivitis sicca. The oral dryness may be

Surgical removal with preservation is recommended during a noninfectious period. All surgery in the region of the parotid, particularly when a congenital anomaly is suspected, must be planned for a facial nerve exposure and dissection. The initial presentation may appear to be directly under the skin and give the surgeon an impression of limited surgery. The surgeon approaching this area must be prepared to deal with any possibility.

A variety of other cysts may occur and appear to be related to the basic obstructive disease process with the cyst forming secondarily.

SYSTEMIC MANIFESTATIONS IN THE SALIVARY GLANDS

The salivary glands may present manifestations not only of local disease but also of systemic diseases. These may be immunologic, endocrine, drug-related, and infectious.

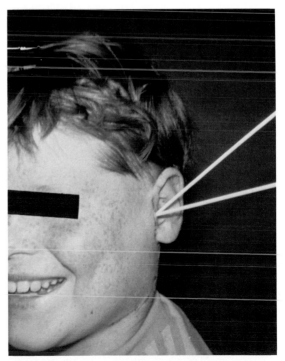

Figure 33–12. Presentation of a first branchial sinus in the ear canal. Probes demonstrate the canal and the sinus extending into the parotid region.

described by the patient as difficulty swallowing or chronic sore throat, halitosis, or ductal problems. There are no convenient tests for quantifying the oral secretions.

Enlargement of the parotid glands can usually be seen and palpated (Fig. 33–13). Most often the enlargement is asymptomatic and may not bother the patient or be a cosmetic concern. The enlargement is diffuse and nontender. There is a diffuse glandular firmness to the process. The submandibular gland may be involved and noticeably enlarged.

Specific diagnosis is usually obtained from biopsy material from the lower lip. A good correlation among parotid, submandibular, and lower lip diseases has been shown previously. The biopsy of the lower lip is simple and should cause few problems. The pathologic findings of Sjögren's syndrome show acinar atrophy, destruction, and lymphoid infiltrate.

The eye dryness manifests as burning and light sensitivity. Slit-lamp examination shows superficial keratosis and pericorneal debris. Schirmer's test indicates the degree of involvement.

Secondary Sjögren's syndrome may have a variety of systemic diseases such as rheumatoid arthritis, scleroderma, lupus erythematosus, and polymyositis. Symptoms associated with these problems must be evaluated and correlated because the patient may make no such association. The appropriate serum protein analysis must be ordered.

Treatment of Sjögren's syndrome is supportive in most instances; it consists of oral saliva substitutes and periodic examinations. On occasion, the gland enlargement may be a significant cosmetic concern, and surgical removal is indicated.

Acquired Immunodeficiency Manifestations

It is known that patients carrying the human immunodeficiency virus commonly have parotid swelling caused by cystic lesions. Fine-needle aspiration of the lesions has shown benign lymphoepithelial and inflammatory disease in most instances. There are documentations in the literature of the lesions that are associated with a B-cell lymphoma in a patient with acquired immunodeficiency syndrome. Although the lesions may be handled surgically, conservative treatment with needle aspiration may be the most advisable. For diagnosis of cystic involvement of the parotid, a computed tomography scan and fine-needle aspiration are very helpful. Indeed, the fine-needle aspiration may be the preferable way of managing the cystic enlargements over a period of time.

Bulimia

Salivary gland enlargement has been seen in patients suffering from bulimia. It is reported to occur in approximately 30% of patients with bulimia, usually in females, and is transient. Once the disease is controlled, the salivary gland enlargement subsides.

Treatment is supportive in all instances. Certainly the most important aspect of recognizing the correlation between bulimia and salivary gland enlargement is the possibility of early identification and control of the primary problem.

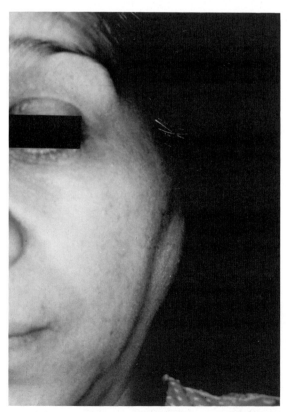

Figure 33–13. Diffuse parotid enlargement as seen with Sjögren's syndrome.

Gustatory Sweating

Gustatory sweating, Frey's syndrome or auriculotemporal lacrimation, is a frequent sequela to surgery in the parotid or neck region. Any surgery or injury that interrupts the autonomic fibers of the auriculotemporal nerve may lead to this phenomenon. This includes parotidectomy, radical neck dissection, and facial lacerations. During the healing process, the autonomic fibers that originally stimulated the salivary system are redirected into the sweat glands of the skin. Once this route is established, normal sialagogues then stimulate sweating instead of salivation.

Careful history taking or physical examination shows this to occur in the majority of parotidectomy patients, but only 10% to 15% find that it is a disability. Of this group, only a few require treatment.

Treatment is usually conservative and consists of antiperspirant application to the skin involved. Surgical procedures that interrupt the nerve and prevent regrowth of the fibers into the glands have been advocated. One method of accomplishing this has been to place a dermal graft over the parotid region. Some surgeons believe that a thicker flap prevents these problems.

SUGGESTED READINGS

Alappatt JL, Ananthachari MD: A preliminary study of the structure and function of enlarged parotid glands in chronic relapsing pancreatitis by sialography and biopsy methods. Gut 8:42–45, 1967.

Batsakis JG: Tumors of the Head and Neck, 2nd ed. Baltimore: Williams & Wilkins, 1988.

Bloch KJ, Buchanan WW, Wohl MJ, et al: Sjögren's syndrome. A clinical, pathological and serological study of sixty-two cases. Medicine (Balt) 44:187–231, 1965.

Borsanyi SJ: Chronic asymptomatic enlargement of the parotid glands. Ann Otol 71:857–867, 1962.

Chisholm DM, Mason DK: Labial salivary gland biopsy in Sjögren's disease. J Clin Pathol 21:656–660, 1968.

Colebunders R: Parotid swelling during human immunodeficiency virus infection. Arch Otolaryngol Head Neck Surg 114:330–332, 1988.

Cummings CW, Fredrickson JM, Harker LA, et al: Otolaryngology—Head and Neck Surgery, vol 2. St. Louis: CV Mosby, 1986.

Eversole LR: Oral sialocysts. Arch Otolaryngol Head Neck Surg 113:51–56, 1987.

Finfer MD: Cystic parotid lesions in patients at risk for the acquired immunodeficiency syndrome. Arch Otolaryngol Head Neck Surg 114:1290–1294, 1988.

Geterud A: Follow-up study of recurrent parotitis in children. Ann Otol Rhinol Laryngol 97:341–346, 1988.

Gullane PJ, Havas TJ: Facial nerve grafts: effects of postoperative irradiation. J Otolaryngol 16:112–115, 1987.

Jones AR, Mason DK: Oral Manifestations of Systemic Disease. Philadelphia: WB Saunders, 1980.

Mason DK, Chisholm DM: Salivary Glands in Health and Disease, pp 92–105. Philadelphia: WB Saunders, 1975.

Nash L, Morrison LF: Asymptomatic chronic enlargement of the parotid glands; review and report of case. Ann Otol Rhinol Laryngol 58:646–664, 1949.

Ogren FP: Transient salivary gland hypertrophy in bulimics. Laryngoscope 97:951–952, 1987.

Olson NR: Atypical mycobacterial infections of the neck. Laryngoscope 77:1376–1389, 1967.

Paparella MM, Shumrick DA: Otolaryngology: Head and Neck, 1st ed, vol. 3. Philadelphia: WB Saunders, 1973.

Pinelli V: The pathogenesis of chronic recurrent parotitis in infants: a study of 93 cases including an analysis of the vascular and glandular changes before/after parasympathectomy. Clin Otolaryngol 13:97–105, 1988.

Rontal M: The use of sialodochoplasty in the treatment of benign inflammatory obstructive submandibular gland disease. Laryngoscope 97:1417–1421, 1987.

Shearn MA: Sjögren's Syndrome. Philadelphia: WB Saunders, 1971.

Work WP: Newer concepts of first branchial cleft defects. Laryngoscope 83:1581–1593, 1972.

Work WP, Hecht DW: Non-neoplastic lesions of the parotid gland. Ann Otol 77:462–467, 1968.

Work WP, Hecht DW: Inflammatory diseases of the major salivary glands. In Paparella MM, Shumrick DA (eds): Otolaryngology, pp 258–265. Philadelphia: WB Saunders, 1973.

Work WP, Johns ME (eds): Salivary gland diseases. Otolaryngol Clin North Am, 1977.

Work, WP, McCabe BF: The salivary glands. In Maloney WH (ed): Otolaryngology, vol IV (chapter 9). Hagerstown: Harper & Row, 1975.

Work WP, Proctor CA: The otologist and first branchial cleft anomalies. Ann Otol 72:548–562, 1963.

CHAPTER 34

Neoplasms of the Salivary Glands

Dale H. Rice, MD

The major salivary glands and the minor salivary glands of the oral cavity are believed to be derived from ectoderm; the remaining glands are believed to arise from endoderm. Nevertheless, there are no histologic differences between the disease processes involving these glands in their various locations. The majority of tumors in all locations are of epithelial origin (Table 34–1). For the parotid gland, the ductal branching and facial nerve migration as well as the association of lymph nodes occur before the condensation of the intervening mesenchyme, ensuring an intimate relationship among these structures. Thus numerous lymph nodes develop within and adjacent to the parotid gland, and salivary gland tissue has been found within these nodes. This is thought to explain the origin of Warthin's tumor and may well explain other entities that occur in the parotid gland nearly exclusively.

The parotid acini are largely serous, whereas the submandibular acini are seromucous and the minor salivary glands may be serous, mucous, or mixed. Myoepithelial cells are located around the periphery of the acini and the intercalated ducts and appear to have the ability to contract, thus expelling saliva from the acini. Current knowledge implicates the myoepithelial cell as an important contributor to neoplasms of the various salivary glands. The parotid, the largest salivary gland, lies anterior and inferior to the ear, overlying the upper fourth of the sternocleidomastoid muscle and much of the posterior part of the masseter muscle. Common usage designates the portion of the gland extending medially between the ascending ramus of the mandible and the mastoid process as the deep lobe. In addition, there is also tissue medial to the facial nerve on the masseter muscle, which is also considered deep lobe. The parotid duct passes forward from the anterior margin of the gland and across the masseter muscle approximately midway between the zygomatic arch and the oral commissure, turning medially at the anterior border of the masseter to penetrate the buccinator muscle and open into the oral cavity opposite teeth 2 and 15 on the right and left, respectively. The major structure of concern in the parotid gland is the facial nerve, which exits the temporal bone via the stylomastoid foramen, crosses the posterolateral aspect of the styloid process, and enters the gland. The nerve initially divides into the temporofacial and cervicofacial branches, which then further subdivide in a variable pattern to supply the mimetic muscles of the face.

The submandibular gland occupies much of the submandibular triangle. The lateral surface of the gland is crossed by the anterior facial vein and, in approximately 10% of people, the marginal mandibular branch of the facial nerve. The nerve is at greater risk in that percentage of patients, however, because in the surgical position the branch is typically pulled down to a more inferior location. Deep to the gland lie the lingual and hypoglossal nerves as well as the hyoglossus muscle. The submandibular duct passes an-

TABLE 34–1. Epithelial Tumors: World Health Organization Classification

Adenomas
  Pleomorphic adenoma
  Monomorphic adenoma
    Adenolymphoma (Warthin's)
    Oxyphilic adenoma
    Other types

Mucoepidermoid Tumors

Acinous Cell Tumors

Carcinomas
  Adenoid cystic carcinoma
  Adenocarcinoma
  Epidermoid carcinoma
  Undifferentiated
  Carcinoma ex-pleomorphic adenoma

Nonepithelial Tumors

Unclassified Tumors

teriorly between the mandible and the hyoglossus and genioglossus muscles. It is crossed first laterally and then medially by the lingual nerve.

The sublingual gland lies beneath the mucosa of the floor of the mouth, between the submandibular duct and the mylohyoid muscle. Sublingual ducts are approximately 12 in number and empty either directly into the floor of the mouth or into the submandibular duct.

IMAGING TECHNIQUES

Computed tomography (CT) is considered to be the most reliable current examination for tumors in and around the parotid and submandibular glands. Spray artifact from dental amalgams may still occasionally cause problems, but usually not insurmountable ones (Fig. 34–1). The attenuation of the glands varies considerably but is always greater than that of fat and less than that of muscle, which generally makes the gland readily visible. Most benign lesions have well-defined borders, but so do many low-grade malignant lesions. Lesions with irregular or indistinct margins are more characteristic of malignancy and also suggest aggressive behavior. Multiple masses, particularly if they are bilateral, are highly suggestive of metastatic tumor, lymphoma, or the lymphadenopathy associated with acquired immunodeficiency syndrome. One particular strength of CT scanning is differentiation between deep lobe

parotid and parapharyngeal space tumors. Parapharyngeal lesions are usually separated from the parotid gland by a layer of normal body fat. If this layer of fat is not present, it is probable the lesion is a parotid tumor of the deep lobe.

CT scanning is also of value in distinguishing between intrinsic and extrinsic parotid masses. In general, benign tumors show high to moderate attenuation regardless of their histologic type, whereas malignant tumors show a low-to-moderate attenuation. The important additional signs of malignancy include lesions with irregular margins, extension beyond the gland capsule, erosion of bone, obliteration of fat planes, and metastatic deposits. CT is also useful in determining the relationship of the tumor to the facial nerve. It has been shown that the nerve can be represented on a CT scan by an arch of radius 8.5 mm, the center of which is the most posterior point of the ramus of the mandible. The arch extends from directly lateral to directly posterior.

Magnetic resonance imaging (MRI) in some respects may supplant CT scanning for imaging the head and neck. It is particularly useful in salivary gland disorders, partly because it is unaffected by dental amalgams

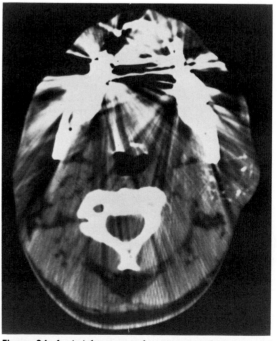

Figure 34–1. Axial computed tomogram of patient with pleomorphic adenoma of left parotid partially obscured by dental amalgams.

and partly because tissue contrast resolution is better with MRI than it is with CT (Fig. 34–2). This allows the viewer to better distinguish the parotid gland from surrounding structures. Further work is needed to determine the precise place of MRI in the workup of salivary gland neoplasms.

FINE-NEEDLE ASPIRATION CYTOLOGY

Fine-needle aspiration cytology has gained increasing support as individual institutions have increased their experience. Fine-needle aspiration cytology is highly accurate when performed by experienced clinicians, and studies show the rate of misleading reports to be under 10%. Because benign and malignant tumors of the salivary glands are relatively uncommon and have diverse and overlapping morphologic patterns, an individual pathologist with little experience may have difficulty distinguishing these lesions. An experienced pathologist, however, should be able to diagnose lesions accurately a high percentage of the time, particularly the most common neoplasms. These include the pleomorphic adenoma, the mucoepidermoid carcinoma, Warthin's tumor, and the adenoid

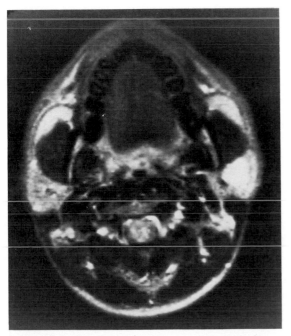

Figure 34–2. Axial magnetic resonance imaging of same patient as in Figure 34–1.

cystic carcinoma. The cytologist, however, is unable to classify mucoepidermoid lesions as to grade. This also cannot be done on frozen-section diagnosis and requires multiple sections through the entire tumor mass. In a comparison of fine-needle aspiration cytology with frozen-section diagnosis, fine-needle aspiration cytology was found to be correct in 16 of 21 tumors; frozen section was found to be correct in 15 of 21.

BENIGN NEOPLASMS

General Considerations

Salivary gland neoplasms account for less than 3% of all tumors but produce a larger variety of neoplasms than does any other organ system in the body (Table 34–1). Approximately 75% to 85% of all salivary neoplasms occur in the parotid gland, whereas most of the remainder are equally divided between the submandibular gland and the minor salivary glands. The most common location for minor salivary gland tumors is in the oral cavity; 50% occur on the palate. Eighty percent of parotid gland, 65% of submandibular gland, 50% of minor salivary gland, and 20% of sublingual gland tumors are benign. The incidence rate is approximately 43 cases per million. The incidence of salivary gland tumors in the White population is essentially the same worldwide. African Blacks have an increased incidence of pleomorphic adenomas in the minor and lesser major salivary glands. The only known risk factor for salivary gland tumors is previous exposure to radiation. In the United States, a significant source of this radiation is dental x-ray examination. It appears that the salivary glands behave not unlike the thyroid gland in that a low dosage of radiation is sufficient to cause tumors with a long latency and an increase in both benign and malignant tumors.

Benign salivary gland tumors usually manifest as an asymptomatic, slowly enlarging mass below intact skin or mucosa. The rate of growth is variable, and there is often considerable delay by both patient and physician in seeking medical attention. As many as 25% of the patients may be told by the initial examining physician that the swelling is nothing to be concerned about. For the parotid gland, approximately 80% of the tumors arise in the inferior aspect of the superficial lobe beneath the ear lobe. Thus every subcutaneous mass in the region of the inferior attachment of the ear should be considered a parotid neoplasm. The parotid gland is superficial to the sternocleidomastoid muscle; the cervical nodes are deep to the muscle. Symptoms are usually absent. The presence of pain does not necessarily signify malignancy because 5% of benign and 6% of malignant tumors produce pain.

Pleomorphic Adenoma

This neoplasm was originally designated the benign mixed tumor in 1866. The classical microscopic description was first reported in 1874. It was suggested in 1948 that the name be changed to pleomorphic adenoma to better fit its suspected unicellular origin. Additional, more recent ultrastructural study suggests that the tumor arises from the intercalated duct reserve cell, although there is some evidence that the myoepithelial cell is responsible for the stromal component of the tumor.

This neoplasm is the most common of all salivary gland tumors and alone accounts for 65% of parotid gland, 50% of submandibular gland, and 30% of minor salivary gland tumors. It accounts for 93% of all benign tumors in the minor salivary glands. However, 90% of all pleomorphic adenomas occur in the major salivary glands; 5% to 6% arise in the oral cavity, the palate being the most common site and the tongue being second. For uncertain reasons, the incidence of involvement of the submandibular gland is higher in Africa.

In the major salivary glands, the pleomorphic adenoma most commonly appears in the fifth decade of life; in the minor glands, it appears a decade later. There is a slight predominance among females, and the average duration before medical attention is sought is 6 years. The usual clinical presentation is that of a slow-growing, round, smooth, firm, asymptomatic, mobile mass. However, the tumor may become lobulated if it is left untreated. True multicentricity is rare, occurring in 0.5% of all pleomorphic adenomas, and there have been only six reported cases of multiple pleomorphic adenomas in a single parotid gland. A small percentage of these tumors undergo malignant change if they are left untreated or if they are recurrent. This change usually occurs an average of 10 years after presentation, and the rate of the transformation varies from 3% to 15%. Signs of malignant degeneration include sudden rapid growth, facial paralysis, development of irregular margins, fixation to surrounding tissues, and skin ulceration.

Gross examination of a typical pleomorphic adenoma reveals an ovoid, smooth, and firm encapsulated mass. The capsule is of varying thickness; the apparent satellitosis is really an outgrowth of the main mass, which can be demonstrated on serial sections. Compression of surrounding tissues is expected and should not be misinterpreted as a sign of malignancy. The cut surface is moist and gray-white and may have areas of cartilage. Capsules with a myxoid stroma may have a slimy consistency. Cystic spaces may be present.

On microscopic examination, pleomorphic adenomas are morphologically complex and diverse. There is an epithelial component and a stromal component, and both can be remarkably pleomorphic (Fig. 34–3). The epithelial component consists largely of epithelial and myoepithelial cells, which are classically arranged in a tubular pattern with an inner row of epithelial cells and an outer row of myoepithelial cells. However, the epidermoid cells may show keratinization, and the two cell types may occur in a wide variety of other patterns. The stroma is also pleomorphic and consists of mixtures of mucoid, myxomatous, and fibrous areas with chondroid areas. Ossification is rare. Thyrosine crystals may be found in the nonepithelial areas; these appear to be unique to pleomorphic adenomas. There is an equal distribution of myxoid and acellular components in 36%; 22% are predominantly cellular; and 12% are extremely cellular.

The treatment of pleomorphic adenoma, wherever it occurs, is complete excision with a cuff of normal tissue around it. Adherence to this policy produces a recurrence rate of less than 5%. For the parotid gland, this requires a minimum of superficial parotidectomy with preservation of the facial nerve. A recommendation of enucleation followed by postoperative radiation is mentioned only to be condemned. Subjecting a patient to the risks and complications of two modalities of tumor treatment when one carefully applied modality suffices seems irrational. There is excellent evidence that a well-performed par-

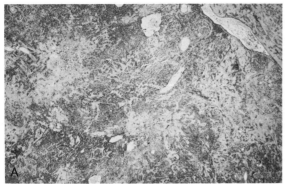 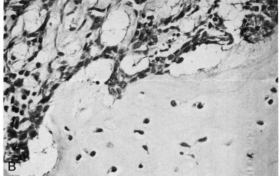

Figure 34–3. *A*. Low-power view of pleomorphic adenoma (magnified 25 times). *B*. High-power view of pleomorphic adenoma (magnified 250 times).

otidectomy yields the smallest recurrence rate and the least morbidity. In the parotid gland, it is often difficult to obtain a 360° cuff of normal tissue around the tumor because the closest margin is virtually always some branch of the facial nerve that passes very close to the capsule. Despite this drawback, the recurrence rate with careful superficial parotidectomy is low.

The recurrent pleomorphic adenoma deserves special mention. When enucleation is performed, recurrence rates as high as 50% have been reported, as have delays as long as 30 years. The recurrence rate after formal excision with generous margins is generally under 5%. In either case, repeat excision is the treatment of choice and may be a demanding operative procedure. Care must be taken at every step, for the nerve may be damaged at the time of flap elevation or at any time thereafter because the previous procedure, particularly if it was a superficial or total parotidectomy, and subsequent scarring may have displaced the nerve from its normal location.

The nerve stimulator and the operating microscope may be invaluable in identifying the nerve in the midst of scar and recurrent tumor. The surgeon should be prepared to dissect the nerve in either an antegrade or a retrograde manner. On rare occasions, en bloc removal of the recurrent tumor and the involved portion of the facial nerve may offer the only reasonable chance for cure. If this is necessary, the resected branch of the facial nerve should be repaired immediately. If, in this situation, resection would require removal of the main trunk of the facial nerve, if the tumor burden is small, and if the patient is not young, consideration should

be given to employing radiation therapy before the nerve is sacrificed. There is some evidence that radiation may halt the growth of some pleomorphic adenomas. If radiation fails, the main trunk can still be resected, particularly because it has been shown that radiation does not interfere with nerve regeneration.

Benign pleomorphic adenomas of the salivary glands are rare in children. In all reported series, the tumors were small, and in all cases they were more common in the parotid gland than in other sites. All the patients presented with an asymptomatic mass in the salivary gland that had existed for months to years. Two cases have been reported in which the patients' recurrent neoplasms eventually developed malignant degeneration.

Warthin's Tumor

This entity was first described in Europe in 1910 by H. Albrecht and L. Artz. In 1929, in the United States, Warthin reported the first two cases in the American literature. The disease has been named adenolymphoma by the World Health Organization. Common usage in the United States pays homage to Warthin. In addition, the term *adenolymphoma* carries a connotation of malignancy, which does not exist with this entity. The tumor is thought to arise from heterotopic salivary tissue entrapped within lymph nodes during embryogenesis, and there is a considerable body of evidence in support of this theory. Despite a few unquestioned exceptions occurring in the lip and the palate, Warthin's tumor should be considered as an almost exclusively parotid disease. Most cited exceptions to this location are suspect.

Warthin's tumors are reported in the age range from 2.5 to 92 years; 82% occur between the ages of 41 and 70 years. It has long been said that there is a 5:1 predominance in males. The author's personal experience and a report suggest that this ratio is changing dramatically. The authors of the report found a decreasing male-to-female ratio of less than 2:1. It is hypothesized that the reason for this change is an increased incidence of smoking by women, which may be responsible for the increasing incidence of Warthin's tumor among females. In the study of decreasing male predominance, 93.8% of the patients with Warthin's tumor were smokers. The tumor is rare in Blacks and Asians, however. It is bilateral in 5% to 10% of cases. It accounts for 6% to 10% of parotid tumors and is the second most common benign tumor in the parotid gland. Approximately 5% of tumors may be multicentric within the same gland.

The clinical presentation is usually that of a well-defined, soft-to-firm mass in the tail of the parotid, frequently under the ear lobe. It is generally 3 to 4 cm in diameter and asymptomatic. However, as many as 18% of patients may complain of pain. In addition, there have been three reported cases of facial paralysis associated with Warthin's tumor and 15 reported cases of malignant Warthin's tumor. The average duration of the mass on presentation is 3 years.

On gross inspection, the tumor is usually encapsulated, round or oval, cystic, and compressible. Upon sectioning, the tumor contains a mucoid brown- to gray-tinged fluid.

The cut surface has multiple irregular cystic spaces with papillary projections.

Microscopic examination shows a double layer of epithelial cells with a lymphoid stroma containing mature follicles (Fig. 34–4). The inner row of epithelial cells has nuclei that are vesicular, whereas those in the outer layer are pyknotic and located toward the luminal surface. Epithelial cells contain abundant mitochondria typical of oncocytes.

The treatment of Warthin's tumor is excision, which usually means a superficial parotidectomy. Recurrence rates are essentially unavailable, partly because of the multicentricity possible in a single gland. In various series, the recurrence rate ranges from 9% to 12%.

Involvement of Warthin's tumor by lymphoma has been reported, and it has been shown to be composed of B cells. There have, however, been only nine reported cases of non-Hodgkin's lymphoma in Warthin's tumor. There have been 17 reported cases of epithelial malignancies in Warthin's tumors. Two cases occurred in patients who had received previous radiation therapy to the area for benign conditions 8 and 13 years earlier.

Oncocytoma

Oncocytes were originally believed to be degenerative epithelial cells from either the acini or interlobular ducts, but electron microscopic studies have refuted this belief. The cells contain an abundance of mitochondria but have an increase in abnormal metabolism, with production of only small amounts of adenosine triphosphate. In addition, on-

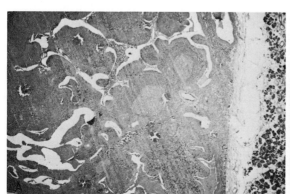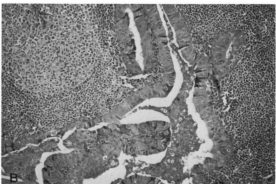

Figure 34–4. *A.* Low-power view of Warthin's tumor (magnified 25 times). *B.* High-power view of Warthin's tumor (magnified 100 times).

cocytes appear to be the consequence of an acquired disturbance of the mitochondrial enzyme organization. Oncocytes are normal findings in aging salivary tissue, particularly in the parotid gland. Oncocytes are rarely seen in salivary tissue before the age of 50 years but are seen nearly 100% of the time in patients over 70 years of age. Because other cells can give a staining appearance similar to that of the oncocyte, the precise documentation of mitochondria must be done by histochemical or electron microscopic means. To further complicate the matter, the criteria for the separation of neoplastic and hyperplastic lesions have not been set. However, most oncocytic lesions are probably hyperplastic rather than neoplastic.

The oncocytoma was first described in 1875 and probably accounts for less than 1% of all salivary gland tumors. It most commonly occurs in the parotid gland and is unusual in other sites. In report series, bilaterality and multicentricity have been conspicuous. In concert with the appearance of the oncocyte, most tumors occur in the sixth decade, and there is a 2:1 female-to-male ratio. On close examination, the tumor is encapsulated, lobular, and usually less than 5 cm in diameter. On cut section, it may be solid or papillary. Under microscopic examination, the tumor consists of large cells with an oxyphilic granular cytoplasm. It is currently impossible to differentiate the benign from the malignant oncocytoma on microscopic examination alone, but malignant tumors are usually solid. The treatment is complete excision. Recurrences are uncommon and should be viewed with suspicion because they may herald a malignant biologic course. Thus recurrences should be treated quickly and aggressively.

Monomorphic Adenomas

The World Health Organization and the Armed Forces Institute of Pathology classify Warthin's tumor and the oncocytoma as monomorphic adenomas, but most of the world's literature limits discussion of monomorphic adenomas to the basal cell adenoma, the membranous adenoma, the salivary duct adenoma, the sebaceous adenoma, the clear cell adenoma, the hybrid basal cell adenoma, and the myoepithelioma. Some articles are more restrictive.

The characteristics of monomorphic ade-

nomas are a monomorphic cellular composition, probable origin in the intercalated duct reserve cell, common multicentricity in the major salivary glands, common occurrence in the minor salivary glands, and benign biologic course. In many monomorphic adenomas, there are histologic features that recall stages in the embryologic development of dermal adnexa as well as salivary glands. The closest anlage among skin tumors is the dermal eccrine cylindroma.

The basal cell adenoma is an uncommon tumor; there are fewer than 200 cases in the world's literature. The average age is 60 years, and there is an equal sex distribution. There is a distinct predilection for the parotid gland and for the minor salivary glands in the upper lip; 80% of minor salivary gland tumors occur in the upper lip. Some authors consider the lesion to be the benign variant of the adenoid cystic carcinoma or a nonpleomorphic form of the pleomorphic adenoma. Treatment is excision, and recurrences are unexpected. The hybrid basal cell adenoma is a rare form of basal cell adenoma with histologic features that suggest an evolution toward pleomorphic adenoma or adenoid cystic carcinoma.

The myoepithelioma, a rare tumor, is probably a monomorphic variant of the pleomorphic adenoma. The diagnosis is difficult to make and requires electron microscopic demonstration of myoepithelium.

Ectopic sebaceous glands occur in 33% of parotid glands in adults but are less common in the other salivary glands. Three types of sebaceous cell neoplasms can occur: the sebaceous lymphadenoma, the sebaceous carcinoma, and the sebaceous adenoma.

Hemangioma

The hemangioma accounts for 50% of all parotid growths in children. It is uncommon in the salivary glands in adults. The exact nature is unclear, but capillary hemangiomas are probably neoplasms or vascular malformations, whereas cavernous hemangiomas are best regarded as a reaction to trauma or as a vascular malformation. Capillary hemangiomas are the most common; 61% are present at birth, and 86% appear within the first month of life. They manifest as a discrete mass of variable consistency and growth rate. A period of rapid growth, during which the mass may be quite hard, is common at 4 to

6 months of age. The mass is generally painless, transluminates poorly, and does not compress. There may be an associated cutaneous hemangioma that lends strong circumferential evidence to the diagnosis. On roentgenologic examination, 50% show phleboliths. On clinical presentation, it is generally quite characteristic. Should there be any doubt, CT or MRI can reliably establish the vascular nature of this lesion. In general, no treatment is necessary because more than 90% of hemangiomas undergo spontaneous involution within the first 5 years of life. If a cutaneous hemangioma is present, the two involute simultaneously, and this involution is heralded by a central graying of the cutaneous mass. Thus treatment is not necessary in the absence of a complication. In one series in which treatment was necessary, the mortality was 4.3%, and the incidence of facial paralysis was 23%.

Submandibular, Sublingual, and Minor Salivary Gland Tumors

The same benign tumors that occur in the parotid gland also occur in the other salivary glands. The statistics in these glands, however, are dominated by the pleomorphic adenoma and the basal cell adenoma. Other benign tumors are exceedingly rare. For these tumors, the biologic behavior remains benign, and complete excision is curative. The submandibular gland is the site of 10% of all salivary gland neoplasms; of these, 40% are pleomorphic adenomas, and there is a 2:1 female-to-male predominance. The tumors are often inconspicuous and asymptomatic as well as slow-growing. Thus the duration of the mass before treatment often exceeds 5 years. CT or MRI generally shows a smooth mass within the body of the submandibular gland. Complete excision of the submandibular gland is usually curative. The rate of recurrence is 5% to 6%, and this invariably follows inadequate excision. The sublingual gland is the site of 0.5% to 4.5% of all salivary gland tumors. Fewer than 50 cases of benign tumors have been reported, which underscores the fact that at least 80% of the sublingual gland tumors are malignant. The benign tumors are virtually exclusively pleomorphic adenomas and manifest as an asymptomatic mass under the anterior tongue in the floor of the mouth. CT scan or MRI is quite helpful in this area and generally delineates the

boundaries of the mass well. Complete excision of this gland is curative, and no recurrences have been reported.

Although minor salivary glands are distributed widely in the upper respiratory tract, at least 50% of all minor salivary gland tumors occur in the oral cavity; of these, 50% occur on the palate, followed in frequency by the upper lip and the buccal mucosa. In the palate itself, the most common location is the posterior third of the hard palate and the soft palate. This corresponds to the location of the minor salivary glands, which are uncommon anterior to a line connecting the first molars. Benign tumors in all locations appear as asymptomatic submucosal swellings that are usually present for months. Except for those in the palate, they are generally mobile. Pleomorphic adenomas account for 56% of all minor salivary gland intraoral tumors. Second in frequency is the basal cell adenoma. Management is by wide excision.

Minor salivary gland neoplasms account for 4% to 8% of all neoplasms in the nose and paranasal sinuses. Most of these tumors are malignant; the pleomorphic adenoma is third in frequency, following the adenoid cystic carcinoma and the adenocarcinoma. All of the benign neoplasms are quite rare. The pleomorphic adenoma is usually intranasal rather than intrasinus and most often arises from the nasal septum; 20% arise from the lateral nasal wall. The larynx and trachea are uncommon sites for benign salivary gland neoplasms, and essentially all reported cases are pleomorphic adenomas.

MALIGNANT NEOPLASMS

General Considerations

Malignant neoplasms are much less common than are benign neoplasms. Approximately one of six parotid, one of three submandibular, one of two minor salivary gland, and four of five sublingual gland neoplasms are malignant. If specific histologic types are disregarded, the prognosis is most favorable for neoplasms located on the palate, slightly less favorable for those in the parotid, and least favorable for those in the submandibular gland. Because malignant tumors of the salivary glands often have a protracted course, the success of any treatment program is best evaluated at 20 years rather than at 5 years or 10 years. The majority of malignant salivary gland neoplasms occur in the fifth and sixth decades; 2% occur in children 1 to 2 years of age, and 16% occur in people under 30 years of age.

Like benign tumors, 60% to 85% of malignant neoplasms appear as asymptomatic masses. In the minor salivary glands, the most common location is the palate, followed by the tongue, as is the case for benign tumors. The presence or absence of pain does not help in distinguishing the benign from the malignant; 5% of the benign and 6% of the malignant salivary neoplasms are associated with pain. Curiously, however, if the tumor is malignant, the presence of pain considerably worsens the prognosis. For those malignant tumors with pain, the overall 5-year survival is 33%, whereas for those without pain, it is 66%. Facial nerve paralysis on presentation portends a grave prognosis and occurs in 12% to 14% of parotid carcinomas. The 5-year mortality approaches 100% for this presentation. The incidence of distant metastases increases with increasing follow-up; the lungs are the most common site of metastasis, followed by bone. The overall recurrence rate for all salivary gland carcinomas varies from 27% to 50%. The only known risk factor for malignant tumors is previous radiation exposure. There is some controversy concerning the association of malignant salivary gland tumors with breast cancer, but this association has been reported. Additional reports have shown a positive correlation between malignant salivary gland tumors and skin carcinoma, which suggests some etiologic role for ultraviolet radiation exposure. As many as 11% of patients with a salivary gland cancer present with a simultaneous second malignancy.

In general terms, the lower the stage, the better the prognosis. The finding of decreasing survival with increasing stage has led some investigators to recommend planned combined therapy for high-grade tumors and for large tumors. Numerous studies have shown that planned combined therapy with surgery followed by postoperative radiation therapy improved survival over surgery alone. In one study, primary tumors in the parotid gland were controlled by surgery alone in 24%, by radiation alone in 15%, and by surgery and radiation combined in 74%. Primary submandibular tumors were controlled by surgery alone in 29%, by radiation alone in 0%, and by surgery combined with radiation in 70%. In another study, local control rate was improved from 20% to 70% by the addition of postoperative radiation therapy.

Mucoepidermoid Carcinoma

The mucoepidermoid carcinoma was first reported in 1895 and is a specific type of adenocarcinoma. This neoplasm received its current name in 1945 based on the two main cellular components seen on microscopic examination, mucous cells and epidermoid cells (Fig. 34–5). Mucoepidermoid carcinoma accounts for 3% to 9% of all salivary gland tumors, 7% to 29% of all malignant salivary gland tumors, and 10% to 20% of parotid neoplasms. More than 60% of all mucoepidermoid carcinomas occur in the parotid gland. The palate is the second most common location.

Mucoepidermoid carcinomas are currently divided into low, intermediate, and high grades on the basis of microscopic appearance. Low-grade tumors have numerous mucous cells and cystic spaces, whereas high-grade tumors resemble squamous cell carcinomas with few mucous cells. Both intracellular and extracellular keratinization may occur. In general, biologic behavior parallels the microscopic appearance. Seventy-five percent of mucoepidermoid carcinomas are low grade. On close examination, the tumors are unencapsulated; the low-grade tumors usually are well circumscribed, and the high-grade tumors are less well defined.

Most low-grade mucoepidermoid carcinomas appear as masses indistinguishable from

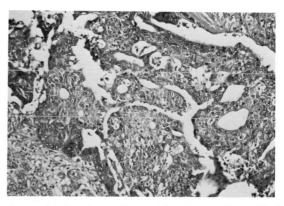

Figure 34–5. Mucoepidermoid carcinoma (magnified 100 times).

pleomorphic adenomas. The majority occur in the fourth to sixth decades with a history usually months to years long. The MRI or CT scan usually shows a well-circumscribed mass within the parotid gland. Fewer than 10% ever develop metastases. In general, adequate treatment is by wide excision, with a recurrence rate of approximately 15%. Recurrences should be treated aggressively because the biologic behavior may belie the benign microscopic appearance. For low-grade tumors, the overall 5-year survival is 90%.

The high-grade mucoepidermoid carcinoma usually has a shorter history. On clinical examination, the margins are usually less distinct. As many as 25% of patients have preoperative facial paralysis, and up to 50% have cervical metastases. CT scan or MRI may also show ill-defined borders in this tumor. Current data show that adequate surgical resection, followed by routine postoperative radiation, is the treatment of choice. The 5-year survival is 45%. According to reports of survival rates by stage, the 5-year survival is 100% for stage 1, 65% for stage 2, and 10% for stage 3 regardless of histologic grade.

Adenoid Cystic Carcinoma

The adenoid cystic carcinoma has been recognized since 1853 as a specific variant of adenocarcinoma of the salivary and mucous glands. The tumor was given the name cylindroma in 1857 by Billroth, but this term has proved to be too nonspecific and should be discarded. It accounts for 4% of all neoplasms of the major salivary glands and 2% to 5% of

all parotid tumors; it comprises 35% of all malignant minor salivary gland tumors and 40% to 60% of all sublingual gland tumors. It is the most common malignant tumor of the submandibular gland. The mean age at presentation is 45 years; there is an equal sex and racial distribution. The majority appear as asymptomatic masses with a history of duration of 4 weeks to 20 years; 20% of patients present with paresthesias, whereas 30% have partial or total facial paralysis. This high percentage of early facial paralysis graphically demonstrates the propensity to perineural invasion, which is the hallmark of this tumor (Fig. 34–6).

Like the high-grade mucoepidermoid carcinoma, the adenoid cystic carcinoma often has indistinct margins, which are well appreciated both on clinical examination and on CT scan or MRI. The diagnosis can usually be made by fine-needle aspiration cytology with a high degree of accuracy. The tumor is unencapsulated with microscopic extensions that belie its appearance of being circumscribed. There is considerable controversy over whether the survival rate can be related to histologic appearance in this tumor. Survival is dependent on site, with 15-year survival rates of 38% for the palate, 21% for the parotid, 10% for the submandibular gland, and 8% for tumors of the maxillary sinus area. Regardless of histologic type, the best prognosis is for patients whose tumors are less than 4 cm in diameter. Patients with this disease are at lifelong risk of recurrence. In one study at 20 years, 48% of the survivors had metastases and local recurrence. This tumor tends to metastasize hematogenously, unlike most salivary gland tumors, and spreads most commonly to the lungs and to

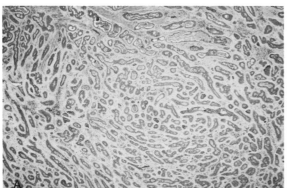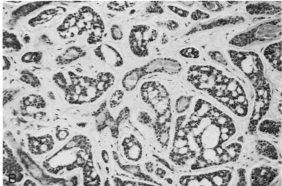

Figure 34–6. *A.* Low-power view of adenoid cystic carcinoma (magnified 25 times). *B.* High-power view of adenoid cystic carcinoma (magnified 100 times).

bone. Whereas approximately one third of patients with pulmonary metastases die within 1 year, 20% live 5 years or more. Lymph node involvement is uncommon, resulting usually from direct extension rather than embolic metastases. According to a review of 52 published studies in the literature, the 5-year and 10-year survival rates for adenoid cystic carcinoma were 62% and 39%, respectively. It is now generally agreed that planned combined therapy is the treatment of choice for adenoid cystic carcinoma. In one study, tumors treated with radiation alone recurred in 100% of patients. Of the patients who were treated with planned combined therapy, 50% relapsed locally within 5 years. There was, however, a small subgroup whose field size exceeded 8 cm by 8 cm and whose dose exceeded 4500 cGy; 88% of these patients remained disease free at 5 years, in comparison with only 22% of those whose dose or field size or both were inadequate by comparison.

Malignant Pleomorphic Adenoma

Three neoplasms are included under the generic term malignant pleomorphic adenoma. The overall frequency of these malignant pleomorphic adenomas is low, accounting for less than 2% of all pleomorphic adenomas. The great majority of these are carcinomas arising in or from a pre-existent benign pleomorphic adenoma, the so-called carcinoma ex-pleomorphic adenoma. One of the other two histologic types is malignant from the beginning and contains both components of a mixed tumor, epithelial and mesenchymal. In one variant there is a synchronous, biphasic malignant neoplasm, a carcinosarcoma whose metastases contain both carcinoma and sarcoma; this is exceedingly rare, and only a few cases have been reported. The third type is the very rare metastasizing benign pleomorphic adenoma. This represents a situation in which a histologically completely benign pleomorphic adenoma metastasizes.

The preferred terminology for the most common variant is carcinoma ex-pleomorphic adenoma, which was coined in 1970. Most commonly the carcinoma ex-pleomorphic adenoma arises in a pleomorphic adenoma of long duration, as a consequence either of no treatment or of recurrence. The risk of carcinomatous transformation appears to increase as the age of the tumor increases, and this is supported by deoxyribonucleic acid (DNA) analysis, which shows that there is an increasing DNA content in pleomorphic adenomas with short in comparison with long preoperative duration. This neoplasm is most common in the fifth and sixth decades, and the average age is 10 years older than the average age of presentation of benign pleomorphic adenoma. The classical history is that of a long-standing asymptomatic mass that suddenly manifests rapid growth, often with associated pain. This tumor is more malignant than are the more common salivary gland carcinomas. Nodal metastases have developed in 25% of patients on initial presentation. Local recurrence after initial resection occurs in 30%, and perineural invasion occurs in up to 50%. The treatment of this tumor is wide excision. A radical neck dissection should be performed if there is cervical lymphadenopathy, and it should be considered even if there is not. Patients should also undergo postoperative radiation. Reported 5-year survival rates vary from 48% to 77%; 20-year survival rates approach 0%.

Acinous Cell Carcinoma

This neoplasm was classified as a benign adenoma until 1953, at which time it was demonstrated that with sufficient follow-up, some of these neoplasms behaved in a clearly malignant manner. The majority of investigators now believe that all are malignant, some being of low grade and some high. The high-grade carcinomas manifest intravascular extension, fingerlike invasion, and medullary, ductuloglandular, or primitive tubular growth patterns. More than 90% occur in the parotid gland; the second most common location is the oral cavity, in which 66 cases have been reported. This tumor accounts for 2% to 5% of all parotid neoplasms and 17% to 19% of all malignant parotid neoplasms; 3% are bilateral.

Most cases occur between the fourth and fifth decades, but the incidence of this tumor is second only to that of the mucoepidermoid carcinoma of malignant tumors in children. In most series there is a 2:1 female predominance. This tumor generally manifests as an asymptomatic, slowly growing mass. Biologic behavior cannot be predicted from the histomorphologic pattern or by cell type. In one large study of 244 cases, the recurrence rate was 12%, the metastatic rate was 7.8%, and the death rate was 6.1%. Recurrences have been reported from 1 to 50 years after initial treatment, the average duration to time of recurrence being 14 years. Metastases tend to be hematogenous to the lungs and bone, particularly the vertebral column. Treatment is complete excision, in general with sparing of the facial nerve. Recurrences should be treated aggressively; numerous reports attest to successful salvage.

Adenocarcinoma

Adenocarcinomas are those primary glandular malignant neoplasms that cannot be classified as adenoid cystic, acinous cell, or mucoepidermoid carcinomas. They account for 2.8% of all parotid neoplasms and 15% of all parotid carcinomas. They most often occur in the fourth to sixth decades. Presentation with facial paralysis occurs in 22%; 25% have regional metastases, and 20% have systemic metastases. Treatment is wide excision. Radical neck dissection should be performed if there is cervical adenopathy, and many surgeons would perform a prophylactic neck dissection. Postoperative radiation should be given because the development of recurrence carries a grave prognosis. Five-year survival rates range from 49% to 78%.

Squamous Cell Carcinoma

Primary squamous cell carcinoma in the salivary glands is unusual. To make the diagnosis, the examiner must exclude (1) the high-grade mucoepidermoid carcinoma, (2) metastatic squamous cell carcinoma to the gland or nodes within the gland, (3) invasion of the gland from contiguous structures, and (4) squamous metaplasia within the gland. In a number of large series, this tumor accounts for 0.3% to 3.4% of parotid tumors. There is a 2:1 male predominance, and the patient is usually over the age of 60 years. Most authors recommend total parotidectomy with sacrifice of the facial nerve and immediate repair as initial treatment. A radical neck dissection should be performed if there is cervical adenopathy and given serious consideration even if there is not. Most authors would follow with postoperative radiation therapy. In one large series, the 5-year and 10-year determinate survival rates

by stage were 83% and 75% for stage 1 and 14% and 11% for stage 2 and stage 3.

Undifferentiated Carcinomas

The undifferentiated carcinomas are those tumors that cannot be classified as adenocarcinomas or squamous cell carcinomas. They are uncommon and account for less than 3% of all salivary gland neoplasms and for 1% to 4.5% of all malignant parotid tumors. They most commonly occur in the seventh and eighth decades. One third appear to arise in a pre-existing pleomorphic adenoma, usually of long duration; 33% of patients have partial or total facial paralysis, and 40% extend beyond the parotid on presentation. The recommended treatment is wide excision followed by postoperative radiation. The 5-year survival is the lowest for all salivary gland tumors at 25% to 30%.

Metastatic Disease to the Parotid

Approximately 20 lymph nodes are associated with the parotid gland. They are divided into the intraglandular and paraglandular lymph nodes, which communicate freely with each other. The intraglandular nodes are located within the portion of the gland lateral to the facial vein. Afferent channels drain the nose, the eyelids and the conjunctiva, the frontotemporal scalp, the external auditory meatus, the middle ear, the lacrimal gland, and the sinonasal, nasopharyngeal, and oropharyngeal cavities. The paraglandular nodes lie in the subcutaneous tissue and are largely pretragal and supratragal in location. They drain the lateral surface of the auricle and the adjacent scalp and cheek. Both groups drain to the cervical chain.

Metastatic carcinoma must be in the differential diagnosis of any parotid mass. Metastatic carcinoma to the parotid is almost always the result of lymphatic embolic spread to the lymph nodes. Contiguous spread and hematogenous spread to the parenchyma are uncommon. Thus patients at high risk are those with deeply invasive melanoma or with poorly to moderately differentiated squamous cell carcinoma of the eyelid, conjunctiva, frontotemporal scalp, posterior cheek, or anterior ear. Fifty percent of these lesions metastasize at some time in the course of the disease, and 33% of patients have parotid metastases as the first manifestation of metastatic disease. The treatment plan must be aggressive if any hope is to be offered for cure. Excision should include the primary lesion, in continuity with the parotid gland, and a radical neck dissection should be performed if possible. Postoperative radiation should be used. The usual 5-year survival rates are 12.5% overall and 11% for melanomas and 14% for squamous cell carcinomas. Infraclavicular primary tumors with metastases to the parotid gland are quite rare, and the sites in descending order of frequency are the lungs, the breasts, the kidneys, and the gastrointestinal tract.

Submandibular, Sublingual, and Minor Salivary Gland Carcinomas

Fifty percent of submandibular gland tumors are malignant. They are the same histologic type that occur in the parotid gland but, in general, are more aggressive. The relative frequency is also different. In a literature review involving 632 cases, the most common was adenoid cystic carcinoma, followed by mucoepidermoid carcinoma; most of the remainder were equally divided among undifferentiated carcinoma, squamous cell carcinoma, carcinoma ex-pleomorphic adenoma, and adenocarcinoma. Five-year survival rates are poor, being approximately 10% for adenoid cystic carcinomas, 17% for mucoepidermoid carcinoma, and 0% for adenocarcinoma. Contemporary thinking favors a composite resection, and many authors would include a radical neck dissection and postoperative radiation therapy.

Tumors of the sublingual gland are unusual. Eighty percent are malignant; the adenoid cystic carcinoma and the mucoepidermoid carcinoma account for approximately 40% each. The presenting symptom is always a submucosal mass under the anterior tongue. Treatment and survival figures are similar to those for the submandibular gland.

The frequency of minor salivary gland tumors is equal to or more than that of tumors of the submandibular gland; 50% to 65% are malignant. The majority occur in the oral cavity; 50% of these occur on the palate. Most manifest as a mass only, although 18%

are also painful, and these are always adenoid cystic carcinomas. In all locations, the adenoid cystic carcinoma predominates and accounts for 35% to 40% of all malignant tumors. The preferred treatment is the widest possible excision. Strong consideration should be given to postoperative radiation because the overall 5-year survival rate with excision alone as primary therapy is 8%. Next in frequency is the adenocarcinoma, and third is the mucoepidermoid carcinoma. These are also marked by aggressive behavior with regional spread. Wide excision is the recommended treatment with postoperative radiation. The overall survival rates as reported are usually 44% at 5 years and 32% at 10 years.

MALIGNANT NEOPLASMS IN CHILDREN

In children, 25% to 35% of salivary gland tumors are malignant. All are rare; the mucoepidermoid carcinoma is the most common, followed by the acinous cell carcinoma. However, in one large study, the adenocarcinoma was second most common. Treatment should be the same for children as it is for adults, although radiation therapy should be used with some discretion.

SUGGESTED READINGS

Armstrong JG, Harrison LB, Spiro RH, et al: Malignant tumors of major salivary gland origin. Arch Otolaryngol Head Neck Surg 116:290–293, 1990.

Batsakis JG: Tumors of the Head and Neck. Baltimore: Williams & Wilkins, 1979.

Conley J: Salivary Glands and the Facial Nerve. New York: Grune & Stratton, 1975.

Eneroth CM: Incidence and prognosis of salivary-gland tumors at different sites. A study of parotid, submandibular and palatal tumors in 2632 patients. Acta Otolaryngol (Stockh) [Suppl] 263:174–178, 1969.

Johns ME, Coulthard SW: Survival and follow-up in malignant tumors of the salivary glands. Otolaryngol Clin North Am 10:455–460, 1977.

Rice DH: Surgery of the Salivary Glands. Philadelphia: Raven Press, 1986.

Spiro RH: Salivary neoplasms: overview of a 35-year experience with 2,807 patients. Head Neck Surg 8:177–184, 1986.

CHAPTER 35

Tonsillectomy and Adenoidectomy

Orval E. Brown, MD   Scott C. Manning, MD

Tonsillectomy and adenoidectomy are among the most commonly performed surgical procedures in the pediatric age group. These procedures have been the source of great controversy regarding indications and efficacy. Only in the 1980s did well-designed scientific studies begin to provide evidence on which to base rational indications for surgery. Tonsillectomy was described as a surgical procedure as early as A.D. 50 by Celsus. Adenoidectomy was probably initially described in the late 1800s by Wilhelm Myer of Copenhagen. Early surgical indications were diverse, and in the 1930s the medical community began to question whether children should be subjected to tonsillectomy and adenoidectomy for poorly defined indications. This climate of questioning the indications for tonsillectomy and adenoidectomy has probably been one of the major factors in the decrease in incidence of these procedures from approximately 2 million procedures in 1970 to approximately 260,000 in 1987. Reasonable and rational indications for surgery have been developed as a result of completed research and the climate of careful evaluation of surgery of the tonsils and adenoids.

Tonsillectomy and adenoidectomy should be regarded as separate procedures with separate indications. The major indications for removal of lymphoid tissue of the upper airway are recurrent or persistent infection, airway obstruction, and middle ear disease.

INDICATIONS

The indications for tonsillectomy and adenoidectomy are reviewed separately. The indications are still primarily clinical in basis, although some studies provide a stronger foundation on which to recommend surgical therapy.

Tonsillectomy

Indications for tonsillectomy can be divided into definite and relative indications (Table 35–1). Definite indications are primarily based on hypertrophy of the tonsils, which causes airway obstruction. Lymphoid hypertrophy is the most common cause of upper airway obstruction during sleep in children. Grundfast and Wittich (1982) noted that the incidence of upper airway obstruction secondary to tonsil and adenoid hypertrophy had increased in recent years. Upper airway obstruction is becoming the most common indication for tonsillectomy and adenoidectomy. Other definite indications include cor pulmonale secondary to tonsil hypertrophy, dysphagia for solid food, speech distortion, suspicion of malignancy, and uncontrollable tonsillar hemorrhage. Relative indications include recurrent tonsillitis, tonsillitis with complicating medical factors, and peritonsillar abscess.

Obstructive sleep apnea can be defined as a cessation of air flow during sleep for longer

TABLE 35–1. Indications for Tonsillectomy and Adenoidectomy

Definite Indications	Relative Indications
Tonsillectomy	
Airway obstruction	Recurrent tonsillitis
Obstructive sleep apnea	Tonsillitis with
Cor pulmonale	Complicating medical
secondary to tonsillar	factors
hypertrophy	Rheumatic fever
Dysphagia for solid food	Peritonsillar abscess
Speech distortion	
secondary to tonsillar	
hypertrophy	
Suspicion of malignancy	
Uncontrollable tonsillar	
hemorrhage	
Adenoidectomy	
Nasal airway obstruction	
secondary to adenoidal	
hypertrophy	
Otitis media with effusion	
unresponsive to medical	
therapy	
Chronic adenoiditis	

than 10 seconds. However, the manifestations of upper airway obstruction can range from simple snoring without airway obstruction to severe obstructive sleep apnea with associated heart failure, altered growth and development, and behavior changes. It is the responsibility of the treating physician to decide when airway obstruction is significant enough to warrant tonsillectomy and adenoidectomy. This is best determined with a complete history and a thorough physical examination. Snoring that is not significant is associated with orderly and regular respi-

rations. Snoring with obstructive apnea with cessation of air flow and paradoxical chest and abdominal movements followed by gasping for air is indicative of significant obstructive sleep apnea. Associated problems can include enuresis, frequent awakenings, restless sleep, sweating, excessive daytime sleepiness, mouth breathing, and behavior problems.

Physical examination should include observation of the patient's breathing and of the pharyngeal tonsils. Mouth breathing is frequently found, and the size of the tonsils should be assessed. The authors use a clinical grading system for assessing tonsillar size that includes grades 1 through 4. Grade 1 tonsil tissue is very small and insignificant. Grade 2 tonsil tissue is normal and nonobstructive. Grade 3 tonsils are large and appear to crowd the oropharynx, and grade 4 tonsils completely fill the oropharynx with flat medial surfaces opposing each other. These tonsils may hide the uvula (Fig. 35–1). Alternatively, Brodsky (1990) developed a system in which the tonsil size is graded on a 0 to +4 range. Grade 0 tonsils do not encroach upon the airway. Grade +1 tonsils include less than 25% of the airway. Grade +2 tonsils are readily apparent and obstruct 25% to 50% of the airway. Grade +3 tonsils obstruct 50% to 75% of the airway, and grade +4 tonsils are massive and obstruct more than 75% of the airway.

With both a history of obstructive sleep apnea and a physical examination result that are consistent with tonsillar hypertrophy in a healthy patient, the authors recommend

Figure 35–1. Grade 4 tonsils with flat medial surfaces obstructing the oropharynx.

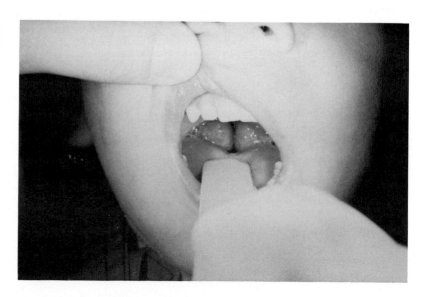

tonsillectomy. Lateral adenoid films are not made because the adenoids are evaluated at the time of surgery. If the adenoids are hypertrophic and obstructing the nasal airway, adenoidectomy is performed simultaneously. Adenoidectomy is not performed for small adenoids that do not obstruct the nasal airway.

Polysomnography has come into increasing use as the "gold standard" for the diagnosis of sleep apnea. The study consists of many different simultaneous recordings, which often include electrocardiogram, nasal and oral air flow assessment, pO_2 and pCO_2 monitoring, abdominal and chest breathing measurements, and electroencephalogram. Polysomnography is expensive and requires overnight hospital admission. It is a valuable diagnostic tool but is not indicated in all patients. The authors perform polysomnography in patients who have a history of obstructive sleep apnea but whose physical examination results are not consistent with this condition, or in patients who have no history of obstructive sleep apnea but whose physical examination reveals hypertrophic tonsils that should produce it. In addition, the authors often recommend polysomnography in very young patients or in patients with underlying medical diseases that complicate tonsillectomy, such as hematologic problems, severe anemia, bleeding disorders, neurologic problems such as cerebral palsy, or craniofacial disorders. Polysomnography allows determination of the severity of obstructive sleep apnea and can be valuable in directing therapy in these special patient groups. The authors recommend polysomnography in a distinct minority of patients seen for tonsil and adenoid problems.

In some patients, prolonged obstructive sleep apnea can result in elevated pCO_2 levels and hypoxia, which can progress to chronic hypercapnia with a respiratory center that is primarily driven by hypoxia. This can lead to cor pulmonale. Severe upper airway obstruction leading to cor pulmonale is the result of decreased respiratory minute volume from apnea, which leads to chronic alveolar hypoventilation. The resultant hypercapnia and hypoxia cause pulmonary artery vasoconstriction, leading to increased right ventricular work and eventual cardiac hypertrophy. When prolonged, this can cause right ventricular dilation that leads to cor pulmonale. Cor pulmonale can be divided into two groups: mild and severe.

Patients with mild cor pulmonale have only abnormal electrocardiographic or chest x-ray findings. Severely affected patients have elevated pCO_2 levels and are regarded as critically ill patients from both medical and surgical standpoints.

All patients undergoing tonsillectomy and adenoidectomy for obstructive sleep apnea are screened with a chest film and electrocardiogram. If the results of these studies are normal, the patient is managed routinely. Patients who have an abnormal chest film or electrocardiogram are admitted to the hospital on an urgent basis, and the cardiology service is consulted. Arterial blood gases are drawn, and an echocardiogram is performed. Patients are treated appropriately by the cardiology service, and those who are found to have normal pCO_2 without severe cor pulmonale are managed with tonsillectomy and adenoidectomy and with intensive postoperative observation. Patients who have an elevated pCO_2 level undergo tonsillectomy and adenoidectomy after medical stabilization in concert with cardiologic consultation. Intubation is maintained in the intensive care unit postoperatively. The patients are monitored until they can successfully maintain a normal pCO_2 level, which often takes between 2 and 5 days; they are then carefully extubated. Patients with chronic hypercapnia who breathe on hypoxic drive may suffer respiratory arrest upon administration of oxygen and removal of the airway obstruction. Accordingly, patients with cor pulmonale must be managed extremely carefully in order to prevent the postoperative complication of respiratory arrest.

Patients with tonsils large enough to cause dysphagia for solid food or poor weight gain have definite indications for tonsillectomy. Often these patients are affected by obstructive sleep apnea, and this must be taken into account. Other rare indications for tonsillectomy include a unilaterally enlarged or ulcerated tonsil in which there is a suspicion of malignancy. In children, the most common malignancies are those of mesodermal origin, such as lymphoma or Hodgkin's disease. In rare cases, a patient suffers uncontrollable hemorrhage from bleeding tonsil vessels. This condition is a definite indication for tonsillectomy. Patients who have speech distortion secondary to tonsillar hypertrophy should be strongly considered for tonsillectomy. As in patients with dysphagia for solid food, not only are the tonsils often large enough to cause speech disorder with hyponasal speech, but these patients also often have obstructive sleep apnea.

Relative indications for tonsillectomy are primarily those of infectious problems of the tonsils. Tonsillitis is one of the most common infections in the pediatric age group and probably is experienced by almost all people. The timing of and the need for tonsillectomy for recurrent tonsillitis are questions that have been facing physicians since the advent of tonsillectomy. Until the 1980s, the only indications were those of considered opinion. Paradise and coworkers (1984) found, in a study including both randomized and nonrandomized trials, that patients severely affected with tonsillitis benefited from tonsillectomy. They found that patients who suffered at least three episodes of documented streptococcal tonsillitis in each of 3 years, five episodes in each of 2 years, or seven episodes in 1 year had a significantly lower incidence of throat infection after tonsillectomy during 2 years of follow-up. The third-year follow-up differences were not statistically significant, although they did favor the surgical group.

Whereas this study provides evidence that recurrent tonsillitis is a disease process that, when severe, can be ameliorated by tonsillectomy, the authors did not feel that this study mandated surgical treatment. The management of each patient must be individualized, and the indications from this study are not to be taken as a "gold standard" for indicating surgery. It is the authors' recommendation that children who have five to six episodes of documented tonsillitis in a year or, occasionally, four episodes in 6 months, be considered reasonable candidates for tonsillectomy. Occasionally tonsillectomy may be indicated with a lower number of infections in patients with complicating medical factors. Patients who have rheumatic heart disease with the possibility of developing subacute bacterial endocarditis or other cardiac infection from a head and neck infection should be considered for tonsillectomy. These cases must be considered carefully, with the risk from the altered cardiac status and the relative risk to the patient's health from recurrent tonsillitis taken into account.

Peritonsillar abscess is the most common deep infection of the head and neck and has been traditionally considered an absolute indication for tonsillectomy. Children presenting with peritonsillar abscess are often ill and febrile with decreased oral intake and volume depletion. The bacteriologic study is usually that of a mixed flora; predominantly streptococcal, staphylococcal, and mixed anaerobes cause the infection. Patients with acute peritonsillar abscess are admitted to the hospital for intravenous administration of fluids and volume repletion, and the authors believe that the antibiotic treatment of choice is clindamycin. Because children do not protect their airways as well as adults do, patients under the age of 12 years who are not completely cooperative are often taken to the operating room for a careful incision and drainage of the peritonsillar abscess. The authors prefer not to perform an immediate tonsillectomy for quinsy because of the increased risk of bleeding, not primarily in the side on which the peritonsillar abscess is, but in the contralateral tonsillar fossa. Older patients who are cooperative can be managed with needle aspiration or careful incision and drainage with local anesthesia.

Schechter and associates (1982) found, in contrast to previous belief, that patients with one peritonsillar abscess are not necessarily prone to have recurrent peritonsillar abscesses. In view of this finding, tonsillectomy is recommended as an interval procedure when there is a history of other tonsil disease, such as recurrent tonsillitis, a previous peritonsillar abscess, or hypertrophy of the tonsils with obstructive sleep apnea.

Adenoidectomy

Adenoidectomy should be managed as a procedure separate from tonsillectomy; the indications are similar for both: lymphoid hypertrophy with airway obstruction or chronic infection. Indications for adenoidectomy include nasal airway obstruction secondary to adenoid hypertrophy with obstruction of the nasopharynx, otitis media with effusion, and chronic adenoiditis.

The adenoids are located in the nasopharynx proximal to the eustachian tube orifice. Middle ear disease with resultant otitis media with effusion is hypothesized to result either from chronic infection with inflammation of the eustachian tube orifice or from obstruction of the orifice; poor function of the eustachian tube results from hypertrophy of the adenoids. Enlargement of the adenoids with nasal airway obstruction results in mouth breathing, snoring, nasal discharge, and hy-

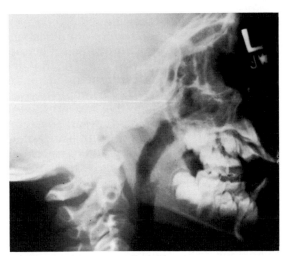

Figure 35–2. Lateral adenoid radiograph revealing a normal nasopharyngeal airway.

ponasal voice. Patients with hypertrophied adenoids and nasal airway obstruction often present with a long history of mouth breathing, snoring, and hyponasal speech. Other signs and symptoms related to adenoid hypertrophy include sleep disturbance, headaches, problems with cognitive and psychosocial development, and occasionally nocturnal enuresis.

Severe and long-term nasal airway obstruction, particularly in younger children, can result in delayed growth and development and occasionally in right-sided heart failure and cor pulmonale. Occasionally, older patients can be seen with so-called

adenoid facies, which consists of a long, narrow face, an open-mouthed appearance with an anterior open bite deformity, and a narrow high-arched protruding maxilla. The development of this craniofacial abnormality is somewhat controversial, and it is not entirely clear whether nasal airway obstruction from hypertrophic adenoids alone causes this or whether it is simply an accompaniment of abnormal facial development. Nevertheless, when confronted with this abnormality, the examining physician must look for adenoid hypertrophy and nasal airway obstruction. After other causes of nasal airway obstruction are ruled out, adenoid hypertrophy can be evaluated by mirror examination of the nasopharynx or by direct visualization by rigid or flexible fiberoptic instrumentation. The newer endoscopes can be used after careful application of topical decongestants and analgesics, and the posterior choana and nasopharynx can be directly evaluated. Adenoid hypertrophy obstructing the posterior choana can be clearly seen and the diagnosis confirmed.

A lateral neck or adenoid radiograph can be very helpful in evaluating children for nasal airway obstruction. In patients with nasal airway obstruction and no other evident cause of the problem, a lateral adenoid radiograph is usually obtained by the authors. Although some limitations can be present, the film is often diagnostic because it either is normal (Fig. 35–2) or shows hypertrophic adenoids obstructing the nasal airway (Fig. 35–3). When hypertrophy with nasal

Figure 35–3. Lateral adenoid radiograph revealing obstruction of the choana by hypertrophic adenoids.

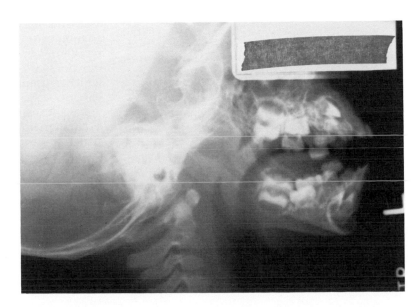

airway obstruction is diagnosed and confirmed, adenoidectomy is recommended.

The effect of adenoidectomy on ear disease, particularly otitis media with effusion and recurrent acute otitis media, has long been controversial. Two well-controlled trials have strongly indicated that adenoidectomy is beneficial in the treatment of middle ear effusion. Gates and colleagues (1987) studied 491 children 4 to 8 years old and found that patients undergoing adenoidectomy with simple myringotomy or with tympanostomy tube placement had a better 2-year outcome than did children who received myringotomy or tympanostomy tube placement without adenoidectomy. Patients undergoing adenoidectomy and tympanostomy tube placement had 47% less time with recurrent effusion than did patients receiving myringotomy alone. Gates and colleagues recommended adenoidectomy and myringotomy with removal of middle ear effusion as initial treatment for persistent otitis media with effusion. They also recommended insertion of tympanostomy tubes if effusion should recur after this medical treatment.

Paradise and associates (1990), in a randomized and nonrandomized trial of children undergoing a second tympanostomy tube insertion, found that adenoidectomy subjects had 47% less time with otitis media than did control subjects in the randomized trial and 28% fewer episodes of acute otitis media in the first year of follow-up. In the second year of follow-up, patients undergoing adenoidectomy had 37% less time with otitis media and 35% fewer episodes of acute otitis media than did control subjects. The study population ranged in age from 1 to 15 years; however, only seven patients were within the 1- to 2-year age group. Paradise and associates believed that adenoidectomy was effective for 2 years, and perhaps a third year, in reducing the overall occurrence of otitis media. The effect of adenoidectomy seemed greater with regard to time with middle ear effusion than to the incidence of acute middle ear infection, although this also seemed clinically improved. Paradise and associates concluded that adenoidectomy was warranted on an individualized basis for children who developed recurrent otitis media after extrusion of tympanostomy tubes.

In view of this information, the authors believe that adenoidectomy is beneficial in older patients with persistent otitis media with effusion unresponsive to medical therapy. In Gates and colleagues' study, the youngest age was 4 years; the youngest age group with significant numbers in Paradise and associates' study was 3 years. Routine adenoidectomy is not recommended for recurrent acute otitis media; Paradise and associates' study is suggestive but not definitive in the authors' opinion. Adenoidectomy is indicated in patients 3 years of age or older undergoing tympanostomy tube placement for persistent otitis media with effusion. Adenoidectomy evidently has a beneficial effect on eustachian tube function, which the authors infer from the results of these studies. Precisely what this effect is, whether removal of chronic infection or provision of better ventilation to the eustachian tube, is as yet unclear.

A few patients have "chronic" adenoiditis. These patients may not have significant hypertrophy of the adenoid pad, but they have persistent and recurrent purulent nasal discharge that recurs quickly after medical therapy. They are usually younger children in whom the paranasal sinuses are small and not clinically significant. Very occasionally, adenoidectomy can be indicated as a clinical trial in these patients for removing a chronic focus of infection and decreasing episodes of purulent rhinorrhea. A full work-up including immune studies is indicated before adenoidectomy in this small group of patients.

RISKS AND BENEFITS

It is the responsibility of the physician in assessing each patient for tonsillectomy and adenoidectomy to determine the individual risks and benefits to the patient. Included in the risks are considerable costs of surgery, which are approximately $2000 to $3000 per patient at major hospitals across the United States. Anesthesia risks, complications such as malignant hyperthermia or airway obstruction, and risks such as velopharyngeal insufficiency or nasopharyngeal stenosis must be weighed against the potential benefits to the patient. Improvement in the patient's airway, reduction in episodes of otitis media and improved hearing, less time in the physician's office, better sleep with improved psychosocial development and behavior, and normal craniofacial growth are all potential benefits. Although money is certainly not the determining factor, all these risks must be weighed carefully in the physician's attempt to fulfill the responsibility to do the very best for each patient. To have reasonable indications for surgery, the impact of the disease process must be severe enough to warrant the procedure, which in turn must be efficacious and as safe as possible in treating the disease process.

PREOPERATIVE WORK-UP

In the evaluation of patients for tonsillectomy and adenoidectomy, a careful, comprehensive history must be taken. A history for recurrent tonsillitis is relatively straightforward. In discussions of obstructive sleep apnea, a careful history of mouth breathing, snoring, and other sleep disturbances such as restless sleep, gasping, coughing, and choking should be established. The authors often demonstrate to the parents how a child with obstructive sleep apnea breathes, with obstruction and gasping at night, to be sure that they understand what obstructive sleep apnea is. Parents frequently identify these signs and confirm the diagnosis. A careful history for bleeding disorders must be obtained; the family history must be looked into, and a history of easy bruising or easy bleeding must be taken. A history of other medical problems, including congenital heart disease, cerebral palsy, or other high-risk states, must be investigated.

A careful physical examination must be performed, including a complete examination of the ears for associated otologic disease, nose and nasal cavity examination for nasal problems, and neck examination. For further diagnosis of nasal airway obstruction, the authors often apply topical decongestants and analgesics to the nose and do a fiberoptic examination. Nasal cavity abnormalities and adenoidal hypertrophy are readily demonstrable.

Radiographic and laboratory studies are indicated in some patients. The authors obtain a lateral adenoid radiograph if they are considering adenoidectomy alone. If tonsillectomy is performed, the adenoids are evaluated at surgery; if they are hypertrophic, they are removed. A lateral adenoid radiograph is generally not made if tonsillectomy is to be performed. A chest film and electrocardiogram are indicated in all patients with obstructive sleep apnea. If findings are ab-

normal, these patients are managed as described previously. Prothrombin time and partial thromboplastin time coagulation studies are usually not performed preoperatively. With a careful history for bleeding disorders and a normal physical examination, the screening prothrombin time and partial thromboplastin time have no predictive value for surgical bleeding. Manning and associates (1987) found that the prothrombin time has little value in detecting patients with inherited coagulopathies because these are usually abnormalities of the intrinsic clotting system. The partial thromboplastin time measures intrinsic clotting system function; however, it is insensitive when factor XIII, IX, or XI deficiencies are above 10% of normal. Because patients with mild classical hemophilia may have factor VIII levels of 5% to 25%, the partial thromboplastin time is insensitive to these disorders as well. It is likewise insensitive for detecting von Willebrand's disease, which is the most common single bleeding disorder.

A careful history of aspirin use should be taken, and aspirin must be stopped at least 1 week before surgery. Polysomnograms or sleep studies are not performed routinely in all patients undergoing tonsillectomy and adenoidectomy. Patients with recurrent tonsillitis without a history of obstructive sleep apnea generally do not require a polysomnogram. Normal, healthy patients with a positive history for obstructive sleep apnea and a physical examination consistent with hypertrophic tonsils do not usually undergo polysomnography. Polysomnography is reserved for patients with significant underlying disease processes, such as congenital heart disease or cerebral palsy, which increase the risk in these patients. Sleep studies are indicated in patients who have a positive history for obstructive sleep apnea but whose physical examination results are not consistent with this, or in a patient with no history for obstructive sleep apnea but very hypertrophic tonsils and adenoids. The polysomnogram is used to sort out difficult and problem cases.

CONTRAINDICATIONS AND HIGH-RISK PATIENTS

Contraindications for tonsil and adenoid surgery can be divided into three groups: hematologic problems, palatal problems and velopharyngeal insufficiency, and infection. Hematologic considerations are made for patients with anemia or bleeding disorders. In general, patients presenting with hematocrit of less than 30%, which has not been previously evaluated, require a medical and hematologic work-up for assessing the cause of the anemia. Surgery should be canceled and deferred until the cause of this problem can be assessed. The single most common cause of anemia in patients with tonsil and adenoid disease in the authors' practice is sickle cell anemia. Patients with sickle cell anemia commonly have hematocrit levels in the 25% to 30% range but are relatively stable. Patients with the sickle cell trait usually have hematocrit levels that are near normal and generally do not require special treatment. Patients with sickle cell anemia, however, must be very carefully managed because of the potential for sickle crisis, sickle chest syndrome, and stroke. All patients with sickle cell anemia are managed in concert with the hematologist. These patients are usually not transfused before surgery in the authors' practice, which is a controversial issue in pediatric hematology. All of these patients have a chest film and electrocardiogram preoperatively to assess their cardiac status. These patients are often hospitalized the night before surgery for intravenous hydration for ensuring volume repletion at surgery. After surgery, the patient is kept under intense observation, intravenous fluids and hydration are given, oxygen is administered to prevent sickling, and temperature is monitored to keep the patient warm. Periodic measurements of the hemoglobin level are obtained. If patients with sickle cell anemia are kept well hydrated, oxygenated, and warm, the incidence of serious complications in tonsillectomy and adenoidectomy is very low. However, some complications can occur independently, such as sickle chest syndrome, which resembles a severe pneumonia, or stroke.

The most common bleeding disorders in the authors' practice are von Willebrand's disease and hemophilia A or factor VIII deficiency. Patients with these disorders are managed in concert with the hematologist. Patients with mild to moderate hemophilia A or von Willebrand's disease can be managed with administration of desmopressin. This drug decreases the bleeding time by causing a transient twofold to threefold increase in plasma factor VIII complex levels. Desmopressin can be used on an every-other-day basis but should not be used daily so that tachyphylaxis is prevented. It is extremely safe, and because the risk of bleeding in tonsillectomy can be up to 2 weeks, the authors usually administer desmopressin on an every-other-day basis for at least 7 to 10 days postoperatively. Desmopressin can be given on an outpatient basis. Patients with more severe von Willebrand's disease, hemophilia A, or other hematologic diseases are managed in an individualized fashion with the hematologist.

A major consideration in adenoid surgery is the condition of the palate abnormalities that can result in hypernasal speech after adenoidectomy. Cleft palate or repaired cleft palate, submucous cleft with bifid uvula (Fig. 35–4), or relatively short palate in a large pharynx can result in nasal emission after adenoidectomy. Careful examination and palpation of the palate should be performed preoperatively, and if abnormalities are present, consideration should be given to consultation with a team expert in cleft palate and speech management. Occasionally, a careful anterior adenoidectomy can be undertaken to clear the posterior choana, but with a posterior adenoid pad left for velar closure.

Acute infection is a contraindication to tonsillectomy because its presence may increase the risk of postoperative bleeding. Therefore, the authors do not perform tonsillectomy on an acute basis in the presence of acute tonsillar infection. Acute tonsillectomy is usually deferred in the case of peritonsillar abscess, and patients with acute mononucleosis and airway obstruction can usually be managed with steroids and a nasal airway rather than acute tonsillectomy.

Certain patients can be considered to be at extremely high risk for tonsillectomy. Patients with cor pulmonale can develop respiratory arrest if they are not carefully managed with preoperative cardiac consultation and postoperative airway management. Patients with neurologic disorders such as cerebral palsy are at increased risk with tonsillectomy and adenoidectomy because of their altered neurologic status. These patients often have poor coordination of their airway swallowing mechanism and cough; they can have problems with aspiration and develop aspiration pneumonia postoperatively, and they are also at risk for airway obstruction

Figure 35–4. Child with bifid uvula and submucous cleft palate.

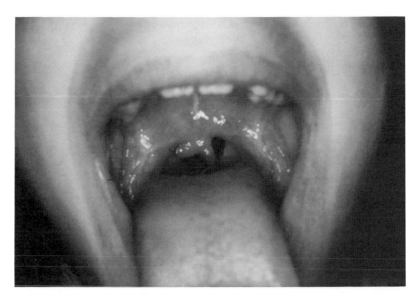

postoperatively. These patients are similar to patients with Down's syndrome, who have similar problems resulting from the floppiness and poor neurologic tone. Down's syndrome patients may refuse food and drink for prolonged periods and require prolonged hospitalization with intravenous fluids or nasogastric feedings until they eat postoperatively. Patients with craniofacial abnormalities, such as Treacher Collins syndrome or Crouzon's disease, should be managed very carefully because their airways are usually abnormal and they can have obstructive problems in the postoperative period. Extremely young patients, such as those under 2 years of age undergoing tonsillectomy and adenoidectomy, should be considered high-risk patients. Young pediatric patients do not maintain an airway as well as older children do, and the smaller size of the airway places them at greater risk for airway obstruction problems with the swelling that goes with tonsillectomy. These patients may require observation in the intensive care unit and management with a nasopharyngeal airway postoperatively.

COMPLICATIONS

Complications associated with tonsillectomy and adenoidectomy can be divided into those occurring early and those occurring late. Early complications consist primarily of hemorrhage and dehydration or volume depletion. The risk of postoperative hemorrhage ranges from about 3% to 5%. Handler and colleagues (1986) found a 2.62% incidence of postoperative bleeding, which was divided into primary hemorrhage (within 24 hours) of 0.14% and delayed hemorrhage of 2.48%. Although some authors recommend postoperative antibiotics for prevention of bleeding, no good controlled studies supporting the use of antibiotics in prevention of postoperative bleeding are available. The major methods used to prevent immediate postoperative bleeding include a thorough history and physical examination, for ruling out bleeding disorders and the use of aspirin, and meticulous hemostasis at the time of surgery. Some surgeons inject a local anesthetic with a vasoconstrictor at the time of surgery; however, it is not clear whether this form of therapy decreases the rate of postoperative hemorrhage. Delayed hemorrhage can occur anytime from 24 hours to 2 weeks postoperatively. Most commonly, delayed hemorrhage occurs 7 to 10 days postoperatively when the tonsillar eschar is shed. Patients with this complication can often be managed with observation if the bleeding stops spontaneously. Patients with significant bleeding or recurrent bleeding, however, may require general anesthesia to facilitate hemostasis. External carotid artery ligation is rarely indicated.

Because of pharyngeal pain, patients undergoing tonsillectomy and adenoidectomy often have poor fluid intake. This may resolve after 24 hours, but some children have problems lasting for 2 to 3 days. Pain relief in the immediate postoperative period can improve fluid intake, and the surgeon, in an effort to provide such relief, can inject a local anesthesia agent such as bupivacaine into the tonsillar fossa. The authors routinely recommend acetaminophen elixir for relief of pain during the postoperative period. Chewing gum can also reduce pain by relieving muscle spasm and improving swallowing. Steroids have no place in the postoperative management of patients undergoing tonsillectomy and adenoidectomy. Day-surgery patients are usually kept in the extended care unit postoperatively; intravenous fluid administration ensures hydration before discharge. These patients are observed to ensure that fluid intake is adequate before discharge. The patient should be carefully hydrated intraoperatively, and the fluid loss from preoperative restrictions must be replaced. However, the surgeon and anesthesiologist must be careful to avoid giving too much fluid because of the risk of pulmonary edema.

A prominent late complication for tonsillectomy and adenoidectomy is nasopharyngeal stenosis. This problem usually occurs when tonsillectomy and adenoidectomy are performed in concert and removal of mucosa from the palate and posterior pharynx results in extensive cicatrix development with fusion of the soft palate and tonsillar pillars to the posterior pharyngeal wall. This complication should be a rare occurrence if careful attention is paid to technique and to preservation of palatal and posterior pharyngeal mucosa. When this complication does occur, however, surgical correction is indicated. There are multiple methods of correction, including Z-plasty flaps, hard palate or retropharyngeal flaps, and laterally based pharyngeal flaps. This complication is difficult to manage and is better prevented.

Mortality from tonsillectomy and adenoidectomy is very uncommon, and the incidence of mortality from tonsil and adenoid surgery as a result of faulty surgical technique or postoperative complications is extremely low. Paradise (1990) reported no mortalities among 35,710 children undergoing tonsil and adenoid surgery at Pittsburgh Eye and Ear Hospital between 1954 and 1974. The risk of anesthesia is probably the major concern in tonsil and adenoid surgery, and mortality from this aspect of the procedure probably ranges from approximately 1 in 15,000 to 1 in 50,000 patients.

OUTPATIENT TONSILLECTOMY AND ADENOIDECTOMY

An increasing trend in medical practice is to perform surgery on an outpatient or day-surgery basis. The appropriateness of tonsillectomy and adenoidectomy as outpatient surgery is a source of controversy. Many physicians are reluctant to discharge patients after tonsillectomy and adenoidectomy because of the risk of postoperative complications. However, hospitals, patients, and physicians are under increasing demands from third-party payers to control costs. Whereas certain patients can be managed safely on an outpatient basis, others are inappropriate candidates for ambulatory tonsillectomy and adenoidectomy. It is the physician's responsibility to carefully identify patients who are candidates for ambulatory surgery. In an extensive review, Carithers and coworkers (1987) found that 98.2% of patients undergoing tonsillectomy and adenoidectomy who were candidates for outpatient surgery could be released 10 hours after surgery with less than a 10% chance of subsequent complications. They believed that their study indicated that patients undergoing tonsillectomy and adenoidectomy should be kept at least 8 to 10 hours after surgery for minimizing the risk of complications after discharge. However, Helmus and coworkers (1990) reviewed 1088 patients undergoing tonsillectomy and adenoidectomy and found a very low incidence of complications.

Shott and associates (1987) reviewed 491 patients undergoing tonsil and adenoid surgery and developed guidelines for outpatient surgery. They believed that inappropriate candidates for outpatient tonsil and adenoid surgery are very young patients (under 3 years of age), patients who live more than an hour's drive from the hospital, patients with obstructive sleep apnea, and patients with other medical problems. Occasionally, social circumstances with perceived inadequate postoperative observation may indicate that the patient should be hospitalized. If it appears that adult supervision will be inadequate, with inadequate communication or transportation between home and hospital, hospitalization after tonsillectomy and adenoidectomy should be strongly considered. Patients who are very young—under 3 years of age according to Shott and associates, and under 5 years of age in the authors' experience—are not reasonable candidates for outpatient tonsillectomy and adenoidectomy. Very young patients have smaller airways and are at greater risk for airway obstruction and postoperative volume depletion. Patients who live a long distance from the hospital may have complications that cannot be adequately treated in time, particularly if significant postoperative hemorrhage occurs. Patients with a history of obstructive sleep apnea are not discharged on the same day as surgery because of the risk of postoperative airway obstruction. Patients with coexisting medical problems, such as congenital heart disease, craniofacial abnormalities, Down's syndrome, or neurologic problems, are not candidates for outpatient tonsillectomy.

SURGICAL TECHNIQUE

There are two basic surgical techniques for performing tonsillectomy and adenoidectomy. In one technique, sharp dissection of the tonsils is performed after the mucosa is incised with a knife. Blunt dissection with Metzenbaum scissors and a Fisher knife is then used to free the tonsil from the fossa. The tonsil is amputated with a snare, and hemostasis is obtained with use of an electrocautery. For the second technique, the Bovie cautery is used to dissect the tonsil from its fossa. This technique has the advantage of better hemostasis, but there may be more problems postoperatively with pain, volume depletion, and somewhat delayed healing. The authors prefer to use the sharp dissection technique for most patients. The Bovie cautery technique is reserved for patients with bleeding disorders or for patients in whom excessive blood loss is an absolute contraindication. Such patients include those with sickle cell anemia or very young patients in whom the blood volume is very small.

Adenoidectomy is usually undertaken with use of curettes for tissue removal and packing for hemostasis. The authors prefer to use the Bovie cautery exclusively for adenoidectomy because it is a quick and safe technique that produces excellent hemostasis. This technique is not used if a biopsy procedure is indicated and tissue is needed for pathologic examination. Occasionally, a patient who has had repair of a submucous cleft or a complete cleft palate has associated hypertrophic adenoids and nasal airway obstruction. In these cases, a very careful anterior adenoidectomy at the posterior choanae can be undertaken with use of the Bovie cautery. This limited adenoidectomy can improve the nasal airway and, with a posterior adenoid pad left for velar closure, limits velopharyngeal insufficiency. This technique has the advantage of accurate tissue removal and hemostasis, and so partial adenoidectomy can be confidently undertaken.

SUGGESTED READINGS

Brodsky L: Tonsillitis/adenoiditis: the clinical work-up. J Resp Dis 11:19–26, 1990.

Brown OE: The use of desmopressin in children with coagulation disorders. Int J Pediatr Otorhinolaryngol 11:301–305, 1986.

Brown OE, Manning SC, Ridenour B: Cor pulmonale secondary to tonsillar and adenoidal hypertrophy: management considerations. Int J Pediatr Otorhinolaryngol 16:131–139, 1988.

Carithers JS, Gebhart DE, Williams JA: Postoperative risks of pediatric tonsilloadenoidectomy. Laryngoscope 97:422–429, 1987.

Colclasure JB, Graham SS: Complications of outpatient tonsillectomy and adenoidectomy: a review of 3340 cases. Ear Nose Throat J 69:155–160, 1990.

Crysdale WS, Russel D: Complications of tonsillectomy and adenoidectomy in 9409 children observed over night. Can Med Assoc J 135:1139–1142, 1986.

Gates GA, Avery CA, Prihoda TJ, Cooper JC Jr: Effectiveness of adenoidectomy and tympanostomy tubes in the treatment of chronic otitis media with effusion. N Engl J Med 317:1444–1451, 1987.

Grundfast KM, Wittich DJ: Adenotonsillar hypertrophy and upper airway obstruction in evolutionary perspective. Laryngoscope 92:650–656, 1982.

Handler SD, Miller L, Richmond KH, Baranak CC: Post-tonsillectomy hemorrhage: incidence, prevention, and management. Laryngoscope 96:1243–1247, 1986.

Helmus C, Grin M, Westfall R: Same-day-stay adenotonsillectomy. Laryngoscope 100:593–596, 1990.

Koopman CF: Avoiding the complications of tonsillectomy and adenoidectomy. J Resp Dis 9:84–98, 1988.

Madderr BR: Snoring and obstructive sleep apnea. In Bluestone CD, Stool SG (eds): Pediatric Otolaryngology (pp 927–934). Philadelphia: WB Saunders, 1990.

Manning SC, Beste D, McBride T, Goldberg A: An assessment of preoperative screening for tonsillectomy and adenoidectomy. Int J Pediatr Otorhinolaryngol 13:237–244, 1987.

Paradise JL: Tonsillectomy and adenoidectomy. In Bluestone CD, Stool SG (eds): Pediatric Otolaryngology (pp 915–926). Philadelphia: WB Saunders, 1990.

Paradise JL, Bluestone CD, Bachman RZ, et al: Efficacy of tonsillectomy for recurrent throat infection in severely affected children: Results of parallel randomized and nonrandomized clinical trials. N Engl J Med 310:674–683, 1984.

Paradise JL, Bluestone CD, Rogers KD, et al: Efficacy of

adenoidectomy for recurrent otitis media in children previously treated with tympanostomy-tube placement: Results of parallel randomized and nonrandomized trials. JAMA 263:2066–2073, 1990.

Potsic WP, Pasquariello PS, Baranak CC, et al: Relief of upper airway obstruction by adenotonsillectomy. Otolaryngol Head Neck Surg 94:476–480, 1986.

Rowe LD: Tonsils and adenoids: when is surgery indicated? Primary Care 9:355–369, 1982.

Schechter GL, Sly DE, Roper AL, Jackson RT: Changing face of treatment of peritonsillar abscess. Laryngoscope 92:657–659, 1982.

Segal C, Berger G, Basker M, Marshak G: Adenotonsillectomies on a surgical day-clinic basis. Laryngoscope 93:1205–1208, 1983.

Shott SR, Myer CM, Cotton RT: Efficacy of tonsillectomy and adenoidectomy as an outpatient procedure: a preliminary report. Int J Pediatr Otorhinolaryngol 13:157–163, 1987.

PART FIVE

Larynx and Neck

CHAPTER 36

Anatomy of the Neck and the Larynx

Gayle E. Woodson, MD, FACS

The intricate anatomy of the neck is a source of fascination and a challenge to surgeons. Many vital connections pass between the head and the body, and these structures are compressed into a narrow structure that flexes and twists to permit variation in head position with respect to the body. The posterior neck is composed of the spinal cord, the spinal column, and supporting muscles. The anterior neck contains the pharynx, the larynx, and the cervical esophagus. The configuration of the upper aerodigestive tract is precarious because both food and air must enter the body via the pharynx. Because of this, swallowing is a hazardous process, and precisely coordinated action of the larynx and the pharynx is necessary for preventing the aspiration of ingested food or water into the lungs. The complex anatomy of the neck, the pharynx, and the larynx can be best understood by considering the embryologic development of this region. This chapter is a review of the embryology and functional anatomy of the anterior neck.

EMBRYOLOGY

The embryonic respiratory system arises from the digestive tract, and this ontogenetic relationship accounts for the common upper aerodigestive tract (Fig. 36–1). The respiratory diverticulum first appears at 3 weeks of gestation as an outpouching of entoderm from the primitive foregut. This structure subsequently elongates to form the trachea and the lung buds. The larynx arises from the endoderm of the opening between the respiratory diverticulum and the foregut as well as from mesodermal elements of branchial arch origin.

The locations of structures in the head and neck are greatly influenced by their origin from the embryonic branchial arch system (Figs. 36–2, 36–3). Branchial structures first appear in the fourth or fifth week of gestation, when the fetal pharynx forms several outpouchings. At the same time, four grooves known as pharyngeal clefts appear on the ectodermal surface. The surface grooves deepen as the pouches expand laterally so that endoderm and ectoderm approximate very closely, pushing aside the intervening mesoderm. This results in the formation of five strips of mesoderm between the clefts known as branchial arches. The embryonic arterial system also develops as five aortic arches; each is associated with one of the branchial arches, and each has a segmental nerve. This association is preserved throughout development as the arches differentiate into the musculoskeletal and connective tissue elements of the upper aerodigestive tract, so that the structures arising from each arch are associated with the corresponding nerve and blood supply (Fig. 36–4).

The first arch forms the mandible and middle ear ossicles. The second, third, fourth, and sixth arches all contribute to formation of the larynx. The hyoid bone arises from the second and third branchial

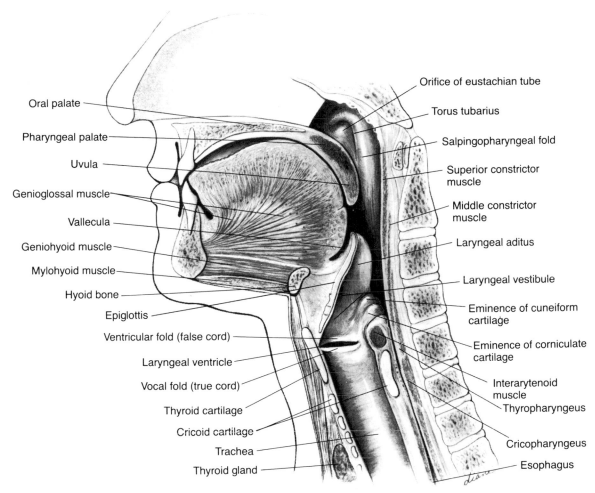

Figure 36–1. Sagittal view of the upper **aerodigestive** tract. (From Bosma J: Functional anatomy of the upper airway during development. *In* Mathew DP, Sant'Ambrogio G [eds]: Respiratory Function of the Upper Airway [p. 51]. Baltimore: Johns Hopkins University Press, 1986.)

arches. The nerve of the second arch, the facial nerve, supplies two of the muscles that attach to the hyoid bone, the stylohyoid, and the posterior portion of the digastric muscle. The fourth arch forms the thyroid cartilage; its related muscle, the cricothyroid, is supplied by the superior laryngeal nerve. This segmental nerve also contains most of the sensory fibers from the larynx. The recurrent laryngeal nerve is the segmental nerve of the sixth arch, which develops into the cricoid cartilage and the intrinsic laryngeal muscles.

SURFACE ANATOMY

Surface landmarks of the neck include the airway column in the anterior midline and the spinal column in the posterior midline. The surface contour of the posterior neck is primarily defined by the trapezius muscle. Anteriorly, the thyroid cartilage is the most prominent feature. This is the chief skeletal element of the larynx. Caudal to the thyroid cartilage, it is possible to palpate the rounded bulge of the cricoid cartilage and the tracheal rings, which become deeper and less easily palpated lower in the neck. Above the larynx is the hyoid bone. This structure is quite rostral with respect to the skull and the spinal column in infancy and gradually descends with advancing age. The sternocleidomastoid muscle traditionally divides the neck on each side into anterior and posterior triangles. This division is more a convention of terminology than an anatomic fact, but the concept

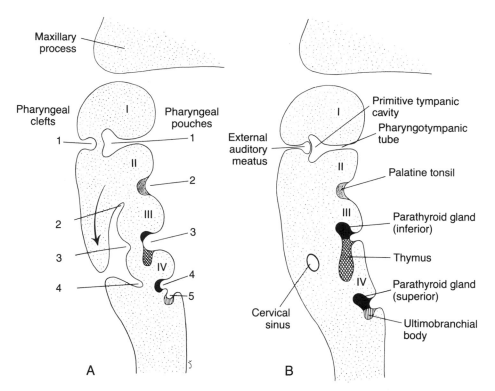

Figure 36–2. Diagram of the branchial arch system. (From Langman J: Medical Embryology. Baltimore: Williams & Wilkins, 1969.)

is useful clinically. The internal jugular vein and carotid arteries, for much of their length, are deep to the sternocleidomastoid muscle, but the arteries are easily palpable. The pulsation of the external jugular vein is usually visible low in the neck. The thyroid gland and lymph nodes are not easily palpable in the normal neck.

THE LARYNX

The larynx is located at the intersection of the upper respiratory and digestive tracts, at the caudal end of the pharynx. It is just anterior to the upper end of the esophagus and serves as a valve in the opening between the pharynx and the trachea. The larynx is best known for its role as the sound source in speech production, but its most vital function is protection of the lower airway from aspiration, particularly during the act of swallowing. The larynx is important in coughing, a mechanism for cleaning the lungs. An effective cough requires the glottis to close

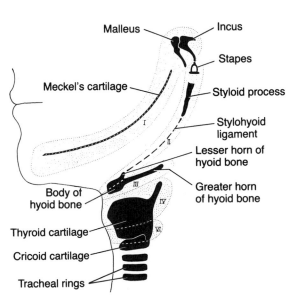

Figure 36–3. Structures formed by the branchial arches. (From Langman J: Medical Embryology. Baltimore: Williams & Wilkins, 1969.)

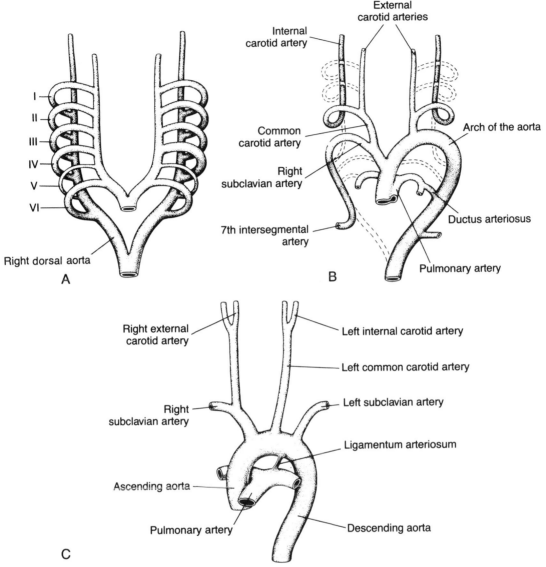

Figure 36–4. Embryonic aortic arches (A), their derivatives (B), and the mature aortic arch system (C). (From Langman J: Medical Embryology. Baltimore: Williams & Wilkins, 1969.)

tightly during the preparatory phase and to open widely and rapidly during the expulsive phase. The larynx also plays a role in regulating the rate of breathing by modifying the rate of exhalation.

Skeletal Structure

The larynx has a skeleton made up of several cartilages and one bone strung together in series by ligaments, joints, and sheets of connective tissue and suspended from the mandible and the base of the skull (Fig. 36–5). The most cephalad component of the laryngeal skeleton is the hyoid bone, which lies in the axial plane and is roughly U-shaped. The two free ends project postero-laterally as the greater cornua. Two small bumps on the superoanterior surface are the lesser cornua. The hyoid bone supports the larynx and maintains patency of the hypopharynx. The inferior edge of the hyoid bone is connected to the thyroid cartilage by the broad thyrohyoid membrane.

Below is the thyroid cartilage, which is narrower and taller than the hyoid; it also opens posteriorly. The two halves of the thyroid cartilages fuse anteriorly to form a

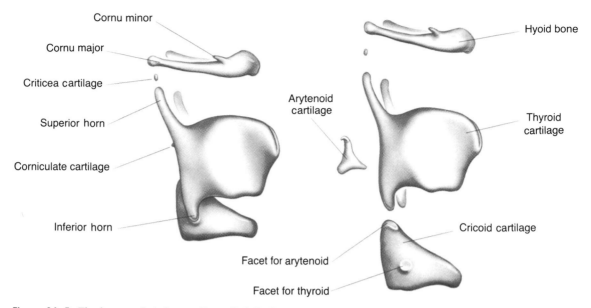

Figure 36–5. The laryngeal skeleton. (From Fink R, Demarest R: Laryngeal Biomechanics. Cambridge, MA: Harvard University Press, 1978.)

sharp angle (90° in males, 120° in females). This prominence is commonly referred to as the Adam's apple. Posteriorly, the edges of the cartilage project as the superior and inferior cornua. The thyrohyoid ligament connects the superior cornu of the thyroid cartilage to the hyoid bone; the inferior cornu articulates with the cricoid cartilage. After the age of 20 years, the thyroid cartilage begins a gradual process of ossification. The resultant increase in rigidity of this structure accounts for much of the age-related changes in pitch and resonance of the voice.

The epiglottis is a leaf-shaped piece of fibroelastic cartilage. The stem of this "leaf" points inferiorly and is attached to the inner surface of the thyroid cartilage in the superior midline. The hyoepiglottic ligament runs from the inner anterior surface of the hyoid bone to the anterior upper epiglottis. The superior, free end of the epiglottis projects into the hypopharynx, just behind the base of the tongue, and forms the upper boundary of the larynx.

The cricoid cartilage, caudal to the thyroid, is a complete ring, wider in back than in the front. Anteriorly, it is a few millimeters high and has a smooth, curved surface. It is 2 to 3 cm high posteriorly, where the superior surface is flattened centrally for providing an area of articulation for the arytenoid cartilages. There are superior facets posterolaterally for articulation with the inferior cornua of the thyroid cartilage. The cricothyroid

joints allow the cricoid cartilage and the thyroid to rotate with respect to each other in a sagittal plane, opening or closing the anterior cricothyroid space.

The two arytenoid cartilages are the most mobile portions of the laryngeal framework. Each is a roughly pyramidal or pear-shaped mass, with a wide base for articulation with the posterosuperior surface of the cricoid cartilage. The cricoarytenoid interface is a complex synovial joint; it permits both rotation of the arytenoid cartilage in a roughly axial plane and gliding medially or laterally along the facet of the cricoid. Posteriorly, the firm cricoarytenoid ligament tethers the arytenoid cartilage. The base of the arytenoid cartilage projects anteriorly and medially as the vocal process, which attaches to the posterior end of the vocal fold. The vocal folds extend from the thyroid cartilage anteriorly to the vocal processes of the arytenoid cartilages posteriorly. Movement of the arytenoids results in vocal fold abduction or adduction. The corniculate and cuneiform cartilages are two small sesamoid masses located superior to the arytenoid cartilage, under the same mucosal cover. These cartilages may serve to support the arytenoepiglottic folds.

Connective Tissue

The thyrohyoid membrane is a sheet of fibroelastic tissue that extends from the posterior surface of the hyoid bone to the superior edge of the thyroid cartilage. It does not attach directly to the hyoid bone but is connected by an interposed bursa. This connection enhances vertical mobility of the larynx. The lateral edges of this membrane form the thyrohyoid ligaments (Fig. 36–6).

The quadrangular membrane, which supports the superior larynx, stretches from the epiglottis to the arytenoid and the corniculate cartilages. Its free edges form the arytenoepiglottic fold, superiorly, and the false vocal fold, inferiorly.

The conus elasticus supports the caudal larynx. It extends from the midline of the lower border of the thyroid cartilage anteriorly to the vocal process of the arytenoid posteriorly. Its lateral edge is attached along the superior surface of the cricoid; its free, medial edge forms the vocal ligament of the true vocal fold.

Laryngeal Muscles

Intrinsic laryngeal muscles both arise and insert on laryngeal cartilages and open and close the glottis by abducting or adducting the vocal folds. There are five pairs of intrinsic muscles and one unpaired midline muscle, the interarytenoid (Fig. 36–7). Opening of the glottis can also be effected by traction along the rostral-caudal axis, as during inspiration, because of the way the skeleton is interconnected. Extrinsic laryngeal muscles can also alter glottic posture and dimensions.

The posterior cricoarytenoid muscle is the only muscle that abducts the vocal folds. It originates from the posterior surface of the cricoid cartilage and inserts onto the muscular process, on the posterior surface of the arytenoid cartilage. Contraction of this muscle rotates the vocal process laterally and also produces lateral and posterior gliding displacement of the arytenoid cartilage, thereby

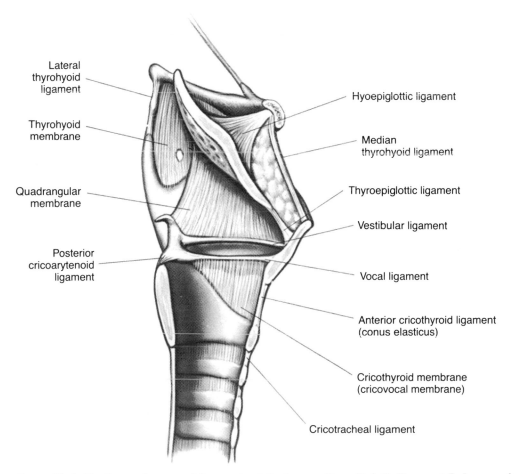

Figure 36–6. Elastic membrane and ligaments of the larynx. (From Fink R, Demarest R: Laryngeal Biomechanics. Cambridge, MA: Harvard University Press, 1978.)

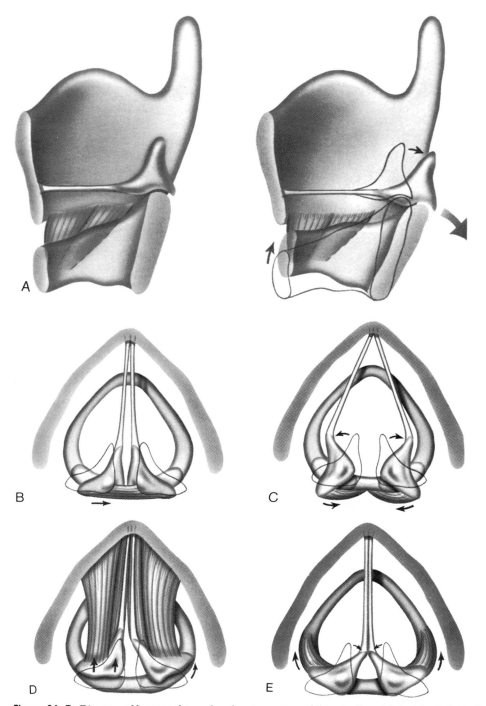

Figure 36–7. Diagram of laryngeal muscles showing action of the cricothyroid muscles *(A)*, the interarytenoid muscle *(B)*, the posterior cricoarytenoid muscles *(C)*, the thyroarytenoid muscles *(D)*, and the anterior cricoarytenoid muscles *(E)*. (From Tucker HM: The Larynx. New York: Thieme Medical Publishers, 1987.)

abducting the vocal fold. The lateral cricoarytenoid muscle originates on the lateral aspect of the cricoid cartilage, and it inserts on the posterior muscular process of the arytenoid cartilage. When it contracts, the mus-

cular process is pulled forward, with rotation of the vocal process medially and adduction of the vocal folds. The thyroarytenoid muscle arises from the anterior inner surface of the thyroid cartilage and inserts on the vocal process of the arytenoid cartilage. When this muscle contracts, it pulls the vocal process anteriorly to adduct the vocal folds. It also increases vocal fold tension and stiffness, which is important in determining vocal pitch. The thyroarytenoid muscle may be divided into two separate muscles: the medial thyroartenoid (vocalis) and the lateral thyroarytenoid. The cricothyroid muscle connects the anterior surface of the cricoid muscle to the thyroid cartilage, so that contraction of this muscle pulls these two cartilages together anteriorly, lengthening and tightening the vocal fold. The effect of cricothyroid contraction on abduction or adduction of the vocal folds is controversial. Contraction of the cricothyroid at physiologic levels does not significantly affect vocal fold position. The interarytenoid muscle, the only unpaired intrinsic laryngeal muscle, connects the posterior and medial borders of the arytenoids so that contraction adducts the vocal folds. A very small band of muscle fibers, originating from the lateral epiglottis and attaching to the contralateral arytenoid, can constrict the supraglottic laryngeal inlet.

Extrinsic laryngeal muscles connect the laryngeal skeleton to other structures. The mylohyoid, digastric, and stylohyoid muscles suspend the larynx from the base of the skull. The cervical strap muscles include the omohyoid, sternohyoid, sternothyroid, and thyrohyoid. Contraction of extrinsic muscles can produce elevation or depression of the larynx or movement anteriorly or posteriorly.

Subdivisions of the Larynx

The skeleton and intrinsic muscles of the larynx are draped in mucosa to form a system of folds. The glottis, or laryngeal valve, is made up of the true vocal folds. The portion of the larynx above the vocal folds is referred to as the supraglottis; the area below is the subglottis.

The superior extent of the supraglottis is the epiglottis, which consists of the epiglottic cartilage covered with mucosa on both sides so that its superior free margin projects into the lumen of the pharynx. The vallecula is the pouch between the base of the tongue and the epiglottis. Bands of mucosa-covered tissue that extend from the epiglottis to the arytenoid cartilage on both sides form the arytenoepiglottic folds. Lateral to the arytenoepiglottic folds, but still medial to the thy-

roid cartilage, are the piriform fossas, recesses that extend downward and open posteriorly at the esophageal inlet. During a swallow, the larynx is pulled upward and anteriorly. This pulls the larynx out of the direct path between the mouth and the esophagus and also opens the piriform fossas, which permits ingested food to pass through these lateral channels en route to the esophagus. The epiglottis serves as a baffle for diversion of food around the glottis. The false vocal folds are inferior and medial to the arytenoepiglottic folds.

The glottis is made up of the true vocal folds, those parts of the larynx that vibrate to produce sound during phonation. These structures are composed of muscle stretched across the laryngeal opening from anterior to posterior and draped in mucosa. In females, the anterior point of attachment is about midway along the vertical dimension of the cartilage. In males, the point is about one third up from the inferior edge. The posterior ends of the vocal folds rotate in an axial plane to open or close the glottis.

The ventricle is a pouch between the true and false vocal folds that ascends laterally to the false fold. It functions as a resonator in some lower animals, but its function in humans is not known. It may serve as a reservoir for mucus for lubrication of the glottis.

The subglottis is the portion of the larynx caudal to the glottis but above the trachea. Because the cricoid cartilage, the skeletal support of the subglottis, is the only complete ring in the human respiratory tract, it is the only point at which the lumen is fixed, changing only with swelling of the lining mucosa. It is also the level of the respiratory tract with the smallest cross-sectional area; although individual bronchioles and alveoli are smaller, they are much more numerous, so that total area is greater.

Mucosal Cover

The larynx is covered mostly by respiratory epithelium, with numerous mucous glands (Fig. 36–8). The mucosa over the free edge of the vocal fold, however, is highly specialized for vibration. It is composed of squamous epithelium, without mucous glands, and is very loosely connected to the underlying muscle, thus permitting a wide range of movement. The junction between the epithelium and the muscle is often referred to

Figure 36–8. Mucosal cover of the larynx. (From Isshiki N: Phonosurgery, Theory and Practice. Tokyo: Springer-Verlag, 1989.)

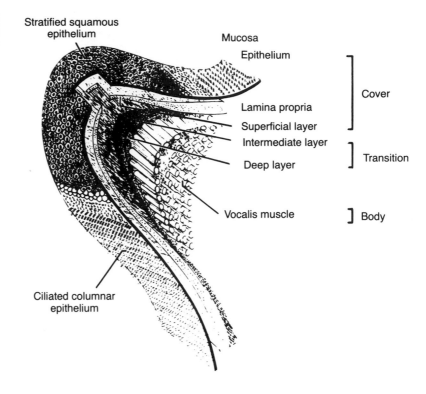

as Reinke's space, although it really consists of the lamina propria and is not a potential space. The lamina propria of the vocal fold contains three layers (superficial, intermediate, and deep), which have different mechanical properties as a result of varying densities of elastic and collagenous fibers. The deep layer, known as the vocal ligament, is continuous with the conus elasticus. The deep layer is the stiffest because the concentration of collagen fibers is greatest in that layer. The density of elastic fibers is greatest in the intermediate layer and gradually decreases toward the epithelium as well as toward the muscle. The superficial lamina propria has the least impedance to vibration because it has the lowest concentration of both elastic and collagenous fibers.

The transition between layers is gradual, not sharp, which allows impedance matching between the epithelium and muscle. Thus vibration of the low-density, flexible epithelium is not really constrained by the stiffness and mass of underlying muscle tissue.

Laryngeal Nerves

The nerve supply to the larynx is provided by the superior laryngeal nerve and the re-

current laryngeal nerve, both of which are branches of the vagus. The superior laryngeal nerve leaves the vagus below the nodose ganglion and divides into an internal sensory and external motor branches. The internal branch carries afferent fibers from receptors in the supraglottis and the vocal folds. The nerve enters the larynx laterally through the thyrohyoid membrane. The external branch supplies innervation to the cricothyroid muscle; it may also contain sensory fibers from receptors in the cricoarytenoid joint. Such a sensory component of the external branch has been demonstrated in cats.

The recurrent laryngeal nerve carries motor fibers to all intrinsic muscles of the larynx except the cricothyroid muscle. It mediates sensation from the larynx below the vocal folds and from the trachea. The nerve follows a long and circuitous route from the vagus to the larynx, traveling farther on the left than on the right. On the right side, the recurrent laryngeal nerve leaves the vagus in the upper mediastinum and curves around the subclavian artery. The left recurrent laryngeal nerve separates from the vagus at a lower point, curving up around the ligamentum arteriosum, a fibrous band connecting the aortic arch to the pulmonary artery. Both nerves ascend in the tracheoesophageal groove and enter the larynx behind the cricothyroid joint.

The descent of the embryonic arches into the thorax during development is responsible for the long route of the recurrent laryngeal nerve. This sixth segmental nerve follows its segmental artery, whereas the branchial arches remain cephalad. The sixth aortic arch on the left forms the fetal ductus arteriosus, which connects the pulmonary artery to the descending aorta. The recurrent laryngeal nerve is pulled down into the thorax because it curves around this structure. After birth, this vessel degenerates but persists as a fibrous band between the two great vessels, the ligamentum arteriosum. On the right, the embryonic sixth arch totally disappears, so that the sixth segmental nerve is subject only to the pull of the fourth arch artery, which becomes the subclavian artery.

THE TRACHEA

The cervical trachea descends from the larynx in the midline, anterior to the esophagus, to enter the mediastinum. Its lumen is maintained by the support of a series of incomplete cartilaginous rings, which open posteriorly. It is lined by respiratory mucosa. Its sensory innervation is via the recurrent laryngeal nerve, and its chief blood supply is from the inferior thyroid artery.

THE PHARYNX

The pharynx is a roughly tubular structure attached to the cervical vertebrae posteriorly and extending from the base of the skull, behind the nose, to the esophageal inlet, just behind the larynx. The walls of the pharynx are composed of three pharyngeal constrictor muscles lined by mucosa. Another muscle on each side, the stylopharyngeus, connects the styloid process to the lateral pharynx between the superior and middle constrictors. The pharynx opens anteriorly into the nasal cavity and into the mouth, and it may be considered to have three segments: the nasopharynx, the oropharynx, and the hypopharynx. Transoral inspection of the throat reveals only the posterior wall of the oropharynx, and so a complete examination re-

quires the use of mirrors or endoscopic instruments (Figs. 36–9, 36–10).

The superior constrictor muscle is suspended from the base of the skull, the medial pterygoid plate, the pterygomandibular raphe, the mylohyoid line of the mandible, and the lateral tongue. There is a gap between the upper border of the superior constrictor muscle and the base of the skull between the posterior midline and the pharyngeal tubercles. This space is filled by the pharyngobasilar fascia, which is pierced by the eustachian tube on each side. The tensor veli palatini and levator palatini muscles are superficial and deep, respectively, to this fascia. The anterior attachments of the middle constrictor are the hyoid bone and the stylohyoid ligament. The inferior constrictor muscle attaches to the thyroid and cricoid cartilages. The lower part of this muscle, known as the cricopharyngeus, is functionally although not grossly anatomically distinct.

The nasopharynx can be sealed off from the oropharynx by simultaneous elevation of the soft palate and formation of a fold in the pharyngeal walls known as Passavant's ridge. This process is important during speech as well as deglutition. During a swallow, sequential activation of the constrictor muscles propels food through the pharynx into the esophagus. Coordinated activity of the palate, the tongue, and the tonsillar pillars is necessary for preventing reflux into the mouth or nose. In contrast to the rest of the pharynx, the cricopharyngeus is normally in a state of tonic contraction, relaxing only at the end of the pharyngeal phase of a swallow. The muscle serves to prevent suction of air into the esophagus and is a second barrier against reflux of stomach contents into the pharynx.

THYROID AND PARATHYROID GLANDS

The thyroid is a butterfly-shaped endocrine gland located anterior to the trachea; its isthmus is usually at the level of the second to fourth tracheal rings. The gland moves up and down with swallowing because it is attached to the trachea by fibrous tissue, called Berry's ligament. The recurrent laryngeal nerve is almost always just deep to this ligament; hence it can be injured during

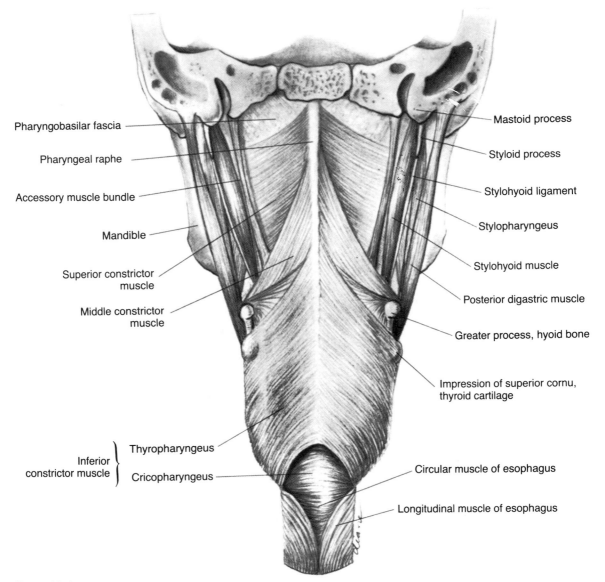

Pharyngobasilar fascia

Pharyngeal raphe

Accessory muscle bundle

Mandible

Superior constrictor muscle

Middle constrictor muscle

Inferior constrictor muscle {

Thyropharyngeus

Cricopharyngeus

Mastoid process

Styloid process

Stylohyoid ligament

Stylopharyngeus

Stylohyoid muscle

Posterior digastric muscle

Greater process, hyoid bone

Impression of superior cornu, thyroid cartilage

Circular muscle of esophagus

Longitudinal muscle of esophagus

Figure 36–9. Posterior view of the constrictor and posterolateral muscles of the pharynx. (From Bosma J: Functional anatomy of the upper airway during development. *In* Mathew DP, Sant'Ambrogio G [eds]: Respiratory Function of the Upper Airway [p. 59]. Baltimore: Johns Hopkins University Press, 1986.)

thyroidectomy if care is not taken to identify the nerve lower in the neck. Sometimes a pyramidal lobe arises from the isthmus and ascends in midline. When present, this structure is a reminder of the embryologic origin of the gland. Thyroid tissue arises from the foramen cecum of the tongue. The tract that it follows in its descent is usually obliterated, but it may persist as a thyroglossal duct, a thyroglossal duct cyst, or a pyramidal lobe.

The parathyroid glands are usually four in number: an upper pair and a lower pair. The superior pair arise from the fourth branchial pouch and migrate with the thyroid gland, usually settling in the posterior capsule of that gland. The inferior pair arise from the third branchial pouch and are therefore associated with the thymus. The location of the inferior parathyroid glands is much more variable than that of the superior parathyroid glands. The inferior glands are most often associated with the lower thyroid, but they may be lower, even in the mediastinum, or in some other ectopic site.

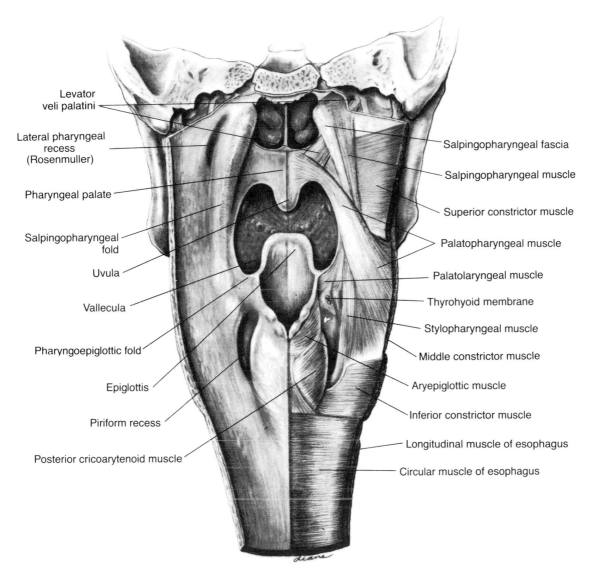

Levator veli palatini

Lateral pharyngeal recess (Rosenmuller)

Pharyngeal palate

Salpingopharyngeal fold

Uvula

Vallecula

Pharyngoepiglottic fold

Epiglottis

Piriform recess

Posterior cricoarytenoid muscle

Salpingopharyngeal fascia

Salpingopharyngeal muscle

Superior constrictor muscle

Palatopharyngeal muscle

Palatolaryngeal muscle

Thyrohyoid membrane

Stylopharyngeal muscle

Middle constrictor muscle

Aryepiglottic muscle

Inferior constrictor muscle

Longitudinal muscle of esophagus

Circular muscle of esophagus

Figure 36–10. Posterior view of anterior pharyngeal structures. (From Bosma J: Functional anatomy of the upper airway during development. *In* Mathew DP, Sant'Ambrogio G [eds]: Respiratory Function of the Upper Airway [p. 57]. Baltimore: Johns Hopkins University Press, 1986.)

BLOOD VESSELS

The common carotid artery arises from the innominate artery on the right and the aortic arch on the left and enters the neck deep to the sternocleidomastoid muscle. It divides into internal and external branches. The carotid sinus located at this bifurcation is a baroreceptor organ that senses blood pressure. Compression of this structure can lead to hypotension and bradycardia. The adjacent carotid body is sensitive to blood levels of carbon dioxide and oxygen. Both the carotid sinus and body are innervated by the

nerve of Hering, a branch of the glossopharyngeal nerve. The internal carotid continues up into the skull without branching; the external carotid branches into the superior thyroid and the ascending pharyngeal, the lingual, the facial, the occipital, the posterior auricular, the superficial temporal, and the internal maxillary arteries.

The vertebral artery is the first branch of the subclavian artery. It joins the spinal column at the sixth cervical vertebra and ascends in the foramina of the vertebral processes to enter the foramen magnum.

The thyrocervical trunk is the second

branch of the subclavian and divides immediately into inferior thyroid, transverse cervical, and transverse scapular arteries. The transverse cervical artery is of particular significance because it supplies the trapezius muscle. The trapezius musculocutaneous flap is a useful tool in head and neck reconstructive surgery. Therefore, care must be taken to preserve this artery during neck dissection because sacrifice would limit later options for reconstruction.

The internal jugular vein is a direct continuation of the sigmoid sinus, which exits the skull behind the mastoid. The internal jugular vein descends within the carotid sheath and empties into the subclavian vein. Tributaries of the internal jugular vein are variable. It is normally joined by the facial vein at the level of the hyoid and often receives the middle thyroid vein. Other tributaries may include the superior thyroid, pharyngeal, or laryngeal veins. The superficial venous system of the neck is even more variable. The external jugular vein originates from one or some combination of a number of veins, including the posterior facial, posterior auricular, facial, or maxillary veins. It descends over the sternocleidomastoid muscle and then receives as tributaries the transverse cervical and suprascapular veins as well as, when present, the anterior jugular vein.

LYMPHATIC DRAINAGE

The lymphatic system serves both immunologic and circulatory functions. Interstitial fluid, which may contain bacteria, viruses, or tumor cells, is returned to the blood circulation via the lymphatic channels. En route, the fluid is filtered by lymph nodes, where foreign particles are trapped and interact with lymphocytes. Lymph nodes may become enlarged as a result of this immunologic function or because their defense systems become overwhelmed, so that they become infected or the focus of metastatic cancer.

Collection of lymph begins in blind-ended capillaries that drain into collecting trunks of the afferent vessels of regional lymph nodes. Efferent lymphatic vessels leave the nodes and join larger channels, which eventually coalesce to form two large collecting trunks: the thoracic duct and the right lymphatic duct. The thoracic duct receives lymph from the entire left half of the body and from below the diaphragm on the right. The right lymphatic duct drains only the right side of the body above the diaphragm. The thoracic duct empties into the venous circulation at the junction of the internal jugular and subclavian veins on the left. The right lymphatic duct empties into the same junction on the right. Lymphatic vessels are delicate and not as easily identified as are arteries and veins during surgery, but transection of smaller channels is of no clinical significance. However, transection of larger vessels, particularly the thoracic duct, must be repaired. Otherwise, serious leakage of fluid can result in a subcutaneous seroma or even a fistula through the skin.

The lymphatic drainage of the neck can be divided into superficial and deep groups of lymph nodes. Superficial nodes include occipital, retroauricular, parotid, submandibular, and submental nodes. Deep nodes include retropharyngeal, internal jugular, supraclavicular, and subclavian nodes. The nasal cavity, the paranasal sinuses, and the pharynx drain first into retropharyngeal nodes; the mouth, the lips, and the external nose are drained by submandibular nodes. The tongue is richly supplied with lymphatics. Tongue lymphatics drain from the tip to submental nodes, from the sides to submental nodes, and from the back to cervical nodes.

NERVES

The facial nerve (cranial nerve VII) supplies motor input to the posterior belly of the digastric, the stylohyoid, and the platysma muscles. The only branch of cranial nerve VII supplying facial muscles that dips into the neck is the marginal mandibular branch. This nerve exits the parotid gland, descends to travel in the fascia over the submandibular gland, and then ascends to supply muscles controlling the lower lip.

The glossopharyngeal nerve (cranial nerve IX) is not commonly encountered during neck operations because it runs deep to the carotid artery and the stylopharyngeus muscle. It carries motor fibers to the stylopharyngeus muscle and sensory fibers from the carotid body and sinus as well as from the pharyngeal plexus and the posterior tongue. The glossopharyngeal nerve enters the skull through the jugular foramen along with the vagus and the spinal accessory nerve.

The cervical portion of the vagus nerve travels in the carotid sheath and lies between the glossopharyngeal and accessory nerves as it passes through the jugular foramen in the base of the skull. The pharyngeal branch of the vagus arises from the upper nodose ganglion; the superior laryngeal nerve arises from the lower end. The courses of the superior and recurrent laryngeal nerves have been previously described in this chapter.

The spinal accessory nerve (cranial nerve XI) carries motor fibers to the sternocleidomastoid and trapezius muscles. It exits the skull through the jugular foramen and then runs posteriorly. Initially it is in the anterior triangle, and so it can be injured during dissection around the upper jugular vein. It then passes deep to the sternocleidomastoid, supplying it with a branch, and emerges at Erb's point to enter the posterior triangle en route to the trapezius muscle.

The hypoglossal nerve (cranial nerve XII) exits the skull through its own canal, medial to the internal carotid artery and the internal jugular vein, and receives "hitchhiking" fibers from the second and sometimes the first cervical nerves. The hypoglossal nerve then travels inferiorly and laterally to pass between the jugular vein and the carotid artery and deep to the posterior belly of the digastric muscle. At this point, cervical fibers exit to form the ansa cervicalis, which supplies motor fibers to the sternohyoid, thyrohyoid, and sternothyroid muscles. The hypoglossal nerve then loops around the occipital artery near that vessel's origin from the carotid artery and continues under the submandibular gland to reach the tongue.

The cervical sympathetic trunk lies on the longus muscle, behind the carotid sheath, and contains three or four ganglia: the superior cervical, middle cervical, vertebral ganglia, and sometimes a separate inferior cervical ganglion. More often, the inferior cervical ganglion fuses with the first thoracic ganglion to form the stellate ganglion.

The cervical plexus, made up of the anterior rami of the first four cervical nerves, transmits sensory fibers from the greater auricular, small occipital, cervical cutaneous, and supraclavicular nerves. The cervical cutaneous branches run anteriorly through the fibrofatty tissue of the neck, where they are routinely encountered during neck dissection. Motor fibers of spinal regions C1 and C2 innervate the cervical strap muscles via the ansa cervicalis. Some of these fibers hitchhike with the hypoglossal nerve and then exit as the descendens hypoglossi to form the superior limb of the ansa cervicalis; other fibers form the inferior limb. Motor fibers from regions C3 to C5 form the phrenic nerve, which descends from lateral to medial on the surface of the anterior scalene muscle. The last four cervical nerves, along with the first thoracic nerve, form the brachial plexus.

FASCIAL PLANES AND SPACES OF THE NECK

The neck is subdivided into compartments by layers of fascia (Fig. 36–11). These divisions are clinically relevant, not only because they help to distinguish the relative locations of structures, but also because the spread of infections in the neck is determined by these divisions.

The superficial fascia, just deep to the subcutaneous tissue, surrounds the entire neck. It encases the trapezius muscles posteriorly and the sternocleidomastoid muscles anteriorly, with a single layer of fascia between the muscles. It also encases the submandibular and parotid glands. Inferiorly, it is attached to the scapula, to the clavicle, and to both the anterior and posterior surfaces of the sternum. Anteriorly, it is attached to the hyoid and the mandible. The pretracheal fascia surrounds the median visceral column, including the trachea, the thyroid, the larynx, the pharynx, and the esophagus. Anteriorly and superiorly, this fascia terminates at its attachment to the oblique line of the thyroid cartilage. Posteriorly, the fascia continues superiorly to become continuous with the buccopharyngeal fascia. Inferiorly, the pretracheal fascia extends into the superior mediastinum to merge with the adventitia of the great vessels. The prevertebral fascia surrounds the spinal column and associated muscles. Superiorly, the fascia attaches to the skull. However, the anterior prevertebral fascia extends down into the mediastinum.

Retropharyngeal Space. This space lies between the pretracheal and prevertebral fascia. It extends from the base of the skull into the mediastinum, where the two layers of fascia fuse at the level of the first thoracic vertebra.

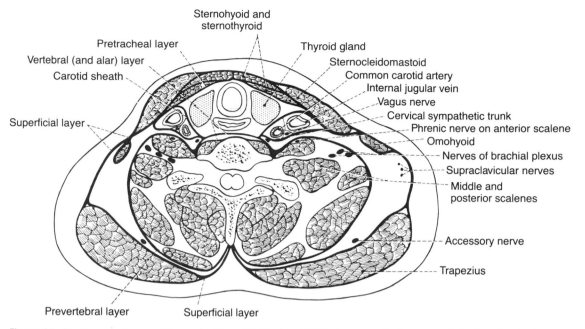

Figure 36–11. Fascial planes of the neck. (From Hollinshead WH: Anatomy for Surgeons, 3rd ed, vol 1. Philadelphia: Harper & Row, 1982.)

Prevertebral Space. This space is between the prevertebral fascia and the bodies of the vertebrae. It extends from the base of the skull all the way to the coccyx.

Parapharyngeal Space. This is the most clinically significant space. It is shaped roughly like an inverted pyramid or a cone; its apex is at the hyoid bone. It is bounded laterally by the superficial fascia and medially by the pretracheal fascia. Its posterior limit is the prevertebral fascia, and this space may communicate with the prevertebral space. The styloid process and associated muscles divide this space into anterior and posterior compartments; the posterior compartments contain the carotid sheath as well as cranial nerves IX through XII. Infections can spread to the parapharyngeal space from the tonsils, the teeth, the parotid gland, or the mastoid process.

Carotid Sheath. This is a fibrous tube that invests the internal jugular vein, the common carotid artery, and the vagus nerve. Its anteromedial wall is the pretracheal fascia. Posteriorly, it is bounded by the prevertebral fascia. Its lateral limit is the superficial cervical fascia.

Submandibular Space. This space lies in the anterior neck, deep to the superficial fascia, and superior and anterior to the hyoid bone. The mylohyoid muscle lies between the two component subdivisions: the *sublingual* and *submaxillary* spaces. The *submental* space is the portion of the submaxillary space ventral to the anterior belly of the digastric muscle.

Infections in the submandibular spaces typically arise from dental infections. When the sublingual space is involved, the tongue may be pushed rostrally and dorsally, impinging on the airway. Such an infection, referred to as Ludwig's angina, can progress very rapidly and requires prompt surgical drainage.

SUGGESTED READINGS

Hirano M, Kakita Y, Ohmary K, Kurita S: Structure and mechanical properties of the vocal fold. Speech Language: Adv Basic Res Pract 7:271–297, 1982.

Hollinshead W: Anatomy for Surgeons, 3rd ed. Hagerstown, MD: Harper & Row, 1982.

Levitt GW: Cervical fascia and deep neck infection. Laryngoscope 80:409–435, 1972.

Woodson GE: The larynx. *In* Dulbecco R (ed): Encyclopedia of Human Biology, vol 4. San Diego: Academic Press, 1991.

CHAPTER 37

Physiology of Pharynx and Larynx

David G. Hanson, MD   Jeri A. Logemann, PhD   Malcolm H. Hast, PhD

The larynx and pharynx, key components of the upper aerodigestive tract, play major roles in respiration, deglutition, and human speech production. The pharyngeal musculature guards the entry to both the alimentary and respiratory tracts.

THE PHARYNX

The pharynx is a muscular, fibrous, cone-shaped tube that forms a mutual passage for both air and food. It extends from the base of the skull, to which its cone-shaped base is attached, to the cricoid cartilage, its apex. At the lower border of the cricoid, the laryngo-pharynx joins the esophagus, and the larynx continues the airway through the trachea. At the lower apex of the pharynx, both the esophagus and the upper airway are narrowest. In the adult, the pharynx is approximately 13 cm long and narrows from 3.5 cm in width superiorly to 1.5 cm inferiorly.

The pharynx lies behind the nose, the mouth, and the larynx; it communicates with each and thereby is divided into the naso-pharynx, the oral pharynx, and the laryngo-pharynx (hypopharynx). Its lateral walls are attached to the medial pterygoid plate, the side of the dorsal tongue, the inner surface of the mandible, the hyoid bone, and the thyroid and cricoid cartilages. The pharyn-gotympanic tube, the tensor veli palitini, and the levator veli palatini muscles pass through an interval in the lateral pharyngeal wall.

Posteriorly, the pharynx is attached to the basioccipital bone and lies in front of the upper six cervical vertebrae. It is separated from the vertebrae by the prevertebral muscles and fascia and by the loose areolar tissue of the retropharyngeal space.

The wall of the pharynx is composed of four layers: (1) the innermost mucous membrane, (2) the pharyngobasilar fascia, (3) the middle layer of striated muscle that is absent anteriorly, and (4) an outermost covering of buccopharyngeal fascia. The muscular layer is composed of both circular and longitudinal fibers and consists of three pairs of muscles.

The circular muscles are organized into the superior, middle, and inferior constrictors. The superior constrictor arises from the medial pterygoid plate, the posterior border of the pterygoid mandibular raphe, the side of the last mandibular molar, and the side of the tongue. The fibers of this muscle pass backwards to be inserted into the pharyngeal tubercle of the occipital bone and the median raphe of the pharynx to form the upper portion of the conical tube. The triangular middle constrictor originates from greater and lesser horns of the hyoid bone and from the stylohyoid ligament; the fibers also pass backwards to be inserted into the median raphe. The upper fibers overlie the superior constrictor muscle, and the lower fibers are overlapped by the inferior constrictor muscle. The stylopharyngeus, the glossopharyngeal nerve, and the stylohyoid muscle pass through a fascia-filled muscular gap formed by the lower border of the superior constrictor and the upper border of the middle constrictor muscles. The inferior constrictor muscle originates from the oblique line of the thyroid cartilage, the side of the cricoid cartilage, and the fascia on the lateral aspect of the cricoid cartilage. Its upper fibers pass upward to insert into the median raphe of the pharynx and overlap the middle constrictor muscle. Through an anterior gap between the origins of the middle and inferior constrictor muscles and the thyrohyoid muscle, the internal laryngeal nerve and the superior laryngeal vessels pierce the thyrohyoid membrane. The lowermost fibers of this muscle pass horizontally backwards, from the cricoid cartilage, to form the cricopharyngeus muscle. Through a gap between the inferior fibers of the inferior constrictor muscle and the upper border of the esophageal musculature, the recurrent laryngeal nerve and the inferior laryngeal vessels pass. All constrictor muscles are innervated by the pharyngeal vagal plexus of nerves; the cricopharyngeus receives additional innervation from the recurrent laryngeal nerve.

Like the inferior constrictor muscle, the three pairs of longitudinal muscles of the pharynx—the stylopharyngeus, the palatopharyngeus, and the salpinopharyngeus—have a direct mechanical effect on the larynx. Arising from the styloid process, the stylopharyngeus inserts on the posterior border of the thyroid cartilage. From its attachment at the posterior border of the palate and the palatine aponeurosis, the palatopharyngeus forms an arch with its opposite mate and inserts inferiorly on the posterior border of the thyroid cartilage. Fibers of the salpinopharyngeus originate from the cartilaginous part of the auditory tube, pass downward, and blend with the muscle fibers of palatopharyngeus. With the exception of the stylopharyngeus muscle, which is innervated by the glossopharyngeal nerve, the longitudinal muscles also receive their supply from the pharyngeal vagal plexus.

The interior or cavity of the pharynx is subdivided into the nasopharynx, the oral pharynx, and the laryngopharynx. The nasopharynx is the widest part of the pharynx, lying behind the nasal cavities and above the soft palate, its floor. The nasopharynx is lined by pseudostratified ciliated columnar epithelium. On the lateral side of the nasopharynx is the orifice of the pharyngotympanic tube. At the level of the inferior tubinate, it is defined by the area of the tubal elevation, a rounded prominence of cartilage. In the area of the tubal elevation, there is a variable amount of lymph tissue, the tubal tonsil, that merges posteriorly with the pharyngeal tonsil (adenoids). Just below the tubal opening, there is a bulge formed by the levator palatini muscle. A pharyngeal recess, behind the tubal elevation, passes posterolaterally below the petrous part of the temporal bone. The roof and the posterior wall of the nasopharynx lie against the occipital and sphenoid bones and the arch of the atlas. The pharyngeal tonsil is an accumulation of lymph tissue that increases in mass up to the age of 6 years and atrophies gradually with age. This enlarged mass of lymph tissue results in folds of mucous membrane that radiate anteriorly from a blind recess, the pharyngeal bursa. This part of the pharynx, which has solely a respiratory function, communicates with the oral pharynx by way of the pharyngeal isthmus that is posterior to the soft palate.

The oral pharynx extends from the soft palate to the superior border of the epiglottis. It opens anteriorly into the mouth through the oropharyngeal isthmus. This isthmus, the theoretic division between the oral pharynx and the mouth, lies between the lateral palatoglossal arches. These arches extend downward from the interior surface of the soft palate to the mucous membrane on the posterior aspect of each side of the tongue. Just behind the palatoglossal arch is the palatopharyngeal arch. From the posterior portion of the soft palate, this arch passes backwards and downward into the side wall of the pharynx. Between the palatoglossal arch and the palatopharyngeal arch is the triangular tonsilar fossa.

Lying within each fossa is the palatine tonsil, an aggregation of lymphoid tissue. The pair of tonsils are present at birth, grow rapidly until about age 6 years, begin involuting at puberty, and finally atrophy in old age. The lymphoid tissue in the nasopharynx, in the oral pharynx, and in the base of the tongue (lingual tonsil) constitute Waldeyer's ring, a front line aggreggation of the immune system's defense against infection.

The main arterial supply to the palatine tonsil is from the tonsilar branch of the facial artery and feeds primarily into the external palatine (paratonsillar) vein and the facial vein. Efferent lymphatic vessels drain the palatine tonsils through the jugulodigastric nodes and the upper deep cervical chain. The tonsil receives its nerve supply from the glossopharyngeal and lesser palatine nerves. The tonsils and tonsillar crypts, like the mucous membrane of the oral and laryngopharynx, are covered by stratified squamous epithelium because these portions are functionally subject to mechanical stress by the passage of food.

The laryngopharynx (hypopharynx), which lies behind and incompletely around the posterior larynx, extends from the superior border of the epiglottis to the lower border of the cricoid cartilage, where it becomes continuous with the esophagus. With the exception of the region of the vermiform appendix, this cricoid portion of the esophagus is the narrowest portion of the alimentary canal. The anterior wall of the laryngeal pharynx is formed by the posterior surface of the epiglottis and the laryngeal inlet, bounded by the arytenoepiglottic folds that unite the epiglottis to the arytenoid cartilages superiorly and by the mucous membrane of the posterior arytenoid and cricoid cartilages. On the lateral side of the glossoepiglottic fold, arytenoepiglottic folds, and arytenoid cartilages is the piriform fossa, or recess. This fossa is bounded medially by the arytenoepiglottic folds and laterally by the medial surface of the thyroid cartilage and the thyrohyoid membrane. The posterior wall of the laryngopharynx lies in front of the third to sixth cervical vertebrae.

The pharynx receives its arterial supply from branches of the ascending palatine, maxillary, facial, and lingual arteries. Pharyngeal veins form a plexus that drains into the pterygoid plexus superiorly and into the internal jugular and facial veins inferiorly. Lymphatic drainage is through the deep cervical nodes and, in particular, the jugulodigastric node. The pharyngeal plexus, formed by the glossopharyngeal plexus, is derived from the cranial part of the accessory nerve, traveling to the pharynx by branches of the vagus nerve. All muscles of the pharynx are supplied by this plexus, with the exception of the stylopharyngeus, which is supplied only by the glossopharyngeal nerve, and the tensor veli palatini, which is innervated by the mandibular nerve. Sensory supply of the mucous membrane of the nasopharynx is from the maxillary nerve; that of the oropharynx is from the glossopharyngeal and lesser palatini nerves; and the laryngopharynx receives its sensory supply from the internal and recurrent laryngeal branches of the vagus nerve.

THE LARYNX

The primary role of the larynx is in respiration. It protects the airway, influences airway resistance during respiration, aids in air mixing within the alveoli, and contributes to the regulation of breathing. The larynx, which extends from the root of the tongue to the trachea, is situated from the level of approximately the disk of the third cervical vertebra to the disk of the sixth cervical vertebra of the superior third of the body of the seventh cervical vertebra. Anteriorly, it is covered by the sternohyoid, sternothyroid, thyrohoid, and omohyoid muscles. Laterally, it provides attachment for the inferior constrictor muscle, which also encloses the larynx posteriorly. The superior part of the larynx is continuous with the trachea from below and opens into the pharynx above.

The skeleton of the larynx is composed of the thyroid, cricoid, and epiglottic cartilages and of the paired arytenoid, corniculate, and cuneiform cartilages. The larynx is suspended superiorly from the hyoid bone by the strap muscles and the thyrohyoid ligaments, the thyrohyoid membrane, and the hypoepiglottic membrane. The hyoid bone forms the anterior and superior boundaries of the pre-epiglottic space, where a depression from the back of the tongue, the vallecula, is formed. The vallecula is divided in the midline by the glossoepiglottic fold.*

Cartilages

The thyroid, the largest cartilage of the larynx, is composed of two alae that have posterior hornlike extensions called the superior and inferior thyroid cornua. Anteriorly, the alae are fused in the midline, at an angle of approximately 90° in the male. The fused anterior borders form the laryngeal prominence, or Adam's apple. Because the angle formed by the two laminae is wider in the female, about 120°, the prominence is usually absent in the female. The alae are not fused superiorly but are separated by the thyroid notch. The posterior portion of the thyroid cartilage, the superior horn, is suspended from the hyoid bone by the lateral thyrohyoid

---

*This section on the anatomy of the laryngeal organ was largely taken from Hast MH: Anatomy of the larynx. *In* English GM (ed): Otolaryngology, vol 4. Philadelphia: Harper & Row, 1987.

ligament. The conus elasticus extends from a tubercle projecting downward in the middle of the thyroid cartilage to the anterior superior border of the cricoid cartilage. On the external surface of each thyroid ala, an oblique line runs downward and forward from the superior cornu to the inferior thyroid tubercle at the lower border of the lamina. The thyrohyoid, the sternothyroid, and the inferior constrictor muscles attach on this ridge. Muscle fibers from the stylopharyngeal and palatopharyngeal constrictor muscles insert on the posterior border of the thyroid cartilage.

The thyroepiglottic, vestibular, and vocal ligaments and the thyroarytenoid and vocalis muscles are attached at the angle formed by the thyroid alae, at a point halfway between the thyroid notch and the inferior border of the anterior thyroid cartilage. The thyroid cartilage is composed of hyaline cartilage, which begins to ossify at approximately the age of 25 years.

The thyroid cartilage articulates with the smaller, signet-ring–shaped cricoid cartilage. The anterior arch of the cricoid cartilage is about 5 to 7 mm in height, and posteriorly the ring expands to 20 to 30 mm in height. The anterior arch of the cricoid cartilage forms the lower portion of the larynx, and its high posterior lamina forms a major part of the posterior wall of the larynx. The almost horizontal inferior margin of the cricoid cartilage suspends the first ring of the trachea by the cricotracheal ligament. Approximately midway between the superior and inferior borders on the posterior lateral aspect of each side of the cricoid cartilage, a small, raised facet articulates with the inferior thyroid cornu. Convex, oval-shaped facets facing upward and laterally form the articulation with the base of the arytenoid cartilages. Longitudinal fibers of the esophagus are attached by a tendon to a median vertical ridge on the posterior surface of the cricoid cartilage. The posterior cricoarytenoid muscles originate on the posterior surface of the cricoid lamina in a shallow depression on each side of the vertical ridge. The lateral cricoarytenoid muscle attaches to the superolateral edge of the arch. The cricothyroid muscle attaches to the external anterolateral surface of the arch. The inferior constrictor muscle attaches to the posterolateral part of the arch. The superior margin of the cricoid cartilage attaches to the conus elasticus and is suspended by the cricothyroid ligament.

The paired pyramid-shaped arytenoid cartilages sit on the lateral part of the superior border of the lamina of the cricoid cartilage. Each arytenoid cartilage has three side surfaces, a base, and an apex. The posterior surface is smooth, concave, and triangular and forms the attachment of the transverse interarytenoid muscle. The medial surface of the arytenoid cartilage is flat, smooth, and narrow and is covered with mucous membrane; its lower margin is the lateral boundary of the cartilaginous part of the rima glottidis. The smooth and concave base articulates with the posterior lamina of the cricoid cartilage. The muscular process projects laterally and backward. The posterior cricoarytenoid muscle inserts posteriorly, and the lateral cricoarytenoid muscle inserts anteriorly. The anterior pointed vocal process provides the attachments for the vocal ligament and thyroarytenoid muscle. The apexes of the arytenoid cartilages curve backward. The apexes and vocal processes consist of elastic fibrocartilage, and the remainder of the arytenoid cartilage is composed of hyaline cartilage.

Small, paired nodules of elastic fibrocartilage, the corniculate cartilages, articulate with the apex of the arytenoid cartilage in the posterior part of the arytenoepiglottic folds. The cuneiform cartilages are small, paired, elongated, rodlike structures of elastic fibrocartilage embedded in the margin of the arytenoepiglottic folds in front of the corniculate cartilages.

The epiglottis, a thin, leaflike, flexible, elastic fibrocartilage, projects upward behind the tongue and the body of the hyoid bone at the entrance of the larynx. Its narrow inferior portion, the petiole, is attached to the medial surface of the thyroid cartilage by the thyroepiglottic ligament, inferior to the thyroid notch and superior to the anterior commissure. The epiglottis is attached to the arytenoid cartilages by the arytenoepiglottic folds. The lower part of the epiglottis is connected to the hyoid by the elastic hyoepiglottic ligament. On its lower part, there is an elevation known as the tubercle. The lower part of the epiglottis has severe small pits that contain vessels and mucous glands.

The inferior cornua of the thyroid cartilage articulate with the cricoid cartilage along its posterolateral sides. The cricothyroid joints are synovial, and the capsular ligaments are strengthened by anterior, lateral, and posterior ligaments. At these articulations, the cricoid cartilage rotates on the inferior horns of the thyroid cartilage about an axis passing transversely through the joints; some gliding movement of the cricoid can also occur anteriorly.

The arytenoid cartilage also articulates with the cricoid cartilage by means of a synovial joint. The capsular ligament is strengthened by a strong posterior cricoarytenoid ligament. This complex joint permits two types of movement. The first is a rotation of the arytenoid cartilage around an axis that runs obliquely from a dorsomediocranial to a ventrolaterocaudal position, permitting movement of the vocal process medially or laterally. The joint also allows gliding movement by the arytenoid cartilages toward or away from each other. Because the movements of rotation and gliding are associated, medial rotation occurs with medial gliding and lateral rotation with lateral gliding. Forward movements of the arytenoid cartilages occur but are limited by the posterior cricoarytenoid ligaments.

The mucosa-covered lumen of the larynx is supported by fibroelastic membranes. Above the ventricle, the quadrangular membrane extends from the lateral margins of the epiglottis to the arytenoid and corniculate cartilages; the inferior boundary of the upper portion is thickened to form the vestibular ligament (false cord). The lower portion of this fibroelastic membrane forms the conus elasticus. The anterior median cricothyroid ligament extends from the lower border of the thyroid cartilage to the upper border of the cricoid cartilage; this strong, thick ligament is narrow above and broad below. The lateral part of the cricothyroid membrane is thinner; it extends from the superior inner border of the cricoid cartilage to the inner surface of the thyroid angle and posteriorly to the tip of the vocal process of the arytenoid cartilage. The superior edge of the lateral part of the cricothyroid or cricovocal membrane is free and is suspended from the angle of the thyroid lamina anteriorly to the vocal process of the arytenoid cartilage posteriorly to form the vocal ligament of the vocal fold.

The lumen of the larynx is divided by two muscular valves. The vestibule of the larynx, the portion above the ventricle, is closed off by contraction of the vestibular, or false vocal, folds. The vestibular folds are separated from the true vocal folds by the ventricles, which allow for free vibration of the upper surface of the vocal folds. At the anterior end of each ventricle is a narrow diverticulum, the laryngeal saccule, which extends upward between the vestibular folds and the inner surface of the thyroid cartilage. Within the fibrous capsule of the saccule are a large number of mucous glands whose secretions lubricate the vocal folds when the saccule of the larynx is compressed by fibers of the thyroepiglottic muscle.

The vestibular folds are a pair of thick folds of mucous membranes that enclose a narrow bank of fibrous tissue, the vestibular ligament; they are attached to the angle of the thyroid cartilage in front and to the anterolateral surfaces of the arytenoid cartilages behind. The vestibular folds are approximated in forced closure of the glottis. The opening between the vestibular folds, the rima vestibuli, is wider than the opening of the glottis.

The true vocal folds extend from the anterior commissure at the thyroid cartilage to the vocal processes of the arytenoid cartilages and include the vocal ligament, which is the thickened upper margin of the conus elasticus, and the thyroarytenoid muscle. In cross-section, the vocal folds are triangular, with their inferior borders angled medially. The opening between the vocal folds is named the rima glottidis, or glottis. Approximately two thirds of the anterior rima glottidis is intermembranous and muscular; the posterior third, which lies between the vocal processes and the bases of the arytenoid cartilages, is intercartilaginous. The average lengths of the glottis are 23 mm in the adult male and 17 mm in the adult female.

The infraglottic larynx extends from the level of the vocal folds to the lower border of the cricoid cartilage. It widens downward toward the cavity of the trachea and is lined with respiratory mucous membrane.

Muscles

The function of the extrinsic muscles is to elevate, to depress, or, acting synergistically, to fix the larynx during deglutition, respiration, and phonation. The elevators of the larynx are the digastric, stylohyoid, geniohyoid, mylohyoid, stylopharyngeal, and thyrohyoid muscles. The depressors of the larynx are the sternohyoid, omohyoid, and sternothyroid muscles. The middle and inferior constrictor muscles of the pharynx are extrinsic laryngeal muscles that play an important role during swallowing. The principal function of the depressor group of muscles is the vertical displacement of the larynx downward during inspiration. During the normal expiratory cycle, there is a slight vertical elevation of the larynx.

The intrinsic muscles are the cricothyroid, posterior cricoarytenoid, lateral cricoarytenoid, transverse interarytenoid, oblique interarytenoid, arytenoepiglottic, thyroarytenoid, and thyroepiglottic muscles. With the exception of the transverse interarytenoid muscles, the intrinsic muscles are paired.

The posterior cricoarytenoid muscle arises from the posterior surface of the cricoid lamina in a broad depression just lateral to the median vertical ridge; its fibers, which run upward and laterally, converge to insert into the posterior surface of the muscular process of the arytenoid cartilage. The lowest and almost vertical fibers insert on the anterolateral surface of the arytenoid cartilage. This muscle is the main abductor of the vocal folds. Its primary function is to open the glottis by rotating the arytenoid cartilages laterally around an axis passing through the cricoarytenoid joints; the lateral fibers of the muscle draw the arytenoids laterally, thereby separating the vocal processes and vocal fold. The more horizontal and middle oblique fibers assist the cricothyroid muscle in tensing the vocal fold by pulling back the arytenoid cartilage.

The lateral cricoarytenoid muscle is smaller. Its fibers arise from the superior border of the arch of the cricoid cartilage and pass obliquely backward and upward to insert into the anterior aspect of the muscular process of the arytenoid cartilage. This muscle closes the glottis (adducts the vocal folds) by rotating the arytenoid cartilages medially. Medial rotation is limited by approximation of the vocal processes.

The transverse arytenoid (interarytenoid) muscle is a single muscle whose fibers arise from the muscular process and the lateral border of the arytenoid cartilage of one side to insert into the corresponding surfaces of the arytenoid of the opposite side, thereby bridging and filling the space between the posterior concave surfaces of the arytenoid. The function of this muscle is to approximate the arytenoids, which results in the closing of the cartilaginous rima glottidis.

The oblique arytenoid muscle is composed of two fasciculi posterior to the transverse arytenoid muscle, which cross each other in passing from the back of the muscular process of one arytenoid cartilage to the apex of the opposite cartilage, forming an X. Superiorly, at the apex of each arytenoid cartilage, fibers continue laterally into the arytenoepiglottic fold to form the arytenoepiglottic muscle. This muscle acts as a sphincter of the inlet of the larynx, adducting the arytenoepiglottic folds and approximating the arytenoid cartilages to the tubercle of the epiglottis.

The thyroarytenoid muscle is a broad, thin muscle that arises from the inner surface of the lower half of the angle of the thyroid cartilage. Its fibers pass backward laterally and upward to be inserted into the anterolateral surface and the vocal process of the arytenoid cartilage. This muscle, the median thyroarytenoid ligament, and the cover of laryngeal mucous membrane constitute the vocal folds. Anatomically and functionally, the thyroarytenoid muscle can be subdivided into three parts: the more lateral and superficial fibers compose the thyroarytenoid externus; the lower and deeper fibers of the muscle, which are parallel and just lateral to the vocal ligament, compose the thyroarytenoid internus or vocalis; and fibers from the thyroarytenoid externus, which pass backward and upward to be inserted into the arytenoepiglottic fold and margin of the epiglottis, form the third part, the thyroepiglotticus. There are also some crossing fibers that can act to change the shape of the glottis. Contraction of the thyroarytenoid externus draws the arytenoid cartilages forward toward the thyroid, thus shortening the vocal ligaments and relaxing the covering mucous membrane; with the lateral cricoarytenoid muscles, the arytenoid cartilages are rotated medially to approximate the vocal fold. Contraction of the vocalis portion of the muscle produces shortening and graded internal tension of the vocal cord. Acting as a synergist, contraction of the cricothyroid muscle increases the length, the tension, and the extent of adduction of the vocal fold for the production of middle- and high-pitched vocalizations; the cricothyroid also increases the area of the glottic opening during inspiration. The thyroepiglottic muscle widens the inlet of the larynx by acting on the arytenoepiglottic fold.

The cricothyroid muscle is a triangularly shaped muscle that arises, in two parts, from the anterior lateral part of the external surface of the arch of the cricoid cartilage. Its anterior fibers, the straight part, run upward and backward to insert into the lower border of the lamina of the thyroid cartilage; its lateral fibers, the oblique part, run backward and laterally to insert into the anterior border of the inferior horn of the thyroid cartilage. The medial borders of this paired muscle are separated by the triangular cricothyroid ligament. The cricothyroid muscle produces elongation and tension of the vocal fold ligament (and the vocal fold) by elevating the arch of the cricoid cartilage and tilting back the superior border of the cricoid lamina; the cricothyroid space is thus narrowed, and the distance between the vocal processes and the angle of the thyroid is increased, and the vocal ligaments are thereby lengthened and stretched. The oblique portion of the cricothyroid muscle also pulls the thyroid cartilage forward in relation to the posterior lamina, thereby additionally stretching the vocal folds.

Vascular and Lymphatic Systems

The arterial blood supply to the larynx is derived from the laryngeal branches of the superior and inferior thyroid arteries and from the cricothyroid branch of the superior thyroid artery. The superior laryngeal artery, along with the internal branch of the superior laryngeal nerve, enters the larynx through the thyrohyoid membrane. The superior laryngeal artery runs downward beneath the mucosa of the lateral wall and the floor of the piriform fossa to supply the muscles and mucous membranes in the superior portion of the larynx; it also anastomoses freely with branches of the artery of the opposite side and with those of the inferior laryngeal artery. The inferior laryngeal artery ascends on the trachea, together with the recurrent laryngeal nerve, and enters the larynx beneath the lower border of the inferior constrictor muscle along with the inferior laryngeal nerve. The inferior laryngeal artery supplies the mucous membrane and the muscles of the lower part of the larynx. The cricothyroid artery, a branch of the superior thyroid artery, passes across the superior portion of the crocothyroid ligament and anastomoses with the branch of the other side. Accompanying the arteries, the superior and inferior laryngeal veins join their respective superior and inferior thyroid veins.

The lymphatics of the larynx are divided into a superior group and an inferior group. Except in the area of the vocal folds, they are quite numerous. The area of the larynx above the vocal cords is drained by the superior group, which pierces the thyrohyoid membrane in the company of the superior laryngeal artery, and ends in the upper deep cervical nodes. The part of the larynx below the true vocal folds is drained by the inferior group of vessels, which pierce the cricothyroid membrane, pass to the pretracheal laryngeal nodes, and end in the lower deep cervical nodes. Additional lymphatics pass below the cricoid cartilage and above the first tracheal ring to join the deep cervical nodes directly. Although there is minimal lymphatic drainage from one side of the larynx to the other, contralateral drainage can occur when the ipsilateral drainage is obstructed. The true vocal cords appear to be devoid of lymphatic channels in the region of their free margin.

Nerve Supply

The nerve supply to the larynx is derived from the internal and external branches of the superior laryngeal nerve, from the recurrent laryngeal nerve, and from the autonomic nervous system. The internal laryngeal nerve, which is mostly sensory, enters the larynx through the posterior and inferior parts of the thyrohyoid membrane, above the superior laryngeal artery, to supply the upper half of the larynx to the level of the vocal folds. The external laryngeal branch supplies the cricothyroid muscle, entering the muscle laterally after piercing the inferior constrictor muscle.

Although principally derived from the inferior ganglia of the vagus, the superior laryngeal nerve does receive a branch from the superior cervical sympathetic ganglion. The inferior laryngeal nerve, from the recurrent nerve, divides into a motor branch and a sensory branch before entering the larynx at the posterior aspect of the cricothyroid joint. The sensory branch of the inferior laryngeal nerve supplies the mucous membrane of the larynx below the level of the vocal folds; it unites, within the piriform fossa, with the descending sensory branch from the internal laryngeal nerve. With the exception of the cricothyroid muscle, the inferior laryngeal nerve supplies all intrinsic muscles of the same side and the transverse arytenoid muscle bilaterally. The internal branch of the superior laryngeal nerve and the recurrent nerves also carry afferent fibers from neuromuscular spindles and other stretch receptors in the larynx.

The Esophagus

The esophagus extends from the inferior portion of the laryngeal pharynx to the stomach. This muscular tube of 25 cm begins in the midline at the caudal border of the cricoid cartilage, central to the sixth cervical vertebra, and follows the curvature of the vertebral column. It usually deviates slightly to the left as it descends until the level of the fourth thoracic vertebra, where it returns to the midline. At the level of the seventh thoracic vertebra, the esophagus moves forward and again to the left, piercing the diaphragm at the level of the tenth thoracic vertebra.

Posterior to the trachea and ventrally applied to the prevertebral fascia, the esophagus is flanked by the left and right recurrent laryngeal nerves, which lie in a groove formed by the trachea and esophagus. In the thorax, the esophagus passes through the superior and posterior mediastina. In its descent, it comes in contact with the following structures: (a) to the right, the mediastinal pleura, the azygos vein, and the right vagus nerve; (b) to the left, the subclavian artery, the thoracic duct, the mediastinal pleura, the aortic arch, the left vagus nerve, and the descending aorta; (c) anteriorly, the trachea and the left recurrent nerve, the left bronchus, the pericardium posterior to the left atrium, and the diaphragm; (d) posteriorly, the vertebrae, the longus cervicis muscle, prevertebral fascia, the thoracic duct, the azygos vein and its connection to the hemiazygos veins, the posterior intercostal arteries, and the descending thoracic aorta.

As the esophagus enters the abdomen, it turns sharply to the left; its right border becomes continuous with the lesser curvature of the stomach, and its left border forms an acute angle, the cardiac notch, with the fundus. Posteriorly, the esophagus lies on the left crus of the diaphragm and anteriorly on the esophagus impression of the left lobe of the liver. Left vagal fibers, forming the anterior vagal trunk, are carried on its anterior surface, whereas fibers derived from the right vagus, forming a posterior trunk, are carried on its posterior surface. The esophagus is constricted at four points: (1) 15 cm from the incisor teeth, (2) where it is crossed by the arch of the aorta, (3) where it is crossed by the left principal bronchus, and (4) where it pierces the diaphragm.

Structurally, the wall of the esophagus adheres to the pattern of the alimentary canal. It consists of four layers, which are, from within outwards, the mucous membrane (or mucosa), the submucosa, the muscularis externa, and the adventitia (or serosa). It is lined with nonkeratinized stratified squamous epithelium and is continuous with the pharynx above and at the gastroesophageal junction with the gastric mucosa. Its muscularis externa consists of inner circular and outer longitudinal muscle fibers. The upper third of the esophagus is composed of striated fibers; the lower third, of smooth fibers; and the middle third, of a mixture of both smooth and striated muscle fibers. The longitudinal muscle is more developed than the circular muscle, and its superior portion forms two diverging longitudinal bands that are attached to the posterior surface of the cricoid cartilage. The layer of circular muscle fibers is continuous with the cricopharyngeal muscle superiorly and with the circular and oblique muscle fibers of the stomach inferiorly. Two types of glands are found in the esophagus: esophageal glands proper and cardiac glands. They are composed of mucus-secreting cells and have ducts that open onto the surface of the epithelial lining.

The vascular supply to the esophagus comes from branches of the inferior thyroid, bronchial, thoracic aorta, left gastric, and left inferior phrenic arteries. Esophageal veins begin in a submucosal plexus, pass through the esophageal wall, and terminate in the inferior thyroid and vertebral veins superiorly, in the azygos and hemiazygos veins inferiorly, and in the left gastric vein in the abdomen. The left gastric vein, a branch of the portal vein, communicates with the azygos vein by way of anastomatic channels in the lower esophageal submucosa, forming a connection between the portal and systemic venous systems. Lymph vessels from the esophagus drain to the cervical, the posterior mediastinal, and the left gastric lymph nodes.

The esophagus receives vagal fibers from the recurrent laryngeal nerve and from sympathetic fibers accompanying the inferior thyroid artery. The thoracic esophagus receives its nerve supply from the esophageal plexus, the thoracic sympathetic trunk, and the greater splanchnic nerves. The abdominal esophagus is supplied by the anterior and posterior vagal trunks and is reconstituted from the esophageal plexus and from branches of the greater splanchnic nerves. Parasympathetic neurons are found within the walls of the esophagus as a myenteric plexus.

Central Neural Control

Comparative anatomic studies indicate that the primary role in the development of laryngeal structures was to separate the airway from the alimentary canal and protect the respiratory organ from foreign substances. This view helps to explain some apparent priorities in the organization of neural control of the larynx. Most of the muscular activities of the larynx are not consciously controlled. Even in speech the fine motor coordination necessary for intelligible language production is not conscious, and intended speech utterances may be interrupted for breathing, coughing, or gagging. In order for more volitional functions, such as phonation, to take place, respiratory and airway protection reflexes must be inhibited.

Volitional control of laryngeal function originates in the cortex. Electrical stimulation studies indicate that motor and sensory cortex areas that inhibit laryngeal action are as numerous as loci that facilitate vocalization. In the presence of extensive diffuse bilateral cortical damage with loss of voluntary phonation, the vocal folds may remain in spastic hyperabduction during respiration, but movement elicited by reflex coughing, gagging, laryngospasm, and even emotional cries remains intact. When there is progressive damage to supranuclear tract inputs to the laryngeal motor neurons, as seen in Steele-Richardson-Olszewski syndrome, olivopontocerebellar atrophy, and some progressive supranuclear palsies, loss of inhibition of laryngeal reflexes may be a prominent part of the symptoms. Such patients demonstrate poor volitional control of speech movements and decreased control over emotional crying, but, most distressing, they may be subject to prolonged laryngospasm with almost any stimulation of the laryngeal area, even by swallowing or phonation.

Injury to the corticobulbar motor connections to the laryngeal lower motor neurons results in spastic posture and slowed movements of the involved muscles, but generally cortical or corticobulbar injury does not result in paralysis. The primary connections of the important life-sustaining laryngeal reflexes are localized in the brain-stem and remain intact with higher level disease. The lower motor neuron cell bodies that control the pharyngeal and laryngeal muscles lie in a rostral extension of the lateral horns, the nucleus ambiguus. There is a rostral-to-caudal order of motor neuron cell bodies for the pharyngeal and laryngeal muscles. In order, progressing caudally, are cell bodies for upper and lower pharyngeal constrictor, thyropharyngeus, cricopharyngeus, cricothyroid, arytenoepiglottic, posterior cricoarytenoid, thyroarytenoid, lateral cricoarytenoid, and interarytenoid muscles.

The afferent sensory fibers responsible for reflex regulation of the larynx and pharynx are carried in all of the nerves that supply the larynx and a majority of these fibers synapse in the nucleus tractus solitarius, which has extensive interconnections with the nucleus ambiguus. The nucleus parabranchialis in the pons also provides many connections to the nucleus ambiguus, and there is important input to the nucleus ambiguus from the reticular formation, the basilar nuclei, and the cerebellum as well. It appears that the periaqueductal gray matter is an important area in which the extrapyramidal interconnections converge to influence laryngeal function.

Damage to extrapyramidal input to the laryngeal motor neuron nucleus is associated with difficulties in fine motor control of the laryngeal muscles that may significantly interfere with normal speech. Yet basic respiratory and airway protection reflexes remain intact. Examples of extrapyramidal diseases that affect laryngeal function include Parkinson's disease, choreas, tremors, vagal myoclonus, dystonias, and ataxias. Although these dysfunctions provide some clues toward understanding of the neural organization of laryngeal and pharyngeal motor control, relatively little is known about the central neuroanatomic structure of laryngeal and pharyngeal physiology.

VALVE FUNCTIONS IN PHARYNX AND LARYNX

The pharynx and the larynx each incorporate several muscular valves whose physiologic structures are integral to all of the functions of the upper aerodigestive tract. The pharynx includes two valves: (1) the velopharyngeal port, which controls the entrance to the nasal cavity, and (2) the cricopharyngeal region, or upper esophageal sphincter, which serves as the valve into the cervical esophagus. The larynx contains three valves: (1) the true vocal folds and the arytenoid cartilages, (2) the false vocal folds, and (3) the epiglottis; these valves serve to protect the trachea and the lower airway during swallowing. The physiologic structure of each of these valves is complex and is described first, followed by a discussion of the coordination of these valves with other movements of the pharynx and larynx during respiration, deglutition, and phonation.

Velopharyngeal Sphincter

When viewed superiorly, the velopharyngeal port consists of the velum anteriorly, the lateral pharyngeal walls laterally, and the posterior pharyngeal wall and adenoid pad posteriorly. Usually the sphincter is open during respiration. Velopharyngeal closure occurs momentarily during speech production and swallowing. On occasion, closure occurs pathologically during respiration in patients with patent eustachian tubes. The anatomic and physiologic mechanisms contributing to velopharyngeal closure are intricate and highly varied among individuals. Elevation and retraction of the velum is usually the largest contributor to velopharyngeal closure. This movement of the velum results largely from vector action created by contraction of two muscles: the levator veli palatini and the palatopharyngeus. The levator veli palatini pulls the palate upward, whereas the palatopharyngeus retracts and lowers the palate. The combined contraction of the two muscles results in an upward and backward vector of palatal movement.

The uvular muscle and the tensor veli palatini stiffen the palate and thus also contribute to velopharyngeal closure. In some people, the lateral pharyngeal walls, which are composed of the superior constrictor at the level of the soft palate, move medially to meet the elevating and retracting soft palate and thereby contribute significantly to velopharyngeal closure. In other people, selected fibers of the posterior pharyngeal wall contract and move anteriorly (Passavant's pad)

to meet the retracting velum, or the posterior and lateral pharyngeal walls move forward and inward together, like a purse string, to surround the retracting soft palate. An enlarged and anteriorly protruding adenoid pad may contribute to velopharyngeal closure by projecting anteriorly toward the soft palate, narrowing the anteroposterior dimension of the nasopharynx. The adenoid pad can become so enlarged and protrude so far anteriorly that it completely occludes the velopharyngeal port so that no velar or pharyngeal wall movement is needed to create velopharyngeal closure. To understand velopharyngeal dynamics in a given patient, videonasendoscopy or multiview videofluoroscopy is usually required. These techniques are particularly important in the planning of treatment for a malfunctioning velopharyngeal mechanism.

Cricopharyngeal (Upper Esophageal) Sphincter

During respiration and speech production, the cricopharyngeal region is closed to prevent the inhalation of air into the esophagus. During swallowing, the opening of the upper esophageal sphincter, or cricopharyngeal region, is a complex biomechanical event. Because the sphincter is a musculoskeletal structure composed of the cricopharyngeal muscle attached to the lateral aspects of the cricoid lamina, the opening of the sphincter requires both muscle relaxation and anterosuperior movement of the hyolaryngeal complex. During the pharyngeal swallowing sequence, the cricopharyngeal muscle (which is in a contracted state during respiration and speech) relaxes approximately 0.1 second before the upward and forward movement of the hyoid bone, and the larynx opens the sphincter. When the cricopharyngeal or upper esophageal sphincter is opened, the pressure exerted by the food or liquid bolus increases the width of the opening as the bolus moves through the sphincter. As larger volumes of material are swallowed, the cricopharyngeal region opens wider and for longer periods of time. The width of the cricopharyngeal opening is modulated by the intrabolus pressure, which increases with larger volumes. After the bolus has passed, the cricopharyngeal region closes as the hyoid bone and the larynx descend to their rest positions and the cricopharyngeal muscle contracts.

Laryngeal Valves

The three valves of the larynx are open during respiration. During speech production, the true vocal folds close (adduct), whereas the false vocal folds remain open and the epiglottis remains upright. Occasionally, in some speakers who pathologically use extreme, excessive laryngeal tension to produce the voice, false vocal fold closure may be observed during phonation. During swallowing, all three laryngeal valves close to protect the airway from the entry of food or liquid. Closure of these valves during swallowing progresses inferiorly to superiorly: the true vocal folds close first, followed by the false vocal folds and the epiglottis.

Closure of the larynx involves direct neural control as well as biomechanical closure. The *true vocal folds* close or adduct by contraction of the lateral cricoarytenoid muscle and the interarytenoid muscles, which rotate the vocal processes of the arytenoid cartilages medially, bringing the arytenoid cartilages and the true vocal folds together anteroposteriorly. Contraction of the thyroarytenoid muscle pulls the vocal process toward the anterior commissure, if unapposed, and thereby increases the muscle mass and decreases effective length. When the contraction is isometric, thyroarytenoid contraction increases the intrinsic stiffness and mass of the vocal fold. Opening, or adduction, of the vocal folds is accomplished actively by the contraction of the posterior cricoarytenoid muscle in combination with relaxation of the adductors.

Musculature in the arytenoepiglottic folds contracts to move the *false vocal folds* medially and tilt the arytenoid cartilages anteriorly. During swallowing, the arytenoid cartilages tilt anteriorly to contact the base of the epiglottis. Closure of the airway at this level during deglutition increases in duration with larger bolus volumes.

The epiglottis closes over the airway only during swallowing. It folds over the top of the airway as the biomechanical result of (1) elevation and anterior movement of the hyolaryngeal complex and (2) retraction of the tongue base. As the larynx and the hyoid bone elevate and move anteriorly during deglutition, the epiglottis, which is attached to both the hyoid bone and the larynx by ligaments, is folded downward from its resting position to horizontal. The tongue base then begins retracting toward the pharyngeal wall, carrying the epiglottis backward with it until the tip of the epiglottis contacts the posterior pharyngeal wall. As the tip of the epiglottis contacts the posterior pharyngeal wall and the tongue base continues to retract toward the pharyngeal wall, the epiglottis is squeezed below horizontal until it reaches its maximal lowering at the time when the tongue base achieves its maximal contact with the posterior pharyngeal wall. At the end of the swallow, as the tongue base retracts away from the pharyngeal wall toward its relaxed resting position, the epiglottis is carried anteriorly until it is no longer in contact with the posterior pharyngeal wall. The instant that the tip of the epiglottis is relieved of contact with the posterior pharyngeal wall, the epiglottis springs back to its resting position within 0.06 seconds; this action reflects the elasticity of this cartilage.

Closure of the true vocal folds and closure at the level of the false vocal folds with anterior tilting of the arytenoid are elicited as a part of the pharyngeal swallowing reflex programmed in the swallowing center in the medulla, whereas epiglottic movements are secondary biomechanical effects of hyolaryngeal elevation and tongue base retraction. Failure of the airway to close at the epiglottis results in penetration of food or liquid into the airway during the swallow. Penetrating material is usually squeezed out of the airway as the swallow progresses. Failure of the larynx to close below the epiglottis results in aspiration during the pharyngeal stage of swallowing and in the entering of food into the trachea below the vocal folds.

INTERACTIVE PHYSIOLOGY OF PHARYNX AND LARYNX

The three functions of the pharynx and the larynx are different in their relative physiologic importance, the nature of neural control, and the strength of muscle contraction. The relative importance of respiration, swallowing, and phonation is reflected in their frequency of occurrence. Respiration occurs approximately 900 times per hour in the average adult, whereas swallowing occurs only 10 to 15 times per hour. Speech is an

connected speech, pitch and intensity are exquisitely regulated by changes in mass and tension of the vocal folds in combination with modulations in air flow from below. During articulation of voiceless consonants, the vocal folds are partially abducted.

The vibration that produces voice occurs in the membranous portions of the vocal folds anterior to the vocal process. Ultra–high-speed cinephotographic studies and stroboscopic examinations demonstrate that in modal phonation, the vocal folds are parted from below by air pressure until the forces holding together the upper edges of the folds are overcome; at that point, the vocal fold edges separate relatively rapidly. They may open from anterior to posterior or from posterior to anterior, or inital opening may occur at midfold.

When the vocal folds separate, air flow through the glottis suddenly accelerates. The opening of the glottis is reflected in a wave-like movement of the vocal fold epithelial cover; this movement spreads laterally until the aperture of the opening between the vocal folds reaches a maximum. With the air flow through the glottis, Bernoulli's effect occurs as air flow velocity increases across the glottis. Also, subglottic pressure drops and the inferior portions of the bodies of the vocal folds begin to return to midline. As the bodies of the vocal folds fall toward each other, the glottal aperture narrows. The epithelial wave of the upper epithelial cover is usually still traveling laterally. As subglottal pressure continues to decrease, the bodies of the vocal folds contact and closure of the glottis occurs relatively abruptly. The epithelial waves on the upper edges of the folds return to the midline and mound up at the center of the glottis until vocal fold contact area is maximal. Subglottal pressure again begins to rise as soon as the vocal folds are closed.

The duration of the closed period is determined by relative balance of the resisting mass and elasticity of the folds pitted against the force of subglottic pressure. When subglottic pressure reaches a level to overcome the resistance of the closed lower vocal folds, the bodies of the folds are again forced apart from below, and another glottal cycle occurs.

Variations from the modal vibratory pattern occur with modifications of the mass and the tension of the vocal fold body, and the relative elasticity of its epithelial cover. In general, as body muscular tone increases, the body of the folds becomes less elastic. With extreme rigidity in the vocal fold musculature, such as that seen in Parkinson's disease, vibration may be confined to the epithelial cover. In this case the relatively isometric contraction of muscle fibers causes an increase in mass and stiffness.

As the vocal folds are passively stretched by cricothyroid contraction, there is progressively less distinction between the mass and elastic characteristics of the epithelium in comparison with those of the vocal fold bodies until the mode of vibration changes to falsetto mode. With elongation of the vocal folds in falsetto mode, the tissues of the vocal folds are stretched passively, their relative elastic and mass characteristics become more similar, and the tensed epithelial cover and body vibrate more as a single unit. The fundamental frequency of vibration is thus determined by several factors, not just by the length of the vibratory portions of the vocal folds. For example, it is possible with training to produce a limited range of fundamental frequencies in both modal and falsetto modes of vibratory pattern.

Position of the valves and folds of the pharynx and the larynx during phonation, connected speech, and singing can be controlled by voluntary cortical influence, and this conscious control can be increased with learning. Inhibitory influence over reflex effects such as gagging and coughing can also be enhanced by training in the normal neural system. In the presence of either anatomic or neurologic disease, compensatory adjustments may be made in the coordination of the laryngeal muscles. This may occur at both a conscious level and an unconscious level. It is important in assessing the pathophysiologic processes of the system to recognize the contributing role of compensatory effects. Such factors complicate the study of laryngeal physiology.

The exact nature of neural control of vocalization and the relationships of neural control for respiration, deglutition, and speech production are incompletely understood. From electromyographic studies, it is known that the thyroarytenoid muscles are most active during phonation and relax during respiration. The lateral cricoarytenoid muscle is also active during phonation and even more so during sphincteric closure of the larynx. The ventricular fold muscle fibers are most active during glottic closure, but they may also be active in phonation to varying degrees. The arytenoepiglottic fibers are active primarily in glottic closure for gagging and swallowing. The interarytenoid fibers are active during phonation and during glottic closure. The posterior cricoarytenoid muscle is the sole abductor of the vocal processes and shows its greatest activity during the inspiratory phase of the respiratory cycle. The cricothyroid muscles are most active during elevation of fundamental frequency but are also active in deep inspiration. This, with maximal abduction of the vocal folds, has the effect of further enlarging the glottal aperture.

Production of low-pitched sounds or sounds of high intensity is also associated with increased motor unit activity in the sternothyroid muscle. In the production of high-pitched or low-intensity vocalizations, there is increased motor unit activity in the thyrohyoid muscle and inhibition of the sternothyroid muscle.

Activity of the intrinsic laryngeal muscles is varied in pulmonary disease, and partial closure of the glottis during expiration may be a compensatory factor in adapting to obstructive pulmonary disease. Feedback from mucosal pressure receptors appears to be an important factor in the control of laryngeal movements during respiration. Disturbance of the normal balance of sensory feedback influence can result in inappropriate movements during the respiratory cycle. Thus if sensory input is pathologically sensitive to air flow or pressure, the glottis may close during inspiratory efforts. In such cases the inappropriate closure may be aggravated by decreasing airway pressure during inspiration and may be relieved by increasing airway pressure during inspiration. In instances associated with inflammation of a reactive airway, the pathologic respiratory movements may disappear with resolution of the inflammation of the airway epithelium.

LOWER MOTOR NEURON INJURIES

The history of laryngology has witnessed some controversy about the specific physiologic effects on laryngeal function when there is injury to the peripheral innervation. Recurrent laryngeal nerve section results acutely in loss of adduction and abduction of the vocal folds, loss of tone in the thyroarytenoid muscle, and loss of muscular fixation of the arytenoid muscle. Immediately after injury, the vocal fold is situated in an intermediate position between full adduction and full abduction. Over time, the vocal fold becomes positioned more medially as a result of the continued effects of intact interarytenoid muscle contraction and also as a result of passive tension effects on the arytenoid cartilage from cricothyroid action. The paralyzed muscles demonstrate fibrillation potentials on electromyography. The clinical situation is complicated by the fact that some reinnervation occurs over time. Because nerves in the immediate area have different functional characteristics, the effects of reinnervation may be variable, depending on which nerves provide the reinnervating fibers. Muscle fiber twitch and contraction characteristics are determined by the nature of the motor innervation and may therefore change with reinnervation by a new source of neural input. Relatively little is known about the complex effects of reinnervation in the laryngeal musculature.

Paralysis of one vocal fold from recurrent laryngeal nerve section causes alterations in vibratory pattern as a result of decreased mass in the body of the paretic cord. If the vocal folds are approximated in phonation, the two folds vibrate in phase with one another. The pattern of vibration in the paretic cord differs in that the slack muscular body yields relatively quickly to subglottic pressure, and glottic opening occurs relatively early. Thus even when voice quality in modal range is fairly normal after recurrent paralysis, it is difficult for the patient to produce elevated intensities.

Superior Laryngeal Nerve Injury

Superior laryngeal nerve section results in acute loss of motor input to the cricothyroid muscles and, possibly, also the supraglottic muscles, the ventricular fibers, and the arytenoepiglottic fibers. Superior laryngeal nerve section also results in acute loss of sensory feedback from the innervated area. When there is unapposed contraction of the cricothyroid muscles on one side of the larynx, their actions result in a rotation of the thyroid cartilage in relation to the cricoid cartilage as the muscles contract at the onset of phonation. The inferior horn of the thyroid

There is a delay between the opening of the lower and upper margins of the vocal fold referred to as a phase delay. Viewed on high-speed film or by stroboscopy, this fluid-like movement of the vibrating vocal folds appears as a traveling mucosal wave. It is important to realize that this wave motion is the primary influence on the rise and fall in the amount of air flowing through the glottis during voicing. The shape of the air flow puff results in the acoustic pressure wave, which in turn is used in the perception of voice—that is, fundamental frequency and associated harmonics of varying amplitudes. Thus the traveling wave of the vocal folds profoundly affects the sound produced by the larynx. A number of factors are pertinent to the characteristics of the traveling wave. Minoru Hirano proposed the body/cover theory of vocal fold vibration. It suggests that the layer structure of the vocal fold divides into two groups that have different rheologic properties. The cover is composed of squamous epithelium and the superficial and intermediate layers of loose connective tissue or lamina propria. Thus it is pliable but has no intrinsic contractile properties. Conversely, the inner group or body is composed of the deep layer of the lamina propria and the thyroarytenoid muscle. Cricothyroid muscle contraction produces a stretching of the cover, and thyroarytenoid muscle contraction produces stiffening of the body. The combined stiffness of the entire vocal fold would then be determined by the extrinsic longitudinal tension on the cover and the internal stiffening of the body. In this theory, vocal fold vibration—that is, traveling wave motion—occurs primarily in the cover.

Changes in the stiffness or tension of the vocal folds may affect traveling wave motion. This is because the velocity of a traveling wave in an elastic medium, such as the vocal folds, is directly related to the stiffness of the medium and inversely related to the density of the medium. Thus as the tension in the vocal folds increases as a result of muscular contraction, the traveling wave velocity also increases and the pitch rises.

LESIONS AFFECTING THE TRAVELING WAVE

Lesions that affect traveling wave motion produce aberrations in the modulation of the air flowing through the glottis. These include vocal fold edema, mass lesions, asymmetric stiffness lesions, and symmetric stiffness lesions.

Inflammation and Mass Lesions

Inflammatory disorders associated with edema of the vocal folds may produce restriction in the traveling wave motion and thus diminish the ability of the vocal folds to modulate the air flow and excite harmonics in the upper frequencies. Mass lesions or vocal fold scarring may produce irregular vibration of the vocal folds; these have been associated with the appearance of energy at inharmonic frequencies—that is, noise in the source spectrum. In general, mass lesions affect vibration by preventing the vocal folds from touching. This results in the escape of unmodulated air flow through the glottis. Mass lesions may also alter the viscoelastic characteristics of the vocal cords. For example, patients with microinvasive carcinoma involving the epithelium and the lamina propria often exhibit loss of traveling wave motion because of the increased stiffness imparted by the cellular density of the neoplasia.

Asymmetric Stiffness Disorders

Asymmetric stiffness occurs in states of vocal fold paresis or paralysis. Changes in stiffness characteristically affect the amplitude and velocity of the traveling wave. It can be generally stated that the more forcefully the vocal folds close during vibration, the more energy is imparted to the higher frequencies and the more normal or bright the voice sounds. Conversely, in paralysis states, because the vocal folds close more slowly and with less force, less energy is imparted to the higher harmonics, and the voice frequently sounds soft or breathy. Furthermore, because asymmetric stiffness and paralysis states are often associated with large leaks of unmodulated air flow, the perception of breathiness is often associated with a perception of hoarseness because of the white noise produced by the unmodulated leaky air. Most laryngologists accept that the fundamental unit of laryngeal vibration is at the level of the traveling wave; that is, the wave is the vibration. Typically, entrainment (the simultaneous opening and closing of the left and right vocal folds) occurs through tissue proximity and air flow. However, when asymmetric conditions are associated with decoupling caused by wide glottal gaps, the left and right traveling wave velocities may diverge, producing serious aberrations in vibration and acoustics. Both vocal folds may actually vibrate at different frequencies, which results in the acoustic perception of diplophonia. Subharmonic frequencies (below the fundamental frequency) may also be generated. Both diplophonia and subharmonic frequencies may have the perception of roughness or harshness.

Symmetric Hyperfunctional and Hypofunctional Disorders

In contrast to asymmetric flaccid laryngeal states, other patients demonstrate symmetric hyperfunctional or hypofunctional voice disorders. Spasmodic dysphonia is a hyperfunctional disorder in which the normal neuromuscular reflex loops controlling intralaryngeal medial adductory compression are disturbed; this results in a mismatch between the glottal resistance, which must be overcome to initiate phonation, and the pulmonary driving pressure. When this occurs, glottal resistances are too high to sustain uniform vibration, and the voice often sounds harsh with a strained quality associated with it. Other patients demonstrate symmetric weakened closure. Elderly patients frequently lose muscular tone and strength, which results in vocal fold bowing or the appearance of a sulcus in the mucosal cover. These forms of glottal insufficiency produce soft and harsh voices.

OBJECTIVE MEASURES OF HOARSENESS

Because laryngeal vibration typically occurs at frequencies between 100 and 300 cycles per second and is thus too rapid to be appreciated by the human eye, a number of objective measurement systems that permit evaluation of laryngeal function for the purposes of documentation and quantification have been developed. Being able to quantify hoarseness is useful because untrained listeners often judge the same patient's degree of hoarseness differently. These objective measurement systems include glottography, stro-

boscopic imaging, and aerodynamic and acoustic measurements.

Glottography

Glottography is an objective measurement system in which physiologic sensors are used to record the amount of light transilluminated by the larynx during vibration, termed *photoglottography* (PGG), or the degree of vocal fold contact exhibited by the larynx during vocal fold vibration, termed *electroglottography* (EGG). PGG and EGG signals are complementary; PGG measures the degree of vocal fold opening, whereas EGG measures the degree of vocal fold closure. Changes in glottographic waveforms have been observed to reflect changes in laryngeal vibration associated with mass lesions or states of asymmetric stiffness that produce hoarseness. The advantage of glottography is that it is a noninvasive test, and the analysis of signals can be automated through computerized programs. The disadvantage is that because the output is the sum total of vibration from both the right and left vocal cords, it is frequently difficult to tell, on the basis of PGG and EGG signals alone, the precise nature of the anatomic lesion.

Imaging

Laryngeal imaging by cine or video recording has proved to be helpful in documenting and clarifying a wide variety of laryngeal abnormalities. Although indirect laryngoscopy has the advantages of low cost, widespread availability, and ease, it has the disadvantage of examining only the static position and gross adductory and abductory movements of the vocal folds. Laryngeal stroboscopy has been successfully used to examine the detailed vibratory nature of the vocal folds during phonation. The principles of stroboscopy have been known since about 1930. Modern laryngostroboscopes use flashes of light to create a montage of the vibrating folds; the synchronization of the flashes is controlled either by the fundamental frequency of phonation of the examined subject or by a frequency generator. Stroboscopy has been used in the diagnosis of phonatory disorders and in the early detection of invasive glottic cancer. Because stroboscopy samples images

death in the delivery room. Rare newborns have been saved by astute neonatologists and anesthesiologists who have placed large-bore needles in the cervical trachea to ventilate the patient until a tracheotomy could be performed. However, most infants die within the first few minutes of life from asphyxia.

Laryngeal atresia is a result of lack of recanalization of the airway after the development of the epithelial plug. Laryngeal atresia has been classified into three types by Smith and Bain. The different types are based on which portion of the epithelial plug is reabsorbed and which remains (Table 39–1). Repair of an atresia has rarely been attempted, and therefore there is no uniform technique for reconstruction of this complicated defect. Each case has to be individualized, and the parents should be forewarned that a completely successful result is very unlikely.

Laryngeal webs can also be thought of as the mildest form of laryngeal atresia and probably represent the almost complete reabsorption of the superior and inferior portions of the epithelial plug. Only a portion of the epithelium remains, which gives rise to a thin membrane most frequently at the level of the vocal folds, although the web can be located both supraglottically and infraglottically. There can be variable degrees of webbing from the persistence of only a small pharyngotracheal opening, which would give rise to severe airway distress, to a very minimal web, of which hoarseness may be the only symptom.

The treatment of the patient with a web is dependent on the degree of airway distress. If the patient has an inadequate airway (even after bronchoscopy to dilate the web), tracheotomy is indicated. However, a more conservative approach can be taken with the patient who has a satisfactory airway. The web traditionally has been approached externally through a laryngofissure with lysis of the web and placement of a stent. However, if the web is thin, an endoscopic approach with the laser can be used. An endoscopic stent or keel can be placed so that external surgery may not be necessary.

Clefts

A posterior laryngeal cleft results from the failure of complete upward migration of the tracheoesophageal septum. There is failure of closure of the posterior lamina of the cricoid, which may extend variable distances into the trachea as well. In the most severe form of this anomaly, the larynx, the trachea, and the esophagus are one common cavity with no separation whatsoever.

The most common symptom is coughing and respiratory distress upon feeding secondary to aspiration. A barium swallow may demonstrate the abnormality, but in mild deformities, only aspiration may be noted. The diagnosis is made at endoscopy, although small defects can be missed by the unsuspecting clinician. To rule out a small cleft, the laryngoscope should be placed in the endolarynx and gentle pressure applied in an attempt to separate the posterior aspect of the cricoid. If a significant cleft is found, the child should be intubated and a gastrostomy placed before repair. The defect is closed in layers by way of a thyrotomy or lateral pharyngotomy.

Cysts

Cysts of the larynx may be present at birth or may develop shortly thereafter and cause significant airway problems. The most common site for the cyst is in the false vocal fold. The etiologic origin of these cysts has been debated, and there is still no answer as to whether they represent congenital cysts (perhaps of minor salivary gland origin) or are internal laryngoceles that fail to communicate with the airway. In either case, the symptoms are a hoarse cry and airway distress. Treatment can usually be carried out endoscopically and consists of marsupialization of the cyst, usually by use of the CO_2 laser. It is unusual for these children to require tracheotomy because the airway can usually be established with an endotracheal tube. The airway is usually quite good after marsupialization of the cyst.

Hemangiomas

Capillary hemangiomas of the subglottic space can be insidious in growth and devel-

TABLE 39–1. Classification of Laryngeal Atresia

	I	II	III
Vestibule	Absent	Normal	Normal
Sinuses	Absent	Normal	Normal
Arytenoid cartilages	Fused	Separate	Fused
Cricoid cartilage	Conical shape	Dome shape	Normal

opment. The child, usually female, may be perfectly normal at delivery, but over the succeeding weeks, the hemangioma enlarges, producing stridor and airway distress. Some patients have cutaneous hemangiomas, which should make the clinician even more suspicious of the presence of a subglottic hemangioma. The natural history of capillary hemangiomas is gradual or rapid enlargement during the first year of life, at which time the size of the lesion stabilizes. The hemangiomas then regress and disappear over the next 2 to 3 years. Unfortunately, because of the small size of the neonatal subglottic airway, even the slightest enlargement causes symptoms.

The diagnosis is made through endoscopy. Subglottic hemangiomas tend to occur more frequently on the posterior or lateral walls, but they can completely encircle the airway. The lesions may be bluish but may also appear as normal mucosa. The lesion is compressible, and the slow refilling of the vascular channels and re-expansion of the lesion can be observed by passing a bronchoscope through the subglottic area and withdrawing it until the tip is at the level of the glottis.

In the past, children with subglottic hemangiomas were treated with tracheotomy until the hemangioma regressed. However, other options are now available. If a child has a subglottic hemangioma that is symptomatic, systemic steroids can be helpful in achieving a rapid decrease in the size of the lesion. However, the long-term administration of steroids is probably not a suitable treatment for this condition because of the myriad side effects of steroids. Tracheotomy can frequently be avoided and the hemangioma removed completely by use of the CO_2 laser endoscopically through a subglottoscope. Small lesions can be vaporized during one procedure, whereas the removal of larger ones should be staged to avoid circumferential laser burns, which predispose the area to stenosis. Bleeding is minimal because hemangiomas have a very slow blood flow.

Vocal Cord Paralysis

Vocal cord paralysis in newborns is quite different from that in adults. There is a predominance in males, and bilateral paralysis is more common than is unilateral paralysis. The most common symptom of unilateral paralysis is hoarseness, although stridor is not unusual. Stridor is the most common symptom of bilateral paralysis. Although birth trauma is not an unusual etiologic factor, in most cases it is either idiopathic or related to an Arnold-Chiari malformation with hydrocephalus (Table 39–2). The diagnosis can be made in the neonatal intensive care unit through flexible laryngoscopy. The advantage of flexible laryngoscopy over direct laryngoscopy in evaluating vocal cord movement is twofold. First, the patient can be examined for extended periods of time very easily with the flexible scope, which permits an adequate time for study. Second, movement of the vocal cords can be accidently impaired by the rigid laryngoscope in the larynx.

Children with a unilateral paralysis rarely require tracheotomy because they have an adequate airway. Tracheotomy is difficult to avoid in the child with bilateral paralysis. Occasionally, a child with an Arnold-Chiari malformation with hydrocephalus can be treated with a cerebrospinal fluid shunt, which results in a return of vocal fold function and thereby eliminates the need for a tracheotomy. The long-term outlook for children with vocal paralysis is fairly good, and lateralization procedures should be deferred until at least 5 years of age because many of the paralyses spontaneously resolve during the first 5 years of life.

Laryngomalacia

Laryngomalacia is the most common congenital laryngeal abnormality. Initially it was thought that laryngomalacia was caused by an immaturity of the laryngeal cartilages, particularly the corniculate cartilage, which

TABLE 39–2. Vocal Cord Paralysis

Etiology	Unilateral Paralysis	Bilateral Paralysis
Idiopathic	4	2
Birth trauma	1	4
Arnold-Chiari malformation with hydrocephalus	1	4
Surgery	4	0
Syphilis	0	1
Encephalocele	0	1

Number of patients less than 1 year of age by etiology and type of paralysis. Adapted from Gentile RD, Miller RH, Woodson GE: Vocal cord paralysis in children less than one year of age and younger. Ann Otol Rhinol Laryngol 95:622, 1986.

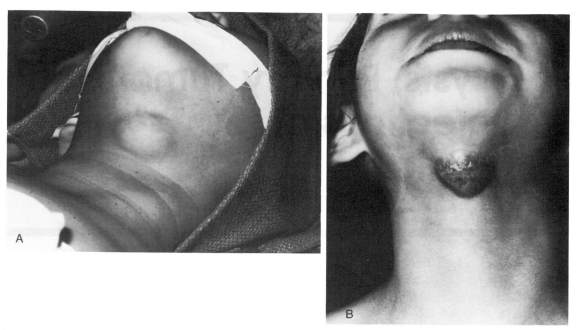

Figure 40–1. *A.* Thyroglossal duct cyst deep to the skin, at the hyoid level slightly to the left of the midline. *B.* Thyroglossal duct cyst with a large area of skin involvement and discoloration. (From Hawkins DB, Jacobson BE, Klatt EC: Cysts of the thyroglossal duct. Laryngoscope 92:1254–1258, 1982.)

1*B*). A draining sinus tract is sometimes present. The cysts usually contain clear, thick, mucoid fluid. Thyroglossal duct cysts are lined by either respiratory epithelium or squamous epithelium, which may be obliterated by granulation tissue in patients with chronic inflammation. Islands of thyroid tissue or lymphoid tissue are found within the wall of some cysts. On examination, a thyroglossal duct cyst is a soft to relatively firm rounded mass that moves upward with swallowing. It usually consists of one rounded mass, but an occasional cyst is lobulated. Thyroglossal duct cysts are almost always associated with a patent thyroglossal duct proximal to the cyst.

The differential diagnosis of thyroglossal duct cyst includes any localized soft tissue swelling that develops in the anterior midline of the neck. Submental lymph nodes can usually be differentiated by clinical examination and ectopic thyroid gland by radionuclide thyroid scan. Lesions such as lipomas, deep hemangiomas, dermoid or epidermoid cysts, and thyroid nodules may be differentiated on clinical examination but occasionally require surgical exploration in order to differentiate them from thyroglossal cysts. Branchial cleft cysts lie more laterally

and usually are easily differentiated from thyroglossal duct cysts.

Surgical Indications and Technique

Surgical excision of a thyroglossal duct cyst is usually indicated because the cyst is cosmetically undesirable or because of previous or persistent infection. Another relative indication is the slight possibility of malignant change. This has been reported occasionally in adults and also in children as young as 9 years of age. Small cysts, especially in very young children, that are not noticeable and have not been infected do not necessarily require surgery.

Although computed tomographic (CT) scans or magnetic resonance imaging (MRI) scans may be of interest, they are not necessary in the preoperative evaluation of a thyroglossal duct cyst. A radionuclide thyroid scan, although not absolutely necessary in all cases, is helpful in documenting the location of the thyroid gland. It is the author's policy to obtain thyroid scans preoperatively on all suspected thyroglossal duct cysts.

The standard technique for excision of thyroglossal duct cyst was described by Sistrunk (1928): excision of the cyst and duct, including a central portion of the hyoid bone and a 5- to 10-mm core of tissue proximal to the hyoid at a 45° angle with lines drawn perpendicular and horizontal to the hyoid bone. This corresponds to a line drawn from the center of the hyoid bone to the foramen cecum of the tongue and should contain the duct. The tissue excised proximal to the hyoid should contain portions of the raphe of the mylohyoid muscle and portions of the geniohyoid and genioglossus muscles. Sistrunk was not the first to advocate excision of the central portion of the hyoid; that was first suggested in the 1890s. He apparently was the first to advocate excision of a core of muscle tissue proximal to the hyoid bone. He emphasized that the duct is small, delicate, and difficult to locate. Even if it is located, it may break during dissection and be lost. An additional reason for excising a core of tissue is that multiple ducts with outpouchings containing mucus-secreting glands have been found in some surgical specimens.

If the cyst does not involve overlying skin, the surgical incision can be made directly over the cyst or in a skin crease below the cyst. If the cyst involves overlying skin, with or without a draining sinus, it is usually necessary to remove the involved skin in an ellipse with the incision. A well-delineated cyst usually can be dissected to the hyoid bone relatively easily. On some occasions, the cyst cannot be delineated well from surrounding soft tissue. In these instances, it is advisable to remove the cyst and a cuff of surrounding soft tissue en bloc to the hyoid bone. Care must be taken not to rupture the cyst. Once a cyst has ruptured and deflated, it may be difficult to differentiate from surrounding tissues. This increases the chances of leaving a portion of cyst wall, which increases the chances of recurrence. In removal of the central portion of the hyoid bone, it should not be skeletonized or the duct may be dissected away from it. The core of soft tissue proximal to the hyoid bone should be removed almost to the foramen cecum, without opening into the pharynx. Finger pressure intraorally to the foramen cecum helps identify the level and depth of dissection, but this is awkward to perform, and the author has found it to be unnecessary in most cases. Once the muscle core dissection has reached the desired depth, the core is clamped and removed. The stump is closed with a pursestring suture of 2–0 or 3–0

chromic catgut, which is then oversewn by one or two figure-of-eight sutures. The wound is then closed with a drain, which is left in place for 48 hours postoperatively, and a pressure dressing is applied. If the cyst has recently been infected and residual infection is suspected at the time of surgery, an antibiotic is used prophylactically.

The recurrence rate for thyroglossal duct cyst excision without removal of the hyoid bone is stated to be over 50%. Removal of the hyoid bone without excision of a proximal core of tissue by the Sistrunk technique results in a recurrence rate of over 20%. Excision by Sistrunk's method should result in recurrence rates of less than 10%.

MIDLINE CERVICAL DEFECT

This rare midline cervical anomaly is often mistaken for an abnormality of the thyroglossal duct. However, it probably results from a failure of the branchial arches to merge completely in the midline. It typically consists of four components: a vertical strip of tissue devoid of skin, a skin tag at the upper end, a superficial dimple at the inferior aspect (Fig. 40–2), and a subcutaneous fibrous cord beneath the defect that may extend to the mandible. The treatment is excision of the defect and the immediately underlying fibrotic tissue. The length of the defect often requires a single or double Z-plasty closure.

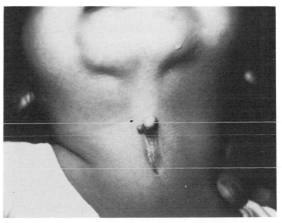

Figure 40–2. Midline cervical defect: a vertical strip of tissue devoid of skin with a skin tag at the upper end and a superficial dimple at the inferior aspect. A subcutaneous fibrous cord can be seen extending from the defect up to the chin.

BRANCHIAL CLEFT CYST AND FISTULA

Embryology

The branchial or pharyngeal arches appear in the fourth and fifth weeks of embryonic development. They consist of five bars of mesoderm separated externally by branchial or pharyngeal clefts and internally by branchial or pharyngeal pouches. The clefts and pouches approximate each other but do not have open communications. A detailed description of the arches, clefts, and pouches and their derivatives is beyond the scope of this chapter. Briefly stated, the first cleft is the only one giving rise to a definitive structure, the external auditory canal. Active proliferation of the second arch results in its overlapping the third and fourth arches and thereby obliterating the second, third, and fourth clefts. Temporarily, the clefts form a cavity, the cervical sinus of His. With normal development, this sinus usually disappears. Branchial cleft cysts are thought to be remnants of this cervical sinus. They may have external or internal fistulous connections or both, or they may have neither external nor internal connections. Also, a branchial fistula without a cyst may be present. Because the mesoderm that gives rise to the sternocleidomastoid muscle is in the epicardial ridge that lies caudal to the arches, the cyst lies beneath the sternocleidomastoid muscle, and any external fistulous opening lies along its anterior border. Theoretically, remnants of the cervical sinus could communicate with the second, third, or fourth pouch. In reality, those with internal connections usually communicate with the tonsillar fossa, the remnant of the second pouch. (A first cleft cyst that communicates with the external ear canal is found occasionally. Such cysts are much rarer than those arising from the cervical sinus and are not the subject of this discussion.)

Clinical Characteristics

Fistulas with internal and external communications usually manifest themselves during infancy as a small opening, just anterior to the sternocleidomastoid muscle, that drains saliva or mucus. There may or may not be a cystic component deep to the sternocleidomastoid muscle. Branchial cleft cysts that do not have internal or external openings usually appear in the teenage years or early adulthood as a swelling beneath the upper portion of the sternocleidomastoid muscle. Needle aspiration of the cyst obtains milky fluid that contains an abundance of cholesterol crystals. The demonstration of cholesterol crystals on a smear is virtually pathognomonic of a branchial cleft cyst. CT or MRI scan, helpful but not essential, reveals a rounded cystic mass beneath the sternocleidomastoid muscle. Neither scan will identify or rule out an internal fistula of the cyst. If an external opening is present, radiopaque contrast material injected into the opening may demonstrate a tract extending to the pharynx (Fig. 40–3). On the other hand, the failure of such a contrast "sinogram" to demonstrate a tract does not prove that one does not exist.

Branchial cleft cysts are lined by squamous or respiratory epithelium or both and have lymphoid tissue within the cyst wall. With repeated infections, the epithelium may be replaced by granulation tissue.

Surgical Indications and Technique

Branchial Fistula

The indication for surgical excision of a branchial fistula is the undesirable constant drain-

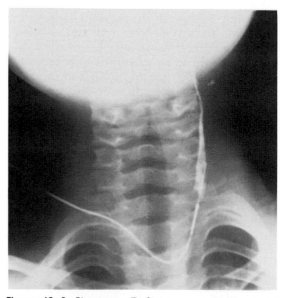

Figure 40–3. Sinogram. Radiopaque contrast material injected into the external opening of a branchial fistula low in the neck demonstrates a tract extending superiorly to the pharynx.

age of saliva or mucus from the fistula opening in the neck. The tract connected to the external opening may extend all of the way to the tonsillar fossa, or it may extend only part of the way. Surgery can be performed at any age. The smaller the patient is, the shorter the dissecting distance of the tract is. As the infant grows, the tract lengthens along with the neck. On the other hand, the tract is likely to be stronger and more easily dissected in a larger patient. The author prefers to excise fistulas late in the first year of life.

A horizontal elliptical incision is made around the external opening of the fistula. The tract usually is easy to identify and dissect; there is no need to inject substances such as methylene blue to identify the tract. The author has on occasion passed a 3-French diameter Fogarty catheter into the lumen of the tract to aid in stabilizing it. This is not necessary, however, in most cases. The tract is dissected upward with blunt and sharp dissection. The tract is closely related to the internal jugular vein and the carotid arteries; however, if the dissection is kept directly on the tract, these vessels will not be injured and do not have to be identified. With tracts that extend from low in the neck to the tonsillar fossa, it is necessary to make a second, higher incision for adequate exposure of the superior dissection (Fig. 40–4). The digastric muscle is identified as the tract courses beneath it. After retraction of the digastric muscle, the tract is noted to course

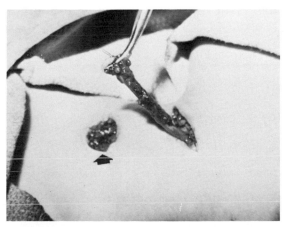

Figure 40–4. Excision of a branchial cleft fistula by use of two incisions. When the upper limit of exposure through the lower incision (arrow) is reached, a second horizontal incision is made in the submandibular area. The lower portion of the tract is brought out through the second incision, and the upper portion is dissected to the pharynx.

superficially to the hypoglossal nerve and then enter the pharyngeal wall. It is ligated at this point with a suture or with a vascular clip, which is easier. The wound is closed with a drain and a pressure dressing. The drain can be removed on the first or second day after operation.

Branchial Cleft Cyst Without External Fistula

The indication for surgery is the presence of an undesirable lateral neck mass that may or may not have been the site of previous infection.

A horizontal incision is made in the skin of the anterior triangle of the neck overlying the cyst and is extended posteriorly over the anterior portion of the sternocleidomastoid muscle. The sternocleidomastoid muscle is dissected from the superficial surface of the cyst and is retracted posteriorly. Unless significant scarring from prior infections exists, the cyst can usually be excised intact by blunt dissection close to the cyst wall. This is best started at the lower aspect of the cyst. The deep superior portion should be the last area dissected. At this point, the surgeon should look for a possible internal fistula to the pharynx. The internal jugular vein, the carotid artery, the common facial vein, and the spinal accessory nerve are proximal to the deep portion of the cyst and should be avoided. The wound is closed with a drain and pressure dressing. The drain is removed in 24 to 48 hours. Prophylactic antibiotics are used in the same manner as described for thyroglossal duct cyst.

CYSTIC HYGROMA

Embryology

Two theories of lymphatic development have been debated over the years. The most widely accepted theory is that the lymphatic system originates from five primordial lymphatic sacs from which lymphatic vessels sprout centrifugally to form the peripheral lymphatic system. The five sacs are the two jugular sacs lateral to the jugular vein on each side of the neck, the two paired sacral sacs, and an unpaired retroperitoneal sac. The other theory is that peripheral lymphatics develop in mesenchymal clefts and join together to form continuous channels that develop in a centripetal direction to join the venous system. Cystic hygromas apparently develop from portions of the lymphatic system that become separated from the primary sacs during embryonic development.

Cystic hygromas are generally considered to be lymphangiomas. In the most quoted classification of lymphangiomas (Landing and Farber, 1956), they are divided into broad categories on the basis of size of the lymphatic spaces; lymphangioma simplex is made up of many small lymphatic vessels, cavernous lymphangioma is made up of larger lymphatic vessels, and cystic lymphangioma is the same as cystic hygroma. In reality, there is considerable mixing and overlapping of these three categories, and it has been suggested that the nature of the surrounding tissue determines to some extent the physical nature of a lymphangioma. More recently, Mulliken and Young (1988) objected to the terms *lymphangioma* and *cystic hygroma*. They stated that all of these abnormalities should be called *lymphatic malformations*. They cited the term *lymph cyst* as being more accurate than *cystic hygroma*, but the latter term is of historic significance and undoubtedly will be preserved.

Clinical Course and Management

Sixty-five per cent to 75% of cystic hygromas are diagnosed at or shortly after birth, and 85% appear by the third year of life. Seventy-five per cent to 90% of cystic hygromas are found in the neck. The next most common site is the axilla. Other areas in which they are found are the shoulder and back, the mediastinum, the pectoral region, the retroperitoneal area, the pelvis, and the groin. Of those that arise in the neck, 2% to 3% extend into the axilla or the mediastinum. The most common site of origin in the neck is the posterior triangle, although hygromas often grow to involve both anterior and posterior triangles. They may be unilateral or bilateral. Those that are present at birth often are quite large and diffuse (Fig. 40–5). Those that appear later in life, after 3 years of age, often seem to be more localized and often arise in the anterior triangle.

The usual sign of a cystic hygroma is that of a mass that is soft, doughy, and freely mobile. Larger hygromas are often associated with enlarged lymph nodes, and these may give rise to areas of palpable firmness. Hygromas may be single or multiple, interconnected or separate. Those involving the floor of the mouth and the tongue may cause respiratory obstruction, but hygromas involving only the neck seldom do so. Sudden increase in size may occur with hemorrhage into the cysts or with infection. Although hygromas may fluctuate in size, they seldom disappear spontaneously. The author has seen spontaneous regression once in the case of a premature neonate of 1100-g birthweight born with a large unilateral cervical hygroma; operation was delayed while the patient was growing. When the patient was approximately 1 month of age, the mass became infected, which resulted in a septic course for the patient. As the infection subsided, the cystic hygroma regressed and disappeared. At 3 years of age, the patient still

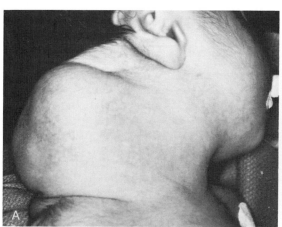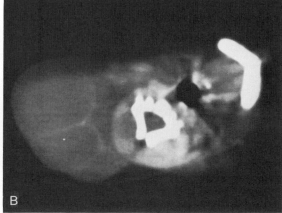

Figure 40–5. *A.* A massive cystic hygroma in the neck of a neonate. This was excised at 5 days of age. *B.* Computed tomography scan of the large cystic hygroma shown in *A.*

showed no sign of recurrent hygroma. Because of low incidence of regression and the tendency to increase in size, surgical excision is the treatment of choice. Neonates with large hygromas (Fig. 40–5*A*) should undergo surgery as soon as they are stable and of sufficient weight. Preoperative evaluation should include either CT (Fig. 40–5*B*) or MRI scan for help in delineating the relationships of the mass.

Cystic hygromas tend to expand along tissue planes and usually involve the adjacent vital structures. Any nerve or vessel in the vicinity may be intimately involved with the tumor. The spinal accessory nerve in particular is almost always involved with hygromas. Hygromas low in the neck are in close relationship to the brachial plexus as well as the subclavian vein and its junction with the internal jugular vein. The marginal mandibular branch of the facial nerve and the hypoglossal nerve are in jeopardy when hygromas involve the submandibular area. The entire facial nerve is endangered if the parotid gland is involved. The carotid arteries, the internal jugular vein, and the vagus nerve may also be involved. Preservation of these structures requires very careful dissection. Excision of a cystic hygroma is tedious and time consuming. Although it is virtually impossible to keep from rupturing some of the smaller peripheral cystic components, an effort should be made to avoid opening into too much of the hygroma because collapse of the cyst walls increases the chances of leaving a portion of the cyst. Excision of large cystic hygromas essentially requires a functional neck dissection with every effort made to preserve important structures. If all of the macroscopically identifiable tissue is dissected away, recurrence is rare, but if portions of obvious hygroma are left behind, the recurrence rate is high. Hygromas lying above the mylohyoid muscle are more difficult to remove and are more likely to recur. With extensive bilateral hygromas, two or more staged excisions may be necessary.

There may be extensive wound drainage. Therefore, a drain is necessary for several days along with a pressure dressing. Antibiotic prophylaxis is advisable.

PRIMARY TUMORS

Many tumors that could be listed in this section are discussed in other chapters. Therefore, this section is devoted to a few primary tumors of the neck that would not be discussed elsewhere.

Sternocleidomastoid Fibroma of Neonates

This is probably the most common lateral neck mass seen in neonates. It is known by several names, such as congenital torticollis, fibromatosis colli, fibrous hematoma of the sternocleidomastoid muscle, or sternocleidomastoid tumor. Sternocleidomastoid fibroma seems to be the best name because histologically the mass consists of atrophic muscle fibers surrounded and entwined by fibrous tissue. It actually is not a tumor but is a swelling or lump within the sternocleidomastoid muscle. The exact cause is unknown, but it is thought to be related to faulty intrauterine positioning or other embryopathies. Up to half of these patients were products of breech or forceps deliveries, which has led to the suggestion of trauma as a contributing factor. Usually the mass is not noticed at birth but is discovered by the parents during the first 4 weeks of the infant's life. It is often mistaken for a tumor beneath the sternocleidomastoid muscle. Careful palpation of both sternocleidomastoid muscles, especially with the patient's neck extended, delineates a mass within the muscle on the affected side. In the majority of cases, the infant's head is turned to the side away from the mass and resists passive rotation toward the affected side.

Sternocleidomastoid fibroma is to be distinguished from a condition referred to as muscular torticollis, which is a tightening of the sternocleidomastoid without a palpable mass. The two lesions are said to be related, however, and it is said that 15% to 20% of patients with sternocleidomastoid fibromas progress to muscular torticollis and develop facial asymmetry. This has not been the author's experience.

The diagnosis is based on clinical recognition by physical examination. Radiographic studies, fine-needle aspiration, or open biopsy usually is not necessary. An actual tumor beneath the sternocleidomastoid muscle must, of course, be ruled out, but this usually can be done by physical examination. The treatment consists of passive cervical stretching by the parent, who is instructed to touch the infant's chin to each of its shoulders five times, three or four times daily. Initially, the infant resists motion toward the affected side. This resistance gradually decreases if the parent persists with the exercises. If this treatment regimen is carried out for the first few months of life, most of the patients recover completely, and no further therapy is necessary.

Lipoma

Ordinary lipomas are composed of mature fat cells containing a large single lipid vacuole that displaces and compresses the nucleus against the cell membrane. Thirteen per cent of all lipomas occur in the head and neck. They are solitary, well-circumscribed, sessile masses that are soft and freely movable; they vary from 2 to 8 cm in diameter. Because of the insulating quality of fat, the skin over a lipoma may feel cooler than the adjacent skin. Although lipomas are more common in patients over 40 years of age, they occasionally occur in children, as shown by the case in Figure 40–6A. The 15-month-old male had a soft, doughy mass in the right supraclavicular area of several months' duration. The clinical diagnosis was cystic hygroma until a CT scan demonstrated that the mass was of the density of fat. The mass was excised (Fig. 40–6B) and found to be a large lipoma. It was in close association with the subclavian artery and vein, which were preserved.

The vast majority of lipomas are benign. If they are cosmetically undesirable or compromise some body function, excision by enucleation with preservation of any adjacent vital structures is the treatment of choice.

Schwannoma

Schwannomas, also called neurilemomas, are relatively rare tumors arising from Schwann's cells that sheath peripheral nerves. They may be found in any portion of the body, but 15% to 45% occur in the head and neck. Schwannomas are slow-growing tumors. The history is usually that of a slowly expanding mass of several months' or years' duration. They are most often found in adults but occasionally are found in children.

The olfactory and optic nerves are extensions of the central nervous system encased by glial cells; they do not give rise to schwannomas. The other cranial nerves, spinal nerves, and most autonomic nerves are sheathed by Schwann's cells. Any of these nerves can be the site of origin of a schwannoma. The acoustic nerve is involved more often than are all other cranial nerves combined. The vagus nerve has been said to be the most commonly involved cranial nerve in the neck. If a schwannoma is situated in the prevertebral area, a dumbbell-shaped tumor arising from a spinal nerve root should be expected. This type of tumor has a larger cervical component connected to a smaller intraspinal component.

Schwannomas are encapsulated tumors usually 1 to 4 cm in diameter but may be as large as 8 cm in the neck. They are quite vascular tumors and often become lobulated

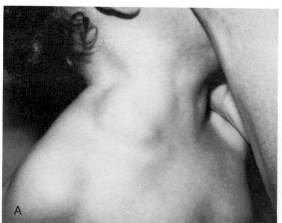
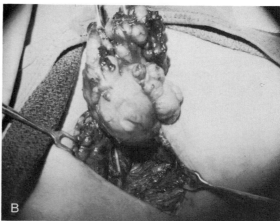

Figure 40–6. *A.* A soft, doughy mass in the supraclavicular area of a 15-month-old child. Originally thought to be a cystic hygroma, it was found to be a lipoma. *B.* The large lobulated lipoma being excised from the supraclavicular area.

as they grow along fascial planes. Their cut surface is gray or tan with irregular yellow areas and cysts. The yellow color is caused by foamy histiocytes and is characteristic of schwannoma. The tissues comprising schwannoma are classified histologically as two types: Antoni-A and Antoni-B. Antoni-A tissue is characterized by compactly arranged spindle cells with long oval nuclei oriented with a long axis parallel to one another. These spindle cell complexes often have nuclei lined up in a row, creating a pattern of palisades. Antoni-B tissue contains spindle cells that are embedded in a loose stroma and form no distinct pattern. Although an entire tumor may be composed of either type of tissue, both types are commonly intermixed. Benign schwannomas seldom if ever undergo malignant change. The rare malignant variety is thought to be malignant from the beginning.

The treatment is surgical excision. Preoperative evaluation may include fine-needle aspiration and CT or MRI scan. Although schwannomas often have lobules extending along fascial planes, they usually can be enucleated surgically with little chance of recurrence. Every effort should be made to preserve important nerves and other structures related to benign schwannomas in the neck. The nerve of origin can be identified in approximately one fourth of cervical schwannomas.

Pilomatrixoma

Pilomatrixoma, also known as calcifying epithelioma of Malherbe, is a benign tumor of hair cell origin. It is an unusual but not particularly rare tumor. Approximately 50% of pilomatrixomas occur in the head and neck. These tumors initially appear as small, firm nodules in the dermis or subcutaneous tissue. At this stage, they may be mistaken for cysts or pimples. They are usually well circumscribed, but with growth they may become multilobular. They often feel stony hard to palpation. In the neck, as they enlarge, pilomatrixomas may be mistaken for lymph nodes, cysts, calcified hematomas, or calcified hemangiomas. In the cheek posteriorly, which is a common location, they may be mistaken for a parotid gland tumor. When removed, the tumor appears grossly to be a calcified mass with a friable granular surface. These tumors may cease to grow while still small or may grow to diameters of up to 15 cm. Occasionally the skin overlying the tumor ruptures, which results in extrusion of calcific material. Pilomatrixomas are considered to be benign tumors, but there have been reports of giant pilomatrixomas with locally aggressive behavior.

The tumor is composed histologically of irregularly shaped islands of epithelial cells surrounded by dense fibrous tissue. Two types of cells make up the epithelial islands: basophilic cells and shadow cells. The basophilic cells have round or elongated, deeply basophilic nuclei with scanty cytoplasm and indistinct cell borders and are arranged predominantly in the periphery of the islands. Inward from the basophilic cells is a transitional zone in which the cells show a gradual loss of their nuclei. On the central side of the transitional zone are the shadow cells, which have distinct borders and a central unstained area as a shadow of the lost nucleus. Calcium deposits are found in approximately 75% of the tumors, and ossification is found in 15% to 20%.

The diagnosis is based on clinical suspicion and physical examination. The treatment is surgical excision. Pilomatrixomas usually can be enucleated from the subcutaneous area easily. Often a 2- to 4-mm ellipse of skin involved with the tumor has to be removed. Recurrence after excision is rare.

INFECTIONS

Deep Fascial Space Infections

A detailed anatomic description of the cervical fascia and its spaces is beyond the scope of this chapter, but a brief description is necessary before consideration of the fascial space infections. All of the structures of the neck are enclosed in connective tissue. The fascial planes are created by condensation of this connective tissue into sheets between adjacent structures. The cervical fascia consists of a superficial fascia and a deep fascia. The superficial fascia is a loose layer that encloses the platysma muscle and the muscles of facial expression and extends inferiorly to the thorax and axilla. The deep fascia is divided into three layers: a superficial or investing layer, a middle layer, and a deep layer. The superficial layer attaches inferiorly to the clavicle and scapula, completely encircles the neck, and attaches to the spines of the vertebrae posteriorly. It envelops two muscles, the sternocleidomastoid and trapezius; two glands, the submandibular and parotid; and two spaces, the suprasternal space of Burns and the space of the posterior triangle. Superiorly, it attaches to the body of the hyoid bone and then ascends to the mandible. It envelops the posterior mandible and splits with the outer layer, which extends over the masseter muscle, zygoma, and temporalis muscle to attach superiorly on a line from the orbital margin to the superior nuchal line of the occiput.

The middle layer of the deep cervical fascia, also called the pretracheal or visceral fascia, envelops the strap muscles, the thyroid gland, the larynx, the trachea, and the esophagus. Anteriorly, its superior extent is its attachment to the hyoid bone; posteriorly, it attaches to the skull base behind the esophagus and pharyngeal constrictor muscles. The deep layer extends around the deep muscular compartment of the neck and the spinal column. Anterior to the spinal column, the deep layer consists of two divisions: the alar and prevertebral layers. The alar layer is anterior to the prevertebral layer and forms the posterior wall of the retropharyngeal or retrovisceral space. It fuses with the middle layer of the deep cervical fascia inferiorly at the level of the first or second thoracic vertebra, thus limiting the inferior extent of the retropharyngeal space. The prevertebral layer of the deep cervical fascia extends from the base of the skull to the coccyx.

The space between the alar and prevertebral layers represents a potential route for spread of infection from the retropharyngeal space into the posterior mediastinum. It is therefore referred to as the "danger space." The carotid sheath enclosing the carotid arteries, the internal jugular vein, and the vagus nerve is derived from all three layers of the deep cervical fascia. It extends from the base of the skull into the chest and also has been considered to be a potential route for spread of infection from the neck to the mediastinum.

The hyoid bone, because of its multiple fascial and muscular attachments, is considered to be the most important structure in the neck in limiting spread of infection. Potential spaces are usually described in relation to the hyoid as suprahyoid, infrahyoid, and those involving the entire length of the neck. Fascial spaces simply consist of potential spaces between the fascial planes. Infections spread along the lines of least resistance, and infection in any one space can spread to involve other spaces. Multiple potential spaces and the symptoms of infections in them have been described. No attempt is made here to discuss infection in all of the spaces. Only those of most clinical significance in the neck are discussed.

Suprahyoid Spaces

Pharyngomaxillary Space

Also called lateral pharyngeal or parapharyngeal space, this is probably the most significant space from a clinical standpoint. It is cone shaped, and its base is located at the base of the skull and its apex at the hyoid bone. Its medial boundary is the lateral pharyngeal wall. Its lateral border is formed by the mandible, the internal pterygoid muscle, and the parotid gland. It is divided into anterior and posterior compartments by the styloid process and its muscles. The anterior portion is in close relationship to the tonsillar fossa medially. The posterior portion contains the carotid sheath and cranial nerves IX to XII. This space communicates inferiorly with the submandibular space and posteriorly with the retropharyngeal space. The sources of infection in this space are most commonly the pharynx, the tonsils and adenoids, the teeth, the parotid gland, and the lymph nodes draining the nose and pharynx.

Submandibular Space

This is the anterior element of the peripharyngeal spaces above the hyoid. It is divided by the mylohyoid muscle into a sublingual space between the mylohyoid and the mucosa of the floor of the mouth and a submaxillary (or submylohyoid) component. The submaxillary space is in continuity with the sublingual space along the posterior edge of the mylohyoid muscle. The submaxillary space may be further divided into a central submental space and a lateral submaxillary space. Most of the infections of this space are of dental origin. This is the site of Ludwig's angina.

Infrahyoid Spaces

Anterior Visceral (Pretracheal) Space

This space is encompassed by the middle or visceral layer of the deep cervical fascia and contains the thyroid gland, the trachea, and the esophagus. It communicates with the retropharyngeal, or posterior visceral, space. Infections in this space usually result from thyroiditis or perforation of the anterior cervical esophagus. Such infection can be serious because of the proximity of this space to the superior mediastinum.

Spaces Spanning the Neck

Retropharyngeal (Posterior Visceral) Space

This space, behind the pharynx and upper esophagus, is the potential space between the posterior visceral fascia and alar fascia. It extends from the base of the skull to the level of T1 to T2, where the visceral and alar fascial layers fuse. The typical infection in this space is a retropharyngeal abscess. This is more prevalent in infants and children under 4 years of age and results from lymphatic drainage from the nose and the nasopharynx. The retropharyngeal lymph nodes that result in abscess formation appear to atrophy after approximately 4 years of age.

Visceral Vascular Space (Carotid Sheath)

The potential space within the carotid sheath may become involved in infection between any of the three layers of deep fascia or from infected lymph nodes. It is most commonly infected secondarily to pharyngomaxillary space infection. Another etiologic factor, relatively prevalent in adult patients at the author's medical center, is intravenous drug use by way of the internal jugular vein. Although this space is considered to be a potential avenue for spread of infection to the mediastinum, the sheath has a compact arrangement, and infections within it usually remain localized. Thrombosis of the internal jugular vein is a relatively frequent occurrence with infections in this space, especially if the source of the infection is intravenous drug abuse. Erosion of the carotid artery with hemorrhage is a rare complication.

Diagnosis and Management

Pain and limitation of jaw or neck motion are present in virtually all deep neck infections. Diffuse swelling, often with pitting edema, is usually present with infections of every fascial compartment. Gross fluctuance is seldom noted because of the deep location of the abscess. The patients usually are febrile, and their blood counts reveal a leukocytosis. Retropharyngeal abscess often is associated with stridorous breathing, dysphagia, and a muffled voice; examination of the pharynx reveals a unilateral bulging of the posterior pharynx. (A midline bulging is suggestive of a prevertebral abscess secondary to cervical vertebral osteomyelitis, possibly tuberculous in origin.) Examination of the pharyngomaxillary space abscess reveals fullness in the retromandibular region and medial displacement of the lateral pharyngeal wall and tonsil.

Infection of the submandibular space results in dysphagia and a muffled voice secondary to tongue immobility. The floor of the mouth is inflamed and edematous. The tongue is pushed upward and backward until airway obstruction develops. Once the infection penetrates the mylohyoid muscle, full-blown Ludwig's angina presents with a "woody" hardness of the submental and submandibular areas.

CT scan is the best radiologic technique for evaluating deep neck infections for the presence of an abscess. Ultrasonography may be of value in some instances, but CT is preferable. Plain lateral neck radiographs may be helpful in evaluating suspected retropharyngeal abscesses but often are difficult to interpret.

All patients with deep neck infections should be hospitalized and placed on intravenous antibiotic therapy that covers the most likely bacterial etiologic agents: *Staphylococcus aureus*, group A beta-hemolytic *Streptococcus*, and a mixture of oral flora, including anaerobic organisms. A mixture of aerobic and anaerobic bacteria may produce an especially virulent type of infection associated with severe systemic toxic effects. This type of infection has been referred to by terms such as necrotizing fasciitis and synergistic necrotizing cellulitis. Oxacillin and penicillin G or ampicillin, often with the addition of gentamicin, clindamycin, or a cephalosporin, are the usual choices for antibiotic coverage. The clinical course must be followed closely. Significant clinical impression of an abscess, demonstration of an abscess by CT scan, or failure of the patient to improve after 24 hours of high-dosage intravenous antibiotic therapy is indication for incision and drainage. This can be done under local or general anesthesia according to the preference of the surgeon for the particular situation. In Ludwig's angina and in retropharyngeal abscess, airway compromise may present problems for general anesthesia. In Ludwig's angina, tracheotomy under local anesthesia may be necessary before general anesthesia is begun. In retropharyngeal abscess, careful and skillful intubation is usually successful in establishing a safe airway before incision and drainage.

Pharyngomaxillary space infections can be approached through an incision beneath the angle of the jaw. Blunt dissection along the medial border of the internal pterygoid process toward the styloid process usually locates the pus. Ludwig's angina is approached through a transverse incision in the submental area extending to one or both lateral submandibular areas if necessary. Blunt dissection opens into the area of cellulitis or phlegmon; usually there is little or no frank pus in this condition. The dissection must extend through the mylohyoid muscle. The mucous membrane of the floor of the mouth may or may not need to be opened, depending on the degree of tension. The anterior visceral space is drained by way of a transverse incision over the area of apparently greatest involvement. Retropharyngeal abscess can be drained adequately through a transoral approach. If it is complicated by extension to other spaces, drainage is best done from an external approach, alone or combined with intraoral drainage.

CERVICAL ADENITIS AND ABSCESS FORMATION

Swelling of lymph nodes in the neck is a relatively common occurrence, especially in young children, as a result of previous nose and throat infections or of infections of the scalp or skin. Once the nodes have been infected, the enlargement may persist for weeks or months. Viral infections of the upper respiratory tract are probably the most common causes of cervical lymphadenopathy. Among the most frequent viral etiologic agents are adenovirus, rhinovirus, enterovirus, and Epstein-Barr virus (infectious mononucleosis). Cervical lymphadenopathy may also develop as a manifestation of acquired immunodeficiency syndrome (AIDS).

Bacterial cervical adenitis, either primary or secondary to viral infection, is relatively common in children aged 5 years or younger, especially between 6 and 12 months of age. This most commonly develops in the submandibular or upper anterior cervical area as a swelling that progresses over several days' duration with or without fever, malaise, or other symptoms of systemic toxic effects. Usually the mass is tender to palpation, and as the confluent nodes break down to form an abscess, the overlying skin becomes reddened and the mass becomes fluctuant. Skin redness and palpable fluctuance vary, depending on the depth of the abscess beneath the skin; the deeper abscesses may exhibit neither redness nor fluctuance (Fig. 40–7). Often no definite source of the infection can be found, but a large number of patients have a history of a recent upper respiratory infection. Dental sources of infection, common in adults, are infrequent in young children. Cervical adenitis and abscesses seem to occur more frequently in children with poor nutrition and lower hemogloblin levels.

Staphylococcus aureus and group A beta-hemolytic streptococci are the most frequently isolated bacteria in cervical abscesses of children. Anaerobic organisms, which are commonly isolated from abscesses of dental origin, are an infrequent etiologic factor in young children. *Haemophilus influenzae* seems to be a very rare pathogen for cervical abscesses in spite of its prevalence in tonsillar cultures as well as in ear and sinus infections.

Abscesses arising from cervical adenitis

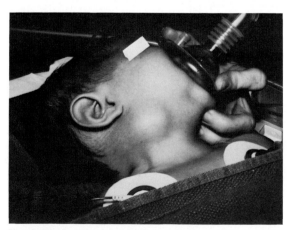

Figure 40–7. This cervical adenitis abscess was relatively firm and not fluctuant at the time of incision and drainage, but yielded 15 mL of pus from which *S. aureus* was cultured.

are sometimes referred to as superficial abscesses for distinguishing them from the deep fascial space infections discussed in the previous section. Some of these abscesses, however, extend quite deeply into the neck.

Diagnosis and Management

Occasional patients with mild bacterial cervical adenitis can be managed as outpatients with oral antibiotics; however, in the author's experience most patients with cervical abscesses require intravenous antibiotic therapy. Adequate antibiotic blood levels for abscess treatment and localization of the infection simply cannot be obtained with oral therapy. Because *Staphylococcus aureus* and group A streptococci are the most common pathogens, an antistaphylococcal penicillin such as oxacillin seems to be the logical first-line antibiotic for treatment. If anaerobic involvement is suspected, an antibiotic effective against anaerobes should be added. CT scan and ultrasonography are not as essential in management of cervical adenitis abscesses as they are with the deep neck infections discussed earlier. Especially in children, the diagnosis of the abscess and its location can usually be determined by physical examination alone. CT or ultrasonography is used by the author in only those patients with deeper infections in which the presence and location of an abscess are in doubt.

An occasional patient with what appears to be early abscess formation recovers with appropriate intravenous antibiotic therapy alone. Most cervical abscesses, however, require drainage. Needle aspiration is less invasive than is incision and drainage and may be effective in some smaller abscesses. On the other hand, needle aspiration may have to be repeated several times; even then, incision and drainage may ultimately be required. The author has found surgical incision and drainage under local or general anesthesia, depending on the situation, to be the most effective treatment for established abscesses. Depending on the severity of the abscess, the drain can usually be removed in 2 to 3 days, and the patient can be discharged on oral antibiotic therapy shortly thereafter.

Airway obstruction, a problem in some of the fascial space infections, is seldom a problem in patients with abscesses arising from cervical adenitis. The possibility of airway obstruction, however, must always be considered in the larger abscesses.

MYCOBACTERIAL CERVICAL ADENITIS

Mycobacteria are being recognized more and more frequently as etiologic agents in cervical adenitis, especially in children. Cervical adenitis may be caused by *Mycobacterium tuberculosis* or by one of the so-called atypical mycobacteria. In areas in which pulmonary tuberculosis is prevalent, such as the Los Angeles area, *M. tuberculosis* is a relatively frequent cause of cervical adenitis. In areas in which *M. tuberculosis* infections are not prevalent, most mycobacterial cervical adenitis is caused by atypical organisms. In a series of 85 pediatric patients with mycobacterial cervical adenitis managed at the Los Angeles County–University of Southern California Medical Center, 36% of those with positive cultures grew either *M. tuberculosis* or *M. bovis*. Sixty-four per cent of cultures grew atypical mycobacteria, and 70% of those were *M. avium-intracellulare*.

Atypical infections usually manifest as unilateral involvement of nodes in the submandibular or mandibular areas, whereas *M. tuberculosis* adenitis tends to be more diffuse in the anterosuperior cervical region, or even the supraclavicular area, and may have bilateral involvement. There are exceptions, however. *M. tuberculosis* infection may manifest as a localized submandibular adenitis, whereas an occasional atypical infection may have more diffuse involvement. Chest radiographs in patients with *M. tuberculosis* adenitis may reveal hilar adenopathy or pulmonary infiltrate, but the films can appear normal. In the natural history of the disease with either etiologic process, the nodes initially are painless, firm, discrete, and nontender. With progression of the disease, the nodes become matted together and adherent to the overlying skin, which becomes discolored (Fig. 40–8) and eventually breaks down to form draining fistulas.

Mycobacterial causes should be suspected when firm, painless lymph nodes progressively enlarge over a period of 2 to 3 weeks or longer, especially if they develop discoloration of overlying skin. A tuberculin skin test (purified protein derivative, or PPD) should be applied. The reactivity rate is ap-

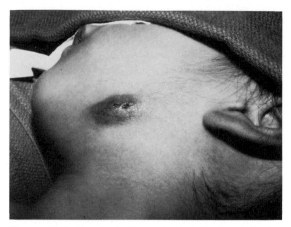

Figure 40–8. An atypical mycobacterial submandibular adenitis with skin involvement and fistula formation.

proximately 97% for *M. tuberculosis* infection and 90% for atypical mycobacterial infection. The reaction size is usually greater than 15 mm with *M. tuberculosis* and 5 to 15 mm with atypical infection. In the presence of signs and symptoms of mycobacterial infection, a PPD reaction of greater than 5 mm is considered to be significant. A chest radiograph should also be obtained. Fine-needle aspiration can be done for the purpose of obtaining smear and culture samples as well as for cytopathologic evaluation. Smears for acid-fast bacilli often are negative in mycobacterial adenitis. Positive smears, therefore, are significant, but negative ones are not. The final results of mycobacterial cultures usually require a minimum of 6 weeks. If neoplastic disease is suspected, open biopsy should be performed without waiting for culture results. On the other hand, children less than 5 years of age with localized cervical adenitis and a positive PPD reaction have a negligible risk for malignant disease.

The otolaryngology literature has emphasized that it is important to differentiate *M. tuberculosis* from atypical infections because the treatment is different; medical therapy is indicated for the former, whereas surgical excision is indicated for the latter. Although that is generally true, it is not that simple. In the author's experience, one cannot always differentiate *M. tuberculosis* and atypical mycobacterial adenitis on initial evaluation, and one must wait several weeks for the culture results. Although most atypical mycobacteria demonstrate in vitro resistance to antituberculosis drugs, some respond to various in vivo regimens, apparently because of synergism of the drugs. Therefore, it is the author's policy in cooperation with the pediatric pulmonology service to institute antituberculous chemotherapy for all patients initially by the regimen recommended in the Joint Statement of the American Thoracic Society and the Centers for Disease Control (1986); that is, a 2-month course of isoniazid, rifampin, and pyrazinamide followed by 4 months of isoniazid and rifampin, with ethambutol included in the initial phase if isoniazid resistance is suspected.

The treatment regimen may be continued longer than 6 months in certain situations. It may also be discontinued earlier than 6 months if the clinical course and culture results indicate an atypical etiologic agent resistant to chemotherapy. The indications for early surgical intervention are suspicion of malignancy or the presence of an abscess that requires drainage. Later surgical intervention may be undertaken for one or more of the following reasons: drainage or excision of an abscess, prevention of skin breakdown, and excision of persistent or enlarging nodes or of draining fistulas. Complete excision of the involved tissues is the preferred surgical approach, but adjacent normal structures should be preserved. In some cases, the large amount of skin involvement or proximity to the marginal mandibular branch of the facial nerve makes complete excision difficult to perform. In these cases, an alternative approach is removal of the purulent fluid and necrotic tissue by suction and curettage through an incision in adjacent normal skin.

CAT-SCRATCH DISEASE

Cat-scratch disease is a relatively common cause of cervical adenopathy that may develop into what can be mistaken for a bacterial or mycobacterial abscess. The etiologic agent is now thought to be a delicate, small, pleomorphic gram-negative bacillus that has been identified within damaged blood vessels and microabscesses of nodes excised from patients with cat-scratch disease. These bacilli are seen with the Warthin-Starry silver impregnation stain. To the author's knowledge, this bacillus has not yet been grown in culture. The typical clinical picture of this condition is that of a scratch from a healthy cat, with an erythematous skin reaction developing at the scratch site. This reaction subsides after several days. Two to 6 weeks after the scratch, one or more regional lymph nodes begin to swell. The nodes are usually tender and may become quite large.

The presumptive diagnosis is made from a history of contact with cats, a positive cat-scratch antigen skin test, a negative PPD reaction, and negative cytologic test results or culture from aspirated material. A specific effective antibiotic for therapy of cat-scratch disease is unknown, and antibiotic treatment usually is ineffective. With the larger inflamed nodes, some type of antibiotic therapy seems to be necessary. Treatment as for bacterial cervical adenitis is reasonable because staphylococcal infection may coexist with cat-scratch disease. If the mass is fluctuant, the temptation is to perform incision and drainage. However, this may result in little improvement and probably will result in persistent drainage from the incision site. Therefore, needle aspiration is preferred to incision and drainage in cat-scratch disease. If the involved nodes can be removed completely, surgical excision may relieve the symptoms. Incomplete excision, on the other hand, often results in poor healing and possible fistula formation. Cat-scratch disease is a benign, self-limiting disease. Unless the nodes are large or causing some type of disability, symptomatic therapy and observation may be all that is necessary.

SUGGESTED READINGS

Cysts

Brock ME, Smith RJH, Parey SE, et al: Lymphangioma; an otolaryngologic perspective. Int J Pediatr Otolaryngol 14:133–140, 1987.

Hawkins DB, Jacobson BE, Klatt EC: Cysts of the thyroglossal duct. Laryngoscope 92:1254–1258, 1982.

Hoffman MA, Schuster SR: Thyroglossal duct remnants in infants and children: reevaluation of histopathology and methods for resection. Ann Otol Rhinol Laryngol 97:483–486, 1988.

Kennedy TL: Cystic hygroma-lymphangioma: a rare and still unclear entity. Laryngoscope 99(Suppl):1–10, 1989.

Landing BH, Farber S: Tumors of the cardiovascular system. In Atlas of Tumor Pathology (section III, fasc 7). Washington, DC: Armed Forces Institute of Pathology, 1956.

Langman J: Medical Embryology, 4th ed (pp 268–282). Baltimore: Williams & Wilkins, 1981.

McNicholl MP, Hawkins DB, England K, et al: Papillary carcinoma arising in a thyroglossal duct cyst. Otolaryngol Head Neck Surg 99:50–54, 1988.

Mulliken JB, Young AE: Vascular Birthmarks; Hemangiomas and Malformations (pp 32–35, 221–222). Philadelphia: WB Saunders, 1988.

Noyek AM, Friedberg J: Thyroglossal duct and ectopic thyroid disorders. Otolaryngol Clin North Am 14:187–201, 1981.

Ravitch MM, Rush BF: Cystic hygroma. In Welch KJ, et al (eds): Pediatric Surgery, 4th ed (pp 533–539). Chicago: Yearbook Medical Publishers, 1986.

Sistrunk WE: Technique of removal of cysts and sinuses of the thyroglossal duct. Surg Gynecol Obstet 46:109–112, 1928.

Soper RT, Pringle KC: Cysts and sinuses of the neck. In Welch KJ, et al (eds): Pediatric Surgery 4th ed (pp 539–552). Chicago: Yearbook Medical Publishers, 1986.

Sternocleidomastoid Fibroma

Jones PG: Torticollis. In Welch KJ, et al (eds): Pediatric Surgery, 4th ed (pp 552–556). Chicago: Yearbook Medical Publishers, 1986.

Tom LWC, Handler SD, Wetmore RF, Potsic WP: The sternocleidomastoid tumor of infancy. Int J Pediatr Otolaryngol 13:245–255, 1987.

Barnes L: Surgical Pathology of the Head and Neck (pp 775–777). New York: Marcel Dekker, 1985.

Lipoma

Barnes L: Surgical Pathology of the Head and Neck (pp 747–753). New York: Marcel Dekker, 1985.

Schwannoma

Hawkins DB, Luxford WM: Schwannomas of the head and neck in children. Laryngoscope 90:1921–1926, 1980.

Maniglia AJ: Schwannomas of the parapharyngeal space and jugular foramen. Laryngoscope 89:1405–1413, 1979.

Pilomatrixoma

Hawkins DB, Chen WT: Pilomatrixoma of the head and neck in children. Int J Pediatr Otolaryngol 8:215–223, 1985.

Stone GE, Donegan JO, Simpson WA: Pilomatrixoma: calcifying epithelioma of Malherbe. Otolaryngol Head Neck Surg 102:751–754, 1990.

Infections

Beck HJ, Salassa JR, McCaffrey TV, et al: Life-threatening soft-tissue infections of the neck. Laryngoscope 94:354–361, 1984.

Brook I: Microbiology of abscesses of the head and neck in children. Ann Otol Rhinol Laryngol 96:429–433, 1987.

Cat-Scratch Disease. Report of the Committee on Infectious Diseases, American Academy of Pediatrics, 21st ed (pp 148–149), 1988.

Dodds B, Maniglia AJ: Peritonsillar and neck abscesses in the pediatric age group. Laryngoscope 98:956–959, 1988.

Hawkins DB, Austin JR: Abscesses of the neck in infants and young children. Ann Otol Rhinol Laryngol 100:361–365, 1991.

Levitt GW: Cervical fascia and deep neck infections. Otolaryngol Clin North Am 9:703–716, 1976.

Stanievich JF: Cervical adenopathy. In Bluestone CD, Stool SE (eds): Pediatric Otolaryngology, 2nd ed (pp 1317–1327). Philadelphia: WB Saunders, 1990.

Tom M, Rice DH: Presentation and management of neck abscesses. Laryngoscope 98:877–880, 1988.

caused by motor vehicle injuries has been dramatically reduced by the widespread use of shoulder harness type restraints and reduced–speed-limit laws, and the growing acceptance of air safety bags should reduce the incidence even further. Normally the caudal projection of the mandible affords bony protection from anterior blows to the region of the larynx. Without shoulder harness restraints, the driver can be thrust forward with the neck in a hyperextended fashion; thus the protection of the mandible is eliminated. The neck is then vulnerable to a direct anterior crushing effect from the steering wheel or the dashboard and is compressed between these objects and the bony cervical vertebrae (Fig. 41–1). These injuries

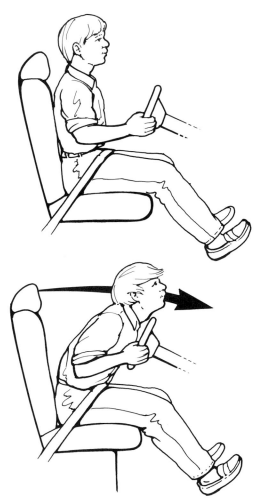

Figure 41–1. With lap belt and without shoulder harness, the neck is extended, which removes the protection that the mandible affords the neck. The larynx is crushed between the steering wheel and the cervical spine.

may range from minor to severe, depending on the speed at impact. Laryngeal injuries may be severe with only minimal damage to the overlying skin. Associated injuries, especially cervical spine and thoracic injuries, are common. Clothesline injuries result when the rider of an unprotected vehicle such as a motorcycle, a snowmobile, or a bicycle strikes a horizontal stationary object such as a clothesline or a tree limb. These injuries direct tremendous forces over a small area and often cause death as a result of massive laryngeal injury, laryngotracheal separation, and resultant loss of airway. The overlying skin usually has marked evidence of trauma, and in severe injury, a laryngocutaneous fistula may be present. Associated trauma is not as common in areas beyond the impact region, although cervical spine injury is frequent. Securing the airway in these injuries is often difficult because of the extent of injury; however, failure to secure the airway shortly after the injury may lead to asphyxiation and death.

Manual strangulation injuries apply low-velocity forces over the laryngeal cartilaginous framework and commonly cause fractures within the larynx without laceration of the overlying mucosa. These injuries include choking by hand or with a blunt object. Attempted hangings with a cloth rope are also typical causes of this type of injury. The overlying skin usually shows ecchymosis or abrasions characteristic of the mechanism used for the attempted hanging. Associated cervical spine injuries are occasionally present. On initial examination, the injury may appear minimal from laryngoscopic examination; however, resultant edema of the mucous membrane hours after presentation may lead to loss of airway and death by asphyxiation.

The severity of penetrating trauma to the larynx is directly related to the energy imparted to the tissue from the penetrating object. High-velocity weapons such as hunting rifles and military weapons may cause massive tissue destruction radiating out from the path of the projectile (Fig. 41–2). Low-velocity weapons, as are commonly used in personal assaults, tend to lack this blast effect. Knife wounds carry the least velocity, and only tissues located directly along the path of penetration are usually damaged.

Inhalation of supraheated air may cause laryngeal mucosal injury. Upon inhalation of supraheated air, a reflex closure of the glottis

Figure 41–2. Penetrating injuries from high-velocity weapons. Note that tissue damage extends beyond the zone of obvious necrosis.

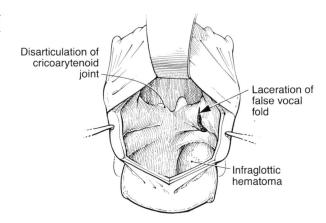

Disarticulation of cricoarytenoid joint

Laceration of false vocal fold

Infraglottic hematoma

occurs which prevents inspiration distal to the level of the larynx. This reflex closure commonly spares the trachea, the bronchi, and the lungs and decreases the amount of air flow and thus injury to the larynx. However, laryngeal injury may still occur, especially in instances involving steam, which has an increased capacity to carry thermal energy, or in cases in which inhalation injury occurs in a closed space. Physical examination is usually most remarkable for burns over other parts of the body. Laryngoscopic and oral cavity examination may reveal erythema in thermal injury only, or carbon flakes may be noted in the instance of smoke inhalation. A dangerous lack of upper airway symptoms is common in a large majority of these patients on initial arrival at the emergency room. However, with the large amount of fluid resuscitation that is often necessary to prevent cardiovascular collapse in the burn patient, any injury to the laryngeal mucosa is rapidly followed by marked edema and possible loss of airway. Treatment, therefore, relies on securing the airway early via endotracheal intubations before laryngeal edema develops if any suspicion of inhalation injury exists. If the patient requires prolonged intubation, the airway is converted early to a formal tracheostomy in order to prevent further mucosal injury to the glottis and subglottis from the endotracheal tube.

Ingestion of caustic substances may cause laryngeal injuries as well as the more common injuries to the oral cavity, the hypopharynx, and the esophageal mucosa. This primarily occurs in the pediatric age group as a result of accidental ingestion of household products. In adults, it usually is the result of an attempted suicide, and the agent is commonly lye or hydrocarbon products. Mucosal injury to the larynx may result from contact with swallowing but is more often the result of contact during regurgitation. Treatments consist of mist humidification and elevation of the head of the bed. Tracheostomy may be necessary to secure the airway and is preferred over orotracheal intubation for prevention of further mucosal injury.

Of special consideration is the pediatric larynx. Situated higher in the neck than the adult larynx, it is afforded greater protection by the mandible from anterior injury. In addition, fractures are less common because of the greater elasticity of the cartilaginous framework. Soft tissue damage is more likely in the pediatric larynx because of the loose attachment of the overlying mucous membrane and the lack of fibrous tissue support. Also, because the area of a circle is determined by the square of the radius of the circle, the cross-sectional area in relation to the size of the larynx is decreased in the pediatric airway, in comparison with the adult airway. This combination of decreased cross-sectional area and increased soft tissue injury can lead to rapid loss of airway, which often may be unappreciated by the medical personnel attending the pediatric patient because of the increased elasticity of the larynx and the resultant lack of fractures.

Diagnosis

The majority of laryngeal injuries are never diagnosed because they often lead to rapid death at the scene of the injury or are so minor as to escape the attention of the attending personnel. In order to diagnose these injuries, therefore, a high index of suspicion must be maintained for all patients with anterior neck trauma. Signs and symptoms of laryngeal dysfunction caused by trauma are all aberrations of laryngeal function: respiration, phonation, and prevention of aspiration.

Alteration in respiration is the most immediately lethal dysfunction of the larynx secondary to trauma. Respiration may be completely and immediately prevented by collapse or near collapse of the laryngeal framework or from cricotracheal separation. More often, the clinician notes a progressive dysfunction of respiration as the laryngeal mucosa becomes progressively edematous after injury. The clinical manifestations of interference of respiration are tachypnea, air hunger, and stridor. Pallor, especially noted in the nail beds and circumoral area, may be present if significant hemoglobin desaturation exists.

If the airway obstruction is slowly progressive, examination of arterial blood gases may reveal a rise in carbon dioxide and a concomitant decrease in pH levels, followed eventually by a fall in arterial oxygen levels. The patient may present clinically in a calm manner, progressing to an agitated state and then to a sense of impending death as the airway obstruction increases. Use of accessory respiratory muscles is common, and the patient may prefer a sitting to a supine position. All of the findings indicate impending loss of airway and mandate immediate steps to secure a safe airway before other diagnostic or therapeutic procedures.

Phonation is determined by the air flow through the lumen of the airway and by stiffness, mobility, and mass of the vocal folds. Edema or hematoma of the vocal folds increases the mass of the vocal folds and thereby alters voice pitch. Injury to the innervation of the larynx may alter phonation by recurrent nerve injury and subsequent vocal fold paralysis or superior laryngeal nerve trauma, giving rise to loss of cricothyroid muscle function with a subsequent change in stiffness of the vocal fold. Cricoarytenoid dislocation or any fracture that decreases vocal fold mobility causes a change in voice. Finally, any obstruction of the airway leads to an alteration of the air flow pattern through the larynx and may manifest as a change in voice.

Although it usually is not of immediate importance or readily obvious in the emergency room setting, laryngeal trauma may cause aspiration. This may result from decreased vocal fold mobility caused by denervation, disarticulation, or framework disruption and the resultant failure of proper vocal fold apposition.

Once an airway has been established, an orderly, complete physical examination is mandatory. In the neck, indications of a vascular injury, such as bruits or an expanding hematoma, should be sought. Deformity of the thyroid or cricoid cartilages and direct exposure of damaged cartilage are the most obvious signs of laryngeal injury. Tenderness on palpation, although not specific for significant injury, is almost always present. Stridor, when present, is usually inspiratory in cases of supraglottic airway obstruction, as occurs with hematomas or soft tissue edema, and expiratory with lower airway obstruction. Examination of the laryngeal mucosa, evaluation of the function of the vocal folds, and search for hematomas or other soft tissue injury may be performed with a direct fiberoptic laryngoscope. If the patient is undergoing surgery for associated injuries, this may be done in the operating room with the use of a direct laryngoscope.

Although history and physical examination remain the mainstay of the diagnostic work-up for laryngeal trauma, CT scanning is useful in specific cases in which the need for operative intervention is undetermined. CT scanning is of limited benefit in cases in which open exploration of the neck is already indicated either for laryngeal trauma, such as exposed cartilage, or for associated injuries, such as an expanding hematoma. In these instances, direct visualization at time of surgery through direct laryngoscopy and surgical exposure of the larynx should be adequate for determining the extent of laryngeal damage. However, if the patient presents with mild signs or symptoms of laryngeal injury, such as hoarseness, or should direct fiberoptic laryngoscopy reveal evidence of injury without absolute indication for surgical repair, such as a hematoma of the true vocal fold, then CT scanning of the larynx is indicated to further define the integrity of the laryngeal framework. CT scanning is also useful as a noninvasive means of examining areas not well seen by direct fiberoptic examination, such as the subglottic area, the anterior commissure, and the cricoid cartilage. The primary usefulness of CT scanning is in identifying patients who may be managed without surgical intervention.

Management

The initial management of the patient with laryngeal injury is securing the airway. Many patients with laryngeal injuries present without airway embarrassment. In those who do present with airway compromise, either endotracheal intubation or tracheotomy must be performed. Although it is advocated by some, orotracheal intubation may cause iatrogenic injury to the larynx and precipitate loss of airway, converting the situation from semiemergent to an emergency. Those patients who by direct fiberoptic laryngoscopy and CT examination are shown to have minimal laryngeal injuries may undergo endotracheal intubation. Otherwise, the most conservative method of establishing the airway is by means of local tracheotomy while the patient is awake.

Patients with nondisplaced thyroid cartilage fractures, mild edema, hematomas with normal overlying mucosa, and small mucosal lacerations without exposed cartilage not involving the anterior commissure may be treated with nonsurgical medical management. This consists of elevation of the head of the bed, a cool-mist face mask, voice rest, and observation for at least 24 hours. The efficacy of steroids is unproved but they may be of benefit if administered immediately after the injury.

Operative Intervention

Those patients who by physical examination and CT assessment have injuries that are not likely to resolve spontaneously without significant functional deficit are taken to the operating room for further assessment and possible surgical intervention. Although some authors recommend waiting several days for the edema to subside so that identification is improved and repair of mucosal lacerations is made easier, immediate surgical intervention is preferred to allow primary closure, decreased infection and granulation, and therefore less scarring and better post-injury function. Once the patient is in the operating room, a tracheotomy is performed. Endoscopy is then performed to further assess the extent of the injuries. Rigid esophagoscopy and bronchoscopy are also per-

formed to rule out associated hypopharyngeal, subglottic, and bronchial tree injuries because these areas are not well seen with direct fiberoptic examination. Finally, direct laryngoscopy is performed to examine the larynx. Care should be taken at this time to palpate the arytenoid cartilages in an effort to detect limitation of normal range of motion.

Of special consideration is the securing of an airway in the pediatric patient. Local tracheotomy is difficult in pediatric patients when they are awake. Should tracheotomy be necessary, rigid bronchoscopy is performed first to secure the airway and induce anesthesia. The tracheotomy may then be performed over the bronchoscope.

After completion of endoscopy, the information found along with the CT scan allows the surgeon to decide whether surgical exploration is warranted. If only small mucosal lacerations without exposed cartilage, edema, and small hematomas are found at endoscopy, and if CT scans reveal no displaced fractures, then the patient will probably do well with conservative management. If vocal fold impairment, large mucosal tears, exposed cartilage, or displaced fractures are present, surgical exploration is indicated.

Surgical exploration is begun with a horizontal skin incision at the level of the hyoid bone membrane, and subplatysmal flaps are raised superiorly to the level of the thyroid cartilage and inferiorly to the level of the trachea. The strap muscles are divided in the midline and retracted laterally. The larynx is entered via a midline thyrotomy approach beginning inferiorly in the cricothyroid membrane and extending superiorly to the thyrohyoid membrane. All mucosal lacerations are meticulously reapproximated with use of absorbable sutures. Any cartilaginous fractures are reduced and internally fixed with use of wire or nonabsorbable sutures. All exposed cartilage must be covered to prevent subsequent granulation tissue and fibrosis. Ideally, this can be achieved with primary closure of the mucosa. In the event primary closure cannot be achieved, mucosal advancement flaps from the adjacent hypopharynx or, less ideally, mucosal or split-thickness skin grafts can be used. Any cartilage denuded of its perichondrial blood supply is removed (Fig. 41–3).

After repair of all laryngeal injuries, the anterior commissure is re-created by suturing the anterior margin of each true vocal fold to

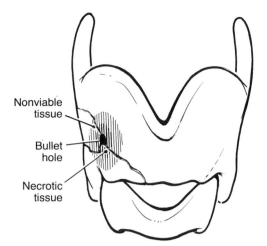

Figure 41–3. Various injuries encountered in the larynx. Note the loss of vertical height of the arytenoid cartilage, which is indicative of dislocation or loss of cricoid support.

the external perichondrium of the thyroid cartilage. The thyrotomy is then closed with wire or monofilament nonabsorbable sutures. The use of stents is controversial: stents improve stabilization and maintenance of the desired shape of the airway during healing; but they also cause additional mucosal damage and eventual scarring. The use of stents is accepted in cases in which the architecture of the larynx cannot be adequately reconstructed and stabilized with open reduction and internal fixation alone, and in cases in which the true vocal folds in the area of the anterior commissure are bilat-

erally denuded of mucosa. The stents should be left in place only as long as necessary to stabilize the larnyx, approximately 2 weeks (Figs. 41–4 to 41–6). Prolonged stenting leads to additional mucosal damage and scarring of the larynx with poorer long-term results. The stent should be designed in the shape of the larynx and secured so that it moves with swallowing and is easily removed by use of endoscopic techniques only. Stents may be purchased from supply companies or created from materials already available in most operating rooms. In either case, the stent should extend superiorly from the arytenoid level to the first tracheal ring inferiorly and be shaped to resemble the laryngeal airway. A 3.5-cm length of Portex endotracheal tube makes an acceptable stent and is readily available (Fig. 41–7). The stent is cut to length and the superior lumen sewn shut to prevent aspiration. Smooth hemostat clamps are then placed to approximate the false and true vocal fold areas, and the entire piece is autoclaved at 180° and then rapidly cooled; this creates a stent permanently molded to the shape of the larynx.

Numerous other problems may be encountered during open exploration of laryngeal trauma. If a recurrent nerve is found to be severed, it should be primarily reapproximated. Although the intricate adductor-abductor innervation will not be restored, reapproximation may help maintain muscle tone and therefore voice strength. If segments of cricoid or tracheal cartilage are missing, these

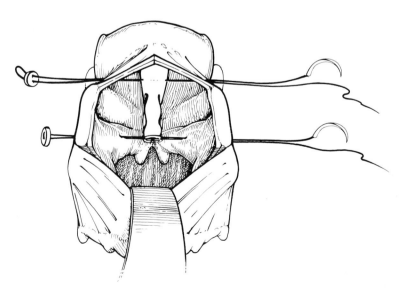

Figure 41–4. Portex stent in place. The stent is secured with either single or double monofilament suture over skin buttons.

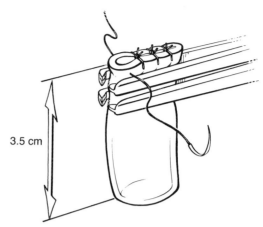

Figure 41–7. Fashioning a stent from an endotracheal tube. The superior lumen is sewn closed to prevent aspiration. The clamps are at the approximate level of the true and false vocal folds.

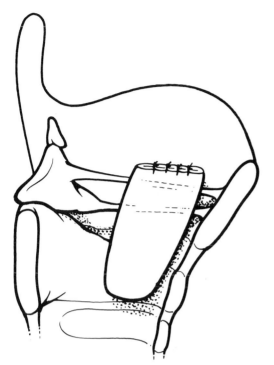

Figure 41–5. Lateral view of a stent within the larynx. Note the position of the apex of the keel in the anterior commissure.

areas should be covered with myofascial flaps from adjacent infrahyoid muscles.

Outcome

The long-term results of laryngeal trauma are dependent on the extent of the original injury and the quality of subsequent repairs. Those

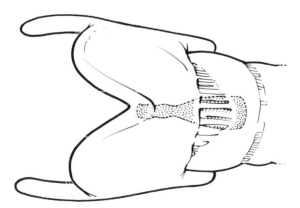

Figure 41–6. Stent in the larynx after closure of thyrotomy. The superior extent is above the arytenoid cartilages; inferiorly, the stent extends to the first tracheal ring.

patients who do not require extensive operative intervention have an excellent prognosis for complete return of laryngeal function.

Patients requiring surgical exploration still have an excellent chance of eventual decannulation with an excellent to good voice. The postinjury complications of granulation tissue and stenosis are best treated with prevention by meticulous repair at the time of surgery and coverage of all exposed cartilage. After surgery, the patient should be followed closely with serial direct fiberoptic examinations. If a stent was placed, direct laryngoscopy and bronchoscopy should be performed at the time of removal in order to assess laryngeal healing and airway. It is important at this time to palpate the arytenoid cartilages to ensure mobility or to ascertain the extent and reason for the decreased range of motion if mobility is limited.

The patient may be decannulated as tolerated as soon as the wounds are healing well or the stent, if placed, is removed. Two common conditions in which decannulation cannot be safely accomplished are subglottic stenosis and vocal fold paralysis. In the instance of subglottic stenosis, no surgical intervention is usually indicated for 6 to 12 months for allowing scar maturation. At this time, repeat direct laryngoscopy and bronchoscopy should be performed to better define the architecture of the stenosis. Short segments of stenosis with normal trachea proximally and distally may be excised with primary closure by use of a suprahyoid release to gain mobility as needed. Longer sections of stenosis may require an anterior and possibly posterior cricotracheal interposition graft, as has been popularized in the treatment of subglottic stenosis on infants.

Vocal fold paralysis may be secondary to recurrent nerve injury, arytenoid dislocation, or loss of cricoid support. When discovered at the time of initial surgery, arytenoid dislocation should be repaired. If it is discovered during the removal of the laryngeal stent, reduction may also be performed with an endoscopic technique. Paresis caused by recurrent nerve injury is followed for at least 6 months. If at that time no improvement has occurred, a medialization procedure for unilateral paralysis or lateralization procedure for bilateral paralysis may be considered.

Finally, associated neurologic damage occurring at the original time of injury may prevent decannulation because of the prolonged need for pulmonary toilet. In these instances, decannulation should occur as the improvement in neurologic states dictates.

NONLARYNGEAL NECK TRAUMA

The same general principles apply for injuries of the neck not affecting the larynx as for those that do. Securing the airway remains the first priority, followed by any supportive measures needed to maintain pulse and blood pressure, the fundamentals of trauma care. A thorough and complete physical examination is mandatory, and any history available from the patient, witnesses, or paramedic personnel is obtained. A cervical collar or a manual cervical traction is used to maintain the neck in a neutral position until a cervical spine injury is ruled out.

Blunt trauma to the neck usually involves the rigid structures present, including the larynx and cervical spine. Unless associated with or a result of rigid structure injury, such as comminuted laryngeal fracture with resultant penetration of the esophagus by laryngeal cartilage, injury to the nonrigid structures of the neck is usually the result of penetrating trauma.

The management of soft tissue neck injury is based on the anatomic division of the neck into three zones. Zone 1 is that area below the clavicles and contains the pleural apices, the subclavian vessels, the trachea, and the esophagus. Injuries to this area are difficult to observe clinically or expose surgically. Repair of injuries in this area may require a thoracotomy and should be undertaken only by someone with this expertise. Zone 2 is the area between the clavicles and the angle of the mandible. Injuries to this area are the most easily observed and exposed when necessary. Zone 3 injuries are those between the angle of the mandible and the skull base. Exposure in this area is the most difficult.

Physical examination should include complete inspection of the patient for other injuries as well as obvious neck trauma. The cervical collar must be removed for inspection of the neck while an assistant holds the patient in a neutral position. Entrance and exit wounds of penetrating injuries are examined, and an attempt is made to identify the type of weapon used. Hematomas, bruits, or profuse bleeding may indicate a major vascular injury. The larynx and trachea should be carefully examined. Cranial nerve dysfunction may reveal nerve injury. Saliva in the wound is indicative of involvement of salivary glands or ducts. Hemoptysis or hematemesis may indicate violation of the mucosal layer of the trachea, the larynx, or the esophagus.

After the initial stabilization and examination of the patient have been achieved, a decision is made as to the patient's ability to undergo diagnostic evaluation. Any patient not stable enough to undergo possibly lengthy radiographic evaluation is taken immediately to the operating room for an open exploration of the neck wound. In addition, any patient obviously requiring surgical exploration, such as the patient with an expanding hematoma, is taken directly to the operating room.

Plain chest films should be the first study performed because these may confirm that the patient is an operative candidate, with relatively little spent in time or money. Pneumothorax may be seen, revealing entrance of the weapon into the pleural space. Mediastinal air may represent esophageal or tracheal injury.

In patients who sustain penetrating trauma proximal to a major vessel but without overt signs or symptoms of vascular injury, arteriography is performed. A four-vessel, multiple-view study is required in zone 2 and zone 3 injuries involving gunshot wounds or stab wounds that cross the midline. In zone 1 injuries, a study of the subclavian and great vessels is also needed. Digital subtraction techniques and image magnification may assist in the identification of subtle injuries.

If the arteriogram is negative, then the possibility of pharyngoesophageal injury must be eliminated. Barium swallow is commonly used for this purpose because it is noninvasive and readily available; however, it may not identify some injuries. Rigid esophagoscopy is more sensitive in the diagnosis of mucosal injury but usually requires general anesthesia and personnel trained in its use. If no injury is found in patients with zone 1 and zone 3 injuries, then simple observation is performed for 24 to 48 hours. Because of the ease of exploration and low associated morbidity in zone 2 injuries, some clinicians have advocated mandatory exploration of all injuries despite normal results of noninvasive studies. This policy results, however, in a 50% to 80% rate of negative results of explorations.

Operative approach to the injury depends on the location and the extent of the injury. An apron flap subplatysmal approach is used if concomitant laryngeal injuries are anticipated. If only vascular or esophageal injuries are present, an incision along the anterior sternocleidomastoid muscle, as is used in carotid endarterectomy, may be substituted.

All vascular injuries are repaired after proximal and distal control is obtained. Esophageal and pharyngeal injuries are closed in layers and drained. Severed cranial nerves should be repaired primarily or, if this is impossible without tension, with the use of an equal-sized nerve graft. Extensive injury to the submandibular gland or duct is best managed with formal excision of the gland. In cases in which pharyngeal or esophageal injury is present, a nasogastric tube is placed for postoperative alimentation.

Of special consideration are esophageal injuries resulting from caustic ingestion. The laryngeal manifestations and treatment are outlined under laryngeal trauma. In addition to the larynx, the esophagus and the stomach must be considered. In the United States, these injuries result primarily from alkali ingestion in the pediatric population, although numerous substances at all ages have been reported. Physical examination is remarkable primarily for oral cavity and oral pharynx mucosal burns. Plain radiographs may demonstrate pneumomediastinum if esophageal perforation is present. Treatment

begins with securing the airway. To prevent further mucosal damage, tracheostomy is preferred over endotracheal intubation if direct fiberoptic laryngoscopy reveals laryngeal injury. Hydration is initiated as needed. Endoscopy is performed to evaluate the need for surgical intervention and also to assess the extent of esophageal and gastric injury. Esophageal and gastric tissue that is obviously necrotic is resected, and a feeding jejunostomy is placed. If minimal esophageal and gastric injury is found, the patient may be managed with nonsurgical support measures. Postinjury stenosis resulting from circumferential scarring may be treated with dilation or, in extreme cases, with interposition grafts.

CONCLUSION

Although management for laryngeal and nonlaryngeal neck trauma now includes more diagnostic evaluation, the reward for this time-consuming and expensive protocol is better selection of patients who are most likely to benefit from surgical intervention. This is not to suggest that all diagnostic modalities available are to be used in the evaluation of every patient. On the contrary, each patient must be individually analyzed, and only tests that are likely to affect the management of the patient are indicated. Cooperation between the various services involved is essential in coordinating the studies needed and avoiding duplications of effort. In addition, the studies needed and the time required in radiology suites for obtaining them must be weighed against the overall condition of the patient and the safety of being away from an acute, critical care area.

SUGGESTED READINGS

Bighora RA, et al: The necessity for mandatory exploration of penetrating zone II neck injuries. Surgery 100:655–660, 1986.

Crumley RL: Experiments in laryngeal reinnervation. Laryngoscope Suppl 30, 1982.

Downey WL, Owen RC, Ward PH: Traumatic laryngeal injury—its management and sequelae. South Med J 60:756–761, 1987.

Gussack GS, Jukovich GJ, Lutermon A: Laryngotracheal trauma: a protocol approach to a rare injury. Laryngoscope 96:660–665, 1986.

Harrison DFN: Bullet wounds of the larynx and trachea. Arch Otolaryngol 110:203–205, 1984.

Kirkorian EA: Laryngopharyngeal injuries. Laryngoscope 85:2069–2086, 1975.

LeMay SR: Penetrating wounds of the larynx and cervical trachea. Arch Otolaryngol 94:558–565, 1971.

Leopold DA: Laryngeal trauma. Arch Otolaryngol Head Neck Surg 109:106–111, 1987.

Lucente FE, Mitrani M, Sacks SH, et al: Penetrating injuries of the larynx. Ear Nose Throat J 64:406–415, 1985.

Lundy LJ, et al: Experience on selective operations in the management of penetrating wounds of the neck. Surg Gynecol Obstet 147:845–849, 1978.

Mancuso AA, Nonafee WN: Computed tomography of the injured larynx. Radiology 133:139–144, 1979.

Meyer CH, Orobello P, Cotton RT, et al: Blunt laryngeal trauma in children. Laryngoscope 97:1043–1048, 1987.

Meyer JP, et al: Mandatory vs. selective exploration for penetrating neck trauma. Arch Surg 122:592–597, 1987.

Nahum AM: Immediate care of acute blunt laryngeal trauma. J Trauma 9:112–125, 1969.

Narrod JA, Moore EE: Selective management of penetrating neck injuries. Arch Surg 119:574–578, 1984.

Olson NR: Wound healing by primary intention in the larynx. Otolaryngol Clin North Am 12:735–740, 1979.

Potter CR, Sessions DG, Ogura JH: Blunt laryngotracheal trauma. Trans Am Acad Ophthalmol Otolaryngol 86:909–923, 1978.

Schaefer SD: Primary management of laryngeal trauma. Ann Otol Rhinol Laryngol 91:399–402, 1982.

Schaefer SD: The acute surgical treatment of the fractural larynx. Oper Tech Otolaryngol Head Neck Surg 1:64–70, 1990.

Schaefer SD, Brown OE: Selective application of CT in the management of laryngeal trauma. Laryngoscope 93:1473–1475, 1983.

Schaefer SD, Close LG: The acute management of laryngeal trauma: an update. Ann Otol Rhinol Laryngol 98:98–104, 1989.

Stanley RB, Hanson DG: Manual strangulation injuries of the larynx. Arch Otolaryngol Head Neck Surg 109:344–347, 1983.

Stanley RB, Cooper DS, FLorman SH: Phonatory effects of thyroid cartilage fractures. Ann Otol Rhinol Laryngol 96:493–496, 1987.

Thomas BK, Stevens MH: Stenting in experimental laryngeal injuries. Arch Otolaryngol 101:217–221, 1975.

Trone TH, Schaefer SD, Carder HM: Blunt and penetrating laryngeal trauma: a 13-year review. Otolaryngol Head Neck Surg 88:257–261, 1980.

CHAPTER 42

Neoplasms and Cysts of Larynx and Cervical Esophagus

Scott P. Stringer, MD

CARCINOMA OF LARYNX

Cancer of the larynx represents approximately 2% of all cancer cases. Except for the skin, it is the most common cancer of the head and neck. There are an estimated 11,000 new cases of laryngeal cancers per year. It occurs at a peak incidence in men in their seventh decade, and it occurs in a male-to-female ratio of about 5:1. Although the number of laryngeal cancers in women has been increasing minimally, it has not increased at the rapid rate of lung cancer in women. The majority of laryngeal cancers (55% to 75%) are glottic. Supraglottic primary tumors account for another 24% to 42%, whereas subglottic tumors are rare, accounting for approximately 1% to 6%.

Cancer of the larynx is overwhelmingly related to cigarette smoking and occurs very rarely in nonsmokers. Laryngeal carcinoma has been reproduced in an animal model with cigarettes. The risk increases with the number of cigarettes smoked per day. Cessation of smoking decreases the risk of tobacco-related upper respiratory cancers after 5 to 6 years, and the risk approaches that of nonsmokers after 10 to 15 years. The use of filters in cigarettes appears to decrease the risk of laryngeal cancer; however, it is unclear whether low-tar and low-nicotine cigarettes result in a lower incidence.

Alcohol appears to play a greater role in supraglottic lesions than in glottic lesions. The effect is independent of but synergistic with tobacco. The combination of the two increases the risk of supraglottic cancer 50% above simple additive effects.

Although exposure to low-dose radiation is usually associated with an increased risk of thyroid and salivary gland malignancies, there are rare reports of laryngeal squamous cell carcinomas, fibrosarcomas, and acinic cell carcinomas after radiation exposure as well.

Anatomy

A review of some portions of the laryngeal anatomy is necessary in order to describe and understand patterns of spread of laryngeal cancer. A more extensive description of laryngeal anatomy is provided in Chapter 36. The larynx is subdivided into the supraglottic, glottic, and subglottic regions. The supraglottis consists of the epiglottis, the false vocal folds, the ventricles, the arytenoepiglottic folds, and the arytenoid cartilages. It is demarcated from the glottic larynx at the apex of the ventricle. The glottis consists primarily of the true vocal folds. Both vocal folds attach to the thyroid cartilage at the anterior commissure. Posteriorly, they terminate at the vocal process of the arytenoid cartilage. The mucosa between the arytenoid cartilages forms the posterior portion of the glottis known as the posterior commissure. The superior border of the subglottic larynx is poorly defined. It arbitrarily begins 5 to 10 mm below the free edge of the true vocal fold and ends more precisely at the inferior border of the cricoid cartilage.

The bony and cartilaginous framework of the larynx includes the hyoid bone along with the thyroid, cricoid, epiglottic, arytenoid, cuneiform, and corniculate cartilages. The hyaline cartilage of the thyroid, cricoid, and arytenoid cartilages may undergo patchy ossification, which makes computed tomographic interpretation of cartilaginous destruction difficult.

This framework is linked together by the thyrohyoid, cricothyroid, and cricotracheal ligaments or membranes. The thyrohyoid membrane is especially thin and, as such, is a poor barrier to tumor spread. A small dehiscence is present in this membrane between the middle and inferior pharyngeal constrictor muscles, where the superior laryngeal neurovascular bundle passes, and thereby provides ready exit for tumors in this area. The epiglottis is attached to the hyoid bone superiorly by the hyoepiglottic ligament and inferiorly to the thyroid cartilage by the thyroepiglottic ligament. An elastic membrane forms a fibrous framework just below the mucosa. It is separated into a superior portion and an inferior portion by the ventricle of the larynx. The superior portion is the quadrangular membrane that extends from the lateral margin of the epiglottis posteriorly to the arytenoid cartilages and inferiorly to the false vocal folds. The inferior portion is the conus elasticus, which connects the upper edge of the cricoid cartilage to the vocal process of the arytenoid cartilage and to the lower thyroid cartilage. Its upper border is thickened to form the vocal ligament.

The pre-epiglottic and paraglottic fat spaces are a single continuous space separately defined by the superior edge of the quadrangular membrane. This space is bounded by the hyoepiglottic ligament superiorly; by the thyroid cartilage, the thyrohyoid membrane, and the hyoid bone anterolaterally; by the conus elasticus inferiorly—the quadrangular membrane medially; and by the piriform sinus posteriorly. The ventricle and saccule form a niche in the paraglottic space. These spaces play an important role in the local spread of laryngeal cancers.

The supraglottis has a rich capillary lymphatic plexus. The collecting ducts pass through the pre-epiglottic space and the thyrohyoid membrane and drain primarily into the jugulodigastric lymph nodes, whereas a few trunks terminate in the middle internal jugular lymph nodes. Lymphatic vessels are present in the true vocal folds but they are sparse. The subglottis also has sparse capillary lymphatic vessels. Those that are present traverse the cricothyroid membrane to the pretracheal nodes or to the lower internal jugular lymph nodes. Lymphatic drainage also occurs posteriorly through the cricotracheal membrane to the paratracheal lymph nodes and again to the lower internal jugular chain.

Pathology

The laryngeal mucosa is pseudostratified, ciliated columnar epithelium except for the laryngeal surface of the epiglottis and the free margin of the true vocal fold, which are lined by squamous epithelium. Therefore, virtually all malignancies of the larynx, specifically squamous cell carcinoma or any one of its variants, are epithelial in origin. Carcinoma of the larynx must be differentiated from fungal, mycobacterial, syphilitic, and granulomatous disorders as well as from benign neoplasia.

Carcinoma in situ and dysplasia are frequently encountered on the vocal folds. Approximately 4% of the hyperkeratotic lesions and 10% to 15% of the carcinomas in situ progress to invasive carcinoma. The majority of the frankly invasive squamous cell carcinomas are either well differentiated or moderately differentiated.

Patterns of Spread

At the time of presentation, about 62% of patients have localized tumors, 26% have regional spread, and 8% have distant metastases. The local patterns of spread of squamous cell carcinoma of the larynx are determined by the normal anatomic boundaries and by the tendency of carcinomas to follow the planes of least resistance initially. Invasion through the pre-epiglottic and paraglottic fat spaces is common. Ligaments and cartilage provide significant deterrence for invasion, but once invasion occurs, the prognosis worsens greatly. Cartilaginous invasion

spac
inva
caus
geal
tum
the e
as w
The
node
with
bene
subtl

Er
unde
tissu
sion,
sions
is a
prim
agos
natio
are u
tract.
prese
trast
Gene
sion
taken

Stagi

Stagir
script
havio
parisc
Joint
for lar

The
the la
ment
early
of the
lesion
growtl
probal

In t
false v
hyoid
aryten
follow

Tis
T1
normal
T2
or sites
T3

begins most commonly at sites of ligamentous insertion and in ossified sections posteriorly in the thyroid and cricoid cartilages. Perineural spread of laryngeal malignancies is uncommon.

Carcinomas of the suprahyoid epiglottis are often exophytic, with minimal cartilage destruction or deep invasion. Occasional lesions may infiltrate the tip of the epiglottis and eventually invade the vallecula, the pre-epiglottic space, the lateral pharyngeal walls, and the remaining supraglottis.

Infrahyoid epiglottis lesions tend to progress through fenestra in the epiglottic cartilage and the thyroepiglottic ligament into the pre-epiglottic space and eventually into the vallecula and the tongue base. Paraglottic extension is common as well. Circumferential mucosal growth leads to involvement of the false vocal folds, the arytenoepiglottic folds, and sometimes the medial wall of the piriform sinuses. Invasion of the vocal folds and thyroid cartilage is uncommon and a late finding.

Carcinomas of the false vocal folds are usually ulcerative and deeply infiltrative. Paraglottic space involvement occurs early with few symptoms; this may lead to clinical understaging. Submucosal involvement of the medial wall of the piriform sinus is frequently seen. These tumors tend to spread submucosally superiorly to the pre-epiglottic space and inferiorly until they encounter the conus elasticus. At this point, penetration inferiorly through the cricothyroid membrane may occur. Thyroid cartilage invasion is a late occurrence.

Initially, lesions of the arytenoepiglottic folds and the arytenoid cartilages are often exophytic. They tend to involve adjacent sites as they grow. Invasion of the cricoarytenoid muscles or joint as well as of the recurrent laryngeal nerve may cause vocal fold fixation. Large lesions may involve the cartilaginous skeleton, the tongue base, or the lateral pharyngeal walls.

Most lesions of the glottis begin on the free edge or the superior surface of the vocal fold. Carcinoma in situ and atypia are often present at the periphery of early glottic lesions. The lesions usually are confined to the vocal fold when diagnosed. The anterior portion of the vocal fold is the most frequently involved site, and extension to the anterior commissure is common. The attachment of the anterior commissure tendon to the thyroid cartilage provides easy access for carti-

laginous invasion. When the anterior commissure is involved, subglottic extension is more prevalent. Carcinomas of the posterior vocal fold tend to spread submucosally to invade the cricoarytenoid joint and the interarytenoid space.

Direct invasion of the thyroarytenoid muscle is the most common cause of vocal fold fixation. In addition, fixation may be caused by involvement of the posterior cricoarytenoid muscle, the cricoarytenoid joint, the paraglottic space, or the recurrent laryngeal nerve.

Larger lesions may extend to the supraglottis and subglottis. Deep infiltration of the vocal ligament and thyroarytenoid muscle allows access to the thyroid cartilage perichondrium. At this point the tumor tends to spread in the paraglottic space rather than invade cartilage. The conus elasticus serves to direct tumor growth to the cricothyroid membrane. Because mucosa is directly applied to the membrane, extralaryngeal spread is common in this area. Eventually, the thyroid and cricoid cartilages are invaded directly.

Subglottic carcinomas are often advanced at the time of diagnosis because of an initial paucity of symptoms; hence they are most often bilateral or circumferential when seen. Invasion of the cricoid cartilage and cricothyroid membrane is common because there is no intervening muscle layer. Invasion of soft tissues of the neck and the thyroid gland occurs with large tumors. Vocal cord fixation resulting from early thyroarytenoid muscle involvement is regularly observed.

The lymphatic anatomy and the location and extent of the primary tumor define the pattern of lymph node metastases. As discussed previously, there is a paucity of lymphatic veins in the glottis, in comparison with the richly supplied supraglottic larynx. The supraglottis arises from the buccopharyngeal anlage (branchial arches III and IV); the subglottic larynx arises from the pulmonary anlage (branchial arch VI). The vascular, lymphatic, and neuroanatomic subdivisions correspond to these boundaries. The supraglottis and the pre-epiglottic space have no well-defined fusion plane, whereas the glottis is formed by two lateral masses. This is reflected by the much higher rate of bilateral neck metastase of supraglottic primary lesions than of glottic lesions. Perineural infiltration and poor differentiation of the primary lesion are associated with a higher

lesion is treated with radiotherapy. If a T3 or T4 lesion is treated with radiotherapy, both sides of the neck are radiated simultaneously. Similarly, a neck dissection is not performed in a neck with no palpable nodal metastases at the time of conservation laryngeal surgery. In the case of early glottic tumors, a neck dissection is typically reserved for palpable nodal metastases.

The majority of advanced glottic carcinomas are treated with total laryngectomy with or without radiation therapy. If the neck is clinically negative for disease and clear indications for postoperative irradiation exists, then both sides of the neck are treated with radiation rather than neck dissection. When malignant nodes exist or if no postoperative radiation is anticipated, a neck dissection is performed on the side of the lesion. Indications for postoperative irradiation include extralaryngeal spread, cartilage invasion, extensive subglottic spread, close or positive margins, multiple malignant lymph nodes, or extranodal spread. Radical radiation therapy for cure may be attempted for patients who refuse surgery or who cannot medically tolerate a surgical procedure.

A near total laryngectomy has been described as a technique to preserve voice in selected patients with advanced laryngeal lesions. Patients with tumors involving the posterior commissure or fixing both vocal folds are not suitable. The resection includes the entire larynx except for a narrow strip connecting the trachea and the pharynx over an uninvolved arytenoid cartilage. In addition, the posterior true and false vocal folds and the hemisubglottis on the uninvolved side are preserved. A tracheoesophageal shunt is formed over the remaining tissue, and the remainder of the pharyngeal wall is closed primarily. Although the patient is able to vocalize through this shunt, the patient is permanently tracheotomy-dependent. There is some debate as to the clear advantage of this procedure over a conventional total laryngectomy with tracheoesophageal puncture for speech rehabilitation.

Most treatment failures manifest within 18 months, but failures may appear up to 5 years later. In the presence of local recurrence of tumor, the risk of cervical metastases increases. Vertical partial laryngectomy may be used for selected radiation failures. Those radiation failures unsuitable for conservation surgery are salvaged with total laryngectomy. The most common sites of failure after total laryngectomy are the tongue base and the parastomal area. Salvage after total laryngectomy and irradiation is difficult.

Surgical complications vary with the extent of removal of laryngeal tissue. Repeated vocal fold stripping may result in a thickened vocal fold with a hoarse voice. Laser endoscopic cordectomy may result in web formation, especially if anterior commissure excision is performed. Laryngofissure with cordectomy may be complicated by local wound problems and laryngeal stenosis. Complications associated with hemilaryngectomy include chondritis, wound infection, glottic incompetency, and laryngeal webs. Near total laryngectomy shares common complications with total laryngectomy, which are discussed in the previous section. In addition, aspiration via and stenosis of the tracheopharyngeal shunt may occur after this procedure.

The primary acute side effects of radiation therapy for glottic lesions are temporary hoarseness and sore throat. Persistent edema of the larynx is the most common long-term complication after radiation. Neck dissection may exacerbate such edema and delay its resolution. Chondronecrosis should occur in less than 1% of treated patients. Hyperbaric oxygen therapy and antibiotics may resolve mild to moderate cases. Many patients with severe cases require total laryngectomy for pain relief and to prevent permanent airway obstruction.

Subglottis

The high incidence of cartilage invasion with subglottic carcinomas limits the use of radiotherapy alone for cure. Early subglottic lesions respond well to irradiation, whereas most T3 and T4 tumors are managed with total laryngectomy, followed by postoperative radiation. On occasion, radiotherapy may be used in advanced stages for patients who refuse surgery or are medically unsuitable for surgery. Conservation surgery is rarely appropriate because of the critical need to preserve the integrity of the cricoid cartilage in order to maintain an airway. Highly selected lesions may be treated with an extended hemilaryngectomy. This involves removal of a portion of the cricoid cartilage along with a standard hemilaryngectomy. The cricoid ring should not be completely disrupted, however. Near total laryngectomy may be used for selected tumors as well. As previously discussed, this procedure has unique benefits and disadvantages.

Although neck nodes are not frequently present at the time of diagnosis, control of occult disease is essential for obtaining acceptable locoregional control rates. When irradiation is used, the paratracheal nodes should be treated. In the case of total laryngectomy, an extensive pretracheal and paratracheal node dissection and a partial thyroidectomy are performed in addition to a standard neck dissection. In the presence of malignant cervical nodes, a combination of nodal dissection and radiotherapy is most effective.

If radiation fails to control early lesions, then total laryngectomy is most commonly required to achieve cure. It is rare that a local subglottic recurrence could be managed by conservation laryngeal surgery. The most common site of failure after total laryngectomy is peristomal, at the tracheal mucosal border or in a paratracheal node. In any event, salvage is difficult. Wide excision with both manubrium resection and mediastinal dissection is rarely successful in obtaining local control. The most effective treatment is prevention, consisting of a thorough paratracheal node dissection and radiotherapy.

Complications after irradiation or surgery are similar to those described for the management of glottic lesions. Airway obstruction may be slightly more common during radiation therapy for subglottic lesions because of local edema within the limiting cricoid cartilage.

Chemotherapy

Chemotherapeutic agents have been employed in a variety of trials in an attempt to improve locoregional control rates and especially overall cure rates for squamous cell carcinoma of the larynx. Historically, methotrexate was the first agent to be used in the management of head and neck cancers. Bleomycin was the next agent to be extensively investigated for this purpose. Its usefulness has been somewhat limited by the side effect of pulmonary toxicity. The agents most commonly used to treat tumors of the larynx currently are cisplatin or one of its derivatives. This is often combined with a second agent such as 5-fluorouracil.

Chemotherapy has several roles in the management of carcinoma of the head and neck. Induction chemotherapy is an attempt to improve the locoregional control rate by cytoreduction and to decrease the incidence of distant metastases. Adjuvant chemotherapy is typically given after traditional surgery or radiation with the same goals as induction treatment. Maintenance chemotherapy is used in hopes of preventing recurrence of distant metastases over a longer period of time. Radiation therapy has been combined with chemotherapeutic agents in hopes of radiosensitizing the tumor. Finally, chemotherapy is used in the treatment of inoperable or metastatic disease for palliation.

Specifically, a multiinstitutional trial of combination chemotherapy and irradiation for the management of stage III and stage IV laryngeal cancers is ongoing. The benefits would be preservation of laryngeal function in advanced disease and, it is hoped, improved overall survival. The results of this study may better define the role of chemotherapy in the treatment of advanced laryngeal lesions. However, to date, the results of chemotherapy in head and neck cancers in general have been disappointing. Despite high initial partial and complete responses, no randomized phase III trial has demonstrated any significant improvement in overall survival time or disease survival time.

Results

Supraglottis

Acceptable survival rates may be obtained with the use of radiotherapy or supraglottic laryngectomy in the treatment of early carcinomas of the supraglottic larynx. Advanced lesions are best managed with surgery or a combination of irradiation and surgery. Surgery alone should achieve a 3-year determinate survival in the 70% to 80% range in the presence of an N0 neck. Survival decreases to 60% to 70% in the presence of clinically malignant nodes. Local recurrences are uncommon (6% to 11%), and salvage is frequently achieved with radiotherapy or total laryngectomy. Total laryngectomy usually is combined with irradiation in the management of advanced lesions; the 5-year survival rate is approximately 70%.

Irradiation is highly effective in the local control of T1 and T2 lesions of the supraglottic larynx. Control rates decrease with increasing stage of the lesion. Local control for all stages has been reported as 67%. In addition, surgical salvage is successful in 60% of cases; the ultimate control rate for all stages is 81%. Ultimate local control rates for early lesions should be in the 90% range. Total laryngectomy is often required to achieve surgical salvage, however.

Glottis

T1 and T2 vocal fold lesions may be effectively treated with irradiation or surgery. Conservation laryngeal surgery, including cordectomy, laser excision, and hemilaryngectomy, should produce disease-free survival rates in the 80% to 95% range for appropriate glottic carcinomas. Local recurrence rates are generally less than 10% to 15%, and approximately 75% of recurrences may be salvaged. Hemilaryngectomy for T3 lesions produces a cure rate of 58%. Of those patients with a positive margin at the time of hemilaryngectomy, about 20% develop a recurrence, as opposed to 6% of patients with negative margins. The majority of T3 and T4 carcinomas treated surgically require total laryngectomy. Local and regional recurrences occur in 20% of patients. Salvage may be obtained in about half the patients; the determinate survival rate is in the 70% range.

Modern-day cure rates for glottic squamous cell carcinoma treated with radiotherapy are in the range of 90% for T1 lesions, 70% for T2 lesions, and 50% to 60% for T3 and T4 lesions. Combining surgical salvages should give a overall cure rate of 90% to 95% for T1 and T2 disease. T2 lesions with impaired vocal fold mobility respond somewhat more poorly to radiotherapy than do those with normal mobility. A highly selected group of T3 lesions as outlined previously may be treated with radiotherapy in an attempt to preserve laryngeal function. A hyperfractionated radiation sequence may provide local control rates of 67%; the ultimate control rate after surgical salvage is 83%. This treatment regimen is associated with a 10% complication rate.

Subglottis

Overall cure rates for all stages of subglottic carcinoma are in the range of 35% for radiation, 42% for surgery alone, and 70% for combined therapy. Postoperative irradiation is especially effective in preventing peristo-

mal recurrence. Peristomal recurrence occurs in approximately 8% of patients. Limited failures may be salvaged and a 2-year survival rate of 45% may be achieved, whereas for more advanced recurrences, the 2-year survival rate is only 10% to 15%.

Voice Rehabilitation

Vocal rehabilitation options after total laryngectomy include mechanical external vibratory devices, esophageal speech, and tracheoesophageal fistula speech. Electrolarynx devices may be cumbersome and are poorly used by a large number of laryngectomy patients. Speech quality is often inadequate. At the present time, these devices serve only as a temporary aid for most laryngectomees, inasmuch as better alternatives are certainly available.

Esophageal speech is produced by swallowing air and belching it out; the pharyngoesophageal segment is used as the vocal generator. Some patients achieve excellent results with esophageal speech. However, the voice achieved is limited with respect to intensity, pitch, and rate. In a comparison of intensity, fundamental frequency, and rate of speech in three groups of patients who used laryngeal, esophageal, and tracheoesophageal fistula speech, tracheoesophageal speech was demonstrated to be significantly more similar to laryngeal speech than was esophageal speech. In addition, in prospectively obtained data, only 12 (26%) of 47 patients were able to acquire esophageal speech; such a low success rate severely limits its effectiveness as a voice rehabilitation technique.

Initial attempts at establishing tracheoesophageal speech consisted of forming a tubed mucosal fistula at the time of laryngectomy. These techniques are rarely used at present because of aspiration, stenosis, and failure to achieve speech. The tracheoesophageal puncture technique is currently the procedure of choice for vocal rehabilitation of most laryngectomy patients. Of 47 patients rehabilitated with the Blom-Singer method, 94% had acquired good to superior speech and 83% continued to use their prosthesis by the end of 1 year. In addition, less than 50% were able to master esophageal speech. Long-term follow-up on 66 patients for 1 to 3 1/2 years demonstrated a 64% success rate. Poor motivation, female gender, and long-term use of a tracheostoma vent were associated with poor maintenance of tracheo-esophageal speech. Criteria for successful establishment of tracheoesophageal speech have been found to be appropriate stomal anatomy, positive results of an insufflation test, an educated and skilled patient, and inclusion of a speech therapist in the vocal rehabilitation team. The team approach to vocal rehabilitation is essential to acquisition and maintenance of tracheoesophageal speech. Finally, a pharyngeal myotomy or a pharyngeal plexus neurectomy at the time of laryngectomy has been reported to improve overall speech acquisition rates with tracheo-esophageal puncture.

The timing of tracheoesophageal puncture, primary versus delayed, remains controversial. A 69% success rate with primary puncture has been reported; this rate improved to 75% with revision surgery. Alternatively, a 79% success rate was demonstrated in a series of 32 patients undergoing puncture as a procedure separate from laryngectomy, with cricopharyngeal myotomy and stoma revision used as necessary. In a series of 21 primary punctures and 15 delayed punctures, 74% and 64% success rates were described, respectively. Finally, in a comparison of primary puncture versus delayed puncture in 26 equally divided patients controlled for age, tumor size, and use of radiation therapy, 10 patients in the primary group achieved excellent to good voices, and 7 patients in the delayed group achieved excellent to good voices. An additional 4 patients in the delayed group developed fair voices. A higher incidence of fistula formation in the primary group and an increased incidence of stent extrusion in the delayed group were found. It appears that depending on the local expertise, acceptable results with low complication rates may be obtained with either technique.

UNUSUAL LARYNGEAL MALIGNANCIES

The overwhelming majority of laryngeal malignancies are squamous cell carcinomas. However, malignancies may be observed in all other cell types in the larynx, including epithelium, neuroendocrine cells, mucous glands, melanocytes, mesenchyme, and lymphoreticular tissue.

Epithelial Tumors

Verrucous squamous cell carcinomas represent less than 3% to 4% of all laryngeal malignancies and are most frequently seen on the glottis and the supraglottis. They are characterized histologically by a proliferation of suprabasal cells that apparently push an intact basement membrane. There is in addition a paucity of cytologic abnormalities and a prominent inflammatory response. The histologic diagnosis is sometimes difficult, and correlation with the gross appearance of the lesion is frequently required. Physical examination most commonly reveals a warty exophytic mass. Lymph node metastases are more uncommon than with typical carcinoma of the larynx.

Verrucous carcinomas of the larynx represent a special case for management. Because of the relative slow-growing and non-aggressive nature of these lesions, surgery is typically more conservative. When suitable, hemilaryngectomy, supraglottic laryngectomy, or an endoscopic excision is the preferred treatment. Recurrence rates after appropriate surgery are in the range of 7%, and death occurs in approximately 4% of all cases.

These tumors are frequently reported to be radioresistant and even to convert to more aggressive anaplastic tumors after radiation. Despite these suggestions, several centers have reported the successful treatment of verrucous carcinomas with radiotherapy. Therefore, when the alternative is a total laryngectomy, radiation therapy may be considered if the patient is informed of the relative risks.

On occasion, an apparent carcinoma and sarcoma may occur together. This condition usually represents a squamous carcinoma with pseudosarcomatous or spindle cell stromal reaction. It may be referred to as pseudosarcomatous carcinoma, carcinosarcoma, spindle cell carcinoma, or pleomorphic carcinoma.

This process is principally thought to be an epidermoid malignancy with pseudosarcomatous stroma. In general, it behaves more aggressively, and the overall prognosis is worse. Radical surgery rather than primary irradiation is associated with higher overall cure rates.

Lymphoepitheliomas are rarely encountered in the larynx. These lesions should be recognized as undifferentiated squamous cell carcinomas with an accompanying lympho-

mass. Valsalva's maneuver performed by the patient may accentuate the physical findings. Diagnosis of a laryngocele is aided by the use of computed tomography and direct laryngoscopy.

Treatment is not necessary unless the laryngocele is symptomatic. The internal type may be marsupialized by microlaryngeal endoscopic techniques. Occasionally, an external approach for excision is required for laryngoceles that extend into the neck.

Saccular Cysts

As previously described, saccular cysts do not communicate with the laryngeal lumen. The cause is either simple congenital atresia of the saccular orifice or acquired obstruction from traumatic, neoplastic, or inflammatory conditions. Saccular cysts are distinctly submucosal, whereas ductal cysts are immediately evident below the mucous membrane. The saccular cyst may protrude posterosuperiorly into the false vocal fold and the arytenoepiglottic fold. Alternatively, the cysts may bulge anteriorly between the false and the true vocal folds overhanging the glottis. Massive saccular cysts may protrude into the neck.

Infants with saccular cysts may present with inspiratory stridor, an abnormal cry, cyanosis, or dysphagia. Adults more commonly present with hoarseness, dysphagia, or a neck mass. Physical examination reveals a small round swelling from the anterior ventricle, a fullness of the arytenoepiglottic and false vocal folds, or a neck mass, depending on the extent of the cyst. Computed tomography and direct laryngoscopy assist with the diagnosis.

Management varies with the location of the cyst and the urgency of the situation. Airway obstruction may be relieved in infants by simple aspiration of the cyst. In adults or children, recurrence is more common after simple aspiration; therefore, endoscopic marsupialization should be considered. Large lateral saccular cysts may necessitate an external approach for submucous excision.

CARCINOMA OF HYPOPHARYNX

Anatomy

The hypopharynx is the portion of the pharynx from the level of the hyoid bone to the beginning of the esophagus at the level of the lower border of the cricoid cartilage. Beneath the squamous mucosa are the pharyngeal constrictor muscles. The constrictor muscles are thin and do not significantly impede tumor growth. Between the muscles and the prevertebral fascia is a layer of loose areolar tissue in what is known as the retropharyngeal space. The parapharyngeal space is located laterally.

The hypopharynx is divided into three main regions: the piriform sinuses, the postcricoid pharynx, and the posterior pharyngeal wall. The piriform sinus is shaped by the intrusion of the larynx into the anterior pharynx. It is made up of an anterior wall, a lateral wall, and a medial wall. The sinus tapers inferiorly to an apex that is near the superior border of the posterior cricoid cartilage. The pharyngoepiglottic fold and the free margin of the arytenoepiglottic fold define the superior borders of the piriform sinus. Anterolaterally, the inner surface of the thyroid cartilage is present; posteromedially, the sinus abuts the arytenoid cartilages and the cricoid cartilage lamina. The postcricoid hypopharynx consists of the posterior mucosal lining of the cricoid cartilage. The posterior hypopharyngeal wall is delimited laterally by the opening of the piriform sinuses.

Epidemiology

Piriform sinus lesions are much more common than either postcricoid or posterior hypopharyngeal wall carcinomas. The incidence of hypopharyngeal malignancies peaks in the sixth decade of life. Lesions of the piriform sinus and the posterior hypopharyngeal wall predominate in men; the incidence of postcricoid tumors is equal between sexes.

Use of tobacco is the prime risk factor for the development of hypopharyngeal malignancies. However, alcohol abuse plays a more significant role in hypopharyngeal carcinoma than in endolaryngeal carcinoma. Northern European women are prone to Plummer-Vinson syndrome, which is characterized by glossitis, spenomegaly, esophageal stenosis, iron-deficiency anemia, and achlorhydria. Patients so affected have an excessively high incidence of postcricoid carcinomas.

Pathology

Well over 95% of hypopharyngeal malignant neoplasms are squamous cell carcinomas. Carcinoma in situ and dysplasia are commonly seen in the hypopharynx at the edge of frank carcinomas or as separate "skip" lesions. Minor salivary gland malignancies, lymphoepitheliomas, and transitional cell carcinomas occur rarely.

Patterns of Spread

As opposed to the larynx, the hypopharynx offers very few barriers to the contiguous spread of carcinoma. Lesions of the posterior hypopharyngeal wall tend to remain on the posterior wall, spreading superiorly and inferiorly rather than laterally. The tumors may spread as high as the nasopharynx but rarely spread below the level of the arytenoid cartilages. There is little resistance to posterior spread until the substantial prevertebral fascia is reached.

Submucosal spread is characteristic of piriform sinus lesions. Carcinomas arising on the medial wall soon involve the arytenoepiglottic fold and the arytenoid mucosa. In addition, deep invasion of the false vocal fold and the arytenoepiglottic fold is common. Advanced lesions may spread superficially across the postcricoid region to the opposite piriform sinus. Infiltration of the cricoarytenoid muscles, the cricoarytenoid joint, the thyroarytenoid muscles, or the recurrent laryngeal nerve may result in vocal fold fixation. Further deep invasion results in involvement of the paraglottic and pre-epiglottic spaces. Growth into the cervical esophagus is a late occurrence. Tumors developing on the lateral wall invade the posterior thyroid cartilage ala and the posterosuperior portion of the cricoid cartilage early in their course. Thyroid gland invasion may occur directly from the apex or through the cricothyroid membrane. Submucosal spread to the contiguous posterior hypopharyngeal wall is common. The most extensive piriform sinus lesions invade all three walls and the soft tissues of the neck.

Postcricoid pharyngeal malignancies tend to invade the posterior cricoarytenoid muscle and the cricoid and arytenoid cartilages before diagnosis. Advanced lesions encircle the hypopharyngeal lumen, enter the esophagus, and invade the piriform sinus.

The hypopharynx, especially the piriform sinus, is profusely invested with capillary lymphatic veins. The jugular chain nodes, particularly the midjugular and jugulodigastric lymph nodes, are the main lymphatic drainage sites for the hypopharynx. Spinal accessory and paratracheal nodes are occasionally involved. Approximately 75% of hypopharyngeal lesions have clinically malignant cervical nodes at diagnosis without regard to T stage; of these, 10% to 20% are bilateral. In addition, there is nearly a 60% incidence of subclinical disease. The thyroid gland is directly invaded in 10% of cases. If clinically palpable nodes are present, there is a 20% to 25% incidence of distant metastases in 1 to 2 years.

Diagnosis

Sore throat, especially unilateral, is the most common symptom of hypopharyngeal malignancies. Dysphagia, odynophagia, referred otalgia, aspiration, and hoarseness appear with progressive disease. Dysphagia may be manifested earlier with postcricoid lesions than with tumors of the piriform sinus or the posterior hypopharyngeal wall. A neck mass may sometimes be the presenting symptom. Weight loss is associated with advanced disease.

Indirect laryngoscopy and rigid or flexible fiberoptic laryngoscopy is used to visualize the hypopharynx. The most inferior aspect of the hypopharynx cannot be visualized with these methods. Phonation and Valsalva's maneuver performed by the patient may improve the examination of the piriform sinuses. Subtle asymmetry and salivary pooling may be clues to a hypopharyngeal mass. Manipulation of the thyroid cartilage laterally against the posterior hypopharyngeal wall typically produces the sound of a click as the superior thyroid horns hit the spine. This click is often lost with postcricoid lesions. Direct extralaryngeal spread may be palpable. A work-up for metastases, including chest radiographs and evaluation of liver function, is usually sufficient for an examination for metastases.

Computed tomography is essential in defining the extent of disease. A barium swallow may help in assessing esophageal involvement or in determining the presence of a second primary lesion in the esophagus.

There is a high incidence of second upper

respiratory and alimentary primary malignancies in the presence of a hypopharyngeal carcinoma. Therefore, endoscopy is essential in planning treatment as well as in obtaining a biopsy and defining the extent of the primary lesion. The apex of the piriform sinus must be evaluated for involvement if conservation laryngeal surgery is to be considered. The cricoid cartilage is likely to be invaded if a tumor is present in the apex of the piriform sinus. In this situation, partial laryngopharyngectomy would be contraindicated.

Staging

The American Joint Committee on Cancer Staging system is most appropriately used for lesions of the piriform sinus. Lesions of the posterior hypopharyngeal wall may be more suitably staged through the use of size limits, as in the oropharynx. The T staging system for the hypopharynx is as follows:

Tis Carcinoma in situ.

T1 Confined to one site.

T2 Extension of the tumor to the adjacent region or site without fixation of the hemilarynx.

T3 Extension of the tumor to the adjacent region or site with fixation of the hemilarynx.

T4 Massive tumor invading bone or soft tissues of the neck.

Treatment

Posterior Hypopharyngeal Wall

Irradiation is the primary modality used for treatment of posterior pharyngeal wall lesions. Cure rates that are similar to those with surgery alone or combined surgery and irradiation with less morbidity may be obtained. Depending on the level of the lesion, one of the following approaches for excision may be performed: transoral excision, midline mandibulolabial glossotomy, lingual release, transhyoid excision, or lateral pharyngotomy. After excision of the mass, the area may be reconstructed with a skin graft, a free revascularized cutaneous flap, or a split jejunal revascularized transfer. More extensive lesions may be resected with a total laryngopharyngectomy, and the area may be reconstructed with a gastric transposition. This obviously results in loss of laryngeal function. In general, there is a high rate of pharyngocutaneous fistula after these procedures. More important, after resection of the posterior hypopharyngeal wall, there is a very high rate of aspiration and dysphagia, which frequently makes permanent enteral feedings necessary. In certain cases, radiation failures may be salvaged with pharyngectomy. Salvage after surgical treatment is unlikely.

Piriform Sinus

Lesions of the piriform sinus classified as T1 have a high cure rate with radiation therapy or partial laryngopharyngectomy. Irradiation has the advantage of leaving the patient's swallowing and speech relatively undisturbed while widely covering the regional lymphatic veins. T2 lesions present a more difficult treatment dilemma. Involvement of the apex of the piriform sinus is a contraindication to partial laryngopharyngectomy, and such patients do not respond well to radiation therapy. If the apex involvement is minimal, a trial of irradiation is possibly curative, and surgery is reserved for salvage. Complications of irradiation most commonly are limited to laryngeal edema and necrosis.

Partial laryngopharyngectomy involves removal of the hyoid bone, the epiglottis, the false vocal folds, the posterosuperior thyroid cartilage, the involved piriform sinus, and one arytenoid cartilage if indicated. The piriform sinus defect is repaired with local tissue, and the base of the tongue is sutured to the thyroid perichondrium. This procedure may be thought of as an extended supraglottic laryngectomy, and it is intended for early lesions in the piriform sinus and selected lesions with minimal invasion outside the piriform sinus. In addition to the previously mentioned contraindication, a fixed vocal fold, bilateral arytenoid involvement, and poor pulmonary reserve are also contraindications for partial laryngopharyngectomy. There is a higher incidence of aspiration after this procedure than after supraglottic laryngectomy. Pharyngocutaneous fistulas and dysphagia also occur in approximately 10% of patients. A cricopharyngeal myotomy may decrease the incidence of dysphagia and aspiration somewhat. A supracricoid hemilaryngopharyngectomy has been used as an extension of the partial laryngopharyngectomy for more extensive lesions of the supracricoid piriform sinus with normal vocal fold mobility. The main difference is that the hemilarynx is included in the resection.

More advanced lesions (T3 and T4) are best treated with total laryngectomy and partial pharyngectomy with postoperative irradiation. This procedure involves removal of the larynx, the hyoid bone, and a sufficient amount of the pharynx to extirpate the tumor. If minimal amounts of pharyngeal mucosa are removed, then primary closure is possible. The resection of extensive pharyngeal lesions requires the use of a musculocutaneous flap for acceptable closure of the pharynx. Attempts to close the pharynx with inadequate tissue result in an extremely high incidence of fistula formation and pharyngeal stenosis. Lesions involving the circumference of the hypopharynx or with significant esophageal extension are best managed with a total laryngopharyngectomy. Reconstruction is then best achieved with either gastric transposition or a jejunal interposition. Tubed cutaneous flaps have an unacceptable rate of stenosis and fistula formation. Several factors, including local skill and expertise of the surgeon, must be considered when the choice is between gastric transposition and jejunal interposition. Both procedures require opening the abdomen, but gastric transposition also violates the mediastinum. Gastric transposition is clearly indicated when substantial esophageal involvement requires an esophagectomy. Either reconstructive option provides acceptable swallowing function; gastric transposition is slightly more likely to allow acquisition of neopharyngeal speech.

Postcricoid Pharynx

Postcricoid carcinomas are generally treated only by total laryngectomy and partial pharyngectomy with musculocutaneous flap closure. As with lesions of the piriform sinus, involvement of the circumferential hypopharyngeal wall and significant esophageal disease require a circumferential total laryngopharyngectomy. Radiation therapy alone is not commonly used for these lesions, but most patients benefit from the addition of postoperative irradiation.

Neck

The choice of treatment of the neck is highly influenced by the preponderance of clinically malignant neck nodes and the significant incidence of occult disease. If radiation alone is to be used for the primary lesion in the absence of positive nodes, then radiation alone is also used to effectively manage occult disease. In the presence of positive nodes, a neck dissection is performed after irradiation. When combined management is to be used, as is the case for all but a few early lesions in the hypopharynx, then a neck dissection is performed in conjunction with the surgical treatment of the primary. Postoperative irradiation is added for the following indications: multiple positive nodes, extranodal spread, close or positive margins, soft tissue extension, or cartilage invasion. In addition, postoperative radiation is effective in controlling occult disease in the contralateral, unoperated side of the neck. Preoperative irradiation is used only in the case of initially unresectable nodes.

Chemotherapy

As in the case of laryngeal carcinomas, there is no indication that chemotherapy in any sequence has significantly altered locoregional control or overall survival rates for carcinomas of the hypopharynx.

Vocal Rehabilitation

The success of vocal rehabilitation after surgery for hypopharyngeal carcinoma is dependent on the extent of pharynx removed and the method of reconstruction used. Speech after partial laryngopharyngectomy is excellent because the vocal folds are preserved. Tracheoesophageal puncture is the most effective means for re-establishing speech after total laryngectomy with partial pharyngectomy. If a musculocutaneous flap is used in reconstruction of the pharynx, the rate of acquisition of tracheoesophageal speech decreases. Tracheoenteral puncture after gastric transposition has limited success in re-establishing speech. Spontaneous gastric speech similar to esophageal speech is possible for a few patients. The acquisition of either of these forms of speech is especially unlikely after jejunal interposition. Most of these patients rely on external vibratory devices for communication.

Results

The results for management of posterior hypopharyngeal wall lesions with radiation are not good. The 5-year determinate survival rates are approximately 29% for stage II lesions, 11% for stage III lesions, and 10% for stage IV lesions. The combination of irradiation and surgery has achieved equally disappointing results. The absolute 5-year survival rate for all stages is in the range of 20%.

The treatment outcome for piriform sinus carcinomas is somewhat better than that for posterior hypopharyngeal wall tumors. The 2-year survival rate for patients with stage I lesions managed with irradiation alone is around 70%. An additional 40% of failures are salvageable with surgery. A similar survival rate is obtainable in early lesions with partial laryngopharyngectomy or total laryngectomy and postoperative radiation therapy. Highly selected T2 and T3 lesions may be treated with irradiation alone; local control rates are around 70%. The most common cause of failure, however, is the inability to control advanced neck disease. Combined surgery and radiation are used most frequently for T2 to T4 lesions; 5-year survival rates are in the 35% range for early stages and the 20% to 25% range for more advanced stages. The most common cause of death in the advanced stages is distant metastases. In general, the best results are obtained with either conservation surgery or irradiation for T1 and selected T2 lesions and with combination therapy for all more extensive lesions.

BENIGN NEOPLASMS OF THE CERVICAL ESOPHAGUS

Benign neoplasms of the esophagus are infrequently encountered; they constitute 0.5% to 0.8% of all esophageal lesions. Leiomyomas are overwhelmingly the most common benign tumor of the esophagus, and yet carcinoma is still 50 times more common. Patients with leiomyomas typically present with dysphagia. An intraluminal mass is detected on barium swallow or at the time of esophagoscopy. Limited lesions may be excised endoscopically; large lesions require a thoracotomy with esophagectomy. Fortunately, only 10% of leiomyomas require removal. Other myomas encountered in the esophagus include fibromyomas and lipomyomas.

A large variety of other benign neoplasms are encountered in the esophagus: hemangiomas, lymphangiomas, reticuloendothelial tumors, lipomas, giant-cell tumors, neurofibromas, osteochondromas, papillomas, polyps, adenomas, gastric mucosal tumors, sebaceous cell tumors, and thyroid nodules. These lesions are all extremely rare. Symptoms and management are determined by the size and the location of the tumors. Granular cell tumors also occur in the cervical esophagus. They should be managed carefully because they typically behave more aggressively than those found in the tongue. There have been rare reports of metastases.

CARCINOMA OF THE CERVICAL ESOPHAGUS

An estimated 10,000 cases of cancer of the esophagus were diagnosed in the United States in 1989. The age-adjusted incidence rates of esophageal cancer were 4.8% and 1.6% for White males and females and 16.9% and 4.5% for Black males and females, respectively. Carcinoma of the cervical esophagus is relatively rare, representing 3.6% to 33% of all esophageal malignancies. Interestingly, cervical esophageal carcinoma, as opposed to all other lesions of the head and neck and of the thoracic esophagus, is more common in women. Affected persons are usually in their sixth or seventh decade of life.

There is a strong history of heavy alcohol use and cigarette smoking in the vast majority of patients with cervical esophageal carcinoma. There are also high incidences of malnutrition, cardiovascular disease, and cirrhosis. Patients with Plummer-Vinson syndrome are at risk for cervical esophageal malignancies as well as hypopharyngeal cancers.

Anatomy

The cervical esophagus is a 6- to 8-cm inferior extension of the hypopharynx, beginning at the level of the sixth cervical vertebra and arbitrarily terminating at the thoracic inlet. This inferior margin is roughly at the level of the superior manubrium. As it progresses inferiorly, the cervical esophagus shifts slightly to the left of the trachea. The trachea and the recurrent laryngeal nerves are anterior. The thyroid gland and the carotid sheath are lateral to the esophagus, and the prevertebral fascia is posterior. The cervical esophagus consists of only squamous epithelium surrounded by an inner circular and an outer longitudinal muscle layer.

Pathology

Squamous cell carcinoma makes up 95% of esophageal cancers; adenocarcinomas represent most of the balance. Adenocarcinoma is especially uncommon in the upper esophagus.

Patterns of Spread

Carcinoma of the esophagus is believed to arise from transition of dysplasia to carcinoma in situ and eventually to frank carcinoma. Submucosal spread beyond the obvious mucosal lesion is extremely common, as are "skip" lesions. Extensive malignancies may extend to involve the larynx, the hypopharynx, the trachea, the thyroid gland, the recurrent laryngeal nerves, and the great vessels of the neck.

The lymphatic veins of the cervical esophagus are relatively abundant. Drainage is to the peritracheal nodes, the periesophageal nodes, the lower internal jugular chain, and the supraclavicular nodes. The upper mediastinal nodes are the next site of drainage for the peritracheal and periesophageal nodal groups. The incidence of lymph node metastases varies upward with increasing length of the lesion: from 50% with tumors less than 5 cm in diameter to 90% with tumors greater than 5 cm in diameter. Distant metastases are common and most often involve the liver and the lungs.

Diagnosis

Dysphagia and weight loss are the two most frequent presenting symptoms. With cervical esophageal carcinomas, dysphagia occurs early as a result of the narrow nature of the lumen, as opposed to that of the pharynx. Direct extension to the larynx or the recurrent laryngeal nerves may cause dyspnea and hoarseness.

Physical findings are usually limited to indirect signs such as pooling of saliva in the hypopharynx, fullness in the lower neck, and vocal fold fixation. Lower cervical metastases may be palpable.

Contrast radiologic examination of the esophagus is usually diagnostic. In addition, a tracheoesophageal fistula may be demonstrated. Computed tomography and magnetic resonance imaging are useful in evaluating soft tissue extension and in identifying nodal metastases.

Esophagoscopy is used to obtain tissue for diagnosis and to delineate the lesion. Great care must be taken in order not to perforate an already weakened esophagus. Bronchoscopy is performed to evaluate possible direct tracheal invasion. A second primary lesion is present in up to 25% of the patients with esophageal cancers.

Staging

The American Joint Committee on Cancer Staging system for primary esophageal tumors is listed as follows:

Tis   Carcinoma in situ.
T1   Tumor invades the lamina propria submucosa.
T2   Tumor invades the muscularis propria.
T3   Tumor invades the adventitia.
T4   Tumor invades adjacent structures.

Treatment

The current treatment options include surgery, irradiation, or combination therapy. The role of chemotherapy is investigational at present.

Irradiation, although rarely curative, is the most simple noninvasive form of palliation for cervical esophageal carcinoma. Selected early lesions in patients who are not candidates for surgery may be treated for cure. The most common acute complications are esophagitis and transient radiation pneumonitis. When the lesion has invaded the trachea or the great vessels, a tracheoesophageal or tracheovascular fistula may develop during irradiation. Late effects of irradiation are limited primarily to esophageal stenosis, but a rare case of radiation myelitis may occur. At present, the most frequent role for radiotherapy is in combination with surgical resection.

Patients who are in reasonable medical condition are treated with a combination of radiotherapy and surgery in hopes of improving the likelihood of local control and in order to obtain an acceptable functional result. Surgery may be viewed as curative or palliative. Only 30% of lesions are initially resectable. Depending on the extent and location of the tumor, a curative resection includes a cervical or total esophagectomy with or without an en bloc laryngopharyngectomy. A neck dissection is included for clinically malignant nodes. The value of a superior mediastinal nodal dissection remains unclear.

A variety of procedures have been used to reconstruct the esophageal site. Pedicled and free skin grafts are mainly of historical interest and are rarely used today. The most commonly used reconstructive methods at present are free jejunal revascularized grafts, gastric transposition, and colon interposition. All of these procedures may be performed in one stage, but they all carry the risk of graft failure, anastomotic leakage, and stenosis. The perioperative mortality may approach 5%, especially in this somewhat debilitated population. Hypocalcemia, dumping syndrome, and regurgitation are commonly associated with gastric transposition. If the larynx is saved, aspiration is a frequent complication no matter which reconstructive technique is chosen.

Palliative surgery is an attempt to allow the patient to swallow his or her own secretions and is most often used if palliative radiotherapy fails. A bypass procedure is frequently successful but carries a significant rate of morbidity and mortality. Placement of esophageal stents and laser debulking of esophageal lesions have met with mixed results in achieving palliation. A gastrostomy or a jejunostomy allows the patient to at least maintain some nutrition.

Recurrence is the rule rather than the exception with cervical esophageal carcinoma and may be at the primary site or in regional nodes. Salvage is rarely if ever practical or successful.

Chemotherapy

Although carcinoma of the esophagus responds impressively at times to various chemotherapeutic agents, there is no evidence at present of an improved cure rate with their use. Currently, several treatment protocols involve the use of chemotherapy as part of combined therapy management.

Results

No randomized trials with which to compare treatment modalities for cervical esophageal malignancies are available. Most series report cure rates of 10% to 20% regardless of the use of radiation, surgery, or combination therapy. Long-term survival rates have in fact not been altered by transcervical esophagectomy and gastric transposition; however, palliation has been achieved.

SUGGESTED READINGS

Bailey BJ, Biller HF (eds): Surgery of the Larynx. Philadelphia: WB Saunders, 1985.

Batsakis JG: Tumors of the Head and Neck. Baltimore: Williams & Wilkins, 1979.

DeSanto LW, Devine KD, Weiland LH: Cyst of the larynx—classification. Laryngoscope 80:145–176, 1970.

Guedea F, Parsons JT, Mendenhall WM, et al: Primary subglottic cancer: results of radical radiation therapy. Int J Radiat Oncol Biol Phys, in press.

Holinger LD, Barnes DR, Smid LJ, Holinger PH: Laryngocele and saccular cysts. Ann Otol Rhinol Laryngol 87:675–685, 1978.

Mendenhall WM, Parsons JT, Brant TA, et al: Is elective neck treatment indicated for T2 N0 squamous cell carcinoma of the glottic larynx? Radiol Oncol 14:199–202, 1989.

Mendenhall WM, Parsons JT, Cassisi NJ, et al: Radiation therapy in the management of early laryngeal and pyriform sinus cancer. In Silver CE (ed): Laryngeal Cancer. New York: Thieme Medical Publishers, in press.

Mendenhall WM, Parsons JT, Devine JW, et al: Squamous cell carcinoma of the pyriform sinus treated with surgery and/or radiotherapy. Head Neck 10:88–92, 1987.

Mendenhall WM, Parsons JT, Mancuso AA, et al: Cancer of the larynx. In Perex CA, Brady LW (eds): Principles and Practice of Radiation Oncology, 2nd ed. Philadelphia: JP Lippincott, in press.

Mendenhall WM, Parsons JT, Stringer SP, et al: T1-T2 vocal cord carcinoma: a basis for comparing the results of radiotherapy and surgery. Head Neck 10:373–377, 1988.

Mendenhall WM, Parsons JT, Stringer SP, et al: Carcinoma of the supraglottic larynx: a basis for comparing the results of irradiation and surgery. Head Neck 12:204–209, 1990.

Million RR, Cassisi NJ (eds): Management of Head and Neck Cancer. Philadelphia: JP Lippincott, 1984.

Million RR, Mendenhall WM, Parsons JT, et al: Irradiation and surgery in the management of neck node metastases from squamous cell carcinoma of the head and neck. In Fee WF, Goepfert H, Johns ME, et al (eds): Head and Neck Cancer, vol 2 (pp 144–150). Toronto: BC Decker, 1989.

Myssiorek D, Persky M: Laser endoscopic treatment of laryngoceles and laryngeal cysts. Otolaryngol Head Neck Surg 100:538–541, 1989.

Parsons JT, Mendenhall WM, Mancuso AA, et al: Twice a day radiotherapy for T3 squamous cell carcinoma of the glottic larynx. Head Neck 11:123–189, 1989.

CHAPTER 43

Intubation, Tracheotomy, and Cricothyrotomy

Donald B. Hawkins, MD

INTUBATION

Of the three methods of airway intervention that are discussed in this chapter, intubation is the least invasive in that it does not require a surgical incision. It is currently the preferred method of airway management whenever possible. Two conditions in which it is not optimal are laryngeal fractures from blunt neck trauma, in which tracheotomy would be the optimal method for establishing an airway, and in patients with suspected cervical spine injuries, in whom extension of the neck is contraindicated and cricothyrotomy is the preferred method of airway intervention. Until the 1970s, intubation was considered to be contraindicated in acute inflammatory obstruction of the larynx except as a prelude to tracheotomy because of the concern that intubation of inflamed larynges would result in laryngeal stenosis. First with acute epiglottitis and later with laryngotracheobronchitis, intubation became the accepted method of emergency airway management even with inflamed larynges during the 1970s.

Intubation for surgical anesthesia under controlled conditions in the operating room is easier than with emergency situations occurring outside of the operating room. In any situation, intubation should be performed in as orderly and controlled a manner as possible. If there is sufficient time to take the patient safely to an operating room, that should be done. If there is not sufficient time

for safe transport, intubation should be immediately performed wherever the patient is. Most emergency rooms or intensive care units are well equipped for emergency intubations.

Insertion of the endotracheal tube into the larynx and trachea should be performed as atraumatically as possible. A variety of intubation laryngoscopes are available, the essential elements of which are a good light and a blade long enough to reach the epiglottis of the patient. Another essential for intubation is good suction. A straight blade is best for intubating children, but curved blades are preferred by some for adults. The author prefers a Jackson laryngoscope with a removable slot for intubation. The endotracheal tube must be straightened to be inserted through a Jackson laryngoscope, whereas it is curved for insertion through the standard intubating laryngoscopes. The endotracheal tube should be large enough to allow adequate ventilation and suctioning but should not be too large for the patient's larynx.

A useful rule for treating children is that the endotracheal tube inner diameter (ID) in millimeters equals the patient's age plus 16 and divided by 4; for instance, a 4-year-old would take a 5.0-mm ID tube. This formula is used if the patient has a normal larynx. Smaller tubes should be used in larynges narrowed by acute inflammatory edema or chronic scarring. Cuffed tubes generally are not used in children under 7 or 8 years of age unless the child's lungs are so noncompliant, or stiff, that a cuff is necessary for adequate ventilation. When a noncuffed tube is used, it is reassuring to have an air leak at respirator pressures that are appropriate for the patient, which indicates that the tube is not too tight in the larynx.

The endotracheal tube can be passed orally or nasally. The oral route is quicker and should be used in emergencies. Once an airway is established by the orotracheal route, another endotracheal tube can be inserted nasally. Under direct vision with a laryngoscope inserted orally, the two tubes can be switched at the larynx. Nasotracheal tubes are more easily stabilized than are orotracheal ones. They are also more comfortable for long-term intubation of adults and children with teeth, who must have an oral airway or bite block taped in their mouths to prevent them from chewing on an orotracheal tube. For long-term intubation of neonates and infants without teeth and for short-term (2 to 4 days) intubation of anyone, the oral route is probably preferable.

Orotracheal intubation obviously avoids the possibility of nasal stenosis that may develop as a complication of nasotracheal intubation. Although the increased stability of a nasotracheal tube makes accidental extubation less likely, it does not make it less likely to injure the larynx. Fixation of the tube at the nose or the lips does not mean fixation in the larynx. Elevation of the larynx with spontaneous swallowing and movement by the patient results in motion of the larynx over the endotracheal tube. It is also possible that the curve, as well as the increased fixation, of a nasotracheal tube may result in more pressure being exerted on the posterior glottic and subglottic larynx than occurs with an orotracheal tube.

Nasotracheal tubes can be passed over a flexible laryngoscope. This is a useful technique in patients whose mouths cannot be opened, those with kyphosis, or those who cannot lie down safely.

Complications

Complications from insertion of the endotracheal tube can be minimized by having adequate equipment as described earlier and by having the patient's head in the proper position. Physicians inexperienced with endoscopy often extend the patient's neck more than is optimal for intubation. The best head position for exposing the larynx is the so-called sniffing position: flexion of the neck on the chest and extension of the head on the neck. Complications that may occur during intubation are injury to the teeth, the lips, and the oropharyngeal structures; perforation of the vallecula or the piriform sinus; intubation of the esophagus; and injury to the arytenoid cartilages or the vocal cords. Subcutaneous emphysema in the neck shortly after a difficult intubation is highly suggestive of a perforation of the hypopharynx or, less likely, perforation of the trachea or the esophagus. In these cases, the patient should be started on intravenous antibiotic therapy, and serial chest radiographs should be taken to search for pneumomediastinum or pneumothorax. Intubation of the esophagus rather than the airway can be fatal if not detected rapidly. Usually it is possible to detect whether the endotracheal tube is in the trachea by auscultation of the breath sounds in the chest. Occasionally, sounds transmitted from the esophagus during vigorous squeezing of the ventilation bag can be mistaken for breath sounds in the lung. If it does not look as if the patient is being ventilated, if the skin is dusky, or if the oxygen saturation is dropping, the larynx must be re-examined immediately to determine the position of the endotracheal tube.

The nursing care that is required for an intubated patient is essentially the same as for a patient with a tracheotomy. Both require increased humidification of the inspired air and frequent suctioning. Patients with tracheotomies can be more mobile and are more comfortable. Once the tract between skin and trachea has formed (between 4 and 7 days postoperatively), tracheotomy tubes are easier than endotracheal tubes to reinsert if either should come out accidentally. Orotracheal intubation prevents oral feeding, and nasotracheal intubation severely limits it.

Postintubation Stenosis

Prolonged endotracheal intubation may result in laryngeal scarring and stenosis. This can occur at the glottic or the subglottic level or both. Ischemia of the tracheal wall from cuff inflation pressure can also cause tracheal stenosis. Airway stenosis develops in a relatively small percentage of intubated patients. Some authors have estimated an incidence of more than 3%, but it probably is less than that. When stenosis does develop, however, it can be a very serious problem.

The factors that contribute to development of glottic or subglottic stenosis in intubated patients include traumatic intubation, prolonged duration of intubation, multiple extubations and reintubations, too large a tube for the larynx, motion of the patient or of the endotracheal tube, local infection, and very low birth weight in neonates. Factors that were important in the 1960s and early 1970s were the composition and shape of endotracheal tubes as well as toxic residue of ethylene oxide sterilization. These are no longer problematic because almost all tubes in use are uniform-diameter disposable tubes composed of tissue-tested polyvinyl chloride. For any patient who develops glottic or subglottic stenosis, several of the preceding factors may have been involved. The common denominator is trauma to the larynx. Prolonged duration of intubation is usually considered to be the most important factor. It alone, without one or more of the aforementioned trauma-related risk factors, does not result in laryngeal stenosis. In addition, if sufficient trauma occurs with the initial intubation, stenosis can develop even though the intubation may be of short duration.

The length of time that an endotracheal tube can remain in the larynx without resulting in stenosis varies with each situation. So many factors are involved that each patient must be considered individually. For instance, if there have been several extubations and reintubations, especially if reintubation was difficult and traumatic, or if the patient is mobile while the tube is in place, the intubation should be converted to tracheotomy relatively early. On the other hand, if the patient is completely immobile, if the intubation was not traumatic, and if the endotracheal tube is not too large, it can be kept in place for an extended period of time. Neonates, especially premature neonates, because of the resilience of their larynges, can often tolerate weeks or months of intubation. The resiliency of the neonatal larynx, however, cannot be duplicated in older patients. The older the patient is, the shorter the duration of intubation should be.

These statements may seem to be inconsistent with the earlier statement that low birth weight is a risk factor for development of subglottic stenosis. The reason that very small premature neonates (under 1000 g) are at increased risk is that their larynges may

be too small for the outer diameter of the smallest functional endotracheal tubes. Also, they often require very prolonged intubation. It is surprising that not all intubated neonates of birth weight under 1000 g develop subglottic stenosis. Some do not because of the resiliency of their immature cricoid cartilages.

As mentioned, neonates can often tolerate intubation of weeks' or months' duration. In the absence of trauma-related risk factors, children under 1 year of age probably can tolerate intubation for 3 or more weeks. Those between 1 and 5 years of age should be allowed less intubation time—for instance, approximately 2 weeks. In those over 5 years of age, shorter periods of intubation, depending on the circumstances, should be considered. Toward the end of these periods, tracheotomy should be considered seriously if the patient still needs respirator support. The assumption of these statements is that the patients had normal larynges before intubation. In patients with inflamed or known stenotic larynges, intubation should be as brief as possible.

TRACHEOTOMY

Tracheotomy was mentioned in medical literature dating back to the second century, and the performance of successful tracheotomies was reported in the 16th and 17th centuries. The procedure increased in popularity and usage in the latter part of the 19th century and first two thirds of the 20th century.

The traditional three categories of indications for tracheotomy are to relieve upper airway obstruction, to assist ventilation, and to facilitate pulmonary or tracheal toilet. Relief of upper airway obstruction appears to have been the only indication until the 1940s, when tracheotomy began to be used for pulmonary toilet and to assist ventilation in patients with bulbar poliomyelitis. Since that time, the application of the three tracheotomy indications has been in a state of constant evolution. In the middle 1960s, most tracheotomies still were being performed for upper airway obstruction. This is shown by the report of Holinger and coworkers (1965), according to which 90% of 86 infant tracheotomies were for upper airway obstruction. Even then, the authors noted that the number of tracheotomies for acute infections of the airway was decreasing "due to earlier diagnosis, the use of high humidity, and antibiotics." Of historical interest is their mention of the early trend toward "prolonged" intubation rather than tracheotomy for ventilation. They stated that tracheotomy is indicated if intubation is required for longer than 12 to 24 hours.

During the 1970s and early 1980s, short-term intubation for airway obstruction from acute infections and long-term intubation for patients on ventilators replaced early tracheotomy for these conditions. Not only has the number of tracheotomies performed to assist ventilation decreased, but those that are done are likely to be of longer duration. Tracheotomies done in earlier years after 48 to 72 hours of intubation often were short-term tracheotomies. Those done currently because of continued ventilatory need after several weeks of intubation may be required for a long time. Upper airway obstruction is still the most common indication for tracheotomy, but the conditions have become more chronic in nature. Instead of short-term tracheotomy for acute upper airway infections, an increase has been seen in the numbers of tracheotomies for postintubation laryngeal stenosis as well as congenital upper airway and mandibulofacial abnormalities. Improvements in the medical management of critically ill, severely injured, and handicapped patients has resulted in their increased survival; some require long-term tracheotomies. The result of all these changes, especially in pediatrics, is that fewer tracheotomies are being performed, and a large percentage of those are long-term tracheotomies. This trend has been reported from several medical centers throughout the world (Wetmore et al., 1982; Carter and Benjamin, 1983; Line et al., 1986; Crysdale et al., 1988).

Terminology

The name that is given to the procedure, *tracheotomy* or *tracheostomy*, is a matter of controversy. Some otolaryngologists insist that the term *tracheostomy* should be used only when the tracheal opening is sutured to the skin as after total laryngectomy. That seems reasonable, but Dorland's Illustrated Medical Dictionary (1985) does not agree completely. It defines tracheostomy as "the surgical creation of an opening into the trachea through the neck, with the tracheal mucosa being brought into continuity with the skin" and states that "the term is also used to refer to creation of an opening in the anterior trachea for insertion of a tube." *Tracheotomy* is defined simply as "incision of the trachea." From those definitions, it seems that although the dictionary prefers tracheostomy, either term should be appropriate for the procedure discussed in this chapter. In the reality of common usage, that is the way it is. The author prefers to use the "-ostomy" term as in its first definition and to use "-otomy" for opening the trachea and inserting a tube. Also, dropping the "s" seems to make the word less cumbersome.

Surgical Technique

The surgical technique of tracheotomy has undergone many variations by individual physicians. The following description makes no attempt to describe all of those variations but is intended to be a general discussion.

If an endotracheal tube or a bronchoscope is in place, the procedure can be done under general or local anesthesia. If an airway is not established before tracheotomy, the procedure usually must be done while the patient is under local anesthesia. Most tracheotomies since 1975 have probably been performed over indwelling endotracheal tubes. Either a midline vertical incision or a horizontal incision is made in the lower portion of the neck. A vertical incision gives a better view of the vertical anatomic landmarks and perhaps makes midline dissection easier. In small children, it allows the tracheotomy tube to better settle into proper alignment between skin and trachea. A horizontal incision ultimately heals with less of a scar, and it is better for suturing an inferiorly based tracheal flap. After the skin incision, the trachea is approached by blunt dissection in the midline.

Each new tissue layer that is opened by the dissection is retracted on each side by the surgeon and assistants standing on each side of the patient. In children, bleeding is minimal with blunt dissection in the midline. Seldom is ligation of vessels or much cautery necessary. In adults, ligation of prominent vessels may be necessary. Bleeding should be controlled before the trachea is opened. The isthmus of the thyroid gland is identified lying anterior to the first two or three tracheal rings. The cricoid cartilage may or may not be identified. The thyroid isthmus may or may not be transected, depending on the judgment of the surgeon. Openings into the trachea are usually made in the area of rings three, four, or five. When the tracheal opening is made, the endotracheal tube is slowly withdrawn until it is slightly superior to the opening. The tracheotomy cannula is then inserted. The endotracheal tube should not be removed until it can be determined that the patient is being ventilated well bilaterally through the tracheotomy tube.

In adults and older children, the author constructs an inferiorly based flap of anterior tracheal wall that is sutured to the lower skin flap. In children under the age of approximately 8 years, a vertical incision is made through two or three tracheal rings. In these younger children, traction sutures are often placed through the anterior tracheal wall lateral to the incision. The author has mixed feelings about these sutures. They provide a safety feature in the case of accidental decannulation, but it is suspected that they may contribute to development of tracheomalacia in some patients. The inferiorly based tracheal flap technique makes replacement of the cannula easier in the event of accidental decannulation, but the author hesitates to use it in young children because of concern regarding possible development of tracheomalacia. Another concern is that in young children who are on respirators and have noncuffed tracheotomy tubes, there is a larger leakage from the stoma of a flap tracheotomy than from one made with a vertical incision. With either method, the flanges of the tracheotomy cannula are sutured to the skin, and tracheotomy ties are secured around the neck. The flange-to-skin sutures and the traction sutures are removed in approximately 7 days. The incision is sutured loosely or not at all.

Posttracheotomy Care

Postoperatively the patients are kept in either an intensive care unit or a step-down unit with constant nursing care and observation. A chest film is taken to check the cannula position in relation to the carina and to look for pneumomediastinum or pneumothorax. Frequent suctioning of the cannula and continuous mist to the tracheotomy are the two essentials of postoperative care for preventing tracheal cannula obstruction from crust-

ing and mucus plugs. If the tracheotomy tube has an inner cannula, it should be removed and cleaned at set intervals, usually every 2 hours initially and every 4 hours later.

It is difficult to state an exact schedule for suctioning, but the routine for children is to suction every 30 minutes, and more frequently as needed, for the first 12 hours postoperatively. After 12 hours, the time interval for routine suctioning is increased to 1 hour with more frequent suctioning as necessary. As the postoperative time increases, the intervals between routine suctioning may increase further, depending on the needs of the particular patient. In general, the smaller the tracheal cannula is, the more frequently it needs to be suctioned. Mist is applied to the tracheotomy continuously for 48 hours postoperatively and at least 50% of the time after 48 hours. Increased humidification of the inspired air is especially critical for the smaller tracheotomies, which can easily become obstructed with drying of secretions. On the other hand, too much mist delivered to the younger patients may induce bronchospasm and compromise their lower respiratory tract function.

Tracheotomy Tubes

The tracheotomy tubes that the author uses are the Shiley pediatric and adult plastic tubes and the Jackson and Holinger metal tubes. Shiley tubes are used in almost all cases in children. Shiley pediatric tubes come in sizes 00 to 4. The 00 and 0 sizes also have a neonatal design that has a shorter cannula and a shorter flange than the pediatric design.

Table 43–1 shows the comparative outer diameters of the three types of tracheotomy tubes. The metal tubes are consistent in outer diameters through size 6, after which the Holinger tubes are larger. The Shiley plastic tubes have the same outer diameter as the metal tubes through the pediatric size 4, which is 8.0 mm. Above that, Shiley tubes vary. There is a cuffed adult size 4 whose outer diameter is 8.5 mm. Shiley tubes with cuffs and inner cannulas are available in even-numbered sizes only. Those with cuffs but no inner cannula are available in all sizes 5 through 10. As shown in Table 43–1, the single-cannula tubes have smaller outer diameters than the double-cannula tubes do, except for size 10. The metal Jackson and

TABLE 43–1. Tracheotomy Tube Outer Diameters (in Millimeters)

Size	Jackson	Holinger	Shiley
000	—	4.1	—
00	4.5	4.5	4.5
0	5.0	5.0	5.0
1	5.5	5.5	5.5
2	6.0	6.0	6.0
3	7.0	7.0	7.0
4	8.0	8.0	8.0—Pediatric
			8.5—Adult
5	9.0	9.0	7.0*
6	10.0	10.0	8.3*
			10.0†
7	11.0	12.0	9.6*
8	12.0	13.6	10.9*
			12.0†
9	13.0	14.0	12.1*
10	14.0	14.3	13.3*
			13.0†

*Single cannula; †double cannula.

Holinger tubes do not have cuffs but have inner cannulas in all sizes.

Without an inner cannula to be removed and cleaned at intervals, a metal tracheotomy tube would become occluded by crusting within the inferior aspect of its lumen. Because of decreased surface tension, Shiley pediatric tubes are less likely to become occluded, making an inner cannula unnecessary. The absence of an inner cannula makes nursing care easier and provides a larger lumen for breathing and clearing of secretions. A disadvantage of not having an inner cannula is that the entire tracheotomy tube must be removed and replaced if it becomes obstructed. That, however, seems to be a very rare occurrence with Shiley pediatric tubes. Another disadvantage is that the flaccidity of Shiley pediatric tubes possibly makes accidental decannulation more likely to occur.

Complications

The most frequent early complication, defined as that noted within 24 hours of tracheotomy, is pneumomediastinum. This often is asymptomatic unless it is associated with a large pneumothorax. The most serious early complications are cannula obstruction, accidental decannulation, and tension pneumothorax. Any of these three can result in rapid death of the patient, and this is the reason why all new tracheotomy patients need constant observation. Cannula obstruction can

be prevented by applying mist and frequently suctioning the tracheotomy. Decannulation can be prevented by tying the tracheotomy tape snugly around the neck and suturing the flanges to the skin. Pneumomediastinum and pneumothorax can be prevented or minimized by having an endotracheal tube or bronchoscope in place for an airway before the tracheotomy and by careful dissection in the pretracheal area. General anesthesia or local anesthesia combined with muscle paralysis prevents movement of the patient during the procedure and makes pneumomediastinum or pneumothorax less likely to develop.

In an immediate posttracheotomy patient on a respirator, careful attention to the respirator pressures may prevent or help detect a tension pneumothorax. Excessively high pressures and restlessness of the patient may contribute to development of a pneumothorax. Also, a need for increasing pressures over a short period of time in order to accomplish ventilation may indicate that a tension pneumothorax is developing. If a pneumothorax is suspected, an x-ray film of the chest must be obtained immediately. Other early complications, usually more annoying than serious, are subcutaneous emphysema and bleeding from the wound. Subcutaneous emphysema may occur along with pneumomediastinum from surgery or may result from closing the wound too tightly. The bleeding usually is persistent, slow oozing. Seldom is a major vessel involved at this stage. It usually can be controlled by packing the wound with a hemostatic substance such as absorbable knitted fabric (Surgicel). Packing too tightly, however, can contribute to the development of subcutaneous emphysema or pneumomediastinum.

The most common serious late complications are also obstruction of the cannula and accidental decannulation. Obstruction of the cannula from crusting, with possible fatal results, is a possibility as long as the tracheotomy is in place, especially with small children. For this reason, patients with chronic tracheotomies should have added humidification of inspired air when they are sleeping. Suctioning in long-term tracheotomies obviously is not necessary every hour, but it should be done routinely several times a day and more often as needed. A useful technique for dislodging mucus is to instill 1 or 2 mL of saline into the tracheotomy before suctioning. Accidental decannulation may not create an acute emergency if the patient has a normal airway but needs the tracheotomy for periodic respirator use. On the other hand, a patient with significant airway stenosis above the tracheotomy may die within minutes of accidental decannulation if the tracheotomy is not replaced. Medical and nursing personnel too often consider all tracheotomy patients as similar, but it is important to differentiate the two categories.

Another serious but, fortunately, rare late complication is hemorrhage from the innominate artery, which is fatal if it is not detected and managed immediately. Pneumomediastinum and pneumothorax occasionally occur as late complications from difficulty with changing of the tracheotomy tube or excessive respirator pressures. Infection to some degree occurs in almost every tracheotomy stoma, but this usually is not a significant problem. Granulation tissue develops on the anterior tracheal wall just above the tracheotomy stoma in most long-standing tracheotomies. Occasionally, a large granuloma forms and requires endoscopic removal. A depressed anterior tracheal flap above the stoma can become fibrosed to the adjacent trachea, resulting in stenosis. The destruction of too much tracheal cartilage, surgically or by pressure necrosis from the cannula, may result in a localized area of tracheomalacia. Necrosis of skin, either of the posterior neck or of the suprasternal area, may occur in neonates or infants with Shiley tracheotomy tubes in whom the tapes have been tied too tightly to prevent accidental decannulation. Tracheocutaneous fistula may also result after decannulation in long-standing tracheotomies.

Decannulation

The author's usual routine for decannulation is to remove the tracheotomy after the patient has tolerated plugging of a noncuffed cannula for 24 hours. A smaller size than the patient was wearing is often used for the purpose of plugging. Occasional children tolerate plugging of Holinger metal cannulas even though they could not tolerate plugging of the same-sized Shiley cannulas. Failure to tolerate plugging of even a small Holinger tracheotomy is usually caused by some persistent anatomic obstruction and must be investigated.

Home Care

With the increased incidence of long-term tracheotomy, there has been an increased emphasis on home care. Patients with tracheotomies should be discharged only after the parents have undergone training in tracheotomy care and cardiopulmonary resuscitation and have been provided with all of the necessary equipment to care for the tracheotomy, including suction equipment, humidification equipment, and an apnea-bradycardia monitor. Whereas adults with tracheotomies can often care for themselves, children cannot care for themselves. For children, there should be at least two adults in the home who are skilled with tracheotomy care because this is a 24-hour, 7-day-a-week job.

CRICOTHYROTOMY

Considerable debate ensued in the later 19th century and the early 20th century over whether high or low tracheotomy should be performed. Openings into the airway above the thyroid gland isthmus, including those through the cricothyroid membrane, were called high tracheotomies and were considered to be easier to perform. Low tracheotomies were more difficult to perform but were thought to be safer for long-term use. Either approach in those days had a high complication rate. The controversy over high and low tracheotomy was put to rest by Jackson's classic paper in 1921 in which he reported 158 patients with laryngeal stenosis secondary to high tracheotomy. He stated that "high tracheotomy should never be done" and that only low tracheotomy should be taught. For over 50 years after Jackson's paper, cricothyrotomy, which is a type of high tracheotomy, was in disrepute. It was considered to be indicated only when rapid access to the airway was necessary in extreme emergencies. Even then, the general teaching was that it should be converted to a standard low tracheotomy as soon as possible.

The controversy of the early 1900s was reopened by a landmark paper in 1976 by two cardiothoracic surgeons, Brantigan and Grow. They reported an astounding total of 655 patients in whom they had performed cricothyrotomies and left the tube in place for periods varying from a few days to several months. The overall complication rate of their series was 6.1%, and they reported that no patients developed subglottic stenosis. They concluded that the simplicity of the procedure, the absence of cross contamination of median sternotomy incisions, and the safety documented by their study recommend routine use of cricothyrotomy instead of tracheotomy in patients whose management required long-term airway support. They felt that Jackson's condemnation of cricothyrotomy was valid for his time but that circumstances had changed. They pointed out that in Jackson's time, most tracheotomies were done as relatively crude operations by a variety of surgeons for infections such as Ludwig's angina, diphtheria, laryngeal tuberculosis, and others. Today, most are performed electively as more precise operations over endotracheal tubes for mechanical ventilation and control of secretions. Other factors are that antibiotics were not available in Jackson's time, and a variety of tracheal cannulas of less physiologic construction were in use.

Brantigan and Grow stimulated a renewed interest in cricothyrotomy. Since their original report, this procedure has been used by various emergency medical departments, cardiothoracic surgery units, and intensive care units. The advantage of cricothyrotomy that makes it appealing is that it is easier and faster to perform than is tracheotomy; it can even be performed if necessary by nonsurgeons with minimal instruments. Of particular importance in cardiothoracic surgery is that a cricothyrotomy wound is less likely than is a tracheotomy wound to cross-infect a median sternotomy wound. Another advantage in trauma situations is that airway access can be gained in patients with suspected cervical spine injury without extending the neck.

Technique

Anatomically, the cricothyroid membrane provides the easiest and fastest avenue for entering the airway by way of a surgical incision. The true vocal cords are approximately 1.3 cm above the membrane, which has a vertical diameter varying from 0.5 cm to 1.2 cm with a mean of 0.9 cm. A tube of less than 9 mm outer diameter theoretically can be inserted with little trauma to the thyroid cartilage above and the cricoid cartilage below. The surgical technique is as follows. The thyroid cartilage is held between the thumb and the second finger of the surgeon's nondominant hand. A vertical or a horizontal skin incision can be used, but a vertical incision maintains dissection in the midline, reduces the risk of venous injury, allows easier identification of the cartilaginous landmarks, and permits rapid extension up or down in the event that initial landmarks are misidentified. The incision in the cricothyroid membrane should always be horizontal and well below the cricothyroid arterial arcade that lies just below the thyroid cartilage. A Trousseau dilator or another instrument is inserted, the incision is spread open, and a tracheotomy tube is inserted.

Complications

With increasing use of cricothyrotomy, an increased incidence of complications has been reported. The data suggest that cricothyrotomy has significant morbidity but that the overall complication rate is no higher than that of standard tracheotomy. The types of complications are different, however. For instance, subglottic stenosis and voice abnormalities are more frequent complications of cricothyrotomy, whereas pneumothorax, major vessel erosion, and tracheal stenosis are more frequent with tracheotomy. Obstruction or displacement of the tracheal cannula is a potential complication with either procedure, as is cuff-induced tracheal stenosis.

The risk of subglottic stenosis secondary to cricothyrotomy appears to be considerably greater than was indicated by Brantigan and Grow's original report. They acknowledged this in a second report (1982), in which they said that the procedure should be avoided in the presence of laryngeal inflammation. It is difficult to determine the exact incidence of subglottic stenosis secondary to cricothyrotomy because this operation is often performed on seriously ill or critically injured patients, many of whom do not survive. The incidence among surviving patients, according to available data, appears to be under 5%. Several authors have identified types of patients and situations that are at high risk for the development of subglottic stenosis. It is recommended that cricothyrotomy as an elective procedure be avoided in these situations: (1) in pediatric or adolescent patients; (2) in elderly patients; (3) in diabetic patients; (4) in the presence of laryngeal inflammation, injury, or obstruction; and (5) after prolonged endotracheal intubation in which trauma from the tube may have been inflicted on the subglottic area.

Cricothyroid cannulation for periods longer than 30 days has also been found to result in a higher incidence of subglottic stenosis and therefore should be avoided.

SUGGESTED READINGS

Intubation and Tracheotomy

Carter P, Benjamin B: Ten year review of pediatric tracheotomy. Ann Otol Rhinol Laryngol 92:398–400, 1983.

Crysdale WS, Feldman RI, Naito K: Tracheotomies: a 10-year experience in 319 children. Ann Otol Rhinol Laryngol 97:439–443, 1988.

Gerson CR, Tucker GF: Infant tracheotomy. Ann Otol Rhinol Laryngol 91:413–416, 1982.

Hawkins DB: Hyaline membrane disease of the neonate. Prolonged intubation in management: effects on the larynx. Laryngoscope 88:201–224, 1978.

Hawkins DB: Pathogenesis of subglottic stenosis from endotracheal intubation. Ann Otol Rhinol Laryngol 96:116–117, 1987.

Holinger PH, Brown WT, Maurizi DG: Tracheostomy in the newborn. Am J Surg 109:771–779, 1965.

Line WS, Hawkins DB, Kahlstrom EJ, et al: Tracheotomy in infants and young children: the changing perspective 1970–1985. Laryngoscope 96:510–515, 1986.

McMillan DD, Redemaker AW, Buchan KA, et al: Benefits of orotracheal and nasotracheal intubation in neonates requiring ventilatory assistance. Pediatrics 77:39–44, 1986.

Rothfield RE, Petruzzelli GJ, Stool SE: Neonatal tracheotomy tube modification. Otolaryngol Head Neck Surg 102:133–134, 1990.

Stool SE: Tracheotomy and/or intubation. *In* Healy GB (ed): Common Problems in Pediatric Otolaryngology (pp 423–429). Chicago: Yearbook Medical Publishers, 1990.

Wetmore RF, Handler SD, Potsic WP: Pediatric tracheostomy—experience during the past decade. Ann Otol Rhinol Laryngol 91:628–632, 1982.

Cricothyrotomy

Brantigan CO, Grow JB: Cricothyroidotomy: Elective use in respiratory problems requiring tracheotomy. J Thorac Cardiovasc Surg 71:72–81, 1976.

Brantigan CO, Grow JB: Subglottic stenosis after cricothyroidotomy. Surgery 91:217–221, 1982.

Erlandson MJ, Clinton JE, Ruiz E, Cohen J: Cricothyrotomy in the emergency department revisited. J Emerg Med 7:115–118, 1989.

Esses BA, Jafek BW: Cricothyroidotomy: a decade of experience in Denver. Ann Otol Rhinol Laryngol 96:519–524, 1987.

Holst M, Hedenstierna G, Kumlien JA, Schiratski H: Elective coniotomy. Acta Otolaryngol 96:329–335, 1983.

Jackson C: High tracheotomy and other errors the chief causes of chronic laryngeal stenosis. Surg Gynecol Obstet 32:392–398, 1921.

Jakobsson J, Andersson G, Wiklund TE: Experience with elective coniotomy. Acta Chir Scand 520(Suppl):101–103, 1984.

Kuriloff DB, Setzen M, Portnoy W, Gadaleta D: Laryngotracheal injury following cricothyroidotomy. Laryngoscope 99:125–130, 1989.

Miklus RM, Elliott C, Snow N: Surgical cricothyrotomy in the field: experience of a helicopter transport team. J Trauma 29:506–508, 1989.

Narrod JA, Moore EE, Rosen P: Emergency cricothyrostomy—technique and anatomical considerations. J Emerg Med 2:443–446, 1985.

O'Connor JV, Reddy K, Ergin MA, Griepp RB: Cricothyroidotomy for prolonged ventilatory support after cardiac operations. Ann Thorac Surg 39:353–354, 1985.

Sisse MJ, Shackford SR, Cruickshank JC, et al: Cricothyroidotomy for long-term tracheal access. Ann Surg 200:13–17, 1984.

Spait DW, Joseph M: Prehospital cricothyrotomy: an investigation of indications, technique, complications and patient outcome. Ann Emerg Med 13:273–285, 1990.

CHAPTER 44

Rigid and Flexible Endoscopy of the Airway

Donald B. Hawkins, MD

HISTORICAL DEVELOPMENT OF AIRWAY ENDOSCOPY

The forerunner of airway endoscopy was the development of the technique of indirect mirror examination of the larynx in 1854 by Manual Garcia, a European singing instructor. Indirect laryngoscopy was first used medically by Johann Czermak in Hungary, then Ludwig Türck in Austria, Charles Elsberg and Jacob Solis-Cohen in the United States, and others. For the first time, physicians had a technique with which they could examine the living and functioning anatomy of the larynx.

Another 40 years passed before the development of methods for obtaining direct access to the airway. This was initiated by the introduction of direct laryngoscopy by Alfred Kirstein in 1894. It is interesting to note that open surgery on the larynx ("laryngotomy") and even total laryngectomy were done years before direct laryngoscopy was developed. In 1897, Gustav Killian demonstrated the feasibility of bronchoscopy for removal of bronchial foreign bodies. His pioneering work in development of both "upper" and "lower" bronchoscopy, as it was then called, earned Killian the title of "Father of Bronchoscopy."

The value of the bronchoscope in removing foreign bodies from the air passages was immediately recognized, and numerous reports of successful removals appeared in the medical literature. The early broncho-scopes had proximal lighting. Instrumentation through the bronchoscope, therefore, tended to obstruct the light. Perhaps the greatest contribution to the early and continued development of bronchoscopy was the development by Chevalier Jackson of the distally lighted bronchoscope in 1905. The distal light provided better visibility, added greater safety, and permitted the use of smaller diameter bronchoscopes. These changes made the procedure applicable in a much wider field.

The value of the bronchoscope in pulmonary diagnosis and therapy other than removal of foreign bodies began to be recognized. In 1923, Kully described its use in benign and malignant neoplasms, tracheobronchial compression, chronic pulmonary suppuration, and other inflammatory conditions. He said that every patient presenting persistent obscure lung signs warranted bronchoscopic investigation. He made the prophetic statement that bronchoscopy, still in its infancy, was destined to develop "vast usefulness."

The advancement of airway endoscopy was carried forward by the work of Gabriel Tucker, Louis Clerf, Chevalier Jackson, Edwin Broyles, and Paul Holinger. Whereas virtually all of the earlier bronchoscopies, and most laryngoscopies, were performed with the patient under local anesthesia, advances in anesthesia in the middle of this century and the development of ventilating bronchoscopes made general anesthesia an attractive alternative. During this same period, fiber-

771

optic lighting replaced lighting by electrical bulbs and batteries for laryngoscopes and bronchoscopes. This provided brighter distal illumination, eliminated the frustration of having to replace burned-out bulbs during a procedure, and made better endoscopic photography possible.

The application of the Hopkins rod-lens optical system to bronchoscopic telescopes in the late 1960s and early 1970s was a significant advance in airway endoscopy, especially in pediatric patients. This was pioneered by George Berci, whose interest in endoscopic optics was initiated by an interest in the endoscopic inspection of the bile ducts. The basic arrangement of the Hopkins rod-lens is the opposite of that in the older endoscopic telescopes, in which small lenses were placed at intervals with air spaces between them. In designing his system, H. H. Hopkins used glass rods to replace the air spaces and used small air spaces to replace the former lenses. The ends of the glass rods were shaped to the form of a lens. This resulted in increased light transmission, excellent optical resolution, and a viewing angle significantly wider than with previous telescopic systems. Because of these qualities, miniaturization was possible, with small telescopes made for pediatric use. This Storz-Hopkins system of bronchoscopes, telescopes, and instruments designed to be used with the telescopes has become very popular. It is used to some degree by almost all pediatric endoscopy services.

Probably the most significant development of the second half of this century in airway endoscopy was the introduction of the flexible fiberoptic bronchoscope in 1968 by Shigeto Ikeda in Japan. Because of the facility and safety with which it could be used and the access that it provided to the more distal subsegmental bronchi, the flexible bronchoscope rapidly became the preferred instrument for diagnostic bronchoscopies in adults.

The earlier generations of flexible bronchoscopes were too large in diameter to be used in pediatric airways. With advances in fiberoptic technology, smaller bronchoscopes gradually became available. Flexible laryngoscopes (nasopharyngolaryngoscopes) were constructed without a suction/instrument channel. They are available in diameters of 4 mm, 3.5 mm, and 3.0 mm, and a 2.2-mm flexible size has become available. The flexible laryngoscopes can be used in adults, but perhaps their most widespread use has been in children.

Flexible laryngoscopy is the use of the fiberscope with the tip above the vocal cords. In this manner, the airway in infants and young children is unlikely to be compromised. Flexible fiberoptic bronchoscopy is more invasive because the bronchoscope is inserted past the vocal cords into the trachea and the bronchi. Unlike rigid bronchoscopy, in which the patient can breathe through the open lumen, the infant or child has to breathe around the flexible bronchoscope. The use of flexible fiberoptic bronchoscopy in children was pioneered in the United States primarily by Robert Wood. By the early 1980s, flexible bronchoscopes with an outer diameter of 3.5 mm and a suction channel of 1.2 mm in diameter had been developed. These instruments were found to be useful and well tolerated even by premature neonates as long as due care was taken to provide adequate topical anesthesia, sedation, and monitoring for airway patency. The smaller premature neonates cannot breathe well around this instrument, however; this limits its usefulness in these patients. Although the 3.5-mm bronchoscope passes through a 4.5-mm inner diameter endotracheal tube, the patient cannot be ventilated around the scope; the patient can barely be ventilated around it through a 5.0 endotracheal tube. Therefore, it is of limited usefulness in children intubated with a 5.0-mm or smaller inner diameter endotracheal tube.

The 3.5-mm bronchoscope is the smallest one with an adequate suction channel. Smaller fiberscopes without suction channels have been developed. These are called ultrathin scopes. Originally, the smallest size with distal tip angulation was 2.7 mm, but a 2.2-mm size has been introduced. Those ultrathin fiberscopes that do not have provision for distal tip angulation are useful only for examining the lower trachea through an indwelling endotracheal tube. Those with distal tip angulation can be used for a more thorough bronchoscopic examination. The 2.2-mm scope can be passed through an endotracheal tube as small as 2.5-mm inner diameter, but the infant cannot ventilate around the instrument. A disposable model that is 1.3 mm in diameter passes more easily through a 2.5-mm inner diameter endotracheal tube, but it cannot be steered.

CONTEMPORARY INDICATIONS AND TECHNIQUES

Since the first recorded direct examination of the airway, bronchoscopy has developed "vast usefulness" far greater than Kully could ever have imagined in 1923. The endoscopist has at his or her disposal a wide variety of instruments, rigid and flexible, for examination of the airway. What are the indications for which instruments in which patients? The following discussion is an attempt to answer that question according to the author's understanding.

Flexible Endoscopy

Flexible Laryngoscopy

Adults and Older Children. Flexible laryngoscopy, or indirect laryngoscopy with a mirror or the indirect laryngoscope designed by George Berci, can be used for adequate examination of the larynx in this age group. The indications for either procedure are to examine the larynx for any reason (hoarseness, stridor, and so on) or simply to perform a complete ear, nose, and throat examination.

The flexible laryngoscope is passed through the nose after application of topical anesthesia. In most patients who can be examined sitting upright in a chair, indirect laryngoscopy through the mouth without anesthesia or with topical anesthesia sprayed orally is more straightforward, is quicker, and provides as good an examination of the larynx. In patients who are bedridden or for those with cervical spine abnormalities or limited jaw opening, flexible laryngoscopy is a better technique for examining the larynx. Another indication for flexible laryngoscopy in these patients is as a guide for inserting endotracheal tubes transnasally.

Younger Children. Children under 6 years of age, and even some considerably older, have difficulty cooperating for indirect laryngoscopy. Before flexible laryngoscopes became available, direct laryngoscopy with or without anesthesia was often necessary for examining the larynx of infants and young children. When a young child with laryngeal symptoms was seen, a decision often had to be made as to whether the symptoms warranted direct laryngoscopy. That concern is relieved with flexible laryngoscopy because it is a relatively noninvasive procedure. The flexible laryngoscope is an excellent method of examination of the pediatric larynx.

As with older patients, the indications for flexible laryngoscopy include any reason why a physician would want to examine the larynx. The most common indications in young children, in the author's experience, are stridor and poor voice.

Flexible laryngoscopy can be performed at any location where suction equipment, oxygen, and resuscitative equipment is available: intensive care units, pediatric wards, outpatient clinics, private offices, emergency rooms, or operating rooms. The author's technique is as follows. The patient is given nothing by mouth for 2 hours before the procedure. The infant or the young child is restrained by being wrapped in a sheet or a papoose board. The thorax is left uncovered so that retractions can be observed. It is helpful to have three persons present in addition to the examiner: one to hold the patient's head, one to hold the patient's shoulders, and one to handle the suction. Most patients are examined in the supine position with the endoscopist at the patient's head, the same position as for direct laryngoscopy. If airway obstruction is a concern in the supine position, the patient is examined in the sitting position.

Topical anesthesia is induced by insertion into one naris of a small cotton pledget soaked with a solution of a half-and-half mixture of 4% lidocaine hydrochloride (Xylocaine) and 0.25% phenylephrine hydrochloride. The cotton is thoroughly soaked with the anesthetic so that, upon insertion into the naris, some of the anesthetic flows through the posterior choana into the pharynx and, it is hoped, the larynx. A useful additional technique, advocated by Wood (personal communication, 1990), is to instill 1 or 2 mL of 1% to 2% lidocaine through one naris with the patient supine. This usually results in delivery of topical anesthesia to the larynx. In some patients, the endolarynx can be examined more easily with a scope in one naris than in the other. In the rare patient whose nose does not permit passage, transoral examination can be attempted, but this usually results in unsatisfactory exposure of the larynx.

In the transnasal examination, once the nasopharynx is reached, the tip of the fiberscope is angled downward (forward in re-measured by pulse oximetry, drops to below 90%, the fiberscope must be withdrawn to above the vocal cords. Supplemental oxygen can be given throughout the procedure by holding oxygen tubing or an oxygen mask adjacent to the patient's mouth.

Bronchoalveolar lavage can be performed for diagnostic purposes or for removal of mucus plugging in patients with atelectasis. The tip of the bronchoscope is wedged as closely as possible into a lobar or segmental bronchial orifice. Three to 10 mL of sterile saline, depending on the size of the patient, is instilled through the suction channel and then suctioned back into a sterile collection chamber; 50% to 70% of the instilled volume usually can be retrieved. This can be repeated several times if necessary, depending on the patient's tolerance of the procedure. The 1.2-mm suction channel of the 3.5-mm fiberscope is too small for adequate biopsy forceps, but brush biopsy specimens can be obtained.

Another technique that can be used, especially in infants, is to perform direct laryngoscopy and insert the flexible bronchoscope through the laryngoscope. This is useful in infants intubated with an endotracheal tube that is too small to permit passage of the laryngoscope through it. The direct laryngoscope is inserted, the endotracheal tube is removed, the fiberscope is inserted, and upon completion of the bronchoscopy, the endotracheal tube is reinserted before the direct laryngoscope is removed. This approach can also be used in patients in whom difficulty is encountered in passing the fiberscope through the glottis by the transnasal approach.

Rigid Endoscopy

Adults

Indications. Since flexible fiberoptic bronchoscopy has become the procedure of choice for almost all diagnostic bronchoscopies in adults, the indications for rigid bronchoscopy have diminished. They include removal of foreign bodies, control of massive hemoptysis, dilation of tracheal or bronchial stenosis, and diagnostic bronchoscopy in a patient with tracheal stenosis such that flexible fiberoptic bronchoscopy would obstruct the lumen. Subglottic stenosis, on the other hand, is a relative contraindication to flexible or rigid bronchoscopy because of the danger of postbronchoscopy edema obstructing the airway.

Direct laryngoscopy indications in adults have changed little. Direct laryngoscopy is still indicated for biopsy and assessment of laryngeal malignancy, removal of benign lesions with forceps or laser, removal of laryngeal foreign bodies, dilation or laser excision of laryngeal stenosis, and evaluation of acute or chronic laryngeal injuries.

Technique. Proper positioning of the patient's head is of extreme importance for any rigid endoscopy. The proper position, referred to as the Boyce or "sniffing" position, is, briefly stated, flexion of the neck on the chest and extension of the head on the neck. This is the anatomically correct position for the introduction of direct laryngoscopes, rigid bronchoscopes, or esophagoscopes. The patient is placed in dorsal recumbency, and the head is elevated until the cervical spine is brought on a line with the upper thoracic spine, and thus the larynx, the cervical trachea, and the cervical esophagus are brought in a straight line with the thoracic trachea and the esophagus. The head is then extended sufficiently on the neck to allow introduction of the direct laryngoscope back to the right side of the base of the tongue. With a gently lifting motion, not by prying on the upper teeth, the epiglottis and the base of the tongue are lifted, and the openings of the larynx and esophagus are brought into view.

Because most adult and pediatric rigid endoscopy at the author's institution is currently performed while patients are under general anesthesia, that technique is described. Direct laryngoscopy can be performed over a previously passed endotracheal tube or by apneic technique. The apneic technique has the advantage of exposure of the larynx unobstructed by an endotracheal tube. Its disadvantage is that the endoscopist has to work in a very limited time frame, usually approximately 2 minutes for each apneic episode.

To facilitate insertion of a rigid bronchoscope, a Jackson slotted laryngoscope is used. Although this may be inserted over an endotracheal tube, it is usually done by the apneic method, which is as follows. The patient is anesthetized and ventilated by mask until the appropriate level of anesthesia is reached. Muscle paralysis is produced with intravenous succinylcholine, atracurium, or vecuronium. The muscle paralysis may be omitted if there is significant airway obstruction and concern regarding the anesthesiologist's ability to ventilate by mask once the patient is paralyzed. Otherwise, the muscle paralysis prevents possible laryngospasm upon passage of the bronchoscope and prevents reflex contraction of the larynx on the bronchoscope during the procedure, thus minimizing the potential for postoperative laryngeal edema.

The Jackson slotted laryngoscope is inserted, and the rigid bronchoscope is inserted through the laryngoscope into the larynx and trachea. Removal of the slotted portion of the laryngoscope allows it to be removed over the bronchoscope. The anesthesia tubing is attached to the ventilating side arm of the bronchoscope, and the patient is ventilated as the bronchoscope is advanced farther into the trachea. After the bronchoscope is in the trachea, the patient's head is lowered to the appropriate level for direct visibility of the tracheal lumen. Small adjustments in the degree of elevation, extension, or lateral deviation of the head may be required as the examination proceeds. The trachea and the carina can be inspected in detail with or without a 0° telescope. Slight deviation of the head to the left allows direct access to the right main stem bronchus. The spur of the orifice of the right upper lobe bronchus, the right middle lobe orifice, and the five segmental bronchi of the right lower lobe can be visualized. Insertion of a 90° telescope allows inspection of the right upper lobe bronchus to its division into its three segmental bronchi. The bronchoscope is withdrawn to the carina, and with deviation of the head to the right, the left main stem bronchus can be entered. The bifurcation of the left upper lobe and left lower lobe bronchi can usually be seen well, and the four segmental bronchial orifices of the left lower lobe can be examined. The left upper lobe bronchus, because it does not arise at as much of an angle as does the right upper lobe bronchus, can often be seen directly to the level of its bifurcation into the upper and the lower (lingular) division. If necessary, a 90° telescope can be used to examine the upper lobe bronchus. Foreign bodies can be removed, suspicious lesions biopsied, or bronchial washings obtained for diagnosis. Tracheal or bronchial stenosis can be dilated with the bronchoscope or, in a relatively new technique, with a balloon catheter inserted through the bronchoscope. Any of these manipulations require close cooperation and coordination between the endoscopist and the anesthesiologist.

Children

Indications. The indications for rigid endoscopy in children include those listed for rigid endoscopy in adults as well as those stated for FFB in children. FFB in children usually does not require detailed examination of the peripheral bronchi. The involved areas of more central bronchi, except the upper lobes, can be examined approximately as well by rigid bronchoscopy with use of the Hopkins rod-lens telescope as by FFB. It therefore becomes a matter of the endoscopist's choice whether to use rigid or flexible bronchoscopy. As mentioned earlier, FFB can be performed in an intensive care unit setting under local anesthesia and can be performed through an endotracheal tube. Rigid bronchoscopy is more effective under general anesthesia in an operating room. Because rigid bronchoscopy provides an avenue for ventilation of a patient during bronchoscopy, it might be the preferred technique for relatively unstable infants requiring bronchoscopy for atelectasis who have endotracheal tubes too small to admit a 3.5-mm flexible bronchoscope. In these circumstances, it can be done in the intensive care unit without general anesthesia.

Technique. The technique and contraindications of rigid bronchoscopy in children are essentially the same as described for rigid bronchoscopy in adults and are not repeated here. Because the pediatric larynx is smaller, subglottic edema that develops postoperatively is more of a hazard than with adults. For this reason, the author usually gives 0.3 to 0.5 mm of dexamethasone intravenously immediately before the bronchoscopy, and patients are kept in a mist tent for 2 or more hours postoperatively. Racemic epinephrine inhalations and repeated doses of dexamethasone are given postoperatively if necessary. The likelihood of postbronchoscopy subglottic edema is minimized by use of an appropriate-sized bronchoscope, avoidance of excessive movement of the scope in the larynx, avoidance of undue prolongation of the procedure, use of muscle paralysis, and avoid-

nodes, and the lower lymphatic veins drain to the lower deep cervical nodes, including supraclavicular, pretracheal, paratracheal, and prelaryngeal nodes.

The nerves of importance in surgery for the thyroid gland are the two recurrent laryngeal nerves (sometimes referred to as the inferior laryngeal nerves) and the superior laryngeal nerves. The right recurrent laryngeal nerve arises from the vagus nerve and then loops around the subclavian artery to course in a medial direction to enter the larynx at the inferior border of the cricothyroid muscle. The left recurrent laryngeal nerve arises from the vagus and passes in front of the aortic arch, looping around it and ascending to the lower border of the cricothyroid muscle, where it enters the larynx. The nerves are not necessarily tucked into the tracheoesophageal groove, but they usually run more lateral than this; the right one is more apt to do so. The most common relationship with the inferior thyroid artery is that in which the right recurrent laryngeal nerve passes between the branches of the artery. The left recurrent laryngeal nerve is usually posterior to the inferior thyroid artery and its branches. However, these relationships are variable.

The right recurrent laryngeal nerve is most apt to be nonrecurrent, and when it is, it is associated with an anomalous origin in which the right subclavian artery courses in a retroesophageal fashion.

Preservation of the recurrent laryngeal nerve is of paramount importance during thyroid surgery. Helpful guides to accomplish this are (1) identification of the recurrent laryngeal nerve at the lower pole of the thyroid; (2) not sacrificing any branches of the nerve, because it may divide outside the larynx; and (3) following the nerve to its entry into the larynx—the thyroid tissue should not be clamped around the upper pole.

The superior laryngeal nerves arise from the caudal end of the nodose ganglion, pass medially and deep to the external and internal carotid arteries, and divide into a smaller external branch and a larger internal branch. The internal branch supplies sensation and parasympathetic secretomotor function to the mucous glands of the interior larynx. The external branch supplies motor power to the cricothyroid muscle, which tenses the vocal cord. In order to preserve the external branch during surgery, it should be found just me-

dial to the superior thyroid artery as it enters the upper pole of the gland.

Physiology and Testing

Starting between the 70th and 80th days of gestation, the follicular cells of the thyroid acquire the unique ability to accumulate iodide from the serum. The iodide is then oxidized to iodine. The iodine is incorporated into amino acid tyrosine residues in thyroglobulin molecules (probably through thyroid peroxidase) to form monoiodotyrosine and diodotyrosine. These couple to form the active hormones thyroxine (T_4) and triiodothyronine (T_3), which in turn form the active hormone thyroglobulin. Thyroglobulin is then hydrolyzed by adenylate cyclase activation, and free T_4 and T_3 are released into the blood stream. This process takes 10 to 30 minutes after exposure to thyroid-stimulating hormone (TSH). The most active of the hormones is T_3, which is estimated to be four times as potent as T_4. A major source of T_3 is conversion of T_4 in the liver, the kidney, and the peripheral tissues. Because T_4 is bound strongly to thyroxine-binding globulin, it is eliminated more slowly than T_3; it has a half-life of 6 to 7 days, whereas the half-life of T_3 is 1 day. Degradation and excretion of thyroid hormone is through the liver, the gastrointestinal tract, and the kidney.

The process of iodination of tyrosine can be blocked by drugs such as methimazole and propylthiouracil, which block the action of thyroid peroxidase. Chlorpromazine and lithium inhibit TSH action and can thus decrease thyroid function.

Thyroid gland function is under the control of a hypothalamic pituitary thyroid feedback mechanism. Thyrotropin-releasing factor is formed in the hypothalamus and stimulates the release of TSH from the pituitary, which acts on the thyroid gland to produce T_3 and T_4. As levels of T_3 and T_4 rise in the blood, there is a negative feedback that shuts off TSH. The reverse process occurs as T_3 and T_4 levels drop in the blood.

For the head and neck surgeon who is evaluating masses in the thyroid gland, it is important to know whether the patient is euthyroid (Fig. 45–1). Tests of a free T_4 level and a sensitive TSH level are the two most sensitive tests of thyroid function status. In the euthyroid state, the free T_4 and TSH

Figure 45–1. Feedback mechanism of thyroid physiology and testing.

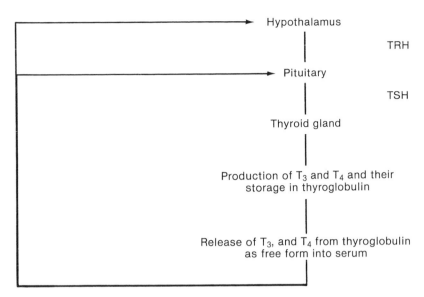

Hypothalamus

TRH

Pituitary

TSH

Thyroid gland

Production of T_3 and T_4 and their storage in thyroglobulin

Release of T_3, and T_4 from thyroglobulin as free form into serum

levels are within the normal range. If the patient is thyrotoxic, the free T_4 level is elevated, and the TSH level is decreased. In primary hypothyroidism, the free T_4 level is decreased, and the TSH level is elevated. If the TSH level is low, the patient may have secondary hypothyroidism as a result of pituitary failure or tertiary hypothyroidism as a result of hypothalamic failure. If the history or the physical examination leads to suspicion of chronic thyroiditis (Hashimoto's thyroiditis), antithyroid microsomal antibody titers should be measured.

Diseases of the Thyroid

Thyroiditis

Acute Thyroiditis. Acute thyroiditis is the most uncommon form of thyroiditis. It can follow an upper respiratory tract infection, and the patient presents with the sudden onset of pain in the anterior neck, dysphagia, fever, and chills and appears to have a toxic condition. This usually is a suppurative process with abscess formation. The most common infecting organisms are *Staphylococcus* and *Streptococcus*, and the treatment is drainage with institution of appropriate antibiotic therapy. In patients with acute suppurative thyroiditis, an internal fistula arising in the piriform fossa should be ruled out as a cause; a barium esophagogram can demonstrate the fistula in a majority of cases.

Subacute Granulomatous (de Quervain's) Thyroiditis. This inflammatory disorder,

which is not of autoimmune origin, is characterized by a giant cell granulomatous reaction in a patient who has a tender thyroid swelling with referral of pain to the ear or other parts of the head and neck and who complains of weakness and malaise. Early in the course of the disease, the serum thyroid tests may show thyrotoxicity, but with time, patients become euthyroid or even hypothyroid. The best way to establish the diagnosis is to obtain a radioactive iodine (^{131}I) uptake test and scan. The uptake is characteristically low—low enough that no appreciable shadow shows on the scan. Salicylates and thyroid replacement alleviate the symptoms. Steroids lead to a dramatic improvement, but a rebound phenomenon can occur when they are stopped, and the steroids may have to be reinstituted; thus steroid administration is reserved for the most severe cases.

Chronic Thyroiditis. Chronic thyroiditis is divided into two categories: Hashimoto's (chronic autoimmune lymphocytic) thyroiditis and Riedel's (struma) thyroiditis.

Hashimoto's thyroiditis is the most common form of thyroiditis and is believed to be an autoimmune disorder. The majority of patients are women between 40 and 60 years of age. They may complain of pain and tenderness in the thyroid region and may have respiratory distress or dysphagia secondary to compression of the trachea or esophagus. Palpation reveals a diffusely enlarged or irregular gland that may be tender. Results of serum thyroid function tests reveal

TABLE 45–2. Thyroid Malignancies

Type	Origin	Proportion
Differentiated	Papillary	60% to 70%
	Follicular	15% to 20%
Undifferentiated	Small cell	10% to 15%
	Giant cell	
Medullary	Familial and sporadic	5%
Lymphoma	Differentiated from small cell by immunocytochemistry	3%
Metastatic	Kidney, breast, and lung	1% to 2%
Squamous	Aggressive tumor	1%

Papillary Thyroid Carcinoma. This is the most frequent of the thyroid cancers (approximately 60% to 70%) and carries the most favorable prognosis. As with other thyroid cancers, papillary thyroid carcinoma is more common in women than in men by a ratio of 3:1. It tends to occur in young patients, although it can occur at any age, and it frequently metastasizes to regional lymph nodes. If the tumor is less than 1.5 cm in size, it is considered occult and offers a better prognosis than do the larger lesions. Papillary cancers are frequently multifocal and bilateral, especially in patients exposed to radiation. If radiograph of the chest shows stippled calcification in the neck, the physician should think of the presence of psammoma bodies, which are calcified deposits scattered throughout the fronds of papillary carcinoma.

Recurrence of the tumor is most often in the central compartment of the neck, but it can metastasize to the lungs, the bones, the brain, and other viscera. When a cervical node contains papillary thyroid tissue, it is considered a metastasis, and a thyroidectomy shows an occult primary lesion in the thyroid gland. A potential of papillary thyroid carcinoma is to change to a more malignant undifferentiated type, and this transition may take 20 to 30 years after initial diagnosis; this is generally believed to result from tumor persistence. Occurrence of this transition is a threat as long as the patient harbors a residual tumor.

Follicular Carcinoma. This is the second most common type of thyroid carcinoma, occurring in about 15% to 20% of patients with thyroid cancer. It is difficult for the pathologist to distinguish a follicular adenoma from a carcinoma unless capsular invasion or angioinvasion is found. Patients with follicular carcinoma are more apt to be older than patients with papillary carcinoma. Follicular carcinoma can metastasize to regional nodes (usually in children, as with papillary carcinoma), and it more often metastasizes hematogenously to the lungs and bones. The majority (75%) of differentiated thyroid cancers, except for Hürthle's cell variant, take up radioactive iodine, and their metastases can be treated with radioactive iodine once the thyroid gland has been removed. Radioactive iodine can also be used to diagnose residual or metastatic disease; however, again, the thyroid gland has to be absent in order to accomplish this method of diagnosis. These tumors do not carry as good a prognosis as does papillary carcinoma, which has a 5-year survival rate of approximately 90%.

Hürthle's Cell Carcinomas. These originate from follicular cells and are more aggressive than either papillary or follicular carcinoma. Hürthle's cell lesions can be benign or malignant; invasion of the capsule and blood vessels characterizes the malignant variety. Hürthle's cell carcinomas are more common in older patients, and there is a relationship of malignancy to size: as the lesion gets larger, it is more apt to be malignant. These tumors can metastasize to bones, the lungs, and other sites, and only a small percentage respond to treatment with radioactive iodine.

Metastatic Lesions. Lesions metastatic to the thyroid gland come most often from hypernephromas, breast cancer, and lung cancer.

Anaplastic Carcinoma. The anaplastic carcinomas can be either small cell or large cell tumors. The small cell variety is easily confused with a lymphoma and has a better prognosis than the giant cell variety. Thyroid lymphomas are often associated with a history of Hashimoto's thyroiditis, occur in older women, and respond well to radiation therapy. Clinically, small cell carcinomas or lymphomas develop as rapidly enlarging, painless, and firm masses. Surgery may be necessary to establish the diagnosis, but sometimes fine-needle biopsy is diagnostic, especially if immunocytochemistry is used.

The anaplastic giant spindle cell carcinoma has the worst prognosis of all the thyroid malignancies; survival is measured in terms of weeks to months. Surgery with resection of as much of the tumor as possible, followed by chemotherapy and radiation therapy, may give the opportunity for longer survival.

Factors Influencing Survival

Prognosis of thyroid carcinoma can be categorized by the acronym AGES:

Age is the most important of the variables; patients over the age of 40 with cancer have an increased rate of mortality.

Grade, or histologic type of tumor, is the second most important factor; the anaplastic tumors have the worst prognosis, and the well-differentiated papillary and follicular types have the best. Medullary carcinomas occupy an intermediate position. Determination of ploidy of deoxyribonucleic acid (DNA) is a new test for determination of prognosis. Euploidy is the situation in which nucleoid DNA amounts are predominantly diploid or tetraploid. Diploid or tetraploid tumors exhibit a better prognosis. Aneuploidy is a chromosome complement that is not an exact multiple of the haploid number of chromosomes, and aneuploid tumors have been shown to be more aggressive and to portend a poorer prognosis because of a higher recurrence rate and incidence of distant metastases.

Extent of the tumor and the presence of distant metastases are significant predictors of increased mortality. Local and regional metastases do not significantly affect survival. Capsular invasion, angioinvasion, and extrathyroidal invasion are factors that predict a poorer prognosis.

Size of the lesion and sex of the patient have been shown to be related to survival. In many reports, men have had a higher mortality rate than have women with a similar presentation. Size of the cancer when occult (i.e., under 1.5 cm in diameter) does not affect survival; however, when the tumor is greater than 2.5 cm in diameter, prognosis is adversely affected.

Treatment of Carcinoma of Thyroid

Surgical management of thyroid cancer has been the subject of considerable controversy for many years. Proponents of total thyroidectomy have been unable to show any significant increase in survival rates over those obtained with subtotal thyroidectomy. Many thyroid cancers have an indolent course: they are often present over more than a 20-year period before an ominous situation occurs, and because the surgeon has usually predeceased the patient, the patient is not aware of the late-onset problems. The majority of thyroid surgeons agree that if the incidence of recurrent laryngeal nerve injury and hypoparathyroidism could be minimized, then total thyroidectomy would be the treatment of choice. There is no doubt in the author's mind that the surgeon who performs total thyroidectomy often has fewer patients with postoperative complications than does the surgeon who performs total thyroidectomy infrequently.

It is generally agreed that total thyroidectomy is the best therapy for carcinoma of the thyroid in the following scenarios:

1. The patient who presents with a carcinoma and a history of previous radiation exposure. Such patients have a higher incidence of multifocal, bilateral disease with capsular invasion and angioinvasion; thus their prognosis is poor if the lesion is not occult (i.e., <1.5 cm).
2. Patients who have had partial resection and return with recurrent disease.
3. When there is extrathyroidal extension of the carcinoma or presence of distant metastases.
4. When gross bilateral disease is present. It then becomes an individual surgical decision as to whether a total or subtotal thyroidectomy should be applied as initial therapy.

Advantages of Total Thyroidectomy

First, total thyroidectomy eliminates the primary tumor and multicentric, bilateral disease, and it eliminates the potential for recurrence in remaining tissue that may appear grossly normal.

Second, the procedure facilitates the postoperative management in which ^{131}I is used for persistent local disease of a microscopic nature and for treatment of recurrent or metastatic disease. It also facilitates the detection of disease with radioiodine scans, inasmuch as all thyroid tissue that would compete for the uptake of the radioiodine has been removed.

Third, the procedure reduces the possibility of transition of a well-differentiated cancer to anaplastic carcinoma.

Fourth, total thyroidectomy facilitates the postoperative follow-up because thyroglobulin increases can be used as a marker for recurrent or metastatic disease.

Fifth, the procedure diminishes the need to rely on rapid frozen-section diagnoses, which may be misleading, at the time of surgery.

Finally, when the procedure is performed frequently, the complications of permanent hypoparathyroidism and recurrent laryngeal nerve paralysis can be similar to those that occur when lesser procedures are performed.

Postoperative Management

When total thyroidectomy has been used for therapy of thyroid carcinoma, the postoperative management includes the following procedures.

Radioiodine Therapeutic Ablation. This is another area of controversy because it has never been definitely established that persistent microscopic disease will be ablated. Many endocrinologists believe that postoperative ^{131}I ablation is helpful. Indications for its use are as follows:

1. Patients over 40 years of age.
2. Children under 20, because pulmonary metastases can be present in as many as 40%. These may be microscopic metastases and not detectable by chest radiography.
3. Patients with capsular invasion, angioinvasion, and lymph node metastases.
4. Patients whose primary tumor exceeds 2.5 cm in diameter.
5. Patients with residual, persistent, recurrent, or distant disease.
6. Patients who refuse operation.

These indications are for both papillary and follicular carcinoma because follicular cancer has a similar low mortality rate in patients under 40 years of age. All patients over the age of 40 with follicular cancer should undergo postoperative ablation because of increased mortality rates and to treat potential metastases before the tumor becomes too large. Older patients with occult papillary thyroid carcinoma probably do not need ablation, but older patients with larger tumors may benefit.

The dose of radioiodine used is 100 to 200 mC, in a single, in-hospital dose. Discharge then is usually 36 to 48 hours after the treatment.

The usual method used at the author's institution is to wait 2 to 3 months after total thyroidectomy, to stop T_3 (liothyronine sodium [Cytomel]) replacement for 14 to 21 days (allowing for maximal TSH stimulation of any microscopic functional foci), and to check TSH levels, which should be above 50 milliunits/L. The therapeutic dose is then administered, and after discharge from the hospital, thyroxine replacement is restarted.

Side effects of this therapy can include temporary nausea, vomiting, radiation sialoadenitis, leukopenia, and platelet depression.

Some Hürthle's cell carcinomas do not concentrate radioiodine and cannot be treated with ^{131}I, as are the papillary and follicular carcinomas.

Levothyroxine. Levothyroxine is used in all patients to replace thyroid follicular function and suppress TSH. The well-differentiated tumors are responsive to TSH, and so TSH levels in the serum must be kept low. In the past, high doses of levothyroxine were used, but it is currently believed that the lowest dose that maintains a low level of TSH (below 0.1 milliunits/mL) is best. Among patients who receive high doses of levothyroxine over a long period of time, there has been an increased incidence of osteoporosis.

Measurement of Serum Thyroglobulin. Serum thyroglobulin levels are measured on a regular basis (every 6 to 12 months) because elevated levels in the presence of low TSH levels signify recurrent or metastatic disease.

Total Body Scans. Total body scans are completed after 1 year and, if negative for metastatic disease, are not taken for 2 to 3 years. The dose of radioiodine used for body scanning is 5 to 9 millicurie because this dose

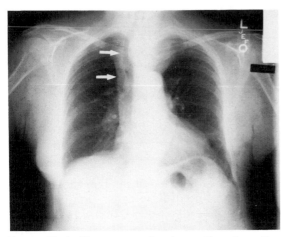

Figure 45–4. Chest x-ray showing widened mediastinum (arrows) with tracheal deviation, compression, and airway distress.

will more likely demonstrate metastatic disease than will a smaller dose.

Annual Chest X-Rays. Radiographs are obtained with the realization that small metastases may not be seen with this examination (Fig. 45–4). However, if serum testing reveals a climbing level of serum thyroglobulin, then a total body scan, a computed tomogram (CT), or magnetic resonance imaging (MRI) scan may be helpful (Fig. 45–5).

The Patient's Account. Of great importance is listening to the patient's complaints and weighing them in relation to the natural history of thyroid cancer and then obtaining appropriate tests to solidify the diagnosis of metastatic disease.

Anaplastic Carcinoma. Anaplastic thyroid carcinomas are among the most aggressive malignancies. Their rapid growth and invasive behavior render surgical extirpation nearly impossible.

The small cell variety may be confused with lymphoma; once a definitive diagnosis is made by either needle biopsy or open biopsy, the tumor may be treated with external radiation therapy with or without chemotherapy. The response is usually good, and the patients are placed on thyroid hormone replacement therapy. However, these tumors are not TSH-dependent. Hashimoto's thyroiditis has been shown to degenerate to small cell anaplastic carcinoma. Surgical intervention is indicated whenever there is a sudden rapid increase in size of the thyroid mass, even when an established diagnosis has been made.

The other type of anaplastic carcinoma is the giant spindle cell variety. Occasionally the transition from a papillary or follicular carcinoma to an anaplastic giant spindle cell lesion can be demonstrated histologically. Immunostaining techniques for thyroglobulin sometimes determine their origin from a follicular cell. Surgery for this condition consists of removal of as much of the tumor as possible, with the realization that it infiltrates the great vessels, the nerves, the trachea, and the esophagus. Combination therapy consisting of external irradiation (6000 to 6500

Figure 45–5. CT scan of patient with substernal thyroid mass in which calcification (arrow) is present: a follicular carcinoma.

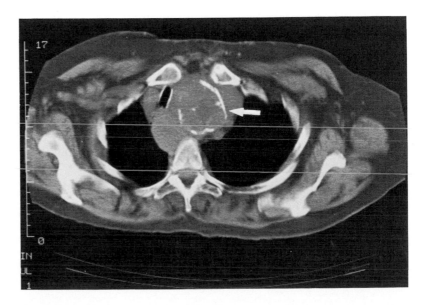

cGy) and chemotherapy with doxorubicin hydrochloride (Adriamycin) has been used as a sensitizer for external irradiation. Unfortunately, the tumor is relentless, and survival is usually measured in months. Radioiodine does not play a role in the treatment of anaplastic carcinoma.

Other Tumors of the Thyroid

Squamous Cell Carcinoma

Squamous cell carcinoma of the thyroid is rare, usually less than 1% of all thyroid tumors. It is an aggressive tumor that can arise from squamous epithelial rests or from degeneration of a well-differentiated tumor. Treatment is total thyroidectomy with or without laryngectomy and radical neck dissection. Postoperative radiation therapy and chemotherapy have been used, but the prognosis is poor.

Medullary Carcinoma

Medullary carcinoma of the thyroid represents approximately 5% of thyroid cancers and arises from the parafollicular C cells that come from neuroectoderm. There is a familial form of the disease that is an autosomal dominant trait and accounts for 10% to 20% of such tumors. The majority of medullary carcinomas (80% to 90%) are of the sporadic variety. The C cells produce calcitonin; this substance can be used as a serum marker not only to diagnose the disease but also to follow its course. All other direct family relatives are screened for elevated calcitonin levels once the diagnosis of medullary carcinoma is established.

Calcitonin has a 32–amino acid chain and decreases osteoclastic activity in bone, thereby decreasing bone, possibly some resorption, and lowering serum calcium. It also causes increased urinary excretion of calcium, phosphorus, sodium, and potassium. In the small intestine it causes an increased secretion of water and electrolytes with decreased mucosal contact time. As a result, some patients present with watery diarrhea, especially in the familial variety (Table 45–3). Other products of the parafollicular C cells are prostaglandins E_2 and $F_2\alpha$, histamine, carcinoembryonic antigen, serotonin, and somatostatin; thus myriad symptoms can be produced, depending on the chemicals produced by the particular tumor.

TABLE 45–3. Conditions Causing Increased Levels of Calcitonin

Medullary thyroid cancer
Chronic renal failure
Pancreatitis
Subacute thyroiditis
Pregnancy
Carcinoid tumor
Oat cell cancer; cancer of the breast, the bladder, the prostate, and the pancreas

Clinical Manifestation. The clinical manifestation of medullary carcinoma is that of a firm, rounded, painless thyroid mass. Approximately 15% of patients present with palpable cervical lymph nodes. Diarrhea may be present in the familial variety.

Diagnosis. The diagnosis is made from findings of elevated serum calcitonin levels in 75% of the patients. Calcitonin stimulations with calcium gluconate and pentagastrin intravenously can be performed with serum testing 0, 1, 2, 3, 5, and 10 minutes after the administration of pentagastrin. Early on there is a marked increase in calcitonin levels, which gradually decrease by the 10-minute mark. On thyroid scans, a cold nodule will be found.

Pathology. The pathologic processes are typified by findings, on gross examination, of a gray-white gritty mass. The sine qua non of making the diagnosis is a histologic finding of amyloid deposits and calcification, which are not typical of psammoma bodies. Immunostaining for calcitonin confirms the diagnosis.

Treatment. Treatment of medullary carcinoma is surgical, with a total thyroidectomy, a bilateral central paratracheal and a superior mediastinal dissection. Radical neck dissection is completed when nodes are found. In some patients, external irradiation has been used to treat hypercalcitoninemia after surgery has been completed. In this situation, the neck, the thyroid bed, and the superior mediastinum are treated. Whether this prolongs survival or not needs to be determined. When gross disease is seen on CT or MRI scans, surgical extirpation is the treatment of choice. For this disease, all surgeons agree that total thyroidectomy is necessary because 90% of patients have bilateral microscopic disease. Medullary carcinoma metastasizes in

70% to 80% of patients to the mediastinum and also to the lungs, the liver, the bones, the brain, the adrenal glands, the ovaries, and the heart. Chemotherapy has not proved helpful, nor has the use of radioiodine.

When surgery has been completed and elevated serum calcitonin level is found, a thorough history should be obtained and a physical examination performed. CT or MRI scans of potential metastatic areas are ordered. A common place for metastasis to be found is the adrenal region, which may be demonstrated by abdominal CT scans. Carcinoembryonic antigen levels need to be checked in these patients; elevation of these levels prognostically marks a more virulent tumor with metastases. Whole body scintigraphy with technetium-labeled dimercaptosuccinic acid has been helpful on occasion in demonstrating either neck recurrence or distant metastasis. Another test, radioimmunoimaging of metastatic medullary carcinoma with an indium-111–labeled monoclonal antibody to carcinoembryonic antigen, has also shown some promise in detecting regional and metastatic disease.

Both of these tests need further evaluation with larger trials of patients with hypercalcitoninemia before either is considered a reliable means of detecting recurrent disease.

The 5-year survival rate is better for the familial variety (75% to 80%) than for the sporadic form (50% to 60%). The increased survival rate in the familial type is probably related to earlier diagnosis made on the basis of familial calcitonin screening.

Multiple Endocrine Neoplasia

The MEN syndrome is a genetically autosomal dominant disorder with high penetrance and protean manifestations (Table 45–4). Two subsyndromes, MEN type I (Wermer's)

and MEN type II (Sipple's), have been identified.

Wermer's Syndrome

This syndrome attacks the parathyroid in 85%, the pancreas in 65%, and the pituitary in 40% of patients. The thyroid gland can be involved not with medullary cancer but with other thyroid carcinomas. The parathyroids are involved with either hyperplasia or an adenoma, and the pancreas is involved with insulinomas or gastrinomas. The pituitary, when involved, most often has a chromophobe adenoma that can produce acromegaly.

MEN Type II: Sipple's Syndrome

The type II syndrome is subdivided into a type A and a type B; the main difference between the two is that in type B, there is no hyperparathyroidism.

Type II-A is characterized by the presence of medullary carcinoma in nearly 100% of patients. Bilateral pheochromocytomas are found in 10% of patients, and hyperparathyroidism is found in 60%. The important thing for a head and neck surgeon to remember is that the diagnosis and treatment of a pheochromocytoma take precedence over the treatment of the neck disease, in order to avoid a hypertensive crisis.

Type II-B is characterized by the absence of hyperparathyroidism and the presence of medullary carcinoma and pheochromocytoma associated with multiple neuromas in the conjunctiva, the lips, and the buccal mucosa. Marfanoid habitus without the cardiovascular defects has been reported.

Complications of Thyroid and Parathyroid Surgery

The possibility of complications in thyroid and parathyroid surgery is high, but the

TABLE 45–4. Multiple Endocrine Neoplasia Syndromes

Type of Malignancy	Type I	Type II-A	Type II-B
Parathyroid	X	X	
Pancreas	X		
Pituitary	X		
Nonmedullary thyroid tumors	X		
Medullary thyroid cancer		X	X
Pheochromocytoma		X	X
Mucosal neuromas			X
Marfanoid habitus			X

actual rate of occurrence is low. With proper preoperative evaluation, well-planned and meticulously performed surgery, and thorough postoperative care, the complication rate can be minimized.

The postoperative complications are related to (1) wound complications, (2) hemorrhage, (3) injury to the recurrent and or the superior laryngeal nerves, (4) hypoparathyroidism, and (5) hypothyroidism.

Wound Complications

These are exceedingly rare and usually are related to edema of the flaps and a small hematoma. Infections are unusual unless the operation is being performed on an infected gland. With the use of suction drains, fluid collections that can lead to infections are minimized. When an infection does occur, culture and sensitivity tests, wound drainage, and the administration of antibiotics are appropriate treatments.

Hemorrhage

This is probably the most life-threatening complication of thyroid and parathyroid surgery. Its occurrence is unusual when meticulous technique is adhered to during surgery. The hemorrhage is arterial or venous in origin and usually occurs immediately after the patient awakens from anesthesia, which is when coughing and straining are most commonly seen, or within the first 8 hours after operation. The symptoms of neck swelling, stridor, tightness of the neck, and hypoxia usually are present with hemorrhage. It is worthwhile to have a tracheostomy set at the bedside or nearby so the wound can be quickly opened and the bleeding controlled under aseptic conditions. When there is time, the patient should be returned to the operating room, where while he or she is under anesthesia and in a sterile environment, the wound can be explored. To avoid hemorrhage, double ties of nonabsorbable sutures are used on all major arteries and veins during surgery, and postoperatively the patient is placed in a head-up position, without the application of occlusive dressings (which may obscure the impending crisis). With the use of suction drains (which are not a substitute for careful technique) that are removed when the wound drainage

is less than 20 mL over a 24-hour period, serum accumulations are minimized.

Nerve Paralysis

Two nerves are intimately associated with thyroid and parathyroid surgery. The recurrent laryngeal nerve is the one most often injured during this surgery. Cardiothoracic surgery around the aortic arch has replaced thyroid surgery as the most common cause of recurrent laryngeal nerve injury. Unplanned injury to the recurrent laryngeal nerve should occur in 1% or less of patients of experienced surgeons.

Injury to the superior laryngeal nerve is less often recognized and occurs less often. The best method of avoiding damage to this nerve and its external branch, which supplies the cricothyroid muscle and causes tensing of the vocal cord, is to isolate the superior pole vessels and individually ligate them as they enter the upper pole of the thyroid gland (see Anatomy section).

Injury to the recurrent larygeal nerve can be minimized by identifying the nerve inferiorly and following it superiorly to where it enters the cricothyroid membrane. In this fashion, a right nonrecurrent laryngeal nerve is more easily identified as it crosses either anterior or posterior to the common carotid artery above or below the inferior thyroid artery. The most common vascular abnormality would be a dorsal origin of the right subclavian artery from the aortic arch. Another surgical principle to be followed is not to disturb any branches of the recurrent laryngeal nerve on its way to entering the larynx. There can be two or more major divisions of the nerve extralaryngeally that need to be dissected and preserved.

If the nerve is damaged during operation, an immediate end-to-end reanastomosis is probably the best treatment. When bilateral nerve injury occurs, the patient has marked airway retraction, and tracheotomy is necessary. The long-term management of vocal cord paralysis with thyroplasty, polytef (Teflon) paste injections, reinnervation procedures, and electrical pacing is not discussed in this chapter, and the reader is referred to the current literature for more information.

At the author's institution, patients undergoing thyroid and parathyroid surgery also routinely undergo direct laryngoscopy at the conclusion of surgery as the endotracheal tube is removed, in order to document vocal cord mobility. If paralysis is noted a week or so later, it is more likely to be of a temporary nature.

Hypoparathyroidism

During thyroid and parathyroid surgery, the parathyroid glands can be injured, devascularized, or removed. During surgery, the parathyroids are identified, and the inferior thyroid artery, which is the major source of nourishment to both the superior and inferior glands, is preserved; its branches are ligated as they enter the thyroid substance. When clinical conditions do not permit use of this technique, as when so-called midline cleanout is performed for extensive carcinoma, the parathyroids are dissected off the specimen and autotransplanted.

The incidence of hypoparathyroidism ranges from 1% to 30% in patients undergoing total thyroidectomy, and its occurrence is indirectly proportional to the experience of the surgeon doing total thyroidectomy.

The symptoms of hypoparathyroidism include anxiety, paresis, and numbness of fingers, toes, and lips with the presence of Chvostek's or Trousseau's sign if the calcium level is low enough. With severe hypocalcemia, carpopedal spasm, laryngeal stridor, convulsions, and death can occur.

Treatment should begin before severe symptoms occur. Depending on the degree of damage to the parathyroids, hypocalcemia usually develops within 24 to 72 hours after surgery. Acute treatment is completed with the intravenous use of 10% calcium gluconate, which is stocked in 10-mL vials and contains 1 g of calcium. The usual dose used in cases of severe damage is 12 to 16 g a day in divided doses every 6 hours in 100 mL of saline or dextrose and water over a 45-minute period. When able, the patient is started on oral supplements and calciferol (vitamin D), which will enhance the absorption of calcium. Daily serum calcium (ionized) determinations are obtained and then monitored closely until supplementation is no longer necessary.

Hypothyroidism

Myxedema is expected after all total thyroidectomies, and so administration of levothyroxine is begun postoperatively. In older patients and in patients with a cardiac history, the initial dose is low with gradual increments every 3 weeks until the lowest dose that will maintain a normal T_4 level and a low TSH blood level is reached. Usually this is 0.1 to 0.15 mg. High doses of levothyroxine are no longer used because they seem to enhance osteoporosis and demineralization of the skeleton.

In the surgical management of hyperthyroidism when less than a total thyroidectomy is performed, the size of the remnant determines function. To avoid recurrent hyperthyroidism and the need for secondary operations or use of radioactive iodine, 1- to 2-g remnants of thyroid tissue on either side as described by some surgeons can be retained.

Decreased thyroid function occurs after laryngectomy, partial thyroidectomy, and postoperative irradiation. It also occurs in all patients followed for many years who have had radioactive iodine therapy.

The symptoms of hypothyroidism are myriad: intolerance to cold; thickness and dryness of the hair and skin; edema of face, eyelids, and hands; tendency to be overweight; feeling weak and tired; and sometimes cardiomegaly, bradycardia, and a cardiomyopathy. For the otolaryngologist–head and neck surgeon, sleep apnea and obesity-hypoventilation syndromes have been associated with hypothyroidism. It would be efficacious to obtain serum studies to define thyroid function because the patients who are hypothyroid often dramatically improve with thyroid replacement therapy and weight loss. Hearing loss, both conductive and neurosensory, can be seen, and the patients may have tinnitus and vertigo. Nasal obstruction secondary to turbinate enlargement can also be seen. Some patients with hypothyroidism have hoarseness of the voice and thickened vocal cords. Two syndromes that otolaryngologists may encounter that are associated with hypothyroidism are Pendred's syndrome, which is autosomal recessive and is associated with a goiter and deafness of a neurosensory variety, and Ascher's syndrome, which is an autosomal dominant condition characterized by a nontoxic nodular goiter, blepharochalasis, and a double-lip deformity.

PARATHYROID GLANDS

History

In 1800, Ivar Sanstrom of Sweden discovered the parathyroid glands. The name was well chosen, inasmuch as *para* is the Greek prefix meaning "alongside of."

In the United States, the first surgery for primary hyperparathyroidism was carried out at the Massachusetts General Hospital in 1926. The patient had six operations over a 7-year period, including total thyroidectomy, before the ectopic offending gland was found in a substernal, superior mediastinal location.

The majority of patients with hyperparathyroidism in the early years of discovery had osteitis fibrosa cystica, renal stones, or both. The diagnosis of hyperparathyroidism was uncommon until the 1960s, when autoanalyzers were used for screening serum calcium levels. Now patients with hyperparathyroidism rarely have osteitis fibrosa cystica, and the incidence of renal stones is approximately 10%. This is all attributable to early diagnosis and, perhaps, better treatment.

Calcium Metabolism

Calcium homeostasis is dependent on release of parathyroid hormone (PTH) and, to a lesser degree, small amounts of vitamin D and calcitonin. The function of the parathyroid glands is to maintain calcium and phosphorus homeostasis. Calcium is important for the formation of intercellular ground substance, teeth, and bones. At the membrane level it affects neuromuscular irritability, muscular contractility, and cardiac rhythmicity. Lack of calcium to be carried across cell membranes causes tetany and ultimately death if not corrected.

Calcium when needed is pumped from the extracellular compartment to the intracellular level. Calcium circulates in the extracellular compartment in three forms:

1. Ionized (47%): the free and active form that is readily used.
2. Protein-bound calcium (47%): bound to albumin and globulin and fluctuates especially as the serum protein level goes up and down.
3. Calcium bound to anions (6%): such as bicarbonate, phosphate, and citrate.

When the serum calcium level falls, the parathyroids release PTH, which causes (1) increased osteoclastic activity, which in turn causes resorption of bone and release of calcium; (2) increased resorption of calcium at the renal tubular cell; (3) increased absorption of calcium from the gastrointestinal tract;

(4) stimulation of renal-1-hydroxylase that allows 1-hydroxylation of vitamin D in the kidney; and (5) increased excretion of phosphorus in the urine, which thus decreases the serum phosphorus level.

In the average 70-kg male, there is a little more than 1000 g of calcium, which is divided into (1) bone, which contains 1000 g, is stable and solid, and is broken down only by osteoclastic activity; (2) calcium that is exchangeable in the bone (4 g); (3) intracellular calcium (approximately 11 g); and (4) extracellular fluid calcium (1 g).

Dietary calcium is provided by dairy products, green vegetables, nuts, and fish, as well as by calcium supplements. Approximately 1 g of calcium is ingested per day, and most of this is absorbed in the duodenum and the upper jejunum. At the brush border of the intestine, 1,25-dihydroxy-calciferol vitamin D increases the uptake of calcium by increasing cellular adenosine triphosphate and alkaline phosphatase content. At the other end of the cell, calcium is extruded into the extracellular fluid in exchange for sodium.

Vitamin D is obtained from sunlight or dietary components. This inactive vitamin D is transported via carrier protein to the liver, where it is 25-hydroxylated. It is then transported to the kidney, where 1-hydroxylation takes place, and it becomes activated to perform its function in maintaining calcium homeostasis by increasing calcium absorption and increasing calcium release from bone by osteoclastic activity.

Parathyroid hormone is an 84–amino acid peptide with an active amino terminal end and an inactive carboxyl terminal end. Its secretion by the parathyroid glands is enhanced by a low level of ionized serum calcium and a high phosphate level.

Calcitonin, a 32–amino acid peptide produced by the parafollicular C cells of the thyroid, contributes to calcium homeostasis by suppressing osteoclastic activity in bone and thereby decreasing the amount of calcium that could be available to the extracellular space.

Hyperparathyroidism, the most common cause of hypercalcemia (Table 45–5), is classified into three categories: primary hyperparathyroidism (when either an adenoma or hyperplasia of the glands exists); secondary hyperparathyroidism (when the glands are hyperplastic as a result of malfunction of another organ system; usually this results from renal failure but also can occur in osteo-

Th
the

say
tw
ter
ass
fra
bo
ag
spe
ass
hy
gui
this
but

vat
eas
The
pos
sup
ske
ske
siu
be
bec
nes
irri

S
ph
ele
ure
chl
dec
kidr
res
rem

B
nin
mea

U
Mor
is e
Wit
not
diag

Ra

X-r
bros

TABLE 45–5. Causes of Hypercalcemia

Primary hyperparathyroidism: most common cause for
    hypercalcemia
Malignancy: second most common cause related to
    metastatic bone disease from carcinoma of breast,
    lung, kidney, prostate, and thyroid
Other endocrine disorders
    Hyperthyroidism
    Adrenal insufficiency
    Pheochromocytoma
    Pancreatic islet cell tumors
Granulomatous diseases
    Sarcoidosis
    Tuberculosis
    Histoplasmosis
    Coccidioidomycosis
    Leprosy
Lymphomas: with ectopic production of 1,25-
    dihydroxycalciferol vitamin D
Drugs: thiazide diuretics
    Lithium
    Estrogens/antiestrogens
    Milk-alkali syndrome
    Vitamin A and vitamin D toxicity
Immobilization
Acute and chronic renal disease
Benign familial hypocalciuric hypercalcemia

genesis imperfecta, Paget's disease, multiple myeloma, carcinoma with bone metastasis, and pituitary basophilism); and tertiary hyperparathyroidism (when PTH production is irrepressible, or autonomous, in patients with normal or low serum calcium levels).

The hypercalcemia of malignancy usually occurs as a result of five carcinomas that commonly metastasize to bones: prostate, thyroid, breast, lung, and kidney. However, squamous cell carcinoma, cholangiocarcinoma, bladder cancer, pancreatic islet cell tumors (vasoactive intestinal peptide syndrome, or VIP), and ovarian tumors have produced hypercalcemia in the absence of bone metastases.

The following substances have been shown to be able to increase serum calcium levels either by increasing osteoclastic activity or by secreting amino acids that are similar but not identical to PTH: (1) prostaglandins, (2) transforming growth factor, (3) white blood cells or production of interleukin-1, and (4) lymphotoxin.

Clinical Manifestations of Hyperparathyroidism

In more than 50% of patients, the only manifestation of hyperparathyroidism is hyper-calcemia found on a routine serum chemistry profile.

The symptoms present when the diagnosis is not made early are predominantly related to osteitis fibrosa cystica and nephrocalcinosis. Bone and joint pains and renal stones with hematuria were commonly found in the early days (the 1940s) of Fuller Albright's evaluation of patients who had hyperparathyroidism.

Many of the symptoms seen in the 1980s are nonspecific. Fatigue is a very common presenting symptom. Bone, joint, and muscle pains followed by symptoms of peptic ulcer, cholelithiasis, pancreatitis, renal disease, and hypertension then follow. Approximately 10% of patients are completely asymptomatic. Headaches and mental confusion, even hallucinations, can be seen when serum calcium levels exceed 15 mg.

Embryology and Anatomy

During the fifth week of gestation, the parathyroid glands form from the ectoderm of the dorsal third and fourth branchial pouches. The third arch also forms the thymus gland. In its descent, the parathyroid is brought along and comes to lie near the lower portion of the thyroid gland. The fourth arch parathyroid does not migrate, and so it becomes the upper glands.

Aberrant parathyroids from the third and fourth arches occur in 15% to 20% of people. With a knowledge of the derivatives of these arches, the surgeon can be assisted in finding the ectopic gland (Table 45–6). Surgeons have found hyperfunctioning glands as high as the level of the internal carotid artery and as low as the level of the aortopulmonary window, anterior or posterior to the aortic arch.

There are usually four parathyroid glands, but six or more may be present. Each gland

TABLE 45–6. Aberrant Sites for Parathyroid Adenomas and Hyperplasia

Anterior mediastinum: usually in the thymus, a third
    arch derivative
Posterior mediastinum: a fourth arch derivative
Aorta pulmonary window: in the middle mediastinum;
    may be third or fourth arch in derivation
Retroesophageal prevertebral
Tracheoesophageal
Intrathyroidal
Carotid bifurcation

5 mm in diameter); and (3) its cost, which is higher than that of radionuclide scans. Its advantages are that it is noninvasive and fast to perform.

CT scans (1) are more expensive to obtain, (2) provide poor resolution of glands less than 1 cm in diameter, and (3) do not usually distinguish between parathyroids that are intimately associated with the thyroid.

The invasive tests of angiography and selective venous catheterization for PTH should be reserved for the patient in whom exploration has been inconclusive. The technique is dependent on the skill of the angiographer; the tests are time consuming (3 to 5 hours), expensive, and uncomfortable for the patient. If any of the veins have been ligated during previous surgery, the tests can be nonlocalizing but may lateralize the offending gland to a particular site.

Medical Management of Hypercalcemia

When an identifying cause for the hypercalcemia that is surgically correctable is found and the surgical procedure is completed, the patient has a 95% chance of cure as long as chronic renal failure is not the cause. In patients with renal failure, surgical cure rates are from 50% to 85%.

Hypercalcemia that is related to sarcoidosis and to other granulomas responds to steroids. The steroids blunt the synthesis and effects of elevated 1,25-dihydroxycalciferol vitamin D.

When confusion, delusional behavior, and mental deterioration are associated with hypercalcemia, more aggressive therapy with a saline furosemide diuresis may be helpful. Four to 10 L of saline per 24 hours with 40 to 80 mg of intravenous furosemide every 4 to 6 hours is given to prevent hypernatremia.

To reduce bone resorption and hypercalcemia, mithramycin and calcitonin can be given. Mithramycin in a dose of 25 μg/kg causes a rapid fall in serum calcium in 1 to 3 days. However, if multiple infusions are necessary, toxicity to the bone marrow, kidney, and liver can occur.

Gallium nitrate has been shown to block the effect of PTH on bone and to lower serum calcium levels in patients with intractable hypercalcemia associated with parathyroid carcinoma.

Surgical Management of Hyperparathyroidism

Patients with symptomatic hyperparathyroidism and serum calcium levels 1 mg above the upper limit of normal should undergo parathyroidectomy, as long as there are no mitigating circumstances to suggest a nonoperative approach. Patients who are asymptomatic and have mildly or intermittently elevated serum calcium levels also benefit from parathyroidectomy. With knowledge of the natural history of hyperparathyroidism, it is known that the longer the pathologic process functions are unchecked, the more severe the demineralization of the skeleton, nephrocalcinosis, and other symptoms become. Again, the surgeon needs to use discretion in treating elderly patients and poor-risk patients because the surgical approach may not be of great benefit.

Most patients operated on by experienced head and neck surgeons for hyperparathyroidism have a 95% or better cure rate.

Patients undergoing parathyroid surgery are prepared in the same fashion as those undergoing thyroid surgery. Indirect laryngoscopy to document normal vocal cord motion is carried out. If the alkaline phosphatase level is elevated on the chemistry profile, the surgeon is alerted to the fact that the patient may need calcium or magnesium supplementation, or both, during the postoperative period as bone metabolism equilibrates. Patients with mild or moderate azotemia need adequate hydration preoperatively to avoid worsening of renal function. Several generalities when performing parathyroid surgery should be considered:

1. It has always been said that at least four glands must be identified during the neck exploration. With the advent of more accurate preoperative localization tests, some surgeons advocate removal of the localizing gland and biopsy identification of one other normal gland. The surgeon needs to develop a keen sense of judgment in performing these surgeries and must be prepared to resect a spectrum of one gland to three and one half glands to total parathyroidectomy and auto-transplantation of 20 mg of tissue into a muscle bed.

2. If results of the neck exploration are normal, the thymus and the superior mediastinum are examined. It is assumed that the surgeon has already examined the thy-

roid gland and made the decision that there is no intrathyroidal parathyroid tissue, which is present in approximately 2% to 5% of patients.

3. The superior parathyroids are more constant in their position. They are located in the posterior aspect of the thyroid lobe at the point where the recurrent laryngeal nerve passes under the cricothyroid muscle or just posterior to this, where the inferior constrictor muscle fibers are found. This necessitates a medial rotation of the upper pole, which can be done while the superior parathyroid artery and vein are preserved.

4. The inferior parathyroids can usually be found within 1 to 2 cm of the inferior thyroid artery where it enters the body of the thyroid gland. However, they can be located anywhere in the tracheoesophageal sulcus, in paratracheal fat, or within the thymus, with which they have a common embryologic origin.

5. The main blood supply to the parathyroids is from the inferior thyroid artery. In general, the superior parathyroid artery also arises from branches of the inferior thyroid, but it can arise from the superior thyroid artery. To avoid devascularizing normal parathyroid tissue, the inferior thyroid artery should be preserved. If the vessel is ligated, it is done as it enters the thyroid gland.

6. No parathyroid that appears normal should be removed unless a frozen-section biopsy proves that it is hyperplastic. Anatomically, the parathyroids are ovoid, are pale to dark tan, and turn a deep red-brown with manipulation. They are approximately 8 mm in diameter, are encapsulated from the thyroid gland, and are surrounded by a rim of fat. If at the completion of the exploration a gland has turned blue-black, it most likely has been devascularized and should be diced for transplantation to either the sternocleidomastoid muscle or the brachioradialis muscle in the forearm.

7. If a definite adenoma is located, a small biopsy specimen from one other gland should be used for comparison to help the pathologist distinguish adenomas from hyperplasia. The sine qua non for diagnosing parathyroid adenomas is to find a rim of normal parathyroid tissue being encroached upon by the adenoma.

Operative Technique

A low cervical incision is used. The strap muscles are either retracted or divided, depending on individual anatomic variations. The middle thyroid vein is secured after adequate inspection and palpation of the thyroid gland. If the preoperative localization test identifies the side of the lesion, the search for the parathyroid is begun inferiorly on the side of localization, even though the inferior glands are the ones most apt to be aberrant. The inferior laryngeal nerve and recurrent thyroid artery are identified. If no parathyroid is found in this location, the exploration is continued in a superior direction toward the upper pole of the thyroid; branches of the inferior thyroid artery that do not enter the thyroid parenchyma should be preserved.

The dissection is carried out on the capsule of the thyroid gland, and with medial rotation of the gland, the recurrent laryngeal nerve is followed, and the anterior branches of the superior thyroid artery are ligated. The posterior vessels are preserved until either the parathyroid is identified or a branch from the inferior thyroid to the parathyroid is detected. A common location for the superior parathyroid is within 1 cm of where the recurrent laryngeal pierces the cricothyroid membrane. If the inferior parathyroids have not been identified, dissection is performed between the carotid artery and the trachea in a systematic fashion to include the superior mediastinum. If necessary, the prevertebral-retroesophageal tissue is carefully inspected, as is the retrotracheoesophageal compartment. When an inferior gland is missing, it frequently is found within the thymus, whereas if the upper parathyroid is missing, it can be in a more posterior position and frequently in the posterior mediastinum.

If one enlarged gland is found, it is removed and sent for frozen-section diagnosis. If the diagnosis is adenoma, biopsy of one other gland is performed; if it is normal on frozen section, the surgery is completed. If the enlarged gland is adenoma and biopsy of another gland demonstrates hyperplasia, then three and one half glands are removed with the option of autotransplanting half a gland to the forearm or the sternocleidomastoid muscle. Another option is that of cryopreserving one gland (which can be stored for up to 18 months in this fashion) and, if necessary, transplanting it at a later date.

If the patient has all hyperplastic glands, familial hyperplasia, or multiple endocrine adenomatosis, removal of three and one half glands or total resection is performed with autotransplantation. Parathyroid tissue can also be cryopreserved for an 18-month period of time and, when needed, transplanted as discussed.

Patients with renal failure and parathyroid hyperplasia probably are best treated with total parathyroidectomy and autotransplantation of approximately 20 mg of parathyroid tissue to the brachioradialis muscle in the forearm. This spot is recommended over a cervical transplantation because of the ease of excising the transplanted tissue when it hyperfunctions.

If parathyroid tissue has been cryopreserved and the patient remains hypoparathyroid 2 months after surgery, the tissue can be thawed and transposed to the forearm muscular bed while the patient is under local anesthesia; in that location, it stands a better than 50% chance of maintaining calcium homeostasis.

Primary hyperparathyroidism in pregnancy is uncommon; only 100 cases have been reported to date. Surgical exploration should be conducted during the second trimester (16 to 26 weeks) to minimize the complications of neonatal tetany, stillbirth, and spontaneous abortion. Surgery could be reserved for a postpartum date as long as the surgeon and the physicians involved in the care of the mother and the child are aware of the potential complications. Neonatal tetany can occur in mothers with hyperparathyroidism because calcium crosses the placental barrier but parathyroid hormone (PTH) does not. Therefore the child has neonatal hypercalcemia that precipitously drops during the first 24 to 48 hours of life, as the placental source of calcium has been cut off. It usually takes 7 to 10 days for the child's own parathyroid glands to recover normal function; this process necessitates careful monitoring and supplementation.

Primary hyperparathyroidism in infancy can be a fatal disorder. These infants usually display hypercalcemia, respiratory distress, muscular hypotonia, and skeletal demineralization. Surgical exploration with removal of the adenoma if present, or total parathyroidectomy with autotransplantation of a portion of one gland if four-gland hyperplasia is present, affords the best opportunity for eucalcemia.

Children with hypercalcemia should be checked for familial hypercalcemic hypocalciuria. Low levels of urinary calcium excretion establish the diagnosis in this disorder.

Most often, these patients do not develop the same complications that patients with hyperparathyroidism do; therefore, no treatment may be necessary. Patients with familial hypercalcemic hypocalciuria who have surgery require a total parathyroidectomy. Cryopreservation of one gland that could be transplanted at a later date, if necessary, may be worthwhile in the treatment of this particular syndrome.

Parathyroid Carcinoma

This disease is rarely encountered in clinical practice; the incidence is 0.5% to 4% of cases of primary hyperparathyroidism. The surgeon's index of suspicion rises when the serum calcium level is exceptionally high, when there is a palpable neck mass, or when high serum calcium levels persist or recur after surgery.

During surgery, a reliable sign of malignancy is the dense fibrous reaction that surround the tumor, making it adhere to other neck structures. It is essential that a wide excision of the tumor be completed because the local recurrence rate is approximately 30%. Regional and distant metastases to the lungs, the liver, and the bones occur in 25% to 30% of patients. In addition to removal of the parathyroid gland, ipsilateral thyroid lobectomy, skeletonization of the tracheoesophageal groove, excision of paratracheal lymph nodes, and keeping the tumor intact during the removal provide the best chance for long-term survival. Radical neck dissection is reserved for only those patients with palpable lymph nodes. Resection of the recurrent laryngeal nerve may be necessary if the tumor is intimately associated with it.

Radiation therapy is not used as primary treatment because the results are disappointing and discouraging. It may be of some benefit in a postoperative setting in the presence of microscopic disease.

Persistent Hyperparathyroidism

Recurrent or persistent hyperparathyroidism is seen in approximately 5% of patients. Reoperation for persistent or recurrent hyperparathyroidism after a surgical exploration is difficult and increases the risks of complications. Most surgeons agree that localization of the offending gland or glands is critical to developing a sound surgical plan. Use of noninvasive thallium-technetium scans and of invasive arteriography with selective venous sampling for parathyroid hormone is helpful. These two examinations have uniformly identified the site of the residual disease in the series of patients whom the author has treated. Unfortunately, performance of angiography and venous sampling requires skill, and it is time consuming as well as expensive. Usually in this setting the offending parathyroid gland is in an ectopic position, and localizing it makes the surgery safer.

Autotransplantation of Parathyroid Tissue

Parathyroids in patients without renal failure and without parathyroid hyperplasia are not destroyed. If during the removal of a parathyroid adenoma a normal parathyroid gland appears to be devascularized, it will develop a deep blue-black discoloration. That gland is removed and placed in a sterile iced saline bath until the time for autotransplantation to a muscular bed. This technique is also used in other aspects of head and neck surgery: when thyroid surgery is being performed and a parathyroid appears devascularized; when a midline cleanout for carcinoma of the larynx, the pharynx, or the cervical esophagus is being conducted; or when parathyroids are identified and, if they cannot be preserved on their vascularized pedicle, are autotransplanted.

The parathyroid is removed from the iced saline bath and cut into 1- to 2-mm pieces; usually 10 to 20 sections are obtained from the average-sized gland. A separate muscle bed is created for each piece of tissue, which is then transplanted deep in the muscle. This pocket is then sutured or clipped with a hemoclip that holds it in position. An area of muscle averaging 2 to 3 cm in diameter is adequate for the transplanted tissue. Within 2 to 3 months, the graft is neovascularized and functioning. As the serum calcium level begins to rise, the calcium supplements are decreased gradually and then discontinued as the monitored calcium level is maintained in the normal range. Venous samples can be taken from a proximal vein, close to the transplant (to avoid dilution) and can be compared for PTH levels with a venous sample from the other arm. A thallium-technetium parathyroid scan of the forearm can also

be used to establish whether this transplanted parathyroid gland definitely has function.

Complications

The complications—(1) hypocalcemia (temporary or permanent), (2) vocal cord paralysis, and (3) hematoma—are more specific to parathyroid surgery and can be minimized by adequate preoperative planning, by following basic surgical techniques, and by exercising good judgment. Complications can arise, however, even when all these procedures are performed well.

Approximately 20% to 30% of patients develop temporary hypoparathyroidism; many of these patients do not need supplemental calcium or vitamin D. An asymptomatic low serum calcium level can develop within a few hours after parathyroidectomy, but usually the lowest levels are reached between 1 and 3 days after operation. Calcium levels then start to return to a normal range. A serum calcium level that is in the low normal range (i.e., 2.2 mEq/L or around 2.0 mEq/L) provides stimulation of the remaining parathyroids to function. However, if the patient is symptomatic with signs of muscular irritability, as reflected by a positive Chvostek's or Trousseau's sign, then supplementation with calcium and vitamin D is started.

A positive Chvostek's sign is a grimacing of the face when the facial nerve is tapped through the skin as it exits the stylomastoid foramen. A positive Trousseau's sign is obtained when blood pressure is measured and the blood pressure cuff is maintained above the systolic pressure for 3 to 4 minutes: the patient, if hypocalcemic, develops carpopedal muscle spasms. Under these circumstances, 2 to 4 g of calcium gluconate diluted in dextrose and water or saline can be administered intravenously every 6 hours and given slowly over a 30- to 45-minute period. Oral calcium supplements in four equally divided doses of 8 to 16 g with either 0.2 mg of dihydrotachysterol or 50,000 units of vitamin D_2 are also begun. As the serum calcium level begins to rise and the symptoms abate, the intravenous form is decreased and stopped. It is not unusual to need to maintain supplemental calcium and vitamin D for 2 to 6 months in some patients. In patients receiving long-term therapy with calcium supplements, serum levels are monitored on a weekly basis.

If the patient continues to be symptomatic and the serum calcium level is normal, the surgeon needs to consider the need to replace magnesium because hypomagnesemia can cause a positive Chvostek's sign and other signs of increased muscular irritability. Especially in patients with bone-wasting hyperparathyroidism, it is more likely that magnesium supplements are necessary because magnesium and calcium are being returned to bone at a rate higher than usual in these cases.

Vocal cord paralysis occurs in less than 1% of patients who have undergone parathyroid surgery; this is discussed in the section on thyroid disease.

Wound collections of blood and serum are controlled by the use of functioning suction drains.

SUMMARY

Primary hyperparathyroidism can be caused by a solitary parathyroid adenoma, by hyperplastic parathyroid glands, by multiple adenomas, or occasionally by a carcinoma. The diagnosis in most patients is made tentatively by chemistry profile with elevated serum calcium levels and is confirmed by repeated serum calcium and PTH determinations. A parathyroid adenoma can usually be localized preoperatively by thallium-technetium scan, by ultrasonography, by CT scan, or, in the case of persistent disease with hypercalcemia, by angiography with selective venous sampling for PTH. Both sides of the neck may need exploration, or a unilateral exploration may be sufficient if the preoperative localization tests are confirmatory and biopsy of another "normal" gland yields normal histologic findings. During the postoperative period, suction drains lessen the likelihood of hematoma formation, and serum calcium levels are monitored for the first 3 to 5 days. Patients who have low calcium levels and are symptomatic receive supplementation not only of calcium but also of vitamin D until the serum levels are brought to the low normal range, at which time oral supplements are continued until eucalcemia is maintained. Most patients who undergo parathyroid surgery benefit both symptomatically and metabolically.

SUGGESTED READINGS

Thyroid Physiology and Testing

Beenken S, Guillamondegui O, Shallenberger R, et al: Prognostic factors in patients dying of well-differentiated thyroid cancer. Arch Otolaryngol Head Neck Surg 115:326–330, 1989.

Beierwaltes WH: The treatment of thyroid carcinoma with radioactive iodine. Semin Nucl Med 8:79–94, 1978.

Brown JS, Steiner AL: Medullary thyroid carcinoma and the syndromes of multiple endocrine adenomas. DM 28(11):1–37, 1982.

Chonkich GD, Petti GH Jr, Goral W: Total thyroidectomy in the treatment of thyroid disease. Laryngoscope 97:897–900, 1987.

Eisenberg BL, Hensley SD: Thyroid cancer with coexistent Hashimoto's thyroiditis. Clinical assessment and management. Arch Surg 124:1045–1047, 1989.

Falk SA, Birken EA, Baran DT: Temporary postthyroidectomy hypocalcemia. Arch Otolaryngol Head Neck Surg 114:168–174, 1988.

Grant CS: Diagnostic and prognostic utility of flow cytometric DNA measurement in follicular thyroid tumors. World J Surg 14:283–290, 1990.

Hamming JF: The value of fine needle aspiration biopsy in patients with nodular thyroid disease. Arch Intern Med 150:113–116, 1990.

Harvey HK: Diagnosis and management of the thyroid nodule. Otolaryngol Clin North Am 23:303–337, 1990.

Hay ID: Prognostic factors in thyroid carcinoma. Thyroid Today 12(1):1–9, 1989.

Ingbar S: The thyroid gland. *In* Williams RH (ed): Textbook of Endocrinology, 6th ed (pp. 117–247). Philadelphia: WB Saunders, 1981.

Keller MP, Crabbe MM, Norwood SH: Accuracy and significance of fine-needle aspiration and frozen section in determining the extent of thyroid resection. Surgery 101:632–635, 1987.

Kodama T, Okamoto T, Fujimoto Y, et al: C cell adenoma of the thyroid: a rare but distinct clinical entity. Surgery 104:997–1003, 1988.

Loré JM: An Atlas of Head and Neck Surgery, 3rd ed. Philadelphia: WB Saunders, 1988.

Loré JM: The thyroid gland. *In* Lee KY, Loré JM, Milley PS (eds): Advances in Otolaryngology—Head and Neck Surgery (pp 261–294). Chicago: Yearbook Medical Publishers, 1988.

Mazzaferri EL: Papillary thyroid carcinoma: factors influencing prognosis and current therapy. Semin Oncol 14:315–332, 1987.

Mazzaferri EL, Young RL, Oertel JE, et al: Papillary thyroid carcinoma: the impact of therapy on 576 patients. Medicine (Baltimore) 57:171–196, 1977.

McCall AR, Ott R, Jarosz H, et al: Improvement of vocal cord paresis after thyroidectomy. Am Surg 53:377–379, 1987.

McHenry C, Jarosz H, Lawrence AM, Paloyan E: Improving postoperative recurrence rates for carcinoma of the thyroid gland. Surg Gyn Obst 169:429–434, 1989.

Miller JM, Hamburger JI, Kini SR: The needle biopsy diagnosis of papillary thyroid carcinoma. Cancer 48:989–993, 1981.

Miyauchi A, Matsuzuka F, Kuma K: Piriform sinus fistula: an underlying abnormality common in patients with acute suppurative thyroiditis. World J Surg 14:400–405, 1990.

Modan B, Baidatz D, Mart H, et al: Radiation-induced head and neck tumours. Lancet 1:277–279, 1974.

Noyek AM, Greyson ND, Steinhardt MI, et al: Thyroid tumor imaging. Arch Otolaryngol 109:205–224, 1983.

Ozoux JP, de Calan L, Portier G, et al: Surgical treatment of Graves' disease. Am J Surg 156:177–181, 1988.

Perzik SL: The place of total thyroidectomy in the management of 909 patients with thyroid disease. Am J Surg 132:480–483, 1976.

Ram MD: Apudomas. Curr Surg 38:230–233, 1981.

Samaan NA, Schultz PN, Hickey RC: Medullary thyroid carcinoma: prognosis of familial versus sporadic disease and the role of radiotherapy. J Clin Endocrinol Metab 67:801–805, 1988.

Sawin CT, Geller A, Hershman JM: The aging thyroid. The use of thyroid hormone in older persons. JAMA 261:2653–2655, 1989.

Shapiro MJ: Medullary carcinoma of the thyroid gland. Laryngoscope 86:1375–1385, 1976.

Surks MI, Chupra IJ, Mariash CN, et al: American Thyroid Association guidelines for use of laboratory tests in thyroid disorders. JAMA 263:1529–1532, 1990.

Thompson NW: Current diagnostic techniques for single thyroid nodules. Curr Surg 40:255–259, 1983.

Tollefson HR, Shah JP, Huvos AG: Papillary carcinoma of the thyroid: recurrences in thyroid gland after initial surgical treatment. Am J Surg 124:468–472, 1972.

Wartofsky L: Osteoporoses: a growing concern for the thyroidologist. Thyroid Today 11(4):1–11, 1988.

Bibliography

Albright F: A page out of the history of hyperparathyroidism. J Clin Endocrinol 8:637–657, 1948.

Bergman DA: Disorders of calcium metabolism. Med Times 116(5):85–96, 1988.

Brennan MF, Brown EM, Spiegel AM, et al: Autotransplantation of cryopreserved parathyroid tissue in man. Ann Surg 189:139–142, 1979.

Burtis WJ, Brody TG, Orloff JJ, et al: Immunochemical characterization of circulating PTH-related protein in patients with humoral hypercalcemia of cancer. New Engl J Med 322:1100–1105, 1990.

Davidson J, Noyek AM, Gottesman I, et al: The parathyroid adenoma—an imaging/surgical perspective. J Otolaryngol 17:282–287, 1988.

Falk SA, Birken EA, Baran DT: Temporary post-thyroidectomy hypocalcemia. Arch Otolaryngol Head Neck Surg 114:168–174, 1988.

Garabedian M, Holick MF, Deluca HF, et al: Control of 25-hydroxycholecalciferol metabolism by parathyroid glands. Proc Natl Acad Sci USA 69:1673–1676, 1972.

Halstead WS, Evans HM: The parathyroid glandules, their blood supply and their presentation in operations of the thyroid gland. Ann Surg 46:489, 1907.

Harris SS, D'Ercole AJ: Neonatal hyperparathyroidism: the natural course in the absence of surgical intervention. Pediatrics 83:53–56, 1989.

Higgins RV, Hisley JC: Primary hyperparathyroidism in pregnancy. A report of two cases. J Reprod Med 33:726–730, 1988.

Kaplan RA, Snyder WH, Stewart A, et al: Metabolic effects of parathyroidectomy in asymptomatic primary hyperparathyroidism. J Clin Endocrinol Metab 42:415–426, 1976.

Keyes GR, Tenta LT: Diagnosis of parathyroid disorders. Otolaryngol Clin North Am 13:127–135, 1980.

Lowe DK, Orwoll ES, McClung MR, et al: Hyperparathyroidism and pregnancy. Am J Surg 145:611–614, 1983.

Kristoffersson A, Dahlgren S, Lithner F, Järhult J: Primary hyperparathyroidism in pregnancy. Surgery 97:326–330, 1985.

Mashburn MA, Chonkich GD, Chase DR, Petti GH Jr: Parathyroid carcinoma: two new cases—diagnosis and treatment. Laryngoscope 97:215–218, 1987.

Nussbaum SR, Zahrodnik RJ, Lavigne JR, et al: Highly sensitive two site immuno-radiometric assay of PTH and its clinical utility in evaluating patients with hypercalcemia. Clin Chem 33:1364–1367, 1987.

Petti GH Jr: Hyperparathyroidism: a study of 100 cases. Otolaryngol Head Neck Surg 90:413–418, 1982.

Prinz RA, Paloyan E, Lawrence AM, et al: Radiation-associated hyperparathyroidism: a new syndrome? Surgery 82:296–302, 1977.

Ross AJ 3d, Cooper A, Attie MF, Bishop HC: Primary hyperparathyroidism in infancy. J Pediatr Surg 21:493–499, 1986.

Scholz DA, Purnell DC: Asymptomatic primary hyperparathyroidism. 10-year prospective study. Mayo Clin Proc 56:473–478, 1981.

Thompson NW, Carpenter LC, Kessler DL, Nishiyama RH: Hereditary neonatal hyperparathyroidism. Arch Surg 113:100–103, 1978.

Voorman GS, Petti GH Jr, Schulz E, et al: The pitfalls of technetium Tc 99m/thallium 201 parathyroid scanning. Arch Otolaryngol Head Neck Surg 114:993–995, 1988.

Warrell RP Jr, Issacs M, Alcock NW, Backman RS: Gallium nitrate for treatment of refractory hypercalcemia from parathyroid carcinoma. Ann Intern Med 107:683–686, 1987.

Wells SA Jr, Ross AJ 3d, Dale JK, Gray RS: Transplantation of the parathyroid glands: current status. Surg Clin North Am 59:167–177, 1979.

PART SIX

Disorders of Soft Tissue and Skeleton

CHAPTER 46

Cutaneous Lesions

Carolyn B. Lyde, MD   Forrest C. Brown, MD   Paul R. Bergstresser, MD

From the dermatologist's point of view, two elements are key in the management of cutaneous lesions: first, a careful examination of the skin in order to formulate an appropriate differential diagnosis, and second, a reliance on clinicopathologic correlations between what is seen clinically and subsequent (and inevitable) histopathologic examinations. The ultimate question in this regard concerns how the histopathologic observations support or deny what is seen clinically. After this question is resolved, appropriate therapy can be planned. Thus dermatologists are biased by their knowledge of the physical examination and by their reliance on histopathologic examination. Moreover, with experience, it is possible to predict, with a high degree of accuracy and on clinical grounds alone, both the histopathologic changes and the ultimate diagnosis.

Although it is inappropriate to excise incompletely or to treat insufficiently a malignant skin tumor, the requirement for complete treatment cannot justify excessive or exuberant treatment for the numerous benign and premalignant lesions that also occur commonly in skin. Once again, the formulation of an appropriate differential diagnosis is the first task. This task is facilitated by an understanding of the structure and function of skin.

STRUCTURE AND FUNCTION OF SKIN

Three compartments—epidermis, dermis, and subcutis—make up skin. Epidermis, the outermost portion, consists of a cellular aggregate of cells, primarily keratinocytes (95%), melanocytes (2%), and Langerhans' cells (2%). It is important to recognize that the vast majority of cutaneous malignancies originate from two of these epidermal cells, keratinocytes and melanocytes. Separating the epidermis from dermis is a complex structure termed the basement membrane, which is important for this discussion only because the breaching of this membrane by invading cells represents the fundamental event in the development of an epidermal malignancy.

Finally, an underlying dermis, composed of collagen, elastin, nerves, and blood vessels, provides strength and nutrition to skin as a whole. Although skin cancers ordinarily do not originate in the dermis, its stromal and vascular support is required for tumor growth. Moreover, dermis can serve as an attractive site for the lodging of metastatic carcinomas (from a variety of origins) as well as the site of direct invasion.

The major function of skin is to establish and maintain an effective barrier between a person and his or her many environments. This barrier prevents entry and destructive effects of a variety of environmental factors, including toxic chemicals, infectious agents, heat, and ultraviolet radiation. Skin also prevents the loss of fluids and soluble materials from the inside. This barrier to chemical and infectious assault resides in the outermost layer of skin, the stratum corneum, which is a laminated and adherent product of proliferation and differentiation among the underlying keratinocytes. The barrier to ultraviolet radiation resides in the capacity of stratum corneum to scatter light as well as in the capacity of melanin, within underlying keratinocytes and melanocytes, to absorb much of the radiation that is not scattered. Since 1970, a number of therapeutic techniques have been devised to retard and to facilitate percutaneous penetration; more important, the penetration of ultraviolet radiation is retarded through the use of sunscreens.

TERMINOLOGY

Appropriate use of terms simplifies and makes more accurate the description of lesions that are seen in skin. First, a distinction is made between an initial lesion, termed *primary*, and a subsequent change, termed *secondary*. These terms are used throughout the chapter, and their use emphasizes the need to formulate a precise and accurate clinical diagnosis before diagnostic and therapeutic procedures are considered.

Primary Lesions

A *macule*, a circumscribed, flat defect in the skin, is visible primarily because of color differences. Most freckles, lentigines, and junctional nevi are macules.

A *papule*, a small lesion (less than 1 cm in diameter), produces distinct elevation of the skin surface. A papule may or may not have overlying scale. Most warts, seborrheic keratoses, compound nevi, and actinic keratoses are papules.

A *nodule* is a larger, elevated skin lesion (greater than 1 cm in diameter). Basal cell and squamous cell carcinomas and, unfortunately, some melanomas that have been ignored become nodules.

Secondary Lesions

Erosion, a superficial discontinuity in the epidermal covering of skin, usually is associated with an exudate that forms a crust or a scale crust. Granulation tissue is ordinarily not present. Erosions may involve large areas of skin, and they ordinarily, in the absence of bacterial infection, heal without scar formation.

An *ulcer*, a relatively deep discontinuity in the skin surface, involves both epidermis and dermis, with underlying granulation tissue formation. Ulcers may result from trauma to the skin, from underlying vascular insuffi-

ciency, or in the context of a destructive cutaneous carcinoma.

A *scar* is a visible discontinuity in the dermis, often with a depression in the skin surface; the overlying epidermis is intact. Scars assume many forms, which are usually dependent on the cause of a previous ulcer or on treatment.

PIGMENTATION

Freckle

Freckles (ephelides) are discrete, small macules in which melanocytes produce excessive amounts of melanin, primarily in response to ultraviolet light. Freckles do not have increased numbers of melanocytes; rather, they represent areas of functionally overactive melanocytes, which become homogeneously brown upon exposure to sunlight. Freckling occurs primarily in fair-skinned people who do not tan well; therefore, freckles serve as a marker for increased susceptibility to skin cancers of all types.

On histopathologic examination, one sees increased pigment and normal numbers of melanocytes along the dermal/epidermal junction.

Avoidance of ultraviolet light exposure permits freckles to fade with time, and this process may be enhanced by the judicious use of hydroquinone-containing products or tretinoin (Retin-A) applied topically.

Freckles that appear before the age of 2 years should alert physicians to the possibility of *xeroderma pigmentosum*, an inherited defect in deoxyribonucleic acid (DNA) repair that follows ultraviolet light injury. This defect leads to the development of multiple, aggressive skin cancers. Finally, axillary freckling is a sign of *neurofibromatosis* and calls for further search for café au lait spots and neurofibromas.

Lentigo

A *lentigo (lentigines)* is a common, flat, hyperpigmented macule that is attributable to an increase in the number of normal melanocytes at the dermal/epidermal junction. Lentigines rarely become more than a few millimeters in size, and they are usually round or polycyclic in shape. Of importance is that surface epidermal markings are completely preserved. Lentigines may be divided broadly into two types: *lentigo simplex* and *solar lentigo*. The simplex lentigenes occur singly and are often found in children with a distribution that is unrelated to sun exposure or to the degree of pigmentation. The natural history of lentigo simplex is not known, although it may "disappear" with age, as family photographs often demonstrate. Acral and mucosal lentigines are common, especially in darkly pigmented persons, and they are probably inherited in an autosomal dominant fashion. Although few investigators contend that some lentigines are precursors to junctional nevi (Stegmaier and Montgomery, 1953), their malignant potential remains uncertain.

By contrast, solar (formerly called senile) lentigines occur on sun-exposed areas in elderly patients. These macules make up the majority of what are commonly called "liver spots" in the vernacular. (Seborrheic keratoses with their granular surfaces, plane warts, and junctional nevi account for the remaining majority of "liver spots.") Solar lentigines often fade with time if ultraviolet light is avoided.

A special category of solar lentigines, termed PUVA lentigines, is induced in patients treated therapeutically with a photoxic compound, such as psoralen, and ultraviolet light from spectrum A (UVA). PUVA lentigines are similar in appearance to solar lentigines, although some data suggest that these iatrogenic hyperpigmented macules have a higher frequency of atypical melanocytes (Rhodes et al., 1983).

Finally, *lentigo maligna*, a special form of melanocytic hyperplasia, occurs on the faces of chronically sun-exposed, elderly patients. Lentigo maligna may become quite large, attaining a diameter of several centimeters and exhibiting uneven pigmentation and uneven borders. As noted subsequently, a significant proportion of these lentigines develop a melanoma in situ, which in turn may become an invasive melanoma.

Although histopathologic variation occurs among these forms of lentigines, they all exhibit the general feature of elongated rete ridges with club ends where melanocyte proliferation may be found.

The cosmetic removal of lentigines can sometimes be accomplished with a light liquid nitrogen freeze, because melanocytes are relatively more sensitive to cold. Trichloroacetic acid peels and tretinoin (Retin-A) applied topically have also been useful. These techniques have invariably yielded incomplete results when applied to lentigo maligna.

Excessively dark lentigines in elderly patients, or a lentigo maligna that exhibits palpability or surface marking changes, should be histopathologically evaluated for melanoma. Whenever possible, a complete excisional biopsy should be performed, although a large lentigo maligna on the face may leave a defect that is difficult to repair. A reasonable compromise would include incisional biopsy of the darkest or thickest portion.

Several autosomal dominant, neuroectodermal syndromes include multiple lentigines. The LEOPARD syndrome includes thousands of *l*entigines, *E*lectrocardiographic abnormalities, *o*cular hypertelorism, *p*ulmonary stenosis, *a*bnormality of genitalia, *r*etardation of growth, and neural *d*eafness. Moynihan's syndrome includes growth and mental retardation and hypoplastic genitalia along with a multitude of lentigines. Peutz-Jegher syndrome includes intestinal polyposis along with generalized lentigines that evolve into persistent oral lentigines.

MELANOCYTIC NEVI

Melanocytic nevi, or "moles," are exceedingly common. These ordinarily benign collections of melanocyte-like cells arise from the neural crest and migrate to skin during embryogenesis.

Junctional nevi predominate in children, and they appear as sharply circumscribed, darkly hyperpigmented macules or barely perceptible papules. Epidermal surface markings are seen to be slightly distorted when examined closely with oblique lighting. The corresponding histopathologic examination reveals epithelioid nevus cells, which are very similar to normal melanocytes, nesting along the dermal/epidermal border. For simplicity, these melanocytic nevus cells are referred to as melanocytes.

Compound nevi have a more papular clinical component, and they tend to be lighter in color. On histopathologic examination, melanocytes are seen not only at the dermal/epidermal junction but also extending more deeply into the dermis to form cords and strands.

Finally, intradermal nevi are the common nevi of older adults. They are dome-shaped, smooth or verrucous, and often flesh colored; they may contain large terminal hairs (Figs. 46–1, 46–2). Histopathologic examination reveals that the melanocytes occur primarily within the dermis, and they exhibit a "mature" phenotype; that is, the superficial cells (type A) are more epithelioid, mid-zone cells (type B) are more lymphoid, and the deepest cells (type C) are quite neuroid and spindle-shaped in appearance.

It is clear that at least some moles begin their existence as junctional nevi in children and progress with time to compound nevi and, finally, to intradermal nevi in older adults. The melanocytes seem to multiply and drop deeper into the dermis as the lesion clinically becomes correspondingly lighter in color and more palpable.

The peak mole-forming period is late teens and early adulthood, at which time each person has an average of 30 to 40 nevi (Nicholls, 1973); people with fair skin have the largest numbers of nevi. The number and location of nevi are determined on a genetic basis, although environmental factors such as ultraviolet light increase their number. Hormonal changes, such as those in puberty and pregnancy, also increase the number of nevi as well as cause a darkening of existing ones. Any person with more than 50 moles is at increased risk for melanoma (Holly et al., 1987). Because acquired melanocytic nevi are very rare in persons more than 80 years old, all new dark moles in an elderly adult are suspect for melanoma.

Common melanocytic nevi may be viewed largely as a cosmetic nuisance by patients, but of more concern is their limited but real malignant potential. Most malignant melanomas arise either de novo or from preexisting melanocytic nevi, usually nevi with junctional cells. Although the vast majority of nevi evolve through their life span without malignant transformation, certain changes may signal that event. The need for biopsy is signaled by growth after age 30 years; a size greater than 6 mm; sudden and uneven darkening; uneven white, pink or black pigmentation; bleeding; ulceration; or irritation. As noted previously, complete excisional biopsies are most often preferred when a melanoma is suspected.

Certain subtypes of melanocytic nevi carry a higher risk for transformation into melanomas. Congenital nevi, which are present at or shortly after birth, and especially large nevi (greater than 20 cm in diameter) have rates of malignant degeneration that have been estimated variously from 2% to 20% (Pack and Davis, 1961; Reed et al., 1965; Greely et al., 1965; Lanier et al., 1976; Lorentzen et al., 1977). Dysplastic nevi are greater than 6 mm, are somewhat asymmetric, have a macular component and a papular component, and tend to exhibit shades of pink along with brown. There is general agreement that possession of many dysplastic nevi, in the setting of two or more first-degree family members with a history of malignant melanoma, places the patient at virtually 100% lifetime risk for developing a melanoma. Whether melanomas arise directly from dysplastic nevi or whether these nevi are simply markers is a debated point.

Thus the management of these patients is controversial with regard to excision of the dysplastic nevi. Removal of dysplastic nevi prophylactically in patients who do not have a family history of melanoma is even more difficult to justify because their risk for melanoma is probably much lower. However, at

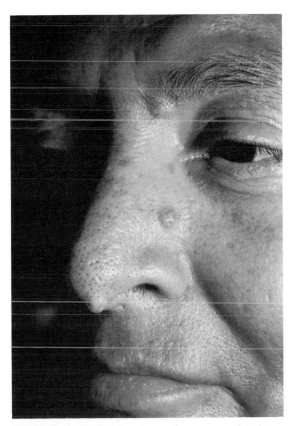

Figure 46–1. Flesh-colored papules representing intradermal nevi. Patients often wish these removed for cosmetic reasons.

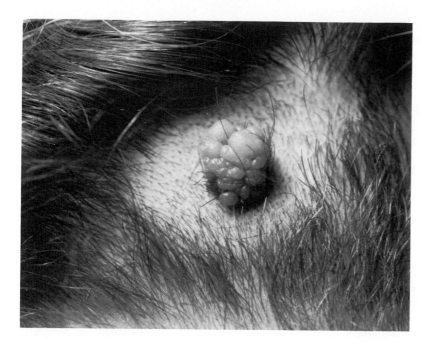

Figure 46–2. This scalp lesion represents a "cerebroid" intradermal nevus, named for its distinctive topographic features.

least three strategies have been used. First, warning about possible additional promoters of melanoma, such as ultraviolet light, coupled with scheduled follow-up examinations, is a prudent course to take. Second, a high index of suspicion should be maintained for early melanoma, especially in patients with familial melanoma, and excisional skin biopsies should be obtained. A skilled dermatopathologist is invaluable in the management of these patients. Finally, total body photographs may aid in detecting changes in existing lesions and are routinely used in some dermatology centers.

For the most part, nevi are removed for reasons other than strong suspicion for melanoma. There are several methods, but only those that yield tissue for histopathologic examination are recommended.

Facial nevi should probably be excised and sutured along the maximal skin tension lines. Most nevi are less than 6 mm in diameter and are amenable to removal by round Key's punch. This method quickly and neatly removes the lesion to subcutaneous fat. This yields the best cosmetic result and provides the best chance for complete removal; therefore, there is less chance of recurrence. Unfortunately, recurrent nevi may mimic melanoma histologically.

Pedunculated nevi may be shaved at the base slightly below skin level and left to heal by secondary intention. A sterile, double-edged blade broken lengthwise becomes a sharp and easily manipulated cutting tool when bent into a bow.

Again, all removed nevi should be submitted for histopathologic examination. Basal cell carcinomas, melanomas, neurofibromas, adnexal tumors, and infectious granulomas may all closely mimic the common mole.

BENIGN CUTANEOUS TUMORS OF KERATINOCYTE ORIGIN

Warts

Warts result from DNA papilloma virus infection of keratinocytes. They occur most commonly in children and young adults, and they assume a variety of clinical appearances. Their typical appearance on the head and neck is the focus of this discussion.

Flat (plane) warts occur on the face as flesh-colored, tan, or brown, polygonal, flat-topped papules and plaques that range from a small dot to more than a centimeter in diameter. They may occur in great numbers, often grouped in a linear array, from autoinoculation of virus along scratch lines. *Filiform (digitate) warts* occur commonly as horny projections of one to several millimeters around the eyelids, the corners of the mouth, and the nasal rim or in the beard area. *Common warts* occur mostly on the hands of children and young adults as rough, round papules a few millimeters in diameter.

Different types of human papilloma virus have been identified by DNA hybridization techniques in the various forms of warts. Flat warts include mostly types 2 and 3; warts in epidermodysplasia verruciformis are primarily type 5; and common warts are primarily types 1, 2, and 4. Indeed, typing is more important in the context of genital warts in which types 6, 11, 16, and 18 are associated with the development of squamous cell carcinomas. Finally, typing of genital warts in children may soon be used for medical-legal purposes when child abuse is suspected.

Epidermodysplasia verruciformis is a rare autosomal recessive disorder in which myriad flat warts cover primarily the extremities. Not only are they refractory to treatment, but malignant degeneration occurs on sun-exposed sites in one third of these patients.

Histopathologic examination of common and filiform warts reveals acanthosis (thickening of the epidermis), hyperkeratosis (thickening of the stratum corneum), and papillomatosis (undulation of the epidermal surface) of the epidermis. Rete ridges curve inward at the periphery, and vacuolated cells, representing keratinocytes with viral infection, are seen in upper portions of the epidermis (Fig. 46–3). Flat warts have much less hyperkeratosis, but the vacuolated cells are sufficient for diagnosis.

More than 66% of warts disappear spontaneously (Massing and Epstein, 1963), but others remain frustratingly recalcitrant to all of the many treatments. Immunity, especially cellular immunity, is thought to play a large role in eradication of warts, and one unproved hypothesis is that warts, found often in children, are rejected as the immune system matures and recognizes warts as foreign. On the other hand, there is no disputing the high frequency of warts found in patients treated with immunosuppressive drugs to protect transplanted organs (Spencer and Andersen, 1970) or in patients with acquired immunodeficiency syndrome, who also have suppressed cellular immunity.

The large number and the great variety of treatments for warts indicate that there is no perfect treatment, and it is important to avoid modalities that may cause scarring in this ordinarily self-limited cutaneous disorder.

Filiform or digitate warts may be removed with a sharp blade, followed by hemostasis with ferric subsulfate solution (Monsel's), aluminum chloride (Drysol), or light electrocautery at the base. Cryotherapy with liquid nitrogen in several "fast freeze, slow thaw" cycles is also commonly used. This technique may be repeated every 2 weeks until each lesion disappears.

Salicylic acid in colloidin suspension or impregnated into plasters, coupled with paring of common warts, is often effective and less painful than are most treatments. A combined regimen of cryotherapy followed by salicylic acid resulted in a 72% cure rate, in contrast to about 57% for either modality alone (Bunney et al., 1976).

Figure 46–3. Hyperkeratosis, acanthosis, and virus-infected vacuolated cells are seen in this photomicrograph of a wart.

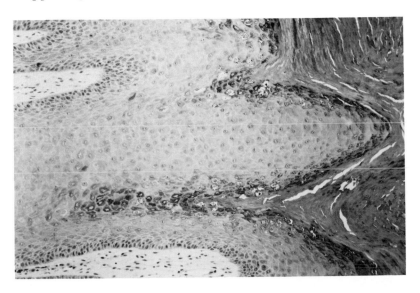

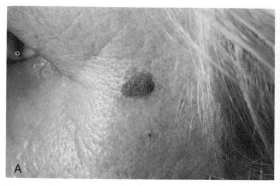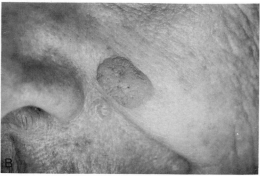

Figure 46–4. *A.* The temple region is a common site for seborrheic keratoses. Note the furrowed surface on this plaque. *B.* This well-circumscribed plaque with a furrowed surface appears to sit atop the epidermis. Most seborrheic keratoses possess these features. Note the umbilicated pearly papule inferior to the seborrheic keratosis. A biopsy revealed basal cell carcinoma.

Flat warts of the face are more difficult to treat, but they may respond to twice-a-day application of 1% to 2% topical 5-fluorouracil. Topical application of tretinoin (Retin-A 0.1% cream twice daily) may be useful in eradication of these lesions, although this modality may require several weeks of treatment. Reports of 10 mg of isotretinoin (Accutane) orally twice a day for flat warts indicate prompt and complete clearing, although systemic side effects limit this treatment mode (White, 1988).

Other treatments used commonly for warts outside of the head and neck include podophyllin, alpha-hydroxy acid paste application, formaldehyde or glutaraldehyde soaks, cantharone (from the blister beetle), dinitrochlorobenzene contact sensitization, the carbon dioxide laser, or injections of alpha-interferon or bleomycin.

Molluscum Contagiosum

Molluscum contagiosum results from pox virus infection of keratinocytes. These firm, smooth, dome-shaped papules, with a central plug, are most often found on the trunk, the extremities, and the face of children. They have distinct histopathologic features; infected keratinocytes penetrate into the dermis, forming saccules of eosinophilic inclusion bodies composed of virus and cellular debris.

A useful treatment for this benign condition consists of cryotherapy with liquid nitrogen, followed by flicking off with a sharp curet. Removing the central core with a No.

11 blade hastens involution of each papule and is somewhat less traumatic than cryotherapy.

Lesions of *Cryptococcus* (a deep fungus), or even metastatic carcinoma, may mimic molluscum contagiosum. A punch biopsy or a shave biopsy that includes adequate tissue settles the issue.

Seborrheic Keratosis

Seborrheic keratoses are very common epithelial tumors with no malignant potential. They usually begin to appear after the age of 30 years, and it is thought that the tendency to develop them is autosomal dominantly inherited. The underlying etiologic factor remains a mystery for the common seborrheic keratosis; viral infection, sunlight, pre-existing inflammatory disease, and estrogens have all been suggested.

Seborrheic keratoses occur on hair-bearing areas, especially the trunk, on temple areas on the face, and on the hands. They appear first as subtle, flesh-colored, slightly granular-surfaced papules and, with time, grow in circumference and in number. Uneven pigmentation is usually present; the overlying surface is greasy and slightly verrucous or furrowed and may be seen to contain small keratin plugs and pits (Fig. 46–4). Seborrheic keratoses may appear as dark, warty growths that are stuck on the skin; often they are dislodged easily with the flick of a fingernail. Inflammation frequently occurs around seborrheic keratoses, and it may indicate low-grade trauma or an intrinsic immunologic response. The diameter of each lesion ranges from a few millimeters to several centimeters, and some lesions may even be pedunculated, especially when they occur on the eyelids.

Because of their size and dark color, seborrheic keratoses are most often confused with melanomas. A careful study of the topography of the lesion with magnification ordinarily differentiates the two, and a careful dermatologist can tell the difference in the great majority of cases. On the other hand, any doubt mandates a biopsy.

On histopathologic examination, seborrheic keratoses are composed of squamoid and basaloid keratinocytes that lie above a straight line drawn from one side of the normal epidermis to the other. A papillomatous surface and hyperkeratosis, and even horn cysts (round swirls of keratin within the epidermis), may be evident (Fig. 46–5).

The literature cites several cases in which the sudden appearance of numerous eruptive seborrheic keratoses on normal skin was associated with internal malignancy. This is called the sign of Leser-Trelat and may well represent the effect of tumor-derived growth factors that act on the immature keratinocytes or fibroblasts within each lesion.

Another pertinent variant of the common seborrheic keratosis is found on the face of highly pigmented persons. Dermatosis papulosa nigra consists of 1- to 5-mm, flat or pedunculated, small papules clustered on the cheeks; these closely resemble seborrheic keratoses histologically (Fig. 46–6).

Treatment of the seborrheic keratosis is often effective. A light freeze with liquid nitrogen causes most seborrheic keratoses to

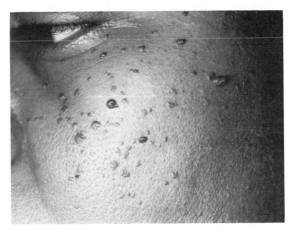

Figure 46–6. Dermatosis papulosa nigra is probably a form of seborrheic keratosis. These dark, pedunculated papules may be removed in a variety of ways, but scissor clipping may leave less postinflammatory hyperpigmentation.

desquamate over the ensuing several days, although hypopigmentation may remain at the site of treatment. Scraping with a sharp curet also removes these tumors effectively because they are limited to the epidermis. Electrocautery may be used but is more likely to produce a scar. For numerous flat lesions of the skin, trichloroacetic acid, glycolic acid, or even tretinoin (Retin-A) may have some efficacy. The individual lesions of dermatosis papulosa nigra should be clipped with scissors, or curetted, because liquid nitrogen tends to cause dyspigmentation, especially on darker skin.

Keratoacanthoma

Keratoacanthomas are benign, self-healing, epithelial tumors thought to arise from hair follicles. They occur primarily on sun-exposed skin of patients more than 60 years old; cheeks, nose, ears, and eyelids are most commonly involved. The clinical and histopathologic resemblances between keratoacanthomas and squamous cell carcinomas may make differentiation quite difficult. Similarities between these tumors extend to their postulated etiologic factors, which include ultraviolet light, tar and pitch, cigarette smoking, viral infection, pre-existing inflammatory skin diseases, and various types of skin trauma. Host immune status may also play an important role because immunosuppressed transplant recipients have higher incidences of many epithelial neoplasms, in-

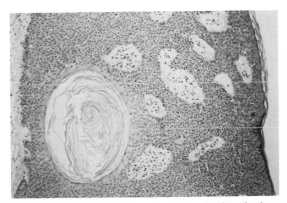

Figure 46–5. Laminated keratin is seen within the horn cyst of this seborrheic keratosis. Horn cysts may be seen clinically as pits in the surface of the plaque.

cluding keratoacanthomas (Washington and Mikhail, 1987).

Typically, each keratoacanthoma begins as a solitary, small papule on sun-damaged skin; it grows rapidly over several weeks to attain a size of 1 to 3 cm. This rapid growth phase helps distinguish it from a squamous cell carcinoma, which tends to grow much more slowly. Each keratoacanthoma is dome-shaped, with a slightly reddish, telangiectatic surface, and it appears to be stretched around a central plug of keratin (Fig. 46–7). This plug often dislodges, leaving a crateriform center. Spontaneous involution usually occurs after several months, occasionally leaving a disfiguring scar.

On histopathologic examination the key observation is an overall cup-shaped pattern of epidermal invagination that is filled with keratin (Fig. 46–8). Keratinization of cells yields a homogeneous, eosinophilic, glassy appearance of the tumor. Individual cells during growth phase may exhibit sufficient nuclear atypia to mimic those found in a squamous cell carcinoma. It is wise to obtain an incisional wedge biopsy through the center and the edge of the lesion to establish diagnosis before any treatment with the exception of complete surgical excision.

Several less common varieties of keratoacanthoma warrant mention. Giant solitary keratoacanthomas may grow to 3 to 5 cm or even larger. Their growth can be quite destructive, an unfortunate circumstance because they occur most commonly on the nose or central face. Although giant keratoacanthomas may also involute spontaneously,

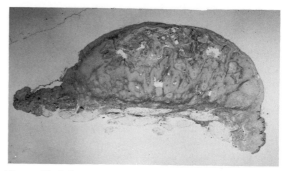

Figure 46–8. Low-power magnification of this keratoacanthoma reveals a hyperplastic cup-shaped epidermis with intact keratin plug.

early surgical, intralesional, antimetabolic, or oral retinoid therapy is recommended to prevent scarring.

Keratoacanthoma centrificum marginatum, or multinodular keratoacanthoma, occurs commonly on the upper extremities; it is characterized by multiple, expanding, peripheral nodules, also with central scarring. These lesions can attain a large size and usually do not regress completely; thus surgical excision is required. Finally, syndromes of multiple keratoacanthomas include a familial self-healing type (Ferguson-Smith); an adult-onset, nonfamilial eruptive type (Grzybowski); and a combination of both (Witten and Zak). Multiple keratoacanthomas may be seen in Muir-Torre syndrome, which also includes sebaceous adenomas, basal cell epitheliomas with sebaceous differentiation, and low-grade visceral carcinomas.

Treatment of keratoacanthomas must take into account their self-limited nature. First, complete surgical excision is favored because it not only removes the lesion (with a recurrence rate of less than 5%) but also provides adequate tissue for histopathologic examination. In several case reports, biopsy-confirmed "keratoacanthomas" later metastasized; this points out the importance and difficulty of histopathologic differentiation from squamous cell carcinoma. Deep fungal infections, such as chromoblastomycosis or atypical bacterial infections, may also mimic keratoacanthoma. These cases make complete excision of keratoacanthomas an even more attractive alternative when feasible.

Other distinctive methods of treatment have been applied to keratoacanthomas of unusual size, location, or number. These include curettage (with or without electro-

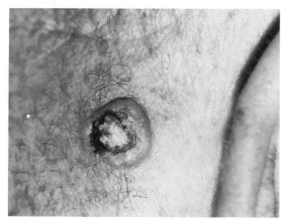

Figure 46–7. This postauricular keratoacanthoma nicely demonstrates a central keratin plug. Upon dislodging, a volcano-like crater is seen.

desiccation), liquid nitrogen cryotherapy, or radiotherapy. More recently, topical 5-fluorouracil applied twice daily, or weekly intralesional 50 mg/mL of 5-fluorouracil with 1 to 3 mL total volume per treatment, has been used with good results (Parker and Hanke, 1986); these are most effective during the tumor's growth phase. Finally, oral retinoids (isotretinoin at 1 mg/kg/day for 12 weeks) have been used successfully for multiple lesions found in the Grzybowski type of keratoacanthoma (Shaw et al., 1985; White, 1988).

Mohs micrographically controlled surgical excision may give the yield result for keratoacanthomas, leading to a low 2% recurrence rate (Larson, 1987).

Actinic Keratosis

Actinic keratoses are probably the most sensitive indicator of lifetime sun exposure. Not only do a high percentage of elderly people with light complexions have actinic keratosis, but younger adults who live in areas of high solar exposure are also commonly found to have them. For example, more than 50% of Australians, age 40 years or above, have actinic keratosis (Marks et al., 1983). This also seems to be true in "sun-belt" states such as Texas, where sun-worshipping teenagers have even been found with actinic keratosis.

Like basal cell carcinomas and squamous cell carcinomas, actinic keratoses represent a disordered growth of keratinocytes. It has been proposed that malignant squamous cell carcinomas may arise from actinic keratoses, and although some sources cite occurrence rates as high as 12%, the actual rate is probably far less (Marks et al., 1986). On the other hand, the etiologic factors for actinic keratoses and squamous cell carcinomas are identical, which is not surprising inasmuch as the two conditions are different degrees of the same pathologic process. This means that patients with actinic keratoses are clearly at risk for subsequent malignancies.

The typical solar-induced actinic keratoses occur within the milieu of sun-damaged skin, including exaggerated skin lines, elastosis, dyspigmentation, and telangiectasia. Initially, most actinic keratoses are felt as rough spots more easily than they are visualized. With time, however, keratotic scale thickens and enlarges to several millimeters in size, becoming yellow-brown in color, with or without surrounding erythema. Occasionally, exuberant growth of overlying scale forms a cutaneous horn that may reach a centimeter in size.

Actinic keratoses that are accompanied by any of the following developments should be biopsied to rule out a squamous cell carcinoma: induration at the base, progressive erythema or enlargement, a cutaneous horn, or ulceration.

On histopathologic examination, differences between actinic keratoses and squamous cell carcinomas are mostly that of degree. In actinic keratoses, keratinocytes, starting at the basal layer, appear dysplastic; that is, they vary in size and shape, or exhibit polar disorientation. They are also more eosinophilic and have enlarged or multiple nuclei. The overlying stratum corneum is thickened and contains residual keratinocyte nuclei (parakeratosis). Of importance is that these changes spare adnexal structures, such as hair follicles and sweat glands. On the other hand, when these dysplastic changes include the entire epidermis, the lesion is likely to have become a squamous cell carcinoma in situ (Bowen's disease), and when keratinocytes invade the dermis, a diagnosis of squamous cell carcinoma can be made. Obviously, the distinction between actinic keratosis and squamous cell carcinoma may at times be arbitrary, and thus it is always wise to consult a pathologist who examines skin biopsies frequently.

Although as many as 25% of actinic keratoses resolve spontaneously, and often within 1 year if sun exposure is reduced (Marks et al., 1986), most dermatologists treat them because of their unsightly appearance, pruritus, and the small but definite potential for malignancy.

Ultraviolet light exposure, especially in the B or tanning range of 290- to 300-nm wavelength, is undoubtedly the primary etiologic factor for actinic keratoses. Hydrocarbons, in tar for example, are another class of carcinogen that may induce premalignant epithelial keratoses. Keratoses induced by x-rays are, fortunately, not commonly seen now because of x-ray therapy for acne is no longer used. Organic arsenic induces keratoses that resemble actinic keratoses, as well as inducing squamous cell carcinomas. In the past, arsenic-containing medications were an important consideration, but now the more common scenario is a history of arsenic contamination in drinking water or previous

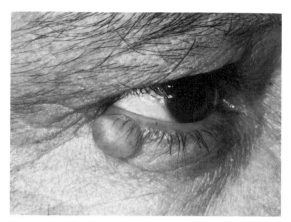

Figure 46–10. This translucent, cystic hidrocystoma mimics an adenoid basal cell carcinoma clinically. Hidrocystomas frequently occur around the eyelids.

may mislead a pathologist who is not accustomed to viewing many skin slides. Light electrocautery, or caustic chemical application, may successfully remove syringomas.

Each of these benign adnexal tumors lends itself to simple excision, although the great number of lesions seen in trichoepitheliomas and syringomas makes alternative techniques more satisfactory.

COMPLEX BENIGN TUMORS

Acrochordon

Acrochordons are the common benign "skin tags" that occur in up to 40% of middle-aged and older patients (Banik and Luback, 1987). Frequency increases with obesity, and common sites of involvement include flexural areas such as the axilla, neck, and groin,

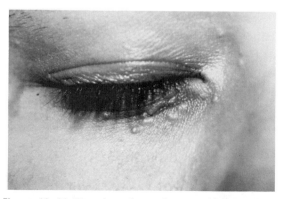

Figure 46–11. Tiny dermal papules around the eye are seen in this patient with benign syringomas.

which are prone to chronic low-grade friction. Each papule or nodule is soft and pedunculated and usually measures no more than 2 to 3 mm in length. A smooth to pebbly surface with hyperpigmentation is common.

On histopathologic examination, acrochordons have a slightly hyperplastic epidermis, a papillated surface, and an underlying loose connective tissue that contains no adnexal structures. Larger pedunculated lesions that contain fat are referred to as skin polyps.

Many patients want these cosmetic nuisances removed, and it is easy enough to accommodate them. A simple clip with small iris scissors at the base followed by coagulation, with aluminum chloride solution (Drysol) or ferric subsulfate solution (Monsel's), is sufficient. Light electrodesiccation or cryotherapy at the base also removes them. Patients should be warned that new lesions tend to develop over time.

Keloids

Keloids contain an overabundance of dermal connective tissue that usually forms in response to injury. The tendency to form keloids has a hereditary basis; autosomal dominant and autosomal recessive inheritance patterns are recognized, and keloids occur with high frequency in persons of African descent.

Clinically, each keloid appears initially as a firm scar. An exaggerated repair mechanism soon overgrows the boundaries of original injury, growing in some circumstances to gigantic proportions. Keloids are different from hypertrophic scars, which are also elevated but remain confined to the original site of injury. Keloids may itch or be painful, especially during their growth phase; spontaneous resolution occurs only rarely.

Keloids are firm and rubbery, and the overlying epidermis is usually thinned, appearing shiny and without epidermal markings. No adnexal structures are present within the keloid. Coloring progresses from reddish to red-brown to pale (Fig. 46–12).

Common scenarios in keloid formation include (1) firm papules adjacent to pierced earlobes, (2) spontaneous midchest plaques at the site of increased skin tension lines on previous acne scars, (3) myriads of 2- to 3-mm round papules at the base of the skull associated with ingrown hairs and pustules

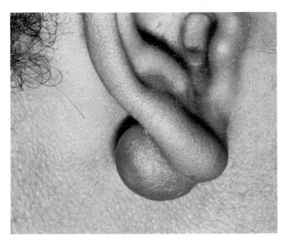

Figure 46–12. A common site for keloid formation is the earlobe after cosmetic ear piercing. The nodule is quite firm to touch.

(acne keloidalis nuchae), and (4) neck papules secondary to folliculitis.

Several factors may influence the formation of keloid nodules. Trauma almost certainly plays a role; thermal injuries appear to be more provocative than cutting injuries. Also, the presence of a foreign body within skin tends to provoke keloid formation.

By histopathologic examination, thick, glossy collagen bundles with numerous associated mast cells are easily identified.

The best treatment for keloids is to avoid the precipitating trauma. Nonessential surgery should be avoided if possible; when surgery is necessary, closure should be with minimal tension and along the maximal skin tension lines. People with keloids in their earlobes should be warned not to have their children's ears pierced.

Injecting existing keloids with a steroid suspension is useful to decrease the symptoms of itching and pain as well as to flatten the plaque. Five to 10 mg/mL of triamcinolone acetonide is a good treatment to start with; concentrations as high as 20 mg/mL are reserved for recalcitrant lesions. Injections should be made every 2 to 4 weeks. Many keloids become softer and may even flatten out to an acceptable degree with this modality alone. Freezing of lesions with liquid nitrogen before injection causes slight edema, which facilitates penetration of the steroid throughout the nodule (Hirshowitz et al., 1982). Posttreatment hypopigmentation may result either from the cryotherapy injury to melanocytes or from the steroid

itself. Also, the usual systemic side effects of steroids are possible when large concentrations or many areas are injected.

Surgical removal of keloids may be attempted, but there is a high rate of recurrence. Simple excision of pedunculated nodules, such as those that occur on earlobes, with primary closure under minimal tension (without buried sutures) may suffice. Success is more certain when the operative site is injected with a small volume of triamcinolone acetonide at concentrations of about 520 mg/mL at the time of surgery. Monthly follow-up for injection of triamcinolone acetonide at lower concentrations is also advised for the next several months to help prevent recurrence. Pressure at an operative site may keep the area flat as well, and clip earrings are recommended.

Excision, with use of the carbon dioxide laser, was initially thought to be associated with less frequent recurrences, but this no longer appears to be the case (Henderson et al., 1984).

As more investigation uncovers the pathogenesis of these lesions, better treatment aimed at inhibiting the function of dermal fibroblasts will surely follow. For acne keloidalis nuchae, the first goal is to control the inflammatory pustular reaction with antibiotics, such as tetracycline or one of the oral retinoids.

VASCULAR TUMORS

Telangiectasia

Small, dilated, superficial vessels occur in several forms. Linear and spider telangiectasias represent the most common forms, although these vessels may also form arborizing, punctate, mat, or nodular telangiectasia. In general, all show superficial dilated vessels on pathologic examination.

Linear telangiectasias are single or branched, reddish-blue vessels that are found commonly on the face, especially the nose. In the majority of cases, they carry no medical significance and simply represent a degenerative process after solar exposure. Besides actinic damage, however, the examining physician should be aware of several disease associations. In children, telangiectasias may indicate ataxia-telangiectasia, Bloom's syndrome, or xeroderma pigmentosum. In adults, they may indicate rosacea, lupus erythematosus, dermatomyositis, scleroderma, CREST syndrome (calcinosis cutis, Raynaud's phenomenon, esophageal dysfunction, sclerodactyly, and telangiectasia), or radiation dermatitis. The telangiectasias may even form a mat of tiny linear vessels as occurs in collagen vascular diseases such as scleroderma.

Spider telangiectasias, actually arterial in origin, may be seen to pulsate. A central red papule with leglike projections radiates to the periphery; filling occurs from the center toward the periphery after blanching. Such "spiders" occur in the normal population but are often seen in pregnancy and in alcoholic cirrhosis of the liver. Increased levels of circulating estrogen are thought to permit the growth of ectatic vessels. Hereditary hemorrhagic telangiectasia (Osler-Weber-Rendu disease), with its associated bleeding gastrointestinal lesions, may also manifest with multiple spider or nodular angiomas on the face and mucous membranes.

Eradication of telangiectasias on the face from whatever cause is fairly straightforward. Electrocautery with a fine needle tip usually destroys the lesion, although great care must be taken to prevent visible scarring. The newer dye lasers also eradicate superficial vessels after several treatments with much less overlying epidermal damage.

The use of sclerotic agents on the face does not yield the same gratifying results as are obtained in leg telangiectasias treated with the same agents.

Venous Lakes

Venous lakes are common vascular lesions in elderly men and are frequently found on the ear rim, the face, or the lip. These soft elevations measure a few millimeters in diameter and exhibit dark blue to almost black coloration. Blood can easily be expressed to leave a saucerlike depression with lax skin overlying. On histopathologic examination, there is a dilated venule with little, if any, surrounding smooth muscle or elastic tissue support. Liquid nitrogen therapy and blade excision have been used successfully to eradicate these lesions. A more sophisticated removal technique involves use of an argon laser to selectively coagulate the lesion. A glass slide is used to press out blood as the

laser beam is directed through the glass (Dover and Arndt, 1990).

MALIGNANT SKIN TUMORS

Basal Cell Epithelioma

Basal cell epithelioma (basal cell carcinoma, or BCE) is the most common skin cancer; about 500,000 new cases are identified each year (Skouge and Tromovitch, 1988). The malignant epithelial cells (keratinocytes) are morphologically similar to basal cells in the epidermis, and they probably arise from pluripotent cells in this region. Although rates of metastases are extremely low for this common tumor, it may, through local destruction and invasion, have serious consequences.

The common BCE manifests clinically as a pearly papule with overlying telangiectasia (Figs. 46–13, 46–14). Areas of frequent occurrence include periorbital, postauricular, and paranasal regions of the head, whereas lesions on the cheeks, the forehead, the scalp, and the trunk are considerably less common. In early phases, tumor growth rates are slow, perhaps 1 mm per year. Tumor enlargement is accompanied by accelerated growth with central ulceration, and neglected tumors may show extensive local destruction, ulceration, and a rolled, translucent border. These tumors have been given the colorful name

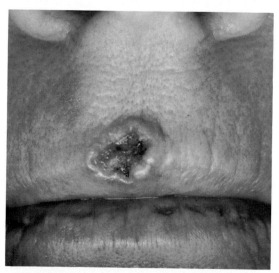

Figure 46–13. This basal cell carcinoma has the characteristic pearly, rolled border. The central necrotic portion of the tumor probably appeared simply umbilicated during the early growth period.

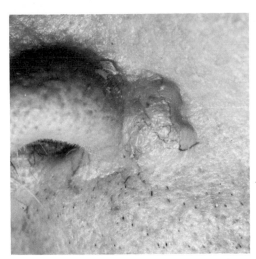

Figure 46–14. Alar fold basal cell cancers may be extensive, perhaps because they lie over an embryonal plane. Note the telangiectasia on the surface of this nodular basal cell carcinoma.

"rodent ulcer" to convey the appearance of an area gnawed by a rat. Neglect for many years has even led to death from local invasion into the orbits, the meninges, or the large vessels. Pigmentation occurs commonly in nodular BCEs on highly pigmented patients and sometimes mimics a malignant melanoma. A BCE most often assumes one of three clinical forms: superficial, nodular, or sclerosing. Nodular BCEs, the most common, exhibit a typical, pearly, translucent nodule with visible telangiectasia; they occur in all sites of predilection. Superficial BCEs occur most often on the trunk and mimic tinea corporis, psoriasis, or eczema. When they are examined carefully, a flattened, scaly plaque is found to have a characteristic pearly border. Morpheaform BCEs are difficult to diagnose because they look like waxy plaques or depressed scars. As discussed later, treatment is also difficult because the extensive fibrous tissue and slender tumor strands make margin evaluation a challenge, and curettage is ineffective because the scarlike tissue cannot be scraped out as can the large masses of tumor in nodular BCEs. Finally, metatypical BCEs have features of both basal cell epithelioma and squamous cell carcinoma. Both a pearly papule and hyperkeratosis with ulceration may be seen. These tend to be more aggressive tumors than are common nodular BCEs.

BCEs exhibit histopathologic variations that correspond to their clinical appearance.

Nodular BCEs exhibit dark blue masses of large cells with large nuclear-to-cytoplasmic ratios. These masses show no intracellular bridging and appear to drop into the dermis from the overlying epidermis. Cells at the boundary between dermis and tumor mass line up in parallel or "palisade" fashion. A common retraction artifact at this boundary gives nodular BCEs a characteristic spacing between tumor and stroma. The surrounding dermal connective tissue stroma appears to proliferate and interdigitate among the basaloid cells (Fig. 46–15). A variant of nodular BCE, termed adenoid, has a lacy, pseudoglandular appearance; it resembles nodular BCEs clinically and prognostically. Superficial BCEs show budding of darker basaloid keratinocytes from the lower surface of the epidermis with modest invasion into the dermis. Sclerosing BCEs exhibit isolated strands of basaloid cells in a dense connective tissue stroma (Fig. 46–16). Metatypical BCEs show some features found in squamous cell carcinomas. These features include atypical keratinocytes with intercellular bridging, keratin horns or pearls, and hyperkeratosis. Pigmented BCEs simply have more melanin, so much that it may even obscure cellular characteristics.

Ultraviolet light exposure in light-skinned people is thought to be the major etiologic factor in the development of BCEs. Despite good epidemiologic evidence to support this statement, other factors must also play a role. For example, BCEs frequently occur behind the ear, in the inner canthus, and in the alar fold, areas that do not correspond to sites of maximal solar intensity. Equally important, BCEs rarely occur on the forearm or dorsum

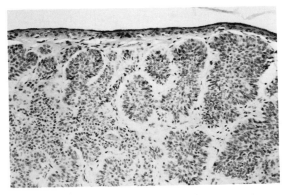

Figure 46–15. Nodules of basaloid cells are seen in the dermis in this nodular basal cell cancer. Cells at the edge of each mass line up (palisade).

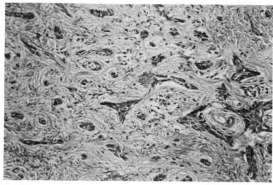

Figure 46–16. Cords and strands of basaloid cells are embedded in a dense stroma in this sclerosing (morpheaform) basal cell carcinoma. This histopathologic pattern has therapeutic implications (see text).

of the hand, where ultraviolet light exposure is maximal. This is in contrast to squamous cell carcinomas, which form most frequently in these areas of maximal solar intensity. Regional differences, such as density of pilosebaceous units, may permit the growth of BCEs. Although formal studies have not been done, it is possible that intermittent sunburning of these relatively non–sun-hardened areas might also play an etiologic role. Finally, previous ionizing irradiation and arsenic exposure definitely predispose a person to the development of BCEs.

Although BCEs do occur relatively commonly in younger patients, their appearance should prompt the examining physician to consider the possibility of one of the genetic predisposing disorders such as xeroderma pigmentosum, basal cell nevus syndrome, or Bazex's syndrome.

Xeroderma pigmentosum is a disorder of defective DNA repair that translates clinically into the development of cutaneous malignancies of all types during childhood. In the basal cell nevus syndrome, an autosomal dominant disease, numerous BCEs develop even before the age of 20 years. Pitted palms, mandibular bone cysts, bifid ribs, hypertelorism, and partial agenesis of the corpus callosum are associated entities. Finally, Bazex's syndrome is a rare disease that includes BCEs and follicular atrophoderma.

Treatment of the potentially highly destructive, even fatal skin cancer is, for the most part, very gratifying. Rowe and colleagues published in 1989 an extensive review of the treatment of primary and recurrent BCEs. Recurrence rates at 5 years, for

TABLE 46–1. Recurrence Rate for Treatment of Primary Basal Cell Epithelioma at 5 Years

Treatment Modality	Recurrence Rate
Surgical excision	10.1%
Radiation	8.7%
Electrodesiccation and curettage	7.7%
Cryotherapy	7.5%
Mohs micrographic surgery	1.0%

Modified from Rowe DE, Carroll RJ, Day CL: Long-term recurrence rates in previously untreated (primary) basal cell carcinoma: implication for patient follow-up. J Dermatol Surg Oncol 15:3, 1989.

each treatment modality, are shown in Tables 46–1 and 46–2.

Details of the different types of treatment for BCEs and squamous cell carcinomas are discussed in the treatment section. For all treatment modalities, follow-up for more than 5 years yields an overall recurrence rate for primary tumors of 8.7% (Rowe et al., 1989).

Squamous Cell Carcinoma

Cutaneous squamous cell carcinomas (SCCs) are malignant tumors derived from epidermal keratinocytes. Like actinic keratoses, they are strongly linked to ultraviolet light exposure and occur most commonly in fair-skinned people. Ultraviolet light not only damages DNA of the keratinocyte, which becomes the aberrant cell, but also damages the adjacent Langerhans' cells, which are thought to be relevant antigen-presenting cells in immunosurveillance against tumors.

SCCs occur most commonly on the head and neck on a background of sun-damaged skin. The ears, the nose, the neck, the hands, and the forearms are particularly susceptible, and examining physicians must inspect all surfaces and skin folds in these regions. Most

TABLE 46–2. Recurrence Rate for Treatment of Recurrent Basal Cell Epithelioma at 5 Years

Treatment Modality	Recurrence Rate
Electrodesiccation and curettage	40.0%
Surgical excision	17.4%
Cryotherapy	13.0%
Radiation	9.8%
Mohs micrographic surgery	5.6%

Modified from Rowe DE, Carroll RJ, Day CL: Mohs surgery in the treatment of choice for recurrent (previously treated) basal cell carcinoma. J Dermatol Surg Oncol 15:424–431, 1989.

commonly, SCCs manifest as firm, red, scaly nodules. Induration at the base of the lesion is emphasized as a sign of distinguishing actinic keratoses from SCCs. SCCs may attain a size of several centimeters over several months (a pace that helps distinguish them from the more rapidly growing keratoacanthomas). They almost always have keratotic scale. As the nodule grows, it becomes firm with irregular borders. Ultimately, central ulceration may leave a shallow ulcer with a friable base that bleeds easily.

In the United States, about 100,000 patients develop SCC of the skin each year (Scotto et al., 1974). As might be expected, incidences are higher in regions with greater solar intensity, such as Texas and Florida. Because chronic exposure to ultraviolet light over years plays such an important role in the development of SCCs, behavioral factors such as occupation, clothing style, hair style, and leisure activities also determine who will develop skin cancer.

Ultraviolet light is not the only relevant etiologic factor. Exposure to organic hydrocarbons, such as coal tar, or to arsenic may also cause aggressive squamous cell carcinomas. Sources of arsenic include medications, industrial exposure, well water, and insecticides. X-ray radiation, often in repeated small doses, may give rise many years later to aggressive carcinomas. Documented SCCs have also arisen in areas of chronic osteomyelitis, nonhealing burn scars (Marjolin's ulcer), chronic ulcers and sinuses, and chronic inflammatory skin diseases such as chronic cutaneous lupus erythematosus, sarcoidosis, lichen planus, warts, or even herpes simplex. Pipe smoking or chewing tobacco also predisposes a person to SCC of the lip or the mouth. Finally, phototherapy with ultraviolet radiation or with ultraviolet and a sensitizing drug therapy, such as for psoriasis, increases the incidence of cutaneous SCC. It is certain that altered immune responses play an important role in the development of SCCs because immunosuppressed patients tend to develop them with more frequency and because the clinical course of SCCs is often more aggressive.

The anatomic location and etiologic processes of SCCs are important predictors of behavior. For example, SCCs that arise on mucosal surfaces or on the lip are often aggressive, metastasizing through lymphatic veins relatively early (Fig. 46–17). By contrast, SCCs arising in sun-damaged skin have

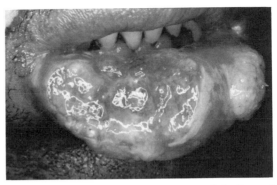

Figure 46–17. Squamous cell carcinomas of the lip tend to be more aggressive than those arising from actinic keratoses on nonmucosal surfaces. This large lesion most likely has already metastasized.

a low (less than 1%) incidence of local, nodal, or distant metastasis (Lund, 1965). SCCs that arise apparently de novo, or from chemical exposure or chronic scarring disease, may have rates of metastasis approaching 20% to 40% (Rowe et al., 1989).

Three factors influence prognosis at the time of treatment: depth of invasion, cell cytology, and anatomic location. Studies of SCCs on the trunk reveal depth of tumor greater than 4 mm to be an indicator of recurrence or metastasis. Similarly, invasion below dermal eccrine glands is a poor sign. Lesions on the head and neck are known to be more likely to recur or spread at relatively thinner tumor stages than are lesions on the trunk or the extremities. SCCs are notorious for perineural spread, and death may result from intercranial invasion. Areas of embryonal fusion planes, such as the alar fold and auricular sulcus, permit greater invasion of the tumor.

Anaplastic cellular morphology is associated with higher frequencies of recurrence and metastasis. For example, SCCs arising in old burn scars or sites of x-irradiation have less differentiated cellular architectures. The malignant keratinocytes in these tumors are more likely to exhibit atypical nuclei, mitotic figures, absence of intercellular bridges, individually keratinized cells, loss of polarity, and variable sizes and shapes. Keratin horn pearls often form in more differentiated tumors. A parakeratotic scale or an erosion often overlies the tumor.

Broder's grading system for SCCs helps establish prognosis on the basis of cellular

frequently administered in the office setting; more and more physicians defer to a clinic-based radiologist. Scarring and necrosis have been decreased significantly by the abandonment of the single-dose treatment and the adoption of modern techniques of dividing the dose into a number of small fractions over several weeks. However, even with the most careful "fractionation," atrophy of some degree is inevitable and tends to become more prominent as time passes (Albright, 1982). Although lack of response and recurrence in the treatment area are unusual, the usual precautions must be considered. Diagnosis must be the first consideration because skin tumors vary in their radioresponsiveness; the type of lesion as well as its histologic subclass must be established. Location becomes very important for the standard areas of high recurrence and, in addition, those areas in which radiation itself seems to be associated with a high failure rate or with significant long-term side effects must be considered (Albright, 1982). Age of the patient is very important because of the long-term effects of radiation; this treatment is believed to be best suited for the elderly and those for whom the strain of surgery might prove to be too great. However, many patients have found that the numerous visits to the radiologist for fractionated therapy also prove to be a significant stress. Finally, radiotherapy should not be used a second time to treat recurrent tumors because of cumulative long-term radiation effects on normal tissue (Orton, 1978).

The actual techniques of treatment by ionizing depend on the characteristics of the source of the radiation and are beyond the scope of this chapter. The reader is referred to the standard textbooks in the field.

Immunomodulation

Immunomodulation is another area in which new research may lead to alternative therapy benefits in selected cases. Intralesional human recombinant alpha$_2$-interferon was injected into eight biopsy-proved basal cell carcinomas with complete success (Greenway et al., 1986). Biopsies 8 weeks after the 3-week course of therapy showed no residual tumor. Local and systemic side effects were those consistent with the injection of interferon and were considered at worst moderate in severity, transient, and reversible. The mechanism

for this antitumor response may be on the basis of suppression of proliferation of cancerous cells, triggering the body's immune systems, or both. Increased numbers of Leu-2 positive cells and OKT-6 positive cells have been noted in the lesion after treatment (Morito and Haneda, 1986).

Retinoids

So far, most beneficial effects of these vitamin A derivatives seem to be seen in the premalignant actinic keratoses; in one crossover 4-month study of 44 patients, 84% of these patients demonstrated complete or partial response (Kingston et al., 1983). However, in basal cell carcinoma, Peck's study of 12 patients with a total of 270 lesions had only a 16% regression rate (Peck, 1985). Two retinoids, isotretinoin and etretinate, have been used orally in dosages of about 1 mg/kg for large squamous cell carcinomas with a response rate as high as 70% (Lippman et al., 1988). Retinoids may replace radiation as palliative treatment for inoperable squamous cell carcinomas. The side effects associated with the present generation of retinoids make general use both impractical and unacceptable, but it is likely that the development of newer compounds will overcome this barrier. When that barrier is passed, it is likely that these compounds will find major use in patients in whom the immune system is depressed and who can no longer manage the usual cutaneous population of subclinical malignant and premalignant tumors.

Photodynamic Therapy

In photodynamic therapy, a light-absorbing drug such as hematoporphyrin derivative is administered intravenously and accumulates preferentially in the tumor. Selective absorption of the delivered ultraviolet light leads to necrosis of the tumor, presumably as the basis of singlet oxygen generation (Carruth, 1986).

Surgical Excision

Surgical excision is by far the most popular and widest used means of extirpating tumors. However, a few simple points must be borne in mind before the human skin is cut. How often is a beautiful plastic excision done with ample margins for what is reported to be a benign lesion? In consideration of cost containment, it becomes more and more likely that payment will be determined by final pathologic diagnosis, and it behooves all physicians to expend time and efforts wisely.

The second point is location. For benign-appearing lesions, a thorough knowledge of the usual location of congenital remnants and abnormalities will prevent what was to be a simple removal from turning into a major and, perhaps, even disastrous event. For malignant lesions, location can be of tantamount importance; from the Mohs surgery literature, it has been shown that several areas are associated with significantly higher recurrence rate (Berg et al., 1975; Salasche and Amonette, 1981; Roenigk, 1988). High-risk sites for recurrence include the midfacial triangle (eyes, nose, upper lip) and the auricular and preauricular areas.

The third point concerns histologic confirmation of complete removal. Even with the technique of multiple-step sections (bread-loafing), routine sectioning may miss as much as 35% of cases of residual tumor. These three points, then, must be weighed carefully along with all the others listed so that the appropriate decision about surgical therapy is made (Abide et al., 1984).

A useful and underutilized technique for identifying tumor margins at the time of excision is curettage. Because a tumor mass varies in consistency from surrounding normal skin, it has a different feel when probed and scraped with a curet. Because lesions often extend beyond visible surface borders, the curet has become invaluable in helping to delineate margins at the time of surgery. In one scenario, a 2- to 3-mm border is drawn around the defect after curettage of a small BCE, and a scalpel is then used to excise the remaining tissue. Primary closure is then performed along maximal skin tension lines.

Basal cell epitheliomas greater than 2 cm ideally are treated with Mohs micrographic surgery, but when this technique is not available, a margin greater than 3 mm is recommended. Although there are no absolute guidelines regarding the margin of excised normal skin, 3 to 5 mm for lesions smaller than 1 cm in diameter is reasonable. Special circumstances, such as lesions greater than 2 cm, a location on the lips or the ears, a poorly differentiated appearance, or previous treatment, require wider margins. (Referral for Mohs micrographically controlled surgery should also be considered.) Depths of excision should be at least to the subcutaneous fat and deeper if the lesion penetrates through dermis. Although undermining of the wound edges allows a more attractive closure, some investigators believe that disturbing fascial planes may permit residual tumor cells to metastasize locally.

In any event, it is especially important to ensure that margins are clear before any major tissue movement for covering surgical defects. Not only will the graft or flap have to be sacrificed when residual tumor is removed, but the presence of this tissue will delay recognition of the recurrent tumor.

Follow-up examination after tumor destruction is important for two reasons: not only will possible recurrence be detected early, but patients with one skin cancer are at risk for developing more. Most recurrences of old tumors occur within 5 years; however, a significant proportion, up to 20%, may occur after 5 years (Rowe et al., 1989). Careful follow-up must include a diligent examination of sites of previous treatment with palpation for changes in scar and subcutaneous tissue and observation for topographic and pigmentary changes as well as the standard signs of tumor growth. Avoidance of causative factors, especially ultraviolet light, is a key element in the management of patients after treatment. The use of a waterproof sunscreen with a sun protection factor of 15 or higher should become routine for the skin cancer patient. An examination of sun-exposed areas every 6 months to yearly is also imperative for treatment of precancerous lesions and diagnosis of skin cancers in their early curable stages. Finally, adequate examination of the lymphatics draining the area of previous tumor is important for detecting metastatic disease.

Mohs Surgery

The most reliable way of removing malignant lesions and troubling growths of questionable malignancy while preserving the greatest amount of normal tissue was developed by Fredrich Mohs from what was a medical school research project (Mohs, 1941). Working with various metallic ions to discover their effect on tumors in rats, Mohs found that zinc chloride, when applied to a visible tumor, would produce necrosis of the tumor while preserving tissue architecture that

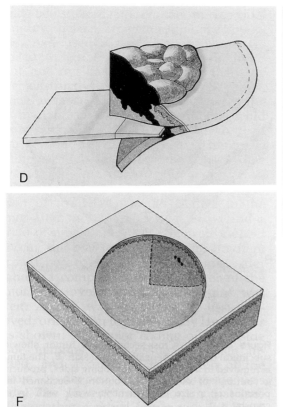

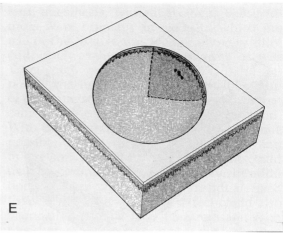

Figure 46–21 *Continued D.* Inverting the tissue on the stage of the cryostat allows a flat sample section to be taken of the outermost surface of that portion of the tissue. *E.* For the positive area, a new flat section is taken. This is repeated until all sections are free of tumor.

tumors must be put aside to encourage proper therapy for each specific lesion.

SUGGESTED READINGS

Abide JM, Nahai F, Bennett RG: The meaning of surgical margins. Plast Reconstr Surg 73:492, 1984.

Albright SD: Treatment of skin cancer using multiple modalities. J Am Acad Dermatol 7:143–171, 1982.

Baker SR, Swanson NA: Management of nasal cutaneous malignant neoplasms: an interdisciplinary approach. Arch Otolaryngol 109:479, 1983.

Balch CM, Soong SJ, Murad TM, et al: A multifactorial analysis of melanoma. Ann Surg 193(3):377–388, 1981.

Balch CM, Soong SJ, Murad TM, et al: A multifactorial analysis of melanoma. IV. Prognostic factors in 200 melanoma patients with distant metastases (Stage III). J Clin Oncol 1:126–134, 1983.

Banik R, Luback D: Skin tags: localization and frequencies according to sex and age. Dermatologica 174:180–183, 1987.

Bennett RG: Fundamentals of Cutaneous Surgery. Washington, DC: CV Mosby, 1988.

Berg G, et al: Histographic surgery: accuracy of visual assessment of the margins of basal cell epitheliomas. J Dermatol Surg 1:21, 1975.

Breslow A: The prognosis of cutaneous melanoma. Ann Surg 172:903–908, 1970.

Breza T, Taylor JR, Eaglstein WH: Noninflammatory destruction of actinic keratoses by fluorouracil. Arch Dermatol 112:1256–1258, 1976.

Briele HA, Walker MJ, DasGupta TK: Melanoma of the head and neck. Clin Plast Surg 12:495–504, 1985.

Bunney MH, Nolan MW, Williams DA: An assessment of methods of treating viral warts by comparative treatment trials based on a standard design. Br J Derm 94:667–679, 1976.

Callaway MP, Briggs JC: The incidence of late recurrence (greater than 10 years); an analysis of 536 consecutive cases of cutaneous melanoma. Br J Plast Surg 42:46–49, 1989.

Carruth JAS: Photodynamic therapy: the state of the art. Lasers Surg Med 6(4):404–407, 1986.

Clark WH Jr, Reimer RR, Greene M, et al: Origin of familial malignant melanomas from heritable melanocytic lesions. Arch Dermatol 114:732–738, 1978.

Day CL Jr, Lew RA, Mihm MC Jr, et al: The natural break points for primary-tumor thickness in clinical stage I melanoma. N Engl J Med 305:1155, 1981.

Demis DJ: Clinical Dermatology, vol 1–4, 17th rev. Philadelphia: JB Lippincott, 1990.

Diwan R, Skouge JW: Basal cell carcinoma. Curr Probl Dermatol 2:70–91, 1990.

Dougherty TJ: Photodynamic therapy: an effective and less toxic therapy in cancer treatment. Primary Care Cancer 10R–130R, 1986.

Dover JS, Arndt KA: Illustrated Cutaneous Laser Surgery. Norwalk, CT: Appleton & Large, 1990.

Elder DE: Dysplastic nevi: their significance and management. Dermatol Clin 6:257–269, 1988.

Elliott JA: Electrosurgery. Arch Dermatol 95:340, 1966.

Epstein E, Epstein E Jr: Skin Surgery, 6th ed. Philadelphia: WB Saunders, 1987.

Fitzpatrick TB, Eisen AZ, Wolff K, et al (eds): Dermatology in General Medicine, 3rd ed. New York: McGraw-Hill, 1986.

Friedman RJ, Rigel DS, Heilman ER: The relationship between melanocytic nevi and malignant melanoma. Derm Clin 6(2):249–256, 1988.

Gallagher RP: Epidemiology of Malignant Melanoma. New York: Springer-Verlag, 1986.

Greeley PW, Gilman AG, Curtin JW: Incidence of malignancy in giant pigmented nevi. Plast Reconstr Surg 36:26–31, 1965.

Greenway HT, et al: Treatment of basal cell carcinoma with intralesional interferon. J Am Acad Dermatol 15:437, 1986.

Henderson DL, Cromwell TA, Mes LG: Argon and carbon dioxide laser treatment of hypertrophic and keloid scars. Lasers Surg Med 3:271–277, 1984.

Hirshowitz B, Lerner D, Moscona AR: Treatment of keloid scars by combined cryosurgery and intralesional steroids. Aesthetic Plast Surg 6:153–158, 1982.

Holly EA, Kelly JW, Shpall SN, Chiu SH: Number of melanocytic nevi as a major risk factor for malignant melanoma. J Am Acad Dermatol 17:459–468, 1987.

Jackson R: Basic principles of electrosurgery: a review. Can J Surg 12:354, 1970.

Kaplan EN: The risk of malignancy in large congenital nevi. Plast Reconstr Surg 53:421, 1974.

Kingston T, Marks R: The effects of a novel potent oral retinoid (R013-6298) in the treatment of multiple solar keratoses and squamous cell epithelioma. Europ J Cancer Clin Oncol 19:1201–1205, 1983.

Knox J, Lyles TW, Shapiro EM, Martin RD: Curettage and electrodesiccation in the treatment of skin cancer. Arch Dermatol 82:197, 1960.

Lanier VC Jr, Pickrell KL, Georgiade NG: Congenital giant nevi: clinical and pathological considerations. Plast Reconstr Surg 58:48, 1976.

Larson PO: Keratoacanthomas treated with Mohs' micrographic surgery (chemosurgery). J Am Acad Dermatol 16:1040–1044, 1987.

Lederman JS, Sober AJ: Does wide excision as the initial diagnostic procedure improve prognosis in patients with cutaneous melanoma? J Dermatol Surg Oncol 12:697–699, 1986.

Lever WF, Schaumburg-Lever G (eds): Histopathology of the Skin, 6th ed. Philadelphia: JB Lippincott, 1983.

Lippman SM, Shimm DS, Meyskens FL: Nonsurgical treatments for skin cancer: retinoids and α-interferon. J Dermatol Surg Oncol 14:862–869, 1988.

Lorentzen M, Pers M, Bretteville-Jensen G: Incidence of malignant transformation in giant pigmented nevi. Scand J Plast Reconstr Surg 11:163, 1977.

Lund HZ: How often does squamous cell carcinoma of the skin metastasize? Arch Dermatol 92:635–637, 1965.

Marks R, Foley P, Goodman G, et al: Spontaneous remission of solar keratoses: the case for conservative management. Br J Dermatol 115:649–655, 1986.

Marks R, Ponsford MW, Selwood TS, et al: Non-melanotic skin cancer and solar keratoses in Victoria. Med J Aust 2:619–622, 1983.

Massing AM, Epstein WL: Natural history of warts. Arch Dermatol 87:306–310, 1963.

McCaughan JS Jr, Guy JT, Hicks W, et al: Photodynamic therapy for cutaneous and subcutaneous malignant neoplasms. Arch Surg 124:211–216, 1989.

Mohs FE: Chemosurgery: Microscopically Controlled Surgery for Skin Cancer. Springfield, IL: Charles C Thomas, 1978.

Mohs FE: Chemosurgery: a microscopically controlled method of cancer excision. Arch Surg 42:279–295, 1941.

Mohs FE: The versatile curette. J Dermatol Surg Oncol 4:106, 1978.

Morito H, Haneda T: OKT-6 positive cells and lymphocyte subsets within skin tumors before and after therapy with local injections of interferon alpha. Acta Dermatol (Kyoto) 81:241–246, 1986.

Moschella SL, Hurley HJ: Dermatology, vol 1 and 2. Philadelphia: WB Saunders, 1985.

Nicholls EM: Development and elimination of pigmented moles, and the anatomical distribution of primary malignant melanoma. Cancer 32:191–195, 1973.

Orton CI: The treatment of basal cell carcinoma by radiotherapy. Clin Oncol 4:33–34, 1978.

Pack GT, Davis J: Nevus giganticus pigmentosus with malignant transformation. Surgery 49:347, 1961.

Parker CM, Hanke CW: Large keratoacanthomas in difficult locations treated with intralesional 5-fluorouracil. J Am Acad Dermatol 14:770–777, 1986.

Peck GL: Retinoids and cancer. J Invest Dermatol 85:87–88, 1985.

Peck GL, Gross EG, Butkus D, et al: Chemoprevention of basal cell carcinoma with isotretinoin. J Am Acad Dermatol 6:815–823, 1982.

Peck GL: Topical tretinoin in actinic keratosis and basal cell carcinoma. J Am Acad Dermatol 15:829–835, 1986.

Raderman D, Giler S, Rothem A, Ben-Bassat M: Late metastases (beyond ten years) of cutaneous malignant melanoma. J Am Acad Dermatol 15:374–378, 1986.

Reed WB, et al: Giant pigmented nevi, melanoma, and leptomeningeal melanocytosis: a clinical and histopathological study. Arch Dermatol 91:100, 1985.

Rhodes AR, Harrist TJ, Momtaz TK: The PUVA-induced pigmented macule: a lentiginous proliferation of large, sometimes cytologically atypical, melanocytes. J Am Acad Dermatol 9:47–58, 1983.

Roenigk RK: Mohs micrographic surgery. Mayo Clin Proc 63:175–183, 1988.

Ronan SG, Eng AM, Briele HA, et al: Thin malignant melanomas with regression and metastases. Arch Dermatol 123:1326–1330, 1987.

Rook A, Wilkinson DS, Ebling FJ, et al (eds): Textbook of Dermatology, 4th ed, vol 1–3. Oxford: Blackwell Scientific Publications, 1986.

Rowe DE, Carroll RJ, Day CL Jr: Mohs surgery is the treatment of choice for recurrent (previously treated) basal cell carcinoma. J Dermatol Surg Oncol 15:424–431, 1989.

Rowe DE, Carroll RJ, Day CL Jr: Long-term recurrence rates in previously untreated (primary) basal cell carcinoma: implications for patient follow-up. J Dermatol Surg Oncol 15:315–328, 1989.

Rowe DE, Carroll RJ, Day CL Jr: Long-term recurrence rates for squamous cell carcinoma of the skin: implications for treatment modality selection. J Dermatol Surg Oncol 16:1, 1990.

Salasche SJ, Amonette RA: Morpheaform basal cell epitheliomas: a study of subclinical extension in a series of 51 cases. J Dermatol Surg Oncol 7:387–393, 1981.

Scotto J, Kopf AW, Urbach F: Non-melanoma skin cancer among caucasians in four areas of the United States. Cancer 34:1333–1338, 1974.

Shaw HM, Beattie CW, McCarthy WH, Milton GW: Late

maxillary and mandibular ridges arise from remnants of the dental lamina. Those cysts associated with the midpalatine raphe are probably the result of epithelial inclusions in the line of fusion of the palatine processes. These cysts are common in the newborn but tend to regress spontaneously during the first few months of life and are quite rare after 3 months of age.

Clinical Features. Gingival cysts of infants appear as raised, white or pink nodules that range from 1 to 5 mm in diameter (Fig. 47–1). They may be solitary but are often multiple.

Histopathology. Gingival cysts of infancy are lined by stratified squamous epithelium, which is usually parakeratinized. The cyst cavity, in most cases, is filled with keratin. The epithelial lining lacks the coronal basal layer with the corrugated appearance that is commonly seen in odontogenic keratocysts.

Treatment. The majority of gingival cysts of infancy are discharged shortly after birth and require no immediate surgical intervention.

Gingival Cysts of Adults. Gingival cysts in adults are uncommon. This developmental lesion is defined as an epithelium-lined cyst that occurs in the gingival soft tissue and may cause superficial bone erosion, but it does not arise within bone. Gingival cysts in adults form as slow-growing, painless swellings of the free or attached gingiva. They appear to occur with increased frequency in the interdental papilla. The pathogenesis is not known, but suggested origins include odontogenic rests derived from dental lamina and traumatic implanting of surface epithelium.

Clinical Features. Gingival cysts are more common in the mandible. The most common location is the canine or first premolar region, usually on the facial surface of the gingiva. The lesions appear as painless, circumscribed swellings in the gingiva and are white, red, or bluish-gray. They are usually less than 1 cm in diameter and, when palpable, are soft and fluctuant. Pressure resorption of underlying bone results in saucerization of the cortical surface; this may or may not be evident radiographically as a radiolucency.

Histopathology. Most gingival cysts of the adult are lined by thin, nonkeratinized squamous epithelium devoid of rete peg formation, which ranges from one to three cells in thickness. There is usually inflammation of varying degrees in the fibrous wall.

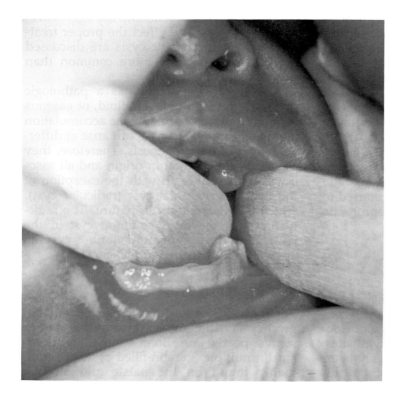

Figure 47–1. Gingival cysts of infants (clinical features).

Treatment. The gingival cyst of adults tends to grow slowly and does not have a tendency to recur. Therefore, simple surgical excision is curative.

Lateral Periodontal Cysts. Various forms of odontogenic cysts, such as the odontogenic keratocysts and the radicular cysts, may be related to lateral root canals. Therefore, they may occasionally manifest on the lateral aspect of a tooth as related to lateral root canals and are referred to as lateral periodontal cysts. A lateral periodontal cyst is likely to be discovered on a routine radiograph and to appear as a well-defined area of lucency on the lateral aspect of a root. The developmental type of lateral periodontal cyst is characterized by location (generally lateral to the tooth root and above the root apex of a canine or premolar tooth), size, shape, and radiographic appearance. The pathogenesis of lateral periodontal cysts is speculative. It is generally accepted that they are derived from reduced enamel epithelium after the tooth has erupted.

Clinical Features. Lateral periodontal cysts are usually found in the canine to premolar region and are rare before 20 years of age. The adjacent teeth are vital, and the lesion is frequently asymptomatic. The associated teeth are vital and should not be extracted. The characteristic radiographic appearance is that of a round or oval lucency with sharply defined margins of less than 1 cm in diameter (Fig. 47–2*A*).

Histopathology. Like the gingival cyst of the adult, the lateral periodontal cyst is nearly always lined by thin, nonkeratinizing squamous epithelium only one to four cells in thickness. The characteristic histologic feature is formation of epithelial plaques in the lining (Fig. 47–2*B*).

Treatment. The lateral periodontal cyst does not have a tendency to recur. When possible, it is treated by surgical excision without damage to adjacent tooth roots.

Dentigerous Cysts (Follicular). The dentigerous cyst is a developmental cyst that encompasses the crown of an unerupted tooth. Essentially a cystic enlargement of the dental follicle, it develops after the crown of the tooth has completely formed as fluid accumulates between the reduced enamel epithelium and enamel. The dentigerous cyst is one of the most common odontogenic cysts, secondary in frequency only to the radicular cyst.

Clinical Features. Dentigerous cysts are twice as common in men as in women. The cysts are most frequently detected in the second, third, and fourth decades of life. These cysts are frequently asymptomatic and may be discovered initially during routine radiography. The third molar region of the mandible and the canine region of the maxilla are the two most common sites for development of a dentigerous cyst. This is followed by the mandibular premolar and maxillary third molar areas. The pressure of pain and

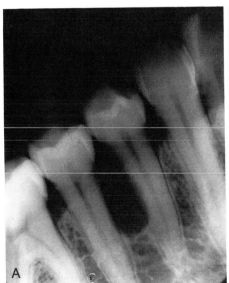
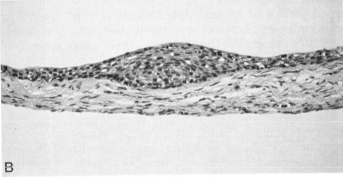

Figure 47–2. Lateral periodontal cyst. *A.* Radiographic features. *B.* Histologic features. (*A* and *B* courtesy of Dr. John M. Wright.)

the follicular pattern is more common. Malignant ameloblastomas with evidence of metastasis are rare.

Treatment. The conventional ameloblastoma has the capacity for continued growth and the tendency to infiltrate between bony trabeculae. Ameloblastomas in the posterior part of the maxilla should be treated more radically than are similar lesions in the mandible because the tumor may spread to the pterygopalatine fossa, base of skull, or temporal fossa. A marginal resection of the mandible is indicated when a tumor-free margin of bone can be preserved at the inferior border. The procedure can usually be accomplished by use of an intraoral approach. The teeth immediately involved with the ameloblastoma should be removed with the tumor, and a primary closure of the soft tissue should be obtained. In large, recurrent tumors involving the ramus or angle region of the mandible, extraoral hemimandibulectomy is indicated (Fig. 47–7E, 47–7F). The involved teeth and bone are removed with at least a 1-cm margin of uninvolved bone on the proximal and distal ends of the lesion. If the ameloblastoma is in the mandibular ramus, the posterior border and condylar process should be saved, if possible, to aid in immediate or delayed reconstruction of the mandible (Fig. 47–7G to 47–7I). The recurrence rate for ameloblastomas treated by enucleation or curettage alone is reported to be between 60% and 90%.

Adenomatoid Odontogenic Tumor. The adenomatoid odontogenic tumor is an uncommon epithelial tumor formerly known as the adenoameloblastoma or ameloblastic adenomatoid tumor.

Clinical Features. The adenomatoid odontogenic tumor is usually asymptomatic, but there may be a localized painless swelling. The tumor characteristically affects younger patients than does ameloblastoma. Most lesions are located in the anterior part of the mandible (Fig. 47–8A, 47–8B). In contrast, the ameloblastoma is located most often in the posterior ramus or angle region. Two thirds of adenomatoid odontogenic tumors are discovered in the second decade of life. Two thirds occur in the maxilla, two thirds are seen in females, and two thirds are associated with an impacted tooth, two thirds of which are canines. Radiographs of the adenomatoid odontogenic tumor show a well-defined area of radiolucency containing radiopaque foci of calcified tissue (Fig. 47–8C). Rare extraosseous examples of the adenomatoid odontogenic tumor have been described in the literature.

Histopathology. On a microscopic level, the adenomatoid odontogenic tumor has a well-defined fibrous capsule containing cystic spaces filled with blood-stained fluid (Fig. 47–8D). One or more teeth may be attached to the tumor or encased within its substance. Additional microscopy shows epithelium in a scanty, but vascular, connective tissue stroma. In addition, there are more solid areas where much of the epithelium is in whorls or rosettes of cells devoid of central spaces; calcified material is present in both epithelium and stroma.

Treatment. The adenomatoid odontogenic tumor is benign, and many pathologists consider it to be a hamartoma rather than a true neoplasm. Enucleation is curative, and associated impacted teeth should be removed during enucleation of the lesion. Recurrences have not been reported, even after incomplete removal.

Calcifying Epithelial Odontogenic (Pindborg's) Tumor. The calcifying epithelial odontogenic tumor, or Pindborg's tumor, is a distinctive and rare neoplasm of the jaws. It is thought to arise from the epithelial elements of the enamel organ. In comparison with other types of odontogenic tumors, the calcifying epithelial odontogenic tumor is relatively uncommon and comprises only 1% of all odontogenic tumors.

Clinical Features. The lesion is a slow-growing, painless swelling. The average age of presentation is approximately 40 years; there is no sexual predilection. Seventy percent are found in the mandibular premolar region. Depending on the stage of development, Pindborg's tumors manifest variable radiographic appearances (Fig. 47–9A, 47–9B). Approximately one half of the cases are associated with an unerupted tooth.

Histopathology. The calcifying epithelial odontogenic tumors have a characteristic microscopic appearance (Fig. 47–9C, 47–9D) of sheets or islands of polyhedral epithelial cells with prominent cellular borders, intracellular bridges, and occasional ringlike calcifications (Liesegang's rings).

Treatment. Pindborg's tumors behave similarly to ameloblastomas and are locally in-

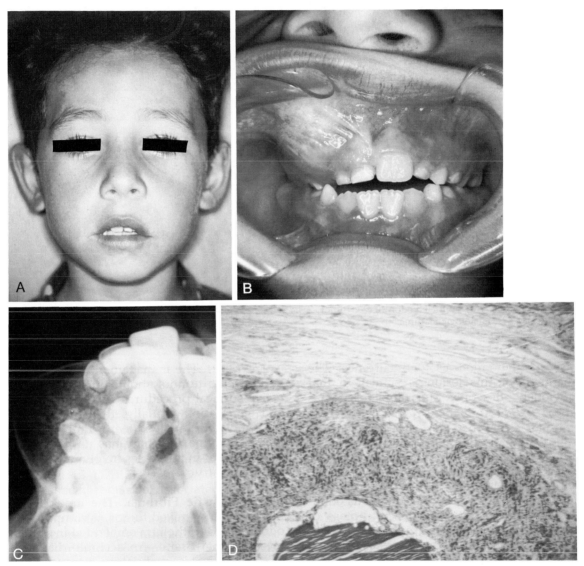

Figure 47–8. Adenomatoid odontogenic tumor. *A, B.* Clinical features of right maxillary swelling. *C.* Radiographic features. *D.* Histologic features.

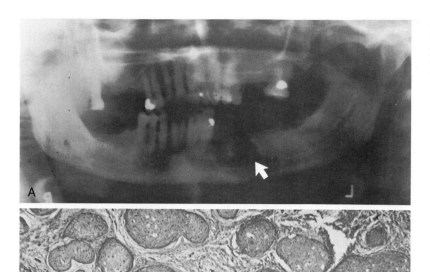

Figure 47–10. Squamous odontogenic tumor. *A.* Radiographic features (marked by arrow). *B.* Histologic features. (*A* and *B* courtesy of Dr. John M. Wright.)

Histopathology. The ameloblastic fibro-odontoma is a tumor that represents a more mature form of the ameloblastic fibroma. In other words, this mature form has histodifferentiated, resulting in the formation of enamel and dentin (Fig. 47–12B).

Treatment. During surgery, the ameloblastic fibro-odontoma is found to have a well-defined connective tissue capsule and is easily enucleated. After enucleation, the surgical bed should undergo thorough curettage.

Odontomas (Complex and Compound). Odontomas are the most frequently encountered odontogenic tumor. Although classified as odontogenic tumors, they may be more accurately defined as malformations or hamartomas composed principally of mature dentin and enamel. Two subcategories of odontomas are generally recognized: the complex and compound odontomas. The complex odontoma is a malformation in which all the dental tissues are represented. The individual tissues are generally well formed but occur in a disorderly pattern. On the other hand, the compound odontoma is a malformation in which all the dental tissues are represented in an orderly pattern; this lesion contains many toothlike structures (Fig. 47–13A). Therefore, when the dental tissues are deposited in the form of structures that resemble normal small teeth (denticles), the lesion is referred to as a compound odontoma. If the dental tissues are irregularly arranged throughout the lesion, it is referred to as a complex odontoma. Of all the odontogenic hamartomas and tumors, the compound odontoma achieves the highest degree of differentiation.

Clinical Features. Although odontomas can arise at any age, they are usually associated with the permanent dentition of children and young adults. These lesions are asymptomatic and rarely expand the jaw. Complex odontomas are slightly more common in the mandible and usually occur in the posterior regions. Compound odontomas show a marked predilection for the maxilla in the anterior region. On radiographic examination, odontomas possess a densely radiopaque solitary mass, as seen with complex odontomas, or a number of denticles, as seen with compound odontomas. Both complex and compound odontomas are usually surrounded by a thin radiolucent zone and are associated with an unerupted tooth (Fig. 47–13B, 47–13C).

Histopathology. Odontomas manifest as a mixture of enamel, enamel matrix, dentin, pulp tissue, and cementum. This may be arranged in an orderly or a haphazard fashion. Histopathologic examination of a complex odontoma shows an irregular arrangement of the dentin, enamel, cementum, and

pulp with formation of an irregular mass enclosed in a fibrous capsule. A compound odontoma generally consists of an encapsulated mass of separate denticles in a fibrous stroma (Fig. 47–13D).

Treatment. Treatment for odontomas, whether complex or compound, is identical to that for an impacted supernumerary tooth. Early removal is usually indicated in order to prevent interference with adjacent tooth development. Surgical removal of these benign tumors is conservative: removal of overlying bone and enucleation of the calcified mass with associated surrounding soft tissues (Fig. 47–13E, 47–13F). Growth potential for odontomas is usually limited, and recurrence is very uncommon.

Mesenchymal Tumors

Odontogenic Fibroma. The odontogenic fibroma, a fibroblastic tumor, is thought to

Figure 47–11. Ameloblastic fibroma. *A.* Radiographic features of lesion, keeping third molar depressed (marked on right by arrow). *B.* Histologic features.

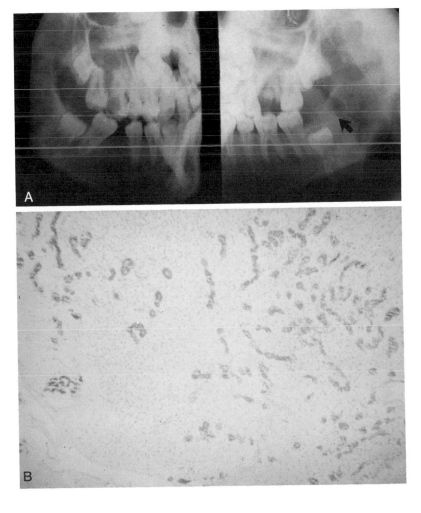

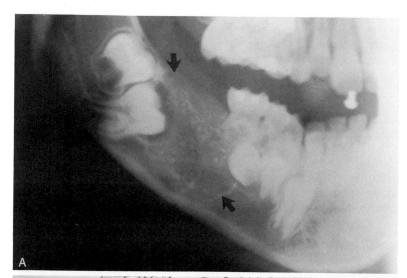

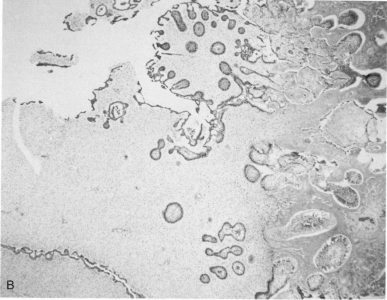

Figure 47–12. Ameloblastic fibro-odontoma. *A.* Radiographic features (marked by arrows). *B.* Histologic features. (*A* and *B* courtesy of Dr. John M. Wright.)

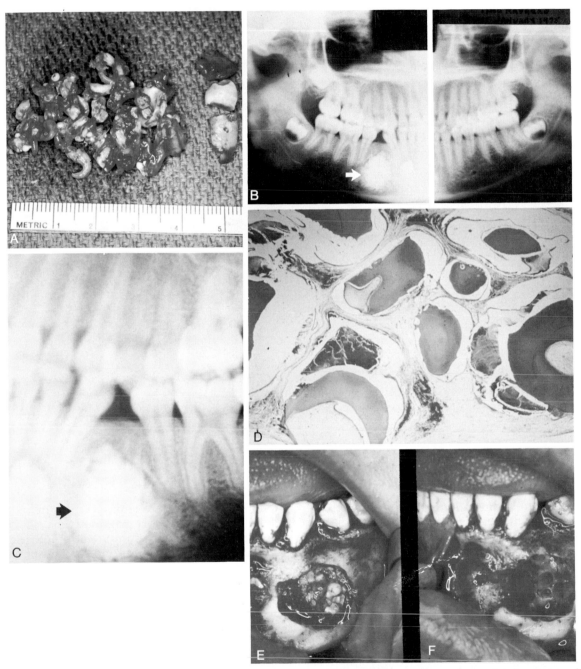

Figure 47–13. Compound odontoma. *A.* Surgical specimen of impacted premolar and associated compound odontoma. *B, C.* Radiographic features (marked by arrows). *D.* Histologic features. *E, F.* Surgical exposure and enucleation.

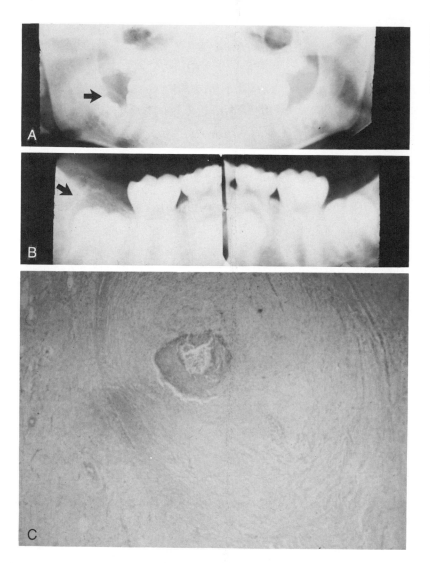

Figure 47–14. Odontogenic fibroma. *A, B.* Radiographic features of lesion (marked by arrows) associated with crown of impacted molar. *C.* Histologic features.

originate from odontogenic mesenchyme. The odontogenic fibroma is an uncommon and poorly understood lesion.

Clinical Features. The odontogenic fibroma forms a circumscribed mass within the jaw associated with the root or crown of an impacted tooth. The age at which the odontogenic fibroma manifests ranges from 11 to 80 years; the average age is 35 years. The odontogenic fibroma is a slow, persistent mass producing an asymptomatic cortical expansion. This lesion appears radiographically as a radiolucency associated with an impacted or displaced tooth (Fig. 47–14A, 47–14B).

Histopathology. Lesions similar to the odontogenic fibroma in the gingiva are termed *peripheral odontogenic fibromas.* The odontogenic fibroma is composed of scat-

tered rests of odontogenic epithelium in a dense collagenous stroma; there may exist numerous strands of odontogenic epithelium and calcifications in a stroma that resemble dysplastic cementum or dentin (Fig. 47–14C).

Treatment. Complete removal by enucleation or curettage is generally curative.

Odontogenic Myxoma. The odontogenic myxoma is a locally aggressive tumor that does not possess metastatic potential. It is thought to arise from odontogenic mesenchyme.

Clinical Features. The myxoma is a rare tumor seen most commonly in patients below the age of 20 years. This lesion generally involves the maxilla or the mandible and forms a slow-growing swelling of the involved bone (Fig. 47–15A, 47–15B). The posterior regions of both jaws are the sites most commonly affected. The main symptom associated with the odontogenic myxoma is a slow, progressive swelling with associated bone expansion; facial asymmetry becomes quite prominent. On the other hand, pain or paresthesia is very rare. A multilocular (soap-bubble or honeycombed) radiolucency with a radiopaque sclerotic margin, similar to that seen in ameloblastomas or central giant cell granulomas, is often seen radiographically (Fig. 47–15C, 47–15D). The gross specimen consists of gelatinous tissue that may be completely or partially encapsulated. An impacted tooth may be associated with this gross specimen.

Histopathology. On microscopic examination, stellate-shaped cells are sparsely distributed in a mildly basophilic stroma. Thin bundles of collagen are variable features, and mitotic figures are rarely seen (Fig. 47–15E).

Treatment. Because of the loose, gelatinous nature of this lesion, it is quite difficult to remove through enucleation. Incomplete removal is frequently followed by a recurrence rate of 10% to 30%. The prognosis of this lesion is good, but recurrent rates are high. Small lesions are best treated by vigorous curettage, followed by electrical or chemical cauterization, cryotherapy, or mechanical fulguration with an acrylic bur. Larger lesions usually require en bloc resections followed by immediate reconstruction (Fig. 47–15F to I).

Benign Cementoblastoma. The benign cementoblastoma is the only true neoplasm of cemental origin. The World Health Organi-

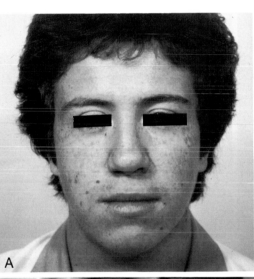
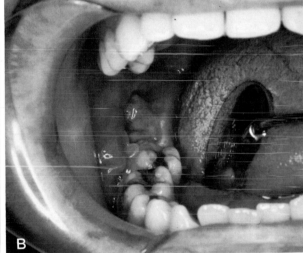
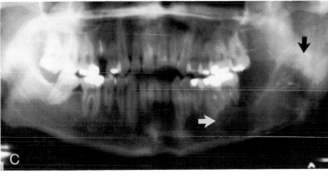
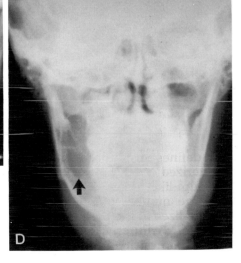

Figure 47–15. Odontogenic myxoma. *A, B.* Clinical features. *C, D.* Radiographic features (outlined by arrows).

Illustration continued on following page

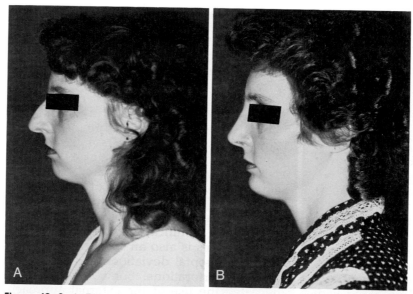

Figure 49–8. *A.* Preoperative view of dorsal hump and underrotated nasal tip. *B.* Postoperative result.

ously described approaches. The typical deformity is a dorsal convexity or hump (Fig. 49–8), which is usually caused by excessive bone or cartilage (upper lateral and septum). Occasionally, a surgeon encounters a dorsal concavity, or a saddle nose. This has several possible causes. Most often the saddle deformity is posttraumatic with the loss of septal cartilage from a septal hematoma, a fracture, or an abscess. The saddle may be iatrogenically caused by excessive dorsal resection in a previous rhinoplasty or septoplasty. The saddle may also be caused by granulomatous disorders of the septum such as Wegener's granulomatosis. These causes must obviously be ruled out before any rhinoplasty surgery. Most often, however, a dorsal hump will need to be reduced.

The initial step is to elevate the skin and soft tissue off the dorsum through any of the preceding approaches. One must be careful not to separate the attachment of the upper lateral cartilage and the nasal bones. The dorsum is then incrementally lowered as needed. This may be done by use of osteotomes, rasps, or saws at the surgeon's discretion. Portions of the nasal bones, the upper lateral cartilages, and the nasal septum can be removed as needed. The surgeon must strive not to lower the dorsum excessively, which leads to a "ski jump" appearance. This is particularly important in males and in patients from ethnic groups possessing a strong dorsal profile. The surgeon should carefully determine the patient's de-

sired profile preoperatively, rather than impose his or her own standards. In the case of the saddle deformity, augmentation rather than reduction of the dorsum is needed (Fig. 49–9). This can be performed with a variety of materials such as autograft cartilage (septal, conchal, or rib), autograft bone (cranial or iliac crest), homograft irradiated cartilage, or alloplastic materials. The augmenting material should be selected according to the severity of the defect and the surgeon's expertise.

After the removal of a dorsal hump, the nose is typically left with an "open roof" deformity. This is then closed by mobilizing the nasal bones with osteotomies (Fig. 49–10). Medial osteotomies serve to separate the nasal bones from the bony portion of the nasal septum. They may not be necessary if a large bony hump was previously removed. When needed, the medial osteotomies are performed with a sharp osteotome and can be either straight or curved slightly laterally. Lateral osteotomies are then performed to separate the nasal bones from the maxilla. The lateral osteotomies are usually performed in the nasal process of the maxilla, rather than in the nasal bones themselves (Fig. 49–10). This maneuver allows the nasal bones to be "infractured," thus closing the open roof and narrowing the bony pyramid. The lateral osteotomies can be performed either intranasally or percutaneously. Either way, it is advisable to preserve an inferior triangle of bone so that the attachments of

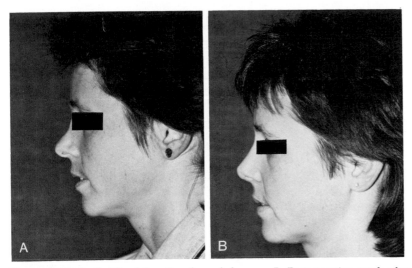

Figure 49–9. *A.* Saddle deformity of nasal dorsum. *B.* Postoperative result after correction with conchal cartilage graft.

the lower lateral cartilages to the maxilla are undisturbed (Fig. 49–10). Intranasal osteotomies are done with use of either straight or curved osteotomes as desired by the surgeon. Percutaneous lateral osteotomies can be performed with a small 2-mm osteotome through a small stab incision without fear of visible scarring in the nasal skin. It is important to obtain complete mobilization of the nasal bones so that the open roof can be fully closed and the dorsum adequately narrowed.

If a deficient chin projection was identified

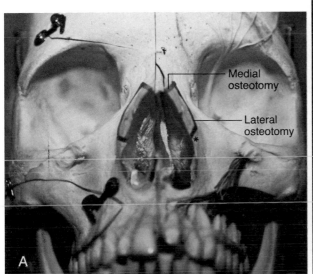

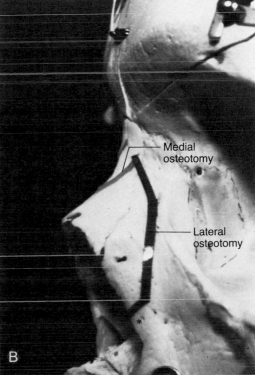

Figure 49–10. *A.* Frontal view of placement of osteotomies shown on human skull. The triangle of bone to preserve (see text) is marked with an asterisk. *B.* Lateral close-up view of osteotomy position. Note that the lateral osteotomy is in the nasal process of the maxilla, not in the nasal bone itself.

preoperatively, then it should be corrected at the time of rhinoplasty. Chin augmentation can be performed either intraorally or extraorally through a small incision in the submental crease. A variety of alloplastic materials have been used for this purpose. The implants are usually placed in a subperiosteal pocket overlying the symphysis. Alternatively, a forward sliding genioplasty can be done to move the mandibular bone forward.

At the conclusion of the rhinoplasty, the dorsum of the nose is usually covered with carefully applied tape and a plaster, aluminum, or thermoplastic splint. Loose intranasal packs of nonadherent material are placed and removed as soon as possible. Intranasal septal splints are occasionally used to help prevent synechiae between the septum and lateral nasal structures. Perioperative antibiotics are not usually needed. Intraoperative corticosteroids have been shown to help reduce postoperative pain and edema. The external and internal splints are usually removed in 1 week's time. The patient is advised to avoid strenuous activities for several weeks and all contact sports for at least 6 weeks. Postoperative photographs are usually taken after 6 or 12 months.

Fortunately, complications occur infrequently in rhinoplasty. They include infection, hematoma (especially septal), epistaxis, and a poor cosmetic outcome. Many cosmetic complications have been described, but only a few of the more common ones are described here (Fig. 49–11). Bossing or asymmetries of the nasal tip can occur if the alae are excessively weakened or resected. A supratip fullness ("pollybeak") can form if the cartilaginous dorsum, particularly the septal angle and upper lateral cartilages, is inadequately lowered. An open roof deformity can occur if the infracture of the nasal bones is inadequate. If asymmetries of the nose exist preoperatively, they should be pointed out to the patient during the preoperative counseling; otherwise, the patient may assume that they were caused by the surgery. Again, the importance of careful photographic documentation is obvious. If, however, a careful surgical approach has been employed and the patient has been counseled well, a successful result can be expected. Experience remains the single most important factor in obtaining a good outcome. Revision rhinoplasty is well beyond the scope of this text and is not discussed.

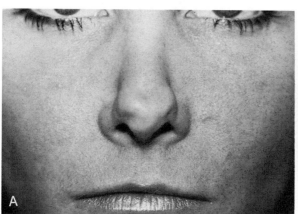
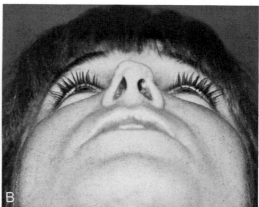
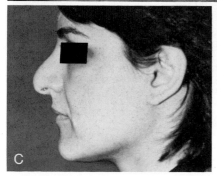

Figure 49–11. Rhinoplasty complications. *A.* Nasal tip bossing. *B.* Asymmetry. *C.* Pollybeak deformity resulting from excessive supratip fullness.

Figure 49–12. Anatomy of musculature of the forehead and brow. The natural rhytids in this area are at right angles to the direction of contraction of the muscles. The frontalis is partially removed on the left to demonstrate the corrugator muscle.

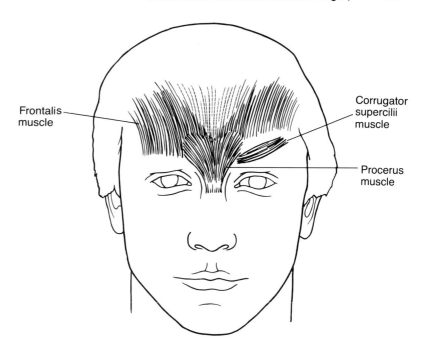

Frontalis muscle

Corrugator supercilii muscle

Procerus muscle

SURGERY ON THE AGING FACE

As the population of elderly persons increases and life expectancy grows, so will the demand for surgery on the aging face. It is also becoming more apparent that younger people are seeking rejuvenation surgery as well. The most commonly performed procedure for changes in the aging face is blepharoplasty, followed by face lift, collagen injections, chemical peel or dermabrasion, and liposuction. As with all other facial cosmetic procedures, it is crucial to thoroughly evaluate the patient preoperatively. It is important to define what the patient wants to change about his or her appearance and to determine whether those changes are realistic. Surgery on the aging face does not offer a "fountain of youth." Rather, it can provide a means to lessen the impact of aging on one's facial appearance.

Surgery of the Upper Third of the Face

There are two basic goals of surgery of the upper third of the face: one is to efface rhytids in the forehead, and the other is to correct ptosis of the brows. Not all patients require both to be corrected. Forehead rhytids form principally because of the action of the underlying muscles; namely, the frontalis muscle causes the horizontal rhytids of the

forehead, the corrugator supercilii the vertical glabellar lines, and the procerus the horizontal lines of the nasal root (Fig. 49–12). This is well illustrated in patients with a facial nerve palsy, who also have a marked reduction in forehead wrinkles. The position of the brow should be carefully assessed before any eyelid surgery is performed. Brow ptosis is frequently unrecognized by patients and surgeons alike. The ideal position of the brow is somewhat different for males and females. In the woman, the brow should lie at or slightly above the supraorbital rim. It should have an arching appearance with the peak of the brow at a point above the lateral canthus or slightly medial to it (Fig. 49–13). In the

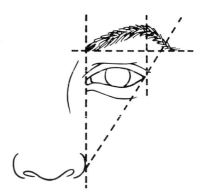

Figure 49–13. Ideal position of the brow in a female. A male brow has a less curved profile.

male, the brow should be at or slightly below the supraorbital rim, and it should have a flatter contour. The medial end of the club-shaped eyebrow is usually above the medial canthus.

Brow ptosis should be carefully ruled out in all patients who are candidates for blepharoplasty because brow ptosis frequently manifests as excess upper eyelid skin. Forehead and brow surgery should *always* be performed before any eyelid procedures. There are four principal approaches to the aging forehead and brow: coronal, pretrichal, midforehead, and direct browplasty (Fig. 49–14). These are each discussed in turn.

The standard photographic views employed are full-face frontal, lateral, and three-quarters; close-up of the eyelids in lateral and frontal views with the patient looking straight ahead, looking up, and with eyes closed; and full-face animation (smiling, elevating brows) views as needed to demonstrate rhytids. Most brow or forehead procedures are performed while the patient is under local anesthesia, although a general anesthetic may be chosen for the coronal technique.

The coronal brow lift entails a bicoronal scalp incision from ear to ear with the creation of a subgaleal scalp/forehead flap. The major indication for this approach is in females with low frontal hairlines and in patients whose primary concern is the forehead rhytids. This approach is contraindicated in males with androgenic pattern baldness and in females with a high frontal hairline. It is not a good choice for patients with severe brow ptosis. The principal advantages of this technique are the hidden scar in scalp, access to frontal musculature, and preservation of forehead length. The principal disadvantages are elevation of the frontal hairline, risks of hematoma, anesthesia of the scalp and forehead, and difficulties in suspending and positioning the brows accurately. The facial nerve is also at risk during the elevation of the flap in the region of the lateral canthus and zygomatic arch. The basic technique involves making an incision parallel to and 5 to 7 cm behind the frontal hairline. A subgaleal flap extending down to the supraorbital rims and zygomatic arches is then elevated. The frontalis, corrugator, and procerus muscles are resected as indicated. It is wise to limit frontalis muscle resection to the area medial to the pupils so that some natural motion of the brow is preserved. The scalp is resected as needed (typically 1 to 3 cm) and closed. Drains are usually placed under the flaps.

The pretrichal brow lift is principally indicated for the female with a high frontal hairline or a long forehead. This approach is not good for male patients in general and is

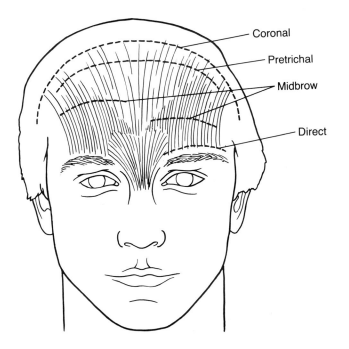

Figure 49–14. Location of the incisions for the various surgical approaches to the aging brow. See text for details.

Coronal

Pretrichal

Midbrow

Direct

contraindicated in those with male pattern baldness. The advantages of this technique are the same as those of the coronal lift with preservation of the position of the hairline. The principal disadvantage is the possibility of a visible scar if it is not performed properly. There is also an increased possibility of greater scalp anesthesia. In this technique, an incision is made 2 to 3 mm behind the frontal hairline. This incision should be beveled so that hair follicles are left on the scalp side of the incision deep to the cut (Fig. 49–15). Such beveling will enable hairs to grow up through the scar and help to camouflage it. The remainder of the procedure is similar to the coronal lift.

The midforehead brow lift is indicated in those patients who primarily need correction of brow ptosis. It is not used for the effacement of forehead rhytids; however, it can provide access to the corrugator and procerus muscles to reduce the rhytids that they produce. The principal advantage of the midforehead brow lift is that it allows the surgeon to precisely correct brow ptosis and accurately position the brow. The brow elevation is likely to be very long-lasting because suspension sutures are used. The incision is hidden in natural skin creases, and skin excision does not distort the appearance of the brow. The main disadvantage is the potential for a visible scar in an area that is difficult to hide. This technique is also excellent for patients with a facial nerve paralysis and unilateral brow ptosis.

The technique is as follows. The optimal position of the brow is first marked while the patient is sitting upright. The amount of skin to be excised is determined by how much elevation of the brow is needed. An appropriate skin crease is selected above each brow, usually at different levels to aid camouflage. The skin excision is centered over the rhytid, and a skin flap is elevated superficial to the frontalis muscle down to the orbicularis muscle. The orbicularis is suspended with sutures up to the periosteum of the forehead, thereby precisely positioning the brow. The skin is then closed carefully to evert the skin edges.

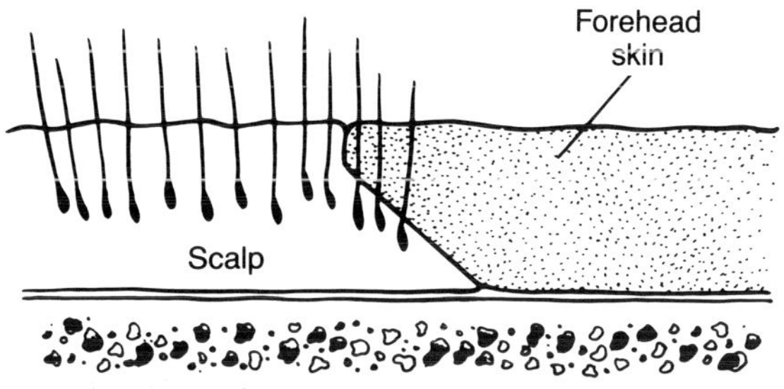

The direct brow lift is indicated primarily in elderly patients with brow ptosis and a deep suprabrow crease. It offers no obvious advantage over the midforehead lift except its technical simplicity. The major disadvantages are cosmetic: the scar is visible and difficult to hide; the superior brow hairs may be lost, which leads to a sharply demarcated eyebrow margin; and brow positioning is less precise, especially medially. The technique basically involves direct excision of an appropriate amount of skin directly above the brow. The brow is then suspended with sutures to the periosteum at the superior margin of the skin excision. The skin edges are then carefully closed.

Complications of brow and forehead lifts are rare and vary according to the procedure selected. Hematomas can occur, especially with the coronal and pretrichal lifts. Facial nerve injury is rare but is most likely to occur also in coronal and pretrichal lifts. Scarring is primarily an issue in midforehead, direct, and pretrichal approaches. Anesthesia of the scalp or the forehead from injury to the supraorbital or supratrochlear nerves can occur with any of the approaches but is most likely in those techniques in which a subgaleal flap is used. Perhaps the most troublesome problem occurs when the brow is excessively elevated, which leaves the patient with a surprised look. Certainly, all of these problems can be avoided with careful surgical technique.

Blepharoplasty

Blepharoplasty is the most commonly employed procedure for the aging face. A brief review of pertinent terminology and anatomy is provided before the surgery itself is discussed. A distinction should be made between dermatochalasis and blepharochalasis of the eyelids. *Blepharochalasis* is a rare, familial disorder usually with an onset in adolescence. It is characterized by unpredictable, recurrent attacks of eyelid edema that eventually leads to thinning of the skin and orbital

Figure 49–15. Cross-sectional anatomy of a pretrichal incision. This design allows hairs to grow up through the scar, which helps camouflage it.

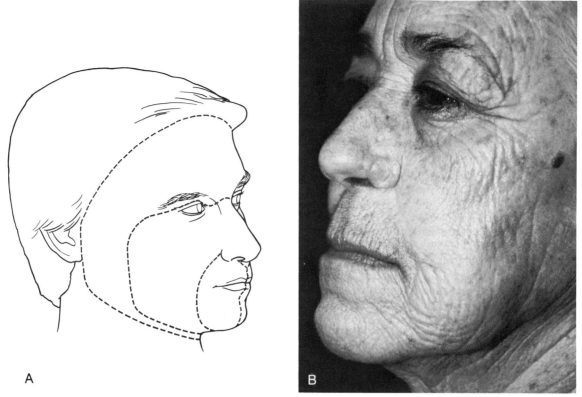

Figure 49–26. *A.* Diagramatic representation of relaxed skin tension lines (RSTL). *B.* Photograph demonstrating well the RSTL in an elderly patient.

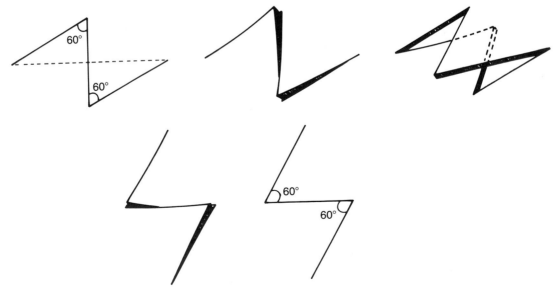

Figure 49–27. A 60° Z-plasty. Left to right: design, elevation, transposition, and closure. Note how the central vertical segment becomes horizontal and how the overall vertical length is increased.

Figure 49–28. Examples of running W-plasty (left) and geometric broken line closure (right). Note the relationship to the RSTL.

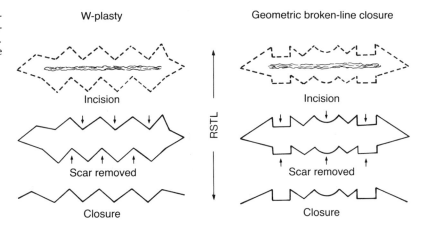

Z-plasty is that the overall scar length is three times that of the initial scar. When it is properly applied, the benefits of the Z-plasty usually justify its use nonetheless.

Another commonly employed scar revision technique is the running W-plasty. The geometric broken-line closure is a variant of this. In general, straight lines on the face are very visible and noticeable. In contrast, a complex line is less noticeable and difficult for the eye to follow. Both of these techniques create scars with a complex contour and thereby camouflage the scar. A further benefit is that a portion of the length of the scar can be reoriented along RSTLs. Examples of these techniques are shown in Figure 49–28. The major disadvantage of these methods is that the overall scar length is increased.

Dermabrasion also plays a vital role in scar revision surgery. Most patients who are candidates for scar revision surgery should be advised at the outset that dermabrasion will likely be indicated. Dermabrasion is frequently the final step in scar revision after any of the preceding techniques. In the case of acne "ice-pick" scars, dermabrasion is the treatment of choice and can be used to treat the entire face if needed. Dermabrasion helps blend scars into the surrounding skin and helps minimize pigmentary discrepancies in the face. The technique, postoperative care, and complications of dermabrasion have been discussed previously.

Finally, brief mention should be made of the role of intralesional corticosteroids in scar revision. Corticosteroids have profound anti-inflammatory effects in healing soft tissue, and they also may help reduce fibrosis in the final wound. Corticosteroids also help soften and flatten scars during the maturation phase. These medications are the mainstay of treatment of hypertrophic and keloid scars. Potential undesirable effects of their use are a reduction of wound strength, delayed healing, and epidermal thinning. There is also a risk of localized necrosis, dermal atrophy, and adrenal suppression. Most of these problems are dose-related, however. Triamcinolone is most commonly used in a concentration of 10 to 20 mg/mL. The drug is injected directly into the scar with a syringe and a 30-gauge needle or with a pressurized needleless injector. The scar is usually injected every 4 to 6 weeks until the desired effect is obtained.

CONGENITAL ANOMALIES

Congenital anomalies of the head and neck encompass a staggering array of defects. These range from small vascular cutaneous lesions to massive craniofacial syndromes. Only a few examples are discussed here for illustrative purposes.

Cutaneous vascular lesions of the head and neck can range from simple, small capillary hemangiomas to grotesquely deforming port wine stains. It is important to clinically distinguish capillary from cavernous hemangiomas whenever possible. Hemangiomas with principally capillary components are more likely to involute than are cavernous lesions. Whenever possible, it is best to allow hemangiomas to regress spontaneously and to reserve treatment for those lesions that bleed, interfere with feeding, and cause airway difficulties or other clinical problems.

Developments in cutaneous laser treatments have enabled many of these lesions to be well treated and eradicated. Perhaps the most promising new laser is the flashlamp-excited tunable dye laser (Candela Corp.). This allows photocoagulation of the superficial vascular lesion without damage to the overlying epithelium. The lesions can be treated without any anesthesia (except in young children). When these lesions are treated properly, the risk of scarring is negligible. This laser appears to be best for low–blood-flow lesions such as port wine stains, capillary hemangiomas, and telangiectasias. Even young children with extensive lesions can be safely treated. Other vascular lesions such as arteriovenous malformations and cavernous hemangiomas may also be amenable to neodymium:YAG, argon, or copper vapor laser therapy. Angiographic embolization is frequently used to facilitate treatment of these high-flow lesions.

Otoplasty is a commonly performed procedure for congenital auricular deformities. The most common defects seen are excessive protrusion of the auricle (large conchal-mastoid angle) and absence of an antihelical fold (Fig. 49–29). The otoplasty should thus be designed to correct the individual patient's deformity. Three principal techniques are employed in otoplasty. One involves the placement of horizontal mattress sutures (Mustarde sutures) to recreate an antihelical fold. Another involves a set-back procedure by excising skin and soft tissue from the postauricular surface and over the mastoid process. Finally, sutures are occasionally placed from the conchal bowl to the mastoid periosteum (Furnas sutures). These three techniques can be employed alone or in combination as indicated. The most common complication of all types of otoplasty is an auricular hematoma. These should be quickly drained so that an abscess does not form and to reduce the likelihood of auricular perichondritis, which can lead to severe deformation of the auricle.

Cleft lip and palate is another commonly seen deformity of the face. This obviously is a complex subject that has received much attention in the literature through the years. Developmentally, the palate is divided into a primary palate and a secondary palate. The incisive foramen separates the palate into a primary and secondary palate (Fig. 49–30). The primary palate (alveolus) and the lip develop first, and the secondary palate (hard and soft palates) forms later. Clefts of the lip and the primary palate are thought to result from a failure of migration or proliferation of mesenchyme from the midline frontonasal and lateral maxillary processes. Clefts in this area are not caused by the failure of tissue groups to fuse. In contrast, the secondary palate forms by the fusion of the palatal processes of the maxilla with the developing

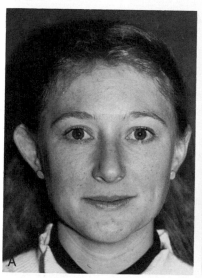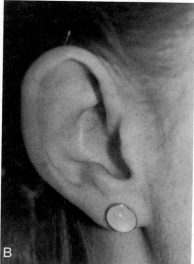

Figure 49–29. Typical deformity seen in a patient desiring otoplasty. *A.* Frontal view demonstrating excessive protrusion of the right auricle (large conchal-mastoid angle). *B.* Close-up of the right ear. Note the absence of the superior antihelical fold.

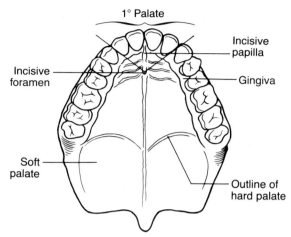

Figure 49–30. Anatomy of the primary and secondary palates.

nasal septum. Thus clefting of the secondary palate may in fact be a failure of the tissue fusion process.

Cleft lip and palate represents a spectrum of deformities ranging from an isolated unilateral incomplete cleft lip to bilateral complete cleft lip and palate. The most common finding is a combined cleft of the primary and secondary palate (35% to 50%), followed in frequency by cleft secondary palate only (30% to 45%), and isolated cleft lip (10% to 30%). The etiologic process of clefting is usually multifactorial. It is only rarely inherited in a straightforward mendelian fashion. Increasing paternal age has a greater impact than does maternal age. Race also plays a significant role: clefts are more common in whites than in blacks. Because of the complex nature of cleft lip and palate genetics, all families of children with cleft lip and palate should undergo genetic counseling. It should be remembered that cleft lip and palate causes a wide spectrum of clinical and social problems. These patients frequently have hearing, speech, and feeding problems. Thus all these patients should ideally be treated by a team composed of surgeons, speech pathologists, dentists or orthodontists, social workers, audiologists, geneticists, and nurses. Only through a group effort can optimal care be given.

Surgery of cleft lip and palate is done in stages. The lip is repaired first, usually at the age of 2 to 3 months. The palate is then repaired between the ages of 12 and 24 months. Further scar revision can be done any time after the age of 4 years or so.

Definitive nasal surgery is usually done in the early teens, although some nasal repair is typically done at the time of the lip surgery. The cleft lip repair (Figs. 49–31, 49–32) has several goals: to restore a complete orbicularis oris muscle sphincter, to realign the vermilion and the Cupid's bow, to normalize the height of the lip, and to restore the nostril sill. Cleft palate repair also has several major goals: to close the oronasal fistula, to lengthen the palate to reduce the velopharyngeal incompetence, and to realign and reattach the muscles of the soft palate (intravelar veloplasty). Repair of the cleft nose deformity (Fig. 49–33) is an attempt to raise the dome on the cleft side and make the domes symmetric, to elevate the depressed ala on the cleft side, to medialize the alar base on the cleft side, and to lengthen the columella (especially in bilateral clefts). The technique of external rhinoplasty has proved to be very beneficial in cleft lip nasal surgery. Various techniques for accomplishing these goals have been described by D. R. Millard, T. Skoog, and others. A description of these techniques is beyond the scope of this chapter. Surgery for cleft lip and palate can offer dramatic improvement in terms of function and cosmesis for those patients afflicted. The emotional and psychologic support offered by the team approach can lessen the ordeal

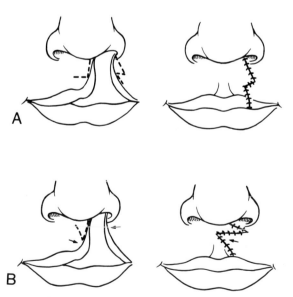

Figure 49–31. Schematic representations of cleft lip repairs. *A.* Triangular flap technique. *B.* Rotation-advancement technique. Both techniques reorient the orbicularis oris muscle and repair it as a separate layer.

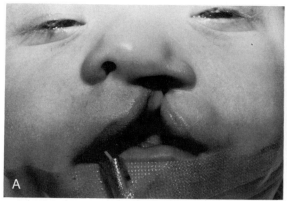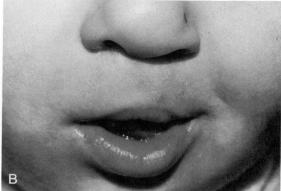

Figure 49–32. *A.* Preoperative appearance of a complete cleft of the lip and palate. Note the nasal deformity (see Fig. 49–33). *B.* Postoperative appearance after repair with a triangular flap technique.

of the surgery and help ensure a successful outcome.

MAXILLOFACIAL TRAUMA

All patients who sustain injuries to the head and neck require extensive evaluation so that the extent of injury can be ascertained and other associated injuries identified. A patent and secure airway is of the utmost concern in these patients. Those who sustain complex mandibular fractures and midface injuries are at the greatest risk for airway compromise. Endotracheal intubation, tracheostomy, or cricothyrotomy should be done to protect the airway when indicated. Bleeding from head and neck lacerations can be dramatic and life threatening, particularly when the scalp is involved. Massive bleeding should be con-

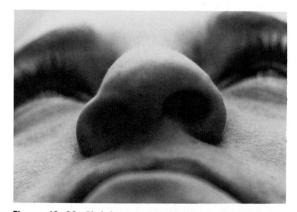

Figure 49–33. Cleft lip nasal deformity in an adult. On the cleft side (left) the alar base is lower and laterally displaced. The columella is relatively short, and the tip is broad and flattened on the cleft side.

trolled acutely by whatever means until the definitive repair can be done. The patient's tetanus immunization status should be ascertained and treated if needed. Any related injuries should be sought in these patients and identified at the initial presentation. Injuries most commonly associated with maxillofacial trauma are cervical spinal, thoracic or pulmonary, intracranial, ocular, and cervical visceral (trachea, larynx, great vessels, thyroid) injuries. Once the patient has been thoroughly evaluated and stabilized, management of the maxillofacial injury can proceed.

Maxillofacial injuries are assessed with a combination of history taking, physical examination, and radiographic studies. A thorough history is essential, with particular emphasis on the mechanism of injury. If the injury was related to a motor vehicle accident, the speed of the vehicles, the position of the patient in the vehicle (i.e., driver or passenger), and whether restraints were used are all important facts to know. If the injury was sustained in an assault, the weapons used should be identified if possible. These details all help direct the examination and help the clinician to choose appropriate imaging studies. The patient's visual acuity should be tested and documented. Cranial nerves should be assessed, including all branches of the trigeminal nerve. Facial nerve function should be assessed if possible; however, facial edema may make this difficult. The temporozygomatic and marginal mandibular are the branches most commonly injured because they are superficially located over the zygomatic arch and mandible, respectively. The patient's dental occlusion

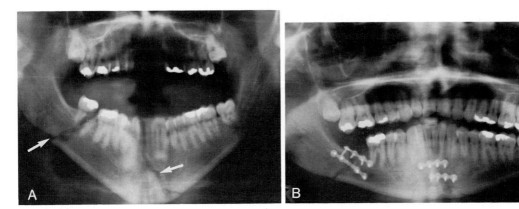

Figure 49–34. Panorex of bilateral mandibular fracture. *A.* Before reduction: a right angle fracture and a left parasymphyseal fracture are seen (arrows). *B.* Postreduction Panorex view of plate and screw fixation of the reduced fractures.

should be carefully checked and compared with the preinjury occlusion if possible. If trismus is present, it may indicate entrapment of the coronoid process by a depressed zygoma. The major bony prominences of the orbit, the zygoma, the nose, and the mandible should be palpated in order to help identify fracture lines. Radiographic imaging of facial fractures includes standard multiple-view x-ray films and computed tomographic (CT) scanning. The Panorex view is the single best study for mandible fractures (Fig. 49–34). CT scans should be done in both the axial and the coronal planes with thin

sections (Fig. 49–35). These studies are particularly helpful in delineating fractures in the naso-orbito-frontal region. Radiographic studies are unnecessary in patients with isolated nasal fractures. Magnetic resonance imaging is usually of little benefit in maxillofacial injuries because of the lack of bony detail that it provides (it may be of use in evaluating any intracranial injury, however). Complete photographic documentation is essential and should include close-up views of different anatomic areas involved (e.g., eyelids, lips).

Management of maxillofacial injuries can proceed as soon as the patient's condition is

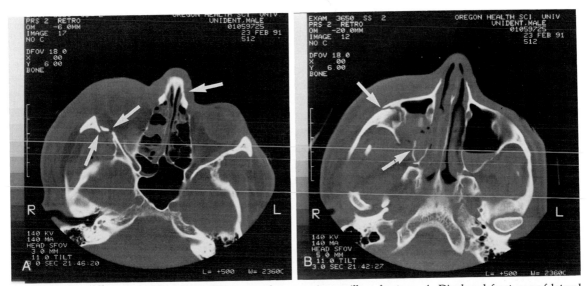

Figure 49–35. Axial computed tomographic scans of zygomaticomaxillary fracture. *A.* Displaced fractures of lateral orbital wall and rim and nasal bone fractures are well demonstrated (arrows). *B.* Fractures of anterior and posterior walls of the maxillary sinus are seen (arrows). The fluid in the sinuses is blood.

stable and when the facial edema no longer obscures the pertinent anatomy. Most patients benefit from use of perioperative antibiotics and perhaps corticosteroids as well. Repair of soft tissue injuries should follow thorough wound cleansing and irrigation. Normal saline is the only solution that should be used to irrigate wounds. Other agents such as hydrogen peroxide or antimicrobial solutions offer no advantage over saline alone and may be detrimental to the tissue. Debridement should be very conservative and limited to frankly necrotic tissue. The deeper soft tissue injuries (muscle, nerve, salivary gland) should be addressed first. If the facial nerve has been severed or avulsed, it should be repaired at the same time as the initial repair if possible. This may entail direct microsurgical repair or cable grafting as needed. Excision of injured salivary tissue may be necessary as well. The same meticulous techniques of handling soft tissue that are used in the closure of elective incisions should be employed when traumatic wounds are repaired. Judicious undermining of the wound edges and primary closure of lacerations should be done whenever feasible.

Several important facial landmarks should be carefully preserved and aligned: the cutaneous-vermilion border of the lips; eyelid margins; eyebrows and hairlines; alar and columellar margins; auricles; and melofacial and sublabial creases and folds. Any deformity or misalignment of these is quite visible and disturbing to the patient and may be difficult to correct later. The surgeon's goal should be to preserve the soft tissue and to cover the underlying bone and cartilage. Scar revision and camouflage should be left for a later procedure. It is always wise to advise the patient at the time of the *initial* repair that revisions may be needed at a later date.

Repair of maxillofacial bone injuries involves reduction of the fractures and then rigid fixation of those fractures. It is beyond the scope of this chapter to address all of the various fractures and their treatments; rather, basic principles are discussed. The fractures may be exposed either through existing lacerations or with appropriate incisions. The entire facial skeleton can be exposed with a combination of bicoronal, sublabial, and periorbital incisions (Fig. 49–36). The surgeon should attempt to return the bone fragments to their normal anatomic locations. A stable point that is not involved in the fracture should be sought and exposed. The surgeon then works away from this point, reducing and fixating fragments as they are encountered. For example, in midface fractures, the mandible might be a stable inferior reference point, and the zygoma and frontal bones may be superolateral reference points.

In many cases, restoration of proper occlu-

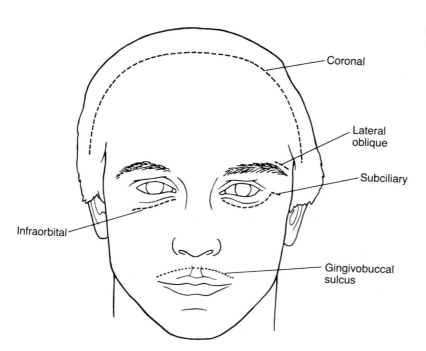

Figure 49–36. Various incisions used to approach facial fractures.

Coronal

Lateral oblique

Subciliary

Infraorbital

Gingivobuccal sulcus

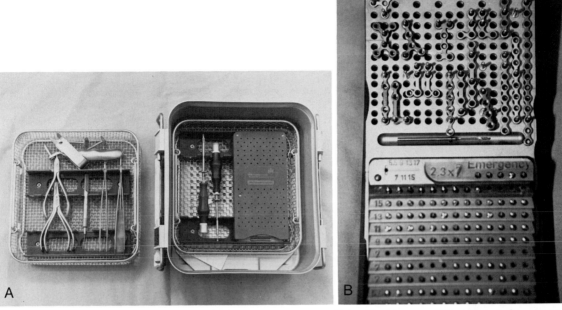

Figure 49–37. An example of a maxillofacial plating instrument set. It is critical to use a fully integrated screw and plate system so that all instruments are compatible with one another. *A.* The complete instrument tray. *B.* Various plates and screws available.

sal status with intermaxillary fixation is the initial step. Once the fragments of bone have been reduced, rigid fixation should be achieved. This can be accomplished with interfragmentary wires or, preferably, with screw and plate fixation (Fig. 49–37). Several maxillofacial plating systems are now available. All maxillofacial trauma surgeons should be well versed in their use and application. On occasion, primary bone grafting to the midface may also be needed to replace bone lost in severely comminuted fractures. The reader is referred to the suggested readings at the conclusion of the chapter for more information.

FACIAL RECONSTRUCTION

Facial reconstruction may be needed after cancer removal, traumatic tissue loss, or burns of the head and neck. The reconstruction may involve the replacement of bone, soft tissue, or both. CT scanning may be invaluable in evaluating what bone defects are present. Because many reconstructive efforts entail staged, multiple procedures, ex-

tensive preoperative counseling is essential. Complete photographic documentation aids the surgical planning, assists patient counseling, and is essential for medicolegal purposes.

Reconstruction of bone defects typically requires either bone grafting, bone-containing flaps, or alloplastic implants. Bone grafts may be membranous (e.g., calvarial) or cancellous (e.g., iliac crest, rib). Membranous bone has been shown to have less resorption than cancellous bone grafts have in both animal models and in clinical practice. However, the thinness of calvarial grafts may limit their application. Bone-containing vascularized pedicled or free flaps have been employed in head and neck reconstruction, particularly for the mandible. Radial forearm, fibular, and scapular free flaps have all been used with excellent results. Free nonvascularized bone grafts have also been employed for many years with good results, especially in the midface and the orbit. Rigid fixation of bone grafts with plates and screws can enhance bone grafting techniques and allow even broader application of bone grafting. Alloplastic materials such as silicone, hydroxyapatite, and others also have a role in reconstruction of bone defects. However, alloplasts should be used principally to fill in areas of bone loss and should not be used where function and structural support are needed. In addition, alloplastic materials should be employed only where thick, healthy soft tissue coverage is available.

Soft tissue reconstruction ranges from simple scar revision to microvascular free tissue transfer. Whenever possible, it is best to use adjacent soft tissue to fill a defect. Numerous local flaps are available for repair of facial defects (see Jackson, 1985; Salasche et al., 1988; Becker, 1985). When planning these flaps, the surgeon should choose a flap that provides skin of similar texture and color. In addition, the flap should be designed so that the incisions lie in natural creases or along relaxed skin tension lines. Whenever possible, reconstructions should not cross different esthetic areas of the face. If a local or adjacent tissue flap is not feasible or does not provide sufficient tissue, then a regional flap may be needed. Examples of these include pectoralis major myocutaneous flaps and deltopectoral flaps. If these are inappropriate, then a microvascular free flap can be used. Commonly used free flaps in the head and neck are the radial forearm flap, the latissimus dorsi flap, and the groin flap. Many other examples are in the literature, and more are likely to be introduced in the future. As can be seen, facial reconstruction is a diverse and challenging field that has stimulated surgeons' imaginations and skills for many years.

Acknowledgments

The authors wish to express their sincere appreciation to Lynn Kitagawa for her expertise in the preparation of the illustrations.

SUGGESTED READINGS

Anderson JR, Ries WR: Rhinoplasty: Emphasizing the External Approach. New York: Thieme Medical Publishers, 1986.

Baker SR (ed): Microsurgical Reconstruction of the Head and Neck. New York: Churchill Livingstone, 1989.

Becker FF: Facial Reconstruction with Local and Regional Flaps. New York: Thieme Medical Publishers, 1985.

Brent BD: Surgical treatment of congenital disorders of the external ear. *In* Serafin D, Georgiade NG (eds): Pediatric Plastic Surgery (pp 655–664). St. Louis: CV Mosby, 1984.

Colton JJ, Bekhuis GJ: Blepharoplasty. *In* Cummings CW, et al (eds): Otolaryngology—Head and Neck Surgery. St. Louis: CV Mosby, 1986.

Doxanas MT, Anderson RL: Clinical Orbital Anatomy. Baltimore: Williams & Wilkins, 1984.

Furnas DW (ed): Facial aesthetic surgery: Art, anatomy, anthropometrics and imaging. Clin Plast Surg 14(4), 1987.

Habal MB, Ariyan S: Facial Fractures. Toronto: BC Decker, 1989.

Jackson I: Local Flaps in Head and Neck Reconstruction. St. Louis: CV Mosby, 1985.

Kellman RM (ed): Facial plating. Oto Clin North Am 20(3), 1987.

Kerth JD, Toriumi DM: Management of the aging forehead. Arch Otolaryngol Head Neck Surg 116(10):1137, 1990.

Krause JL, Nelson GD: Clinical Photography in Plastic Surgery. Boston: Little, Brown, 1988.

Maniglia AJ (ed): Trauma to the head and neck. Oto Clin North Am 16(3), 1983.

McCarthy JG: Plastic Surgery, vols 2, 3, 4. Philadelphia: WB Saunders, 1990.

McCollough EG, Langsdon PR: Dermabrasion and Chemical Peel. New York: Thieme Medical Publishers, 1988.

McKinney P, Cunningham BL: Rhinoplasty. New York: Churchill Livingstone, 1989.

Nordstrom REA (ed): Hair replacement. Facial Plast Surg 2(3), 1985.

Parkin JL (ed): Lasers in otolaryngology. Oto Clin North Am 23(1), 1990.

Peck GC (ed): Rhinoplasty. Clin Plast Surg 15(1), 1988.

Rees TD: Aesthetic Plastic Surgery. Philadelphia: WB Saunders, 1980.

Rhys-Evans PH (ed): Otoplasty. Facial Plast Surg 2(2), 1985.

Salasche SJ, Bernstein G, Senkarik M: Surgical Anatomy of the Skin. Norwalk, CT: Appleton and Lange, 1988.

Sheen J: Aesthetic Rhinoplasty, 2nd ed. St. Louis: CV Mosby, 1987.

Tardy ME (ed): The aging face. Oto Clin North Am 13(2), 1980.

Tardy ME: Surgical Anatomy of the Nose. New York: Raven Press, 1990.

Thomas JR (ed): Facial plastic surgery. Oto Clin North Am 23(5), 1990.

Thomas JR, Holt GR: Facial Scars, Incision, Revision & Camouflage. St. Louis: CV Mosby, 1989.

Tobin GR (ed): Refinements in flap reconstruction. Clin Plast Surg 17(4), 1990.

Trier WC (ed): Cleft lip and cleft palate. Clin Plast Surg 12(4), 1985.

Walter C (ed): Face lifts. Facial Plast Surg 4(2), 1987.

CHAPTER 50

Orthognathic Surgery

Douglas P. Sinn, DDS   G. E. Ghali, DDS

The objectives of orthognathic surgery are to attain optimal functional and esthetic results for patients who have acquired, developmental, or congenital deformities of the facial bones and jaw. In performing this type of surgery, one must be properly prepared to understand the anatomy and physiologic function of the jaws, dentition, and associated masticatory structures. The surgeon must also be current in the diagnosis and design of the orthognathic surgical procedures and possess a good understanding of occlusion and orthodontics. In addition, one must have the expertise to analyze cephalometric and panoramic radiographs and dental study models. The proper execution of orthognathic surgical procedures is predicated on the ability of the surgeon to perform definitive model surgery, help the orthodontist establish treatment objectives, and prepare surgical prediction tracings and surgical treatment plans. In order to maximize surgical predictability and shun potentially vexatious results, a thorough knowledge of the surgical procedures and an appreciation of operative complications are mandatory. Regardless of the specific dentofacial deformity, complications may occur during the preoperative, intraoperative, or postoperative period. In general, most orthognathic surgical cases are divided into three treatment phases: (1) presurgical orthodontic phase, (2) surgical phase, and (3) postsurgical orthodontic phase. In this chapter, the basic principles common to all orthognathic surgical procedures are reviewed.

EVALUATION OF THE PATIENT

Clinical Evaluation

The single most important presurgical aspect to be evaluated is the patient's pre-existing facial morphologic characteristics. This esthetic facial evaluation is accomplished while the patient comfortably sits or stands with the head in a natural, relaxed position. The only essential instrumentation required for this clinical examination is a millimeter ruler. In general, it is preferable to divide the clinical portion of such evaluations into a frontal, a profile, and a three-quarter profile evaluation. Regardless of which part is initially examined, it is essential that the patient's head be properly oriented with the Frankfort plane parallel to the floor and in centric occlusion with the lips in repose in order to evaluate the osseous and soft tissue structures. A good understanding of normal anatomy and its millimetric values, facial balance, and those factors that deviate from this normality is essential. Factors such as centric relation–centric occlusion shifts, mucogingival problems, jaw posturing, and pre-existing temporomandibular joint problems should be assessed presurgically and incorporated into the treatment plan; unrecognized temporomandibular joint disorders may worsen as a result of orthognathic surgery.

Frontal

In general, the frontal evaluation is considered balanced when the upper, middle, and

909

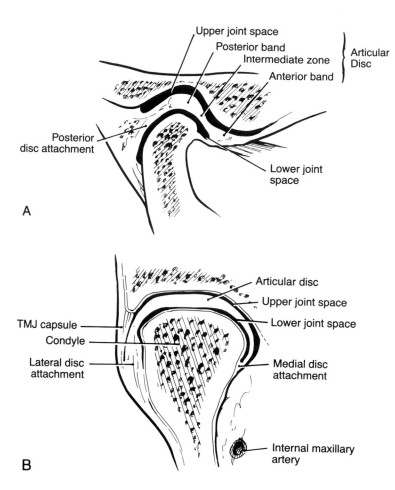

Figure 50–3. *A.* This illustration depicts the major anatomic structures seen on a sagittal view of the temporomandibular joint. *B.* This illustration reinforces the anatomic structures seen on a coronal section through the temporomandibular joint.

Figure 50–4. Lateral cephalometric radiograph represents a lateral soft tissue film that is taken at a standard distance with the head in a standard fixed position.

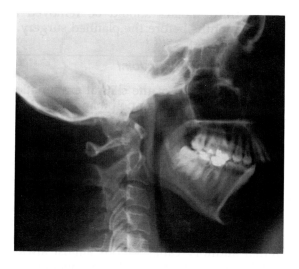

Figure 50–5. A tracing of the lateral cephalometric radiograph is superimposed onto acetate tracing paper. With one or a combination of several available cephalometric analyses, anatomic landmarks are identified, labeled, and connected by straight lines so that their relationships may be precisely measured. (From Burstone CJ, et al: Cephalometrics for orthognathic surgery. J Oral Surg 36:269, 1978.)

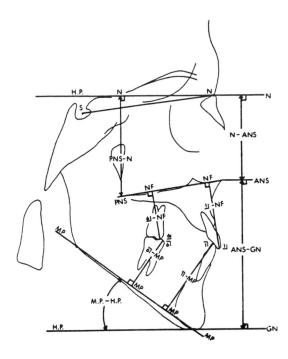

with which he or she is most comfortable. Table 50–1 summarizes common measurements used in the cephalometric analysis for orthognathic surgery. These measurements are related to the cephalometric tracing to aid in the determination of the nature of the skeletal deformity. It is beyond the scope of this chapter to discuss the specifics of any single analysis; one should refer to the suggested readings for detailed discussions on cephalometry. A panoramic radiograph is evaluated for visible bone, TMJ, dental, periapical, periodontal, or sinus disease (Fig. 50–6). In addition, the position of tooth roots in relation to planned interdental multisegment osteotomies is grossly evaluated on the panoramic radiograph. A further detailed assessment, particularly in cases of interdental osteotomies, may require periapical radiographs (interdental radiographs).

Occlusal Evaluation

Most occlusal evaluations are subdivided into intraoral and dental model phases. An intraoral evaluation is performed to compare centric relation–centric occlusion compatibility and assess attrition of the dentition. On the other hand, a dental model evaluation allows the clinician to directly assess intraarch relations and tooth mass discrepancies.

TABLE 50–1. Orthognathic Cephalometric Analysis

	Standard (Male)	Standard (Female)
Horizontal (Skeletal)		
N-A-Pg (angle)	3.9°	2.6°
N-A (‖ HP)	0.0°	−2.0°
N-B (‖ HP)	−5.3°	−6.9°
N-Pg (‖ HP)	−4.3°	−6.5°
Vertical (Skeletal, Dental)		
N-ANS (HP)	54.7 mm	50.0 mm
ANS-Gn (HP)	68.6 mm	61.3 mm
PNS-N (HP)	53.9 mm	50.6 mm
MP-HP (angle)	23.0°	24.2°
1-NF (NF)	30.5 mm	27.5 mm
1-MP (MP)	45.0 mm	40.8 mm
6-NF (NF)	26.2 mm	23.0 mm
6-MP (MP)	35.8 mm	32.1 mm
Maxilla, Mandible		
PNS-ANS (‖ HP)	57.7 mm	52.6 mm
Ar-Go (linear)	52.0 mm	46.8 mm
Go-Pg (linear)	83.7 mm	74.3 mm
Ar-Go-Gn (angle)	119.1°	122.0 °
Dental		
OP upper-HP (angle)	6.2°	7.1°
OP lower-HP (angle)	—	—
A-B (‖ OP)	−1.1 mm	−0.4 mm
1-NF (angle)	111.0°	112.5°
1-MP (angle)	95.9°	95.9°

N, nasion; A, subspinale point; Pg, pogonion; B, supramentale point; ANS, anterior nasal spine; Gn, gnathion; PNS, posterior nasal spine; MP, mandibular plane; HP, hard palate; NF, normal face; Ar, articulare; Go, gonion; OP, opisthion. (Modified from Burstone CJ, et al: Cephalometrics for orthognathic surgery. J. Oral Surg 36:269, 1978, with permission.)

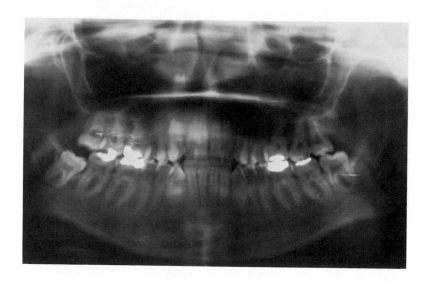

Figure 50–6. Panoramic radiographs are considered essential in the evaluation of orthognathic surgery patients. This extends to the assessment of available space between adjacent teeth for interdental osteotomies as well as to the assessment of the position of the inferior canal relative to planned mandibular osteotomies.

The failure to recognize a tooth mass discrepancy may result in a late functional compromise. During the evaluation of intra-arch relations on the models, the desired postsurgical cuspid-molar relationship should be determined. It is most desirable to establish, when feasible, an Angle class I molar and canine relationship (Fig. 50–7). Correlation of the dental model analysis with the cephalometric analysis helps the orthodontist and

Class I-Neutroclusion

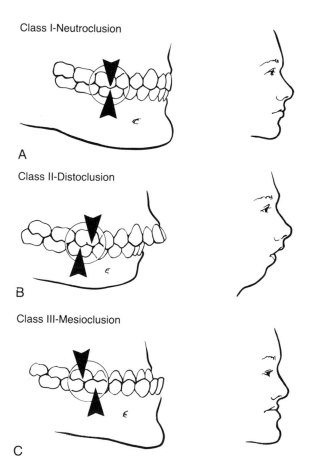

A

Class II-Distoclusion

B

Class III-Mesioclusion

C

Figure 50–7. *A.* Class I occlusion generally results in a harmonious facial profile. *B.* Class II malocclusion results in a retrognathic profile. *C.* Class III malocclusion results in a prognathic profile. Skeletal malocclusions result from the abnormal development of the mandible or maxilla or both.

surgeon determine whether tooth extractions are indicated. In addition, this correlation helps determine which type of orthodontic mechanics and surgical procedures are necessary for providing the patient with the optimal functional and esthetic result without compromising stability.

SURGICAL TREATMENT PLANNING

Esthetic Treatment Objectives

The primary surgical procedure chosen for the correction of any specific maxillofacial deformity is predicated upon the existing facial esthetics and the patient's desired changes. There exist numerous surgical procedures that may be used for the correction of dentofacial deformities. In general, the authors choose from four major procedures for the correction of these deformities: (1) sagittal split-ramus osteotomy, (2) vertical subcondylar ramus osteotomy, (3) osteotomy of the inferior border of the mandible (genioplasty), or (4) total maxillary osteotomy (Le Fort I). One-jaw surgery is the surgical repositioning of either the maxilla by a Le Fort I osteotomy or the mandible by some type of ramus osteotomy. Two-jaw surgery is the surgical repositioning of both the maxilla by a Le Fort I osteotomy and the mandible by some type of ramus osteotomy. Three-jaw surgery is the surgical repositioning of both jaws and an osteotomy of the inferior border of the mandible. A significant number of patients require a combination of these procedures in order to achieve the desired esthetic results.

For the patient in whom more than one surgical procedure is needed to achieve the desired facial alterations, the surgeon should carefully analyze the patient's existing occlusion. In this instance, the choice procedure is the one that will produce the most ideal occlusal result. For example, in a patient with microgenia, for whom the treatment plan would include an increase in chin prominence, there are a couple of considerations. If this patient possesses a stable class I occlusion, an osteotomy of the inferior border of the mandible with advancement of menton is the treatment of choice. Conversely, as is most often the case, the microgenia is accompanied by a class II malocclusion, and a mandibular advancement with or without an

advancement genioplasty becomes the treatment of choice. In review, most decisions regarding the selection of a specific orthognathic surgical procedure are predicated on existing facial esthetics in conjunction with occlusal and cephalometric predication tracing analyses.

Available Surgical Procedures

Sagittal Split Ramus Osteotomy

A paramount leap in the development of intraoral mandibular surgery occurred with the conception of the sagittal split ramus osteotomy (Fig. 50–8), described first by K. Schuchart in 1942 and then modified and reported in English by R. Trauner and H. Obwegeser in 1957. Refinements by Obwegeser involved extension of the medial osteotomy to include the posterior border of the mandible and extension of the vertical component to the region of the antegonial notch. In 1961, G. DalPont contributed to the evolution of this technique by extending the osteotomy anterior to the antegonial notch to include a greater segment of the body of the mandible. In describing a modified intraoral splitting technique for correction of mandibular prognathism, Hunsuck noted that it was not essential to carry the medial cut to the posterior border as described by Obwegeser. Consequently, Hunsuck proposed that the medial cut be carried only to the retrolingular fovea. B. N. Epker suggested limiting the extent of the soft tissue dissection as a further modification. L. M. Wolford introduced a modification in which a saw blade is used to facilitate controlled inferior border splitting, which has gained some popularity because it allows a more predictable split of the inferior mandibular body.

In the current practice of orthognathic surgery, there exist multiple indications for the modified sagittal ramus osteotomy of the mandible. In general, the four major indications for this procedure are (1) symmetric mandibular setbacks, (2) minor asymmetric mandibular setbacks, (3) symmetric and asymmetric mandibular advancements, and (4) vertical lengthening of the ascending mandibular ramus. In addition, if properly executed, this procedure provides wide bony contact for rigid internal fixation and avoids condylar rotation in the horizontal axis. Some disadvantages to this technique are related

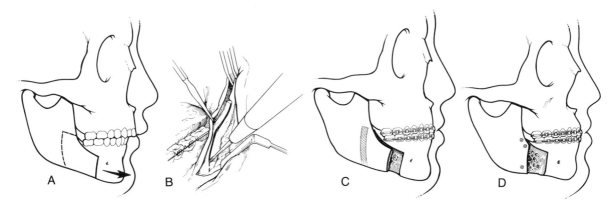

Figure 50–8. *A.* This simplified illustration demonstrates a class II malocclusion and associated mandibular retrognathia. Outlined is a planned bilateral sagittal split-ramus osteotomy with mandibular advancement. The goal of this procedure is to maintain presurgical positioning of the proximal segment while establishing unrestricted movement of the distal segment. *B.* An incision is made on the lateral aspect of the anterior border of the ramus in the region of the external oblique ridge. For optimal visibility, this should extend from midway up the ascending ramus inferiorly to approximately the mandibular first molar in the depth of the vestibule; all dissection is done subperiosteally. Dissection is carried medially just posterior and superior to the lingula and inferior alveolar neurovascular bundle. The medial soft tissues are retracted, and the medial (horizontal) bone cut is made into only the lingual cortex approximately 1.5 to 2 cm from the anterior border of the ascending ramus and 2 mm superior to the lingula. Subsequently, the bone cut is extended down the lateral aspect of the anterior border of the ascending ramus to the region of the second or first molar. The lateral (vertical) bone cut is completed at this point just through the lateral cortex in order to avoid the inferior alveolar neurovascular bundle. When the cortex of the inferior border has been reached, the cut is buried into only the buccal cortex. The inferior border bone cut is accomplished with use of a specially designed saw blade. All bone cuts are checked for completeness with osteotomes, and the segments are levered while the entire osteotomy site is carefully observed. *C.* The mandible is advanced the predetermined amount, as predicted from cephalometric tracings and model surgery, to achieve optimal occlusion and facial esthetics. *D.* This illustration demonstrates rigid fixation of the advanced mandible by placement of two bicortical bone screws at the superior border and a single screw at the inferior border. All incisions are closed in a single layer with absorbable gut suture. Advances in rigid internal fixation have significantly decreased the length of maxillomandibular fixation.

to the risk of serious injury to the inferior alveolar and mental nerves and the need for precise proximal segment fixation for positioning the condyle.

Vertical Subcondylar Ramus Osteotomy

The vertical subcondylar ramus osteotomy (Fig. 50–9) can be performed by either an intraoral or an extraoral approach. The impetus for general acceptance of this operation by American surgeons came from a paper published in 1954 by J. B. Caldwell and G. S. Letterman. As a means to set the mandible back, they thoroughly reviewed the procedure's history and described in detail the diagnostic and technical aspects of surgery in the ramus of the mandible through a submandibular skin incision. The vertical ramus osteotomy of the mandible was performed exclusively through an extraoral approach until reports in 1964 by S. M. Moose described an intraoral technique that was

performed from the lingual aspect of the mandible. Four years later, R. P. Winstanley described the intraoral vertical osteotomy from the lateral aspect of the mandible. Further refinements in the procedure followed, and in 1987, H. D. Hall and S. J. McKenna advocated retaining a portion of the attachment of the medial pterygoid to the distal tip of the proximal segment. They contended that this modification completely eliminated condylar sag, anterior open bites, and ischemic necrosis of the tip of the proximal segment. Currently, the subcondylar vertical ramus osteotomy is used for both mandibular setbacks and minor advancements.

With refinements in intraoral osteotomies of the ramus, an extraoral approach is seldom indicated. One relative indication for the extraoral approach is when wide exposure of the lateral aspect of the ramus is necessary. This is often the case when the mandible is set back more then 1.5 cm. Another uncommon indication for an extraoral approach exists when the mouth is very small or the soft tissues are inelastic; visualization may be restricted because of extreme bowing of the vertical rami. The extraoral vertical ramus osteotomy has also been advocated when severe dentofacial asymmetries exist or when reduction of an obtuse gonial angle is indicated. A surgeon may choose between the intraoral and extraoral approaches on the basis of personal preference in relation to the patient's deformity.

In review, the three major indications for the intraoral vertical subcondylar osteotomy are (1) vertical shortening of the mandibular ramus, (2) minor mandibular setbacks (<15 mm), and (3) minimal asymmetric mandibular setbacks. Advantages to this technique relate to a decreased risk of injury to the inferior alveolar nerve. Some of the cited disadvantages to this procedure are (1) the difficulty in controlling the condylar position in the glenoid fossa, resulting in relapse, and (2) the inability to use the procedure for major mandibular advancements.

Osteotomy of the Inferior Border of the Mandible/Genioplasty

The osteotomy of the inferior border of the mandible, or genioplasty, is one of the most commonly performed orthognathic surgical procedures (Fig. 50–10). It is usually performed in combination with other facial osteotomies. As a sole procedure, the intraoperative complications of the osteotomy of the inferior border of the mandible are relatively few. The genioplasty was first described as an extraoral approach in 1932 by O. Hofer. It was not until the late 1950s that R. Trauner and H. Obwegeser described an intraoral modification of the genioplasty for the correction of mandibular prognathism and retrognathia. Additional contributions to the technique were made by J. M. Converse and D. Wood-Smith in 1964 and by E. D. Hinds and J. N. Kent in 1969. Complications reported with this procedure include unfavorable osteotomies, nerve injuries, bleeding, and malpositioning of the mobilized segment. Basically, the major indications for genioplasties are to advance, reduce, straighten, or lengthen the external chin.

Le Fort I Osteotomy/Total Maxillary Osteotomy

Although maxillary surgery was described in the European literature as early as the 1920s,

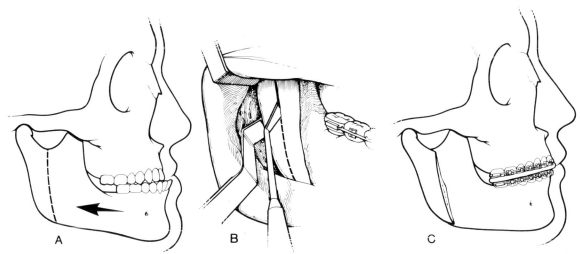

Figure 50–9. *A.* This simplified illustration demonstrates a class III malocclusion and associated mandibular prognathism. Outlined is a planned bilateral intraoral vertical ramus osteotomy (IVRO) with mandibular setback. *B.* The initial incision for the IVRO is identical to that of the bilateral sagittal split ramus osteotomy in establishing access to the ascending ramus. Reflection is carried subperiosteally over the entire lateral, posterior, and inferior borders of the ascending ramus. In addition, the entire temporal muscle is stripped from the coronoid process, and an attempt is made to remove as much of the pterygomasseteric sling as is possible from the distal segment. The bone cut is facilitated by use of a 120° beveled reciprocating saw blade. The bone cut is extended from the sigmoid notch area inferiorly to the region of the mandibular angle. *C.* After completion of the osteotomies, the position of the proximal segments is checked bilaterally. The proximal segments should rest passively lateral to the distal segment of the ascending ramus. Controversy still exists as to the mode of or need for fixation of the IVRO. In general, there appears to be a tendency for relapse into a class II open bite, in the absence of some type of fixation, as a result of the condyles healing anterior and inferior to their normal position within the glenoid fossa. Maxillomandibular fixation is applied, and all wounds are closed with absorbable gut suture.

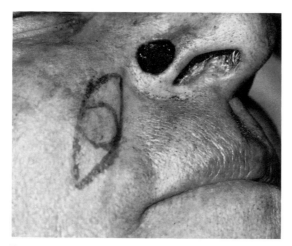

Figure 51–1. Superficial defect of the right lateral ala. Reconstruction of the defect occurs with a full-thickness skin graft from the right melolabial fold. Fusiform excision of skin is accomplished in the relaxed skin tension lines of the melolabial fold. This provides a good color match and good skin thickness.

only the skin and subcutaneous tissues, a full-thickness or split-thickness skin graft may be chosen. Uses for skin grafts in the head and neck include resurfacing of superficial skin or mucosal defects. When defects are deeper, or are composite in nature (e.g., skin and cartilage), skin grafts alone generally do not provide adequate structural support or bulk. In these instances, tissue containing more than one tissue type (composite grafts) must be transplanted for maximal form and function to be achieved.

Split-thickness skin grafts are easily vascularized and may be harvested from any body surface. The precise donor site may be determined by the amount of skin to be harvested, the color of the skin, and whether there is need for hair-bearing. Split-thickness grafts tend to heal somewhat paler in color than surrounding skin and are often not the best cosmetic choice. Survival of full-thickness skin grafts is more dependent on the relative vascularity of the donor tissue. For this reason, full-thickness grafts are usually obtained from the head and neck region. Common sites include the upper eyelid, the pre- and postauricular regions, the melolabial folds, the supraclavicular fossa, and skin from the posterior aspect of the ear lobule (Fig. 51–1).

Split-Thickness Skin Grafts

Split-thickness skin grafts (STSGs) are composed of epidermis and a portion, but not all, of the attached dermis. They may be cut at varying thicknesses, depending on the amount of underlying dermis, and are classified as thin, moderate, and thick (Fig. 51–2). Thin STSGs range from 0.008 to 0.012 inch (0.20 to 0.30 mm) thickness. In general, the thinner the STSGs, the more susceptible it is to the forces of wound contraction. Thinner grafts are also weaker and less resistant to external shearing forces and trauma. Other disadvantages of STSGs are abnormal pigmentation, increased scarring, and lack of growth of the graft.

Split-thickness skin grafts do have certain advantages, however. They are more easily vascularized and have a better overall chance

Figure 51–2. Schematic diagram of the various layers of full-thickness and split-thickness skin grafts. Split-thickness skin grafts can be subdivided into thin, medium, and thick according to the amount of dermis that is taken with the graft.

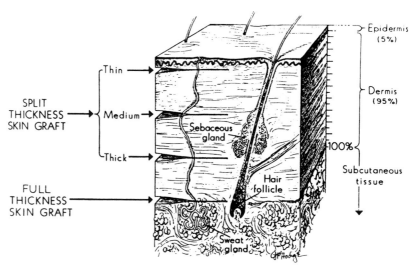

for survival. They are limited in size only by the amount of normal skin available because the donor site from STSGs heals spontaneously. Secondary epithelialization of the donor site results from the deep dermal appendages, which are left intact when STSGs are harvested. With thinner STSGs, more dermal appendages are left intact, and donor site healing occurs more rapidly. They can therefore be taken from almost any location in the body, although broad, flat surfaces are preferable. The donor area most frequently used is the anterolateral surface of the thigh because this area is easily accessible and provides a flat surface with a large surface area, and lesions in this site are usually not cosmetically disfiguring. Skin within the bikini area of the hip or the buttock may also be used.

Split-thickness skin grafts are used in head and neck reconstruction when resurfacing of large areas is required. They may be used for both skin and mucosal surfaces. STSGs provide good lining for resurfacing of cavities such as the mastoid bowl, the maxillary sinus, or the orbit after resection of large amounts of tissue. They can also be used to line the floor of the mouth or in reconstruction of the pharynx, the larynx, or the trachea (Fig. 51–3). However, when used as a resurfacing agent for these types of reconstruction, skin grafts must be supported by local tissues or flaps to prevent contraction and to provide bulk often lost with major cancer resections.

The instruments used for cutting a split-thickness skin graft are power dermatomes, drum dermatomes, and freehand knives. The most commonly used power instrument is the electric Brown dermatome. This allows relatively precise adjustment in the width and thickness of the graft to be harvested. The Davol-Simon dermatome is a rechargeable battery-operated instrument that is preset to harvest small, fixed-thickness (0.015 inch [0.38 mm]) STSGs. The prototype drum dermatome is the Padgett. This dermatome consists of a knife blade attached to a drum, to which the skin is adhered as the drum turns. Various types of freehand knives exist, including the Ferris-Smith knife, the Humby knife, or the Goulian type Weck knife.

Postoperative care of both the donor site and the recipient bed is crucial. Dressings for the donor sites include occlusive types, such as Op-Site (T.J. Smith and Nephew, Ltd, Hull, UK) and Tegaderm (3M Medical/Surgical, St. Paul, MN), and partially occlusive types, such as Xeroform and Adaptic gauze (Johnson and Johnson, New Brunswick, NJ). Occlusive dressings have the advantage of decreasing postoperative pain and crusting. These should remain in place until re-epithelialization has occurred.

Care of the recipient site is perhaps more important because it directly affects the survivability of the split graft. The graft needs to be meticulously sutured into position with maximal contact between the graft and recipient bed. The STSG should be trimmed to match the defect exactly because any skin

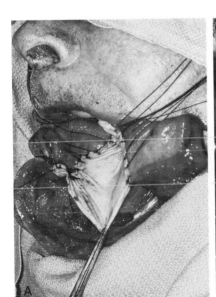
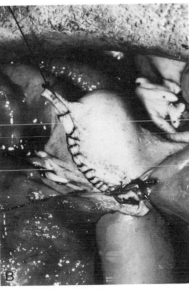

Figure 51–3. *A* and *B*. Intraoperative photographs of reconstruction of the floor of the mouth with a thick split-thickness skin graft. The skin graft is sutured into place and immobilized by use of tie-over sutures over a bolster dressing.

excess or redundancy decreases contact and prevents early graft revascularization. Interrupted sutures should be carefully placed around the periphery for attachment of the STSG to the recipient site. The graft should then be immobilized. This can be accomplished with a bolster dressing. The bolster dressing is generally composed of Xeroform gauze filled with cotton impregnated with mineral oil. The dressing is attached with interrupted tie-over silk sutures. The dressing should remain in place for 5 to 7 days, unless there is evidence of pain, odor, or discharge from the graft site. Early revascularization of the graft should occur within this period of time, and the wound should have early stability. After removal of the bolster dressing, the wound should be cleansed frequently with hydrogen peroxide to prevent crusting and scabbing. If the defect is in a location that precludes the use of a bolster dressing, interrupted basting sutures may be used toward the center of the graft in several locations to attach the graft to the recipient bed. If an accumulation of fluid occurs underneath the graft, several small incisions may be used to assist in removal of serum or blood.

Full-Thickness Skin Grafts

Full-thickness skin grafts (FTSGs) are composed of the epidermis and the entire dermis down to, but not including, the underlying subcutaneous fat. Full-thickness grafts have several advantages over split-thickness grafts when they are used for head and neck reconstruction. They are in general more cosmetically esthetic and afford a better texture and color match than do STSGs. They are relatively resistant to the forces of trauma and wound contraction and therefore less likely to cause cosmetic or functional distortion. FTSGs are also capable of growth as the individual grows. In addition, harvesting of FTSGs is technically easier and requires no special instrumentation. Last, donor site care with full-thickness grafts is minimal.

The primary disadvantage with FTSGs is that the donor site requires closure. This occurs because the donor site, devoid of dermal appendages, is incapable of spontaneous re-epithelialization. Therefore, the donor site must be designed for primary closure or must be resurfaced with a split-thickness skin graft. These procedures may limit the amount of full-thickness donor skin from a given site. Other disadvantages include its lower rate of survival in comparison with STSGs. This decreased survival rate is directly related to the thickness of the grafts. A final drawback related to FTSGs is the prolonged healing time. Although FTSGs often initially appear cosmetically unappealing, most grafts eventually heal with a good result.

Donor sites for FTSGs must be carefully chosen. As a general rule, the best full-thickness skin grafts are those most like the tissue to be replaced in color, consistency, and texture. The thinner and smaller the full-thickness graft is, the greater are the chances of survival of the graft. This makes eyelid, postauricular, and preauricular skin good choices for donor sites. Another good donor site for small grafts is skin from the posterior aspect of the ear lobule (Fig. 51–4). This skin is thin, pliable, and generally a good color match for the skin of the face. Of course, the size of the graft to be taken, and the associated donor site scar, must be considered before a donor site is chosen.

Harvesting of FTSGs is performed with a scalpel and freehand technique. An exact template of the defect is made with paper, foil, or polymeric silicone (Silastic) sheeting. The template is then placed on the donor area, and the periphery of the template is marked with a marking pen or gentian violet. Allowance of approximately 10% to 15% should be made for primary contraction of the graft after it is harvested from the donor site. The donor site incisions should then be planned so that closure will fall in the relaxed skin tension lines. The graft is then harvested by incising through the dermal layer and down to the subcutaneous fat. The graft should then be carefully defatted by use of either a scalpel or a small, sharp scissors. The FTSG should comfortably fit the defect, without bunching or tenting. Meticulous approximation of the graft to the recipient bed should then be performed. Care should be taken to evert the skin edges because postoperative contraction of skin grafts can cause unsightly depressed scars. Interrupted, nonabsorbable sutures should be used. Once again, a bolster dressing or basting sutures should be employed to immobilize the graft postoperatively.

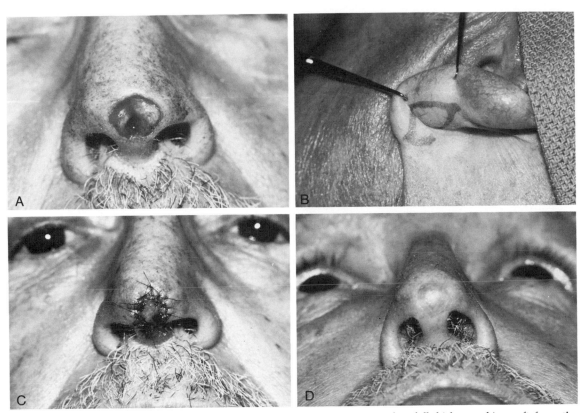

Figure 51–4. Reconstruction of a superficial defect of the tip of the nose with a full-thickness skin graft from the posterior aspect of the ear lobule. *A.* Nasal tip defect after Moh's excision of a basal cell carcinoma. *B.* Fusiform excision of a full-thickness skin graft from the posterior aspect of the ear lobule. *C.* The nasal tip 3 days after operation with suturing of the skin graft in good position. *D.* Appearance of the nasal tip 2 months after operation.

Dermis Grafts

A dermis graft is a split-thickness graft composed of dermis alone. It may be harvested with a power dermatome, a drum dermatome, or a freehand knife after elevation of the overlying epidermis. Closure of donor sites of dermis grafts occurs by mere replacement and reattachment of the overlying epidermis. A dermis graft may re-epithelialize when it is left exposed because it contains all of the epidermal appendages. Dermis grafts may also be buried under skin flaps or used as implants in subcutaneous pockets. When buried, epithelial appendages atrophy or become dormant.

Dermis grafts have been used in head and neck reconstructive surgery to provide protection over a suture line or to provide structure and bulk in the form of filler grafts. They are commonly used to protect the carotid artery from saliva exposure after extensive head and neck cancer resections. They also may be used as subcutaneous filler grafts in depressed areas in the head and neck. Uses as subcutaneous implants include lip augmentation, malar augmentation, and temporal augmentation (Fig. 51–5). They can also be trimmed into thin strips and used to fill linear depressed scars or rhytids.

Dermal-Fat Grafts and Fat Grafts

Grafts composed of fat with or without dermis have been used for both cosmetic and reconstructive purposes in the head and neck. These grafts are generally harvested from the left lower quadrant of the abdomen. Fat grafts are commonly used to obliterate the frontal sinus after surgery for traumatic or infectious disease. Dermal-fat grafts are used as subcutaneous autologous implants to restore normal facial contours. When dermal-fat is used as a filler graft, a variable amount of resorption (between 15% and 30%) may be expected to occur. Therefore, slight overcorrection of facial defects should be employed.

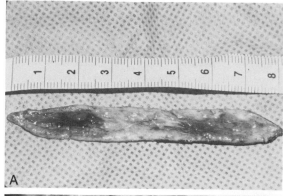

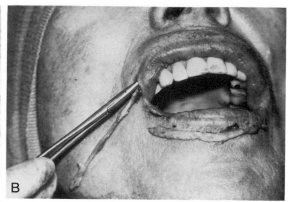

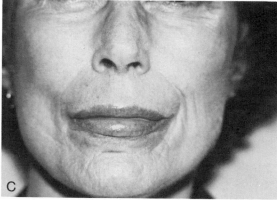

Figure 51–5. Upper and lower lip augmentation with submuscular dermal graft implantation. *A.* Dermal strip harvested from the left lower quadrant of the abdomen. *B.* Intraoperative photographs with strips of dermis graft being tunneled into proposed position for augmentation. *C.* Six-month postoperative result.

Fat grafts may be harvested from either lower abdominal quadrant through a relatively small incision. The incision is closed primarily, and a pressure dressing is applied to the donor site. Dermal-fat grafts require incisions large enough to incorporate the entire graft. The dermis must remain attached to the underlying fat because this attachment aids in revascularization and precise fixation of the graft. The epidermis should be carefully removed from the underlying dermis with a hand-held dermabrader before dissection of the graft. After the graft is removed, donor site closure is performed in layers.

Cartilage Grafts

Cartilage grafts are generally used when structural support is necessary at the defect site. They may be used as simple grafts when only structure is required, or they may be used as composite grafts, with attached skin or mucosa, when both structure and lining are necessary.

Simple cartilage grafts may be harvested from the ear or the nasal septum. The precise location, size, and shape of the graft needed determine the type of cartilage to be obtained. For instance, structural cartilage grafts to fill defects in the nasal dorsum are obtained from the cavum conchae of the ear (Fig. 51–6). Alar cartilage defects may be filled with auricular grafts from the cymba conchae. These areas are used because the curvature and texture of the grafts most closely approximate the cartilage deficiency. In addition, auricular cartilage is morphologic cartilage, which tends to reduce the chance of resorption. Nasal tip cartilage grafts are best obtained from the nasal septal cartilage because this cartilage is thicker, is stronger, and provides more structural support than does auricular cartilage (Fig. 51–7). Other uses for cartilage grafts include reconstitution of the orbital floor after fracture and as a structural batten in the lower eyelid in patients with paralytic ectropion.

Cartilage grafts may also be used in composite form when they are harvested with attached skin or mucosa. Auricular cartilage may be obtained with overlying skin on one or both sides for reconstruction of defects of the nasal tip or the alar (Fig. 51–8). In general, the larger the size of the composite graft,

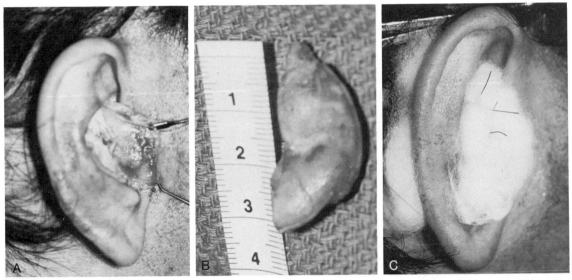

Figure 51–6. Harvesting of auricular cartilage for grafting. *A.* An anterior incision is made just anterior to the antihelical fold. *B.* A large piece of conchal cartilage after harvesting. *C.* A through-and-through bolster dressing placed with cotton or dental rolls to prevent postoperative auricular hematoma.

the less is the chance for survival of the graft. Nasal septal cartilage with overlying mucoperichondrium may also be obtained as a composite graft for use when the defect requires both lining and structural support. An example of this would be a full-thickness defect of the lower eyelid, where skin, tarsal plate, and conjunctiva are all deficient. After harvesting of auricular cartilage grafts, the donor defect is closed primarily. A pressure dressing is applied to the ear with cotton or dental rolls to prevent hematoma or seroma formation. Nasal septal donor defects are closed with through-and-through quilting su

tures when cartilage only is obtained. When composite nasal septal grafts are obtained, the donor site is allowed to heal by secondary intention.

Bone Grafts

Bone grafts have become increasingly more popular for use in head and neck reconstruction. They are usually obtained from the calvarium of the skull, the iliac crest, or the rib. Other sources such as the vomer or the anterior surface of the maxilla may also be used. Bone grafts are used in two basic ways.

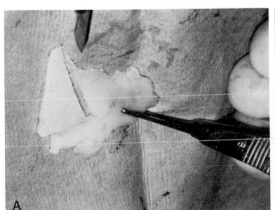
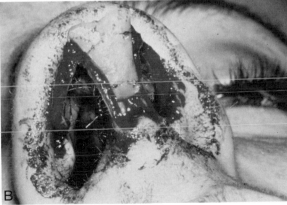

Figure 51–7. Nasal septal cartilage used for nasal tip grafting. *A.* A piece of nasal septum being carved after being harvested from the nasal septum. *B.* After sculpting, the nasal septal cartilage is sutured into position to provide structural support and definition to the nasal tip.

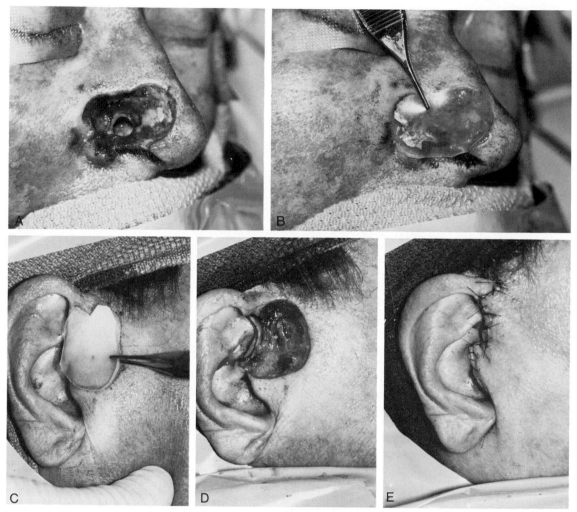

Figure 51–8. Reconstruction of a full-thickness defect of the alar rim with a composite graft from the ear. *A.* Right nasal alar defect after Mohs' excision of a sclerosing basal cell carcinoma. The lateral crus of the right lower lateral cartilage has been removed, and there is a full-thickness defect in the center of the wound. *B.* A polymeric silicone (Silastic) template of the wound is made for use as an exact outline of the defect. *C.* A template is then used to outline the size of the donor graft exactly. The donor graft will be mostly skin, but a small portion will also contain both skin and cartilage. The cartilage is taken from the root of the helix. *D.* The donor defect after removal of the graft. *E.* Closure of the donor defect after skin advancement.

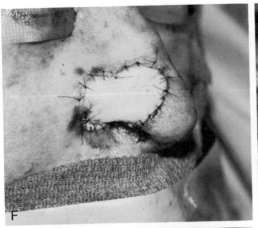

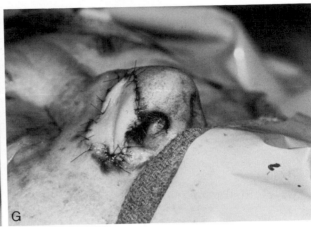

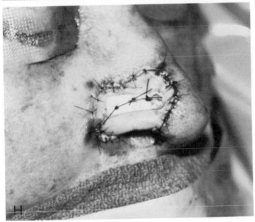

Figure 51–8 *Continued F.* Oblique view of the wound after careful suturing of the graft into position. *G.* Basal view of the immediate postoperative appearance. *H.* Placement of a fine bolster to recreate the nasal alar groove.

The first use is as a structural graft. These grafts are harvested from the rib or the skull as sheets or strips of bone (Fig. 51–9). They are used in areas such as the zygoma, the mandible, the orbit, or the dorsum of the nose as structural grafts. They are integrated into the facial skeleton and are usually fixed into position with interosseous wires or plate fixation. The second type of grafts are harvested from the medullary aspect of bone and are used as filler grafts. An example of this would be cancellous bone from the iliac crest. This bone is harvested as bone paté or bone chips and is used to fill areas such as maxillary alveolar clefts, or to fill trays in mandibular reconstruction.

LOCAL SKIN FLAPS

When a surgical defect in the head and neck cannot be closed primarily, the area may be allowed to re-epithelialize, or it may be skin grafted. In many instances, however, these reconstructive options produce suboptimal esthetic and functional results. In these cases, a local skin flap provides the best reconstructive option.

A local skin flap is a segment of skin and subcutaneous tissue that is released from its donor site and transferred to and incorporated into the recipient site. The tissue initially derives its nutrient supply through an attached neurovascular pedicle. This supply is conveyed through the base of the flap. After transfer, revascularization of the flap occurs at the recipient site. In some instances, after flap revascularization, the pedicle is transected.

Local flaps can be used to correct defects by providing resurfacing, bulk, and structural support. They may be composed of skin, subcutaneous tissue, cartilage, muscle, and bone. The facial plastic surgeon must consider the size, composition, and location of the defect before selecting a flap donor site. After selection, the flap must be accurately designed and constructed. Finally, the

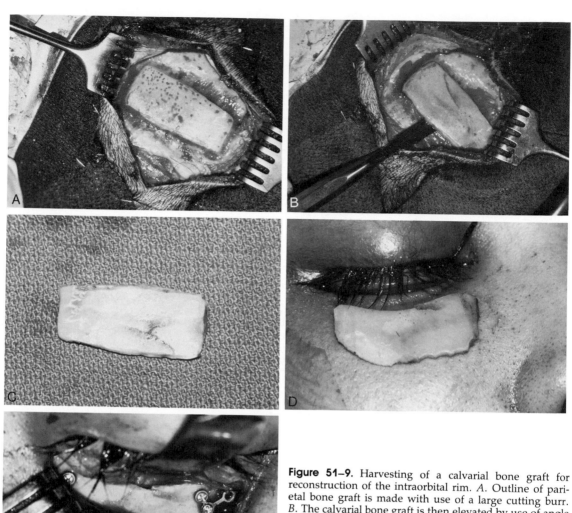

Figure 51–9. Harvesting of a calvarial bone graft for reconstruction of the intraorbital rim. *A.* Outline of parietal bone graft is made with use of a large cutting burr. *B.* The calvarial bone graft is then elevated by use of angle osteotomes and the angled Stryker saw. *C.* After harvesting, the cranial bone is ready to be sculpted and contoured for use in the infraorbital rim. *D,E.* After sculpting, the cranial bone is fixed into position with microplate fixation.

flap must be successfully transferred to the recipient defect.

Flaps may classified in a variety of ways (Table 51–1), such as by site of origin, composition, morphologic characteristics, and construction. Most commonly, however, they are categorized by their method of transfer from donor site to recipient site. When a margin of the donor site is adjacent to the recipient site, the flap is termed *local.* All other flaps are termed *regional* or *distant.* Flaps may be described as *homogeneous,* or simple, when they are derived from a single tissue type. When more than one tissue type is incorporated into the flap, it is said to be *heterogeneous,* or composite. Flaps may also be designated according to their morphologic characteristics. A *monopedicle* flap contains tissue with a single neurovascular pedicle. Tissue may also derive its blood supply from more than one pedicle, as in the *bipedicled* lower lateral cartilage flaps in the delivery approach in rhinoplasty. Flaps may also be described as *open* when the flap is maintained in its original plane or *tubed* when the edges of the flap are approximated to one another. Flaps may also be described as *primary* when the flap is designed, constructed, and trans-

TABLE 51–1. Classification of Flaps

Site of origin	Local
	Regional
	Distant
Composition	Homogeneous (simple)
	Heterogeneous (composite)
Morphology	Monopedicle/bipedicle
	Open
	Tubed
Construction	Primary
	Delayed (staged)
Transfer	Advancement
	Rotation
	Transportation
	Free

Modified from Tenta LT, Keyes GR: Biogeometry: the logic in the process of selection, siting, design, construction, and transfer of flaps. Clin Plast Surg 12:423–452, 1985.

ferred in one maneuver. When the flap is designed and incised, but not transferred, the flap is described as *delayed*. Flap transfer is then accomplished during a second stage. The delay is made to ensure adequate vascular supply to the flap when there is question of the viability of the flap during single-stage transfer.

Flaps are most commonly classified according to their method of transfer (Table 51–2). Four basic types of flap transfer exist: advancement, transposition, rotation, and free flaps. These terms describe the action imparted on the pedicle during transfer of the flap. Often, more than one action is imparted on the flap during transfer. When this occurs, the transfer is designated by the most predominating form of transfer.

Advancement Flaps

Advancement flaps impart a linear action to the pedicle (Fig. 51–10). They are often used to close rectangular defects. No secondary defect is developed when an advancement flap is used because the flap itself advances over the defect. Advancement flaps are very helpful in areas in which vertical distortion

of local anatomy would cause cosmetic or functional impairment. Examples of these areas are the forehead, the lateral lip, and the eyelid (Fig. 51–11). Maximal tension on advancement flaps in these regions occurs in a horizontal direction, parallel to the relaxed skin tension lines. This avoids vertical distortion of the eyebrow, the lip, or the eyelid margins. Movement of advancement flaps and closure of defects can be facilitated by excision of one or more Burow's triangles (Fig. 51–12). These may be created anywhere along the long side of the incision (Fig. 51–13).

Transposition Flaps

Transposition flaps are commonly used for local reconstruction in the head and neck. The action imparted on the pedicle by a transposition flap is an angular one (Fig. 51–14). The pivot point for the pedicle of the flap is at one end of the base of the flap. These flaps may occur at local or distant sites. A secondary defect is always created with a transposition flap, and this defect is usually closed primarily with local advancement flaps.

Many of the local skin flaps commonly used in the head and neck are transposition flaps (Fig. 51–15). These include rhombic flaps, Z-plasty flaps (which are two transposition flaps), the flap of Dufourmentel, midline forehead flaps, and the note flap. All of these flaps impart an angular motion to the pedicle.

The classical rhombic flap as described by Limberg (1984) consists of a rhombus with two 60° and two 120° angles. Many variations on Limberg's classical rhombic flap have been made, including the 30° transposition flap and the flap of Dufourmentel. It is important when designing these flaps to understand the areas of maximal closing tension. Maximal closing tension always occurs across the donor site in rhombic flaps or variations of these. Donor closure should therefore lie in the relaxed skin tension lines to minimize

TABLE 51–2. Characteristics of Flaps (Classified by Method of Transfer)

Type	Action on Pedicle	Secondary Defect	Site	Design
Advancement	Linear	None	Local	Quadrilateral
Transposition	Angular	Always	Local or distant	Quadrilateral
Rotation	Radial	Rarely	Local	Semicircle

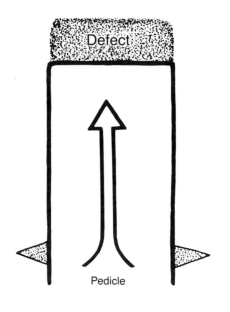

Advancement flap

Figure 51-10. Schematic diagram of an advancement flap. The action imparted on the pedicle is a linear one.

scarring. Rhombic flaps are particularly useful in the cheek, the temple, and the medial canthal regions.

Midline forehead flaps and melolabial flaps are versatile transposition flaps used in reconstruction of the nose and cheek. Melolabial flaps may be inferiorly or superiorly based and can be designed and transferred in one stage. They may also be transferred on a subcutaneous pedicle and tunneled subcutaneously to their recipient site. An island pedicled melolabial transposition flap functions well in reconstruction of the floor of the mouth (Fig. 51–16). Although the hearty midline forehead flap is also transferred in one stage, the pedicle of the flap is not transected until a second stage (10 to 14 days later), when revascularization of the flap has occurred (Fig. 51–17).

Rotation Flaps

Rotation flaps impart a radial arcing action to the pedicle (Fig. 51–18). The pivot point for the pedicle is located along the base, but not at the end of the base, as with transposition flaps. The base of the flap is adjacent to the defect. The classical textbook design for this flap is a semicircle, with the defect

being triangular. However, animal studies by Larrabee (1989, 1990) have shown little mechanical benefit in extending rotation flaps past 90°. In addition, few rotation flaps follow the classical pattern with only a rotational (radial arcing) pattern of transfer. Most rotation flaps have varying degrees of advancement and therefore depart from the classical rotation model. A secondary defect is rarely encountered when rotation flaps are used. The major tension when rotation flaps are closed is at the donor site. Again, Burow's triangles may be used anywhere along the longer side of the rotation flap to aid in closure, if necessary.

Examples of rotation-advancement flaps beneficial in head and neck reconstruction include cervicofascial rotation flaps and Mustarde rotation flaps (Fig. 51–19). These flaps are quite helpful in repairing preauricular, cheek, and lower eyelid defects (Fig. 51–20). Rotation flaps are also very helpful in scalp reconstruction. Double rotation flaps can be useful in large circular scalp defects (Fig. 51–21).

Regional Flaps

Regional direct cutaneous flaps and musculocutaneous flaps are frequently used for large defects of the head and neck. These include reconstruction after trauma, but more frequently they are used for reconstructing defects after cancer ablation. Both direct cutaneous and musculocutaneous flaps are usually transposition flaps because the action imparted to the pedicle is an angular one. The secondary defects are often large. The donor defects may be repaired by wide undermining and primary closure, or they may require resurfacing with a split-thickness skin graft. Regional flaps may be used for resurfacing both skin and mucosa. They also have the advantage of providing a large amount of bulk, which is important when the defect involves multiple tissue layers (e.g., after composite resection of the oropharynx).

Direct cutaneous regional flaps were the mainstay of head and neck reconstruction before the advent of musculocutaneous flaps. They work well in reconstruction of the oral cavity, the oropharynx, and the hypopharynx and in resurfacing the skin of the neck. Commonly used direct cutaneous flaps include forehead flaps and deltopectoral flaps. The laterally based forehead flap receives its

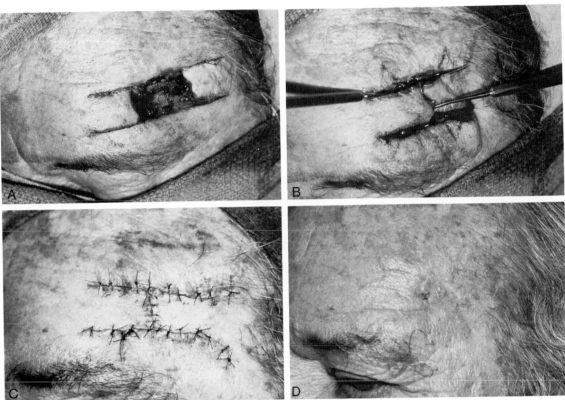

Figure 51–11. Reconstruction of a forehead defect with bilateral advancement flaps. *A.* The defect after Mohs' excision of a basal cell carcinoma. The defect has been trimmed so as to approximate a rectangular shape. *B.* Creation and elevation of bilateral advancement flaps. *C.* Closure of the defect with bilateral advancement flaps with the aid of four small Burow's triangles. *D.* Appearance of the forehead 6 months after operation.

Figure 51–12. Schematic diagram of bilateral advancement flaps depicting the location and closure of Burow's triangle.

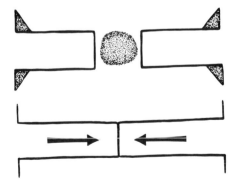

Bilateral advancement flap

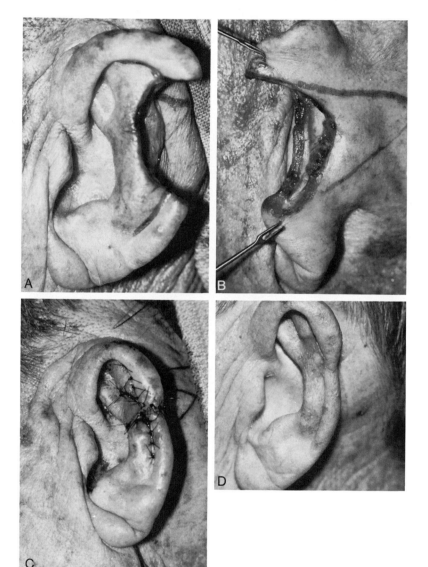

Figure 51–13. Closure of an auricular defect with bilateral chondrocutaneous advancement flaps. *A.* Left ear after Mohs' excision of a large basal cell carcinoma. *B.* Posterior view of this full-thickness defect. *C.* Closure of the defect with two advancement chondrocutaneous flaps facilitated by Burow's triangle excision. *D.* Six-month postoperative appearance.

Figure 51–14. Schematic diagram of a transposition flap. The action imparted to the pedicle is an angular or jackknife action.

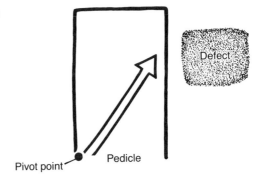

Transposition flap

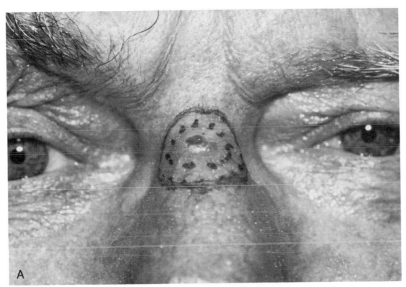

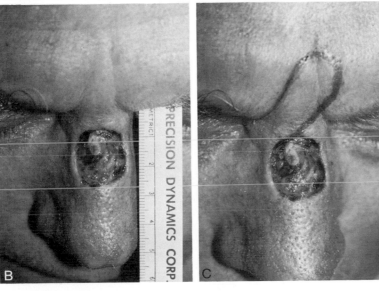

Figure 51–15. Closure of a dorsal nasal defect with a glabellar transposition flap. *A.* Outline of basal cell carcinoma with a 3-mm margin. *B.* Nasal defect after excision with clear margins. *C.* Design of glabellar transposition flap.

Illustration continued on following page

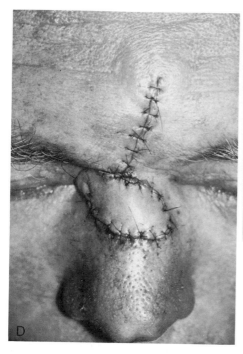

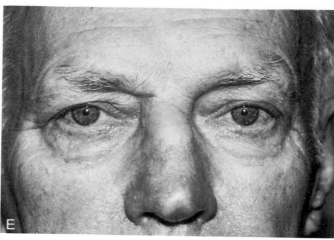

Figure 51–15 *Continued D.* Closure of defect with glabellar transposition flap. *E.* Six-month postoperative result.

blood supply from the posterior branch of the superficial temporal artery. It may be used for reconstruction within the oral cavity, by being passed over or under the zygomatic arch. The forehead donor defect is usually lined with a split-thickness skin graft. The deltopectoral flap receives its blood supply from the first four perforators of the internal mammary arteries. This flap is oriented horizontally, is based medially, and may be transposed to reconstruct defects of the oropharynx, the hypopharynx, and the skin of the neck. The edges of the flap may also be sutured together in a tubed fashion.

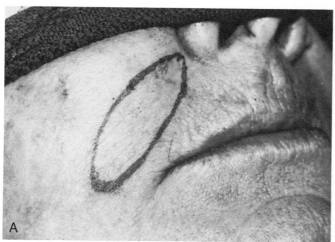

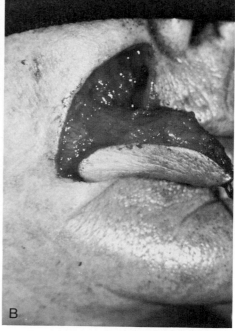

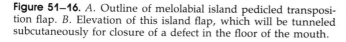

Figure 51–16. *A.* Outline of melolabial island pedicled transposition flap. *B.* Elevation of this island flap, which will be tunneled subcutaneously for closure of a defect in the floor of the mouth.

Figure 51–17. Midline forehead flap used to reconstruct a defect of the lateral aspect of the nasal ala. *A.* Appearance of the defect after Mohs' excision of a basal cell carcinoma. *B.* Silastic template of the defect.

Illustration continued on following page

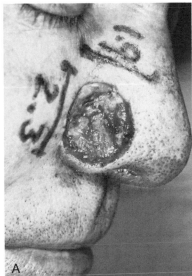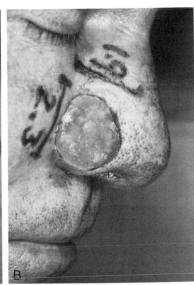

Regional musculocutaneous flaps are widely used today for major reconstruction of the head and neck. They allow single-stage reconstruction, wound control, and safety and are very reliable. They are always thicker than are direct cutaneous flaps because of the thickness of the muscle within the flap. The increased bulk of the muscle of myoepithelial flaps provides good bulk for contour defects and provides vascularized tissue for covering exposed vessels, bone grafts, or reconstruction plates. Disadvantages of musculocutaneous flaps include the increased bulk in intraoral reconstruction, large donor defects, and unwanted hair in recipient areas. In addition, these flaps are adynamic and do not function as normal mucosa does. They may therefore contribute to postoperative swallowing dysfunction. Donor sites of musculocutaneous flaps are generally closed primarily.

The pectoralis major musculocutaneous flap is the most commonly used flap in major head and neck reconstruction (Fig. 51–22). It has excellent reliability and provides a large muscle with an associated large skin paddle for reconstruction of both major skin and mucosal defects. Its primary vascular supply is the pectoral branch of the thoracoacromial artery. The flap may receive a secondary blood supply from the lateral thoracic artery. The pectoralis major flap is elevated off the chest wall and may be tunneled under the upper chest skin for oral and cervical reconstruction. A modified incision may be used to preserve the deltopectoral flap during elevation and transfer of the pectoralis major flap. The flap may also be de-epithelialized and transferred as a muscular flap only.

Trapezius musculocutaneous flaps may be based superiorly or inferiorly. The blood supply to the trapezius muscle comes from several locations, including the transverse cervical artery, the occipital artery, and the paraspinous perforating vessels superiorly. The flap may be delayed or transferred primarily. These flaps may provide tissue for intraoral or cervical reconstruction and may reach the upper aspect of the scalp. Donor closure may require a split-thickness skin graft. Other musculocutaneous flaps used include the latissimus dorsi flap (supplied by the thoracodorsal artery) and the less reliable platysma and sternocleidomastoid flaps.

Free Flaps

In some instances, the pedicle containing the neurovascular supply to the tissue in the flap is totally transected. Revascularization of the flap then occurs by microscopic anastomosis between the transected vessels of the flap pedicle and local recipient vessels. Such flaps, called free or vascularized flaps, have become a useful adjunct in head and neck reconstruction. They can be used when vascularized tissue is needed to replace large composite defects or when local small vessels are inadequate for providing sufficient revascularization of random pattern flaps. The

Text continued on page 946

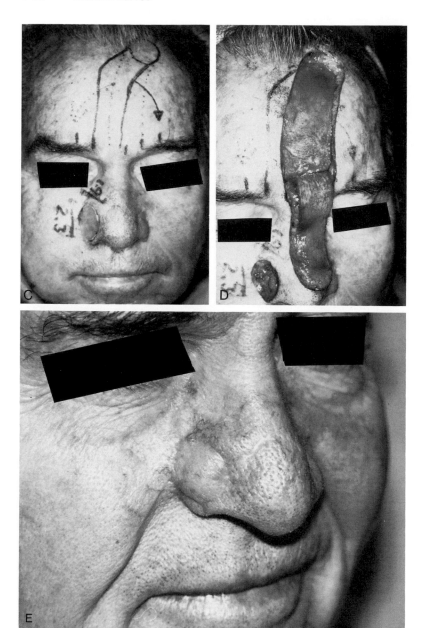

C

D

E

Figure 51–17 *Continued C.* Outline of the midline forehead flap to be used. The flap is taken to the paramedian position superiorly to avoid a hair-bearing portion of the flap. *D.* Elevation of the forehead flap in the subgaleal plane. *E.* Four-month postoperative appearance.

Figure 51–18. Schematic diagram of a rotation flap. The action imparted on the pedicle is a rotational or radial arcing action.

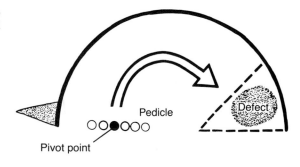

Pedicle

Defect

Pivot point

Rotation flap

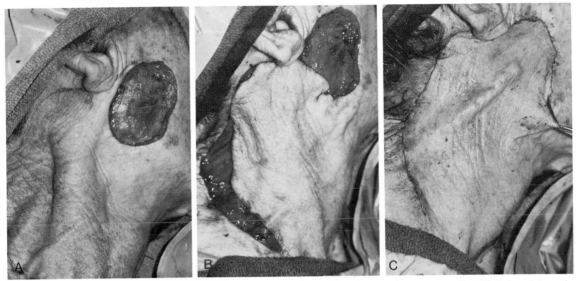

Figure 51–19. Cervical facial rotation flap for closure of a large facial defect. *A.* Appearance after Mohs' excision of a squamous cell carcinoma of the infra-auricular region. *B.* Creation and elevation of a cervical facial rotation flap. *C.* Appearance of the wound after closure of the defect and donor site with a cervical facial rotation flap.

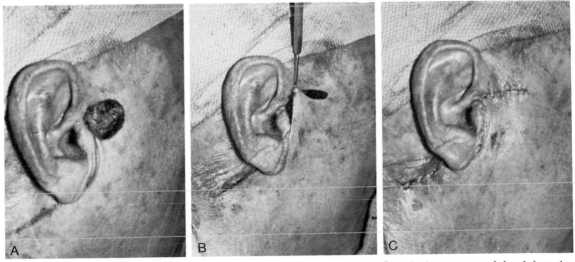

Figure 51–20. Closure of a preauricular defect with a rotation advancement flap. *A.* Appearance of the defect after Mohs' excision of a basal cell carcinoma. *B.* Elevation of a rotation advancement flap. *C.* Closure of the defect with the flap.

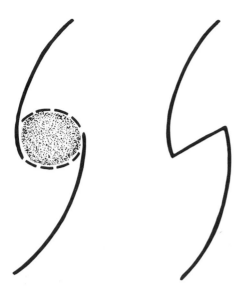

Figure 51–21. Schematic diagram of a double rotation flap often used to close defects of the scalp.

Double rotation flap

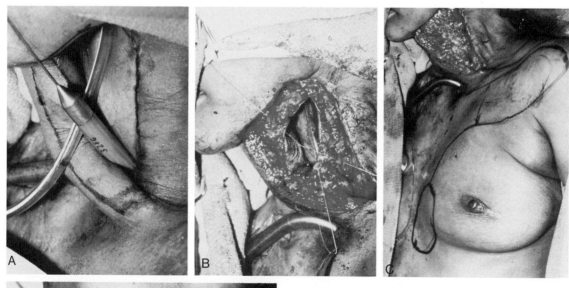

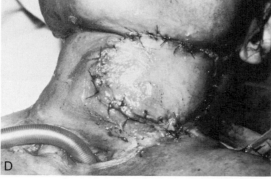

Figure 51–22. Pharyngeal reconstruction with pectoralis major musculocutaneous (PMMC) flap. *A.* Patient after total laryngopharyngectomy and total glossectomy. Nasogastric tube indicates superior aspect of pharynx, and Jackson olive-tipped dilator indicates inferior aspect. (Note: tubed flap is marked for turn-over flaps for inner lining of neopharynx.) *B.* Turn-over flaps used for inner lining of pharynx. *C.* PMMC flap marked out with sparing of deltopectoral flap. *D.* PMMC flap sutured into position.

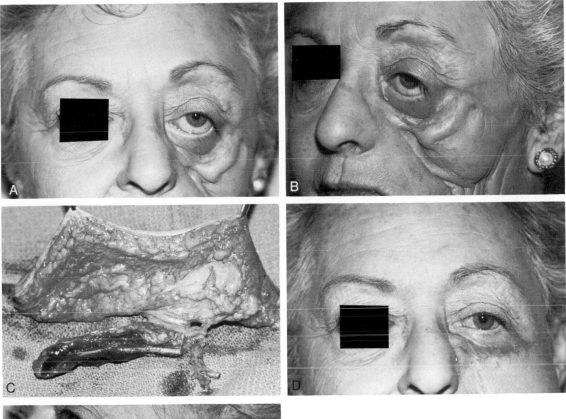

Figure 51–23. Reconstruction of a left orbital and facial defect with an osteocutaneous scapular free flap. *A.* Frontal view of the patient 5 years after maxillectomy and postoperative radiation therapy for a sarcoma of the maxilla. *B.* Oblique view of this patient. *C.* Intraoperative view of the osteocutaneous scapular free flap after transection of the scapular vessels. *D.* Six-week postoperative frontal view of the patient after reconstruction. *E.* Oblique view 6 weeks postoperatively. The patient is scheduled for debulking of the vascularized flap 3 months after the original surgery.

flaps can contain skin, subcutaneous tissues, muscle, bone, or any combination of these tissues. Adequate local recipient vessels are required within the recipient site or adjacent to the defect.

Free flaps can provide tissue to replace the skin of the scalp, the face, or the neck. They can also be used to reconstruct the oral cavity, the oropharynx, the hypopharynx, and the esophagus. In addition, composite vascularized osteocutaneous flaps can replace defects in such areas as the mandible or infraorbital rim (Fig. 51–23). The precise donor tissue to be used depends on the size and location of the defect, the need for bone within the flap, and whether the tissue needs hair-bearing potential. The length of the pedicle required is another important factor in choosing an appropriate donor site. Sources for free flaps include the radial forearm, the scapular and parascapular region, the latissimus dorsi, the lateral thigh, and the iliac crest. Donor sites from free flaps usually can be closed primarily but occasionally require skin grafting.

SUMMARY

Deformities of the head and neck may result from congenital, traumatic, or neoplastic etiologic factors. They may be associated with significant cosmetic and functional impairment. Successful reconstructive surgery for these defects should maximize function and minimize cosmetic deformity.

To determine the best reconstructive option, the facial plastic surgeon must carefully assess the deformity. The reconstructive choice should account for the size, the shape, and the location of the facial defect. Successful reconstruction is then achieved through the use of donor tissue that best approximates the facial defect.

SUGGESTED READINGS

Baker SR, Krause CJ: Pedicle flaps in reconstruction of the lip. Facial Plast Surg 1:61–68, 1983.

Banatt GE, Koopman CF Jr: Skin grafts: physiology and clinical considerations. Otolaryngol Clin North Am 17:335–351, 1984.

Becker FF: Local flaps in facial plastic surgery. J Dermatol Surg Oncol 14:635–647, 1988.

Becker FF: Local tissue flaps in reconstructive facial plastic surgery. South Med J 70:677–680, 1977.

Borges AF: Choosing the correct Limberg flap. Plast Reconstr Surg 62:542–545, 1978.

Burget GC: Aesthetic restoration of the nose. Clin Plast Surg 12:463–480, 1985.

Hirokawa RH, Stark TW, Pruet CW, Stuckey FJ Jr: Skin grafts. Otolaryngol Clin North Am 15:133–145, 1982.

Larrabee WF Jr: Immediate repair of facial defects. Dermatol Clin 7:661–676, 1989.

Larrabee WF Jr: Design of local skin flaps. Otolaryngol Clin North Am 23:899–923, 1990.

Larrabee WF Jr, Sutton D: Variation of skin stress-strain curves with undermining. Surg Forum 32:552–555, 1981.

Limberg AA: The Planning of Local Plastic Operations on the Body Surface: Theory and Practice (translated by Wolf SA). Lexington, MA: Cullamore Press, 1984.

Tardy ME Jr, Sykes J, Kron T: The precise midline forehead flap in reconstruction of the nose. Clin Plast Surg 12:481–494, 1985.

Tenta LT, Keyes GR: Biogeometry: the logic in the process of selection, siting, design, construction, and transfer of flaps. Clin Plast Surg 12:423–452, 1985.

Tromovitch TA, Stegman SJ, Glogau RG: Flaps and Grafts in Dermatologic Surgery. Chicago: Year Book Medical Publishers, 1989.

Walike JW, Larrabee WF Jr: The note flap. Arch Otolaryngol 3:430–433, 1985.

Zitelli JA: The bilobed flap for nasal reconstruction. Arch Dermatol 125:957–959, 1989.

Zitelli JA: Wound healing by secondary intention. J Am Acad Dermatol 9:407–415, 1983.

Allergy and Immunology in the Ear, Nose, and Throat

Abraham M. Majchel, MD   Robert M. Naclerio, MD

Addressing all the issues relating allergy and immunology to otolaryngology is a difficult task because immunologic mechanisms may explain a disease process or may help in its diagnosis. To approach this endeavor, an overview of immunology is given, followed by a brief review of the most frequently used immunologic diagnostic tools that can be applied in the work-up of allergy patients. Many tests have been left out, but the interested physician can find extensive information in more specialized literature. Finally, some diseases that are familiar to the otolaryngologist and have an immunologic basis are discussed. The diseases selected provide examples to illustrate a spectrum of immunologic processes and diagnostic techniques.

UNDERSTANDING THE IMMUNE SYSTEM

The immune system is a complex network of specialized cells and organs that has evolved to defend the body against attacks by foreign invaders. When it functions properly, it prevents infections by bacteria, viruses, fungi, and parasites. When it malfunctions, it can allow infections to progress or it can unleash a torrent of diseases, from allergy to arthritis to cancer to acquired immunodeficiency syndrome (AIDS).

Like humans, microbes are programmed to perpetuate themselves, and the human body provides an ideal habitat for their growth. Because the presence of these organisms is often harmful, the body's immune system attempts to bar their entry or, failing that, to seek out and destroy them.

The immune system displays several remarkable characteristics. It can distinguish between self and nonself. It is able to remember previous experiences and to react more vigorously to subsequent exposure. The immune system displays both enormous diversity and extraordinary specificity: not only is it able to recognize many millions of distinctive nonself molecules, but it also can produce molecules and cells to counteract each of them.

The success of this system in defending the body relies on an incredibly elaborate and dynamic regulatory-communications network. Millions and millions of cells, organized into sets and subsets, pass information back and forth. The result is a sensitive system of checks and balances that produces an immune response that is prompt, appropriate, effective, and self-limiting.

Mounting an Immune Response

The environment contains a large variety of infectious microbial agents that cause pathologic damage and, if allowed to multiply unchecked, may eventually kill their host. However, most infections in a normal person, because of the person's immune system, are of limited duration and leave little if any permanent damage.

The immune system has two functional divisions: the innate immune system and the adaptive immune system. Innate immunity acts as a first line of defense against infectious agents, and most potential pathogens are checked before they establish an overt infection. If these first defenses are breached, the adaptive immune system produces a specific reaction to the infectious agent and normally eradicates that agent. The adaptive immune system also remembers the infectious agent and can prevent it from causing disease later. Thus the two key features of the adaptive immune system are specificity and memory.

The innate and adaptive immune systems consist of a variety of molecules and cells distributed throughout the body. The most important cells are the leukocytes, which are divided into two broad categories: (1) phagocytes, including neutrophils, monocytes, and macrophages, which form part of the innate immune system, and (2) lymphocytes, which mediate adaptive immunity.

The Innate Immune System

The exterior of the body presents an effective barrier to most organisms; in particular, most infectious organisms cannot penetrate intact skin. Most infections enter the body through the mucosal surface of the nasopharynx, the gut, the lungs, and the genitourinary tract. A variety of physical and biochemical defenses protect these areas. For example, lysozyme, an enzyme distributed widely in different secretions, can split a bond found in the cell walls of most bacteria. Other mechanisms of innate immunity are the sebaceous gland secretions, spermine in semen, acid in the stomach, commensal organisms in the gut and vagina, and mucus and cilia covering the upper and lower airways.

If an organism penetrates an epithelial surface, it encounters phagocytic cells. These cells, although of different types, are derived from the bone marrow stem cells and function to engulf and destroy particles. For this purpose, they are strategically located to encounter such particles; for example, Kupffer's cells of the liver line the sinusoids along which blood flows. In the blood, phagocytes include neutrophils and monocytes. Both these cells can migrate from the blood vessels into the tissues in response to a suitable stimulus, but they differ in that the neutro-

phil is a short-lived cell, whereas the monocyte can develop into a tissue macrophage.

Natural killer cells recognize cell surface changes that occur on some virally infected cells and some tumor cells. They bind to these target cells and kill them. This kind of reaction, in which a lymphocyte kills a target cell, is called cytotoxicity. The cells responsible for natural killer activity are primarily large granular lymphocytes, and the target cells may be rendered more susceptible by soluble factors such as interferons.

The serum concentration of a number of proteins, referred to as acute phase proteins, increases rapidly during infection. Concentrations can increase two- to one-hundredfold and remain elevated throughout infection. One example is C-reactive protein, so called because of its ability to bind the C protein of pneumococci. C-reactive protein bound to bacteria promotes the binding of complement, which facilitates their uptake by phagocytes (opsonization).

The complement system, a group of serum proteins, functions to control inflammation. Several of the components are acute phase proteins, which increase in concentration during infection. The components interact with each other and with other elements of the innate and adaptive immune systems. For example, a number of microorganisms spontaneously activate the complement system through the so-called alternative pathway; the system can also interact with antibodies of the adaptive immune system by activation of the classical pathway. The destruction of bacterial cell walls by lysozyme facilitates an attack of the cell membrane by the complement system.

Interferons (IFNs) constitute a group of proteins that are important in defense against viral infections. One type of interferon is produced by cells that have become virally infected; another type is released by certain activated T lymphocytes. IFNs induce a state of antiviral resistance in uninfected tissue cells. They also affect the response to lymphocytes and natural killer cells. IFNs are produced very early in infection and provide the first line of resistance against many viruses.

Adaptive Immunity and Clonal Selection

The specificity of the adaptive immune system is based on the specificity of the antibodies and lymphocytes. Each lymphocyte recognizes only one particular antigen, whereas the entire immune system recognizes many thousands. The lymphocytes recognizing any particular antigen represent a very small proportion of the total. When antigen enters the body, it selects the cells with the best-fitting receptors by binding to and activating them, inducing clonal expansion. This process is called clonal selection. Because fit is a physicochemical concept, it is not surprising that sometimes two quite distinct antigens might have antigenic determinants that fit the same receptor, resulting in cross-reaction. A lymphocyte is not designed to be the cell that reacts with *Treponema pallidum*; it simply bears a receptor with a shape that fits a particular structure in that organism, and the fact that extracts of heart have a similar structure (probably a phosphate ester) is a chance cross-reaction, of which diagnostic advantage was taken many decades ago. More sinister cross-reactions can be imagined: for example, between the human heart and certain streptococci. This occurs both for the B lymphocytes, which proliferate and mature into antibody-producing cells, and for the T lymphocytes, which are involved in the recognition and destruction of virally infected cells.

The innate and adaptive immune systems do not act in isolation. Antibodies produced by lymphocytes help phagocytes recognize their targets. After clonal activation by antigen, T lymphocytes produce lymphokines, which stimulate phagocytes to destroy infectious agents more effectively. The macrophages in turn help the lymphocytes by transporting antigen from the periphery to lymph nodes and other lymphoid organs, where it is presented to lymphocytes in a recognizable form.

The clotting, fibrinolytic, complement, and kinin systems also protect the body from injury by mediating inflammation and resolving tissue damage. Complement components released from sites of inflammation act directly on the local vasculature, and fragments C3a and C5a activate mast cells to release vasoactive substances. The immune system can also interact directly with mast cells through immunoglobulin E (IgE), which binds to crystallizable fragment (Fc) receptors on the mast cell. These diverse systems interact to maintain the integrity of the vascular system and to limit the spread of tissue damage, whether it is caused by physical injury or infectious agents.

Self and Nonself

At the center of the immune system is the ability to distinguish between self and nonself. Virtually every cell carries distinctive molecules that identify it as self. The body's immune defenses do not normally attack its own tissue, and a state of self-tolerance exists.

Any substance capable of triggering an immune response is called an antigen. An antigen can be a virus, a bacterium, a fungus, a parasite, or even a portion or product of one of these organisms. Tissue or cells from another person can also act as antigens.

An antigen declares its foreignness by means of intricate and characteristic shapes called epitopes, which protrude from its surface. Most antigens, even the simplest microbes, carry several kinds of epitopes on their surface; some may carry several hundred. Some epitopes are more effective than others at stimulating an immune response.

In abnormal situations, the immune system can mistakenly identify self as nonself and attack. This results in an autoimmune disease, such as rheumatoid arthritis or systemic lupus erythematosus.

In some people, an apparently harmless substance such as ragweed pollen or cat dander can provoke the immune system to set off the inappropriate and harmful response known as allergy; in this case, the antigens are known as allergens.

Genes and the Markers of Self

Molecules that mark a cell as self are encoded by a group of genes contained in the major histocompatibility complex (MHC). The MHC was discovered in the course of tissue transplantation experiments. Because MHC genes and the molecules that they encode vary widely in structure from one person to another (a diversity known as polymorphism), transplants are likely to be rejected.

Later, it was discovered that the MHC is essential to the immune defenses. MHC markers determine which antigens a person can respond to and how strong the response is. Moreover, MHC markers allow immune cells such as B cells, T cells, and macrophages to recognize and communicate with one another.

One group of proteins encoded by the genes of the MHC (class I MHC antigens) are the markers of self that appear on almost all cells in the body. These molecules alert killer T cells to the presence of body cells that have been changed by infection with a virus or transformed by cancer.

A second group of MHC proteins, class II antigens, are found on B cells, macrophages, and other cells responsible for presenting foreign antigen to helper T cells. Class II products combine with particles of foreign antigen to display the antigen and stimulate helper T cells.

The focusing of T-cell antigen recognition through class I and class II molecules is known as MHC (or histocompatibility) restriction.

Anatomy of the Immune System

Several tissues and organs play roles in host defense and are functionally classified as the immune system. The primary lymphoid organs are the thymus and the bursa of Fabricius in birds and the thymus and the bone marrow (or fetal liver, or both) in mammals. The bone marrow is the source of pluripotent stem cells, which differentiate into lymphocyte, granulocyte, erythrocyte, and megakaryocyte populations. In mammals, the bone marrow also supports the differentiation of lymphocytes. Deficiency or dysfunction of the pluripotent stem cell or of the various cell lines developing from it can result in immune deficiencies of varying expression and severity.

The thymus, derived from the third and fourth embryonic pharyngeal pouches and located in the mediastinum, exercises control over the entire immune system. Its reticular structure permits a significant number of lymphocytes to become fully immunocompetent thymus-derived cells (T cells). However, a large number of cells die within the thymus; this mechanism is postulated to eliminate lymphocyte clones reactive against self-antigens. The thymus also regulates immune function by secretion of soluble hormones. Absence of the thymus or its abnormal development results in T-lymphocyte deficiencies (e.g., DiGeorge's syndrome).

Secondary lymphoid organs in mammals (lymph nodes, spleen, and gut-associated lymphoid tissue) are connected by blood and lymphatic vessels. Through these vessels, lymphocytes circulate and recirculate, responding to antigens and distributing their experiences with antigens to other parts of the lymphoid system.

Lymph nodes attempt to localize antigens and prevent the spread of infection. They have a framework of reticular cells and fibers that are divided into a cortex and a medulla. B cells, the precursors of plasma cells, are found in the cortex (the follicles and germinal centers) as well as in the medulla. T lymphocyte areas are primarily found in the medullary and paracortical areas of the lymph node.

The spleen, functionally and structurally divided into T-cell and B-cell areas, filters and processes antigens from the blood. Gut- and bronchial-associated lymphoid tissue (Peyer's patches of the small intestine, the appendix, and the tonsils) show a similar separation into T-cell–dependent and B-cell–dependent areas. Many lymphocytes are also seen within the lamina propria of the small intestinal villi and between the epithelial cells of the intestinal mucosal surface. Gut-associated lymphoid tissue may play a role in the differentiation of stem cells into B lymphocytes.

Components of the Immune System

Lymphocytes

Lymphocytes initially recognize specific antigens. They are principally divided into B lymphocytes and T lymphocytes on the basis of surface markers and functional tests. The most obvious difference between them is the production of antibody by B cells and cell-mediated cytotoxicity for T lymphocytes. B cells are coated with receptors for complement and the Fc portion of immunoglobulins. Structurally, T and B cells cannot be distinguished from each other under the light microscope. About 80% of circulating blood lymphocytes are T cells, and 10% to 15% are B cells; the remainder are called null cells.

Further separation of T-lymphocyte subpopulations is accomplished by immunofluorescence with monoclonal antibodies that are reactive with individual cell surface antigens. With the use of T cells as antigens, a variety of monoclonal antibodies have been created, enabling identification of T-cell subsets such as helper (CD4), suppressor (CD8), and cytotoxic cells. T4 cells predominate over T8 cells in the circulating blood by a ratio of 2:1. T4 cells provide helper signals for B lymphocytes, T lymphocytes, T8 cell-mediated cytotoxicity, and macrophages. T8 cells, when influenced by T4 cells, suppress B-lymphocyte immunoglobulin production and T-lymphocyte response to major histocompatibility antigens and enhance cytotoxicity and natural killing.

T cells mediate cell-mediated immune responses, such as delayed (tuberculin type) hypersensitivity, graft rejection, and immune surveillance of neoplastic cells.

T cells work primarily by secreting substances known as lymphokines. Lymphokines and monokines, both produced by monocytes and macrophages, are diverse and potent chemical messengers that encourage cell growth, promote cell activation, direct cellular traffic, destroy target cells, and incite macrophages (Table 52A–1).

Null cells probably include a number of different cell types, including natural killer cells. Killer cells are slightly larger, with a kidney-shaped nucleolus, than the typical lymphocyte. Natural killer cells bind IgG through an Fc receptor. When a cell coated with an antibody is destroyed by a natural killer cell, this phenomenon is called antibody-dependent cell-mediated cytotoxicity. Alternatively, natural killer cells can destroy cells without involvement of antibody (e.g., virally infected cells or tumor cells). Other characteristics of these cells include recognition of antigens without major histocompatibility restrictions, lack of immunologic memory, and regulation of activity by interferons and prostaglandins of the E series.

B cells are the direct precursors of mature antibody-secreting cells (plasma cells). Although ongoing investigations indicate an array of complex interactions between B and T cells and tend to obscure distinctions between these two systems, the division into B and T cells with different developmental and functional characteristics allows for an operational understanding of the immune system.

Immunoglobulin Structure. All immunoglobulin molecules share a certain structural similarity: four polypeptide chains divided into two light and two heavy chains linked by disulfide bonds. Disulfide linkages are

TABLE 52A–1. The Major Cytokines

Cytokine	Immune System Source	Other Cells	Principal Targets	Principal Effects
IL-1 alfa IL-1 beta	Macrophages LGLs, B cells	Endothelium, fibroblasts, astrocytes, etc.	T cells, B cells, macrophages, endothelium, tissue cells	Lymphocyte activation, macrophage stimulation, ↑ leukocyte/endothelial adhesion, pyrexia, acute phase proteins
IL-2	T cells	—	T cells	T cell growth factor
IL-3	T cells	—	Stem cells	Multilineage colony stimulating factor
IL-4	T cells	—	B cells, T cells	B cell growth factor
IL-5	T cells	—	B cells	B cell growth differentiation
IL-6	T cells, B cells macrophages	Fibroblasts	B cells, hepatocytes	B cell growth/differentiation "acute phase" response
TNF-α	Macrophages, lymphocytes	Epithelium, fibroblasts	Tissue cells	Activation of macrophages, granulocytes and cytotoxic cells, ↑ leukocyte/endothelial cell adhesion, cachexia, etc.
TNF-β (LT)	T cells	Epithelium, fibroblasts	Tissue cells	Activation of macrophages, granulocytes and cytotoxic cells, ↑ leukocyte/endothelial cell adhesion, cachexia, etc.
IFN-α	Leucocytes	—	Macrophages, granulocytes, tissue cells	MHC class I induction, antiviral effect
IFN-β	—	—	Macrophages, granulocytes, tissue cells	MHC class I induction, antiviral effect
IFN-γ	T cells, NK cells	Epithelium, fibroblasts	Leucocytes and tissue cells	MHC induction, macrophage activation, ↑ endothelial/lymphocyte adhesion
M-CSF	Monocytes	Endothelium, fibroblasts	Stem cells	Stimulate division and differentiation
G-CSF	Macrophages	Fibroblasts	Stem cells	Stimulate division and differentiation
GM-CSF	T cells, macrophages	Endothelium, fibroblasts	Stem cells	Stimulate division and differentiation
MIF	T cells	—	Macrophages	Migration inhibition

tent of recurrence, patients may escape without clinical residual or with a mild nodularity. In pronounced cases, there is a diffuse softening and collapse of the cartilage framework of the ears, including the external auditory canal. Involvement of the nasal cartilages is also clinically sudden and painful but less likely to be recurrent. The only significant cosmetic deformity is a saddle nose. Of a more serious nature is the involvement of the airway. Early signs and symptoms result from a composite of chondritis and edema with inflammation of adjacent soft tissues. Compromise of the airway follows, with stenosis and obstruction at the glottic and subglottic levels. End-stage disease entails dissolution of any or all of the tracheal and bronchial cartilages, obstructive pulmonary disease, and infection.

The clinical course is quite variable. The disease may be relatively indolent, may be rapidly fatal, or may evolve into a chronic, progressive disorder. About half of the deaths are related to the disease process, treatment of the disease, or to an underlying and related connective tissue disorder. Infection is the most common cause of death, and the infection is related statistically to both involvement of the airway and corticosteroid medications. Death from cardiovascular disease, particularly systemic vasculitis, follows infection-related mortality in incidence.

The pathogenesis of the disease remains speculative, although the primary abnormality appears to be the dissolution of the mucopolysaccharide component of the ground substance. Microscopic findings of involved cartilage are a loss of the usual metachromasia, necrosis, calcification, and acute and chronic inflammatory reactions. The destruction of the cartilage may be related to proteases released from leukocytes or perichondral fibroblasts. A possible role of immune complexes is suggested by the immunofluorescent findings of granular deposits of IgG, IgA, IgM, and C3 at fibrochondral junctions. In the occasional case in which the temporal bones have been studied, the findings are similar to those observed in viral endolabyrinthitis, with a preferential degeneration of sensory epithelium, primarily of the cochlea.

Steroids, dapsone, and immunosuppressants constitute the medical treatment of relapsing polychondritis.

Cancer

The most extensive interactions between the disciplines of otolaryngology and immunology are in the area of head and neck cancer. Examples of these interactions are cloning, the use of monoclonal antibodies, the identification of subpopulation of receptors on cancer cells, and the study of immunoregulation, lymphokines, soluble tumor factors, immunodeficiencies, gene abnormalities, and the secretory immune response.

In discussions about patients with cancer, unusual case presentations of malignancies (laryngeal carcinoma in childhood, plasmacytoma of the larynx, primary squamous cell carcinoma of the middle ear invading the cochlea) and infections (*Candida epiglottitis*, parotitis with *Eikenella corrodens*, and *Pseudomonas*-caused rhinosinusitis) lead the authors to think that there is an underlying immunodeficiency. However, AIDS is the only specific example of an immune defect that leads to cancer.

Androgen and progesterone receptors have been identified in head and neck malignancies. The numbers found were small, the responses to antiandrogen therapy were limited, and the response did not correlate with receptor numbers. Although the usefulness of hormonal receptors at present is limited, the advantages of identifying a unique receptor in cancer and other disease processes has obvious diagnostic, therapeutic, and prognostic potential.

Monoclonal antibodies, antibodies produced by single cell hybridoma clones, can be raised against unique, antigenic sites on cancer cells. Monoclonal antibodies coupled with radioactive isotopes or chemotherapeutic agents have been injected into patients with cancer to deliver standard treatment modalities in a more effective manner.

Cloning, the raising of colonies of cells from a single progenitor, has been attempted with head and neck malignancies. Soft agar techniques have been used to grow salivary gland and squamous cell tumors. Squamous cell cancer lines have been established, and tumors have been propagated by injections of cell suspensions into animals. The advantages of this research include in vitro selection of effective chemotherapeutic agents. The studies so far have been limited because of the poor efficiency of growing tumor cells and the lack of ability of the present techniques to predict clinical utility. If the difficulties can be circumvented, a major advance in the treatment of head and neck cancer may occur.

Tumors and their local environments interact in many ways. For example, prostaglandins have been shown to be produced by tumors, and these potent mediators could adversely affect the host's response. This idea led some investigators to study the question of whether lowering prostaglandin production might alter tumor growth. Indomethacin, a prostaglandin synthetase inhibitor, inhibited the growth of epidermoid carcinoma in some rats. In humans, indomethacin induced a reduction in tumor size in a few patients with squamous cell carcinoma. Caution must be used in interpreting these results. Prostaglandins are synthesized by almost every cell in the human body. An inhibitor would affect the production of prostaglandin not just by the tumor but also by other cells, such as macrophages and monocytes. These studies are reminiscent of the early enthusiasm for the use of immunotherapy for cancer. The concept may be correct, but the complexity of the situation has not been fully appreciated at the basic science level. The concept of altering production of tumor factors that adversely affect the host is excellent and should be pursued.

In patients with head and neck cancers, other tumor-host interactions are beginning to be studied. They include immunoregulatory activity in regional lymph nodes, abnormalities in T helper:suppressor cell ratio, natural killer–mediated cytotoxicity in patients with laryngeal carcinoma, suppressor cell activity in patients with laryngeal carcinoma, the level of secretory IgA in secretions of patients with oropharyngeal cancers, and identification of oncogenes, which are genetic segments capable of transforming normal cells into malignant ones.

The ability to detect antibodies in the serum of some patients with nasopharyngeal carcinoma is becoming a useful clinical tool. Antibodies to certain Epstein-Barr virus–associated antigens, IgA antibodies to the viral capsid antigen, and antibodies to early antigen are increased in patients with type II and type III nasopharyngeal carcinoma. Although these increases also occur both in the normal healthy population and in some patients with other head and neck disorders, 85% of patients with type II and type III nasopharyngeal carcinoma have an increased level of these specific antibodies. The measurement of these antibody titers may improve the follow-up condition of patients with nasopharyngeal carcinoma and the identification of nasopharyngeal tumors in patients with unknown primary tumors. The use of the test for antibody-dependent cellular cytotoxicity (ADCC) suggests that a high ADCC titer implies a good prognosis, whereas a low ADCC titer implies poor prognosis. It is hoped that other serum antibodies that are specific markers for other malignancies will be discovered.

Sarcoidosis

Sarcoidosis is a multisystem granulomatous disorder of unknown cause that most commonly affects young adults and manifests most frequently with bilateral hilar lymphadenopathy, pulmonary infiltration, and skin or eye lesions. The diagnosis is established most securely when clinicoradiographic findings are supported by histologic evidence of widespread, noncaseating epithelioid cell granulomaı in more than one organ. Immunologic features include depression of delayed type hypersensitivity and raised or abnormal amounts of immunoglobulins. There may be hypercalciuria with or without hypercalcemia. The course and the prognosis correlate with the mode of onset. An acute onset with erythema nodosum heralds a self-limiting course with spontaneous resolution, whereas an insidious onset may be followed by relentless, progressive fibrosis. Corticosteroids relieve symptoms and suppress inflammation and granuloma formation.

The granuloma of sarcoidosis is the end result of the complex interaction between activated lymphocytic and monocytic cells at the inflammatory site. The circulating blood monocyte leaves the general circulation under the direction of local chemotactic factor, presumably related to unknown triggers of this disease. Once these macrophages appear in the lung or the nasal mucosa, they aggregate into epithelioid cell granulomas. Multinucleated giant cells appear within the tissues. These granulomas are surrounded by a network of lymphatic channels, capillaries, collagen, lymphocytes, fibroblasts, and reticulin. This granulomatous phase may regress, either as part of the natural history of the disease or with therapy, but may also progress to fibrosis.

The initial trigger mechanisms for sarcoidosis (whether immunologic, genetic, infectious, or toxic) stimulate the macrophages to secrete interleukin-1. Interleukin-1 is a potent lymphokine responsible for the migration of T lymphocytes to the site of the disease activity and also activates T cells, increases the interleukin-2 receptors on the T cells, and stimulates T cell release of interleukin-2. The long-recognized peripheral lymphopenia associated with sarcoidosis is caused by the transmigration of T cells from the circulation to the local sites of activity. The local T4:T8 ratio is increased, which is indicative of local enhanced inflammatory activity. The reverse is seen in the peripheral circulation.

The interleukin-2 released by activated T helper cells at the local sites of activity is a T cell growth factor and further amplifies the local inflammatory component of the disease. Similarly, these activated T helper cells secrete chemotactic factors and migration inhibitory factors for monocytes. Alveolar macrophages also spontaneously secrete fibronectin, which enhances fibroblast replication and chemotaxis. Alveolar macrophage–derived growth factor stimulates fibroblasts. Interleukin-1 increases fibroblast replication in response to fibronectin and alveolar macrophage–derived growth factor. Coexisting with these enhancers of fibrosis and inflammation is an opposing system of inhibitors of fibroblast replication, including INF-γ and prostaglandin E_2.

It has long been noted that there is a nonspecific increase of immunoglobulins in sarcoidosis. Activated T4 lymphocytes release B cell growth factor and a B cell differentiation factor, which together increase the production of immunoglobulins at the sites of disease. Thus although the specific etiologic process or immunogenetic trigger of sarcoidosis remains unknown, the cellular and mediator interactions are becoming more fully understood. The clinical importance of such knowledge lies in the identification of sites to modulate the immune and inflammatory amplification cascade in order to control the disease.

The clinical manifestation of sarcoidosis falls into one of three categories: (1) chest x-ray or other laboratory abnormalities in an asymptomatic patient, (2) pulmonary symptoms, and (3) extrathoracic or systemic manifestations. Asymptomatic patients with chest x-ray findings generally belong to the category of stage I disease; bilateral hilar adenopathy is their only manifestation. Patients with radiographic evidence of parenchymal disease are more likely to be symptomatic. The lungs are involved in more than 90% of patients with sarcoidosis, though respiratory symptoms occur in only 40% to 60%. Patients with pulmonary manifestations present with dry cough, chest pain, shortness of breath, hemoptysis, pneumothorax, or a combination of these symptoms.

Approximately 20% of patients present with systemic symptoms such as fever, malaise, or weight loss. Peripheral lymph nodes are affected in 50% to 75% of patients, although less than 5% of these patients are aware of bulky adenopathy. An enlarged peripheral node in a patient with suspected sarcoid provides a low morbidity biopsy site to confirm the diagnosis. Cervical, axillary, epitrochlear, and inguinal are the most frequently involved nodal areas.

Nasal and upper respiratory tract involvement may also be a marker of chronic persistent sarcoidosis (Tables 52A–6, 52A–7). Granulomas may be found anywhere in the upper airway from the nose to the larynx. Symptoms of mucosal involvement, such as nasal stuffiness, occur in 5% of sarcoid patients. Nasal septal perforation occasionally occurs, as does granulomatous invasion through the ethmoid bone into the intracranial cavity. Supraglottic laryngeal involvement can cause hoarseness and upper airway obstruction, even though the true vocal cords are generally spared.

Neural involvement occurs in 5% of people with sarcoidosis. Cranial nerve involvement, particularly the facial nerve, is the most common manifestation, occurring in approximately 50% of neurosarcoid patients. The peripheral nerves are affected, usually

TABLE 52A–6. Involvement of the Head and Neck by Sarcoidosis in 220 Cases

Site	Percentage
Eye and lacrimal gland	40
Skin	26
Nose	13
Peripheral nervous system	6
Larynx	6
Salivary glands	4
Cervical lymph nodes	4
Middle ear	1

From Scully RE (ed): Case records of the Massachusetts General Hospital. N Engl J Med 322:116–123, 1990.

TABLE 52A–7. Manifestations in 17 Patients With Nasal Sarcoidosis

Symptom	No. of Patients	Percentage
Nasal obstruction	14	82
Epistaxis	4	23
Dyspnea	3	18
Cervical mass	2	12
Nasal pain	1	6
Epiphora	1	6
Anosmia	1	6

From Scully RE (ed): Case records of the Massachusetts General Hospital. N Engl J Med 322:116–123, 1990.

in the form of peripheral neuropathy or mononeuritis multiplex. Granulomatous accumulations in the central nervous system may cause masslike lesions, aseptic meningitis, seizures, obstructive hydrocephalus, confusion, and hemiparesis. Psychiatric derangement may occur.

Granulomatous infiltration of the salivary glands causes enlargement, pain, or dry mouth in approximately 5% of patients with sarcoidosis. Involvement is asymptomatic in 30% to 50% of patients with active disease. Biopsy of a minor salivary gland is highly diagnostic regardless of whether there are salivary symptoms. Parotid involvement is frequently accompanied by lacrimal infiltration and keratoconjunctivitis.

The search continues for biochemical markers of sarcoidosis activity. Described markers may correlate with different measures of activity and frequently do not correlate with each other. Levels of serum angiotensin-converting enzyme are elevated in 60% of people with sarcoid granulomas, but this is of low specificity and not predictive of the future course. It tends to correlate with the extent and activity of granulomas in the body. Angiotensin-converting enzyme levels have also been measured in bronchoalveolar lavage fluid, tears, and cerebrospinal fluid. It appears to be secreted from epithelial cells and from sarcoid granulomas. Angiotensin-converting enzyme and other markers, such as lysozyme and beta$_2$-microglobulin, do not yet have a defined role in diagnosis or management of sarcoidosis.

The diagnosis of sarcoidosis depends on a compatible clinical picture, histologic findings, and exclusion of other granulomatous disorders. For the more common clinical presentations, such as bilateral hilar and right paratracheal adenopathy with pulmonary parenchymal infiltrates, these criteria are easy to meet. Because sarcoidosis is defined as a multisystem disease, clinical involvement of more than one system is necessary to support the diagnosis. It is not necessary to have biopsy support from two systems. Local granulomatous tissue reactions to foreign bodies or in nodes draining a tumor must not be misdiagnosed as sarcoidosis. Superficial abnormalities of palpable lymph nodes, skin, or nasal or conjunctival mucosal lesions should always be sought as a source of histologic support. Occasionally a biopsy of buccal, submucosal minor salivary glands may be productive. Other methods used in the diagnosis of sarcoidosis are the Kveim-Stiltzbach reaction, fiberoptic bronchoscopy, bronchoalveolar lavage, computed tomography, and mediastinoscopy.

The management of this disease is beyond the scope of this review. The serial assessments of symptoms, the clinical findings, and the degree of incapacity are the keys to the decision about the need for treatment. The frequency of spontaneous remissions is favorable for a conservative approach to the institution of therapy. When a need for treatment is identified, histologic support is highly desirable. Corticosteroids are the most frequently used treatment and are usually the most effective, except in cases with irreversible scarring. Topical steroids may be helpful in localized nasal disease. Chloroquine and hydroxychloroquine are particularly useful in treating skin and mucosal disease. Immunosuppressive drugs such as cyclosporine and methotrexate have been used, especially because it has been suggested that they have a steroid-sparing effect.

Primary Immunodeficiency Syndromes

Four major immune systems assist humans in the defense against a constant assault by viral, bacterial, fungal, protozoal and nonreplicating agents that have the potential of producing infection and disease. These systems consist of antibody-mediated (B cell) immunity, cell-mediated (T cell) immunity, phagocytosis, and complement. Each system may act independently or in conjunction with one or more of the others.

Deficiency of one or more of these systems may be congenital (e.g., X-linked infantile hypogammaglobulinemia) or acquired (e.g., acquired hypogammaglobulinemia). Deficiencies of the immune system may be secondary to an embryologic abnormality (e.g., the DiGeorge syndrome), may be caused by an enzymatic defect (e.g., chronic granulomatous disease), or may be of unknown cause (e.g., Wiskott-Aldrich syndrome).

In general, the symptoms of immunodeficiency are related to the degree of deficiency and the particular system that is deficient in function. The types of infections that occur can provide an important clue to the type of immunodeficiency disease present. Recurrent bacterial otitis media and pneumonia are common in patients with hypogammaglobulinemia. Patients with defective cell-mediated immunity are susceptible to infection with fungal, protozoal, and viral organisms that may manifest as pneumonia or chronic infections of the skin and the mucous membranes or other organs. Systemic infection with uncommon bacterial organisms, normally of low virulence, is characteristic of chronic granulomatous disease. Other phagocytic disorders are associated with superficial skin infections or systemic infections with pyogenic organisms. Complement deficiencies are associated with recurrent infections with pyogenic organisms.

Numerous advances have been made in the diagnosis of specific immunodeficiency disorders. Screening tests are available for each component of the immune system. These tests enable the physician to diagnose more than 75% of immunodeficiency disorders. The remainder can be diagnosed by means of more complicated studies that may not be available in all hospital laboratories.

In addition to antimicrobial agents for treatment of specific infections, new forms of immunotherapy are available to assist in the control of immunodeficiency or perhaps even to cure the underlying disease. The usefulness of some of these treatment methods, such as bone marrow transplantation, may be limited by the availability of suitable donors. The discovery of enzyme deficiencies (e.g., adenosine deaminase) in association with immunodeficiency offers a potential new avenue of therapy.

X-Linked Infantile Hypogammaglobulinemia

This disease affects male children, who become symptomatic after the natural decay of transplacentally acquired maternal immunoglobulin at about 5 to 6 months of age. They suffer from severe chronic bacterial infections that can be controlled readily with gamma-globulin and antibiotic treatment. Initial symptoms consist of recurrent bacterial otitis media, bronchitis, pneumonia, meningitis, dermatitis, and, occasionally, arthritis or malabsorption. The most common organisms responsible for infections are *Streptococcus pneumoniae* and *Haemophilus infuenzae*; other organisms, such as gram-negative bacteria, are occasionally detected. Although patients normally have intact cell-mediated immunity and respond normally to viral infections such as varicella and measles, there have been reports of paralytic poliomyelitis and progressive encephalitis after immunization with live virus vaccines or exposure to wild virus. An important clue to the diagnosis of hypogammaglobulinemia is the failure of infections to respond completely or promptly to appropriate antibiotic therapy. In addition, many patients with hypogammaglobulinemia have a history of continuous illness. The diagnosis of infantile X-linked hypogammaglobulinemia is based on the demonstration of absence or marked deficiency of all five immunoglobulin classes. Treatment schedules have varied. Commercial gammaglobulin is the mainstay of therapy and is usually given in intravenous starting doses of 100 to 400 mg/kg/month. The final amount given and the frequency of injections should be regulated by the control of symptoms rather than based on a calculated amount or a particular serum level, because metabolism of IgG varies in different individuals.

Common Variable Immunodeficiency (Acquired Hypogammaglobulinemia)

Patients with common variable immunodeficiency present clinically like patients with X-linked hypogammaglobulinemia except that they usually do not become symptomatic until 15 to 35 years of age. In addition to increased susceptibility to pyogenic infections, they have a high incidence of autoimmune disease. These patients also differ from patients with congenital hypogammaglobulinemia in that they have a higher than normal incidence of abnormalities in T cell immunity, which in most instances shows progressive deterioration with time. Acquired hypogammaglobulinemia affects both males and females and may occur at any age. In most instances, the initial presentation of common variable immunodeficiency consists of recurrent sinopulmonary infections. These may be chronic rather than acute and overwhelming, as in X-linked hypogammaglobulinemia. Infections may be caused by streptococci, *H. influenzae*, and other pyogenic organisms. Autoimmune disease has been a presenting complaint in some patients with acquired hypogammaglobulinemia. Immunoglobulin measurements may show slightly higher IgG values than are reported in infantile X-linked hypogammaglobulinemia. Total immunoglobulin levels are usually less than 300 mg/dL, and the IgG level is usually less than 250 mg/dL. IgM and IgA may be absent or may be present in significant amounts. Cell-mediated immunity may be intact or may be depressed, with negative results of delayed hypersensitivity skin tests, depressed responses of peripheral blood lymphocytes to phytohemagglutinin and allogeneic cells and decreased numbers of circulating peripheral blood T cells. B cells may be normal or diminished in number in the peripheral blood. There is occasionally an increased number of null cells—that is, lymphocytes that lack surface markers for either T or B cells. Treatment is identical to that of infantile X-linked hypogammaglobulinemia. Because of the large amounts of gammaglobulin required, intramuscular injections may produce considerable discomfort. Intravenous gammaglobulin is therefore quickly replacing intramuscular preparations. Caution should be exercised in the treatment of associated autoimmune disorders. The use of corticosteroids and immunosuppressive agents in a patient with immunodeficiency may result in markedly increased susceptibility to infections.

Selective IgA Deficiency

This is the most common immunodeficiency. The incidence in the normal population has been estimated to vary between 1:800 and 1:600, whereas among atopic patients, the incidence is 1:400 to 1:200. There is considerable debate about whether people with selective IgA deficiency are "normal" or have significant associated diseases. Results of studies of individual patients and extensive studies of large numbers of patients suggest that the absence of IgA predisposes a person to a variety of diseases. The diagnosis of selective IgA deficiency is established by the finding of an IgA level in serum of less than 5 mg/dL. The most frequent presenting symptoms are recurrent sinopulmonary infections. The absence of serum IgA may result in a significant reduction in the amount of antibody competing for antigens that are capable of combining with IgE. It is also possible that patients who lack IgA in their secretions may absorb intact proteins with an enhanced susceptibility to the formation of allergic responses. Other clinical manifestations of selective IgA deficiency are a high incidence of celiac disease, ulcerative colitis, regional enteritis, pernicious anemia, systemic lupus erythematosus, rheumatoid arthritis, dermatomyositis, thyroiditis, a positive result of Coombs's test for hemolytic anemia, Sjögren's syndrome, and chronic active hepatitis. Patients with selective IgA deficiency should not be treated with gammaglobulin therapy because they are capable of forming normal amounts of antibody of other immunoglobulin classes and may recognize injected IgA as foreign. Patients with recurrent sinopulmonary infections should be treated aggressively with broad-spectrum antibiotics to avoid permanent pulmonary complications.

Acquired Immunodeficiency Syndrome

The human immunodeficiency virus (HIV) causes the clinical manifestations of AIDS. Seroepidemiologic evidence, as well as clinical evidence, suggests that this virus arose as an alteration or mutation in a virus that had been present for a long time in central Africa. The best evidence suggests that this disease began on the west side of Lake Victoria and has since been spreading out in a generally concentric pattern from Africa. However, because of the present mobility of humans, this virus and the diseases that it causes have now essentially been distributed worldwide, although the frequency in countries differs depending on the time of introduction and the prevalence of high-risk practices.

HIV causes disease by two mechanisms. The first is direct viral infection of cells; thus acute viral infection (which is observed in only a small number of HIV-infected persons) similar to that of any acute viremia can occur. The presence of HIV in the central nervous system can result in neurologic illness that is generally manifested as a gradual dementia, although a wide range of neurologic/psychiatric symptoms may ensue. In the central nervous system, the HIV virus appears to infect nonneuronal cells that are CD4 positive. The presence of virally infected cells alters brain function, which leads to the characteristic picture of AIDS encephalopathy and dementia.

The other and more common mechanism by which HIV causes disease is by inducing a profound state of immunosuppression, which results in opportunistic infections or tumors that are then responsible for the fatal outcome of the most advanced stages of HIV infection. This immunodeficiency occurs as a result of the human immunodeficiency virus's infecting cells bearing the CD4 surface molecule, a molecule that is characteristically found on T helper and inducer cells. However, it is now known that this molecule is also found on cells in the monocyte and the macrophage lineage, and such cells may represent a reservoir of viral infection. Exactly how HIV depletes CD4 cells and causes the resulting acquired immunodeficiency disorder is not absolutely clear. One hypothesis is that there is a cytolytic infection of cells. Another hypothesis is that HIV-infected cells bind noninfected cells through the interaction of the viral envelope glycoprotein on the infected cells and the CD4 molecules on uninfected cells to form cell syncytia. In either event, the loss of the infected CD4 T cells and monocytes or macrophages leads to loss of their function with profound depression of responses to cell-mediated immunity.

Although the course of infection is highly variable, many patients develop a chronic lymphadenopathy after months or years as the weakening immune system continues to attack viral antigens on CD4 cell surfaces and in debris floating through the lymphatic veins and the blood stream. CD4 cells are gradually depleted until the immune system can no longer provide an effective defense against disease or an adequate surveillance of potential neoplastic growth of host cells. Patients may complain of extreme fatigue, depression, weakness, drenching night sweats, and weight loss, a syndrome previously labeled AIDS-related complex (ARC) or pre-AIDS. It was estimated that only 20% of these patients would develop opportunistic infections and cancers, but current data suggest that, with time, almost all will progress to AIDS.

The general patterns of presentation of HIV infection are (1) no symptoms; (2) acute HIV disease (acute viral infection); (3) lymphadenopathy; (4) severe opportunistic infections (e.g., *Pneumocystis*, toxoplasmosis, *Mycobacterium avium-intracellulare*); (5) Mild opportunistic infections (mucocutaneous *Candida*, sinus infections); (6) opportunistic tumors (Kaposi's sarcoma, central nervous system lymphomas, squamous carcinoma of the rectum); (7) autoimmune disorders (idiopathic thrombocytopenia purpura, Reiter's syndrome); (8) wasting syndrome; (9) systemic symptoms only (fever, chills, and fatigue); (10) neuropsychiatric symptoms; and (11) renal disease.

Among the recognized opportunistic infections, as well as other infections in general, there are several characteristic features. The first is shortness of breath in otherwise healthy persons. It is not uncommon for previously healthy persons with early onset of *Pneumocystis carinii* pulmonary infection to have several days or even a few weeks of increasing shortness of breath and dyspnea. Such people often have clear chest x-ray films or minimal interstitial infiltrates, although their arterial oxygenation may be significantly depressed. In the absence of a history of bronchospasm and evidence of wheezing, *Pneumocystis* infection in high-risk persons is a consideration.

Nasal and sinus congestion is a common symptom among adult patients with more advanced HIV infection (ARC or AIDS). It is a common and minor complaint, but, in occasional patients, it may be the presenting complaint of HIV infection. This presentation of nasal congestion with recurrent otitis and sinusitis is particularly common in HIV-infected children, and no unusual pathogens are generally identified.

Chronic mucocutaneous candidiasis and persistent generalized lymphadenopathy are quite common in HIV infection and may bring a patient to attention. Clearly, multiple infections, as well as other conditions such as lymphoma and sarcoid granulomatosis, may also manifest with adenopathy. These symptoms and signs are so well recognized as associated with HIV infection that is unlikely that such patients would present first to an otolaryngologist.

In a study of 399 adults with AIDS, 165 (41%) presented with chief complaints referable to the head and neck. Of these 165 patients, 58 (35%) had Kaposi's sarcoma lesions in the mouth, the pharynx, or both; one of these lesions was a primary parotid neoplasm, and the remainder were cutaneous manifestations. Forty patients (24%) presented with oral or pharyngeal candidiasis, eight (5%) had esophageal candidiasis, and three (2%) had laryngeal candidiasis. Thirty-six patients (22%) presented with chronic cough and shortness of breath, of whom 29 (18%) had *Pneumocystis* pneumonia, and seven (4%) had pulmonary manifestations of *Mycobacterium avium-intracellulare.* Thirteen (8%) presented with rapidly enlarging neck masses and had Burkitt's lymphoma. Seven patients (4%), later found to have immunodeficiency, presented with herpes simplex (Table 52A–8). Occasional cases of sudden sensorineural hearing loss, conductive hearing loss, acute otitic infection, chronic sinusitis, and cytomegalovirus parotitis were also seen. In the pediatric population, the presenting finding differs from those of the adults; in a small study done with patients diagnosed with pediatric AIDS, 90% had microsomia; 90% had developmental delay; 80% had acute, chronic, or serous otitis media; 80% had lymphocytic interstitial pneumonia; 80% had mucocutaneous candidiasis; 60% had cortical atrophy; 40% had cervical adenopathy; and 30% had parotid enlargement.

The best test for diagnosing infection is an

HIV antibody test. This test has remarkable specificity and sensitivity. The older antibody tests did have a problem with low-level false-positive reactivity (particularly in multiparous women), which was based on the reactions to the cells used as a substrate for the assay. However, the newer antibody tests with confirmatory Western blot tests have resolved this problem. There is a window of seronegativity in patients acutely infected with HIV that may last up to 2 or more months after infection. However, the ability to screen for circulating viral antigens should reduce this gap and diagnose those patients who fail to make an immune response. The diagnosis of HIV infection in newborns is complicated by the maternal transfer of IgG antibody to HIV. The infected newborn may not proceed to make his or her own IgG to HIV after decay of maternal antibody because of the resulting HIV immunodeficiency. Neither infants nor adults make an IgM anti-HIV response that is useful diagnostically. The availability of HIV-antigen testing for infants provides a way to establish the diagnosis.

Many tests and features appear to correlate with prognosis and survival of patients with HIV infection. They include: (1) hairy leukoplakia; (2) oral and esophageal candidiasis; (3) herpes zoster; (4) shrinkage of previously enlarged lymph nodes; (5) low absolute number of CD4 cells; (6) increased absolute number of CD8 cells; (7) low level of anti-p24 antibody; (8) high level of circulating p24 viral antigen; (9) low level of INF-α production; (10) low level of antibody to reverse transcriptase; (11) high total levels of IgG and IgM; (12) high levels of antibody to cytomegalovirus; (13) high levels of antibody to Epstein-Barr virus; and (14) decreased total lymphocyte count.

The test that appears most relevant at this time is the absolute number of CD4 (T4, helper/inducer T-cell phenotype) cells. The hallmark of HIV infection is the progressive decline in this subset of T cells. In no other acquired condition is there such a profound decrease in absolute number of CD4 cells. This is in contrast to the altered ratios of CD4 and CD8 (T8, cytotoxic/suppressor T-cell phenotype) cells that can be found in numerous diseases. The natural history of HIV infection and disease is a progressive and relentless fall in CD4 cells that does not spontaneously revert toward normal.

Medical research has had limited success

TABLE 52A–8. Presenting Head and Neck Manifestations of AIDS

Site	Number	Percentage
Cutaneous, oral and pharyngeal* lesions of Kaposi's sarcoma	58	35
Aerodigestive lesions of Candida	51	31
Oral and pharyngeal	40	
Esophageal	8	
Laryngeal	3	
Chronic cough and shortness of breath	36	22
Pneumocystis carinii pneumonia	29	
Mycobacterium avium intracellulare	7	
Rapid enlarging neck mass, Burkitt's lymphoma	13	8
Labial oral or pharyngeal lesions of herpes simplex	7	4

*Including nasopharyngeal and hypopharyngeal sites.
From Marcusen DC, Sooy CD: Otolaryngologic and head and neck manifestations of acquired immunodeficiency syndrome (AIDS). Laryngoscope 95:401–405, 1985.

in developing antiviral drugs, and HIV, a retrovirus, has several traits that make potential therapies even more problematic. HIV is an RNA virus that has an extra step in its life cycle in comparison with the normal RNA virus. Rather than simply entering the cell and then reproducing more RNA copies of itself, retroviruses such as HIV use a unique enzyme called reverse transcriptase to make a DNA copy of their RNA. This DNA copy integrates into the host's DNA and persists there. Not only does the inserted DNA copy of the viral RNA persist, but every time the cell divides, the viral information is copied and conferred to the daughter cells. As long as those lymphocytes exist within the host, the virus persists. Currently, there is no way of excising the integrated viral sequence (provirus) from the DNA, nor is there a way to identify and target cells that are carrying the latent provirus. The same enzyme that copies the viral RNA into DNA (reverse transcriptase) is an obvious strategy against HIV, inasmuch as this RNA-dependent polymerase is not found in eukaryotic cells. Thus the first generation of antiviral drugs against HIV has focused on reverse transcriptase with some success (e.g., azidodeoxythymidine). However, this drug also has some ability to interact with normal human cellular polymerases that cause toxic effects on blood-forming elements.

SUMMARY

The interactions between the fields of otolaryngology and immunology are multiple and increasing. Many diseases previously thought to be of infectious or neoplastic nature actually relate to problems in the immune system. This gives physicians the opportunity to intervene more appropriately in the modification of the evolution of a particular disease (e.g., Wegener's granulomatosis). On the other hand, by manipulation of the patient's immune system, the progression of diseases that until now did not have any specific treatment (e.g., use of interferon or monoclonal antibodies against certain cancers) can be changed. As long as research continues to define the pathogenesis of disease, the role of the immune system will increase in importance. A sound knowledge of immunology helps the otolaryngologist understand the pathogenesis, the diagnosis, and the treatment of disease.

SUGGESTED READINGS

Baroody F, Naclerio RM: Allergic rhinitis. In Getchell T, Doty R, Bartoshuk L, Snow J (eds): Smell and Taste in Health and Disease. New York: Raven Press, in press.

deShazo RD, Lopez M, Salvaggio JE: Use and interpretation of diagnostic immunologic laboratory tests. JAMA 258:3011–3031, 1987.

Fahey J, Leonard E, Churg J, Goodman G: Wegener's granulomatosis. Am J Med 17:168–179, 1954.

Harris JP, Sharp PA: Inner ear antibodies in patients with rapidly progressive sensorineural hearing loss. Laryngoscope 100:516–524, 1990.

Johns CJ, Scott PP, Schonfeld SA: Sarcoidosis. Ann Rev Med 40:353–371, 1989.

Karlsson G, Petruson B, Bjorkander J, Hanson LA: Infections of the nose and paranasal sinuses in adult patients with immunodeficiency. Arch Otolaryngol 111:290–293, 1985.

Luetje CM: Theoretical and practical implications for plasmapheresis in autoimmune inner ear disease. Laryngoscope 99:1137–1146, 1989.

Markowitz JC, Perry SW: AIDS: a medical overview for psychiatrists. Rev Psychiat 9:574–592, 1990.

Naclerio RM: Recent advances in immunology with specific reference to otolaryngology. Otolaryngol Clin North Am 18:821–832, 1985.

Roitt I, Brostoff J, Male D: Immunology, 2nd ed. St. Louis: CV Mosby, 1989.

Ruddy S: Hereditary angioedema: undersuspected, underdiagnosed. Hosp Pract [Off] 23(8):91–96, 99–100, 105–106, 1988.

Slavin RG: Nasal polyps and sinusitis. In Middleton E, Reed C, Ellis EF, et al (eds): Allergy: Principles and Practice, 2nd ed (pp 1291–1303). St. Louis: CV Mosby, 1988.

Spaulding WB: Methyltestosterone therapy for hereditary episodic edema (hereditary angioneurotic edema). Ann Intern Med 53:739–745, 1960.

WHO Scientific Group on Immunodeficiency: Meeting report; primary immunodeficiencies. Clin Immunol Immunopathol 28:450–475, 1983.

Otolaryngic Allergy: Evolution of a Discipline

Richard L. Mabry, MD, FACS, FAAOA

Otolaryngology–head and neck surgery, once declared a "dying specialty" after the introduction of antibiotics, survives and continues to expand. Areas of surgical advance that have changed the field include facial plastic and reconstructive surgery, microscopic otologic (and skull base) surgery, the use of lasers, and endoscopic surgery of the sinuses. In addition, it has become increasingly evident that the proper diagnosis and treatment of allergy play a significant role in the management of otolaryngic disorders. Although not as appealing to many otolaryngologists as the surgical side of the specialty, otolaryngic allergy has been an integral part of the practice of many otolaryngologists for decades.

MANIFESTATIONS OF ALLERGY IN OTOLARYNGOLOGY

The otolaryngologist entering practice is immediately struck with the number of patients in whom allergy is obviously present or must be considered. In one series, it was estimated that approximately 10% of children and more than 20% of adults in the general population manifest some type of allergic disorder. An estimated 50% of new patients seen in a general otolaryngology practice present with a chief complaint that is attributable in part or whole to allergy.

The symptoms of allergy are readily discernible because they manifest in the ear, nose, and throat. Patients may complain of itching ears or frequent middle ear infections. Studies have linked some instances of Meniere's syndrome to inhalant allergy or food allergy. Nasal congestion, rhinorrhea, and recurrent sinusitis often are caused by allergy. Chronic postnasal drainage, itching nasal and pharyngeal mucosa, repetitive throat clearing, and episodes of hoarseness may have an allergic basis. Allergic manifestations in the eyes (itching, burning, tearing) and the lower respiratory tract (coughing, wheezing) also suggest to the otolaryngologist the need for allergy evaluation.

Examination usually reveals confirmatory signs of allergy. Children may grimace (because of itching mucosa) and use the upward wiping of the nasal tip that has come to be called the allergic salute. Local venous congestion results in dark circles below the eyes. Nasal mucosa is usually pale and boggy, and polyps may be present. Mouth breathing, typical so-called adenoid facies, and a high, arched palate may be results of allergic nasal obstruction. Prominent posterior pharyngeal lymphoid tissue and enlarged lingual tonsils are often caused by postnasal drainage triggered by allergy.

When allergy is suspected on the basis of history and physical examination results, the otolaryngologist must consider further evaluation and appropriate management.

THE ALLERGIC REACTION

In order to properly treat upper respiratory allergy, the nature of the allergic reaction must be understood. Upon exposure to antigens (such as ragweed), sensitive persons produce antibodies (immunoglobulin E [IgE]). These antibodies attach to mast cells in respiratory mucosa and to basophils. Subsequent exposures allow the specific antigen to react with allergen-specific IgE to cause dissolution of the mast cells and basophils and thereby release mediators of inflammation, such as histamine and leukotrienes. These mediators exert their influence on respiratory mucosa (sneezing, itching), mucous glands (rhinorrhea), and stromal vessels (congestion), causing the acute phase of the allergic reaction. Leukocyte migration and mediator release give rise to a subsequent late phase. This IgE-mediated type of reaction, also called a Gell and Coombs type I reaction, is sometimes referred to as anaphylaxis. This is the prototype of the inhalant allergy reaction of the upper respiratory tract (Fig. 52B–1).

MANAGEMENT OF UPPER RESPIRATORY ALLERGY

The management of inhalant allergy involves the triad of avoidance, pharmacotherapy, and (when indicated) immunotherapy. Although pharmacotherapy may be instituted on the basis of only clinical suspicion, some sort of testing may be necessary not only for determining immunotherapy but also to confirm the identity of the provoking allergens so that the patient may use appropriate environmental control. The means for testing are discussed in detail later.

Initial management of inhalant allergy affecting the upper respiratory tract begins with pharmacotherapy. Proper use of the available options requires understanding of the site of action, the benefits, and the potential side effects of the preparations available.

Antihistamines act by occupying H_1-receptor sites on effector cells, thereby preventing (but not reversing) responses mediated by histamine. Because of the nature of their action, antihistamines are more effective when given before allergen exposure than after it. The clinical action of antihistamines is primarily the relief of the "wet" symptoms of nasal allergy, such as sneezing, rhinorrhea, and postnasal drainage. They are less successful in relieving congestion. The primary side effects or adverse reactions associated with antihistamines are sedation (with a tendency to potentiate the depressant effects of alcohol, barbiturates, antidepressants, and similar preparations), gastrointestinal reactions (ranging from nausea and epigastric distress to diarrhea or constipation), and genitourinary effects (mainly dysuria and obstruction of the neck of the bladder). The problem of sedation has been addressed by the development of antihistamines that do not cross the blood-brain barrier. Each of these so-called second-generation antihistamines (terfenadine, astemizole, and so forth) have unique properties, and the prescribing physician should become thoroughly familiar with such new preparations before employing them. Nonsedating antihistamines seem to be less susceptible to the tolerance phenomenon (tachyphylaxis), which inhibits the long-term effectiveness of the older antihistamines.

Decongestants act on alpha-adrenergic receptors in the mucosa of the respiratory tract to produce vasoconstriction, thus temporarily reducing local swelling. Topical decongestants (nose drops and sprays) cause rebound congestion if used longer than 5 to 7 days. Because most allergic situations require therapy for periods longer than this, topical sympathomimetic agents should be avoided in the treatment of allergic rhinitis. Systemic decongestants are usually combined with antihistamines, the stimulatory effect of the

Figure 52B–1. Schematic representation of acute upper respiratory allergic reaction.

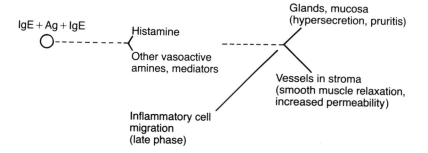

IgE + Ag + IgE

Histamine

Other vasoactive amines, mediators

Inflammatory cell migration (late phase)

Glands, mucosa (hypersecretion, pruritis)

Vessels in stroma (smooth muscle relaxation, increased permeability)

former being balanced somewhat by the sedative action of the latter compounds. Decongestants are potentiated by beta-adrenergic blocking agents, monoamine oxidase inhibitors, and tricyclic antidepressants and should be employed with caution in such circumstances. They also must be used with care in the presence of hypertension, ischemic heart disease, hyperthyroidism, prostatic hypertrophy, and narrow-angle glaucoma.

Cromolyn acts by inhibiting degranulation of sensitized mast cells and thereby preventing the release of histamine and other vasoactive amines. It also prevents the occurrence of late-phase allergic reactions. This property of preventing the allergic event rather than alleviating the symptoms is unique to cromolyn. Cromolyn has no intrinsic antihistamine effect. It is virtually free of side effects, and only 7% of the intranasally administered solution is absorbed, with no significant systemic effects. To be most effective, cromolyn nasal spray must make good contact with nasal mucosa (which requires concomitant use of antihistamines and decongestants in most patients). Nasal cromolyn should be administered four to six times daily during the patient's expected season of allergen exposure, with additional doses before any anticipated heavy exposure. Because of its safety and specificity, cromolyn is a first-line mode of therapy for allergic rhinitis.

Nedocromil, an anti-inflammatory agent similar to cromolyn, requires less frequent use and has other advantages over cromolyn. At the present time, although available in Europe, it is not approved for use in the United States.

Corticosteroids do not prevent the occurrence of acute-phase allergic reactions. They diminish the effects of these reactions by decreasing capillary permeability, stabilizing lysosomal membranes, blocking migratory inhibiting factor, and suppressing the arachidonic acid cascade. Corticosteroids do help prevent late-phase reactions. Systemic corticosteroids must be employed with some degree of caution because their use can be associated with such significant side effects as adrenal suppression, menstrual aberrations, hypokalemia, gastric hyperacidity, central nervous system stimulation, posterior subcapsular cataracts, and aseptic necrosis of the femoral head. To avoid systemic effects, corticosteroid nasal sprays are often used in the management of nasal allergy. However, all nasal corticosteroid sprays currently available may cause local drying, crusting, epistaxis, and even nasal septal perforation. Systemic effects are possible if the preparations are given for prolonged periods, especially at doses higher than those recommended. Corticosteroid therapy for nasal allergy is normally reserved for symptoms that are unresponsive to lesser pharmacotherapeutic measures.

INDICATIONS FOR IMMUNOTHERAPY

The treatment of allergic rhinitis can be thought of as proceeding in a stepwise fashion. All patients suspected of having this disorder should be instructed in general environmental control. First-line pharmacotherapy consisting of antihistamines, decongestants, and nasal cromolyn should be instituted. Severe, persistent, or chronic symptoms may require the use of intranasal or systemic corticosteroids. A constant awareness of complicating factors (infection, rebound rhinitis, rhinitis of pregnancy, and so forth) is necessary. At any point in the treatment of this disorder, testing to determine the presence and the degree of hypersensitivity to specific antigens may be indicated. Indeed, testing is sometimes necessary simply to institute proper avoidance and environmental control measures. In addition, the results of testing allow immunotherapy to be initiated if it is indicated.

In general, immunotherapy is considered in patients whose triggering allergens are not readily avoidable, whose problems are not easily controlled with pharmacotherapy, whose symptoms usually encompass more than a single season, and who are likely to cooperate in a program of immunotherapy injections.

Once immunotherapy is instituted, dosage escalation is continued to the optimal, maximally tolerated dose, and injections are continued for approximately 3 years. Dosage adjustment is necessary throughout this time, depending on allergen exposure and season, and so forth (Table 52B–1).

RESULTS OF IMMUNOTHERAPY

Immunotherapy for inhalant, IgE-mediated allergy is referred to as build-up immuno-

TABLE 52B–1. Guidelines for Immunotherapy

Select appropriate patients
Symptoms are not controlled by pharmacotherapy
Allergen is not readily avoidable
Symptoms are perennial or severe
Patient is likely to comply
Select as a starting antigen dose an amount as high as is likely to be safe
After maintenance dose is reached, continue dosage adjustment as necessary
If immunotherapy is unsuccessful, consider:
Incorrect diagnosis of atopy
Inciting antigens not included in treatment set
Other (noninhalant) triggers, such as food, chemicals, nonatopic factors
Underdosing (shot helps for a few days)
Overdosing (shot makes symptoms worse)
Antigen imbalance in mix
Complication (infection, rebound rhinitis, pregnancy)

From Mabry RL: Pharmacotherapy with immunotherapy for the treatment of otolaryngic allergy. Ear Nose Throat J 69:63–71, 1990.

therapy, in order to distinguish it from neutralization procedures sometimes used to treat food hypersensitivity. In addition to diminishing skin reactivity to injected antigen, and an initial rise followed by a slow decline in allergen-specific IgE, a rise in allergen-specific IgG4 has been demonstrated as a result of immunotherapy. This IgG4 represents a blocking antibody, which occupies mast cell and basophil receptor sites that would otherwise receive allergen-specific IgE and thus prevents the occurrence of an allergic reaction. The formation of blocking antibody is dose dependent and seems to be related to the total dosage of antigen delivered over the entire course of immunotherapy. Other changes occur at the cellular level, including lessening of basophil reactivity, decreased lymphocyte antigen-specific responsiveness, and a change in lymphocyte surface markers. All these effects diminish the severity of the acute- and late-phase allergic reactions.

SPECIFIC TESTING FOR INHALANT ALLERGY

Testing to determine sensitivity to specific antigens can be conducted by several methods. The physician who is treating patients with otolaryngic allergies should be aware that food and chemical hypersensitivity can be manifested in symptoms such as nasal congestion and discharge, headache, and

vertigo. However, all further discussion here is confined to testing for inhalant allergy.

Mucosal Challenge Tests

Perhaps the most direct means of testing is mucosal challenge, or applying antigen directly onto a mucous membrane. Such testing was performed as early as 1911 by Leonard Noon. He quantified the strength of Timothy grass extract used to treat his patients by instilling progressively stronger concentrations into the conjunctival sac and observing the amount with which erythema was produced. Today mucosal challenge is used primarily as a research tool in which measured amounts of antigen are introduced into the nose or the tracheobronchial tree and changes are measured by rhinomanometry, pulmonary function studies, or even direct assay of mediators that appear in nasal secretions. However, mucosal challenge is not an efficient means of allergy testing in everyday practice.

Skin Tests

The most popular diagnostic tool in evaluating for inhalant allergy is some type of skin test. The earliest form of skin test was the scratch test, dating to Charles Blackley's application of pollen directly to his own abraded skin in 1873. Although safe and specific, scratch tests have been shown to be less sensitive, more painful, and less reproducible than other methods. In 1987 the Allergy Panel of the American Medical Association Council on Scientific Affairs failed to recommend the further use of scratch tests.

The next type of skin test to evolve was the prick test. Prick tests are said to excel over scratch testing in their sensitivity, reproducibility, and correlation with intradermal testing. In the typical prick test, a needle is introduced through a droplet of concentrated antigen to a depth of about 1 mm into the skin. The needle enters at a 45° angle, tenting the skin to allow antigen entry. The most common variant of this test is the prick-puncture test, in which a vertical puncture is made through a droplet of concentrated antigen. Because the amount of antigen entering the skin in the prick puncture test is slightly less, this test is somewhat less sensitive than standard prick tests. Yet another variant, often used for screening, is the use of a multiple-prick test device that allows testing simultaneously of up to six antigens plus a positive and negative control. Prick tests are reliable (specific), but lack the sensitivity of intradermal tests.

Intradermal (Intracutaneous) Testing. This type of skin test is said to have been originated by Robert Cooke in 1911. It involves very superficial injection (within the dermis) of a small amount of antigen, usually 0.01 to 0.02 mL, which forms a sharply defined, easily measurable wheal. The concentration of antigen used for intradermal testing is much more diluted than that employed for prick testing. When properly performed, intradermal tests are said to be less painful than prick tests and yet much more sensitive and reproducible. The greater sensitivity of the test is understandable because it is possible to inject larger quantities of antigen intradermally than can be introduced through either scratch or prick tests. The greater accuracy of antigen delivery is said to be responsible for its greater reproducibility. Traditional single-dilution intradermal tests are reported on a scale of 1–4+, depending on the size of the wheal and surrounding erythema (flare) produced. A positive (histamine) and negative (diluent) control are also required.

In Vitro Tests

The latest method developed for allergy testing is the in vitro assay for allergen-specific IgE. This is discussed in a subsequent section.

IMMUNOTHERAPY BASED ON SKIN TESTING

A positive skin test result may not dictate the necessity of immunotherapy. For instance, if testing reveals atopy for readily avoidable antigens (such as certain animal danders or house dust mites), a program of environmental control may be recommended initially. However, immunotherapy may be deemed necessary, and there are differences of opinions regarding how it should be administered. In order to further understand this divergence of opinions, it is necessary to examine how immunotherapy treatment plans have evolved.

Initial Treatment Efforts

The first recorded attempts at immunotherapy were the injections of Timothy grass pollen extract administered by Leonard Noon, an infectious disease specialist, in 1911. He assumed that the extract acted as an antitoxin to toxins released by inhaled pollen.

Early allergists developed many variations of immunotherapy (also referred to as desensitization or hyposensitization), involving different dosages and routes of antigen administration. Of importance is that systemic administration of a substance to which the patient is allergic may produce a worsening of symptoms or even a full-blown, possibly fatal anaphylactic reaction. Therefore, efforts continued in order to develop a treatment schedule that would render the patient less sensitive to allergens without resulting in untoward reactions.

Prick tests and scratch tests confirmed inhalant allergies that were of moderate to marked severity. To avoid systemic reactions during immunotherapy, researchers began treatment by using extremely diluted solutions (in the 1:1,000,000 range), escalating dosage and progressing to more concentrated treatment solutions by an empiric formula.

Using intradermal tests, physicians were able to diagnose allergies of lesser severity. Robert Cooke is said to have been the father of modern intradermal testing. He reviewed the work of Noon and suggested that patients' individual degree of sensitivity could be determined by skin test challenge. He classified patients according to skin reactivity into one of four groups (A to D). Those with minimal skin reactivity started initial immunotherapy with doses of 100 allergy units (100 µg) of the extract. Those with marked skin reactivity started treatment with 5 units. Cooke warned that dosage schedules were advocated as only a rough guide for advancement and that the physician's duty was to monitor the clinical response of the patient to determine the optimal dose.

The Optimum Dose Concept

French Hansel trained as an otolaryngologist at the Mayo Clinic in the late 1920s. He initially followed the prevailing custom of starting immunotherapy with a low to moderate dose of antigen (which did not cause a constitutional reaction) and then increasing it by a fixed schedule to a maximal antigen concentration of 1:100 or even 1:10. However, he observed that many of his patients experienced better relief of symptoms with lower dosage levels (1:1000 or 1:10,000). He began using smaller initial doses and increasing the strength only to the level at which the patient responded best—the optimal dose. This dose was observed to be significantly lower than the usual goal of the maximal dose that could be tolerated without a marked reaction.

The later work of Hansel involving a microdosage regimen is not held to be valid in light of current understanding, but his departure from the traditional concept of immunotherapy set the stage for later work by Herbert Rinkel.

The Evolution of Skin Endpoint Titration

Rinkel, a general allergist from Kansas City, unhappy with his clinical results in patients treated by an empiric dosage regimen, visited Hansel. He was impressed by the results of optimal-dosage therapy and returned to Kansas City to devise a skin titration method in which fivefold dilutions of extracts were used (and thus replaced the tenfold system used by the allergists of the time). He initially called this technique *serial dilution endpoint titration*. It is now known as *skin endpoint titration* (SET). His titration method involved starting testing with an antigen strength predicted to be nonreacting and continuing the testing (using fivefold progressively stronger extracts) until a positive wheal (at least 2 mm larger than the nonreacting wheal) was noted and initiated progressive whealing. This he called the *endpoint for titration*. This bioassay allowed allergenic inhalants to be introduced into extracts at safe and yet potent individualized strengths rather than at an arbitrary and uniform level for all positive reactants (Table 52B–2).

Using this first reacting antigen strength, or endpoint, as the starting point for immunotherapy, Rinkel observed that the "relieving dose" for many of his patients for ragweed was approximately 0.50 mL of the endpoint dilution (what he termed a *50×* *dose*). Modern immunologic methods have shown that blocking antibodies are best formed when doses of between 40 and 1000 µg of antigen are delivered, and current otolaryngologic allergists attempt to advance

TABLE 52B–2. Methods of Skin Testing and Treatment

Semiquantitative Skin Testing Technique; Empiric Immunotherapy
Initially test for inhalants by prick test
  If result is positive (1–4+), treat
  If result is negative or equivocal, go on to next step
Test by intradermal test
  If result is positive, treat
  If result is negative, omit treatment
Treatment regimen
  All antigens are treated at same concentration
  Progression of dosage by schedule
  Dosage is pushed to maximum tolerated without significant local reaction
Skin Endpoint Titration (SET); SET-Based Immunotherapy
Test for inhalants by SET
  Start with anticipated nonreacting dilution
  Apply progressively stronger concentrations until first positive reaction is noted
  Apply next stronger concentration to confirm progressive whealing
  Consider endpoint strength that initiates progressive whealing
Treat on basis of endpoint strength
  Treatment vial made to deliver endpoint strength for every positive inhalant
  Increase dosage to amount that affords relief for longest period while not causing unacceptable local reaction or worsening symptoms

From Mabry RL: Skin Endpoint Titration: History, Theory and Practice. Roundrock, TX: Meridian Biomedical, 1990.

to this level. A review of Rinkel's work indicates that most of his patients had endpoints such that a 50× dose provided approximately this optimal amount. This is a reminder of the clinical acumen of early practitioners, which is often justified by later scientific investigation.

Unfortunately, some physicians still harbor the concept that when immunotherapy is administered on the basis of skin endpoint titration, antigen dosage is advanced only to the 50× level. Actually, Rinkel himself advocated proceeding first to a dose of 0.50 mL of the endpoint dilution for each positive antigen but advancing further as necessary until symptom relief was obtained or unacceptable local reactions occurred. Although the importance of the basic concepts formulated by Rinkel is acknowledged, techniques taught by the American Academy of Otolaryngic Allergy emphasize delivering proper antigen dosage without regard to the 50× concept. The optimal dose is believed to be the one that yields the best relief of symptoms for the longest period of time (usually 1 to 2 weeks), does not produce an unacceptable local reaction (30 mm or larger), and (ideally) delivers between 40 and 1000 µg of antigen.

Advantages of Skin Endpoint Titration-Based Immunotherapy

At the time of Rinkel's experiments and up to the present, the regimen of many allergists was to initially test by using prick tests. If the tests were negative or equivocal and yet allergy to specific antigens was clinically suspected, further testing with the intradermal method was conducted. Treatment was then instituted, initially beginning with very diluted antigen solutions and progressing by an empiric formula to very concentrated ones. In most cases, despite the varying sensitivities for different antigens, treatment was administered at the same concentration for each antigen (Table 52B–2). It is easy to see that if allergens to which the patient was highly sensitive were present in the treatment mixture, local or systemic reactions to these antigens would occur first, often long before effective treatment levels could be achieved for antigens to which the patient was less sensitive.

The advantage of SET lay in the determination not only of the presence or the absence of allergy to given antigens but also of the exact concentration of antigen necessary to first give a positive skin reaction. By the formulation of treatment vials with this endpoint concentration for every antigen, a safe starting point for therapy was determined, even when testing and treating were conducted during the pollinating season for some of the antigens. This determination was accomplished because each antigen had been bioassayed in the patient before therapy was instituted; this indicated their exact sensitivity at that time. Furthermore, progression of therapy was unlikely to be impeded by large local reactions to one antigen because bioequivalent concentrations of all had been included in the mixture, much in the manner of handicapping a race (Table 52B–3).

In Vitro Testing

As previously noted, the typical allergic reaction of the upper respiratory tract involves IgE. Skin tests measure this substance as it is bound to mast cells in the skin. Soon after the discovery of IgE in 1967 by the Ishizakas

TABLE 52B–3. Advantages of Skin Endpoint Titration Technique

Indicates safe, effective starting dose, usually more potent than arbitrary dose chosen after single-dilution testing
Safe for coseasonal testing
Potency for each antigen in set adjusted by bioassay to match patient's sensitivity

From Mabry RL: Skin Endpoint Titration: History, Theory and Practice. Roundrock, TX: Meridian Biomedical, 1990.

in the United States and by S. G. Johansson and H. H. Bennich in Sweden, an in vitro diagnostic assay for serum allergen-specific IgE was developed by L. Wide and colleagues. This assay was the radioallergosorbent test (RAST). The first commercially marketed RAST was the Phadebas RAST (Pharmacia Diagnostics). Because of a very conservative cutoff point separating positive from negative results, a large number of false-negative results, in comparison with skin tests, were noted when it was used. The modified RAST test of Richard G. Fadal and Donald Nalebuff, introduced in 1979, demonstrated two advantages: first, a lower dividing point between positive and negative results yielded a much lower incidence of false-negative results; second, positive results when categorized by RAST classes were shown to correlate closely with skin test results for which the fivefold dilution SET technique had been used.

All in vitro tests for IgE are "sandwich" techniques. An allergen (such as ragweed) is coated onto a paper disc, a well, or some other convenient carrier. It is allowed to react with the patient's serum, which (if the patient is allergic) contains allergen-specific IgE. Further incubation is carried out with human anti-IgE (developed in laboratory animals) and with some type of marker. Washings at each step carry away material that does not enter into the reaction. What is left is a sandwich of the allergen, the allergen-specific IgE from the patient's serum, the anti-IgE, and the marker. Determination of the amount of marker present allows calculation of the amount of IgE in the patient's serum.

In the early 1980s, in vitro IgE determination assays that did not entail use of radioactive markers were developed. Because the marker in these tests was usually linked with an enzyme, they were called enzyme-linked immunosystem assays. These continue to

e
d
b
c
i
h
s
c

c
v
f
c
a
e
a
te
te
a
e
v
m
b
vi
sa
vi
vi
ex

w
te

Im
Sk
l
l
Dr
l

Un
C
A
Cla
Biz
F
Equ
Pre
Pat
a
Sus
Pat
Tes
Con
Tra
in
Tes
Doo

CHAPTER 53

Lasers in Otolaryngology–Head and Neck Surgery

Rarely within the field of otolaryngology has a technology itself been addressed as a separate subject. The science, the applications, and the potential for the use of lasers in otolaryngology–head and neck surgery, however, justify an integrated approach relating the various lasers and associated technology. The American Board of Otolaryngology–Head and Neck Surgery has recognized this relationship and has mandated minimal training standards for exposure to laser use within the subspecialty for resident training. This has come about as lasers have become almost everyday tools in the armamentarium of the head and neck surgeon and have been demonstrated to be the instrument of choice for certain procedures.

The physical principles that constitute the theory behind the operation of the laser were set forward initially by Christian Bohr in the 19th century and more completely elucidated by Albert Einstein in 1917. However, it took until the late 1950s for Arthur Schawlow and Charles Townes to develop the first microwave laser. T. H. Maimon followed soon thereafter, in 1960, with the first visible light laser. In 1961, Johnson developed the neodymium:glass laser, and in 1964, Javan invented the carbon dioxide (CO_2) laser. The same year also saw the development of other gas lasers such as the argon unit, and the field of lasers has been expanding with new types of lasers and output wavelengths ever since.

The first medical procedures with lasers were performed by Leon Goldman in the early 1960s with use of the ruby laser for dermatologic applications. He tried the ruby laser on port wine stains and vascular hemangiomas and for excision of cutaneous lesions with moderate success. Ophthalmologists were among the first to wholeheartedly embrace the technology and apply it to their field. The visible wavelengths had obvious applications within the cornea and the retina.

The first otolaryngologic–head and neck applications were in 1967. At that time, Joseph Sataloff first used the neodymium:glass laser for stapedotomy with limited success, and G. J. Jako began experimentation with the CO_2 laser in the canine glottis. This initiated the application of lasers within the field, and the use of lasers has blossomed since then.

Many lasers are in daily use within the field of otolaryngology. These lasers include the carbon dioxide, neodymium:YAG (yttrium aluminum garnet), argon pumped-dye tunable, helium-neon, potassium titanyl phosphate (KTP), and argon units. For purposes of limiting the length of this chapter, these lasers are the main focus of discussion, but examples of potential applications for other wavelengths are given where appropriate. Lasers are now used within all aspects of otolaryngology–head and neck surgery from intracranial and otologic applications through head and neck tumor resections to endoscopic applications and cutaneous uses. Second only to ophthalmology, otolaryngology is the subspecialty in which lasers are most pervasive.

BASIC PHYSICS OF LASERS

The basic laser phenomenon begins at the atomic/molecular level. Laser is an acronym for *light amplification by stimulated emission of radiation*. This is somewhat inaccurate; a more accurate term would be *light oscillation by stimulated emission of radiation*, but the acronym "Loser" would alienate the unit from many potential patients ("I'm going to use the loser on your port wine stain.").

An atom can be conceptualized as a central core or nucleus of protons, neutrons, and other subatomic particles surrounded by a cloud of electrons. These electrons can exist in any number of potential orbitals surrounding this central nucleus. Each of these orbitals has its own discrete energy content, and in general, the farther out from the nucleus an electron is, the more energy is necessary for maintaining it in these orbitals. When energy is applied to an atom, electrons are elevated to a higher energy status and exist in these more distant orbitals. The lowest orbital is the most stable energy configuration for the atom and is referred to as the ground state. Once energy has been placed into an atom, the energized atom will try to return to its ground state configuration if possible. It can do this through the electron's dropping down to lower energy orbitals in one large step or in several smaller transitions. In the electron's transition to a lower energy state, excess energy must be given off either as a photon or as kinetic energy. This emission of a photon as the electron transits down to the more stable ground state is called spontaneous emission. While in the higher energy state, the electron can be stimulated to undergo a controlled emission by interaction with an incident photon of appropriate energy. This concept whereby an incident photon with the appropriate energy level causes an electron to drop into a lower energy level is known as stimulated emission. The incident photon must have an energy exactly

equal to that of the potential energy drop of the stimulated electron in order for this transition to occur. This fact is dictated by the quantum status of the electron orbitals. Once the electron has dropped down to a lower energy state, the excess energy is yielded up as a second photon equal in energy and direction to the incident photon. This results in two photons of identical directions, wavelengths, and coherences.

Also, the atom has returned to its ground state. The phenomenon of laser output can occur only when enough atoms are maintained in the stimulated state. When more than 50% of the atoms are stimulated, they are in a state of population inversion. A laser requires a constant input of energy to maintain this population inversion. With the foregoing principles in mind, the basic components of a laser thus include the material to generate the laser beam, mirrors (to redirect the photons back into this material for reinforcing the beam and magnifying it), a power source to generate a population inversion, a cooling system to remove excess kinetic energy, and a delivery system to direct the beam for applications. The power supplied is either a 110- or a 220-V current. This power is used to excite the laser material into a state of population inversion and maintain it in this state during operation of the laser. Because this is a very inefficient system, much of the energy is wasted as heat, and a cooling system is necessary. Cooling systems may be either a flowing water radiator system or a closed-loop air-to-fluid radiator system. The cavitary mirrors that redirect and amplify the laser beam are located on the longitudinal ends of the laser medium. One of these mirrors is usually less than 100% reflective. This allows some of the laser beam to be emitted continuously, and this continuous beam is then modified by a shutter system to control application to tissue.

The inciting energy for the generation of the population inversion is applied to the laser media either directly (as electrical current or as radiofrequency energy) or as light energy from a flashlamp tube. This demonstrates that many types of energy input can be used to generate a laser beam. The output of the laser beam is then redirected, by some delivery device, to bring the beam into usable distance for tissue applications. In the visible wavelength lasers, an optical fiber of quartz silica glass may be used. Optical fibers, however, are not yet available for the far infrared applications of the CO_2 laser, and a hollow articulating arm assembly must be employed.

COMMON MEDICAL LASERS

The lasers in common use in otolaryngology–head and neck surgery are the carbon dioxide laser, the neodymium:YAG laser, the Candela flashlamp-excited dye laser, the KTP laser, and the argon laser. The argon pumped-dye laser, which is broadly tunable depending on the dye that is used, is also occasionally used within the field of otolaryngology–head and neck surgery as the light source for photodynamic therapy with hematoporphyrin derivative. Each of these lasers is discussed in regard to its method of operation, power, water requirements, safety requirements, and potential applications.

Carbon Dioxide Laser

The CO_2 laser was among the first to be explored for application within the field of otolaryngology. G. J. Jako used a very early CO_2 laser, coupled to a microscope micromanipulator, to investigate the potential applications of this wavelength for endolaryngeal surgery, and he conducted his first experiments in the canine larynx in the late 1960s. Within several years, Jako and his coauthors had published a series of more than 100 procedures performed in humans demonstrating the safety and efficacy of the CO_2 wavelength applied to laryngeal disorders. Since that time, the CO_2 laser has become the workhorse laser in the armamentarium for otolaryngology–head and neck surgery. Most residents have exposure to this laser through their training program, and the Board of Otolaryngology assumes a minimal competence with this unit as a prerequisite for certification.

The CO_2 laser operates at 10,600 nm in the far-infrared region of the spectrum. This wavelength is highly absorbed by one of the bending frequencies of the water molecule, and because tissue is composed of 75% to 85% water, this wavelength is highly absorbed by tissue. Vaporization occurs quickly, and the steam plume is then ejected from the crater with a velocity of 2 to 6 m/second. Because of the high specific heat necessary to form water vapor, this wavelength causes less thermal damage than do

many of the visible wavelength lasers. Thermal damage on the order of 110 to 250 μm beneath the vaporization impact point is common. This minimal thermal effect means that the CO_2 laser is very effective at causing vaporization but is able only to coagulate and seal small blood vessels. Blood vessels more than approximately 0.5 mm in diameter can bleed with use of the CO_2 laser.

The lasing cavity of the CO_2 laser is a hollow tube filled with a mixture of carbon dioxide, nitrogen, and helium. Energy is initially applied to the nitrogen molecule, which undergoes a transfer of energy to the carbon dioxide molecule that is responsible for the actual laser beam itself. The helium gas acts as a heat sink to dissipate the excess energy within the tube. Energy is applied to the laser cavity either as direct current across electrodes that are placed longitudinally along the cavity or as radiofrequency energy directly into the cavity. The laser beam generated is a true continuous beam, and a shutter system must be used to control the pulsing of the laser beam and its applications to tissue.

The far-infrared wavelength output of the CO_2 laser cannot be transmitted through quartz fibers. The laser beam is redirected as it exits the cavity through a series of hollow tubes joined by mirrored joints. This procedure makes the CO_2 laser slightly less flexible than the other lasers but has not markedly hindered its applications. This hollow articulated arm assembly may be attached either to a focusing handpiece for hand-held laser application or to a microscope manipulator or a bronchoscopic coupler for use endoscopically. New advances in delivery technology for the CO_2 laser have included the development of semiflexible waveguides and the potential for a true optical fiber. The waveguides essentially are small, hollow tubes that are highly reflective on the inside and thus redirect the beam down the length of the tubes. There are practical limitations to the bend radius of these tubes and the amount of power that they are capable of carrying, and the diameter has not allowed applications such as those allowed by a flexible fiber down the side port of a bronchoscope. In addition, many of these waveguides employ purge gases down the length of the tube; the laser plume from tissue vaporization is prevented from coming within the tube itself and being deposited on the mirrored walls. This laser plume that is generated from an impact of the CO_2 laser with tissue also causes a potential problem in the use of CO_2 fibers. Depositing of a laser plume on the end of the fiber would then decrease the amount of energy that may be transmitted through that fiber or, worse yet, may allow the energy to be absorbed at the tip of the fiber, thereby ruining it.

The most common use of the CO_2 laser in the field of otolaryngology is for endoscopic applications. For this, the articulated arm is attached either to a microscope manipulator or to a bronchoscopic coupler for redirection of the CO_2 beam down a rigid bronchoscope. The original microscope micromanipulator has a spot size of well over 1 mm in diameter, and although this was a technologic advance in the late 1960s, newer micromanipulators are able to give spot sizes on the order of 250 μm at a 400-mm focal length, which allows much greater precision. With the option of such high precision, lesions may be either excised or ablated. The small spot size also means a decrease in the area of adjacent thermal injury. This is especially important when the surgeon is working very close to vital structures such as the vocal ligament of the true vocal fold. In this area, thermal coagulation deep to the zone of vaporization is to be avoided because subsequent scarring of the vocal fold to the vocal ligament would alter the mass of the vocal fold and thus change the vocal characteristics of the glottis.

Most CO_2 laser units now have an internal cooling system that makes use of an air-to-water exchange and are powered by a 110-V, 15-A, 60-cycle current. Thus no modifications to the operating room are needed for the instillation of the CO_2 unit.

As with each laser, the CO_2 laser has unique safety precautions that should be followed when it is used. While it is in operation, all room personnel should wear safety glasses. The glasses may be either plastic or glass; either will stop the far-infrared wavelength. The patient's eyes should be taped closed and protected with wet saline gauze pads taped in place; the area surrounding the endoscope should be protected with wet drapes. If the CO_2 laser is used endoscopically and the patient is intubated, a laser-resistant endotracheal tube must be employed. Many laser-resistant endotracheal tubes on the market are acceptable. If the use of an endotracheal tube is to be avoided during this procedure, then venturi jet ventilation may be substituted. Another alter-

native is the apneic technique, in which the endotracheal tube is first removed while the laser is being used and then replaced to ventilate the patient at regular intervals, as monitored by pulse oximeter.

No specific modifications of the instruments are needed as long as they are not mirror surfaced. The surgeon should try to avoid reflecting the CO_2 beam off the surface of shiny instruments, and although the beam may be reflected off internal walls of the laryngoscope, most laryngoscopes have a dull matte finish and are generally safe for laser use. The instruments themselves need not be ebonized, because the concern here is for the reflection of a far-infrared wavelength. This wavelength is as effectively dispersed by a dull matte finish as it is from an ebonized finish. However, some surgeons prefer to use ebonized instruments to cut down on visible light glare from the high-intensity microscope illumination.

Proper laser smoke evacuation should be employed. As mentioned previously, the steam plume from laser impact is ejected from the crater at 2 to 6 m/second. A high-capacity vacuum system should be used to capture this laser smoke. Concerns have been raised about the possibility of the transmission of the human papilloma virus via the laser plume. The status of studies to date has not documented any evidence of direct transmission from patient to surgeon or to operating room personnel through the plume; DNA hybridization studies of the laser plume itself, although showing some segments intact, have failed to demonstrate intact full-strand DNA or intact viral particles. The final recommendation, despite these negative findings to date, must still be to use appropriate draping when operating room personnel are exposed to potential infectious particles.

The CO_2 laser operates in the far-infrared region of the spectrum, and thus the beam itself is invisible to the human eye. In order to make the impact sites visible, an aiming beam is used. The aiming beam is usually a helium-neon laser that is focused coincidently with the CO_2 beam. This procedure occasionally leads to a potential error in focus between the aiming beam and the CO_2 beam; thus another important safety step in the use of the CO_2 laser is to test the laser to ensure alignment of both beams before the patient is brought into the operating room.

Neodymium:Yttrium-Aluminum-Garnet Laser

The neodymium:YAG laser operates in the near-infrared wavelengths at 1064 nm. The neodymium:glass laser was invented in 1960 by L. F. Johnson. The neodymium:glass laser has an operating wavelength of 1060 nm. This difference between the neodymium:glass and neodymium:YAG lasers points out the importance of the surrounding matrixes on limiting the potential energy states for electron clouds surrounding the lasing atom. In a glass matrix, the wavelength constrains the electron transitions and allows production of a beam of only 1060 nm; in the YAG crystal, a wavelength of 1064 nm is allowed. Neodymium is a rare earth metal that is doped into a crystalline garnet matrix of yttrium and aluminum.

Older versions of this crystalline laser had very specific power and water requirements. A 220-V current was necessary to power the flashlamp exciting the crystal, and a flowing water cooling system was required to dissipate the excess heat produced. Newer neodymium:YAG lasers are now air cooled and use a 110-V power supply.

The beam of the neodymium:YAG laser operating in the near-infrared wavelengths can be transmitted through quartz fibers. These fibers are small enough to be used through the operating channel of flexible bronchoscopes and gastroscopes and have wide use for coagulation and hemostasis. These fibers may be used as they are, with nothing on the end of the fibers. This means that the beam rapidly diverges once it leaves the end of the optical fiber, and the fiber must be held close to the operating field in order to achieve a power density high enough for coagulation and vaporization. Contact tips have been developed for the neodymium:YAG fibers. These tips are synthetic sapphire or extruded quartz tips that fit on the end of the flexible fiber. The tips serve to focus the beam energy into a very small spot and decrease the thermal penetration into tissue from the neodymium:YAG laser.

The effects of the neodymium:YAG laser on tissue are directly related to the penetration depth of the near-infrared wavelengths. No tissue chromophores selectively absorb this wavelength, and the 1064-nm beam is able to penetrate several millimeters into tissue before it is attenuated. The clinical effect allows tissue penetration to depths as great as 4 mm, which would allow deep coagulation in the area surrounding the laser impact point. From this it is obvious that the neodymium:YAG laser is very effective at coagulating those vessels that the CO_2 laser has difficulty sealing.

Safety precautions for the neodymium:YAG laser include protection of the endotracheal tube similar to that for a CO_2 laser; appropriate eye protection for the surgeon (with goggles of the appropriate optical density at 1064 nm); eye protection for the patient (to include wet saline gauze sponges and aluminum foil eye shields); and the precaution to be aware of backscatter from tissue surfaces. As much as 20% of the neodymium:YAG beam may be reflected from the surface of the tissue, and if the surgeon's hand is held too close to the end of the optical fiber, some warmth may be experienced from this reflected beam. The neodymium:YAG laser has a problem similar to that of the CO_2 laser in that the operating wavelength is invisible to the human eye and an aiming beam must be employed. Often the aiming beam is an attenuated output of the flashlamp used to excite the neodymium:YAG crystal, but occasionally the aiming beam is a separate helium-neon laser that has been placed into the beam path coincidently with the laser beam itself.

Candela Flashlamp-Excited Dye Laser

The Candela flashlamp-excited dye laser was the first medical laser designed for a specific application. Operating at a wavelength of 585 nm, this laser was designed to decolorize cutaneous vascular lesions. In order to accomplish this, this laser takes advantage of the absorption of hemoglobin at this wavelength with resultant coagulation of the vessels to decolorize port wine stains and hemangiomas.

This laser uses an organic dye that is excited by a flashlamp to provide the laser beam. The organic dye, because of its complex structure, has an almost infinite number of quantumized electron orbitals available to it. When excited with the flashlamp, electrons are elevated to higher energy orbitals and undergo spontaneous emission. The flashlamp is then used to regenerate the excited state in the dye, maintaining the population inversion. By diffraction grating, one of the multiple potential output wavelengths is selected. This laser is set at a 585-nm wavelength. There is a minor Soret band of absorption for hemoglobin in this wavelength region, and the Candela laser is tuned to take advantage of this absorption peak. Whereas there are other, stronger, absorption peaks of hemoglobin in the low 500- and high 400-nm range, there is excessive competition by melanin for absorption at these lower wavelengths. The Candela laser is optimal for hemoglobin absorption through tissue.

The output pulse structure of this laser is also set in a unique pattern. The output pulse is limited to 450 microseconds' duration. The pulse structure is designed so that the hemoglobin absorbs the energy from the laser beam, converting it into heat with enough thermal energy to cause coagulation of the small vessels. Because the duration of the pulse is minimized, the excess thermal energy is also minimized in an attempt to lessen damage to surrounding tissue. Results to date have been very encouraging. Without competition by melanin, the overlying tissue is not damaged by the excess thermal effect, and therefore the textural irregularities that had been seen with the use of the argon and KTP lasers are avoided. The use of the argon and KTP lasers for decolorizing port wine stains were also associated with unacceptable scarring in children under the age of 12 years. This has not been the case with the flash-lamp-excited dye laser.

Potassium-Titanyl-Phosphate (KTP) Laser

The KTP crystal has the unique property of doubling the frequency (halving the wavelength) of a wide range of input beam wavelengths. The KTP laser starts by generating a laser beam from a neodymium:YAG crystal, and the output from this laser is directed through the KTP crystal. This produces a laser output wavelength of 532 nm. The crystal was originally developed by the United States Navy for communications research and was classified for many years. When it was declassified, the crystal was applied to the neodymium:YAG wavelengths so that an output in the visible region in the low 500-nm range could be provided to take advantage of the absorption of hemoglobin. The goal of this laser was the development of a

wavelength similar to that of argon, which is well absorbed by tissue, that would be effective at producing coagulation and, at higher powers, at cutting. An input of 100 W from a neodymium:YAG laser is able to result in an output of 18 to 20 W after the beam is directed through the KTP crystal.

This laser operates in the green region of the spectrum and, as such, serves as its own aiming beam. It is well absorbed by tissue, melanin, and hemoglobin and has been effective at producing coagulation and vaporization (when used at higher powers). This laser, operating in the visible wavelengths, also has the advantage of being able to be transmitted through quartz optical fibers and therefore is able to be transmitted through small diameters and may be used through the side ports of flexible bronchoscopes and esophagoscopes.

Because this laser is well absorbed by melanin and hemoglobin, it generally works better against darker targets than against lighter targets. Although this laser has been recommended for performing stapedotomies, an endogenous absorber must be added to the footplate in order to allow the laser energy to be absorbed. This necessitates placing either a dye or a drop of blood on the footplate, because the beam itself is generally reflected from a smooth white surface as would be encountered on a stapes footplate. However, once the footplate has been heated enough by this laser, and starts to produce a char, the laser energy is then absorbed much faster; the first several impacts from the laser may have no visible effect, but the succeeding impacts may have an unanticipated greater effect.

Safety precautions for this laser include appropriate tinted eyewear for all operating room personnel and for the patients, if they are awake. Potential difficulties arise here in that the tinted eyewear makes visualization of bleeding points somewhat difficult. If the patient is asleep, the eyes must be protected with aluminum foil. In the airway or the oral cavity, an appropriate laser-resistant endotracheal tube or a barrier such as aluminum foil must be used. All operating room windows must be covered because this beam can be reflected off instruments (as can other visible beams). In addition, the earlier models of this laser needed flowing water for cooling, whereas the newer versions are air cooled.

Argon Laser

Early argon lasers were limited to power outputs of 3 to 5 W. This lack of power and inability to vaporize tissue prompted the research and development of the KTP laser. Newer argon units on the market are now capable of producing power in the range of 20-W output, more than enough to coagulate and vaporize tissue.

The argon laser is actually an ion laser. Power input into the system ionizes the argon gas, and more power is applied to place these ions into a population inversion and generate the beam. Consequently, the argon laser is less efficient at converting power to beam output than are lasers such as the CO_2 laser. In addition, because of the high heat generated, all argon lasers to date in these power outputs for medical applications have been cooled with flowing water.

Because the argon laser is an ion laser, a number of very closely spaced potential electron orbitals are available to generate the output wavelength. The argon laser simultaneously produces output at a number of wavelengths, the two strongest of which occur at 488 and 514 nm. The output color is in the blue-to-green range. Output wavelengths can be selected by appropriate filters. Ophthalmologists routinely filter out the shorter wavelengths and use only the 514-nm green band for retinal photocoagulation. Because the argon output is in the visible spectrum, an attenuated portion of the beam is used as the aiming beam of this laser.

The visible wavelength output from the argon laser is capable of being transmitted through quartz optical fibers. Because of the short wavelength output from this laser, fibers as small as 200 μm can be routinely used. These small fibers are especially easy to pass down the side channels of operating bronchoscopes or esophagoscopes.

Appropriate safety precautions include protective eyewear specific for the output wavelengths of the argon laser and protection from reflected beams. When the optical fibers are used through a bronchoscope or an esophagoscope, an electronic shutter employing the proper safety lens must be placed over the eyepiece for the endoscope to protect the surgeon's eyes.

Future Lasers

The number of lasers and their potential wavelength outputs are increasing daily. Many of these lasers will no doubt have medical applications in the future, but their potential has not been fully explored. Excimer lasers operating in the ultraviolet range of the spectrum are especially effective at cutting tissue with minimal thermal effect. These lasers are currently undergoing trials for vascular recanalization in removing atheromatous plaques, but applications to the head and neck have not yet been developed. X-ray lasers have the potential for even more precise cutting with almost no thermal effect at all. However, at the current time, these lasers are exceedingly bulky and are not adaptable for use in the operating room.

Possibly the laser with the most potential is the free electron laser. This laser is a development of the United States' Strategic Defense Initiative program. An electron beam is oscillated by a magnetic field to generate a laser output. The potential for this laser is high because by varying the oscillation of the initial electron beam, output wavelengths from 400 nm to 8000 nm are possible. This truly will be one laser that can do everything from coagulation to cutting to vaporization. At the present time, these lasers are very large, and ongoing research is directed not only at developing applications for this laser but at producing a more compact unit.

LASER-TISSUE INTERACTION

Light Interaction With Tissue

Research into laser-tissue interaction is in a position analogous to that encountered by research on radiation therapy in the 1930s. Current experiments are directed at defining the interaction of light with tissue to yield reproducible results. The use of early lasers in medicine was characterized by the concept of "turn it on and let's see what it does." The newer lasers are now designed with specific applications in mind (i.e., the Candela laser) on the basis of predicted responses within tissue.

Light interacting with tissue may result in one of several outcomes. For example, the light may be transmitted completely through tissue. The only common medical application for this at the present time is pulse oximetry, in which a laser diode is used to transmit light through a finger or the auricle, and the attenuation of this light transmission is related to absorption by oxyhemoglobin.

Light may be scattered within tissue. The light may be reflected off internal structures, or it may be reflected by macromolecules or atoms. Once this light is scattered, one of two reactions may occur. The light may be transmitted deeper through the tissue, which results in diffuse transmission, and must be added to the direct transmission to give the total transmission through tissue. The other reaction that may occur is that the light may be backscattered out from the tissue. This potential reflectance of light from deeper within tissues may have potential diagnostic applications in the future.

The most important interaction that light may have with tissue is that of absorption. Light may be absorbed by macromolecules, small molecules, or atoms. When the light energy is absorbed, the absorbing chromophore is elevated to a higher energy level. This most often results in the conversion of the light energy to kinetic energy. The resultant rise in tissue temperature is the mechanism of action for most laser light interactions with tissue. Occasionally, however, the excess energy is re-emitted as another photon in a process called fluorescence. The concept of fluorescence may have head and neck applications in the use of hematoporphyrin derivative to localize neoplastic tissue in photodynamic therapy.

The absorption of light and the resultant rise in tissue temperature is the basis for most applications of lasers. In general, neoplastic tissue can tolerate temperature rises only to approximately 42°C, whereas normal tissue can tolerate temperature to approximately 45°C. This difference in tolerance is the basis for the concept of hyperthermia treatment of neoplasms. Hyperthermia may be delivered by low-dosage illumination of tissue with a neodymium:YAG laser, but heating is not limited to laser applications. Microwave instruments have also been used to generate this hyperthermic treatment for neoplasms. When tissue is raised above 45°C, several structural, enzymatic, and conformational changes occur. From 45°C to 60°C, enzymes may undergo conformational changes, leading to a slow cell death. From 60°C to 80°C, proteins are markedly denatured with irreversible cell damage. Above 80°C, collagen is degraded and fused, and above 100°C, the tissue is desiccated. Once

tissue is raised much beyond 100°C, the tissue is effectively vaporized.

The laser used in a wide-beam, low-power application to tissue can result in coagulation of or irreversible damage to a large volume of tissue. If the power is increased, then tissue is desiccated and vaporized. In order to cut tissue, very high powers are used in a very small spot size, and the tissue is vaporized along a narrow line. This demonstrates the concept of spot size, which is so important in determining the effects of laser on tissue. In general, the lower powers coagulate, and the higher powers vaporize. The other concept important for the understanding of tissue effects is that of power density. Because power drops off as a function of the square of the radius, it is apparent that if the surgeon wishes to cut along a very narrow line, one power level can be used, but to accomplish the same cutting effect along a very broad front, the power output must be squared.

Clinical Effects

Coagulation and Hemostasis

The most obvious thermal effect resulting from laser-tissue interaction is the coagulation of tissue. Depending on the depth of coagulation, capillaries and small blood vessels up to several millimeters in diameter may be effectively sealed. This depth of coagulation is a function of the wavelength of the laser (and the depth of penetration of this wavelength into the tissue) and the duration of exposure of the laser to the tissue.

Antisepsis

The wide-field vaporization of large volumes of tissues requires a large thermal input. This thermal effect of vaporizing the tissue also causes coagulation of tissue deep to the zone of vaporization. Often, temperatures at the surface of this zone between vaporization and coagulation exceed 100°C and effectively sterilize the area. With bacterial counts reduced to almost nothing, it is only the secondary opportunistic bacteria that may cause wound infections. CO_2 laser mastectomy has been noted to have a lower incidence of postoperative wound infection than does mastectomy with traditional scalpel incision.

Wavelength Dependence of Laser-Tissue Interaction

Each component of tissue has its own visible and infrared absorption characteristics. Absorption spectra for hemoglobin differ from those for bilirubin, melanin, and water. Because of the variation in absorption spectra among tissue components, the interaction of lasers with tissue depends strongly on the summation of absorptions at that operating wavelength.

The CO_2 laser is well absorbed by the bending frequency of water. With the exception of bone, most tissue is 75% to 85% water, which explains the generally good absorption of the CO_2 laser by tissue. Because the absorption is so strong, most of the CO_2 beam is absorbed at the surface of the tissue with very little of the beam penetrating deeper into the tissue. In water, the absorption length for CO_2 laser is on the order of 0.03 mm; in tissue, the absorption and thermal effect is usually less than 0.25 mm.

The neodymium:YAG laser is absorbed by tissue in general; no major chromophore acts as the primary absorber of the near-infrared wavelength. Because of this, the region around the neodymium:YAG wavelength is a relative window into the tissue. The neodymium:YAG wavelength may cause coagulation as deep as 4 mm into tissue because of this great depth of penetration.

The argon and KTP lasers, operating in the blue-green and green portions of the spectrum, are well absorbed by the tissue chromophores hemoglobin, bilirubin, and melanin. Each of these by itself contributes to the absorption, but the depth of penetration of these lasers is still deeper than that from the CO_2 laser. As a consequence, the overall penetration of these wavelengths into the tissue is moderately deeper, and the resulting coagulation is on the order of 2 mm within tissue.

The Candela laser, operating at a yellow wavelength, is absorbed primarily by hemoglobin. This laser is an example of how the design of a unit takes advantage of specific tissue absorption. There is a minor absorption band of hemoglobin near 585 nm; although it is not as strong as the absorption by hemoglobin at 510 and 515 nm, it does not have to compete with the strong absorption by bilirubin and melanin at the shorter wavelengths. This affords a greater tissue precision for the absorption of the Candela

wavelength. This wavelength, absorbed by hemoglobin, induces a thermal effect that results in the coagulation of the vessels. Another characteristic of this laser that was based on experimental design is the pulse structure of 450 microseconds. This pulse structure was designed to heat up the hemoglobin and cause a localized thermal effect without causing extensive thermal diffusion into surrounding tissue. This pulse structure was designed to limit the thermal effect to just the vasculature while preserving intact the surrounding dermis.

Pulse and Spot Size Effect on Tissue Interaction

Power density is the concentration of energy per unit area of the laser beam (expressed as watts per centimeter squared [W/cm^2]). Power density in general determines the tissue effect. Lower power densities gently heat tissue, higher power densities cause coagulation, and much higher power densities cause vaporization. Extremely high power densities over wide areas cause vaporization or ablation. High power in a very narrow focal spot causes ablation in a narrow line—that is, cutting. Thus when the powers used for laser application are specified, it is necessary to specify the spot size as well.

SELECTION OF LASER

The wide selection of medical lasers has made the choice of which laser to use very confusing. Not only must the surgeon decide which wavelength is most appropriate for a particular application, but the delivery mode that is most effective must also be determined.

In general, for vaporization of large areas of tissue, the CO_2 laser is most effective. Limitations to the use of the CO_2 laser, however, include the fact that handpieces must be used attached to an articulated arm, and optical fiber transmission is not yet available.

For coagulation of tissue or vascular lesions, the argon, KTP, and neodymium:YAG lasers are all very effective. The argon and KTP lasers cause thermal coagulation as deep as 2 mm, whereas the neodymium:YAG laser may coagulate as deep as 4 mm.

When tactile feedback is desirable, a contact fiber may be employed. These fibers are available for the neodymium:YAG, KTP, and argon units. The choice then becomes how deep a zone of coagulation lateral to the fiber the surgeon wishes to produce.

Port wine stains and cutaneous vascular malformations are best treated by a laser that is designed to coagulate the vessels with minimal damage to surrounding tissue. This is accomplished with the Candela flashlamp-excited dye laser and other lasers operating in the 570- to 585-nm wavelengths as they are developed.

OTOLOGY

Most medical lasers have been tested for potential applications in the field of otology. Beginning in 1967, Joseph Sataloff first used the neodymium:glass laser for stapedotomy with disappointing results. Each of the current medical lasers has also been used for performing stapedotomies, and each has its proponents. Claims are made for benefits of the noncontact production of the small fenestra and the ease of the learning curve. This "noncontact" claim is somewhat misleading. Each laser functions as a thermal tool, causing charring of the stapes footplate. The char must then be manually removed with a small pick. The pressure involved in removing this char may be somewhat less than that used in performing a stapedotomy with a Buckingham hand drill, but the time and contact with the footplate are approximately the same. An excellent review of the use of lasers for performance of stapedotomy was published by Lesinski and Palmer (1989). They outlined potential difficulties with the use of the argon and the KTP lasers for fenestration of the footplate by highlighting the fact that the visible wavelength of these lasers may be transmitted across the vestibule with the potential to cause damage to the saccule. Gantz (1982) demonstrated ruptured saccules on several cats in which the argon laser was used to perform a stapedotomy. Lesinski and Palmer stated that the CO_2 laser is safer from this standpoint and is their choice of laser for performing laser stapedotomy.

Lasers have also been used to perform a myringotomy. The CO_2 laser was especially effective at vaporizing the tympanic membrane, especially when there was fluid behind the tympanic membrane to protect the promontory. Laser myringotomies maintain patency slightly longer than does a cold-knife myringotomy (3 to 6 weeks versus 48 to 72 hours) but did not prove more efficacious in the management of effusion than did simple myringotomy. The standard of choice still appears to be placement of a pressure equalization tube.

Lasers have also been used to vaporize granulation tissue and adhesions of the middle ear space. The CO_2, because of its limited thermal effect, appears to be the safest for use in this area, but the difficulty of attaching the articulating arm to the micromanipulator and maintaining sterility has precluded its wide acceptance. Handpieces developed for the argon and KTP lasers that may be kept sterile can be inserted into the middle ear space as would any ear instrument and have been used for this application. Lasers have also been used for tissue welding during tympanoplasty. Both the KTP and argon units have been used to anneal the fascia graft to the remaining tympanic membrane. Whereas this procedure is technically feasible, it does not necessarily lead to improved results over a standard medial or lateral graph tympanoplasty.

ENDOSCOPIC APPLICATIONS

The CO_2 laser was the first laser to be used for endoscopic laryngeal work. The CO_2 laser remains the laser of choice within the field of otolaryngology–head and neck surgery for most of these applications. Particular benefits of the CO_2 laser include very efficient vaporization and minimal thermal effect surrounding the vaporization site. This is especially important for work around sensitive areas, such as the vocal ligament or the anterior commissure. Other lasers that have a deeper thermal effect might cause unwanted scarring. However, the CO_2 laser is a "line of sight" laser and is not capable of being transmitted through an optical fiber. This laser cannot be used for flexible bronchoscopic or esophagoscopic applications, and therefore the neodymium:YAG, KTP, and argon lasers all have some application in endoscopy. These other lasers are especially effective when deeper thermal coagulation is desired, such as for oblation or coagulation of intraluminal tumors or vascular lesions.

GENERAL HEAD AND NECK SURGERY

The selection of laser use for general head and neck surgery should be based on the desired tissue effect. When large amounts of tissue are to be removed by vaporization or ablation, the CO_2 laser at high powers in the defocused mode is still among the most effective. When vascular lesions are expected to be encountered, one of the other lasers affording deeper thermal coagulation is a better choice. The neodymium:YAG, with its deepest thermal coagulation, has been used with success for mixed capillary/cavernous hemangiomas and juvenile nasopharyngeal angiofibromas. When intermediate coagulation is desired, the KTP, argon, or neodymium:YAG laser with a contact tip has been shown to be effective. The contact tip has been used in radical neck dissection because it affords the surgeon a tactile feedback in the performance of this procedure.

CUTANEOUS USES

Small vascular malformations with vessels less than 0.2 to 0.5 mm in diameter are best treated with the lasers operating in the wavelength of 575 to 585 nm. The Candela flashlamp-excited dye laser was specifically designed for these applications. Although the argon and KTP lasers have both been used in the past for this, the competing absorption from melanin and bilirubin caused an undesirable thermal effect that led to dermal damage and skin texture changes. In addition, these lasers were not recommended for use in children under 12 years of age because they leave unacceptable scars in this population. For small-vessel cutaneous vascular malformations, the flashlamp-excited dye laser has not caused skin texture changes and has been shown to be safe and efficacious when used in small children.

For cutaneous vascular malformations with large vessels, any of the lasers that afford a deeper thermal coagulation may be employed.

CONCLUSION

The initial development of lasers and their application to medicine in the late 1960s was characterized by a "turn it on and let's see what happens" type of research. In the 1990s, the application of lasers to surgery is directed by the concept of "This is the effect we would like to achieve, which wavelength is most effective to achieve this end result?" To this end, surgeons and researchers have directed the design and development of newer medical lasers. The free-electron laser represents an engineering research tool that is capable of exploring the effects of an infinite range of wavelengths between 400 and 8000 nm and a wide range of pulse structures. Once appropriate wavelengths and pulse structures have been identified, other lasers operating in these regions that are smaller and easier to operate may then be designed.

One final caveat needs to be emphasized. Although lasers are effective at performing many different procedures within the field of otolaryngology–head and neck surgery, they are not the absolute answer. Use of a laser does not turn an average surgeon into a good surgeon, and even good surgeons can encounter problems using lasers. The onus is on the surgeon to intelligently select the laser that is most appropriate for the application or to elect not to use the laser if the laser is not the *best* instrument for that problem.

SUGGESTED READINGS

Anderson RR, Parrish JA: The optics of human skin. J Invest Dermatol 77:13–19, 1981.

Boulnois JL: Photophysical processes in recent medical laser developments: a review. Lasers Med Sci 1:47–66, 1986.

DiBartolomeo JR: The argon and CO_2 lasers in otolaryngology: which one, when and why? Laryngoscope 91:1–16, 1981.

Duncavage JA, Piazza LS, Ossoff RH, Toohill RJ: The microtrapdoor technique for the management of laryngeal stenosis. Laryngoscope 97:825–828, 1987.

Fuller TA: The physics of surgical lasers. Lasers Surg Med 1:5–14, 1980.

Fuller TA: Fundamentals of lasers in surgery and medicine. *In* Dixon JA (ed): Surgical Applications of Lasers (pp 11–28). Chicago: Year Book Medical Publishers, 1983.

Gantz BJ, Jenkins HA, Kishimoto S, et al: Argon laser stapedotomy. Ann Otol Rhinol Laryngol 91:25–26, 1982.

Greenwald J, Rosen S, Anderson RR, et al: Comparative histological studies of the tunable dye (at 577 nm) laser and argon laser: the specific vascular effects of the dye laser. J Invest Dermatol 77:305–310, 1981.

Harris DM, Hill JH, Werkhaven JA, et al: Porphyrin fluorescence and photosensitization in head and neck cancer. Arch Otolaryngol Head and Neck Surg 112:1194–1199, 1986.

Jako GJ: Laser surgery of the vocal cords. Laryngoscope 82:2204–2216, 1972.

Karlan MS, Ossoff RH: Laser surgery for benign laryngeal disease. Surg Clin North Am 64:981–994, 1984.

Landthaler M, Haina D, Brunner R, et al: Effects of argon, dye and Nd:YAG lasers on epidermis, dermis, and venous vessels. Lasers Surg Med 6:87–93, 1986.

Lanzafame RJ, Rodgers DW, Naim JO, et al: The effect of the CO_2 laser excision on local tumor recurrence. Lasers Surg Med 6:103–105, 1986.

Lesinski GS, Palmer A: Lasers for otosclerosis: CO_2 vs. argon and KTP–532. Laryngoscope 99:1–12, 1989.

Lumpkin SMM, Bishop SG, Bennett S: Comparison of surgical techniques in the treatment of laryngeal polypoid degeneration. Ann Otol Rhinol Laryngol 96:254–257, 1987.

Mainster MA: Finding your way in the photoforest: laser effects for clinicians. Ophthalmology 91:886–888, 1984.

McKenzie AL, Carruth JAS: Lasers in surgery and medicine. Phys Med Biol 29:619–641, 1984.

Mehta AC, Livingston DR, Golish JA: Artificial sapphire contact endoprobe with Nd-YAG laser in the treatment of subglottic stenosis. Chest 91:473–474, 1987.

Mihashi S, Jako GJ, Incze J, et al: Laser surgery in otolaryngology: interaction of CO_2 laser and soft tissue. Ann NY Acad Sci 267:263–293, 1976.

Morelli JG, Tan OT, Farden J, et al: Tunable dye laser (577 nm) treatment of port wine stains. Lasers Surg Med 6:94–99, 1986.

Ossoff RH: Bronchoscopic laser surgery: which laser, when, and why. Otolaryngol Head Neck Surg 94:378–381, 1986.

Ossoff RH, Duncavage JA: Past, present, and future usage of lasers in otolaryngology–head and neck surgery. *In* Apfelberg DB (ed): Evaluation and Installation of Surgical Laser Systems (pp 127–149). New York: Springer-Verlag, 1987.

Sataloff J: Experimental use of laser in otosclerotic stapes. Arch Otolaryngol 85:58–60, 1967.

Shapshay SM: Laser application in the trachea and bronchi: a comparative study of the soft tissue effects using contact and non-contact delivery systems. Laryngoscope 97(Suppl 41):1–26, 1987.

Sliney DH: Laser-tissue interactions. Clin Chest Med 6:203–208, 1985.

CHAPTER 54

Staging of Head and Neck Cancer

Dale H. Rice, MD

The TNM (tumor, node, and metastasis) classification and staging system for head and neck cancer has been changed on a number of occasions over the years as more and more knowledge has been gained about the natural history of various tumors in various sites. In addition, there has been some disparity between the American Joint Committee for Cancer (AJCC) Staging and End Result Reporting and the European Union International Contra le Cancrum (UICC) system. The latest changes in the AJCC staging occurred in 1988 and are listed as follows.

NASOPHARYNX

Tis   Carcinoma in situ.
T1   Tumor confined to one site or no tumor visible (positive biopsy only).
T2   Both sites involved (vault and lateral wall).
T3   Skull base extension (bone, cranial nerve involvement, or both).

OROPHARYNX

Tis   Carcinoma in situ.
T1   Tumor 2 cm or less in greatest dimension.
T2   Tumor more than 2 cm but not more than 4 cm in greatest dimension.
T3   Tumor more than 4 cm in greatest dimension.
T4   Massive tumor more than 4 cm in dimension with invasion of bone, soft tissues of neck, or root of the tongue.

HYPOPHARYNX

T1   Tumor confined to the site of origin.
T2   Extension of tumor to adjacent region or site without fixation of hemilarynx.
T3   Extension of tumor to adjacent region or site with fixation of hemilarynx.
T4   Massive tumor invading bone or soft tissue of neck.

ORAL CAVITY

Tis   Carcinoma in situ.
T1   Tumor 2 cm or less in greatest dimension.
T2   Tumor more than 2 cm but not more than 4 cm in greatest dimension.
T3   Tumor more than 4 cm in greatest dimension.
T4   Tumor invading adjacent structures, bone, deep muscles of tongue, maxillary sinus, or skin.

LARYNX

Supraglottis

T1   Tumor confined to site of origin with normal vocal cord mobility.

T2   Involvement of adjacent supraglottic sites without glottic fixation.

T3   Tumor limited to the larynx with fixation, extension, or both to postcricoid area, medial wall of piriform sinus, or pre-epiglottic space.

T4   Massive tumor extending beyond the larynx to involve the oropharynx or soft tissues of the neck or with destruction of the thyroid cartilage.

Glottis

T1   Tumor confined to vocal cord with normal mobility (includes involvement of anterior or posterior commissures).

T2   Supraglottic extension, subglottic extension, or both of tumor with normal or impaired cord mobility.

T3   Tumor confined to larynx with fixation of cords.

T4   Massive tumor with thyroid cartilage destruction, extension beyond the confines of the larynx, or both.

Subglottis

T1   Tumor confined to subglottic region.

T2   Extension of tumor to vocal cords with normal or impaired cord mobility.

T3   Tumor confined to larynx with cord fixation.

T4   Massive tumor with cartilage destruction or extension beyond the confines of the larynx, or both.

CERVICAL ESOPHAGUS

Tis   Carcinoma in situ.

T1   Tumor that involves 2 cm or less of the esophagus and produces no obstruction, is not circumferential, and has no extraesophageal spread.

T2   Any tumor that involves more than 2 cm of esophageal length without extraesophageal spread, or tumor of any size that produces obstruction or involves the entire circumference but without extraesophageal spread.

T3   Any tumor with evidence of extraesophageal spread.

MAJOR SALIVARY GLANDS

T1   Tumor 2 cm or less in diameter without significant local extension.

T2   Tumor more than 2 cm but not more than 4 cm in diameter without significant local extension.

T3   Tumor more than 4 cm but not more than 6 cm in diameter without significant local extension.

T4A   Tumor more than 6 cm in dimension without significant local extension.

T4B   Any size tumor with significant local extension.

REGIONAL LYMPH NODES

N0   No regional lymph node metastasis.

N1   Metastasis in a single ipsilateral lymph node 3 cm or less in greatest diameter.

N2A   Metastasis in a single ipsilateral lymph node more than 3 cm but not more than 6 cm in greatest diameter.

N2B   Metastasis in multiple ipsilateral lymph nodes, none more than 6 cm in greatest diameter.

N2C   Metastasis in bilateral or contralateral lymph nodes, none more than 6 cm in greatest diameter.

N3   Metastasis in the lymph node more than 6 cm in greatest diameter.

DISTANT METASTASIS

M0   No distant metastasis.

M1   Distant metastasis present, specify sites according to the following notations: pulmonary, PUL; osseous, OSS; hepatic, HEP; lymph nodes, LYM; bone marrow, MAR; pleura, PLE; skin, SKI; eye, EYE; other, OTH.

STAGE GROUPING

Stage groupings are designed to group lesions with different TNM scores but with similar survival experience in order to restrict the total number of categories. Stage groupings recommended by the AJCC are as follows.

Stage I   T1, N0, M0

Stage II   T2, N0, M0
Stage III   T3, N0, M0
           T1 or T2 or T3, N1, M0
Stage IV   T4, N0 or N1, M0
           Any T, N2 or N3, M0
           Any T, any N, M1

The TNM category is primarily a clinical determination based on physical examination of the patient, but it may be augmented by additional information obtained by radiologic studies or endoscopy. Any subsequent information obtained at surgery or from the histopathologic examination of the surgical specimen does not alter the TNM category. It is frequently desirable in individual studies to include information based on histologic staging. When patients are classified on this basis, the letter P should be used in place of T. Thus degrees would be P1, P2, P3, and P4 defined so as to correspond with the T category. This classification, however, cannot be compared with the TNM clinical classification for reporting of end results.

tively high dose to the skin and subcutaneous tissues; after one to several centimeters, the dose falls off very rapidly, and the exit dose is quite low. As the energy of the electron beam increases, the surface dose increases and the exit dose increases. Orthovoltage x-ray beams, with energies varying from 100 to 250 kV, deliver a maximal dose at the skin surface, and the depth dose falls off less steeply than that of an electron beam. Orthovoltage radiation is used for the treatment of most skin cancers of the head and neck. An electron beam is preferable for skin cancers on the forehead and the scalp because the dose to the underlying calvarium and the brain may be limited more effectually. Intraoral cone radiation therapy is a form of external-beam irradiation that is given with an orthovoltage or electron beam through a cone placed into the oral cavity or the oropharynx in order to deliver a boost dose to relatively early cancers arising in these sites.

Beams of protons or heavy ions (such as carbon or helium) are produced by a cyclotron and deliver a much more precisely defined high-dose volume with very steep dose falloff in comparison with an x-ray or electron beam. These beams are available for cancer treatment at the Harvard University cyclotron and the University of California Lawrence Berkeley cyclotron; they are useful for management of unresectable cancers adjacent to structures that are sensitive to high doses of radiation (such as chordoma arising in the clivus and cervical spine chondrosarcoma). Neutron beams and pi meson beams have been used experimentally and have no proven advantage over conventional x-ray or electron beams.

Interstitial implants may be used to deliver all or part of the treatment for cancers of the oral cavity and the oropharynx. It is necessary to define the tumor precisely and encompass it with the radioactive sources in order to perform a satisfactory implant. The advantages of interstitial treatment are that the high dose may be limited to a small volume of tissue and the treatment is delivered over a short overall time, producing a high probability of tumor control and a relatively low risk of complications. Radium or cesium needles and iridium hairpins or wires are frequently used for implantation in treating head and neck cancers.

Dose-Fractionation Considerations

Radiation dose is expressed in centigrays (cGy), which are the same as rads (i.e., 5000 cGy = 5000 rad = 50 Gy). The unit of dose specification was changed from "rad" to "gray" to honor L. H. Gray, a distinguished British physicist. In general, the probability of tumor control and complications increases with increasing dose, dose per fraction, and volume irradiated and decreasing overall treatment time. Split-course radiation therapy should be avoided because it is associated with a decreased probability of tumor control and does not appreciably lower the risk of late complications. A conventionally fractionated course of radiation therapy is composed of one treatment per day, 5 days per week, with a fraction size of 180 to 200 cGy. The final dose depends on the volume of tumor irradiated, the radiosensitivity of adjacent normal tissues, and the probability of complications. Acutely responding tissues, such as the normal mucosa, and carcinoma respond similarly to radiation. Therefore, treatment schedules that are associated with a minimum of mucositis and its attendant symptoms have a relatively low probability of eradicating a head and neck cancer.

The probability of late complications is not related to the acute effects of radiation except at the very extremes of acute reactions; it does tend to increase with increasing tumor volume because of destruction of normal tissue by the tumor. It is necessary to accept a low risk ($\leq 5\%$) of severe late complications in order to have a reasonable probability of disease control with treatment. A very low risk (1%) of severe complications is desirable in the treatment of early cancers for which the chance of cure is high and an acceptable treatment alternative exists (e.g., T1 or T2 vocal cord cancer suitable for a hemilaryngectomy). However, a higher risk of severe complications (5% to 10%) is acceptable for more advanced lesions in which the chance of cure is lower or the surgical alternative is associated with a significant functional or cosmetic deficit (e.g., favorable T3 vocal cord cancer requiring a total laryngectomy).

Twice-a-day radiation therapy involving a lower dose per fraction (such as 120 cGy) may be used to increase the probability of tumor control with a similar or a lower risk

TABLE 55–1. Radiation Therapy Alone: Doses and Fractionation Schedules*

| T Stage | Once-a-Day Fractionation | | Twice-a-Day Fractionation |
	180 cGy/Fraction	200 cGy/Fraction	120 cGy/Fraction
T1	6500 cGy	6000 cGy	No data
T2	7000 cGy	6400 cGy	7440 cGy
T3	7000 cGy	7000 cGy	7680 cGy
T4	7500 cGy	7000 cGy	7920 cGy

*These are general treatment schedules and will vary with primary site and tumor cell type.

of late complications in selected patients. Dose-fraction schedules for treatment of various T-stage lesions with external-beam irradiation alone are outlined in Table 55–1; these are approximations and vary according to the primary site and cell type (e.g., lymphoepithelioma requires a lower dose than does squamous cell carcinoma). Twice-a-day treatment schedules usually entail a higher total dose than do conventional treatment schedules.

Preoperative or postoperative radiation therapy is combined with surgery for advanced cancers when the probability for local-regional recurrence is high after surgery or radiation therapy alone. Unless a cancer is not completely resectable, postoperative radiation therapy is preferred because it is associated with a lower risk of postoperative complications. The indications for postoperative radiation therapy include advanced primary lesion, subglottic extension of 1 cm or more, multiple malignant nodes, extracapsular extension, thyroid and cricoid cartilage invasion, bone invasion, close or positive margins, perineural invasion, and extension of the primary tumor into the soft tissues of the neck. Preoperative radiation treatment schedules usually consist of 4600 to 5000 cGy at 200 cGy per fraction over 4½ to 5 weeks; the dose to fixed nodes is boosted to 6000 cGy or more to improve the likelihood of complete resection. Postoperative radiation doses are higher than are preoperative doses because the tumor may be present in a poorly vascularized surgical bed; hypoxic tumor cells are more resistant to radiation, and a higher dose is required in order to achieve the same probability of tumor control. The postoperative dose depends on the suspected amount of residual tumor and is selected on the basis of margins of resection (Table 55–2).

Data Analysis

It is imperative that an accepted staging system (such as that of the American Joint Committee on Cancer [AJCC]) be used when clinical data are collected and reported so that the end results for various treatment modalities can be compared stage for stage. The minimal follow-up necessary depends on how quickly a particular tumor is likely to recur after treatment. Approximately 90% of head and neck squamous cell carcinomas that recur do so within 2 years of treatment, and essentially all recurrences are noted within 5 years of treatment. Therefore, the minimal follow-up for all patients included in reported series analyzing end results should be 2 years. Although survival after treatment is the basic desired outcome, it is also necessary to analyze control of disease at the primary site (local control) and in the neck lymph nodes (neck control) to assess the effectiveness of a local-regional treatment modality such as radiation therapy or surgery. Local-regional control rates should be calculated by excluding from the analysis those patients who die within 2 years of treatment with the site or sites in question continuously disease free, because these patients have not survived long enough for the efficacy of treatment to be determined. Alternatively, the data may be analyzed by use of an actuarial method. All patients should be

TABLE 55–2. Postoperative Radiation Therapy: Doses and Fractionation Schedules (Once-a-Day Fractionation)

Surgical Margins	180 cGy per Fraction	200 cGy per Fraction
No tumor at margins	6500 cGy	6000 cGy
Microscopic residual tumor	7000 cGy	6600 cGy
Gross residual tumor	7500 cGy	7000 cGy

TABLE 55–3. Clinically Negative Neck: Definition of Risk Groups

Group	Estimated Risk of Subclinical Neck Disease	T Stage	Site
I Low-risk	<20%	T1	Floor of mouth, oral tongue, retromolar trigone, gingiva, hard palate, buccal mucosa
II Intermediate-risk	20%–30%	T1	Soft palate, pharyngeal wall, supraglottic larynx, tonsil
		T2	Floor of mouth, oral tongue, retromolar trigone, gingiva, hard palate, buccal mucosa
III High-risk	>30%	T1 to T4	Nasopharynx, piriform sinus, base of tongue
		T2 to T4	Soft palate, pharyngeal wall, supraglottic larynx, tonsil
		T3 to T4	Floor of mouth, oral tongue, retromolar trigone, gingiva, hard palate, buccal mucosa

From Mendenhall WM, Million RR: Elective neck irradiation for squamous cell carcinoma of the head and neck: analysis of time-dose factors and causes of failure. Int J Radiat Oncol Biol Phys 12:741–746, 1986.

included in analyses of complications and survival.

TREATMENT GUIDELINES AND RESULTS

Neck

Clinically Negative Neck. Decisions about management of the neck depend on the plan of management for the primary lesion. The clinically negative neck is treated electively if the anticipated risk of occult neck disease is 20% or greater (Table 55–3). If the primary lesion is to be treated surgically, the neck is electively dissected. If the primary lesion is to be irradiated, the neck is electively irradiated. Resection of the primary lesion should not be combined with radiation therapy for the sole purpose of electively irradiating the neck because radiation therapy may be required at some time in the future for treatment of a second primary head and neck cancer.

Elective neck irradiation and elective neck dissection are equally and highly effective in managing subclinical neck disease (Tables 55–4, 55–5). The morbidity associated with elective neck irradiation is negligible. The likelihood of salvage after neck failure is approximately 50% if the primary site remains continuously disease free.

Clinically Positive Neck. The management of the clinically positive neck depends on the extent of the neck disease and the management of the primary cancer. If there is a single clinically positive node 2.0 cm or less in size or several clinically positive nodes 1.0 to 1.5 cm in size and the primary lesion is to be managed with radiation therapy alone, the neck is also managed with radiation therapy. Other factors that favor the use of radiation therapy alone include location of the nodes within the high-dose field, complete regression at the completion of radiation therapy, a diagnosis of lymphoepithelioma, and poor medical condition of the patient. A neck dissection is performed after radiation therapy in most patients with advanced-stage neck disease. If the primary lesion is to be managed surgically, the neck is treated surgically; the addition of postoperative radiation therapy depends on the pathologic evaluation of the specimen. Patients with more advanced neck disease are treated with the combination of radiation therapy and neck dissection. If the primary

TABLE 55–4. Clinically Negative Neck Nodes: Prevention of Treatment Failure in the Neck by Initial Therapy

Risk Group	No ENI	Partial ENI	Total ENI
I (<20%)	13/15 (87%)	16/17 (94%)	1/1 (100%)
II (20%–30%)	6/9 (67%)	34/38 (89%)	10/11 (91%)
III (>30)	3/4 (75%)	32/33 (97%)	61/62 (98%)

ENI, elective neck irradiation (number controlled/number treated).
From Mendenhall WM, Million RR: Elective neck irradiation for squamous cell carcinoma of the head and neck: analysis of time-dose factors and causes of failure. Int J Radiat Oncol Biol Phys 12:741–746, 1986.

TABLE 55–5. Failure of Initial Ipsilateral Neck Treatment: 596 Patients With Carcinoma of the Tonsillar Fossa, Base of Tongue, Supraglottic Larynx, or Hypopharynx (M.D. Anderson Hospital, 1948–1967)

Treatment	N0			N1	N2a	N2b	N3a	N3b
	No Treatment	*Partial Treatment*	*Complete Treatment*					
Irradiation	—	15%	2%	15%	27%	27%	38%	34%
Surgery	55% (16/29)	35%	7%	11%	8%	23%	42%	41%
Combined	—	1/5	0/6	0	0	0	23%	25%

Adapted from Barkley HT Jr, Fletcher GH, Jesse RH, Lindberg RD: Management of cervical lymph node metastases in squamous cell carcinoma of the tonsillar fossa, base of tongue, supraglottic larynx, and hypopharynx. Am J Surg 124:462–467, 1972.

lesion is to be treated surgically and if the neck disease is completely resectable, surgery is followed by postoperative radiation therapy. If the neck disease is fixed, the patient is treated with preoperative radiation therapy, followed by resection of the primary lesion in conjunction with a neck dissection.

Radiation therapy and surgery are equally effective for early neck disease; for more advanced neck disease, the combination of radiation therapy and neck dissection results in a higher rate of disease control than does either modality alone (Tables 55–5, 55–6). In a series of 143 patients undergoing a course of radiation therapy followed by a unilateral neck dissection, the incidence of postoperative complications necessitating a second procedure was 12%, and the postoperative mortality rate was less than 3%. The likelihood of a postoperative wound complication is reduced when the dose to the skin and subcutaneous tissue is less than 6000 cGy and when the interval between radiation therapy and neck dissection is 6 weeks or less. The use of combined treatment for the neck does not adversely affect the probability of surgical salvage after local recurrence. The probability of a postoperative complication is increased if the neck dissection is performed as a sal-vage procedure after failure of radiation therapy alone or if it is performed in conjunction with resection of the primary lesion after planned preoperative radiation therapy.

After treatment of clinically positive neck disease, the probability of salvage in a patient with recurrence of neck disease is remote, regardless of the initial treatment.

Oral Cavity

Oral Tongue. Early (T1, T2) oral tongue cancer may be treated with either radiation therapy or surgery with an equal likelihood of cure. Although the risk of a significant radiation therapy complication is low, surgery is the preferred treatment in the authors' institution because of the risk of less severe bone exposure or soft tissue necrosis that may persist for months or years after radiation therapy.

Patients are treated primarily with radiation therapy if they decline surgery or are at high risk for operative complications. Patients with T3 oral tongue cancer have a relatively low probability of cure with either radiation therapy or surgery alone and are treated with resection followed by postoper-

TABLE 55–6. Clinically Positive Neck Nodes: Control of Disease in the Neck (459 Patients; 593 Heminecks) at 5 Years*

Stage	RT Alone		RT + Neck Dissection		Significance
	Number of Heminecks	*Control Rate*	*Number of Heminecks*	*Control Rate*	
N1	215	86%	38	93%	$p = 0.28$
N2a	29	79%	24	68%	$p = 0.6$
N2a	138	70%	80	91%	$p < 0.01$
N3a	29	33%	40	69%	$p < 0.01$

RT, radiation therapy.
*Primary site managed with radiation therapy alone; excludes 67 heminecks that had incisional or excisional biopsy before treatment. University of Florida data; patients treated October 1964 to October 1985; analysis December 1988 by Eric R. Ellis, M.D. Control rates calculated by Kaplan-Meir product-limit method.
From Mendenhall WM, Parsons JT, Mancuso AA, et al: Carcinoma of the head and neck: Management of the neck. In Perez CA, Brady LW: Principles and Practice of Radiation Oncology, 2nd ed. Philadelphia: JB Lippincott (in press).

TABLE 55–7. Oral Tongue Cancer: Local Control*

T Stage	Excluded†	Control With Irradiation	Number Salvaged/Number Attempted	Ultimate Control
T1	6	8/10 (80%)	1/2	9/10 (90%)
T2	7	21/35 (60%)	5/10	26/35 (74%)
T3	3	10/24 (42%)	3/8	13/24 (54%)
T4	2	0/5	0/1	0/5

*Treated with interstitial implant and/or continuous-course external-beam irradiation (number controlled/number treated).
†Died within 2 years of treatment with primary site continuously disease free.
University of Florida data; patients treated October 1964 to October 1985; analysis June 1988 by W. M. Mendenhall, M.D.

ative radiation therapy. T4 cancers are rarely curable and are usually managed with palliative, moderate-dose radiation therapy.

Early (T1, T2) oral tongue cancer is irradiated with use of a short, intensive course of external-beam treatment, 3000 cGy in 10 fractions, combined with either an interstitial implant or an intraoral cone boost. The overall treatment time is 3 to 4 weeks. More advanced cancers (T3) that are managed with radiation therapy alone are treated with a higher dose of external-beam radiation combined with an interstitial implant.

The local control rates with radiation therapy alone, as well as the ultimate local control rates (including patients successfully salvaged after a local recurrence), are shown in Table 55–7. Five-year absolute and cause-specific survival rates are shown in Table 55–8. The incidence of severe bone or soft tissue complications necessitating surgical intervention was 5% (5 of 92 patients).

Floor of Mouth. T1 and T2 floor-of-mouth cancers are usually treated surgically, particularly if the tumor abuts the gingiva. Patients who decline surgery or are at high risk for operative complications are treated with radiation therapy. T3 and early T4 cancers are treated with a combination of resection and adjuvant radiation therapy. Patients with advanced T4 cancers are treated palliatively with moderate-dose radiation therapy.

Radiation therapy for T1, T2, and early T3 cancers consists of external-beam treatment, 4600 cGy in 23 fractions, combined with an interstitial implant or an intraoral cone boost. Advanced T3 lesions may be managed either with 5000 to 6000 cGy at 200 cGy per fraction combined with an implant or with high-dose external-beam irradiation alone. In the 1980s, few patients received primary radiation therapy for floor-of-mouth cancer at the authors' institution.

Local control and 5-year survival rates for patients with floor-of-mouth cancer treated with primary radiation therapy at the University of Florida are outlined in Tables 55–9 and 55–10. The incidence of severe bone and soft tissue necrosis was 9% (7 of 81 patients).

Oropharynx

The philosophy at the University of Florida is to treat all oropharyngeal cancer with radiation therapy alone. There is no compelling evidence to suggest that the likelihood of local control or survival is improved by combining surgery with radiation therapy.

Tonsillar Area. T1 and T2 cancers of the anterior tonsillar pillar are treated with external-beam irradiation combined with an intraoral cone or interstitial boost. Early (T1 and T2) cancers of the tonsillar fossa are managed with external-beam irradiation alone. More advanced (T3 and early T4) cancers of both sites are treated with external-beam irradiation alone; a limited interstitial boost may be added if there is 1 cm or greater extension into the adjacent tongue. Patients with advanced T4 lesions are treated with palliative radiation therapy.

The local control rates for tonsillar area

TABLE 55–8. Oral Tongue Cancer: 5-Year Survival*

AJCC Stage	Absolute	Cause-Specific
I	7/13 (54%)	7/9
II	16/22 (73%)	16/21 (76%)
III	8/24 (33%)	8/19 (42%)
IVa	1/11 (9%)	1/8
IVb	1/8	1/5

*Treated with interstitial implant and/or continuous-course external-beam irradiation.
University of Florida data; patients treated October 1964 to June 1986; analysis June 1988 by W. M. Mendenhall, M.D.

TABLE 55–9. Floor of Mouth Cancer: Local Control*

T Stage	Excluded†	Control With Irradiation	Number Salvaged/Number Attempted	Ultimate Control
T1	8	22/27 (81%)	3/4	25/27 (93%)
T2	3	19/27 (70%)	5/7	24/27 (89%)
T3	2	4/9	1/4	5/9
T4	0	2/5	0/1	2/5

*Treated with interstitial implant and/or continuous-course external beam iradiation (number controlled/number treated).
†Died within 2 years of treatment with primary site continuously disease free.
University of Florida data; patients treated October 1964 to June 1986; analysis June 1988 by W. M. Mendenhall, M.D.

primary lesions are shown in Table 55–11. The likelihood of local control for T1 and T2 cancers is higher for lesions arising in the tonsillar fossa than for those arising from the anterior tonsillar pillar. Five-year absolute and cause-specific survival rates are shown in Table 55–12. The overall incidence of severe bone or soft tissue necrosis was 4% (5 of 136 patients): 4% (4 of 93) after external-beam irradiation alone, and 2% (1 of 43) after external-beam irradiation plus an interstitial implant.

Soft Palate. T1 and T2 soft palate cancers are treated with external-beam irradiation combined with an intraoral cone boost or with external-beam irradiation alone. External-beam irradiation plus an interstitial boost is preferred for T3 cancers if the entire tumor volume can be adequately encompassed in the implanted volume. Advanced T3 and early T4 cancers are managed with high-dose external-beam irradiation alone. Advanced T4 lesions are treated with palliative radiation therapy.

The rates of local control are shown in Table 55–13; absolute and cause-specific survival rates are outlined in Table 55–14. The incidence of severe bone or soft tissue necrosis was 2% (1 of 55 patients).

TABLE 55–10. Floor of Mouth Cancer: 5-Year Survival*

AJCC Stage	Absolute	Cause-Specific
I	18/28 (64%)	18/18 (100%)
II	11/18 (61%)	11/14 (79%)
III	9/13 (69%)	9/11 (82%)
IVa	3/11 (27%)	3/10 (30%)
IVb	1/7	1/4

*Treated with interstitial implant and/or continuous-course external-beam irradiation.
University of Florida data; patients treated October 1964 to June 1983; analysis June 1988 by W. M. Mendenhall, M.D.

Base of Tongue. Patients with T1, T2, T3, and early T4 base-of-tongue cancers are treated with high-dose external-beam irradiation alone. The addition of an interstitial implant offers no improvement in local control rates in comparison with external-beam therapy alone. Patients with advanced T4 lesions are treated with moderate-dose, palliative radiation therapy.

The rates of local control with continuous-course, external-beam irradiation at the University of Florida are shown in Table 55–15. Stage for stage, the probability of local control is better for base-of-tongue cancer than for oral tongue cancer. Absolute and relapse-free survival rates for this series of patients are depicted in Figures 55–1 and 55–2. The incidence of severe bone or soft tissue necrosis was 1% (1 of 84 patients).

Larynx

Supraglottic Larynx. T1, T2, and favorable T3 supraglottic cancers may be treated with either radiation therapy alone or a supraglottic laryngectomy. A substantial proportion of patients whose lesions are anatomically suitable for a supraglottic laryngectomy are not candidates for the procedure because of cardiac or pulmonary disease or both; they are best managed with radiation therapy alone. Unfavorable T3 and T4 lesions are endophytic and often associated with airway compromise and a fixed cord or cords; they are best managed with a total laryngectomy. Postoperative radiation therapy may be indicated after laryngectomy, depending on the pathologic findings. Occasionally, a small-volume unfavorable cancer, particularly if the patient is female, may be successfully managed with radiation therapy alone.

Local control rates with radiation therapy alone at the University of Florida are outlined

TABLE 55–17. Supraglottic Larynx Cancer: Local Control With Radiotherapy as Related to Suitability for Operation*

| Stage | Anatomically Suitable for Supraglottic Laryngectomy | | | Anatomically Not Suitable |
	Medically Suitable	Medically Unsuitable	Total	
T1	7/7	5/5	12/12	1/1
T2	14/17 (82%)	8/9	22/26 (85%)	12/16 (75%)
T3	3/5	3/7	6/12 (50%)	19/29 (66%)
T4	1/3	0/1	1/4	2/5

*University of Florida data (number controlled/number treated); 103 patients with 105 evaluable lesions; excludes 26 patients who died within 2 years of treatment with primary site continuously disease-free.

From Mendenhall WM, Parsons JT, Stringer SP, et al: Carcinoma of the supraglottic larynx: a basis for comparing the results of radiotherapy and surgery. Head Neck 12:204–209, 1990.

in Table 55–16. Three of the salvage operations performed were supraglottic laryngectomies; all three were successful. Local control rates versus suitability for a supraglottic laryngectomy are shown in Table 55–17. Of 22 patients whose lesions were anatomically suitable for supraglottic laryngectomy but who were medically unsuitable for the procedure, 16 (73%) were successfully treated with radiation therapy. Similarly, of 51 lesions that were anatomically unsuitable for supraglottic laryngectomy, 34 (67%) were controlled with radiation therapy. Local control as a function of cord mobility for T2 and T3 cancers is shown is Table 55–18. Although impaired cord mobility adversely affects local control rates, three of six lesions with fixed cords were successfully managed with radiation therapy.

Absolute and cause-specific survival rates at 5 years are given in Table 55–19. Severe complications usually consist of chondronecrosis and laryngeal edema that necessitates a tracheostomy. The incidence of severe complications was 6% (8 of 129 patients): 3% (4 of 115) for T1, T2, and T3 lesions, and 29% (4 of 14) for T4 cancers.

Glottic Larynx. T1 and T2 vocal cord cancers may be treated with radiation therapy or a conservative laryngectomy (i.e., cordectomy or hemilaryngectomy) with an equal probability of obtaining local control and cure. A proportion of T1 and T2 vocal cord cancers are unsuitable for a conservative operation because of the anatomic extent of the lesion or the medical condition of the patient. In the authors' experience, 10% of T1 lesions and 56% of T2 cancers were anatomically unsuitable for a conservative laryngectomy. Radiation therapy is the treatment of choice for all previously untreated T1 and T2 vocal cord cancers at the authors' institution because it results in a better voice and is less expensive than conservative surgery.

Favorable T3 lesions are those that involve one cord, are relatively exophytic, and are associated with an adequate airway. They may be treated with radiation therapy alone or a total laryngectomy with an equal probability of cure. Unfavorable T3 and T4 cancers are best managed with a total laryngectomy, often combined with postoperative radiation therapy. The occasional small-volume unfavorable cancer, particularly in a female patient, may be successfully managed with irradiation alone.

Local control rates for T1 and T2 lesions are shown in Table 55–20. T1 lesions were stratified according to whether one (T1a) or

TABLE 55–18. Supraglottic Larynx Cancer: Local Control*

| Stage | Cord Mobility | | | |
	Mobile	Decreased	Fixed	Not Stated
T2	29/33 (88%)	2/5	No data	3/4
T3	18/28 (64%)	3/6	3/6	1/1

*University of Florida data (number controlled/number treated); 83 patients.

From Mendenhall WM, Parsons JT, Stringer SP, et al: Carcinoma of the supraglottic larynx: a basis for comparing the results of radiotherapy and surgery. Head Neck 12:204–209, 1990.

TABLE 55–19. Supraglottic Larynx Cancer: 5-Year Survival*

Modified AJCC Stage†	Absolute	Cause-Specific
I	2/6	2/2
II	10/20 (50%)	10/12 (83%)
III	9/20 (45%)	9/13 (69%)
IVa	4/9	4/6
IVb	7/29 (24%)	7/22 (32%)

*University of Florida data; 84 patients.
†One patient with synchronous primary lesions was staged according to the more advanced lesions.
From Mendenhall WM, Parsons JT, Stringer SP, et al: Carcinoma of the supraglottic larynx: a basis for comparing the results of radiotherapy and surgery. Head Neck 12:204–209, 1990.

both (T1b) cords were involved and by tumor size (in the T1a subset). T2 cancers were stratified according to vocal cord mobility: normal (T2a) and impaired (T2b). The lesions were further stratified by the surgical procedure that would have been necessary had the lesions been initially treated with an operation. Local control with irradiation was obtained in 15 (94%) of 16 T1 cancers and 45 (71%) of 63 T2 cancers that would have initially required a total laryngectomy. Thirty-eight patients underwent a salvage operation for a local recurrence after radiation therapy, and 27 (71%) of these operations were successful: 6 of 10 with a hemilaryngectomy and 21 of 28 with a total laryngectomy. Four patients who had not been suitable for a hemilaryngectomy before radiation therapy later had a hemilaryngectomy for a local recurrence; the procedure was successful in two of four cases. The overall incidence of

local control with voice preservation, which includes as successes those patients who underwent salvage for a local recurrence with a hemilaryngectomy, is shown in Table 55–21. The 5-year absolute and cause-specific survival rates are given in Table 55–22. As in the supraglottic larynx, severe complications usually consist of laryngeal edema and chondronecrosis. Moderately severe and severe treatment complications were noted in 1 (<1%) of 184 T1 cancers and in 4 (3%) of 120 T2 cancers. Three of five complications occurred in patients who would have undergone a total laryngectomy had surgery been the initial treatment.

The results of treatment in a series of patients with T3 vocal cord cancer treated at the University of Florida are outlined in Table 55–23. All but two patients treated surgically underwent a total laryngectomy. Although surgery provides higher initial local and local-regional control rates, the successful salvage of patients who suffer radiation therapy failures results in ultimate local and local-regional control rates that are essentially the same. The 5-year absolute and cause-specific survival rates are virtually identical. Severe complications were noted in 9% of patients treated with radiation therapy alone.

Hypopharynx

Piriform Sinus. T1 and favorable T2 piriform sinus cancers may be managed with radiation therapy alone or with a partial laryngopharyngectomy. Patients with favora-

TABLE 55–20. T1–T2 Glottic Larynx Cancer: Local Control*

T Stage	Subgroup	Size	Excluded†	Local Control	Number Salvaged/Number Attempted Hemilaryngectomy	Total Laryngectomy	Ultimate Local Control
T1a	C	<5 mm	1	12/12 (100%)	No data	No data	12/12 (100%)
		5 to 15 mm	8	73/78 (94%)	3/4	0/1	76/78 (97%)
		>15 mm	2	45/50 (90%)	No data	4/5	49/50 (98%)
T1b	HL	All	0	14/15 (93%)	No data	0/1	14/15 (93%)
	TL	All	2	15/16 (94%)	0/1	No data	15/16 (94%)
T2a	HL	All	5	23/27 (85%)	No data	4/4	27/27 (100%)
	TL	All	2	27/38 (71%)	2/3	7/8	36/38 (95%)
T2b	HL	All	3	13/18 (72%)	1/2	2/3	16/18 (89%)
	TL	All	2	18/25 (72%)	No data	4/6	22/25 (88%)

C, suitable for cordectomy; HL, suitable for hemilaryngectomy; TL, suitable for total laryngectomy.
*University of Florida data (number controlled/number treated); 279 patients.
†Died within 2 years of treatment with primary site continuously disease free.
From Mendenhall WM, Parsons JT, Stringer SP, et al: T1–T2 vocal cord carcinoma: a basis for comparing the results of radiotherapy and surgery. Head Neck Surg 10:373–377, 1988.

patient and those concerning the tumor (Table 56–1). The heavy use of alcohol and tobacco products is a strong predisposing etiologic factor in end organ (for example, pulmonary, cardiac, hepatic, renal, and bone marrow) dysfunction; nutritional status may be adversely affected by the presence of previous surgical therapy or by tumor bulk that prevents mastication or deglutition; and the overall functional status, as a result, may preclude the administration of cytotoxic drugs, which may not be well tolerated. A thorough physical and laboratory evaluation to ensure that treatment-related toxicities will not diminish an already adversely affected quality of life is necessary in the pretreatment work-up.

Conversely, the identification of favorable prognostic factors usually predicts which patients have the best chance of benefiting from treatment, whether it pertains to those with recurrent disease or to those who are potential candidates for initial treatment. These factors include (1) good functional status as defined by the Eastern Cooperative Oncology Group, which includes the maintenance of nutritional status as evidenced by minimal weight loss, (2) small volume of disease, (3) absence of distant metastases, and (4) absence of other active chronic diseases. Age and sex are not absolute prognostic indicators in most studies.

The ultimate goal of therapy is to achieve a complete response, both clinically and histologically, because this is a major determinant of long-term disease-free survival. The intent of this chapter is to review and place into proper perspective chemotherapy studies for the treatment of recurrent and advanced HNSC.

TABLE 56–1. Prognostic Factors in Recurrent or Metastatic Disease

Functional Status
Presence of intercurrent acute or chronic disease
Site of Primary Disease
Site of Recurrent or Metastatic Disease
Local
Regional
Systemic
Previous Therapy
Surgery
Radiotherapy
Chemotherapy
   Adjuvant
   Palliative
Time Interval Since Primary Treatment

CHEMOTHERAPY FOR RECURRENT OR METASTATIC DISEASE

Single-Agent Activity in Recurrent Disease

A number of chemotherapeutic agents have been identified as active in the treatment of head and neck cancer (Al-Sarraf, 1984, 1988). Of these agents, the most active and widely used include methotrexate, bleomycin, 5-fluorouracil, and cisplatin. Because these agents were initially evaluated in the treatment of recurrent disease, the discussion pertains to this setting.

Methotrexate

Methotrexate was the first antitumor agent identified as having antitumor activity in HNSC. As such, it has undergone the most extensive and intensive investigation and generally is considered the standard with which all other drugs are compared for response and survival. Methotrexate is an inhibitor of the enzyme dihydrofolate reductase (DHFR), reducing tetrahydrofolate biosynthesis with subsequent inhibition of deoxyribonucleic acid (DNA) and ribonucleic acid (RNA) synthesis. Lack of response to treatment or development of progressive disease may reflect an acquired resistance. The occurrence of resistance to methotrexate may be produced by an alteration in metabolism of DHFR, either through an increased concentration of DHFR through gene amplification (contained in extrachromosomal DNA, termed *double minutes*, or located in the expanded homogeneously staining regions) or through an altered DHFR gene product.

The cellular uptake and polyglutamation of methotrexate may also be a factor responsible for resistance. To overcome such cellular resistance, high doses of methotrexate with leucovorin are necessary to increase the intracellular concentration and retention caused by the polyglutamylated product. The major toxic side effects consist of myelosuppression, mucositis (oral as well as gastrointestinal), and renal insufficiency.

Oral administration of this agent at low doses (20 to 40 mg/m^2) is possible; however, polyglutamation in the liver results in increasing hepatotoxicity. Various intravenous dosing schedules have been used, from low dosages (40 to 60 mg/m^2/week) to moderate dosages (500 to 1000 mg/m^2/week) to high dosages (up to 7.5 g/m^2/week, made possible with leucovorin rescue), to enhance response rates. In multi-institutional randomized trials, the high-dosage regimen has been devoid of increased therapeutic efficacy and has generally been used at the expense of increased mucosal and myelosuppressive toxicity in comparison with low-dosage regimens (40 to 60 mg/m^2 with weekly escalation by 5 to 10 mg/m^2 to the level of toxicity), which are generally considered the most appropriate methods of administration (Levitt et al., 1973; DeConti and Schoenfeld, 1981). Response rates average 40% (most of which are partial responses); the duration of response is 2 to 4 months, and survival time is 6 months. Previous or concurrent treatment with any potentially nephrotoxic agents may result in enhanced mucosal and bone marrow toxic effects caused by an impaired renal function.

Bleomycin

The bleomycins are a group of antibiotics isolated from *Streptomyces verticillus*, and they consist of 13 species. The primary cytotoxic action of this drug is scission of free bases in the DNA molecule, resulting in strand breaks. Cells in the G$_2$ phase of the cell cycle are most sensitive to its cytotoxic effects. The single-agent activity (complete and partial responses) occurred in the range of 15% to 20% in more than 300 patients studied. Because of its lack of myelosuppressive toxicity, bleomycin is ideal in combination with other, more myelosuppressive agents. Irreversible pulmonary toxicity is a major limitation; the maximal cumulative dose is approximately 300 units. Intramuscular and intravenous administration are equally effective, but when bleomycin is given by a continuous infusion schedule, the adverse pulmonary side effects may be lessened but not totally eliminated.

Cisplatin

Cisplatin (*cis*-diamminedichloroplatinum-II) is currently the most widely used agent in the treatment of both recurrent and previously untreated head and neck cancer. The exact mechanism of action is unknown, but DNA synthesis is inhibited, possibly by the formation of interstrand and intrastrand cross-linking; thus the agent's function is similar to that of an alkylating agent. Despite the similarity to an alkylating agent, there is no evidence of cross-resistance of cisplatin to that class of drugs. This very useful agent was almost discarded until it was discovered that the renal toxicity could be prevented with vigorous hydration and mannitol diuresis. Other acute and chronic toxic effects consist of nausea and vomiting, ototoxicity, and peripheral neuropathy.

A variety of schedules have been tested with the dosage ranging from 80 to 120 mg/m^2 every 3 weeks or 50 mg/m^2 on days 1 and 8 of an every-4-week schedule (Wittes et al., 1977; Hong, 1983). Single-agent activity is 25% to 40%, which is comparable with that of methotrexate; survival time in responders averages 4 to 6 months.

In several randomized studies, researchers evaluated the benefit of a daily low dose (20 mg/m^2/day for 5 days every 3 weeks) as opposed to a high dose (120 mg/m^2/day once every 3 weeks) without demonstrating any significant response difference (26% and 33%). From ovarian and testicular carcinoma trials, there appears to be a dose-response curve for cisplatin. Whereas doses from 60 to 120 mg/m^2 are not significantly different in activity, doses of up to 200 mg/m^2 every 3 to 4 weeks seem to demonstrate a further increase in activity. A single-arm study addressed the dose-response relationship of cisplatin at a total dose of 200 mg/m^2 administered at 40 to 50 mg/m^2 over 4 to 5 days. A 73% objective response rate in recurrent head and neck disease was achieved. Unfortunately, nephrotoxicity, ototoxicity, and neurotoxicity prevailed and limited the dose. Comparisons of high doses (120 to 200 mg/m^2) with standard doses (60 to 100 mg/m^2) of cisplatin have not substantiated these data. Neither the high response rate nor the median survival figures were improved with high doses.

Until successful methods for the amelioration or prevention of platinum-induced neurotoxicity are developed, high-dose studies cannot be recommended. Two compounds have been tested in multiple clinical trials. Diethyldithiocarbamate is a thiol compound that reportedly not only allows administration of higher cumulative doses of cisplatin by preventing renal impairment but also functions as an immunomodulator. Randomized trials have not conclusively substantiated these claims. WR2721 is an organic thiophosphate compound reported to have

TABLE 56–3. Sequence of Combining Chemotherapy, Surgery, and Radiotherapy

Induction (Resectable or Unresectable)
Chemotherapy→radiotherapy (complete responders)
Chemotherapy→surgery plus postoperative
  radiotherapy (complete or partial responders)
Sandwich Technique (Resectable)
Surgery→chemotherapy→radiotherapy
Adjuvant (Resectable or Definitive Radiotherapy)
Surgery plus radiotherapy→chemotherapy
Radiotherapy with or without surgery→chemotherapy
Extended Adjuvant Therapy (Resectable)
Chemotherapy→radiotherapy→chemotherapy
Chemotherapy→surgery plus
  radiotherapy→chemotherapy
Chemoradiotherapy (Unresectable)
Concurrent chemoradiotherapy (radiosensitization)
Concurrent chemoradiotherapy (full dose)
Alternating or interdigitating chemoradiotherapy

For many years, biologic predictors (i.e., mitogen response, cutaneous antigen reactivity) have been reported to correlate with response in other tumor models but have not been universally adopted. C1q binding macromolecules (C1qBA), which are capable of binding the first component of complement, are a circulating immune complex, the measured level of which is capable of predicting not only the development of distant metastases in untreated patients with surgically resectable tumors but also the response to induction chemotherapy (Schantz et al., 1989). In a cohort of 43 patients treated with a cisplatin-based combination, elevated total immunoglobulin and C1qBA levels inversely correlated with complete and partial response. The biologic mechanism for this observation remains to be elucidated. This clinical finding may be a valuable diagnostic as well as prognostic tool but requires confirmation in large clinical trials before acceptance.

The cellular differentiation (well or poorly differentiated) and morphologic characteristics as analyzed by light microscopy and flow cytometry (diploid versus aneuploid) continue to undergo evaluation as they apply to tumor response.

Support of the early treatment of HNSC has its foundation in the Goldie-Coldman hypothesis, which indicates that de novo resistance rapidly develops over a very narrow range of cellular growth with the development of a drug-resistant phenotype. A direct relationship between tumor volume and chemoresistance exists; cell-cycle–de-pendent resistance increases with tumor volume and the loss of exponential growth characteristics. The growth fraction and sensitivity to chemotherapy is higher in the neoadjuvant situation, and de novo resistance is theoretically less.

When treatment is given before surgery or radiotherapy, chemotherapy that was modestly effective against recurrent disease now results in a substantial increase in overall response; 50% or more of patients achieve complete clinical remissions. Selected studies have described histologic complete response in up to 75% of the surgical or biopsy specimens. Altered vasculature after surgery and radiotherapy precludes optimal local drug concentrations, but the growth fraction within the tumor may be higher and drug sensitivity may be enhanced before these treatments.

The presumed reason for recurrence in advanced disease that was treated primarily with surgery and radiotherapy is persistent local microscopic disease or distant micrometastatic disease. The ability of adjuvant chemotherapy to eradicate distant micrometastatic disease is established for certain tumors such as locally advanced breast carcinoma and osteogenic sarcoma, in which it appears to prolong survival by reducing systemic relapse.

The potential advantages of induction therapy include an increased effectiveness in the treatment of advanced locoregional disease by resulting in sufficient cytoreduction to allow surgical resectability, to decrease the extent of local treatment required, and to enhance local and regional control with subsequent surgery or radiotherapy by eliminating disease at the microscopic level. Organ preservation is now in vogue as a prime incentive for this approach.

TABLE 56–4. Prognostic Factors of Response to Induction Chemotherapy

Functional Status
Nutritional Status
Primary Site
Tumor Differentiation
Cellular ploidy
Tumor Burden
Size of primary tumor (resectable versus unresectable)
Extent of nodal disease (resectable versus unresectable)
Biologic Determinants
Cellular immunity
Humoral immunity

Certain disadvantages accompany the clinical course when this treatment is undertaken. Unfortunately, 2 to 3 months of chemotherapy would necessarily precede 2 months of radiotherapy, thereby prolonging an already difficult therapy. Abbreviation of this time frame is possible by a simultaneous chemoradiotherapy combination. A borderline resectable tumor may progress and become unresectable while the patient is receiving chemotherapy. This latter situation is the exception rather than the rule. An enhanced radiosensitivity in residual tumor may be accompanied by enhanced mucosal toxicity. Agents causing this phenomenon are usually well defined, including bleomycin and doxorubicin (Adriamycin). Surprisingly enough, the development of local toxicity has not affected the locoregional therapy in large-scale studies, even when these agents are used. Finally, it is not uncommon for a patient who responds to chemotherapy or for the patient's physician to refuse a planned surgical procedure. Such a change may render the entire treatment ineffective.

Single-Agent and Combination Induction Chemotherapy

Initiated in the early 1960s, single-agent induction chemotherapy trials were proposed to enhance locoregional control by the administration of chemotherapy before or concurrently with radiotherapy, almost exclusively in inoperable cases. Since then, the role of chemotherapy has evolved on the basis of the experience with these agents in treating recurrent disease.

Bleomycin, cisplatin, and methotrexate with or without leucovorin as single agents produce overall response rates of from 20% to 80% (the average is 45%), but complete responses were documented in fewer than 10%. In the late 1970s, a combination of cisplatin and bleomycin by bolus injection or infusion resulted in a 20% complete response rate and overall response rate of 70%. When cisplatin and bleomycin were combined with a *Vinca* alkaloid (vincristine or vinblastine), response rates then approached 90%, with complete responses in up to 28% of patients. In some of these trials, only one cycle of treatment was administered before other definitive treatment.

In the early 1980s, a combination of cisplatin and continuous infusion of 5-fluorouracil was investigated at the Wayne State University in previously untreated patients with encouraging results. For the first time, complete response rates were higher than 50%, and overall response rates averaged 80% to 90% as the number of courses were increased from two to three cycles and as the 5-fluorouracil dosage was escalated from a 4-day to a 5-day infusion schedule. The resultant complete response rate improved from 19% to 54%, and overall response improved from 88% to 93%.

Numerous investigators have confirmed these figures and have made every attempt to improve upon them. Three cycles of therapy seemed to be optimal inasmuch as no further increase in the complete response rate was obtained by adding a fourth cycle of chemotherapy. Modulation of the toxic effects of the 5-fluorouracil with allopurinol did not allow further dosage escalation or improve response.

A number of these patients achieved pathologic complete remissions, which allowed treatment of the primary site with radiotherapy alone, and prolonged disease-free survival rates were obtained. There seems to be a direct correlation between response to chemotherapy and response to subsequent radiotherapy that is independent of the initial stage of the tumor or its histologic differentiation.

Other novel approaches include alternating multiple combinations into an overall intensive regimen that contains non–cross-resistant drugs in hopes of markedly increasing the complete response rate. The Wayne State University group attempted intensification to five cycles of induction therapy by alternating three cycles of 5-fluorouracil/cisplatin combination with three biweekly cycles of high-dose methotrexate with leucovorin and 5-fluorouracil at 28-day intervals. Although toxicity was increased and a dramatic improvement in complete (46%) and overall response (84%) was not forthcoming, this pilot study did demonstrate the feasibility of such an approach. Subsequently, an additional cycle of cisplatin/5-fluorouracil was added, and the cycle intervals were shortened to 21 days. Although a 76% complete response rate was reported, the toxicity was also increased.

As an extension of their recurrent disease trials, Hill and Price's (1987) group continues to test the benefits of a combination without cisplatin. Because there has been minimal

which chemotherapy potentiates the cytotoxic effects of radiation include the inhibition of sublethal damage repair, hypoxic cell sensitization, and cell-to-cell synchronization. These studies have been extensively reviewed (Vokes and Weichselbaum, 1990).

A number of theoretic rationales have been postulated to further explain the interaction between chemotherapy and radiotherapy. These include spatial cooperation (independent action of each modality), toxicity independence (full-dose delivery of each modality without additive toxicity), chemoprotection (protection of normal tissues, which allows higher doses of radiotherapy to be delivered), and chemosensitization or enhancement (increased activity of the chemotherapy and radiotherapy within the treatment field through the use of smaller drug doses, which have less systemic toxicity).

All of the previously mentioned drugs with proven activity (cisplatin, platinum analogs, 5-fluorouracil, bleomycin, hydroxyurea, mitomycin-C, and methotrexate) have been evaluated either as single agents or in multiagent combinations with radiotherapy. Not only do these agents have systemic activity, but they also have documented activity as radiosensitizers (i.e., cisplatin, bleomycin, and 5-fluorouracil). The radiotherapy has been given by a conventional once-a-day fractionation, by split-course technique, or by twice-a-day hyperfractionated schedules. Both randomized and nonrandomized studies have addressed the benefit of this approach (Fu, 1985; Fu et al., 1987). Although an improved local tumor control rate and disease-free survival time have been reported with bleomycin, methotrexate, 5-fluorouracil, and mitomycin-C, an impact on overall survival has not been firmly established.

Cisplatin has been evaluated in a number of schedules and doses in combination with radiotherapy. Early studies reported schedules of weekly infusion of 30 mg/m^2/week of cisplatin throughout the radiotherapy course. Although these doses could provide local radiosensitization, they would be devoid of systemic effect, and those patients would remain at risk for development for metastatic disease. Daily doses of 15 to 20 mg/m^2 on 5 consecutive days every 3 weeks given concurrently with radiotherapy for the duration of therapy provide maximal exposure to the locoregional site and yield a systemic effect. High doses (100–120 mg/m^2) of cisplatin have been given every 3 weeks during the

course of radiotherapy. Patients who have either failed to improve with or are not candidates for induction therapy with 5-fluorouracil and cisplatin have received radiotherapy and concurrent cisplatin on days 1, 22, and 43 with a 40% complete response rate, as well as long-term survival benefit (>30 months) for some. This regimen was reported by the RTOG to be feasible, well tolerated, and effective in 124 patients with advanced disease; a complete response rate was achieved in 69%, and survival at 2 years was achieved by 55%.

The more favorable therapeutic index of second-generation platinum analogs and the similar order of synergism with radiation therapy in comparison with the parent compound encouraged trials of escalating weekly dosages of carboplatin from 60 to 100 mg/m^2 or monthly doses of 400 mg/m^2 in combination with five daily fractions of 1.8 to 2.0 Gy/week for 6 to 8 weeks. In a group of 29 patients with unresectable disease, 15 (52%) were considered to be in complete remission after treatment with a median time to progression of 6 months and survival time of 11 months; 53% of these patients were alive after 8 to 30 months of follow-up. The use of carboplatin is especially attractive in view of its more favorable toxicity pattern. Combination with other drugs without overlapping toxicity in this setting is being pursued.

Optimal integration of 5-fluorouracil and radiotherapy requires a high dose and a continuous exposure for synergy (800 to 1000 mg/m^2/day for 5 days). Complete response rates of up to 50% have been reported in patients with inoperable tumors. The remainder of patients, although classified as partial responders, had survival times equivalent to those of the complete responders. These partial responders reflect the presence of fibrosis or normal tissue edema, which are consequences of the concomitant treatment. The median survival time of all patients was 37 months. When this concept was applied to a small population of patients with advanced laryngeal and hypopharyngeal cancer, 86% had organ preservation and a median survival time of 45 months.

Combination chemotherapy given in conjunction with radiotherapy is not only feasible but also an effective approach. A 5-day continuous infusion of 800 mg/m^2/day of 5-fluorouracil combined with 60 mg/m^2/day of cisplatin can be administered every other week on day 1 in combination with radiotherapy at 2 Gy on days 1 to 5 for a total of seven cycles (70 Gy). Synchronous radiotherapy and infusion of 5-fluorouracil are highly effective in inducing local control, and the cytocidal potential of 5-fluorouracil is increased with the concomitant administration of leucovorin. Another permutation involved the incorporation of accelerated hyperfractionated radiotherapy (Wendt et al., 1989). Actuarial probability of 2-year survival was 52% in this uncontrolled trial. Dosage modification may be necessary, however, to prevent severe mucositis and weight loss. Decrease in the dosage intensity, of both the radiotherapy and the chemotherapy, may render the entire treatment suboptimal.

The concept of delivering chemotherapy alternatively with split-course radiotherapy to further improve the therapeutic ratio has been supported by animal model data and is restated in the mathematical Goldie-Coldman model. Drug sensitivity and, for that matter, radiosensitivity relate to the spontaneous mutation rate. The basic assumption is that responsiveness and curability are achieved if no permanently resistant cell lines are present. Curability rapidly diminishes with the appearance of a single resistant cell if only one effective therapy is available or with the appearance of a doubly resistant line if two equally effective therapies are available, and so on. The implication of this theory is that the most effective mode of therapy would be an intensive front-loaded treatment strategy in which as many effective agents as possible are used. Because radiotherapy is the most efficient and indiscriminant cytotoxic agent, the addition of multiple short courses of radiotherapy to each course of chemotherapy should reduce the probability that drug-resistant clones will emerge during the protracted course of chemotherapy. The overall time course for the completion of treatment would also be considerably shortened.

When a schema of sequential chemotherapy (vinblastine, bleomycin, and methotrexate every 14 days for four cycles) and radiotherapy was compared with a schema of chemotherapy and radiotherapy alternating every 2 weeks to produce a minimal total dose of 60 Gy, progression-free survival rates were higher with the alternating schedule, although there was no survival advantage (Merlano et al., 1988).

In another design, cisplatin and 5-fluorouracil could be employed at full doses on days 1, 28, and 56 alternating with hyperfraction-

ated (twice-a-day) radiotherapy on days 15, 42, and 70.

These studies have illustrated that chemotherapy given in combination with radiotherapy is probably superior to radiotherapy alone, at least for advanced and inoperable head and neck cancer. When the chemotherapeutic agent is used as a single agent, the antitumor activity is less likely because of its inherent activity than because of an additive or synergistic effect in combination with the radiotherapy. Whereas locoregional control may improve, the rate of distant metastases has not been affected.

Use of drugs in systemic dosages is therefore imperative if considerations other than locoregional control are important. Accomplishing this, however, raises the issue of enhanced toxicity. Investigation of an innovative combination is currently evolving. Hydroxyurea and continuous infusion of 5-fluorouracil are both cytotoxic agents and radiosensitizers. Administered concurrently with radiotherapy to 39 patients with inoperable or recurrent disease, the dose of hydroxyurea was escalated safely from 500 to 2000 mg orally with 800 mg/m^2/day of 5-fluorouracil 5 times every other week until the completion of radiotherapy. The activity in these poor-prognosis patients exceeded 90%, and investigation in untreated patients is therefore warranted (Vokes et al., 1989a, 1989b).

In summary, concurrent chemotherapy and radiotherapy with single agents does seem to improve local control and disease-free survival times. Overall survival may not be improved, as yet, but the rate of toxicity has increased, especially in multiagent trials. Careful thought must be given to the choice of drugs to be combined with radiotherapy to allow maximal integration of both modalities. This must be pursued in a phase III format.

ALTERNATIVE APPROACHES FOR DRUG DELIVERY

Regional intra-arterial chemotherapy has the potential advantage of delivering a higher concentration of effective chemotherapeutic agents to the tumor site while minimizing systemic toxic reactions. This technique has been used for more than three decades in various tumor-bearing areas; however, it has not been established in the head and neck as a routine. The regional blood flow to the paranasal sinuses, the tongue, and the buccal cavity makes these areas very accessible to infusion and extends the possibility of organ preservation. Various chemotherapeutic agents have been used for this purpose, including methotrexate, 5-fluorouracil, cisplatin, and bleomycin. Radiotherapy has been used in conjunction with infusions of 5-fluorouracil, but the toxicity is excessive. No controlled trials in which intra-arterial therapy has been compared to intravenous therapy have been reported and unless they are undertaken by a cooperative group, they could not be pursued.

CONCLUSIONS

Each newly published therapeutic approach, regardless of whether it results in an improved overall response rate and survival benefit, provides additional insight into feasible innovations that may ultimately be the key to long-term survival and cure. It must not be forgotten that steady progress in understanding the biologic processes of the disease is being made simultaneously with attempts to treat it. Each published study was designed to evaluate response in a homogeneous clinical setting (advanced, stage IV, operable, inoperable, recurrent, and so forth). Unfortunately, most studies are apt to be otherwise very heterogeneous. More appropriate studies of advanced disease of only one site such as the larynx, the paranasal sinus, or the nasopharynx are being pursued, but accrual of data will depend on availability of sufficient numbers of patients for study.

The optimal regimen and timing of combination chemotherapy for the initial treatment of advanced, recurrent, or metastatic disease has not been defined. Old questions still remain to be answered, and new questions will be raised by future trials:

1. How important is dose intensity, especially as it pertains to multimodality (chemoradiotherapy) and multidisciplinary treatment?

2. How do physicians deal with the increase in toxic effects associated with the ever-increasing use of intensive chemotherapy?

3. What is the future of dose intensification through drug modulation?

4. Is the continued attempt to lessen or eliminate locoregional therapy through preoperative chemotherapy and radiotherapy clinically and biologically sound?

5. Should this approach be applied to all patients?

Only through development of phase III trials on a national or an international level, with sufficient patient populations to withstand rigorous statistical evaluation, will these points be adequately addressed.

SUGGESTED READINGS

Al-Sarraf M: Chemotherapy strategies in squamous cell carcinoma of the head and neck. CRC Crit Rev Oncol Hematol 1:323–355, 1984.

Al-Sarraf M: Head and neck cancer: chemotherapy concepts. Semin Oncol 1:70–85, 1988.

Browman GP, Levine MN, Goodyear MD, et al: Methotrexate/fluorouracil scheduling influences normal tissue toxicity but not antitumor effects in patients with squamous cell head and neck cancer: results from a randomized trial. J Clin Oncol 6:963–968, 1988.

Carboplatin (JM-8). Current Perspectives and Future Directions. In Bunn PA, Canetta R, Ozols RF, Rozencweig M (eds): Philadelphia: WB Saunders, 1990.

DeConti RC, Schoenfeld D: A randomized prospective comparison of intermittent methotrexate, methotrexate with leucovorin, and a methotrexate combination in head and neck cancer. Cancer 48:1061–1072, 1981.

Department of Veterans Affairs Laryngeal Cancer Study Group: Induction chemotherapy plus radiation compared with surgery plus radiation in patients with advanced laryngeal cancer. N Engl J Med 324:1685–1690, 1991.

Dimery IW, Peters LJ, Goepfert H, et al.: Survival in stage IV nasopharyngeal carcinoma after combination chemotherapy and radiotherapy. In Salmon SE (ed): Adjuvant Therapy of Cancer VI (pp 82–91). Philadelphia: WB Saunders, 1990a.

Dimery IW, Legha SS, Shirinian M, Hong WK: Fluorouracil, doxorubicin, cyclophosphamide, and cisplatin combination chemotherapy in advanced or recurrent salivary gland carcinoma. J Clin Oncol 8:1056–1062, 1990b.

Dreyfuss AL, Clark JR, Wright JE, et al: Continuous infusion high-dose leucovorin with 5-fluorouracil and cisplatin for untreated stage IV carcinoma of the head and neck. Ann Intern Med 112:167–172, 1990.

Ervin TJ, Clark JR, Weichelbaum RR, et al: An analysis of induction and adjuvant chemotherapy in the multidisciplinary treatment of squamous cell carcinoma of the head and neck. J Clin Oncol 5:10–20, 1987.

Forestiere AA, Takasugi BJ, Baker SR, et al: High-dose cisplatin in advanced head and neck cancer. Cancer Chemother Pharmacol 19:155–158, 1987.

Fu KK: Concurrent radiotherapy and chemotherapy. In Wittes RE (ed): Head and Neck Cancer (pp 221–248). New York: John Wiley, 1985.

Fu KK, Phillips TL, Silverberg IY, et al: Combined radiotherapy and chemotherapy with bleomycin and methotrexate for advanced inoperable head and neck cancer: update of a Northern California Oncology Group randomized trial. J Clin Oncol 5:1410–1418, 1987.

Greenberg B, Ahmann F, Garawald H, et al: Neoadjuvant therapy for advanced head and neck cancer with allopurinol-modulated high dose 5-fluorouracil and cisplatin: a phase I-II study. Cancer 59:1860–1865, 1987.

Head and Neck Contracts Program: Adjuvant chemotherapy for advanced head and neck squamous carcinoma. Cancer 60:301–311, 1987.

Hill BT, Price LA: The significance of primary site in assessing chemotherapy response and survival in advanced squamous cell carcinomas of the head and neck treated with initial combination chemotherapy without cisplatin: analyses at nine years. *In* Salmon SE (ed): Adjuvant Therapy of Cancer V (pp 111–118). Orlando, FL: Grune & Stratton, 1987.

Hong WK, Schaeffer S, Issel B, et al: A prospective randomized trial of methotrexate versus cisplatin in the treatment of recurrent squamous cell carcinoma of the head and neck. Cancer 44:19–25, 1983.

Johnson JT, Myers EN, Schramm VL, et al: Adjuvant chemotherapy for high risk squamous cell carcinoma of the head and neck. J Clin Oncol 5:456–458, 1987.

Levitt M, Mosher MB, DeConti RC, et al: Improved therapeutic index of methotrexate with "leucovorin rescue." Cancer Res 33:1729–1733, 1973.

Merlano M, Rosso R, Sertoli MR, et al: Sequential versus alternating chemotherapy and radiotherapy in stage III-IV squamous cell carcinoma of the head and neck: a phase III study. J Clin Oncol 6:627–632, 1988.

Pitman SW, Kowal CD, Bertino JR: Methotrexate and 5-fluorouracil in sequence in squamous head and neck cancer. Semin Oncol 10(Suppl 2):15–19, 1983.

Rentschler RE, Wilbur DW, Petti GH, et al: Adjuvant methotrexate escalated to toxicity for resectable stage III and IV squamous head and neck carcinomas—a prospective, randomized study. J Clin Oncol 5:278–285, 1987.

Schantz SP, Savage HE, Racz T, et al: Immunologic determinants of head and neck cancer response to induction chemotherapy. J Clin Oncol 7:857–864, 1989.

Vokes EE, Choi KE, Schilsky RL, et al: Cisplatin, fluorouracil, and high dose leucovorin for recurrent or metastatic head and neck cancer. J Clin Oncol 6:618–626, 1988.

Vokes EE, Moran WJ, Mick R, et al: Neoadjuvant and adjuvant methotrexate, cisplatin, and fluorouracil in multimodality therapy of head and neck cancer. J Clin Oncol 7:838–845, 1989a.

Vokes EE, Panje WR, Schilsky RL, et al: Hydroxyurea, fluorouracil, and concomitant radiotherapy in poor-prognosis head and neck cancer: A Phase I-II study. J Clin Oncol 7:761–768, 1989b.

Vokes EE, Weichselbaum RR: Concomitant chemoradiotherapy: Rationale and clinical experience in patients with solid tumors. J Clin Oncol 8:911–934, 1990.

Wendt TG, Hartenstein RC, Wustrow TPU, Lissner J: Cisplatin, fluorouracil with leucovorin calcium enhancement, and synchronous accelerated radiotherapy in the management of locally advanced head and neck cancer: a phase II study. J Clin Oncol 7:471–476, 1989.

Wittes RE, Cvitkovic E, Shah J, et al: Cis-dichlorodiammine platinum (II) in the treatment of epidermoid carcinoma of the head and neck. Cancer Treat Rep 61:359–366, 1977.

Yabro JW, Bornstein RS, Mastrangelo MJ (eds): Sequential methotrexate and 5-fluorouracil in the management of neoplastic disease. Semin Oncol 10(Suppl 2):1–39, 1983.

CHAPTER 57

General Principles of Skull Base Surgery

Peter S. Roland, MD   Bruce E. Mickey, MD

Many tumors involving the bony skull base were traditionally thought to be unresectable, in part because they traversed the traditional anatomic boundaries separating the surgical specialties of neurosurgery and otolaryngology, and in part because their proximity to cranial nerves, crucial vascular structures, and the basal subarachnoid cisterns rendered such resections hazardous. Advances in imaging technology and surgical technique and a spirit of cooperation among a number of surgical specialties have made possible the exposure and removal of some tumors previously thought to be inoperable and have provided a reduction in the morbidity and mortality previously associated with the removal of others. Although no generally accepted definition of the term *skull base tumor* exists, it has come to refer to tumor involving the bony skull base so that either the tumor or its operative resection places the patient at risk for (1) a cranial nerve injury, (2) a vascular injury, or (3) a cerebrospinal fluid fistula, such that its operative management is benefited by a team approach involving two or more surgical specialties. This chapter is a review of the strategies available to minimize the morbidity of the three most common complications of surgical procedures at the skull base, and the different surgical approaches available to these tumors are outlined.

HAZARDS OF SKULL BASE SURGERY

Cranial Nerve Injuries

When preservation of a cranial nerve is being attempted in the course of resection of a tumor, the most helpful elements in the surgeon's armamentarium are a thorough knowledge of the regional anatomy and the magnification afforded by the operating microscope. Attempts to prove the value of intraoperative monitoring of cranial nerve function have been difficult, although the monitoring process itself is probably beneficial because it serves to heighten the awareness of the surgeon during the tumor resection. Continuous monitoring of the electromyogram of the facial musculature does provide instantaneous evidence of injury to the facial nerve and has facilitated its localization and preservation in the surgery of acoustic neuromas and other tumors involving the cerebellopontine angle. A similar technique has been applied to the extraocular muscles for aiding in the preservation of cranial nerves III, IV, and VI during surgical procedures involving the cavernous sinus and orbital apex. Evoked potential monitoring, for either the optic or the cochlear nerve, has been hindered because information about the integrity of the nerve is delayed. Some surgeons believe that even delayed knowledge of a partial loss of function is of value. Direct recording from the cochlear nucleus has been used in hearing conservation surgery for acoustic neuroma in order to minimize this delay. The degree of adherence to or invasion of a cranial nerve by a given tumor and the biologic characteristics of the tumor itself determine whether it is possible to preserve the nerve in the course of achieving a curative resection. When a cranial nerve cannot be preserved, the proper management of the patient can significantly lessen the morbidity and, in some cases, prevent a mortality related to the ensuing neurologic deficit.

Cranial Nerve I (Olfactory)

In surgical procedures on the anterior skull base, no attempt should be made to spare olfaction if doing so would compromise complete tumor removal or adequate surgical margins. On the other hand, although the small dural cuffs by which the peripheral ramifications of the olfactory bulb pass through the cribriform plate provide a potential route for postoperative cerebrospinal fluid fistulas, the olfactory apparatus should not be sacrificed merely to obtain a watertight dural seal. When sacrifice of olfaction is necessary, the postoperative anosmia that occurs is perceived as a mild to moderate disability by the patient. The ability to enjoy a meal will be impaired, and this may further exacerbate postoperative nutritional problems and postoperative depression. Because the protective function of olfaction will be lost, anosmic patients should be urged to have functioning smoke detectors in their homes and to avoid the use of natural gas appliances. Occasionally, operative trauma to the olfactory nerve leaves the patient with a sensation of unpleasant odors or dysosmia. The incidence of this problem after the deliberate sacrifice of olfaction may be diminished by transecting the olfactory tract posterior to the bulb.

Cranial Nerve II (Optic)

Loss of vision in one eye is relatively well tolerated despite a reduced visual field and the absence of depth perception. In such cases, special care should be given to the preservation of the remaining eye: for example, when postoperative radiation therapy for a malignant tumor is planned.

Cranial Nerve III (Oculomotor)

Injuries to cranial nerve III produce varying degrees of ptosis, mydriasis, and exotropia with diplopia. When the injury is partial, selective eye muscle surgery may be of benefit in restoring binocular vision in some fields of gaze. With a complete loss of function of cranial nerve III, the restoration of any binocular vision is difficult, and the resulting ptosis serves a useful function as a patch; the patient may be counseled that the distressed eye is of little use except to serve as a backup in the case of an injury to the contralateral eye. Although some return of cranial nerve III function has been reported after primary anastomosis or cable grafting of a divided nerve, the synkinesis resulting from aberrant regeneration in such cases may be as disabling as a total paralysis.

Cranial Nerve IV (Trochlear)

A loss of function of cranial nerve IV produces vertical diplopia (one image above the other) and cyclotorsion (image tilting). Tilting the head eliminates the diplopia in primary gaze, and some patients may be satisfied with this method of compensation. A better result may be obtained by surgical procedures on the extraocular muscles, but such procedures should be deferred for 6 to 12 months.

Cranial Nerve V (Trigeminal)

The sensory loss produced by a trigeminal nerve injury, although distressing to the patient, produces little in the way of objective disability unless the cornea is involved or unless the lesion is a bilateral one. When the cornea is anesthetic, the patient is left at risk for the development of exposure keratitis, and the patient and family should be cautioned to inspect the cornea and conjunctiva on the involved side frequently. The combination of an anesthetic cornea and a facial nerve injury places the patient at such a great risk for exposure keratitis that a tarsorrhaphy or some other method of mechanical protection of the cornea is indicated. A bilateral loss of trigeminal sensation is rare, but when it occurs, the resulting intraoral anesthesia produces difficulty manipulating a bolus of food and places the patient at risk for burns when ingesting hot drinks. In some patients, trigeminal sensory loss is associated with uncomfortable or painful dysesthesia, which may be alleviated somewhat from medical therapy with carbamazepine (Tegretol) or other anticonvulsants. Data from patients who have had the sensory portion of the trigeminal nerve sectioned proximal to the ganglion for the treatment of trigeminal neuralgia suggest that 1% to 2% of them eventually develop anesthesia dolorosa, a dreadful central pain syndrome refractory to treatment.

An injury to the motor division of the trigeminal nerve produces a paralysis of the muscles of mastication on that side. The unopposed contraction of the contralateral musculature produces a shift of the mandible, which often results in malocclusion and painful degenerative changes in the temporomandibular joint. The early use of intermaxillary fixation may help prevent this shift, and physical therapy is of benefit in minimizing the secondary temporomandibular joint arthritis.

Cranial Nerve VI (Abducens)

Recovery of cranial nerve VI function after the surgical repair of a transected nerve has been reported, and such a repair is worth undertaking if both ends of the nerve can be identified. The diplopia produced by an ipsilateral rectus palsy can be ameliorated by surgical procedures on the extraocular muscles in patients left with a partial or complete deficit of cranial nerve VI.

Cranial Nerve VII (Facial)

As with any cranial nerve, an important principle in avoiding an inadvertent injury to the facial nerve is its definitive identification in every situation in which it is placed at risk. Such exposure allows the safest resection of a tumor in the vicinity of the nerve and allows the best possible management of a transected nerve with either a primary anastomosis or an interposition graft.

The most urgent consideration in the management of a postoperative facial nerve paralysis is the protection of the cornea, especially if a simultaneous injury to the trigeminal nerve has produced corneal anesthesia. The problem should be addressed in the immediate postoperative period with the frequent instillation of drops and ointment on the paralyzed side. The patient, the family, and the paramedical personnel involved in the patient's care should be educated in the prevention of exposure keratitis. A gold weight implanted in the upper lid or a temporary lateral tarsorrhaphy is often of benefit in the acute postoperative period while the need for longer term protection is being evaluated. The psychologic impact of even a partial facial paralysis should not be underestimated, and these patients often benefit from counseling, psychotherapy, or interaction with support groups such as those organized by the Acoustic Neuroma Association.

Cranial Nerve VIII (Vestibulocochlear)

Unilateral loss of vestibular function is usually well tolerated by younger patients, but older patients may require a prolonged period for recovery and may benefit from physical therapy during the recovery process. Prolonged vertigo in the postoperative period may be the result of a subtotal labyrinthectomy or an incomplete injury to the vestibular division of cranial nerve VIII with the preservation of some vestibular function. In this setting, the presence of residual vestibular function should be confirmed by electronystagmography; if it is present, revision labyrinthectomy or vestibular nerve section should be considered in an effort to control symptoms when they are disabling. Bilateral loss of vestibular function is usually associated with some persistent disability and may require the use of an assistive device such as a cane or a walker.

When useful hearing is present preoperatively, intraoperative monitoring of the auditory brain stem response may be of benefit in its preservation. Lateral to medial manipulation of the nerve seems to degrade the auditory brain stem response more than does medial to lateral manipulation, presumably because of the fragility of the nerve as it enters the cochlea. Most patients tolerate unilateral anacusis so well that they are not interested in overcoming the inconvenience or expense involved in using assistive devices such as the CROS (contralateral routing of signal) hearing aid. Patients with bilateral hearing loss, but a conductive loss only on one side, may benefit from the placement of an implantable bone-conduction device (Xomed Corporation). Patients with bilateral sensorineural hearing loss should be evaluated as candidates for a cochlear implant and may be counseled with cautious optimism that the quality of these devices is improving. An alternative to the use of the cochlear implant is the vibrotactile hearing aid, which translates sound energy into a vibratory signal delivered through the skin.

Cranial Nerve IX (Glossopharyngeal)

An isolated injury of the glossopharyngeal nerve produces little disability and may in some cases be difficult to detect. This loss of function becomes significant when it is associated with an injury to the vagus nerve.

Cranial Nerve X (Vagus)

An isolated injury of the vagus nerve produces an ipsilateral vocal fold paralysis as well as pharyngeal muscle incoordination. The loss of innervation of the stylopharyngeus muscle and of sensation of the posterior and lateral pharyngeal walls produced by an associated glossopharyngeal nerve injury increases the ensuing difficulty with swallowing and the risk of aspiration and pneumonia.

Some patients with tumors that have produced a preoperative deficit of cranial nerves IX and X may have compensated well, especially if the loss of function has been slow and gradual. Other patients with preoperative lower cranial nerve deficits may be debilitated by chronic aspiration; these patients may benefit from an injection of polytef (Teflon) into the paralyzed vocal fold and a 2- to 4-week period of vigorous pulmonary toilet and intense nutritional support in an effort to allow the tracheobronchial tree to recover. Postoperatively, if there is any question as to the ability of the patient to protect the tracheobronchial tree, especially if the patient is older or has an impaired level of consciousness, a tracheostomy should be performed, and careful attention should be paid to nutrition.

In cases in which the vagus nerve is known to have been transected, injection of the vocal fold should be performed at the earliest opportunity. With high transections that have impaired the function of the superior laryngeal nerve, the paralyzed vocal cord will eventually lie at a lower level than the contralateral cord, and a cartilage implantation may be necessary several months later. Many patients with combined vagal and glossopharyngeal injuries also benefit from a cricopharyngeal myotomy. With aggressive rehabilitation, a motivated patient can eventually be decannulated and learn to resume oral nutrition. The rehabilitation process requires the services of a speech therapist or another person trained in the management of swallowing problems and may take several months to complete.

Cranial Nerve XI (Spinal Accessory)

An injury to the spinal accessory nerve produces denervation of the sternocleidomastoid and trapezius muscles. The trapezius muscle deficit results in anterior and inferior displacement of the humeral head within the glenoid fossa, in some cases producing traumatic arthritis of the shoulder and a chronic pain syndrome. The function of the trapezius should be assessed at the earliest possible time after surgical procedures in which cranial nerve XI has been injured or placed at risk, because the early institution of physical therapy will minimize chronic shoulder problems.

Cranial Nerve XII (Hypoglossal)

An isolated loss of hypoglossal nerve function is of little consequence to most patients. When combined with a loss of cranial nerve VII function or with a loss of function of cranial nerves IX and X, a unilateral hypoglossal injury can increase difficulty with chewing or the initiation of swallowing. A bilateral and complete loss of hypoglossal nerve function leaves the patient unable to chew and swallow and usually dependent on chronic enteral nutrition. The resulting deficit also leaves such a patient unable to produce articulate speech.

Vascular Injuries

Internal Carotid Artery

Acute unilateral occlusion of the cervical internal carotid artery produces a cerebral infarction in 20% of patients. Therefore, when a skull base neoplasm lies adjacent to one internal carotid artery or involves its wall, preoperative arteriography should assess the patency and caliber of potential collateral vessels: the anterior communicating artery and the ipsilateral posterior communicating artery. Preoperatively, focal narrowing of the lumen of the internal carotid artery by as much as 50% does not significantly reduce flow and cannot be used to predict tolerance to complete occlusion. Moreover, the demonstration of angiographically patent collaterals does not guarantee tolerance to occlusion of the vessel, so that patients in whom the internal carotid artery must clearly be sacrificed to provide an oncologically sound margin must be further evaluated. Temporary occlusion of the vessel in the conscious patient with a transfemoral balloon catheter, coupled with cerebral blood flow measurement, has been proposed as one method of identifying those patients unable to tolerate internal carotid artery occlusion without a bypass of some kind to provide collateral flow (Sekhar et al., 1987).

In removal of a tumor that involves one wall of the internal carotid artery, consideration should be given to exposing the vessel proximal and distal to the site of involvement before tumor resection. Should the internal carotid artery be inadvertently injured intraoperatively, the temptation to gain hemostasis with hemostats or cautery should be resisted because a minor laceration may thus be rendered irreparable. If possible, adequate hemostasis should be achieved with local pressure while normal vessels are exposed proximal and distal to the site of the injury. Clips or clamps designed for temporary occlusion should be applied, and the injury should be evaluated and repaired.

During temporary occlusion, intravascular volume and blood pressure should be normalized, and barbiturates should be administered for cerebral protection. If the vessel must be sacrificed, it should be occluded as distally as possible, preferably just proximal to the ophthalmic artery, in order to minimize the risk of thrombus formation distal to the occlusion. When the decision is made to sacrifice a vessel, a decision must also be made (on the basis of preoperative evaluation and the overall status of the patient) as to the value of performing a bypass procedure. After occlusion, the patient should receive small amounts of volume expanders and provided with blood pressure support in order to maintain the adequacy of collateral flow.

Vertebral Artery

The vertebral artery is rarely involved with an otherwise resectable skull base neoplasm but is commonly exposed in procedures involving the jugular foramen, such as temporal bone resections and the excision of paragangliomas. Angiographic evaluation of both vertebral arteries is advisable in all such patients because 10% of them will have a unilaterally hypoplastic artery, which mandates preservation of the contralateral vessel.

Sigmoid Sinus, Jugular Bulb, and Internal Jugular Vein

The acute occlusion of one internal jugular vein is almost invariably well tolerated, in part because of the presence of abundant collateral veins at the level of the jugular bulb. When the jugular bulb itself is occluded in a gradual fashion, as is commonly the case with a glomus jugulare tumor or a schwannoma involving the lower cranial nerves, proximal collateral veins develop to compensate for the obstruction. On the other hand, the acute occlusion of a previously patent jugular bulb or sigmoid sinus is not well tolerated by every patient, and in some patients it produces a venous infarction. When the occlusion of a previously patent transverse sinus, sigmoid sinus, or jugular bulb might be required for the exposure or resection of a tumor, it is imperative that the communication of the two transverse sinuses at the torcular Herophili be demonstrated angiographically. One series of angiographic studies documented complete absence of one transverse sinus in 4% of patients and essentially unilateral drainage from the torcular in 24% (Huang et al., 1984). If the surgeon elects to sacrifice a sinus by packing it, care should be taken not to force the packing so far proximally as to occlude potential collateral veins.

Cerebrospinal Fluid Fistulas

Surgical procedures that traverse the nasopharynx, the paranasal sinuses, or the mastoid air cells and the middle ear and then enter the subarachnoid space leave the patient at risk for a cerebrospinal fluid (CSF) fistula and secondary bacterial meningitis. Careful planning of the operative exposure and meticulous wound closure minimize the incidence of these complications, and an understanding of CSF physiology with a systematic approach to the management of those fistulas that do develop allows most wounds to seal without further operative intervention.

CSF Physiology in the Postoperative Period

CSF is formed within the ventricular system at a rate of 0.3 mL/minute, or approximately 500 mL/day, and enters the subarachnoid space in the posterior fossa via midline and the lateral foramina in the fourth ventricle. After circulating within the subarachnoid space, it re-enters the vascular system through arachnoid granulations in the dural venous sinuses, largely in the superior sagittal sinus. The contamination of the CSF circulation by blood or necrotic debris at the time of surgery often impairs CSF resorption, either directly by mechanical interference in the arachnoid granulations or indirectly by inciting an inflammatory response in the subarachnoid space. The resulting syndrome may vary from a brief, asymptomatic elevation of CSF pressure to a clinically manifest aseptic meningitis with fever, severe headache, meningismus, and an elevation of CSF pressure lasting 2 to 3 weeks. The incidence of clinically apparent aseptic meningitis after surgical procedures involving the posterior cranial fossa ranges from 7% to 70%. An awareness of this entity is important for the evaluation of fever and meningeal signs and for the management of CSF fistulas. It is equally important to recognize that it can be minimized by avoiding unnecessary intraoperative contamination of the subarachnoid space with blood, bone dust, and other debris.

Wound Closure

Surgical procedures that have the potential to produce a communication between the subarachnoid space and the nasal cavity or nasopharynx require that the dura be closed in a watertight fashion whenever possible during wound closure. In many situations, a secure dural closure is not possible because of the passage of cranial nerves through the dural defect or because of marked attenuation of the dura at the surgical margins; in these cases, the path of the potential fistula must be obliterated.

Dural defects left by surgical procedures involving the temporal bone may be isolated from the eustachian tube and nasopharynx with a free graft of autologous fat. In a similar fashion, a fat graft is usually sufficient to plug the defect in the floor of the sella left by transsphenoidal surgical procedures that enter the subarachnoid space. Unfortunately, a fat graft does not survive in a grossly contaminated space and is therefore not suitable for repairing a large defect in the dura and skull base that communicates *directly* with the nasopharynx. In this setting, the interposition of a vascularized flap of muscle or muscle and skin between the dural repair and the nasopharynx has proved to be effective in protecting the subarachnoid space from bacterial contamination. With the availability of free tissue transfer by use of microvascular anastomoses, this protection may be extended to any area of the skull base (Fig. 57–1).

Many patients whose dura has not been closed in a watertight fashion develop an extradural collection of CSF, or pseudomeningocele, beneath a scalp or skin flap or

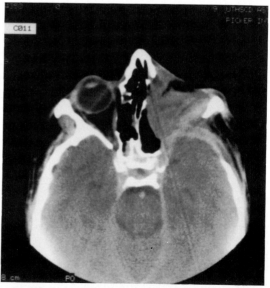

Figure 57–1. Postoperative computed tomographic scan of a 27-year-old woman who had undergone an orbital exenteration as well as a resection of the cribriform plate, the orbital frontal bone, and the greater and lesser sphenoid wings on the left in an attempt to excise an undifferentiated carcinoma arising in the posterior ethmoids on that side. A portion of the rectus abdominis muscle, transferred by use of microvascular techniques, fills the orbital defect and isolates the dural repair from the nasal cavity.

within a defect left by extensive bone or soft tissue resection. The impairment of CSF absorption that underlies such a pseudomeningocele, or a CSF fistula, is usually self-limited. Unfortunately, surfaces that are continuously bathed in CSF soon develop a membranous covering, and a fistulous tract or pseudomeningocele thus lined may remain patent after CSF pressures have normalized. For this reason, the early institution of temporary diversion of CSF may be more effective in producing a well-healed wound than would similar measures instituted after a fistula or pseudomeningocele has been present for 1 or 2 weeks.

Management of CSF Fistulas

If, during the postoperative course, there is a question as to the presence of a CSF fistula, the patient should be observed carefully and repeatedly. If leaking CSF cannot be observed by a physician but is suspected on the basis of testimony from the patient and the nursing staff, it is probably sufficient to nurse the patient with the head of the bed elevated 45° at all times until the question has been resolved. Any patient with a definite fistula should have CSF pressure lowered by one of several measures: (1) multiple lumbar punctures, (2) continuous or intermittent external drainage via a lumbar or ventricular catheter, or (3) permanent CSF diversion by means of an indwelling shunt.

One effective method used for lowering CSF pressure involves the percutaneous placement of a polyethylene catheter in the lumbar subarachnoid space and the establishment of a closed drainage system. The patient is then nursed with the head of the bed slightly elevated (10° or 15°), and the drain is opened intermittently, usually 1 hour out of 3, in an effort to remove 200 to 400 mL of CSF per 24-hour period. It has been empirically noted that the risk of catheter-related infections rises after 5 days, and if prolonged drainage is required, the catheter should be changed on the fifth day. Most patients complain of headache and nausea while the drain is open and should be medicated symptomatically. The decision to re-explore a wound in an effort to directly obliterate the fistula must be individualized, but most patients should receive two 5-day trials of lumbar CSF drainage before re-exploration. Patients with a prolonged or permanent CSF absorptive defect, manifest in some instances by ventricular enlargement on serial computed tomography scans, may require long-term CSF diversion by means of a lumboperitoneal or ventriculoperitoneal shunt.

REGIONAL APPROACHES TO THE SKULL BASE

Frontal-Ethmoidal Region

The most common indication for a resection of the anterior skull base is the involvement of the cribriform plate by a malignant neoplasm arising in the frontal or ethmoid sinuses. The inability to resect these tumors adequately by use of transfacial approaches prompted the development of a combined craniofacial approach (Fig. 57–2), first reported in 1954 (Smith et al., 1954). In the transcranial portion of the procedure, a bicoronal incision is commonly used with preservation of the anterior pericranium as a separate vascularized flap to be interposed at the time of closure between the dura and the nasal cavity. A bifrontal craniotomy is placed as low as possible over the orbital rim in order to minimize the amount of frontal lobe retraction required to expose the cribriform plate and orbital roof. With the exposure thus provided, the cribriform plate and the overlying dura and olfactory bulbs may be resected with the tumor. Inferior exposure must be tailored to the individual tumor, with use of standard approaches to the ethmoid sinuses, the nose, and the orbit.

The resection of the cribriform plate requires the sacrifice of olfaction, which is rarely preserved preoperatively; however, this sacrifice does not threaten other cranial nerve function unless an orbital exenteration is also performed. If the dural resection is anterior to the lesser sphenoid wing, it is usually possible to repair the resulting dural defect in a watertight fashion with use of a free graft of pericranium harvested from posterior to the coronal suture. This repair is then reinforced by the infolding of the attached anterior leaf of pericranium. Some surgeons also repair the bone defect left by the resection with a free graft harvested from the inner table of the bifrontal bone flap. If this bone reconstruction is performed, the graft should be placed superior to the vascularized anterior flap of pericranium to isolate it from the nasopharynx.

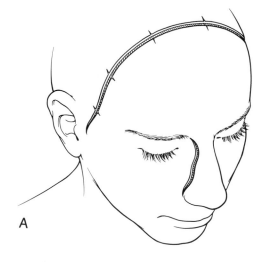

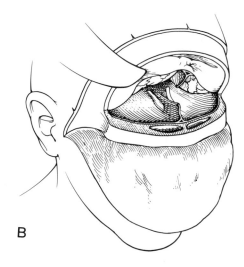

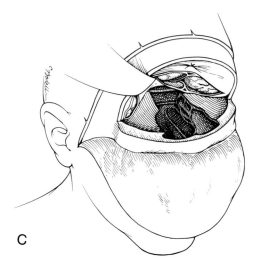

Figure 57–2. A craniofacial approach to the anterior skull base. *A.* A bicoronal incision is used to expose the supraorbital region bilaterally, and a modified Weber-Ferguson incision is used here to expose the ethmoid sinuses and nasal cavity. *B.* The dura is opened, the olfactory tract is sectioned on either side, and the dura is incised circumferentially around the cribriform plate. *C.* The dura is reflected from the floor of the anterior cranial fossa, and the resulting dural defect is repaired with a free graft of pericranium. The anterior dural incision, shown open here, is usually closed prior to the bony resection. The cribriform plate and the tumor are excised en bloc.

The major complications of a craniofacial approach to the anterior skull base are related to local infection. Review of three large series, which include a total of 175 patients, reveals a 3.5% incidence of fatal infectious complications: brain abscess, epidural abscess, and meningitis (Ketcham and Van Buren, 1985; Chessman et al., 1986; Shah et al., 1987). The most common nonfatal complication of the procedure is an epidural infection at the operative site, which despite broad-spectrum antibiotics perioperatively required reoperation for removal of the bifrontal bone flap in 6 of 26 patients in one series (Shah et al., 1987). In view of the fact that most of these patients are elderly, with disease that has proved refractory to previous surgical procedures and radiation therapy, the surgical procedure itself seems to be a safe one.

On the other hand, the value of craniofacial resections for malignant disease involving the anterior cranial fossa remains unclear. Reports of 5-year survival rates of 30% to 50% are meaningless in view of the diversity of the neoplasms included with regard to both their biologic behavior and their degree of skull base involvement. On the basis of experience reported by other researchers, invasion of the brain, involvement of the middle cranial fossa, involvement of both orbits, and the presence of distant metastases appear to be contraindications for surgery. Undifferentiated carcinomas and sarcomas are likely to recur despite an aggressive surgical resection, but well-differentiated adenocarcinomas and epidermoid carcinomas appear to have a low risk for recurrence. Because of the relative rarity of these tumors, a cooperative study involving several institutions is required in order to determine definitive indications for surgery.

Although the exact role of craniofacial resections for the management of malignant neoplasms remains undefined, they are clearly of benefit in the management of benign tumors such as meningiomas that penetrate the cribriform plate to involve the ethmoid sinuses, and some extensive mucoceles of the frontal and ethmoid sinuses that penetrate the dura to involve the frontal lobes.

Sphenoidal Region

The body of the sphenoid bone and the greater and lesser wings that extend laterally from it form the central portion of the skull base. The most common neoplasm involving the body of the sphenoid bone is the pituitary adenoma, a slow-growing neoplasm that may invade the dura and bone of the floor of the sella turcica inferiorly and the dural wall of the cavernous sinus laterally. Farther laterally, en plaque meningiomas of the dura of the middle cranial fossa often invade the bone of the greater and lesser sphenoid wings and may involve the periorbita and the temporalis and pterygoid muscles as well. Juvenile nasopharyngeal angiofibromas arising in the nasopharynx may enter the sphenoid sinus and erode bone to involve the medial aspect of the cavernous sinus, or they may extend laterally through the pterygomaxillary fissure and erode bone to involve the inferior aspect of the cavernous sinus and the floor of the middle cranial fossa. In addition, a number of malignant neoplasms arising from the upper aerodigestive tract may involve the parapharyngeal space and the infratemporal fossa and thus gain access to the body or the greater wing of the sphenoid. Whereas most pituitary adenomas may be adequately managed via a midline transsphenoidal approach, tumors that involve both the floor of the middle cranial fossa and the infratemporal fossa or orbit are best exposed through lateral approaches.

Many variations of the transsphenoidal approach to the floor of the sella have been developed. Although the sphenoid sinus may be well-exposed transethmoidally, most surgeons believe that the midline exposure achieved transnasally can minimize the risk of injury to the laterally placed internal carotid arteries. The transnasal approach may be performed directly through the nostril, but a slightly wider exposure has been claimed for the sublabial approach, which is more commonly performed. When the subarachnoid space is entered in the course of resecting a pituitary adenoma, it is imperative that it be isolated from the nasopharynx at the conclusion of the procedure. Autologous fat is usually placed within the sella, and a piece of the bony or cartilaginous septum is wedged into the defect in the sellar floor to support it. Some surgeons prefer to pack the sphenoid sinus with fat as well, whereas others reserve this maneuver for those cases in which the floor of the sella cannot be repaired directly.

The most common causes of operative mortality, which varies between 0.4% and 2.0%, are meningitis secondary to a CSF fistula, cerebral infarction secondary to injury of the internal carotid artery within the cavernous sinus, and direct injury to the hypothalamus in the course of the removal of the tumor. The reported incidences of CSF rhinorrhea postoperatively vary between 1.5% and 6.5%; most patients respond to a period of temporary CSF diversion via a lumbar subarachnoid catheter. Transsphenoidal excision is curative for pituitary adenomas enclosed within the dural boundaries of the sella; tumors that invade dura may not be amenable to complete resection and may require adjuvant treatment with radiation therapy or antisecretory drugs.

Several combined exposures of both the intracranial and the extracranial aspects of the floor of the middle cranial fossa have been developed. For those disease processes that do not involve the petrous temporal bone, a preauricular incision is preferred. The combination of a frontotemporal craniotomy with lateral displacement of the zygoma allows complete resection of the greater and lesser sphenoid wings and wide exposure of the lateral orbit, the infratemporal fossa, and the middle cranial fossa (Fig. 57–3). Most meningiomas invading the sphenoid wings can be managed without entering the paranasal sinuses or nasopharynx, and a watertight dural closure in these cases is therefore not mandatory.

Most of the morbidity of resecting invasive sphenoid wing meningiomas is related to injury to the cranial nerves traversing the orbital apex, but at least one death caused by injury of the internal carotid artery has been reported. Juvenile nasopharyngeal an-

CHAPTER 58

Management of Patients With Snoring and Obstructive Sleep Apnea

David N. F. Fairbanks, MD   David W. Fairbanks, MD

For more than a century, physicians have observed the coexistence of such common complaints as snoring and excessive sleepiness, but it was not until the past quarter-century that their pathologic interrelationships were recognized. Only in the past decade have effective and acceptable treatment strategies become available.

The patient who snores often finds a visit to the otolaryngologist to be the most logical point of entry into the medical care system. Conversely, excessively sleepy patients tend to seek out neurologists or sleep specialists or diagnostic sleep laboratories initially. When breathing problems are recognized, however, an airway examination, such as otolaryngologists perform, is required.

SYMPTOM EVALUATION

In the patient's interview, notations are made about consistency of snoring (every night? every position?), interruptions to breathing (pauses, gasps, and snorts), quality of sleep, and the impact on the lives of roommates or other household members. A yes-no question about daytime sleepiness is often unrevealing because of the tendency of many males to deny or ignore its presence. More information is discovered by questions about feeling refreshed upon awakening, drowsi-

ness on the job, or difficulty staying awake while driving a motor vehicle or watching a television show. In children, daytime somnolence is manifest as hyperactivity (a frantic effort to stay awake).

Table 58-1 lists the typical symptoms of obstructive sleep apnea. Questions about nasal breathing, alcohol and drug use, and medication consumption are also pertinent. General medical health questions are also vital (i.e., cardiopulmonary disease and blood pressure).

PHYSICAL EXAMINATION

Examination is directed to the upper airway, the objective being an assessment of adequacy of air flow through its entirety. This begins with the nose both in the normal and in the decongested states (after phenylephrine sprays).

In the mouth examination attention is paid to the size of the tongue in relation to the space available for its occupancy. Note is made of narrowing or deformities of the dental arch and especially of a receding mandible.

Special attention is paid to the lowermost border (trailing edge) of the soft palate. In most normal patients, it lies above the horizontal plane of the tongue. In many patients

1061

TABLE 58–1. Signs and Symptoms of Obstructive Sleep Apnea

Loud snoring (notable in all patients)
Abnormal motor activity during sleep
Hypersomnolence (notable in most patients)
Obesity (frequent but not necessary)
Hyperactivity (children)
Personality changes
Hypertension (frequent)
Nocturnal cardiac arrhythmias (frequent)
Cor pulmonale (in advanced cases)

who snore and are apneic, it can be seen only after the tongue is forcibly depressed (the "descending curtain" sign). Tonsils are seen and appear large enough to occupy airway space in one third of adults who snore and are apneic and in almost all children who snore. Other frequent findings in such adults include flabbiness or redundancy of the faucial pillars, vertical folds, or rugae in the posterior pharyngeal mucosa; nasopharyngeal opening narrowed to a slitlike dimension (best seen when the patient is placed supine); and various uvular appearances (long, bulky, flabby, webbed to the pillars, or traversed with horizontal ridges).

The nasopharynx, the hypopharynx, and the larynx can generally be examined well with mirrors, although topical anesthesia is often required (sprayed tetracaine or gargled viscous lidocaine). Flexible endoscopy, which creates added time and cost, is reserved for patients with impossible gagginess. Non-otolaryngologists and physicians not skilled in mirror examinations must also resort to endoscopy, which does not provide natural or life-sized views of the anatomy.

Adenoidal tissue is occasionally found even in middle-aged adults. Tonsil tags in the hypopharynx and lingual tonsils deserve attention. Neoplasms and lingual thyroid tissue have been reported in patients with apnea.

Examination of the hypopharynx through a flexible endoscope during Mueller's maneuver is recommended by a number of investigators as a means of assessing competence in the hypopharyngeal portion of the airway. The collapsed hypopharynx appears more like the interior of the esophagus than an airway. As long as it is recognized that such a maneuver is an artificial event (and may not replicate what occurs during sleep), the information obtained may be helpful.

Cephalometry is another strategy em-ployed to measure airway competence and to localize the area of incompetence. Information obtained is correlated with that of the other physical findings, inasmuch as airway collapse is a three- (rather than a two-) dimensional phenomenon.

Unfortunately, the "site-of-lesion" determination is usually somewhat imprecise because the pathologic state is usually multifactorial: the combined effects of tongue, palatal, mucosal, and nasal problems. Only in some instances is one obvious factor notable (such as large, space-occupying tonsils, in which case the surgical correction yields highly predictable success).

THE NASAL FACTOR

To assess the nasal component of airway compromise, the authors employ a simple at-home test: using a topical nasal decongestant spray on three nonconsecutive nights (nights on which the spray is not used are for "control" observations; Table 58–2). If nasal decongestion brings dramatic relief of snoring (and apnea), then it is predictable that correction, usually surgical, of the nasal airway problem will relieve the snoring (and apnea). If the nose spray gives partial relief of snoring, so will nasal treatments; and if no improvement is obtained, then nasal surgery will likely prove disappointing as a cure for snoring.

Almost half of patients who snore express some complaints about nasal congestion; similarly, about half are found to have some nasal septal or turbinate deformities. However, only about one in ten seems to benefit from the nose spray test or nasal treatments, and they are generally those with the most stuffy noses and with simple snoring or mild to moderate apnea at worst. In patients with

TABLE 58–2. Nose Spray Test for Assessment of Nasal Component of Snoring

Instructions given to patient accompanying sample bottle of oxymetazoline (Afrin) nasal spray.
Nose Spray Test
Three sprays in each nostril
½ hour before bedtime every *other* night this week
Compare snoring on spray nights with snoring on nonspray nights

(This is a test only; the spray is not intended for use as a remedy for snoring or stuffy nose.)

over 100 apnea episodes per night, nasal obstruction is more likely a minor determinant.

The most frequent nasal problem encountered is nasal septal and turbinate deformity, and the authors employ nasal septoplasty with submucous resection of turbinates for the most predictable results.

SLEEP STUDIES

Ideally, every patient with a sleep-related breathing disorder should undergo an overnight sleep evaluation (i.e., polysomnography). In practice, compromises are sometimes made with the recognition that risk is increased with regard to misdiagnosis or failure to appreciate the seriousness of airway compromise or the patient's intolerance to it. Children who snore but are otherwise quite healthy may not require sleep studies, and the same might be said for robust, healthy young adults who snore, who do not suffer from daytime sleepiness, and whose roommates are genuinely competent observers who do not recognize any apneic events after they have been instructed in how to identify them. Unfortunately, some of the reported tragic complications that have followed uvulopalatopharyngoplasty were probably avoidable had the surgeon obtained a sleep study, which would have alerted the surgeon to the surgical and anesthetic risks that would be encountered. Polysomnography quantifies the frequency and duration of apneic events and the impact that such events have on oxygen desaturation and cardiovascular responses thereto. Also, it describes disruption of sleep architecture.

OTHER LABORATORY STUDIES

The patient's general state of health dictates which studies are required; they might include cardiovascular, pulmonary, and neurologic evaluations. Thyroid studies are appropriate for apneic patients because hypothyroidism may create muscular hypotonicity.

NONSURGICAL MANAGEMENT

At the end of the initial visit, the patient is provided with the brochure *Snoring—Not Funny, Not Hopeless* (published by the American Academy of Otolaryngology–Head and Neck Surgery). The self-help remedies contained therein (and listed in Table 58–3) are reviewed with the patient. Unfortunately, very few patients who seek medical consultation are cured by self-help methods alone.

The occasional patient who is hypothyroid can be improved with thyroid replacement medications, but otherwise drug therapy is usually an exercise in frustration. Protriptyline (Vivactil) is a mood-elevating agent that keeps the patient out of the deep stages of sleep, especially rapid eye movement stage, in which apneic episodes are most prevalent. It is given in 5-, 10-, or 15-mg doses about an hour before bedtime, beginning at the 5-mg dose and increasing to larger doses as needed and as tolerated. Side effects include stimulation and sleeplessness with nightmares, urinary retention, and (in men) interference with erections and painful ejaculations. Male patients rarely consider such drug therapy to be satisfactory.

Continuous positive air pressure delivered by a nasal mask serves to keep the airway open, acting as a pneumatic splint. Almost all obstructive sleep apnea patients can benefit from this treatment method—except, of course, those patients whose nasal airways are obstructed. Patient compliance is the other drawback. The prospect of sleeping every night for the rest of one's life with an air pressure pump running and a tightly fitted mask strapped to one's face is incentive

TABLE 58–3. Self-Help Remedies

For adults who are mild or occasional snorers, the following advice is given:

1. Adopt an athletic life-style and exercise daily to develop good muscle tone and lose weight.
2. Avoid tranquilizers, sleeping pills, and antihistamines before bedtime.
3. Avoid alcoholic beverages within 4 hours of retiring.
4. Avoid heavy meals within 3 hours of retiring.
5. Avoid getting overtired; establish regular sleeping patterns.
6. Sleep sideways rather than on the back. Consider sewing a pocket on the pajama back to hold a tennis ball. This helps you avoid sleeping on your back.
7. Try wearing a whiplash collar, one that is wide enough to keep the chin up high.
8. Tilt the entire bed with the head upward 4 inches (place two bricks under the bedposts at the bedhead).
9. Allow the nonsnorer to get to sleep first.

enough for many patients to seek a surgical treatment.

Nevertheless, continuous positive air pressure has almost entirely replaced tracheostomy as treatment for severely apneic patients who are poor surgical risks and for patients who suffer surgical failure. It is also useful for patients who are awaiting surgery or who are unsatisfied with the uncertainty that surgery has to offer; it can also be useful in the postoperative period for maintenance of airway patency.

Of the variety of mouth inserts that are available, the authors have found occasional usefulness from an appliance that advances the mandible into a prognathic state. This pulls the tongue forward a centimeter or so. It is used for postoperative patients who are not fully satisfied with the surgical result but who are not symptomatic enough to accept continuous positive air pressure. An orthodontist can fashion such a device for the patient to wear at night.

UVULOPALATOPHARYNGOPLASTY

Uvulopalatopharyngoplasty, referred to variously as palatopharyngoplasty, uvulovelo-plasty, or uvulopalatoplasty, is an operation that is relatively new to Western physicians. Evolution in the operative technique in any new operation is driven by the need to achieve successful correction of pathologic anatomy as well as to avoid complications (Fairbanks, 1990).

The authors use a technique resembling that originally described by Ikematsu (1964, 1987) and Fujita (1981, 1987), but it is modified to achieve what seem to be some desirable objectives: (1) to maximize the lateralization of the posterior pharyngeal pillars, including submucosal musculature, which would increase the lateral dimension of the oropharyngeal airway; (2) to interrupt some of the sphincteric action of the palatal-naso-pharyngeal musculature, which would increase the patency of the nasopharyngeal airway; and (3) to maximize shortening of the soft palate in the lateral ports while sparing midline musculature (resulting in a "squared-off" soft palate appearance). These objectives are important for prevention of palatal tethering and nasopharyngeal stenosis and for preservation of mobility and function of the palate for purposeful closure.

Technique

Prophylactic antimicrobials are initiated the night before surgery with a single oral dose of dicloxacillin (or equivalent) and 1 hour before surgery with 1 g of nafcillin intravenously. Preoperative sedatives are avoided because patients with obstructive sleep apnea are often overreactive to them, and airway crisis may occur. Likewise, the anesthesiologist should be well aware of the compromised status of the airway in such patients. The orally intubated and anesthetized patient is placed in the head-extended position with the Crowe-Davis tonsillectomy mouth gag and the Ring tongue blade in place.

The areas to be surgically excised are injected with small amounts of epinephrine 1:100,000 solution (usually provided in 1% lidocaine). This is to promote hemostasis, and it is done by earlier agreement with the anesthesiologist, who selects an appropriate inhalation agent (e.g., not halothane).

The mucosa on either side of the uvula is clamped with hemostats and then incised in an oblique direction as in Figure 58–1. This drooping mucosal web between the uvula and the posterior pillars (which is typically found in apneic patients) harbors few muscular fibers of the nasopharyngeal sphincter. Severance increases the mobility of the pillars and prevents soft palatal scar contraction ("tethering").

The palatopharyngeal incision is designed as three sides of a rectangle (Fig. 58–2). It begins at the base of the tongue lateral to the inferior tonsillar pole and extends cephalad in the sulcus or angle formed between the internal surface of the mandible and the anterior tonsillar pillar. At about 1 to 2 cm above the level of the trailing edge of the soft palate, the incision makes a 90° angle, transverses the soft palate horizontally, then angles 90° downward again in a symmetric fashion in comparison with the opposite side. The ideal level for the horizontal palatal incision is at the location of the palatal "dimple" as described by Dickson (1987).

The soft palatal mucosa and submucosa with glands and fat are then stripped away from the muscular layers, beginning at the horizontal palatal incision and moving downward, toward the trailing edge of the soft palate and uvula. One or two brisk bleeders are often encountered near the corners of the incision, and they must be suture-ligated with heavy plain catgut (cautery is inade-

will be encountered, which will inhibit mobilization of the posterior pillars. This fibrous scar should be carefully stripped away from the muscle fibers of the tonsillar fossa (superior pharyngeal constrictor), and the dissection should avoid damage to the underlying musculature or penetration of the muscle into the structures of the carotid sheath.

Dissection should proceed as deep into the hypopharynx as the surgeon can safely reach for fossa closure and for control of any bleeding that may occur. Bleeders are clamped and suture-ligated (which is less traumatic to the musculature than is heavy electrocoagulation); good hemostasis is essential.

The posterior tonsillar pillar is then advanced in a lateral-cephalad direction toward the corner of the palatopharyngeal incision (Fig. 58–4). Contiguous submucosal muscle fibers should be included in this advancement because that inclusion will increase the lateralizing effect and expand the lateral dimension of the pharyngeal airway. This maneuver should flatten out the redundancy (the vertical folds) of the posterior pharyn-

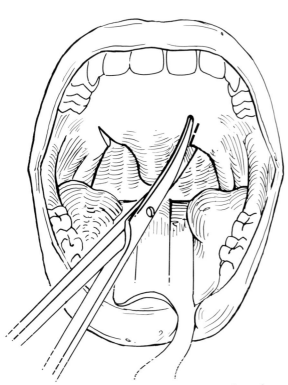

Figure 58–1. Apnea patient with absent tonsils, redundant pharyngeal mucosa with longitudinal folds, and drooping soft palate with webbing between uvula and pillars. Begin procedure by severing the uvulopalatal webs. This mobilizes the posterior tonsillar pillars, releases the contracture, and prevents palatal tethering. (From Fairbanks DNF: Method of Fairbanks. *In* Fairbanks DNF, et al [eds]: Snoring and Obstructive Sleep Apnea [pp 160–167]. New York: Raven Press, 1987.)

quate). The uvula is amputated at the level of the trailing edge of the soft palatal muscle fibers (Fig. 58–3). Traction on the uvula during its amputation should be avoided because that results in excessive shortening of the uvula with interruption of the insertions of the levator palatini muscles into the muscularis uvula. Loss of palatal sphincteric action (required for closure during speech and swallowing) has been attributed to excessive excision of the uvula and midline palatal tissue. A tiny bleeder on each side of the uvula requires electrocoagulation.

Tonsils (present in one third of patients with snoring and apnea) are excised, and other soft tissues between the posterior tonsillar pillars and the lateral incisions are all stripped out, down to the muscular layers. The plane of dissection is the peritonsillar space. However, if a previous tonsillectomy has been performed, dense fibrous scar tissue

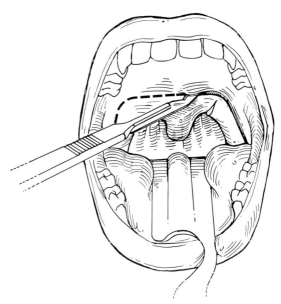

Figure 58–2. Box-shaped incision (through mucosa only) begins at tongue base, ascends in sulcus between anterior pillar and mandible, and then turns medially to cross soft palate about midway between trailing edges of soft and hard palates. (From Fairbanks DNF: Method of Fairbanks. *In* Fairbanks DNF, et al [eds]: Snoring and Obstructive Sleep Apnea [pp 160–167]. New York: Raven Press, 1987.)

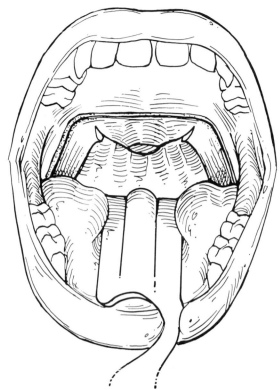

Figure 58–3. Mucosa, glands, fat, and fibrous tissue removed down to—but not through—muscular layers. The uvula is amputated at the trailing edge of soft palatal muscle fibers. (From Fairbanks DNF: Method of Fairbanks. *In* Fairbanks DNF, et al [eds]: Snoring and Obstructive Sleep Apnea [pp 160–167]. New York: Raven Press, 1987.)

geal mucosa. If this does not occur, then a little more of the posterior pillar mucosa should be trimmed.

The pillar is then advanced and fixated into its new lateralized position with multiple sutures of 3–0 polyglycolic acid (Dexon "S"). The sutures pass through the mucosa into superficial muscular layers so that the muscular elements of the pillar as well as the mucosa are lateralized. Furthermore, this eliminates "dead space" in which hematoma might accumulate. The authors prefer to put in the second stitch before tying the first so that the positioning is more visible (Fig. 58–5). Suturing then progresses downward to the tongue base, where a small opening is left unsutured to allow spontaneous drainage. The dissection and closure on the opposite side are identical.

The palatal closure is then accomplished as the nasal surface of the mucosa is advanced to meet the incision on the oral sur-

face (Fig. 58–6). Redundant or flabby mucosa is trimmed, and the sutures are put in place, including a small amount of muscle fiber in the mucosal closure.

POSTOPERATIVE MANAGEMENT

Intravenous antimicrobial prophylaxis is maintained for 48 hours; if swelling or edema begins to be apparent in the operating room or early in the postoperative period, a short course of steroids is given (i.e., 125 mg of Solu-Medrol every 8 hours for three doses).

In patients with simple snoring, postoperative care is the same as in adult tonsillectomy patients. However, in patients with obstructive sleep apnea, pain medication is given more sparingly (i.e., small doses of parenteral morphine or oral elixir of acetaminophen with added codeine: 30 mg/teaspoon), with the recognition that apnea is aggravated by narcotics and that life-threatening loss of airway can be precipitated, especially in the postanesthetic period or the period of postoperative edema of the airway.

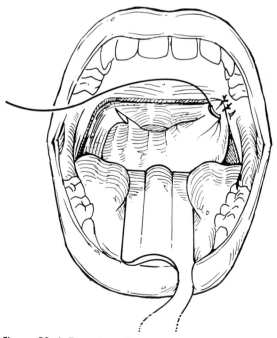

Figure 58–4. Posterior pillar is trimmed and advanced in upward-outward direction to increase lateral dimension of oropharyngeal airway. Note how this tightening maneuver removes redundant pharyngeal folds. (From Fairbanks DNF: Method of Fairbanks. *In* Fairbanks DNF, et al [eds]: Snoring and Obstructive Sleep Apnea [pp 160–167]. New York: Raven Press, 1987.)

Figure 58–5. Sutures pass through mucosal edges and through superficial muscular layers to prevent hematoma formation, maximize lateralization of posterior pillar, and provide mucosal coverage of surgical defect. (From Fairbanks DNF: Method of Fairbanks. *In* Fairbanks DNF, et al [eds]: Snoring and Obstructive Sleep Apnea [pp 160–167]. New York: Raven Press, 1987.)

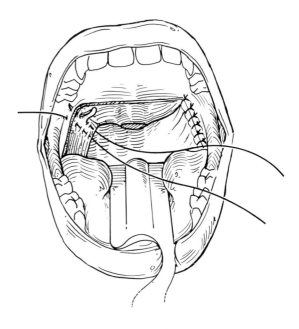

Figure 58–6. Nasal surface of the soft palate is advanced forward to meet the cut edge on the oral surface. This covers the surgical defect on the oral surface and minimizes risk of stenosis. It also expands the anteroposterior dimension of the nasopharyngeal airway. Note squared-off appearance, designed to minimize nasopharyngeal regurgitation. (From Fairbanks DNF: Method of Fairbanks. *In* Fairbanks DNF, et al [eds]: Snoring and Obstructive Sleep Apnea [pp 160–167]. New York: Raven Press. 1987.)

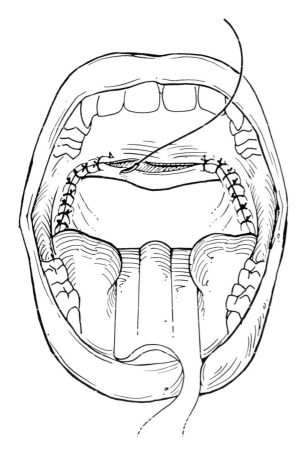

Similarly, antiemetics, sleeping medications, and sedative-tranquilizers can precipitate an apneic crisis; therefore, the authors' nurses are instructed never to accept a telephone order for any of these medications by a physician who is not personally acquainted with the particular patient and is not knowledgeable about the patient's disease.

Any patient with significant apnea preoperatively needs vigilant postoperative monitoring of respiration. The intensive care unit is the ideal place for the first 24 hours after surgery.

Cases of severe apnea that are worrisome to the surgeon and anesthesiologist can be managed with 24 to 48 hours of endotracheal intubation. The oral endotracheal tube is simply left in place with 40% oxygen and mist running over its opening (a bypass connector) and frequent suctioning for secretions. The cough reflex is obtunded with occasional instillations of 2 mL of 4% lidocaine into the tube as necessary. Fortunately, narcotics and hypnotics can be administered more liberally for pain relief in such an intubated patient.

SUGGESTED READINGS

Dickson RI: Determining how much palate to resect. *In* Fairbanks DNF, Fujita S, Ikematsu T, Simmons FB (eds): Snoring and Obstructive Sleep Apnea (pp 167–170). New York: Raven Press, 1987.

Fairbanks DNF: Method of Fairbanks. *In* Fairbanks DNF, Fujita S, Ikematsu T, Simmons FB (eds): Snoring and Obstructive Sleep Apnea (pp 160–167). New York: Raven Press, 1987.

Fairbanks DNF: Uvulopalatopharyngoplasty: complications and avoidance strategies. Otolaryngol Head Neck Surg 102:239–245, 1990.

Fujita S: Method of Fujita. *In* Fairbanks DNF, Fujita S, Ikematsu T, Simmons FB (eds): Snoring and Obstructive Sleep Apnea (pp 134–153). New York: Raven Press, 1987.

Fujita S, Conway W, Zorick F, et al: Surgical corrections of anatomic abnormalities in obstructive sleep apnea syndrome: uvulopalatopharyngoplasty. Otolaryngol Head Neck Surg 89:923–934, 1981.

Ikematsu T: Study of snoring. 4th report. Therapy [in Japanese]. J Jpn Otol Rhinol Laryngol 64:434–435, 1964.

Ikematsu T: PPP and partial uvulectomy method of Ikematsu. *In* Fairbanks DNF, Fujita S, Ikematsu T, Simmons FB (eds): Snoring and Obstructive Sleep Apnea (pp 130–134). New York: Raven Press, 1987.

Additional Readings

Fairbanks DNF: Uvulopalatopharyngoplasty: complications and avoidance strategies. Otolaryngol Head Neck Surg 102:239–245, 1990.

Fairbanks DNF, Fujita S, Ikematsu T, Simmons FB (eds): Snoring and Obstructive Sleep Apnea. New York: Raven Press, 1987. [See especially pp 129–170 regarding techniques of Fujita, Simmons, Ikematsu, and Dickson.]

Koopman CF, Moran WB (eds): Sleep apnea. The Otolaryngologic Clinics of North America, vol 23. Philadelphia: WB Saunders, 1990. [See especially pp 809–826 on maxillofacial surgery by RW Riley and NB Powell.]

CHAPTER 59

Hearing Aids and Aural Rehabilitation

Ross J. Roeser, PhD   Carolyn H. Musket, MA

In 1984 the American Speech-Language-Hearing Association defined aural rehabilitation as the provision of services and procedures for facilitating adequate receptive and expressive communication to people with hearing impairment. Included in the services covered under aural rehabilitation were (1) the identification and evaluation of sensory capabilities; (2) interpretation of results, counseling, and referral; and (3) intervention for communicative difficulties. A major component of any aural rehabilitation program for adults is the evaluation, fitting, and monitoring of appropriate sensory aids.

This chapter is a discussion of aural rehabilitation of the adult with acquired hearing loss. An emphasis of the chapter is on hearing aids and other sensory devices because such instruments are important for most hearing-impaired adults. However, it is important to point out the need for counseling and other rehabilitation strategies for this population.

HEARING AIDS

Historical Development, Styles, and Arrangements

Wearable electronic hearing aids were first made available to the public in the late 1920s and the early 1930s. These instruments were large, heavy, and notorious for their poor performance, especially with regard to fidelity, their high levels of distortion and noise, and their frequent intermittent transmission. Patients with conductive hearing loss benefited most; those with sensorineural loss, virtually not at all. This fact most likely is responsible for the diminishing misconception that patients with sensorineural hearing loss cannot benefit from the use of amplification.

In the mid-1930s, vacuum tubes were miniaturized and made available for use in hearing aids. Hearing aids with vacuum tubes were significantly less noisy, had lower amounts of distortion and greater power output, and were more reliable in performance than earlier instruments.

Although previously in industrial use for quite some time, the first transistors were not applied to hearing aids until the early 1950s. The transistor provided an important technical breakthrough in that it allowed for miniaturization of the amplifier. Transistors are considerably smaller than vacuum tubes, but, more important, they require less power to operate, which eliminates the need for a large battery supply.

Soon after the transistor was introduced into hearing aid technology, the body-borne, pocket type instrument (Fig. 59–1A) was replaced first with eyeglass aids and then with behind-the-ear or postauricular instruments (Fig. 59–1B). Other technologic innovations, such as hybridization of circuits, integrated circuits, smaller batteries, and electret microphones, have even further reduced the size of the modern hearing aid to the point that

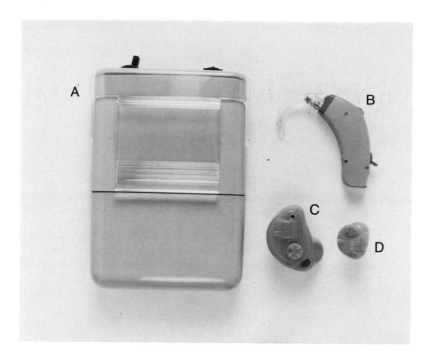

Figure 59–1. Examples of the major styles of hearing aids: *(A)* a body instrument, *(B)* a behind-the-ear (postauricular) or on-the-ear instrument, *(C)* an in-the-ear instrument, and *(D)* a canal instrument. (Photo courtesy of Starkey.)

in-the-ear aids (Fig. 59–1C) and now in-the canal aids (Fig. 59–1D) are available.

At the present time, further miniaturization of hearing aids is no longer an ultimate goal, and there appears to be no real advantage in performance or to the user of decreasing the size of a hearing aid beyond what is currently available. However, the past emphasis on miniaturization has produced a dramatic change in the sales trend of hearing aids.

Before the 1960s, body and eyeglass type instruments led in the number of sales in the United States. In the 1960s, behind-the-ear aids became the most widely used type of instrument. In-the-ear and in-the-canal aids are now the most popular style of instrument, accounting for approximately 79% of the market in 1989.

A unique style of hearing aid is the Contralateral Routing of Signal (CROS) instrument. CROS hearing aids are unique in that the microphone of the hearing aid is located on one side of the head and the signal is delivered to the ear on the opposite side. The original CROS instruments were built into eyeglasses. However, ear-level type CROS aids are now available. The purpose of the CROS hearing aid is to provide sound from both sides of the head to patients with severe unilateral hearing loss. On the basis of known audiometric factors and certain less quantifiable psychologic factors, reports have confirmed that the CROS aid can be beneficial for certain patients with severe unilateral hearing loss.

Several hybrids of the original CROS concept have been described and are used for selected patients. One modification of the CROS principle is the BICROS, a type of hearing aid with two microphones, one on each side of the head, delivering sound input into one ear.

Miniaturization and other advancements in hardware have led to significant improvements in performance. Increased durability, shock resistance, and moisture proofing, as well as prolonged battery life, are all evident. Furthermore, the versatility of hearing aids has increased. In the selection of an aid for a given patient, it is possible to control many electroacoustic performance characteristics, such as frequency response and saturation sound pressure level (SPL), to meet specific desired requirements. Significant progress in all areas of hearing aid technology has been made.

Hearing Aid Components and Controls

The appearance and construction of hearing aids vary considerably, but they operate electronically by similar principles. Differences in hearing aids are a result of how the components of the hearing aid are packaged, the type of amplifier used, and accessories included with the hearing aid.

Figure 59–2 is a block diagram of a hearing aid. The primary components used in this process are an input microphone, amplifier, output receiver, volume/gain control, and battery (power supply).

Input Microphone

The input microphone changes acoustic energy into an electrical signal. Modern hearing aids use electret-condenser microphones. With the introduction of the input type of microphone, it can no longer be said that this component limits the performance of the hearing aid. This contemporary microphone is small in size; has a broad frequency response, ranging from 100 to 10,000 Hz; has a relatively high signal-to-noise ratio; and is mechanically rugged.

Many hearing aid manufacturers offer aids with directional properties; that is, these aids attenuate signals from the rear of the instrument, producing a relative enhancement of signals originating from the front of the instrument. Technically, the way in which the microphone is modified and mounted in the case gives the hearing aid its directional property.

The electroacoustic advantage of a directional hearing aid can be demonstrated by simply measuring the instrument with the input acoustic energy emanating from different locations within the sound field. In such a procedure, as much as a 10- to 15-db intensity advantage can be demonstrated in an anechoic chamber when the sound source is located in the front of the hearing aid; even under reverberant conditions, a 3-db advantage is maintained.

Amplifier

The amplifier is the most complex component of the hearing aid. It takes the weak electrical signal from the microphone and increases its voltage (amplitude). The amplifier is a combination of components (transistors, resistors, capacitors, and so forth) that alter the signal in several stages. The number of stages and the number of components determine the way in which and how much of the signal is modified.

The increase in sound intensity in relation to the input signal (acoustic gain) and the maximal intensity that can be produced in the hearing aid regardless of the input signal (saturation SPL) are determined primarily by the amplifier. However, other components of the system also play a part in determining the acoustic gain and the saturation SPL of an instrument.

Table 59–1 shows the input-output characteristics of a hearing aid and provides an example of how acoustic gain and saturation SPL are calculated. Acoustic gain is determined by simply subtracting the decibel level of the input signal from the output signal—in this example, 40 db. The saturation SPL for this aid is 124 db SPL because increases of the input signal beyond 90 db do not produce an increase in amplification.

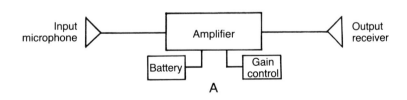

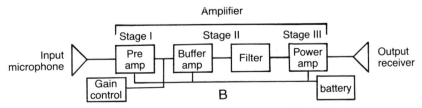

Figure 59–2. Simplified diagram of a hearing aid (top) with additional detail (bottom).

TABLE 59–1. Example of Input Output Function to Demonstrate Calculations of Acoustic Gain and Saturation Sound Pressure Level (SPL)

Input Signal to Microphone (db SPL)	Signal From Output Receiver (db SPL)
Acoustic gain = 40 db	
40	80
50	90
60	100
70	110
80	124
Saturation SPL = 120 db	
90	124

Hearing aid amplifiers operate according to one of two principles: linear or nonlinear. The basic difference between these principles is shown in Figure 59–3. With a linear amplifier, the acoustic gain ratio is 1:1; that is, as the input signal increases, there is an equivalent (linear) increase in the output signal until the saturation SPL is reached. The use of a hearing aid with a linear amplifier is indicated when audiometric studies do not show a critical need to limit the saturation SPL of the instrument; the patient does not have a loudness tolerance problem with a concomitant reduced dynamic range.

Nonlinear amplifiers, or output-limiting amplifiers, operate according to a number of different electronic principles. The two most common types of nonlinear amplifiers have automatic volume control or logarithmic compression. Also, as shown later in Figure 59–3, amplifiers with automatic volume control

limit the output on a linear or a curvilinear principle. Although the operating modes are different, all nonlinear amplifiers are used to control the operating range of the instrument. Hearing aids with nonlinear, output-limiting amplifiers are required for patients who have loudness tolerance problems with accompanying reduced dynamic ranges (i.e., the difference between auditory threshold and level of discomfort).

Some hearing aids have internal adjustments to control the acoustic gain, the saturation SPL, and the amount of compression in the amplifier. Such instruments offer a wide amount of variability and are most useful with fluctuating or progressive hearing losses.

Output Receiver

Once the electrical signal is amplified, it must be reconverted into either an acoustic signal, as in the air-conduction hearing aid, or a vibratory signal, as in a bone-conduction hearing aid. For air-conduction hearing aids, this conversion is accomplished by the output receiver, also known as the earphone, the speaker, or simply the receiver. Bone-conduction instruments use a bone conduction oscillator.

The vast majority of today's hearing aids use air-conduction receivers. High distortion levels and limitations imposed on the power and frequency response characteristics of the amplifier render the bone-conduction type receiver inferior to the air-conduction re-

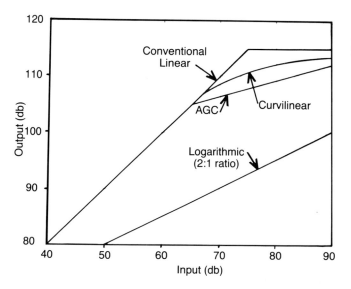

Figure 59–3. Input output function of a conventional, linear amplifier and three types of nonlinear amplifiers.

ceiver, except in rare cases, such as bilateral congenital atresia or severely draining ears.

Current air-conduction hearing aid receivers use a magnetic principle that limits their performance. However, if a broadband receiver is used, hearing aid output can extend to 6000 to 8000 Hz. At present, the output receiver is the most limiting component that restricts the overall performance of the hearing aid system.

An innovation has been the electromagnetically coupled external-to-internal prosthesis (Xomed Audiant Bone Conductor). The ideal candidate for the device is a patient who is unable to use a conventional hearing aid because of malformation or absence of the external ear canal (as a result of disease or congenital cause), chronic infection, or dermatitis of the external ear canal. A limitation of this device is that bone-conduction thresholds must be 25 db or better for the three speech frequencies (500, 1000, and 2000). In the insertion procedure, an internal drive that has a rare earth magnet is surgically placed onto the lateral temporal bone and becomes osseointegrated within several weeks. This internal drive is coupled electromagnetically to an external processor that transforms environmental sounds into an electromagnetic field that passes through the skin, causing the skull and attached structures, including the cochlea, to vibrate. The resulting sensation is a nearly distortion-free sound at normal intensities. By the end of 1989, more than 500 patients had received this device. Although the long-term effects have yet to be determined, the results of preliminary clinical studies of this device have been favorable.

Volume/Gain Control

As listening conditions vary, the amount of amplification required by the hearing aid wearer also varies. The volume control is used by the wearer to adjust the acoustic gain. Thus rather than referring to this component as a volume control, as is typically done, it is technically more correct to refer to it as a gain control. An important point is that although this component adjusts the acoustic gain of the instrument, it typically has no effect on the saturation SPL. However, as the gain control is decreased and the gain is reduced, a higher intensity input

signal is required before the saturation SPL is reached.

The goal of the audiologist is to provide an instrument that is tolerated under typical listening conditions with the gain control at midrange. This enables the wearer to increase or decrease the gain of the instrument as listening conditions vary. It is especially inappropriate to recommend an instrument that is normally worn at full volume because not only is gain adjustment restricted but also high levels of distortion occur within the hearing aid.

Power Supply (Battery)

Small batteries supply the power for the modern hearing aid. They range in size from a penlight battery for use in some body type instruments to less than about one third of the size of a dime for the in-the-ear aid.

Factors such as the type of battery, power of the instrument, type of amplifier, gain control setting used by the wearer, and even the atmospheric conditions in which the aid is worn (temperature and humidity) all affect battery life. However, in general, it is reasonable for a single battery to provide 100 to 250 hours of use in a new aid with 40 to 45 db of gain under normal conditions. Over time, however, as the components of the aid age, battery life expectancy might dwindle to as little as 50% of its original value.

Other Accessories

Additional features included as options on some hearing aids are the telephone pick-up coil and tone/frequency control. Hearing aids with telephone pick-up coils are an advantage because they allow the wearer to use the telephone without interference from ambient background noise. A magnetic induction coil inside the hearing aid picks up signals directly from the receiver of the telephone, which thereby bypass the microphone of the hearing aid. One problem with this method is that newer types of telephones are more efficient and thus radiate an inadequate magnetic field. Because of this, there was a period during the 1970s and the early 1980s when hearing aid telephone coils would not work. However, two laws were subsequently passed to restore telephone compatibility.

The first, PL 97–410, the Telecommunications for the Disabled Act of 1982, requires that all essential telephones, such as coin-operated and emergency-use phones, be hearing aid–compatible. The second, PL 100–394, the Hearing Aid Compatibility Act of 1988, requires that all corded telephones manufactured or imported for use in the United States be hearing aid–compatible after August 1989; the same provisions were effected for cordless phones manufactured or imported after August 1991. The telephone pick-up coil is a very useful option for patients with moderately severe to severe hearing loss who are frequent telephone users.

One way to connect a hearing aid to an external sound source, such as a microphone or a radio signal, is to wire it directly to the hearing aid with a plug by using direct auditory input. Direct auditory input eliminates the distance between the sound source and the receiver's ear, thus improving the signal-to-noise ratio and making the signal easier to perceive.

The tone control changes the gain at the various frequencies being amplified by the hearing aid; that is, it changes the frequency response of the instrument. Tone controls can be discretely or continuously adjustable and are located either externally, for the wearer's control, or internally. The ability to change the tone control externally allows the wearer more acceptable amplification under a variety of listening conditions.

Coupling the Hearing Aid to the Ear

The earmold is a plastic insert that physically attaches the hearing aid to the ear. The earmold directs the amplified sound from the output receiver into the ear canal. Besides acting as a physical coupler, the earmold serves two additional purposes. First, by sealing off the ear canal and preventing the amplified sound from entering the microphone, it helps eliminate acoustic feedback. Acoustic feedback, an annoying squeal sometimes heard from a hearing aid, interferes with speech perception and, if not satisfactorily corrected, can account for rejection by some persons of their hearing aids. Second, the manner in which the hearing aid is coupled affects the acoustic energy reaching the ear; thus the earmold acts as a fine-tuning acoustic control. Attention to both of these functions is important for obtaining a properly fitted hearing aid.

Both the materials used in the construction and the styles of earmolds vary. The list of materials includes lucite, vinyl polyethylene, and silicone for the construction of hard, semihard, or soft earmolds. Nonallergenic material can also be obtained for patients with a history of allergic reactions. The type of earmold material is insignificant with regard to changing the acoustic energy reaching the ear. However, the material used can significantly affect comfort, a factor of utmost concern to the patient.

Because of the varieties of earmold styles and ways of describing them, the National Association of Earmold Laboratories in 1971 agreed to standardize earmold terminology. Figure 59–4 shows six of the most common styles of earmolds as defined by this association. Although not all earmold laboratories adhere to this specific terminology, this figure should provide general information about the styles of molds that are available and the means for describing them.

The standard or receiver type of earmold is used on body style instruments by patients with severe hearing impairment. These patients require powerful aids, and therefore an earmold that helps to reduce unwanted acoustic feedback is needed. The shell or full shell, skeleton, canal, and canal-lock molds are used with most behind-the-ear (postauricular) and eyeglass type aids. In the selection between these types of molds for a given patient, the degree and configuration of the loss are the primary considerations. However, the morphologic characteristics of the auricle and the personal preference of the patient must also be considered.

Only since about 1975 has the importance of the earmold as a fine-tuning acoustic control been realized. Substantial modification of the acoustic output of the hearing aid can be accomplished by the manipulation of various earmold parameters. As such, attention has been focused on the earmold in the hearing aid selection process. The earmold is thought of no longer as a mere accessory to the hearing aid but rather as an intricate component of the total amplification system.

The length of the ear canal, the size of the sound bore, the inner diameter and length of the tubing, the flare, and whether a vent is used all affect the acoustic energy reaching the ear. These parameters have a significant affect on hearing aid output and ultimately on acceptance by the wearer and speech intelligibility. There is a rather complicated

Figure 59-4. Six common styles of earmolds. (Photo courtesy of Westone Earmold Laboratories, Inc.)

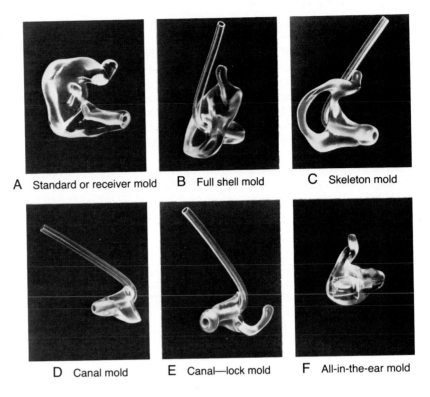

A   Standard or receiver mold

B   Full shell mold

C   Skeleton mold

D   Canal mold

E   Canal—lock mold

F   All-in-the-ear mold

interaction between the physical parameters of an earmold and their effect on sound transmission. However, in general, reduction in the frequencies below 1000 Hz can be accomplished by shortening the canal length and including a vent or increasing the size of an existing vent. A reduction in low-frequency gain can be desirable for two reasons: first, the low-frequency, high-energy vowel sounds no longer mask the high-frequency, low-energy consonant sounds; second, the patient's subjective feeling of fullness or pressure within the ear canal is relieved.

One additional style of earmold frequently used is the free-field, nonoccluding, or open mold. This style of mold is unique in that it consists of a plastic insert that simply holds the tubing from a postauricular aid or an eyeglass aid in the external auditory meatus. This form of coupling provides a minimal amount of occlusion of the external auditory meatus, allowing environmental sounds to enter the ear canal unimpeded and causing a significant loss of low-frequency energy. It has been shown that with this open type system, frequencies above 1000 Hz are enhanced. Open molds are ideal for patients with mild high-frequency loss. This type of

fitting principle is referred to as ipsilateral routing of signal. Open molds are also often used with CROS amplification.

Measuring Hearing Aid Performance

ANSI S3.22 Electroacoustic Measures

Since 1959, standardized procedures have been adopted both to specify the physical measurement of hearing aids and to provide methods for the graphic display of hearing aid characteristics. In 1976, the American National Standards Institute (ANSI) approved ANSI S3.22 (ASA STD7), which has since been revised twice (1982, 1987). This standard expanded the number of measurement procedures to be made on hearing aids and provided tolerance guidelines for hearing aid performance characteristics.

The elaborate procedures for assessing the electroacoustic characteristics of hearing aids are not discussed in this chapter. However, any professional who is engaged in the dispensing of hearing aids must be thoroughly familiar with the standard procedures by which hearing aids are measured and specifications obtained. This knowledge provides a greater understanding of the performance capability of an individual amplification system.

It is possible for a new hearing aid to deviate from its expected electroacoustic characteristics or to completely malfunction even before being worn. Thus it is mandatory that each hearing aid be checked electroacoustically before it is dispensed. Electroacoustic analyses not only identify instruments that do not meet tolerance levels but also allow for systematic manipulation of certain electroacoustic parameters within the hearing aid system in an attempt to provide optimal amplification for the patient.

Hearing Aid Test Sets and 2-mm³ Coupler Measures

Several equipment alternatives are available for measuring electroacoustic parameters of hearing aids. They range from practical, relatively inexpensive hearing aid test sets to elaborate, highly sensitive systems costing many thousands of dollars. A clinical hearing aid test set is shown in Figure 59–5. The basic operating principle of these systems is that a signal, precisely controlled for frequency and intensity, is delivered to the microphone of the hearing aid being measured, which has been placed in an acoustically damped chamber. The output receiver of the hearing aid is coupled to a standard-size (2 mm³) hard-walled cavity and a test microphone. The output from the test microphone provides information on how the in-put signal was changed by the hearing aid. Through use of this system, the basic measures of gain, saturation SPL, frequency response, and distortion are obtained, as are more sophisticated measures when desired.

Gain and saturation SPL have been discussed previously. The frequency response of a hearing aid is a display of the relative gain as a function of frequency with a constant decibel input. Gain varies across test frequencies, depending on the characteristics of the individual hearing aid. Typically, hearing aids can be classified as having flat, high-frequency, or, less commonly, low-frequency response curves. Figure 59–6 shows two common frequency response curves: one for a relatively flat frequency response and one for a high-frequency emphasis.

Distortion occurs when the input signal is not faithfully reproduced; that is, the output signal differs in some way from the input signal, other than in the desired increased amplitude. The only measure of distortion included in the present standard that applies to all hearing aids is harmonic distortion. Harmonic distortion occurs when the output signal contains frequencies that are whole-number multiples of the fundamental frequency of the input signal. When a 1000-Hz pure tone is introduced into the microphone, harmonic distortion causes signals to be produced at 2000 Hz (second harmonic), at 3000 Hz (third harmonic), and so forth. The exact influence of distortion on the performance of hearing aid wearers is not really known. However, studies have shown that excessive

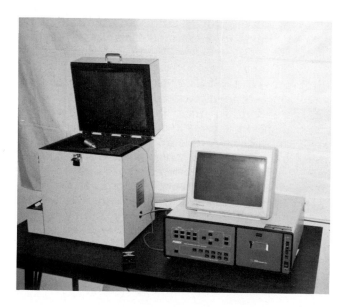

Figure 59–5. Example of a hearing aid test set.

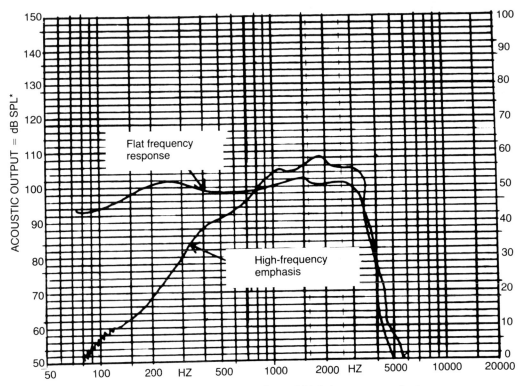

Figure 59–6. Frequency response curves showing flat and high frequency emphasis.

harmonic distortion adversely affects speech perception; thus it is an unwanted characteristic.

Measurements of the electroacoustic performance of a hearing aid obtained through use of standard methods in a hearing aid test set may be compared with the same measurements made and reported by the manufacturer. Thus this information is of great value in determining whether a hearing aid is in good working order. However, the performance of a hearing aid in a 2-mm³ coupler enclosed in a sound chamber is not the same as that obtained when it is actually worn by the user. Important differences are caused by several factors: the acoustic resistance presented to the output of the hearing aid at its receiver is different in the real ear than in a 2-mm³ coupler; placement of the aid on the head (or the chest) results in the reflection and absorption of sound that varies according to frequency and according to the location of the hearing aid microphone. It is possible to determine average correction factors for some of these variables, but there exists a wide range of individual differences. Consequently, measures of aided performance also must be made while the instrument is in

place on the intended user; they cannot be predicted with accuracy from data collected in a hearing aid test set.

Other Considerations

Programmable Hearing Aids. New technology has made it possible to program the desired electroacoustic characteristics into hearing aids; that is, with the same instrument, a wide variety of electroacoustic characteristics is possible. The implications of this capability are profound: one hearing aid would fit all; as hearing loss changed, so would the instrument; stocking numerous models of instruments would no longer be necessary; and so forth. Is it possible that the dispenser of the future will have one or two styles of hearing aids and will be able to adjust the aid to meet the needs of any hearing-impaired patient? With the advances that were made in the 1980s, such a development seems possible in the very near future.

Remote Control Hearing Aids. As with televisions and compact disk players, it is now possible to control several of the operating characteristics of a hearing aid, including turning it on and off, the volume, and the tone control, with a remote control switch. Some hearing aid users find this capability extremely helpful.

Digital Hearing Aids. Digital electronics provide very precise control of the signal, and they are more stable than other forms of hearing aid technology. Hearing aids of today are beginning to be manufactured with digital electronics; without too much question, hearing aids of the future will rely very heavily on digital technology.

Tinnitus Maskers. Although they are housed in behind-the-ear hearing aid shells, tinnitus maskers are not hearing aids. Rather, they produce a sound that is used to cover up, or mask, the tinnitus perceived by the patient. The theory is that the external masking sound produced by the masker is more acceptable than the internal sound of the tinnitus. Some patients do find that tinnitus maskers provide relief from their tinnitus, and as a result, patients troubled by tinnitus should be considered for a trial with a masker. More important, patients with tinnitus who have hearing loss should be considered for hearing aid use because hearing aids also provide a masking signal caused by noise from the amplifier. These patients not only obtain relief from their tinnitus but also experience the benefits of amplification.

Determining Hearing Aid Candidacy

Consideration must be given to many factors when candidacy for hearing aid use is being determined.

Otologic Consultation

In 1977, the federal government, through the Food and Drug Administration, published regulations in the *Federal Register* regarding the labeling and the conditions for sale of hearing aids. This document mandates that a prospective user must receive a medical evaluation from a licensed physician (not necessarily an otologist or an otolaryngologist) within the 6 months preceding the sale of a hearing aid; the dispenser must receive a statement, signed by the physician, indicating that the patient may be considered a candidate for hearing aid use. However, the

regulations permit patients 18 years of age or older to sign a statement waiving this medical evaluation because of religious or personal beliefs.

The Food and Drug Administration's regulations also require dispensers to advise a person to consult a physician, preferably an ear specialist, if any of the following conditions are detected:

1. Visible congenital or traumatic deformity of the ear.
2. History of active ear drainage within the previous ninety days.
3. History of sudden or rapidly progressive hearing loss within the previous 90 days.
4. Acute or chronic dizziness.
5. Unilateral hearing loss of sudden or recent onset within the previous 90 days.
6. Audiometric air-bone gap equal to or greater than 15 db at 500, 1000, and 2000 Hz.
7. Visible evidence of significant cerumen accumulation or a foreign body in the ear canal. (Many audiologists remove cerumen from the ear canal if no medical contraindications are suggested.)
8. Pain or discomfort in the ear.

Medical evaluation by a physician specializing in diseases of the ear for patients who have difficulty hearing should certainly be considered in order to determine whether medical intervention is indicated. In some patients, such treatment may restore or improve hearing to the extent that amplification is no longer needed. In others, medical treatment or surgery may not be indicated or, when completed, does not resolve communicative problems. These patients should be referred to an audiologist for nonmedical management of hearing problems. The physician's diagnosis and prognosis of the disorder may indicate a certain course of action when rehabilitation is planned; for example, a patient with a fluctuating or progressive hearing loss needs a hearing aid that may be adjusted to accommodate changing hearing levels. In addition, the audiologist should know whether hearing aid use is contraindicated in either ear for medical reasons.

Communicative Need

For patients with hearing impairment, there exists a wide array of amplification options as a result of advances in hearing aid design and earmold acoustics. A hearing aid fitting is possible for most types of hearing loss. However, not all potential users are handicapped by their hearing loss or are seeking a solution. Many variables such as lifestyle, job and work settings, and family interactions must be considered. Consequently, it is of primary importance in the assessment of candidacy to determine the extent to which a person is experiencing hearing problems in everyday life. Usually, questions in this area are included as part of the case history.

A more objective and systematic means of assessing the amount of handicap imposed by a hearing impairment is available through the use of questionnaires, either self-report or administered through an interview. Such inventories have been developed, and some have been standardized (e.g., the Hearing Handicap Inventory for the Elderly, Ventry and Weinstein, 1982; the Communication Profile for the Hearing Impaired, Demorest and Erdman, 1987).

Audiologic Evaluation

Information defining the candidacy of a potential hearing aid user is available from a battery of audiometric tests. First, it is evident that an analysis of the pattern of test results, along with the related history and otoscopic inspection, will indicate whether medical referral should be made for those who initially consult an audiologist about their hearing problems.

Next, the magnitude of the hearing loss, which is expressed in decibels by the pure-tone average (500, 1000, and 2000 Hz), speech reception threshold, or both, may be used to estimate the patient's probable difficulty understanding speech at conversational levels and the potential help available from a hearing aid. This system, which is based on the hearing level in the better ear, is not applicable to patients who have hearing losses confined to the high frequencies or unilateral hearing losses. The basic idea is that those with mild hearing losses (26 to 40 db) encounter difficulty hearing only when speech is faint or distant and, therefore, will use a hearing aid on a part-time basis in special situations.

As the degree of hearing loss increases, so does the need for amplification. Patients with moderate losses (41 to 55 db) are likely to have significant listening problems and to use a hearing aid more often. Patients whose hearing losses are more severe (56 to 80 db) are in the so-called region of greatest satisfaction. This term is used because conversational speech cannot be heard unless it is loud, or even shouted, and many environmental sounds of soft to moderate intensity are also not heard; nevertheless, significant benefit is obtained from amplification. Consequently, people with this degree of hearing loss tend to be among the more satisfied hearing aid users.

Although persons whose losses exceed 80 db have a great need for amplification, only partial help in supplementing visual cues and monitoring environmental sounds is available to them from a hearing aid. Undoubtedly, these categories are an oversimplification because use of a hearing aid is dependent on communicative need and other factors. In addition, this classification system ignores the contribution of the frequencies above 2000 Hz to understanding speech, especially in noise. Nevertheless, this format does provide a beginning frame of reference in the description of hearing aid candidacy.

The maximal unaided word recognition score is viewed as an indicator of a person's potential to receive speech clearly through a hearing aid. This factor must be evaluated along with the degree of hearing loss when candidacy for a hearing aid is assessed. For example, patients with mild hearing losses and greatly reduced word-recognition ability may not be good candidates for amplification. However, those with severe hearing losses likely need the auditory cues of speech available with amplification to communicate, even though they may have poor word recognition ability; they must be counseled to understand that help from visual and situational cues is necessary in order to supplement the auditory cues of speech heard with a hearing aid. Also, for patients with high-frequency hearing losses, the word-recognition score may not be an accurate indicator of aided potential. This is because word recognition is measured with the audiometer by means of a broad-band speech signal; with a properly fitted hearing aid, it is possible to amplify only the high frequencies of the speech spectrum, which may result in greater clarity of speech for wearers with losses in this range.

Additional information is available through expanded speech-recognition testing. The relationship between performance-intensity functions for monosyllable words and those for synthetic sentences may be used to identify persons with central auditory dysfunction. It is especially important to include such measures when elderly patients are assessed because the prevalence of central disorders is high in this population and influences expectations from hearing aid use.

Audiometric assessment also provides information on the relationship between ears. This information is needed when the arrangement of wearable amplification—monaural, binaural, or some version of CROS—is determined.

In the audiologic evaluation, the listener's judgments are used to establish the most comfortable listening level and the loudness discomfort level; both speech and frequency-specific stimuli, such as pure tones, may be used. Findings of tests of the loudness discomfort level are compared with the pure-tone thresholds of sensitivity to define the area of residual hearing in each ear. The region between the threshold of sensitivity and the loudness discomfort level is referred to as the dynamic range. The overall goal of a hearing aid is to amplify the sounds of speech for a user so they are perceived at a comfortably loud level but do not exceed the loudness discomfort level. Hearing-impaired patients with a large dynamic range, therefore, are good candidates for hearing aids; special techniques must be used when patients with a reduced dynamic range are being fitted.

Finally, it must be stressed that although the audiometric profile described earlier is important, it is not always an accurate predictor of hearing aid candidacy. Patients with cochlear and neural hearing impairments have disrupted auditory processing capabilities; nevertheless, many aspects of this area are not routinely assessed today. The astute clinician elicits responses to questions such as "What do you hear?" and "How does this sound?" while awaiting the development of objective clinical measures in such areas as frequency resolution, frequency selectivity, and binaural integration.

Motivation

Hearing aid candidacy is more favorable if the hearing-impaired patient has an optimistic outlook on amplification and is genuinely interested in improving communication. Patients who seek evaluation only at the urging of a spouse or other family member are certainly less likely to be successful hearing aid users. It is difficult to overcome the negative connotation associated with hearing aids in society. Physicians who refer patients for consideration of hearing aid use should be supportive of this option and positive about its possible benefit to the user.

Physical Limitations

Several physical attributes should be considered. The size and shape of the auricle and the meatus may dictate use of a certain style of hearing aid, earmold, or both. Prospective hearing aid users must have the manual dexterity as well as the arm and shoulder mobility necessary to position the hearing instrument behind or in the ear; otherwise, a body aid or a personal communication device may be indicated. Patients need sufficient manual dexterity and tactile sensation in the fingertips to operate the controls and switches. Special modifications such as built-up gain (volume) controls, removal knobs for the in-the-ear aids, and a remote control device to govern gain and other functions are available. In addition, vision must be adequate to troubleshoot and care for the aid unless help from other people is available.

Binaural Versus Monaural Fitting

Because practically all hearing aid fittings are ear level, an added goal of an optimal selection procedure is to restore or preserve binaural hearing. Binaural hearing offers several advantages to the listener in comparison with monaural hearing: localization of sound, more perceived loudness of sound (binaural summation), improved speech recognition in a background of noise (the so-called squelch effect), and a subjective experience of more comfort, clarity, and ease of listening. In addition, with binaural hearing aids, the wearer can hear equally well from either side of the body; an aided ear is always directed toward the sound of interest. In a monaural fitting, the user is subject to the "head shadow effect," or the fact that the physical presence of the head reduces the intensity of the desired signal whenever it occurs on the side of the head opposite to the aided ear.

Currently, there is wide support for the use of binaural amplification. Hearing-impaired persons may achieve binaural hearing either through the provision of two hearing aids or, in some cases, through the use of a monaural hearing aid when there is an asymmetric hearing loss and the better ear has normal or nearly normal hearing.

A monaural hearing aid or BICROS may be recommended in cases of bilateral hearing loss when one ear is unaidable because of lack of residual hearing, extremely poor word-recognition ability, poor tolerance for loud sound, the presence of unilateral atresia, or a medical condition that prohibits occlusion of the ear canal. In addition, some persons hear less clearly with binaural aids than with a monaural aid, and some people prefer one hearing aid for other reasons.

Selection of Electroacoustic Characteristics

Some rationale must be used in the selection of the electroacoustic characteristics for a hearing aid that provides optimal amplification for a specific hearing loss. Although no single theoretical approach is generally accepted, several models are in current use.

Prescriptive Procedures

The goal of these methods is to amplify the speech spectrum at average conversational levels so that it falls within the dynamic range of the hearing-impaired user. In prescriptive fitting procedures, it is assumed that there is a predictable relationship between audiometric information and the desired electroacoustic characteristics of the hearing aid. Formulas are used to relate the patient's hearing level at various frequencies—whether at threshold or at comfortable loudness—to the gain and the frequency response of the hearing aid. Other formulas are used to relate the loudness discomfort level to the saturation SPL of the hearing instrument.

For example, an early gain formula that was based on pure-tone thresholds specified that the gain of the hearing aid at each frequency should be equal to half the decibel amount of the hearing loss at the frequency. This formula is logically known as the one-half gain rule. In subsequent versions of this formula, researchers have proposed calculations with variations in the amount of gain needed by frequency; consequently, each approach specifies a different frequency response. At present, it has not been deter-

mined which formula is superior or offers the best amplified signal to the user; each method has its advocates. Through use of a formula, it is possible to plot targets for the amount of gain to be provided by the hearing aid at each frequency; methods of verifying whether these target values are achieved are discussed in a later section of this chapter.

Other procedures involve the use of the intensity of suprathreshold listening levels when the amount of gain needed for a hearing aid is determined. Briefly stated, one prominent theory reasons that if the intensity of speech at average conversational levels is known and the intensity of the comfortable loudness desired by the patient is measurable, the gain of the hearing aid should equal the difference between the two. Prescriptions based on this philosophy of fitting strive to have the hearing instrument amplify the long-term spectrum of speech to the desired listening level in each frequency region available to the user. Similar formulas have been proposed on the basis of various loudness judgments.

Another way to calculate gain by frequency is to predict the desired sensation level for frequencies in the amplified long-term speech spectrum to be presented to the impaired ear. These levels then become the target for aided performance.

In a different category, formulas are available for use in specifying the appropriate maximal or saturation output of a hearing aid. The user's loudness discomfort level, which is obtained in terms of decibel hearing level, must be converted to decibel sound pressure level because hearing aid output is measured with the latter.

Fortunately, prescriptive fitting formulas may be computerized, which thereby makes manipulation of the data involved rapid and accurate. Several computer-assisted hearing aid selection programs have been devised; others are available in dedicated computers that are part of probe-tube microphone measurement systems (described in a subsequent section of this chapter).

Comparative Procedures

A traditional approach to the selection of appropriate amplification for an individual patient emphasizes the use of comparison methods. Rather than determining beforehand the electroacoustic parameters of a fitting, in this paradigm the user may actually try several instruments, may be presented with various frequency responses through a master hearing aid, or may have different adjustments made to one instrument. Then, under each condition, aided performance is compared according to several criteria. Historically, these measures were aided speech thresholds and discrimination scores obtained in quiet conditions and in noisy conditions, as well as aided tolerance for loud sound. It is also possible to elicit judgments from the user as to what sounds best in each condition. This may be accomplished informally or in the format of a paired-comparison procedure.

In the 1980s, there was a decline in the use of comparative trials. Clinicians performing fittings became more sophisticated in the preselection of appropriate electroacoustic parameters; as a result, valid differences in aided performance were not seen in the scores on traditional speech tests. Moreover, the in-the-ear hearing aid, the major style worn today, does not lend itself easily to comparative trials. Different models of this style of instrument usually are not available to be placed in a person's ear; control devices of in-the-ear hearing aids are not as flexible in offering a range of adjustments as are those in other styles.

However, the introduction of programmable hearing aids has caused a resurgence of interest in comparative selection strategies. Some of these instruments offer several frequency responses and output options to accommodate changing listening environments; the user has the ability to select from among those programmed into the hearing instrument. The challenge of fitting thus becomes one of determining the most appropriate electroacoustic characteristics for a variety of settings such as those typical of a quiet room, a party, and the work environment. A single amplified frequency response may not suffice for all listening conditions; it is likely that different frequency responses will be demanded for differing circumstances. One way to approach such a fitting is through comparative trials in which prospective users listen to recordings of speech in quiet and noisy conditions, of music, and even of sounds recorded in their particular job settings while comparing aided frequency responses in each condition.

Verification of Aided Performance

Methods are available to verify whether the goals identified during the preselection process are obtained when the actual hearing aid is worn by the user. Such so-called real-ear assessment is necessary because of anatomic differences in ears and the fact that aided performance cannot always be predicted from unaided information because of factors previously discussed. Also, as mentioned, when describing the hearing aid test set, 2-mm^3 coupler data used by manufacturers to report the electroacoustic capabilities of hearing aids cannot be directly applied to human ears.

Some of these real-ear techniques are especially helpful as follow-ups to prescriptive procedures; they enable the clinician to determine whether predicted target values for gain by frequency and saturation output level have been attained. If they have not, adjustments may be made in the fitting, or, in some cases, another hearing aid may be tried. It is also essential to verify the status of speech as it is heard through the instrument.

Sound Field Measures of Functional Gain

In this procedure, behavioral tests are conducted in a sound-treated room with the acoustic signal, frequency-specific stimuli, presented through a loudspeaker to the subject seated nearby. First, the user's thresholds are measured unaided; then, measurements are repeated with the hearing aid in place and the gain (volume) control adjusted to a comfortable level. The change in thresholds, or the user's ability to respond to tones of lower intensity when aided, is attributed to the gain provided to the stimulus signal by the hearing instrument. Therefore, at each frequency the aided threshold is subtracted from the unaided threshold. These differences, called functional gain, are reported in decibels.

The major advantage of functional gain measures is that they incorporate all factors involved in the psychoacoustic process of hearing; that is, not only is the hearing aid tested in the real ear but the sound also must be perceived by the person involved.

Several disadvantages are associated with this method, however. Measurements are obtained only at limited, discrete frequencies, and, consequently, interpolations based on these points may not represent the true frequency response of the hearing aid. In addition, valid measures of gain are not possible for frequencies at which the user has normal or nearly normal hearing because room noise, the internal noise of the hearing aid, or both obscure the presence of the test tone. Moreover, reliability is a problem if different aids are being compared because of large test-retest variability in aided sound-field thresholds. Finally, as with many behavioral techniques, determining functional gain is a time-consuming task.

Probe-Tube Microphone Measures of Real-Ear Insertion Response

An addition to the armamentarium for verification procedures is a clinically feasible method of measuring the actual SPL present in the ear canal of a person (Fig. 59–7). A slender silicone tube is attached to a miniature measuring microphone and is positioned in the ear canal near the eardrum. The patient is seated, usually facing a loudspeaker. Frequency specific stimuli are then presented through the loudspeaker, and measurements are obtained initially without the hearing aid and then with the aid in place; the probe tube rests between the earmold or the in-the-ear aid and the canal wall during the aided test. Computerized, self-calibrating probe-tube microphone systems for this purpose are available from several manufacturers.

Because probe-tube microphones offer new methodologies and instrumentation in this area, the measurement protocols and associated terminology are still evolving. At this time, the ANSI S3,80 Committee on Probe Microphone Measurements of Hearing Aid Performance has proposed nomenclature for these measures. Accordingly, real-ear insertion response is the difference between the measured frequency response in decibels SPL in the ear canal when a hearing aid is used and the SPL normally there without an aid in place. At any frequency this difference may be calculated in decibels and expressed as real-ear insertion gain.

This instrumentation may also be used to verify the actual saturation SPL present in the aided ear with a precision never before possible. To accomplish this, the real-ear aided response is obtained with an input signal high enough to cause the hearing aid to reach its maximal output level (the saturation SPL).

Probe-tube microphone measures have the advantage of being objective, accurate, and rapid. They may also be performed in any quiet room. Moreover, it is important that a broad range of specific frequencies is measured in a matter of seconds. The clinician may quickly determine real-ear performance and compare results with targets predicted from a formula. Modifications in the hearing aid fitting, if needed, may be performed and the effect determined quickly.

Of course, the disadvantage evident with probe-tube microphones is that these measures offer no information about how a person uses the amplification provided; that is,

Figure 59–7. Example of a probe-tube microphone hearing aid measurement system.

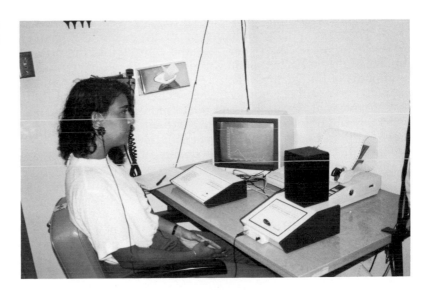

a patient's performance is not assessed. However, where used with a performance measure, probe-tube microphone measures add invaluable information to hearing aid fittings.

Speech Measures

The hearing aid is used in everyday life in communicative situations involving speech. As a result, it is important to verify that the wearer is able to use an aided speech signal. This is especially true for instruments whose selection was based on prescriptive formulas, as opposed to those fittings identified through comparative trials with speech. For such cases, in addition to verification of selection goals through determination of functional gain or real-ear insertion gain, speech stimuli should be presented. Unfortunately, no available single speech-based clinical procedure has been proved to assess everyday communicative efficiency with amplification. Thus clinicians approach measurement in this area a variety of ways.

The amplification system selected should improve speech communication in comparison with the unaided condition. One means of demonstrating this is to present word or sentence recognition tests at an intensity simulating average conversational speech, either in quiet conditions or with competing background noise, and obtain scores both with and without an aid. Such a comparison also is helpful in allowing the user to realize that speech is understood better with a hearing aid than without one.

Judgments of speech intelligibility represent another option. Users listen to segments of recorded continuous speech at conversational levels in quiet conditions or in the presence of noise; then they rate the percentage of the message that they understood. Judgments of the quality of amplified speech may also be obtained; however, researchers have found that these opinions relate more to the amount of low-frequency amplification provided than to the degree of speech intelligibility. It is important that the quality of amplified sound be acceptable to the user.

Validation of Aided Performance

It has been proposed that hearing aid selection and verification procedures may be considered valid if they result in a fitting that is successful in the circumstances of everyday life. Thus follow-up information is needed to determine the amount of benefit achieved on a daily basis with the amplification system recommended. Efforts to establish an accepted protocol in this area have been minimal to date. However, eventually such measures may serve to validate existing or future strategies for fitting.

Frequency of Use Measures

Various methods have been used to establish the amount of time that a hearing aid is being worn on the basis of the rationale that benefit is reflected by regular use. Some investigators have used questionnaires on which respondents rate the percentage of time that they use their aids in various daily activities. Other investigators have employed an indirect measure of use by asking users to report the number of batteries consumed per week or per month.

Self-Report Measures

Self-assessment inventories have been used to quantify aided experiences in various listening situations of everyday life. Respondents answer questions that concern the actual improvement or benefit obtained with amplification.

Reduction of Hearing Handicap

The development of questionnaires designed to measure hearing handicap was discussed in the previous section on communicative need. An additional use of these scales may be to quantify hearing aid benefit by noting the change in handicap scores obtained before the fitting and several months after the fitting. A significant reduction in hearing handicap after the fitting may document a successful fitting.

Hearing Aid Orientation

It is essential that information and counseling be provided to all new users of hearing instruments. As with any electronic device, it is necessary that the user first learn how to operate and care for the hearing aid. A new user must become familiar with the controls, the switches, and the battery requirements of the instrument, as well as with the technique for inserting the earmold or the in-the-ear aid into the ear. In addition, simple troubleshooting methods should be explained. Most failures in this area are caused either by battery problems or by the accumulation of earwax in the sound bore of the earmold or in the receiver port of an in-the-ear instrument. A most annoying recurrent problem is the presence of a high-pitched squealing sound, called acoustic feedback, that occurs whenever the amplified sound coming from the earmold or in-the-ear aid leaks out of the ear and reaches the hearing aid microphone, where it is reamplified. The Food and Drug Administration's regulation regarding the labeling and sale of hearing aids specifies that much of the information just given must be contained in a "User Instructional Booklet" that accompanies every hearing aid.

First-time users must be counseled to develop realistic expectations about hearing aid use. Too many believe they are obtaining new *hearing* instead of a new hearing *aid*. They must be advised to begin a graduated program of listening experiences with the hearing aid, starting with initial trials in a quiet environment with a familiar voice. Users must understand the limitations of hearing aid use, especially in adverse situations such as noisy surroundings. All this information is most effective when shared with family members; the availability of instructional videotapes and manuals makes this feasible (You and Your Hearing Aid: Sound Advice, New York League for the Hard of Hearing, 1989; *The Hearing Aid Handbook*, Wayner, 1990a, 1990b).

ALTERNATIVES TO HEARING AIDS

As stated earlier in this chapter, the vast majority of hearing-impaired patients can benefit from amplification provided by standard hearing aids. However, some cannot. For these patients, alternative devices, including cochlear implants and tactile aids, are available.

Cochlear Implants

For the patient whose hearing loss is in the profound range and who has tried an appropriately fitted hearing aid without success, a cochlear implant should be considered. Cochlear implants provide electrical stimulation to the cochlea through a surgically implanted electrode.

Figure 59–8 illustrates how a cochlear implant functions. Sound is received by the microphone and is sent to the speech processor, where specific components are selected and coded. The coded signal is then sent to the transmitter, where it is relayed across the skin by a magnetic induction coil. The receiver stimulator converts the code into electrical signals that are sent to electrodes that stimulate auditory nerve fibers. These signals are then transmitted to the central nervous system.

The Food and Drug Administration has reviewed cochlear implants extensively and has approved single-channel and multichannel implants for children and adults. The selection criteria for child candidates are as follows.

1. Ages 2 to 17 years.
2. Bilateral profound sensorineural deafness (electrophysiologic assessment must corroborate behavioral evaluation for younger children).
3. Little or no benefit from a hearing (or vibrotactile) aid for a minimum 6 months with appropriate amplification.
4. Motivation and appropriate expectations of families and, if possible, candidates.

The criteria for adults (18 years and older) are as follows.

1. Profound sensorineural deafness.
2. Little or no benefit from a hearing aid.
3. Postlingually deafened.
4. Psychological and motivational suitability.

Contraindications for both groups are as follows.

1. Deafness caused by lesions of the acoustic nerve or the central auditory pathway.
2. Active middle ear infections.
3. Cochlear ossification that prevents electrode insertion.
4. Absence of cochlear development.
5. Tympanic membrane perforation.

Among the adverse effects of cochlear implants are the normal risks of surgery and general anesthesia; infection or bleeding; numbness or stiffness about the ear; injury to or stimulation of the facial nerve; taste disturbance; dizziness; increased tinnitus;

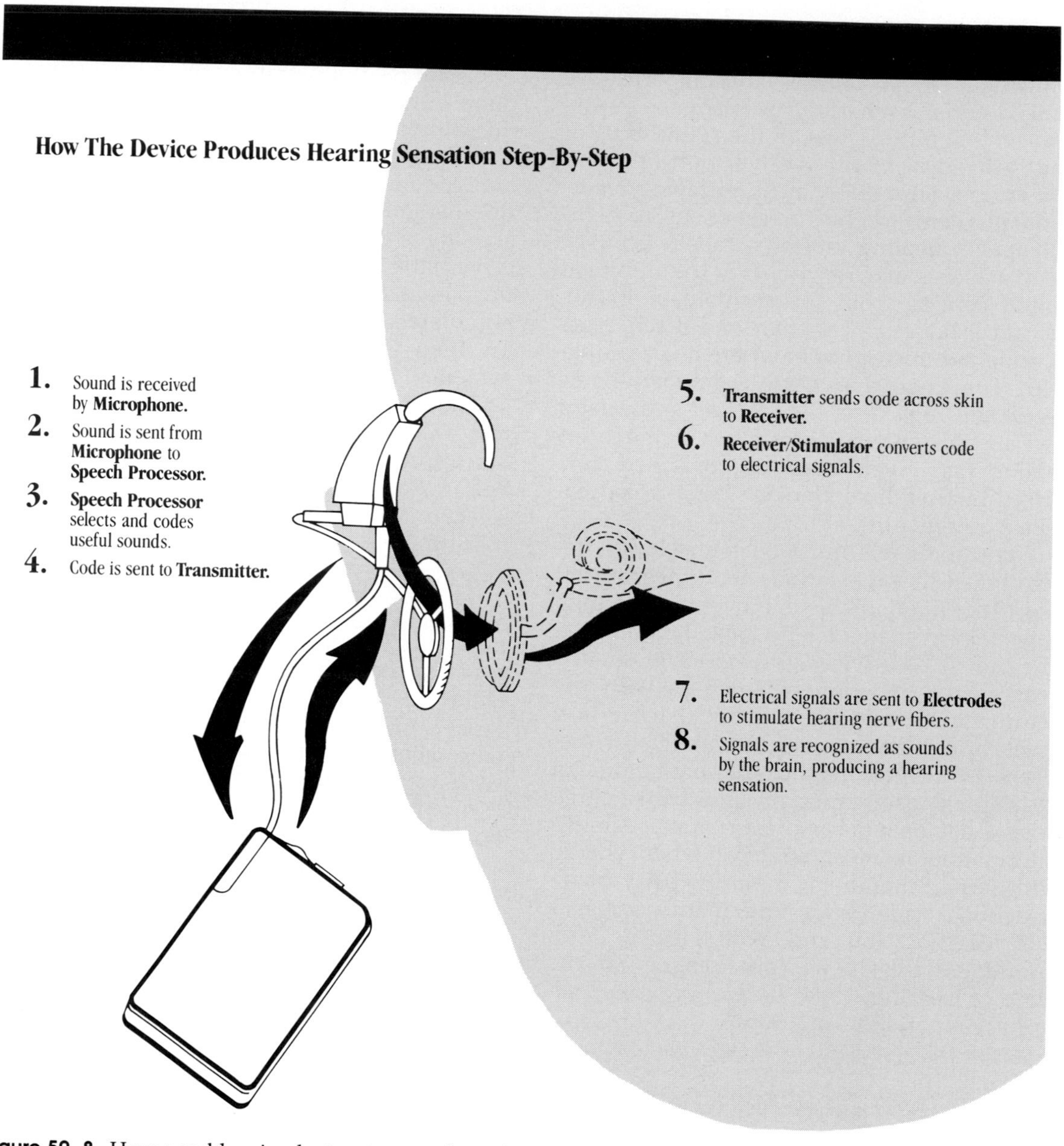

How The Device Produces Hearing Sensation Step-By-Step

1. Sound is received by **Microphone**.
2. Sound is sent from **Microphone** to **Speech Processor**.
3. **Speech Processor** selects and codes useful sounds.
4. Code is sent to **Transmitter**.

5. **Transmitter** sends code across skin to **Receiver**.
6. **Receiver/Stimulator** converts code to electrical signals.

7. Electrical signals are sent to **Electrodes** to stimulate hearing nerve fibers.
8. Signals are recognized as sounds by the brain, producing a hearing sensation.

Figure 59–8. How a cochlear implant system produces hearing sensations. (Photo courtesy of Cochlear Corp.)

neck pain; and perilymph fluid leakage that may lead to meningitis. There will also be a palpable hump behind the patient's ear. Despite early concerns, there are no firm data to suggest that cochlear implants increase the risk for otitis media in children. Moreover, although the long-term effects of chronic electrical stimulation of the cochlea are unknown, histologic reports on the temporal bone of patients using implants for as long as 15 years have to date been favorable.

The most critical aspect of successful coch-lear implant use, especially for children, is the postimplantation rehabilitation process. To be successful, all cochlear implant patients must be managed by a rehabilitation team that must include representatives from the fields of audiology, speech-language pathology, rehabilitation, education, and psychology.

A limited number of cochlear implant users obtain extraordinary benefit from their devices, to the extent that they are able to discriminate open-set speech without visual

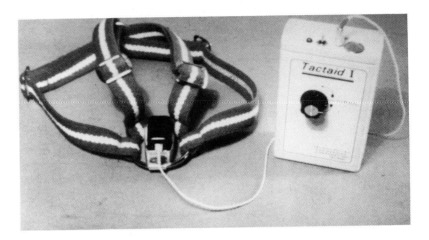

Figure 59–9. Example of a one-channel vibrotactile aid. (Photo courtesy of Audiological Engineering Corporation.)

cues (i.e., communicating over the telephone). However, the majority do not benefit to this extent. Studies on several thousand patients with single-channel and multichannel implanted devices have supported the following expected benefit. The expected benefits for children are as follows.

1. Many (≥52%) can detect medium to loud environmental sounds, including speech, at comfortable loudness levels.
2. Some (>34% to 52%) can identify environmental sounds, chosen from a closed set of alternatives, at comfortable loudness levels.
3. Many (≥52%) can identify timing and rhythm of speech and words from a closed set of alternatives.
4. Some (>34% to 52%) can demonstrate enhancement of their lipreading skills.
5. Many (≥52%) can improve their speech productions after training.
6. A few (>5% to <34%) can recognize speech without lipreading.

Children with congenital or prelingual deafness are less likely to benefit from a cochlear implant.

The expected benefits for adults are as follows.

1. Most (≥52%) can detect medium to loud environmental sounds, including speech, at comfortable listening levels.
2. Some (>34% to 52%) can improve speech recognition with lipreading.
3. A few (>5% to <34%) can improve speech recognition without lipreading.
4. A few (>5% to <34%) can improve in the recognition of environmental sounds.

Currently, data support the notion that expected performance levels are higher for multichannel implants than for single-channel implants. Over time, as the electrical processing strategies improve, the expected benefits from cochlear implants should increase, and larger numbers of hearing-impaired patients will benefit from their use.

Tactile Aids

With tactile aids acoustic signals are transposed into vibratory (vibrotactile) or electrical (electrotactile) patterns on the skin. The goal of a tactile communication system is to extract relevant information from the acoustic signal and to present it to the user in a tactile mode as a means of supplementing or replacing the auditory reception of the acoustic signal, with the successful reception of speech as the ultimate challenge.

Research on tactile aids dates back to the 1920s. Without exception, results have shown that tactile aids are effective in improving communication. However, only since about 1985 have body-worn instruments been available commercially. Several manufacturers currently offer single-channel and multichannel tactile aids. Figure 59–9 is an example of a single-channel vibrotactile aid.

The benefits that can be expected from tactile aid use include detection of medium to loud sounds in the environment; discrimination of loud and soft sounds, continuous and interrupted sounds, and long and short sounds; and differentiation of the number of sounds and syllables in words and different types of sounds in the environment. Unlike the cochlear implant, tactile aids do not pro-

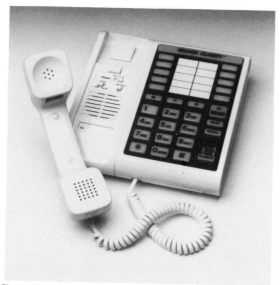

Figure 59–10. Walker Clarity frequency enhancing telephone. (Photo courtesy of Walker Equipment Corp.)

vide open-set discrimination of speech for any wearer.

ASSISTIVE LISTENING DEVICES AND SYSTEMS

Assistive listening devices and systems is a term that refers to a wide variety of equipment,

other than hearing aids, that is designed to improve communication for the hearing impaired. Some devices may be used alone, whereas others supplement hearing aid use in special situations. Demonstrations of these devices along with recommendations concerning their use should be included in aural rehabilitation programs. The following discussion is a brief summary of the type of assistance available in this area.

Telephone

Amplified telephone handsets may be obtained for telephones, or modular in-line amplifiers may be inserted between the handset and base of existing modular telephones. Portable amplifiers, which strap onto a handset, are available for temporary use. In addition, several models of special telephones with built-in amplifiers have been introduced (Figs. 59–10, 59–11). All of these devices intensify the incoming speech signal for the hearing-impaired user.

A telecommunication device for the deaf (TDD), when coupled to the telephone, allows profoundly hearing-impaired persons to communicate. The user types a message on the TDD keyboard that is converted into tones and conveyed over the phone line to another TDD, which transforms the message into printed form on a screen. A software

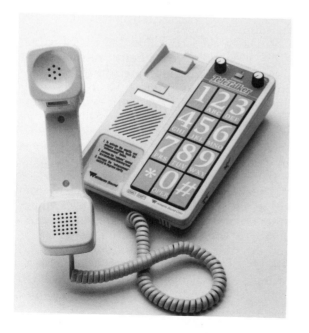

Figure 59–11. Teletalker enhanced telephone. (Photo courtesy of Williams Sound Corp.)

product from IBM, Phonecommunicator, allows a personal computer to interact with a TDD and provides a synthesized speech signal for the user as well.

Television

A variety of arrangements enables the user to receive an amplified auditory signal from the television loudspeaker. A small pick-up microphone may be placed in front of the loudspeaker and its signal transmitted via hardwire or wireless infrared or FM radio transmission to a receiver manipulated by the hearing-impaired person. An alternative method is to place a portable radio that receives the audio portion of television programs near the hearing-impaired viewer.

Closed captioning is a process in which the audio portion of a television program is translated into captions that appear on the screen, much like subtitles in a foreign film. With these captions, a hearing-impaired viewer may read dialogue and narrations to supplement whatever may be heard. The networks and cable systems broadcast closed-captioned programs; however, a small decoder box must be attached to the television set in order to decode the captioning signal (Fig. 59–12). Federal law requires that most television sets sold in the United States after July 1, 1993, have built-in circuitry that allows display of these captions.

Alerting and Warning Signals

In daily life, a person must respond to a variety of environmental sounds; the alarm clock, the doorbell, and the ring of the telephone are the most common. There exist systems that transpose these sounds into flashing lights or vibrotactile stimuli that are meaningful to hearing-impaired persons.

Personal Listening Systems

These individual listening systems are often hardwire and consist of a microphone, an amplifier, and a receiver. These components may be separated, although connected to each other by wires; the microphone may be placed closer to the speaker, which improves listening conditions for the hearing-impaired user (Fig. 59–13). An aided listener may combine one of these systems with a hearing aid by using a neckloop with the receiver and switching the aid to "T," or telecoil. These devices are especially helpful for professionals to use when consulting with hearing-impaired persons who do not have personal hearing aids.

In addition, wireless personal listening systems, which make use of FM radio technology, are available. Such units are extremely flexible and may be used in a variety of situations.

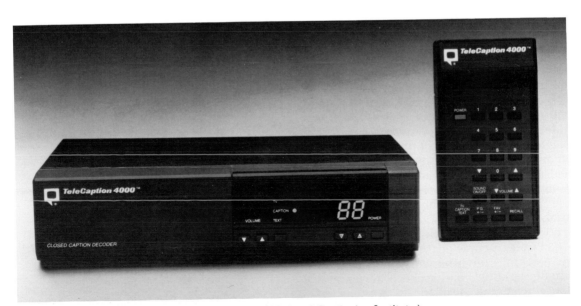

Figure 59–12. Telecaption 4000. (Photo courtesy of National Captioning Institute.)

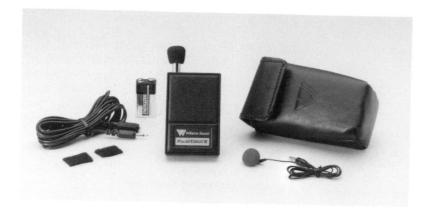

Figure 59–13. Pocketalker. (Photo Courtesy of Williams Sound Corp.)

Large Area Listening Systems

Auditoriums, theaters, and houses of worship may have infrared or FM transmitters added to their existing public address systems to make these facilities accessible to hearing-impaired persons. Special receivers are available to be used by those in attendance with hearing losses.

COMMUNICATIVE TRAINING

Hearing impairment in adults has its greatest impact in the problems encountered when communicating with others. Thus the focus of all aural rehabilitation programs is directed toward improving this communication. Traditional methods emphasize auditory training to extract meaningful information from the audible speech signal and speech reading (lipreading) training to understand the spoken message on the basis of visual information alone. Today most hearing-impaired persons fitted with hearing aids have usable aided hearing; thus a bisensory approach, which combines training in the auditory and visual modes together, is usually recommended.

Newer approaches to improving communication are counseling oriented and are aimed at helping the person accept and adjust to the problems of impaired hearing. These programs stress improving environmental, behavioral, and attitudinal factors that contribute to communicative difficulties. For example, people learn to analyze and alter listening environments in terms of adequate lighting, background noise, and distance from the speaker. Appropriate responses to auditory failures or misunderstandings are discussed so that the hearing-impaired person is prepared to ask for repetitions in a constructive manner. Various coping strategies and assertiveness tactics may be presented through problem-solving sketches of common everyday situations. Training in the use of the telephone may also be included in an aural rehabilitation program.

Speech Conservation

The speech problems associated with acquired hearing loss in adults usually involve errors of articulation and voice. Certain speech sounds tend to deteriorate in the presence of long-standing hearing loss; omissions and distortions of the sibilant sounds are most common because of the reduction of auditory cues for these sounds in people with high-frequency hearing losses. Vocal output may be altered as the ability to monitor oneself auditorily decreases; this is most apparent in people who experience a sudden loss of hearing and, consequently, talk too loudly all the time. The goals of a speech conservation program are to maintain existing speech that might deteriorate and to correct errors that may have developed as a result of the hearing loss.

SUGGESTED READINGS

Alpiner JG, McCarthy P (eds): Rehabilitative Audiology: Children and Adults. Baltimore: Williams & Wilkins, 1987.

Brooks DN (ed): Adult Aural Rehabilitation. London: Chapman & Hall, 1989.

Castle DL: Telephone Strategies: A Technical and Practical Guide for Hard-of-Hearing People. Bethesda, MD: Self Help for Hard-of-Hearing People, 1988.

Castle DL: Telephone Training for Hearing-Impaired Persons: Amplified Telephones, TDD's, Codes, 2nd ed. Rochester, NY: NTID/RIT Press, 1984.

Demorest ME, Erdman SA: Development of the communication profile for the hearing impaired. J Speech Hear Dis 52:129–143, 1987.

Hall RH (ed): Rehabilitative Audiology. New York: Grune & Stratton, 1982.

Hodgson WR (ed): Hearing Aid Assessment and Use in Audiologic Habilitation, 3rd ed. Baltimore: Williams & Wilkins, 1986.

New York League for the Hard of Hearing: You and Your Hearing Aid: Sound Advice. [videocassettes]. New York: New York League for the Hard of Hearing, 1989.

Pollack MC (ed): Amplification for the Hearing-Impaired, 3rd ed. Orlando, FL: Grune & Stratton, 1988.

Sandlin RE (ed): Handbook of Hearing Aid Amplification, Vol. I: Theoretical and Technical Considerations. Boston: College-Hill Press, 1988.

Sandlin RE (ed): Handbook of Hearing Aid Amplification, Vol. II: Clinical Considerations and Fitting Practices. Boston: College-Hill Press, 1990.

Schow RL, Nerbonne MA: Introduction to Aural Rehabilitation, 2nd ed. Austin, TX: Pro-Ed, 1989.

Skinner, MW: Hearing Aid Evaluation. Englewood Cliffs, NJ: Prentice-Hall, 1988.

U.S. Food and Drug Administration: Hearing aid devices: professional and patient labeling and conditions for sale. Fed Reg 42:9286–9296, 1977.

Ventry IM, Weinstein BC: The Hearing Handicap Inventory for the Elderly: a new tool. Ear Hear 3:128–134, 1982.

Wayner DS: The Hearing Aid Handbook—Clinician's Guide to Client Orientation. Washington, DC: Clerc Books, Gallaudet University Press, 1990a.

Wayner DS: The Hearing Aid Handbook—User's Guide for Adults. Washington, DC: Clerc Books, Gallaudet University Press, 1990.

CHAPTER 60

Mohs Micrographic Surgery

Rodney F. Kovach, MD   Richard J. DeAngelis, MD

The incidence of nonmelanoma skin cancer is approaching epidemic proportions, 400,000 head and neck lesions occur annually in the United States (Roenigk, 1988). The majority of these tumors are basal cell carcinomas or squamous cell carcinomas with low metastatic potential that grow by local invasion in a contiguous manner. Although the mortality rate remains low, these cancers have the propensity to develop on sun-exposed areas, and their destructive invasive growth often results in cosmetic and functional morbidity.

Standard treatments such as electrosurgery, cryosurgery, radiation therapy, and excisional surgery have been highly successful in eradicating these neoplastic growths, as pointed out by Swanson and associates (1983). However, another alternative has become available and, in certain instances, is becoming the standard of care. Mohs micrographic surgery, in contrast to other treatment modalities, offers the unique advantage of microscopic aid in tracing out these contiguously growing tumors with their "silent extensions," which are easily missed by other methods of treatment. With such histographic control, a tumor-free plane is achieved regardless of the size, shape, depth, or histologic type of the tumor.

Mohs micrographic surgery has evolved as a reliable and cost-effective treatment offering maximal preservation of normal tissue, an extremely high cure rate, and the assurance of a tumor-free defect that can be reconstructed immediately.

The history, the method, and an illustrative case report are presented, followed by a discussion of the advantages of and indications for the Mohs micrographic technique.

HISTORY

In the mid-1930s, Frederic E. Mohs was studying the inflammatory effects of various chemical irritants on implanted rat sarcoma cells. One of the chemical irritants that he injected was a 20% zinc chloride solution, which was too highly concentrated and caused tissue necrosis. On microscopic examination of the excised tissue, not only was an intense inflammatory infiltrate observed around the tumor, but to his surprise, the microscopic architecture of the killed tissue was preserved, as if it had been removed and immersed in formalin. After much experimentation, he began fixing skin cancers in situ with zinc chloride paste. After this in situ fixation, the tumor-involved area was excised in a saucerlike manner. Horizontal sections were prepared, and the undersurface and periphery were microscopically examined in their entirety. Any areas of residual tumor involvement were then pinpointed and plotted on a reference map corresponding to the wound site while specific anatomic orientation was maintained. This serial process of fixation, excision, microscopic examination, and mapping would be repeated until a tumor-free plane was obtained (Fig. 60–1). Mohs coined the term *chemosurgery* to describe this process.

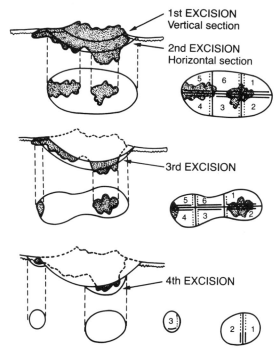

1st EXCISION
Vertical section

2nd EXCISION
Horizontal section

3rd EXCISION

4th EXCISION

Figure 60–1. Schematic diagram of cancer (shaded area, top left) with horizontal projections of the undersurface after each layer of excision. To the right are maps with tumor-positive areas represented in dark. (From Mohs FE: Chemosurgery: microscopically controlled surgery for skin cancer: past, present and future. J Dermatol Surg Oncol 4:41–53, 1978. Copyright 1978 by Elsevier Science Publishing Co., Inc.)

By use of this chemical fixative, bloodless surgery was performed without anesthesia. However, the application of the zinc chloride paste caused pain and edema resulting from tissue necrosis. Such pain experienced by patients was termed *chemomisery.* Another disadvantage of the chemosurgical process was that it allowed excision of only one layer to be performed daily, the reason being that zinc chloride had to "fix" for several hours, and if tumor remained, the fixative had to be reapplied. Large tumors requiring excision of several layers could take longer than a week. Finally, when a tumor-free plane was reached, the remaining fixative would not slough for another 7 to 10 days, thereby preventing immediate reconstruction and closure.

In 1953, Mohs began removing tumors of the eyelid margins without the chemical fixative in order to avoid eye irritation. This major modification was not popularized until 1974 when Tromovitch and Stegman reported that by deleting the fixative, using

local anesthesia, and following the same sequence of events as originally described, they could achieve the same high cure rates. This "fresh tissue technique" allowed excision of multiple layers to be performed in one day, produced less perioperative pain, and permitted immediate reconstruction and closure.

Formerly designated by many synonyms, the term used for the procedure today is *Mohs micrographic surgery,* as adopted by the American College of Mohs Micrographic Surgery and Cutaneous Oncology.

Given its cure rate of 98.2% for primary and 96.6% for recurrent nonmelanoma skin cancers, Mohs micrographic surgery is becoming more popular not only within but also outside the field of dermatology. When it is indicated, other surgical specialists are becoming an integral part of a multidisciplinary team approach, combining their reconstructive skills with the unsurpassed cure rate of Mohs micrographic surgical excision.

METHOD

Mohs micrographic surgery requires personnel specially trained in preparing horizontal fresh-frozen tissue sections. The entire procedure is usually performed in an outpatient setting. Illustrated in Figure 60–2 is a schematic with clinical photographs (Fig. 60–3) of a 45-year-old white male with a 10-year history of a morpheaform basal cell carcinoma of the left cheek. He was referred for micrographic surgery because of the indistinct clinical margins of the lesion.

After the tumor in question has previously undergone biopsy, the following steps are undertaken.

1. The clinical margins of the tumor are outlined.
2. The area is anesthetized by use of 1% lidocaine with epinephrine.
3. The clinically apparent tumor is debulked with a scalpel or dermal curet.
4. The first micrographic layer is obtained by making a saucerized excision (to include a 1- to 3-mm margin) around and beneath the debulked tumor. This excision is performed by beveling the scalpel blade at a 45° angle to the skin surface.
5. Before the excised specimen is detached from the wound bed, several superficial scalpel niches are placed on the excised

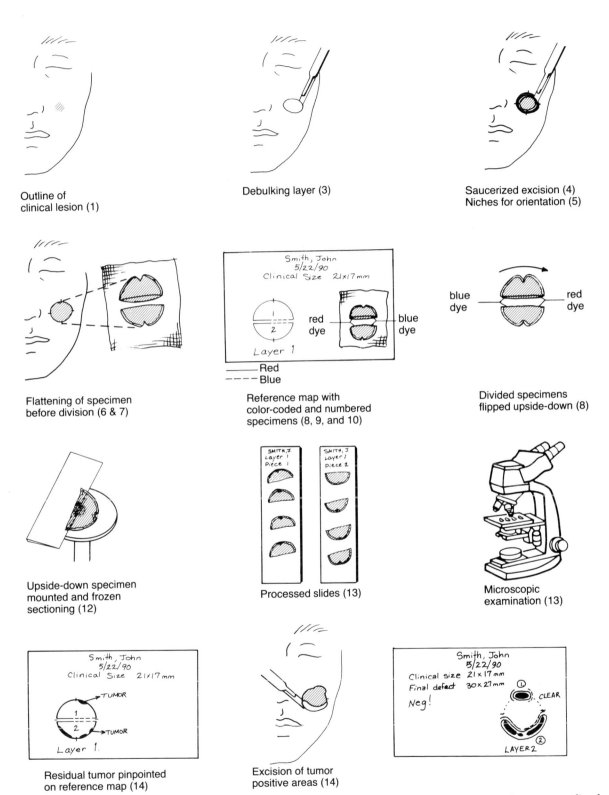

Outline of
clinical lesion (1)

Debulking layer (3)

Saucerized excision (4)
Niches for orientation (5)

Flattening of specimen
before division (6 & 7)

Reference map with
color-coded and numbered
specimens (8, 9, and 10)

Divided specimens
flipped upside-down (8)

Upside-down specimen
mounted and frozen
sectioning (12)

Processed slides (13)

Microscopic
examination (13)

Residual tumor pinpointed
on reference map (14)

Excision of tumor
positive areas (14)

Figure 60–2. Schematic of the Mohs micrographic technique. Numbers in parentheses correspond to steps outlined in the text.

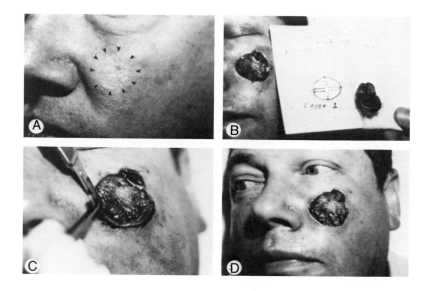

Figure 60–3. *A.* Morpheaform basal cell carcinoma with its indistinct clinical borders before Mohs micrographic surgery. *B.* Defect with excised and divided tissue along with color-coded reference map after excision of the first layer in Mohs micrographic surgery. *C.* Re-excision of tumor-positive areas with 1- to 2-mm margins. *D.* Final defect at the completion of Mohs micrographic surgery.

margin and adjacent normal tissue. These niches are anatomic landmarks that help orient the excised specimen and serve as reference points.

6. While orientation is maintained at all times, the excised specimen is flattened so that the periphery and the undersurface lie within the same plane. This enables the histotechnician to prepare horizontal sections that include both the peripheral skin edge and the deep margin of the specimen.

7. The excised specimen is divided into pieces small enough to fit on a microscope slide. The pieces are divided along specifically oriented scored lines.

8. The pieces are systematically numbered and then turned over so that the undersurface is facing up.

9. The divided edges are then painted (color-coded) with dyes that aid in maintaining orientation during microscopic examination.

10. A map of the corresponding wound site is drawn, including the numbered pieces with their color-codings schematically diagrammed.

11. Significant bleeders are either spot coagulated or suture ligated in order to maximize visualization.

12. The histotechnician prepares multiple horizontally cut frozen sections of each numbered piece from the undersurface to the periphery.

13. Each piece is examined microscopically by the Mohs surgeon with the reference map at hand. Any areas of residual tumor are charted on the map.

14. In turn, the exact location of residual tumor is translated from the reference map to the wound site, guiding the next layered surgical excision.

Between layers, a pressure bandage is applied onto the wound bed while the patient awaits tissue processing and interpretation. This process of serial excisions, mapping, and microscopic examination is repeated until a tumor-free plane is achieved.

WHY IS MOHS MICROGRAPHIC SURGERY UNIQUE?

The vertically cut frozen sections prepared routinely are not equivalent to those obtained by the Mohs technique. By excising tissue in a saucerlike fashion, Mohs micrographic surgery allows the specimen to be flattened out in such a way that horizontal frozen sections can be performed and 100% of the wound margins examined. In comparison with Mohs micrographic surgery, routine frozen sections have been estimated to sample less than 0.1% of all margins. For this reason, the pathology report often reads "Margins appear to be tumor-free." It would be more accurately stated that "sampled tissue margins that were examined show no evidence of tumor" (Fig. 60–4).

Another advantage of Mohs micrographic surgery relates to its precise method of mapping, which allows the surgeon to specifically locate areas of the wound where residual tumor exists (Fig. 60–1). This relatively exact-

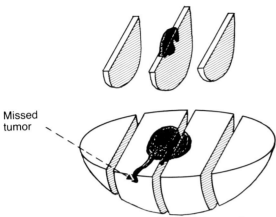

Figure 60–4. "Silent extension" missed by routine vertical sectioning.

ing method avoids the dilemma just described, as illustrated in the case example (Fig. 60–2).

Zitelli (1985) accurately summed up the situation when he stated, "Routine frozen sections neither allow examination of all margins nor provide detailed localization of all remaining tumor; thus the cure rate of excision with routine frozen section control is less than with Mohs surgery."

INDICATIONS

Nonmelanoma Skin Cancers

Mohs micrographic surgery is the treatment of choice for many nonmelanoma skin cancers. Tumors amenable to this technique must grow in a contiguous manner and be easily visualized by frozen-section light microscopy. Basal cell and squamous cell cancers meet these pre-existent criteria, and multiple studies have confirmed the efficacy and statistically unmatched cure rates of Mohs micrographic surgery in the treatment of these neoplasms.

With regard to small (less than 1 cm) well-defined primary nonmelanoma skin cancers, the success rate of conventional therapies approaches that of Mohs micrographic surgery, and therefore conventional therapy is most appropriate. In view of the indications for Mohs micrographic surgery, it must be realized that the procedure can be tedious, time-consuming, and expensive. However, if the patient cannot be assured a 90% chance of cure, or if tissue conservation is impera-

tive, then Mohs micrographic surgery is highly recommended and, in the final analysis, may be most cost effective.

The well-accepted indications for Mohs micrographic surgery are listed in the following sections with this philosophy and these guidelines in mind (Table 60–1).

Recurrent Nonmelanoma Skin Cancers

It has been shown time and time again that once a basal cell or squamous cell cancer recurs, the chance for cure significantly decreases with each additional treatment. Cure rates for recurrent basal cell neoplasms range from 50% to 90% if they are treated by traditional modalities, in comparison with 96% by Mohs micrographic surgery.

Mohs reported an overall 5-year cure rate of 94% from a consecutive series of patients treated chemosurgically from 1936 to 1968 with biopsy-proven squamous cell carcinoma, including squamous cell carcinomas that were early to advanced, primary or recurrent, with or without metastasis. How-

TABLE 60–1. Mohs Micrographic Surgery

Indications	Reasons for Mohs Micrographic Surgery
Recurrent nonmelanoma skin cancers or incompletely excised tumors	Cure rates 96% for Mohs micrographic surgery vs. 40% to 60% by other modalities for recurrent tumors
Location with high rates of recurrence	See Figure 60–5
Large tumors (1 to 2 cm on head and neck)	Cure rates by other methods inversely proportional to tumor size
Maximum tissue conservation	Minimize dysfunction and distortion of critical anatomic areas (e.g., eyes, nose, vermilion border of the lip)
Aggressive histologic tumor subtypes	Cure rates are notoriously lower for morpheaform, metatypical (basosquamous), and infiltrating histologic subtypes
Indistinct clinical margins	Silent extensions easily missed by routine methods
Perineural invasion	Erratic extension beyond main tumor mass
Malignant melanoma	Controversial at this time

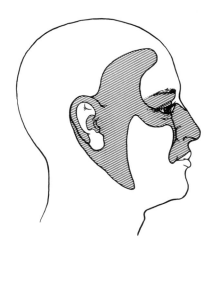
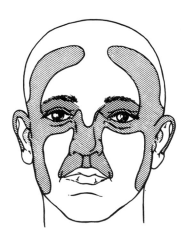

Figure 60–5. "H zone" of face noted for its high recurrence rate and deep extensions of basal cell carcinomas. (From Baker SR, Swanson NA, Grekin RD: An interdisciplinary approach to the management of basal cell carcinoma of the head and neck. J Dermatol Surg Oncol 13:1095–1106, 1987. Copyright 1987 by Elsevier Science Publishing Co., Inc.)

ever, when he specifically compared primary with recurrent squamous cell carcinomas in these patients, the 5-year cure rates were 97.3% and 76.3%, respectively (Mohs, 1978). These cure rates are still superior with those for other comparable reported cases when other ablative treatment techniques are used.

Incompletely Excised Tumors

The definition of "incompletely excised" tumors is often as ambiguous as the pathology report that reads, "Tumor is near one lateral margin." However, if the decision to follow and not to re-excise is made, then the risk of recurrence is significant. Pascal and coworkers (1968) found that of tumors that were present within one high-power field of a surgical margin, 12% recurred. An overall 33% recurrence rate was noted with marginal involvement. In general, as with most tumors, the rate of recurrence of incompletely excised tumors is dependent on size and location. For example, P. Thomas (1970) found that 82% of incompletely excised tumors in the perinasal, periauricular, and periorbital regions recurred. Such tumors would therefore be most amenable to Mohs micrographic surgery.

Locations With High Rates of Recurrence

Tumors situated in the so-called H zone of the face are known to pose an increased risk

of recurrence after standard treatment. This H zone (Fig. 60–5) is composed of the following:

1. The periorbital region, specifically the lower eyelid and inner canthus.
2. The junction of the ala with the nasolabial fold.
3. The nose-cheek angle (nasofacial fold).
4. The nasal ala and the alar crease.
5. The periauricular region extending to the temple.
6. The auricle, the tragus, and the canal of the ear.

In general, tumors tend to spread along paths of least resistance, which accounts for their affinity for embryonic fusion planes, fascial planes, periosteum, perichondrium, and the tarsal plate of the eyelid. Tumors involving these anatomic sites may invade to unusual distances and depths and therefore be difficult to detect and eradicate by any method other than Mohs micrographic surgery.

Large Tumors

In general, the cure rate for nonmelanoma skin cancer decreases as the tumor size increases, regardless of the treatment modality used. Mohs reported a 99.5% cure rate for lesions smaller than 1 cm, but the cure rates with Mohs micrographic surgery begin to decline when the lesion reaches 2 cm in diameter. Basal cell and squamous cell carcinomas between 2 and 3 cm in diameter have cure rates of 98% and 82%, respectively, which are still much better than those obtained with other treatment alternatives.

Tissue Conservation for Functional or Cosmetic Reasons

Approximately 85% of nonmelanoma skin cancers occur on the head and neck. It is no wonder, therefore, that many of these tumors will be located near some important structure. Where tissue preservation is paramount, Mohs micrographic surgery can oftentimes prevent excess tissue loss, thereby minimizing unnecessary dysfunction and distortion. This is particularly important for lesions located on the nose, ears, eyelids, and lips.

Aggressive Histologic Tumor Subtypes

Morpheaform (sclerosing) basal cell carcinomas have indistinct margins and are often clinically mistaken for scar tissue. The standard 4-mm margin recommended for well-defined exophytic lesions by Wolfe and Zitelli (1987) will often be inadequate, resulting in unacceptable recurrence rates. Levine and Bailin (1980) showed that of all the histologic subtypes, morpheaform basal cell carcinomas have the highest recurrence rates. Other histologic subtypes that often warrant initial treatment by Mohs micrographic surgery include metatypical (basosquamous), multicentric, and infiltrating basal cell carcinomas.

Indistinct Clinical Margins

The ambiguity regarding the surgeon's interpretation of pathologist's reports and margin positivity was alluded to earlier. In an article by Abide and colleagues (1984) on the meaning of surgical margins, 14 of 16 plastic surgeons reported that they would re-excise tissue if a squamous cell carcinoma was reported to be close to the surgical margin. However, only 4 of the 16 surgeons would re-excise basal cell carcinoma under the same circumstances (no mention of histologic subtypes was made). In addition, fewer than 1% of all skin edges are examined histologically by routine vertical sectioning; thus there are many opportunities for misinterpretation, error, and incomplete excision.

How does this relate to tumors with indistinct clinical margins? Such tumors are not easily delineated clinically from the surrounding normal skin. In light of the aforementioned ways in which tumor can be "left behind" or incompletely excised, the potential for inadequate removal is even greater when an excision of a tumor with indistinct clinical margins is attempted by routine methods. Therefore, Mohs micrographic surgery is a very viable alternative for tumors with these clinical characteristics.

Perineural Invasion

This is uncommon but more frequent with squamous cell carcinoma than with basal cell carcinoma. Once a nonmelanoma skin cancer spreads along the perineurium, it can travel a long distance from the main tumor mass. Cheek lesions can travel to the base of the brain and can be clinically undetected. Mohs micrographic surgery is the only method that can track these extensions. These patients are frequently treated with an additional tumor-free layer of Mohs surgery or postoperative radiation because of the tenuous nature of the circumstances involved.

Other Nonmelanoma Skin Cancers

As previously mentioned, contiguity of tumor growth and recognition by light microscopy after frozen sections is a prerequisite for treatment by Mohs micrographic surgery. Other tumors that have been successfully treated and fulfill these criteria include Bowen's disease, dermatofibrosarcoma protuberans, extramammary Paget's disease, verrucous carcinoma, and keratoacanthoma.

Is Malignant Melanoma Amenable to Mohs Micrographic Surgery?

At some medical centers, Mohs micrographic surgery is being used for stage I melanoma. Invasive melanoma, however, may exhibit satellitosis and not be in a contiguous growth phase. There is also no unanimity among Mohs surgeons that such tumors are as histologically distinguishable by frozen sections as are basal cell and squamous cell carcinomas. Therefore, it is not surprising that most

Mohs surgeons treat melanoma in a conventional manner.

INTERDISCIPLINARY APPROACH

With the unsurpassed cure rates of Mohs micrographic surgery, other specialists are being incorporated into a team approach with the Mohs micrographic surgeon. Cooperation among colleagues is imperative to ensure that the patient has not only the highest cure rate attainable but also the best chances for excellent cosmetic and functional results. The majority of skin cancers treated by Mohs micrographic surgery are managed by the dermatologic surgeon, but there are times when help is solicited from colleagues in plastic, oculoplastic, and otolaryngologic surgery for the more difficult and extensive cases.

The most common indication for the multispecialty approach involves the reconstruction of large defects created by Mohs micrographic surgery. As tissue sparing as this process can be, difficult reconstructions beyond the expertise of most dermatologic surgeons may in some cases be required.

At other times, tumors may be so extensive that it is unwise to continue in the outpatient department, and the team approach is needed not only for reconstruction but for resection. For example, if skin cancers invade deeper structures such as the parotid gland, the orbit, the sinuses, or the nasal cavity, surgical assistance should be coordinated with the appropriate subspecialist. At this juncture, the patient should be transferred from the Mohs surgical outpatient suite to the operating room. Micrographic margin delineation may still be of benefit, but the deeper the tumor invades the cavities of the head and neck, the more difficult the Mohs micrographic mapping and orientation become. When tissue mapping and orientation become too laborious and obscure, en bloc resections are more practically performed.

Increasing numbers of centers are adopting this multidisciplinary approach for the treatment of selected noncutaneous neoplasms. Examples include squamous cell carcinoma of the tongue, the palate, the floor of the mouth, the tonsillar pillars, and the paranasal sinuses. The primary objective in treating such tumors with Mohs micrographic surgery is preservation of the mandible, the tongue, or the orbit, which may otherwise be sacrificed with treatment by less tissue conservative modalities.

CONCLUSION

Mohs micrographic surgery has stood the test of time and has become the standard with which the success of other treatment modalities is currently being compared. Although it does require specially trained ancillary personnel and at times can be quite tedious and time consuming, it does have distinct advantages.

After tumor extirpation by Mohs micrographic surgery, knowing that all margins have been histologically examined, the surgeon has an increased assurance that the chance of burying incompletely excised neoplasm under flaps or grafts is minimal, and immediate reconstruction can be performed.

The tissue preservative property inherent to the Mohs micrographic serial excisional technique has permitted removal of periorbital tumors, nasal lesions, and other anatomically critical neoplasms while sparing radical procedures such as orbital exenterations and rhinectomies.

When this technique is used for the properly prescribed indications, not only are unsurpassed cure rates obtained but long-term cost effectiveness is achieved.

SUGGESTED READINGS

Abide JM, Nahai F, Bennett RG: The meaning of surgical margins. Plast Reconstr Surg 73:492–497, 1984.

Baker SR, Swanson NA: Management of nasal cutaneous malignant neoplasms: an interdisciplinary approach. Arch Otolaryngol 109:473–479, 1983.

Baker SR, Swanson NA, Grekin RD: An interdisciplinary approach to the management of basal cell carcinoma of the head and neck. J Dermatol Surg Oncol 13:1095–1106, 1987.

Bernstein G, Cottel WI, Bailin PL, et al: Mohs micrographic surgery. J Dermatol Surg Oncol 13:13, 1987.

Borel DM: Cutaneous basosquamous carcinoma. Review of the literature and report of 35 cases. Arch Pathol 85:293–297, 1973.

Ceilley RI, Anderson RL: Microscopically controlled excision of malignant neoplasms on and around the eyelids followed by immediate surgical reconstruction. J Dermatol Surg Oncol 4:55–62, 1978.

Cottel WI: Perineural invasion by squamous cell carcinoma. J Dermatol Surg Oncol 8:589–599, 1982.

Cottel WI, Proper S: Mohs surgery, fresh tissue technique: our technique with a review. J Dermatol Surg Oncol 8:576–587, 1982.

Davidson TM, Naham AM, Haghighi P, et al: The biology of head and neck cancer. Arch Otolaryngol 110:193–196, 1984.

Levine JL, Bailin PL: Basal cell carcinoma of the head and neck: identification of the high-risk patient. Laryngoscope 90:955–961, 1980.

Menn H, Robins P, Kopf AW, et al: The recurrent basal cell epithelioma. Arch Dermatol 103:628–631, 1971.

Mohs FE: Chemosurgery: a microscopically controlled method of cancer excision. Arch Surg 42:279–295, 1941.

Mohs FE: Chemosurgery in Cancer, Gangrene and Infections. Springfield, IL: Charles C Thomas, 1956.

Mohs FE: Chemosurgery for melanoma. Arch Dermatol 113:285–291, 1977.

Mohs FE: Chemosurgery: Microscopically Controlled Surgery for Skin Cancer. Springfield, IL: Charles C Thomas, 1978a.

Mohs FE: Chemosurgery: microscopically controlled surgery for skin cancer: past, present, and future. J Dermatol Surg Oncol 4:41–42, 1978b.

Mohs FE: Chemosurgery. Clin Plast Surg 7:349–360, 1980.

Mohs FE: The width and depth of the spread of malignant melanomas as observed by a chemosurgeon. Am J Dermatopathol 6(Suppl):123–126, 1984.

Mohs FE, Guyer MF: Pre-excisional fixation of tissues in the treatment of cancer in rats. Cancer Res 1:49–51, 1941.

Panje WR, Ceilley RI: The influence of embryology of the midface on the spread of epithelial malignancies. Laryngoscope 89:1914–1920, 1979.

Pascal RR, Hobby LW, Lattes R, et al: Prognosis of "incompletely excised" versus "completely excised" basal cell carcinoma. Plast Reconstr Surg 41:328–332, 1968.

Robins P: Chemosurgery: my 15 years of experience. J Dermatol Surg Oncol 7:779–789, 1981.

Roenigk RK: Mohs' micrographic surgery. Mayo Clin Proc 63:175–183, 1988.

Rowe DE, Carroll RJ, Day CL: Mohs surgery is the treatment of choice for recurrent (previously treated) basal cell carcinoma. J Dermatol Surg Oncol 15:424–431, 1989.

Swanson NA: Mohs surgery: technique, indications, applications, and the future. Arch Dermatol 119:761–773, 1983.

Swanson NA, Grekin RC, Baker SR: Mohs surgery: techniques, indications and applications in head and neck surgery. Head Neck Surg 6:683–692, 1983.

Swanson NA, Taylor WB: Commentary: the evolution of Mohs' surgery. J Dermatol Surg Oncol 8:650–654, 1982.

Thomas JR, Goslen B: Effective use of the team approach in facial malignancy. Fac Plast Surg 5:1–11, 1987.

Thomas JR, Goslen JB, Goebel JA: Mohs excision and immediate reconstruction for cutaneous neoplasms: a multidisciplinary approach. Insights Otolaryngol 3:1–6, 1988.

Thomas P: Treatment of basal cell carcinomas of the head and neck. Rev Surg 27:293–294, 1970.

Tromovitch TA, Stegman SJ: Microscopically controlled excision. Arch Dermatol 110:231–232, 1974.

Weimer VM, Ceilley RI, Babin RW: Squamous cell carcinoma with invasion of the facial nerve and underlying bone and muscle: report of a case. J Dermatol Surg Oncol 5:526–529, 1979.

Wolfe DJ, Zitelli JA: Surgical margins for basal cell carcinoma. Arch Dermatol 123:340–344, 1987.

Zitelli JA: Mohs surgery: concepts and misconceptions. Int J Dermatol 24:541–548, 1985.